Understanding Nutrition

Eleanor Noss Whitney
Sharon Rady Rolfes

SEVENTH EDITION

West Publishing Company
Minneapolis/St. Paul
New York Los Angeles San Francisco

Copyediting: Patricia A. Lewis
Text and Cover Design: Janet Bollow
Dummy Artist: David Farr, ImageSmythe, Inc.
Illustrations: J/B Woolsey Associates
Index: Barbara Farabaugh
Composition: Parkwood Composition
Cover Image: Serotonin; © Michael Davidson

British Library Cataloguing-in-Publication Data. A catalogue record for this book is available from the British Library.

Printed in the United States of America

03 02 01 00 99 98 97 96 8 7 6 5 4 3 2

Library of Congress Cataloging-in-Publication Data

Whitney, Eleanor Noss.
Understanding nutrition / Eleanor Noss Whitney, Sharon Rady Rolfes.—7th ed.
p. cm.
Includes bibliographical references and index.
ISBN 0-314-06385-4 (hc : alk. paper)
1. Nutrition. I. Rolfes, Sharon Rady. II. Title.
QP141.W46 1996 95-47498
613.2—dc20 CIP

Photo Credits

x, x, xi, xii, xiii, xiv, xv © Michael Davidson; **1** © Michael Davidson; **2** © Tom McCarthy/PhotoEdit; **3** © Robert E. Daemmrich/Tony Stone Images; **6** © Felicia Martinez/PhotoEdit; **7** (Top) Thomas Harm and Tom Peterson/Quest Photographic Inc.; **7** (Bottom left) © Tony Freeman/PhotoEdit; **7** (Bottom right) © David Young-Wolff/PhotoEdit; **9** © Tony Freeman/PhotoEdit; **10** © Christopher Bissell/Tony Stone Images; **12** Thomas Harm and Tom Peterson/Quest Photographic Inc.; **14** © Bill Bachmann/PhotoEdit; **22** © Michael Newman/PhotoEdit; **31** © Frank Siteman/Tony Stone Images;

Photo credits continued after index

West's Commitment to the Environment

In 1906, West Publishing Company began recycling materials left over from the production of books. This began a tradition of efficient and responsible use of resources. Today, 100% of our legal bound volumes are printed on acid-free, recycled paper consisting of 50% new paper pulp and 50% paper that has undergone a de-inking process. We also use vegetable-based inks to print all of our books. West recycles nearly 27,700,000 pounds of scrap paper annually—the equivalent of 229,300 trees. Since the 1960s, West has devised ways to capture and recycle waste inks, solvents, oils, and vapors created in the printing process. We also recycle plastics of all kinds, wood, glass, corrugated cardboard, and batteries, and have eliminated the use of polystyrene book packaging. We at West are proud of the longevity and the scope of our commitment to the environment.

West pocket parts and advance sheets are printed on recyclable paper and can be collected and recycled with newspapers. Staples do not have to be removed. Bound volumes can be recycled after removing the cover.

Production, Prepress, Printing and Binding by West Publishing Company.

Printed with Printwise
Environmentally Advanced Water Washable Ink

A Word about Photomicrographs

The photomicrographs in the textbook were made of recrystallized vitamins and other nutrients using a variety of different techniques. Many vitamins can be imaged using the melt-recrystallization process where a few milligrams of the chemical are sandwiched between a microscope coverslip and slide, then heated until melted and allowed to slowly recrystallize. Alternately, for vitamin-salts that will not melt, the chemical is dissolved in a suitable solvent (water or alcohol) and a few microliters of solution are allowed to slowly evaporate between a microscope slide and coverslip. Upon recrystallization, the vitamins are viewed in a microscope using cross-polarized illumination where the crystallites diffract light depending both on the molecular orientation within the crystal and the crystal thickness. The colorful patterns illustrated in this text are a manifestation of both molecular orientation and crystal thickness.

To my husband Tom for the many helpful comments and loving caresses during the writing of this book and to our children Lyle A and Marni Jay who enrich my life daily

Sharon

About the Authors

Eleanor Noss Whitney, Ph.D., R.D., received her B.A. in biology from Radcliffe College in 1960 and her Ph.D. in biology with an emphasis on genetics from Washington University, St. Louis, in 1970. Formerly an associate professor at the Florida State University, she now devotes full time to research, writing, and consulting on nutrition, health, and the environment. Her textbooks include *Nutrition: Concepts and Controversies*, *Nutrition and Diet Therapy*, *Life Choices*, and *Nutrition for Health and Health Care*, among others. She is president of Nutrition and Health Associates, an information resource center in Tallahassee.

Sharon Rady Rolfes, M.S., R.D., received her B.S. in psychology and criminology in 1974 and her M.S. in nutrition and food science in 1982 at the Florida State University. She is a founding member of Nutrition and Health Associates, an information resource center that maintains an ongoing bibliographic data base of research in over 1000 nutrition-related topics. Her other textbooks include *Understanding Normal and Clinical Nutrition*, *Nutrition for Health and Health Care*, and *Life Span Nutrition: Conception through Life*. In addition to writing, she is currently working on a nutrition interactive CD-ROM and is serving on the National Faculty Advisory Committee for a nutrition telecourse being developed by the Dallas County Community College District. She also lectures and has served as nutrition consultant for the Florida House of Representatives, the Florida Department of Education Comprehension School Health Programs, and interactive media science projects funded by the National Science Foundation and developed by the Florida State University. She maintains a professional membership in the American Dietetic Association.

Contents in Brief

Contents

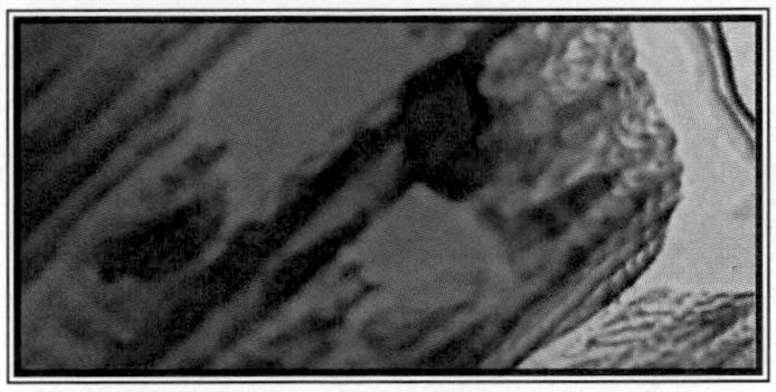

Contents

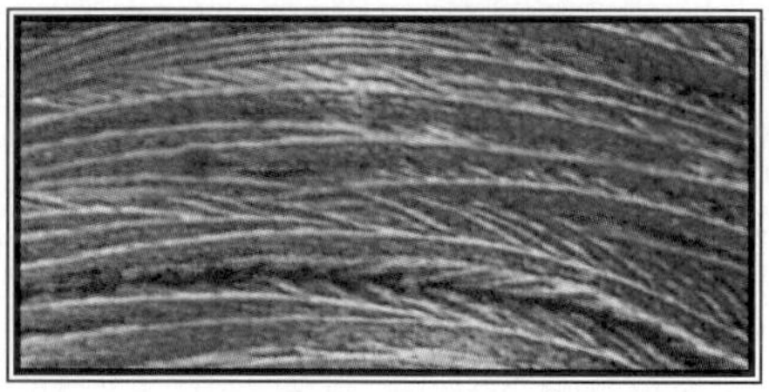

Chapter 5

Chapter 6

Chapter 7

Contents

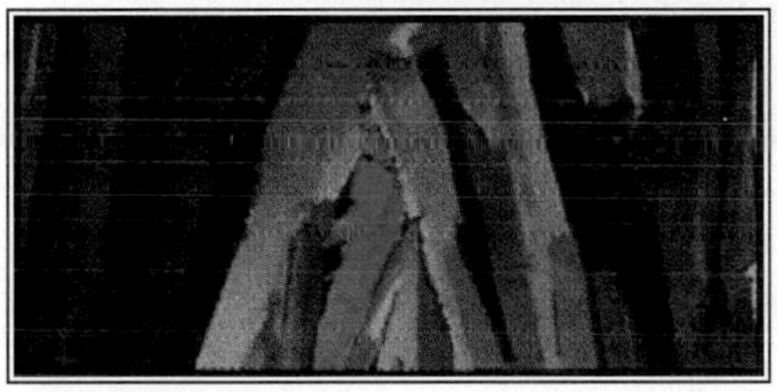

Chapter 10

Contents

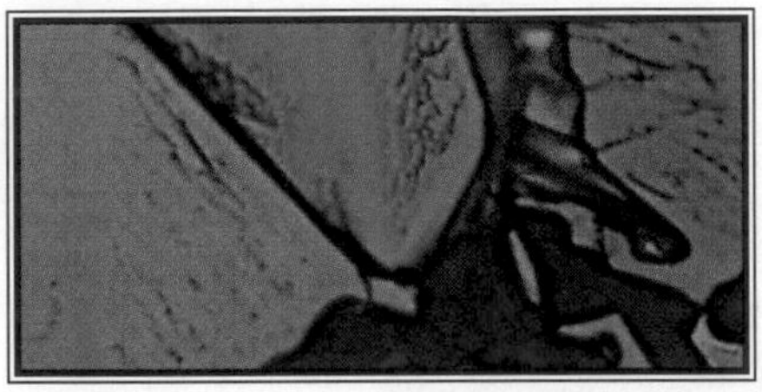

Contents

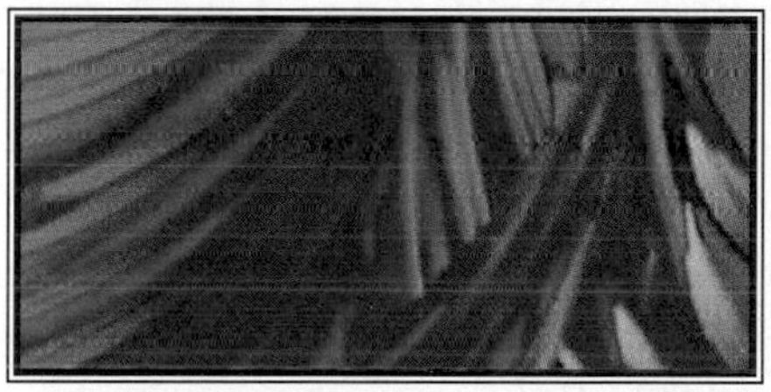

Contents

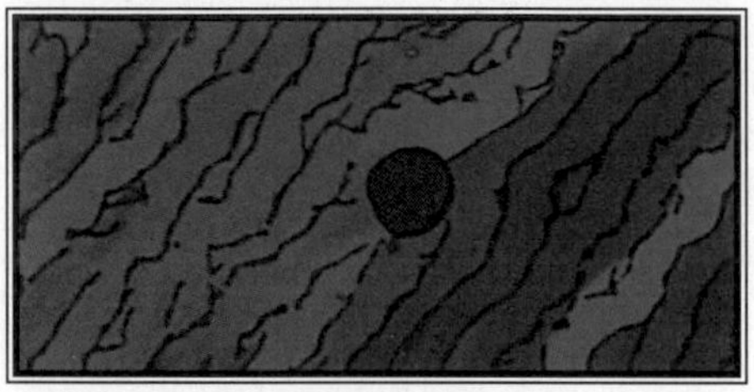

Contents

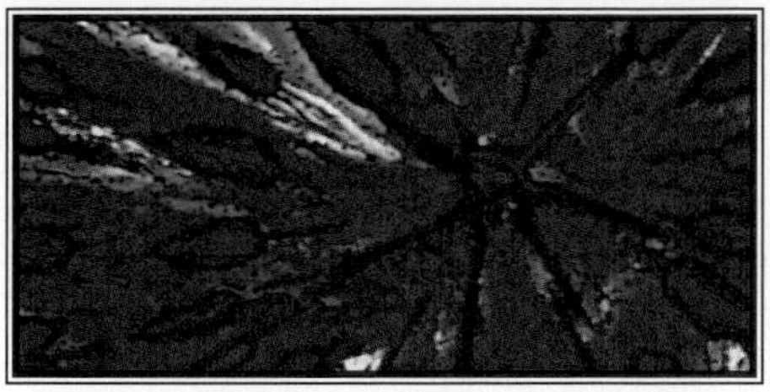

Appendix I

Appendix J

Appendix K

Glossary

Index

Preface

This seventh edition of *Understanding Nutrition* shares the same goals established almost twenty years ago in writing the first edition: to provide a textbook that would both reveal the fascination of the science of nutrition and share the fun and excitement of nutrition with the reader. Readers want more than just facts—they want an understanding of how the scientific facts apply to their daily lives. While the goals for this edition remain unchanged, every chapter has been substantially revised to reflect the many changes that have occurred in the field of nutrition over the years.

This book presents the core information of an introductory nutrition course. Chapter 1 wastes no time in exploring why we eat the foods we do and continues with a brief overview of the nutrients, the science of nutrition, recommended nutrient intakes, assessment, and important relationships between diet and health. Chapter 2 describes the diet-planning principles and food guides used to create diets that support good health and includes instructions on how to read a food label. In Chapter 3, readers follow the journey of digestion and absorption as the body transforms foods into nutrients. Chapters 4 through 6 describe carbohydrates, fats, and proteins—their chemistry, health effects, roles in the body, and places in the diet. Then Chapter 7 shows how the body derives energy from these three nutrients. Chapters 8 and 9 continue the story with a look at energy balance, the factors associated with overweight and underweight, and the benefits and dangers of weight loss and weight gain. Chapters 10 through 13 complete the introductory lessons by describing the vitamins, the minerals, and water—their roles in the body, deficiency and toxicity symptoms, and sources.

The next seven chapters weave that basic information into practical applications, showing how nutrition influences people's lives. Chapter 14 describes how physical activity and nutrition work together to support health. Chapters 15, 16, and 17 present the special nutrient needs of people through the life cycle—pregnancy and lactation; infancy, childhood, and adolescence; and adulthood and the later years. Chapter 18 focuses on the dietary risk factors and recommendations associated with chronic diseases, and Chapter 19 addresses consumer concerns about the safety of the food and water supply. Chapter 20 closes the book with a look at hunger and global environmental problems and offers suggestions for establishing sustainable foodways.

To the person reading this text, it will be obvious that, like most sciences, nutrition possesses no absolute certainties. Nutrition scientists simply do not have all the answers yet; in some cases, we have not even asked all the questions yet. This is true in many areas of nutrition; it is a growing, young science dating only from around the turn of the century. One of the missions of this text, beginning in Chapter 1, is to show readers how researchers ascertain the "facts."

Many of the chapters in this edition include "How To" skill boxes that guide readers through problem-solving tasks. For example, a box in Chapter 1 shows readers how to calculate energy intake from the grams of carbohydrate, fat, and protein in a food; another box in Chapter 13 describes how to calculate iron absorption from a meal.

New to this edition are summary paragraphs, marked with a thin blue bar in the margin. These paragraphs review the contents of the previous section; in some chapters, such as those covering the vitamins and minerals, summaries appear in tables.

Also featured in this edition are the Healthy People 2000 nutrition-related priorities, which are presented wherever their subjects are discussed (Appendix G presents them in full). Healthy People 2000 is a report developed by the U.S. Department of Health and Human Services that establishes national objectives in health promotion and disease prevention for the year 2000.

Each chapter closes with study questions, and many chapters include problem sets. Study questions offer readers the opportunity to review the major concepts presented in the chapters. Problem sets present simple nutrition-related calculations that will prove many of the concepts introduced in the chapter (answers appear in Appendix K).

Highlights on current issues of interest alternate with the chapters. Each highlight provides readers with a brief look at a topic that relates to its companion chapter. New highlights in this edition explore healthy ethnic cuisines (including the Mediterranean diet), the fattening power of fat, the roles of antioxidant nutrients and nonnutrients in disease prevention, childhood obesity and its influence on the early development of chronic diseases, and nutrient-drug interactions.

The appendixes are valuable references for a number of purposes. Appendix A summarizes background information on the hormonal and nervous systems, complementing Appendixes B and C on basic chemistry, the chemical structures of nutrients, and major metabolic pathways. Appendix D assists readers with calculations and conversions. Appendix E provides detailed coverage on nutrition assessment, and Appendix F lists nutrition resources, including book and journal recommendations as well as addresses. Appendix G presents the Recommended Dietary Allowances (1989 RDA), the Daily Values for food labels, the nutrition-related priorities of Healthy People 2000, the United States Exchange System, and recommendations from the World Health Organization (WHO). Appendix H is a 2000–item food composition table made from the latest nutrient data base assembled by ESHA Research, Inc., of Salem, Oregon. Appendix I presents information for Canadians: the Recommended Nutrient Intakes (1990 RNI), the Exchange System, and instructions on reading food labels. Appendix J describes measures of protein quality and Appendix K presents the answers to the problem sets that appear at the ends of chapters.

We have tried to keep the number of footnotes to a minimum. Many statements that have appeared in previous editions with footnotes now appear without them, but every statement is backed by research, and the authors will supply references upon request. We have not provided a separate list of suggested readings, but have tried to include references that will provide readers with additional details or a good overview of the subject.

We hope our informal, conversational writing style makes the study of nutrition an enjoyable experience. Nutrition is a fascinating subject, and we hope our enthusiasm for it comes through on every page.

Eleanor Noss Whitney
Sharon Rady Rolfes
December 1995

Acknowledgments

To produce a book requires the coordinated effort of a team of people—and, no doubt, each team member has another team of support people as well. We salute, with a big round of applause, everyone who has worked so diligently to ensure the quality of this book.

We thank Linda DeBruyne and Yvonne Jones for their valuable contributions to the fitness and hunger chapters, respectively. A million thank yous to Mary Ann Riveccio for her patient attention to manuscript preparation, permissions, and a multitude of other daily tasks. We thank Diane Dziekan for her assistance on the Problem Sets; Sabrina McGriff for her attention to bookkeeping tasks; and Sally Lorch for her help around the office. To Linda Patton, a special thank you for her skilled assistance in library research. We also thank the many people who have prepared the ancillaries that accompany this text: Harry Sitren for writing and enhancing the Test Bank; Lori Turner, Mary Rhiner, and Margaret Hedley for preparing the Instructor's Manual, and Judy Kaufman for providing video disc references in the manual; and Lori Turner for authoring the Student Study Guide. A big thank you to Elizabeth Hands, Bob Geltz, and their staff at ESHA for their meticulous effort in creating the food composition appendix, verifying the data in figures and tables, and developing the computerized diet analysis program that accompanies this book. Our special thanks to the editorial team of Peter Marshall, Becky Tollerson, and Kara ZumBahlen for their conscientious coordination of reviews and production. We also thank John Woolsey and his associates for creating accurate and attractive artwork to complement our writing; Michael Davidson for transforming nutrients into outstanding works of art that grace the cover and chapter opening pages; Tom Harm and Tom Peterson for photographing foods beautifully; and Pat Lewis for copyediting thousands of pages of manuscript. To the many others involved in designing, indexing, typesetting, dummying, and marketing, we tip our hats in appreciation.

We are especially grateful to our associates, friends, and families for their continued encouragement and support. We also thank our many reviewers for their comments and contributions.

Reviewers of *Understanding Nutrition*

Ellen Brennan
San Antonio College

Jim Daugherty
Glendale Community College

Pam Fletcher
Albuquerque Technical Vocational Institute

Betty Forbes
West Virginia University

Eileen Ford
University of Pennsylvania

William Forsythe
University of Southern Mississippi

Julie Friedman
SUNY at Farmingdale

Patty Garrett
University of Tennessee-Chattanooga

Francine Genta
Cabrillo College

Mary Thompson-Gove
Barry University

Leon Hageman
Burlington County College

Charlene Hamilton
University of Delaware

Michael Jenkins
Kent State University

Jayanthi Kandiah
Ball State University

Younghee Kim
Bowling Green State University

Kevin King
Clinton Community College

Kim Kline
University of Texas-Austin

Carolyn Knutson
Clackamas Community College

Margaret Latimer
Delta College

Chunhye Kim Lee
Northern Arizona University

Robert Lee
Central Michigan University

Anne Leftwich
University of Central Oklahoma

Joseph Leichter
University of British Columbia

Janet Levins
Pensacola Junior College

Harriet McCoy
University of Arkansas-Fayetteville

Bruce McDonald
University of Manitoba

Lisa McKee
New Mexico State University

Nina Mercer
University of Guelph

Paula Netherton
Tulsa Junior College

Kitty Hester Ocker
North Harris College

Mary Oleske
Albuquerque Technical Vocational Institute

Linda Peck
University of Findlay in Ohio

Erwina Peterson
Yakima Valley Community College

Janet Sass
Northern Virginia Community College

Ginger Schirmer
Texas Christian University

James Thompson
University of Waterloo

Marie Tymrak
Phoenix College

Anne VanBeber
Texas Christian University

Suzy Weems
Stephen F. Austin University

Lisa Young
New York University

Chapter 1

An Overview of Nutrition

CONTENTS

MICROGRAPH: Carrot

Welcome to the world of nutrition. Nutrition has played a significant role in your life, even from before your birth, although you may not always have been aware of it. And it will continue to affect you in major ways, depending on how you choose your foods.

Every day, several times a day, you make food choices that influence your body's health for better or worse. Each day's choices may benefit or harm your health only a little, but when these choices are repeated over years and decades, the rewards or consequences become major. That being the case, close attention to good nutrition now can bring health benefits later. Conversely, carelessness about nutrition from youth on can be a major contributor to many of today's most prevalent chronic diseases of later life, including heart disease and cancer. Of course, some people will become ill or die young no matter what choices they make; and others will live long lives despite making poor choices; but for the large majority, the food choices they make each and every day will benefit or impair their health in proportion to the wisdom of the choices.

In general, a **chronic** disease is one of long duration that progresses slowly. By comparison, an **acute** disease develops quickly, produces sharp symptoms, and runs a short course.
acute = sharp
chronos = time

diet: the foods and beverages a person eats and drinks.

While most people realize that their food habits affect their health, they often choose foods for other reasons. After all, foods bring to the table a variety of pleasures, traditions, and associations as well as nourishment. The challenge, then, is to combine favorite foods and fun times with a nutritionally balanced diet.

Food Choices

People decide what to eat, when to eat, and even whether to eat in highly personal ways, often based on behavioral or social motives rather than on awareness of nutrition's importance to health. Fortunately, many different food choices can be healthy ones, but nutrition awareness helps to make them so.

Personal Preference One reason people choose foods, of course, is that they like certain flavors. Two widely shared preferences are for the sweetness of sugar and the tang of salt. Other preferences might be for the hot peppers common in Mexican cooking or the curry spices of Indian cuisine. Some research suggests that genetics may influence people's food preferences.[1]

Habit People sometimes select foods out of habit. They eat cereal every morning, for example, simply because they have always eaten cereal for breakfast. Eating a familiar food and not having to make any decisions can be comforting.

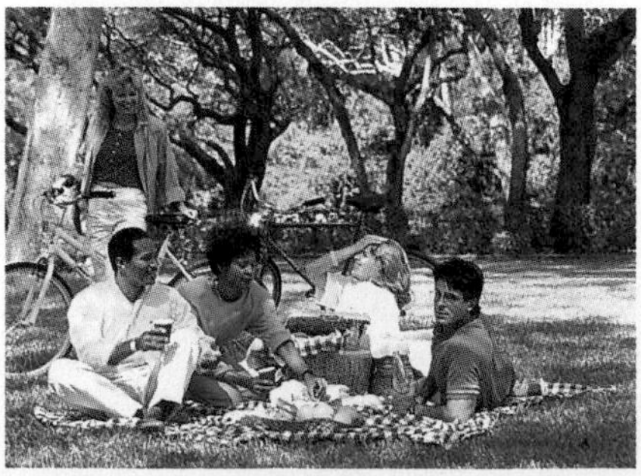
People enjoy companionship while eating.

Ethnic Heritage or Tradition Among the strongest influences on food choices are ethnic heritage and tradition. People eat the foods they grew up eating. Every country—and every region of a country—has its own typical foods and ways of combining foods into meals. Highlight 2 shows how people can make healthful food choices within their own ethnic cuisines.

Social Interactions Food signifies friendliness. Meals are social events, and the sharing of food is part of hospitality. Social customs almost compel people to accept food or drink offered by a host or shared by a group. When your friends are going out for pizza or ice cream, how can you refuse to go along?

Availability, Convenience, and Economy People eat foods that are accessible, quick and easy to prepare, and within their financial means. Consumers today value convenience especially highly, as reflected in their choices of meals they can prepare quickly, recipes with few ingredients, and products they can cook in microwave ovens. Many people frequently eat out or have food delivered, which limits food choices to the selections on the restaurants' menus.

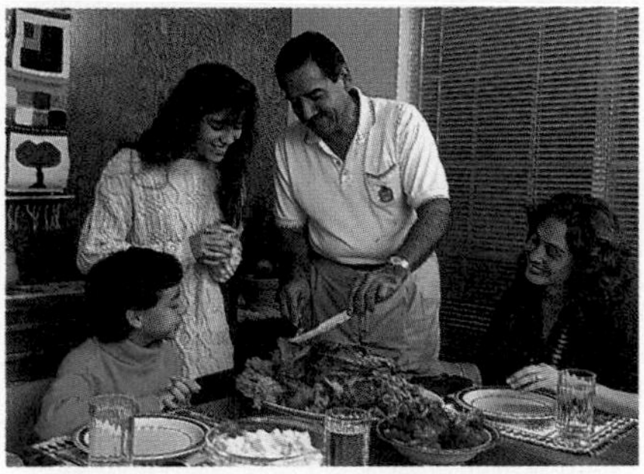

For many people, a special family dinner brings pleasant memories of the holidays.

Positive and Negative Associations People tend to like foods with happy associations—such as hot dogs at ball games or turkey at Thanksgiving. By the same token, people can attach intense and unalterable dislikes to foods that they ate when they felt sick, or that were forced on them when they weren't hungry. Parents may teach their children to like and dislike certain foods by using those foods as rewards or punishments.

Sometimes associations classify foods for certain uses.[2] For example, people may believe that peanut butter is for children, or that lobster is for the rich. Then, depending on whether they permit themselves to be childlike or to indulge in luxuries, they will choose to eat or refrain from eating those foods.

Emotional Comfort Some people eat in response to emotional stimuli—for example, to relieve boredom or depression or to calm anxiety. A lonely person may choose to eat rather than to call a friend and risk rejection. A person who has returned home from an exciting evening out may unwind with a late-night snack. Eating in response to emotions can easily lead to overeating and obesity, but may be appropriate at times. For example, sharing food at times of bereavement serves both the giver's need to provide comfort and the receiver's need to be cared for and to interact with others, as well as to take nourishment.

Values Food choices may reflect people's religious beliefs, political views, or environmental concerns. For example, many Christians forgo meat during Lent, the period prior to Easter, and Jewish law includes an extensive set of dietary rules. A political activist may boycott vegetables picked by migrant workers who have been exploited. People may buy vegetables from local farmers to save the fuel and environmental costs of foods shipped in from far away. Consumers may also select foods packaged in containers that can be reused or recycled.

Body Image Sometimes men and women select certain foods and supplements that they believe will improve their physical appearances and avoid those they believe might be detrimental. Such decisions can be beneficial when based on sound nutrition and fitness knowledge, but undermine good health when based on faddism or carried to extremes.

Nutrition Finally, of course, a valid reason to select certain foods is that they will benefit health. Nutritional and health values have become influential in many consumers' food choices, even when other forces are at work. A person may choose for social reasons to go out "for pizza" with friends, but once there, might eat only one slice with a large salad of fresh vegetables. Food manufacturers have responded to scientific findings linking health with nutrition by offering an abundant selection of health-promoting foods and beverages. Consumers welcome these new foods into their diets, provided that the foods are reasonably priced, clearly labeled, easy to find in the grocery store, and convenient to prepare. These foods must also taste good—as good as the traditional choices. Of course, a person need not eat any of these "special" foods to enjoy a healthy diet; ordinary foods, well chosen, serve just as well.

In summary, a person selects foods for a variety of reasons. Whatever those reasons may be, food choices influence health. Individual food selections neither make nor break a diet's healthfulness, but the balance of foods selected over time can make an important difference to health. For this reason, people are wise to allow nutrition knowledge to play a major role in their food decisions.

Introducing the Nutrients

Do you ever think of yourself as a collection of carefully arranged atoms, molecules, cells, tissues, and organs? Are you aware of the activity going on within your body even as you sit still? The atoms, molecules, and cells of your body continually move and change, even though the structures of your tissues and organs, and your external appearance, remain relatively constant.

Your skin, which seems to have covered you since your birth, is replaced entirely by new cells every seven years. The fat beneath your skin is not the same fat that was there a year ago. Your oldest red blood cell is only 120 days old, and the entire lining of your digestive tract is renewed every 3 days. To maintain your "self," you must continually replenish, from foods, the energy and the nutrients you deplete in maintaining your body.

foods: products derived from plants or animals that can be taken into the body to yield nutrients for the maintenance of life and the growth and repair of tissues.

nutrients: substances obtained from food and used in the body to provide energy and structural materials and to regulate growth, maintenance, and repair of the body's tissues; nutrients may also reduce the risks of some chronic diseases.

THE SIX CLASSES OF NUTRIENTS

Amazingly, the body can derive all the energy, structural materials, and regulating agents that it needs from the foods we eat. The secret lies in the genetic information you inherited from your parents, which gives the instructions for assembling body structures from the nutrients in foods. As long as you give your body the energy and nutrients it needs in sufficient amounts, your genetic blueprints will direct that the pieces be put together and work according to the plan. This section introduces the nutrients that foods bring to the body and shows how they take part in the dynamic processes that keep people alive and well.

Composition of Foods Chemical analysis of a food such as a tomato shows that it is composed primarily of water (95 percent). Most of the solid materials are the compounds carbohydrate, fat, and protein. If you could remove these materials, you would find a tiny residue of vitamins, minerals, and other compounds. Water, carbohydrate, fat, protein, vitamins, and some of the minerals found in foods are nutrients—substances the body uses for the growth, maintenance, and repair of its tissues. Other nutritionally important constituents of foods are the fibers—members of the carbohydrate family that also support good health.

The six classes of nutrients:

- Carbohydrate.
- Fat.
- Protein.
- Vitamins.
- Minerals.
- Water.

The human body, like foods, is composed largely of nutrients.

Composition of the Body A complete chemical analysis of your body would show that it is made of materials similar to those found in foods. A healthy 150-pound body contains about 90 pounds of water and about 30 pounds of fat. The other 30 pounds are mostly compounds containing protein and carbohydrate and the major minerals of the bones. Vitamins, other minerals, and incidental extras constitute a fraction of a pound.

Chemical Composition of Nutrients The simplest of the nutrients are the minerals. Each mineral is a chemical element, which means that its atoms are all alike. As a result, its identity never changes. Iron, for example, remains iron when a food is cooked, when a person eats the food, when iron becomes part of a red blood cell, when the cell is broken down, and when the iron is lost from the body by excretion. The next simplest nutrient is water, a compound made of two elements—hydrogen and oxygen. Minerals and water are inorganic nutrients—they contain no carbon.

The other four classes of nutrients (carbohydrate, fat, protein, and vitamins) are more complex. In addition to hydrogen and oxygen, they all contain carbon, an element that is found in all living things. They are therefore called organic compounds (meaning, literally, "alive"). Protein and some vitamins also contain nitrogen and may contain other elements as well (see Figure 1–1).

Essential Nutrients The body can make some nutrients for itself. The body cannot make all the nutrients, however: some, it cannot make at all; and some, it makes in insufficient quantities to meet its needs. It must obtain these nutrients from foods. The nutrients that foods must supply are *essential nutrients*. When used to refer to nutrients, then, the word *essential* means more than just "necessary"; it means "needed from outside the body"—normally, from foods.

This book focuses mostly on the nutrients, but other constituents also occur in foods and in the body—alcohols, organic acids, pigments, additives, and others. Some are beneficial, some are neutral, and a few are harmful. Later sections of the book touch on these nonnutrients and their significance.

*This definition excludes coal, diamonds, and a few carbon-containing compounds that contain only a single carbon and no hydrogen, such as carbon dioxide (CO_2), calcium carbonate ($CaCO_3$), magnesium carbonate ($MgCO_3$), and sodium cyanide (NaCN).

element: a substance composed of atoms that are alike—for example, iron (Fe).

atom: the smallest component of an element that has all of the properties of the element.

compound: a substance composed of two or more different atoms—for example, water (H_2O).

inorganic: not containing carbon or pertaining to living things.
in = not

organic: a substance or molecule containing carbon-carbon bonds or carbon-hydrogen bonds.* Some farmers call their produce "organic" if it was grown without manufactured fertilizers and pesticides, but by the definition given here, all foods are organic.

molecule: two or more atoms of the same or different elements joined by chemical bonds. Examples are molecules of the element oxygen, composed of two oxygen atoms (O_2), and molecules of the compound water, composed of two hydrogen atoms and one oxygen atom (H_2O).

essential nutrients: nutrients a person must obtain from food because the body cannot make them for itself in sufficient quantity to meet physiological needs; also called **indispensable nutrients**. About 40 nutrients are known to be essential for human beings.

nonnutrients: compounds in foods with no known nutritional value.

	Carbon	Hydrogen	Oxygen	Nitrogen	Minerals
Inorganic nutrients					
Minerals					√
Water		√	√		
Organic nutrients					
Carbohydrates	√	√	√		
Fats	√	√	√		
Proteins[a]	√	√	√	√	
Vitamins[b]	√	√	√		

[a]Proteins also contain the mineral sulfur.
[b]Some vitamins contain nitrogen, some contain minerals.

Figure 1–1

Elements in the Six Classes of Nutrients

Notice that organic nutrients contain carbon.

How to Think Metric

Like other scientists, nutrition scientists use metric units of measure. They measure food energy in kilocalories, people's height in centimeters, people's weight in kilograms, and the weights of foods and nutrients in grams, milligrams, or micrograms. For ease in using these measures, it helps to remember that the prefixes on the grams imply 1000. For example, a *kilo*gram is 1000 grams; a *milli*gram is 1/1000 of a gram, and a *micro*gram is 1/1000 of a milligram.

Most food labels and many recipe books provide "dual measures," listing both household measures, such as cups, quarts, and teaspoons, and metric measures, such as milliliters, liters, and grams. This practice gives people a chance to gradually learn to "think metric."

A person might begin to "think metric" by simply observing the measure—by noticing the amount of soda in a 2-liter bottle, for example. Such experiences allow a person to become familiar with a measure without having to do any conversions.

Many members of the international scientific community have adopted a common system of measurement to facilitate communication—the International System of Units (SI). In addition to using metric measures, the SI establishes common units of measurement. For example, the SI unit for measuring food energy is the joule (not the kcalorie). A joule is the amount of energy expended when 1 kilogram is moved 1 meter by a force of 1 newton. The joule is thus a measure of *work* energy, whereas the kcalorie is a measure of *heat* energy. While many scientists and journals report their findings in kilojoules (kJ), many others, particularly those in the United States, use kcalories. To convert energy measures from kcalories to kilojoules, multiply by 4.2. For example, a 50-kcalorie cookie provides 210 kJ:

$$50 \text{ kcal} \times 4.2 = 210 \text{ kJ}.$$

Exact conversion factors for these and other units of measure are in Appendix D.

- **Volume: Liters (L)**

1 L = 1000 milliliters (mL).
0.95 L = 1 quart.
1 mL = 0.03 fluid ounces.
250 mL = 1 cup.

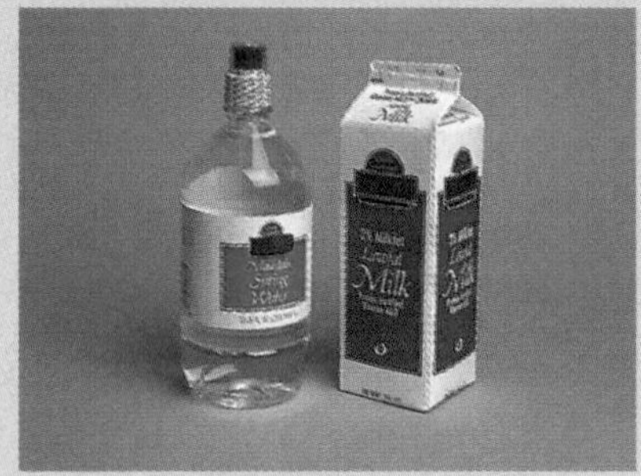

A liter of liquid is approximately one quart. (Four liters are only about 5 percent more than a gallon.)

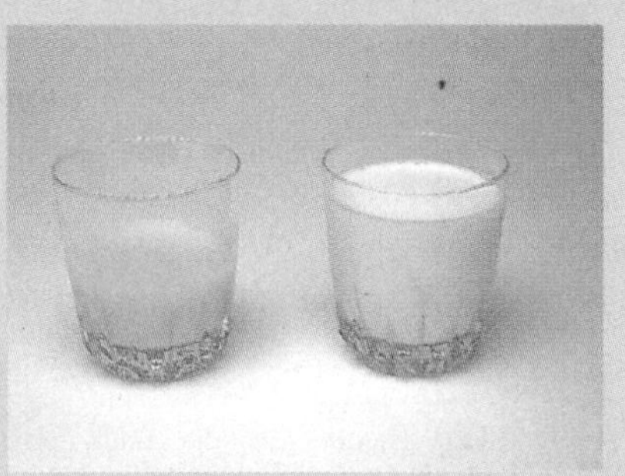

A half-cup of liquid is about 125 milliliters; one cup is about 250 milliliters.

THE ENERGY-YIELDING NUTRIENTS

In the body, three of the organic nutrients are broken down to provide usable energy: carbohydrate, fat, and protein. In contrast, vitamins, minerals, and water do not yield energy in the human body.

energy: the capacity to do work. The energy in food is chemical energy. The body can convert this chemical energy to mechanical, electrical, or heat energy.

energy-yielding nutrients: the nutrients that break down to yield energy the body can use:
- Carbohydrate.
- Fat.
- Protein.

Energy Measured in kCalories The energy released from the energy-yielding nutrients can be measured in calories—tiny units of energy so small that a single apple provides tens of thousands of them. To ease calculations, energy is expressed in 1000-calorie units known as kilocalories (shortened to kcalories, but commonly called "calories"). When you read in popular books or magazines that an apple provides "100 calories," understand that it means 100 kcalories. This

- **Weight: Grams (g)**

1 g = 1000 milligrams (mg).
1 g = 0.04 ounces (oz).
1 oz = 28.35 grams or ≈ 30 grams.
100 g ≈ 3 ½ ounces.

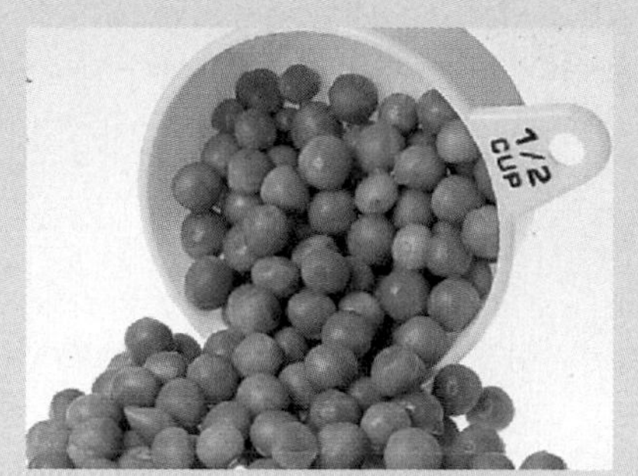

A half-cup of vegetables weighs about 100 grams.

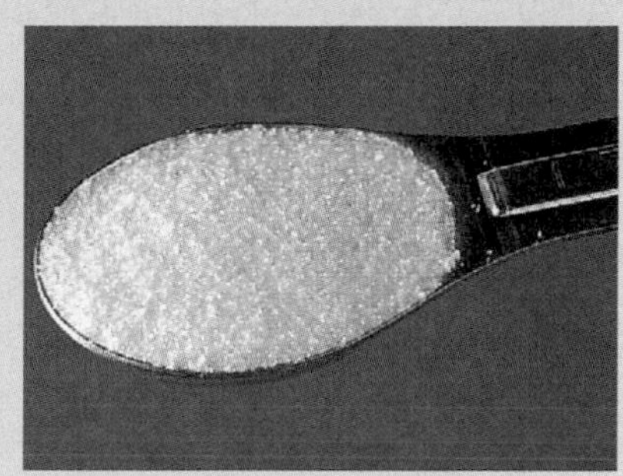
One teaspoon of dry granular powder such as salt or sugar weighs about 5 grams.

1 kilogram (kg) = 1000 grams.
1 kg = 2.2 pounds.
454 g = 1 pound.
A kilogram is slightly more than 2 pounds; conversely, a pound weighs about ½ kilogram.

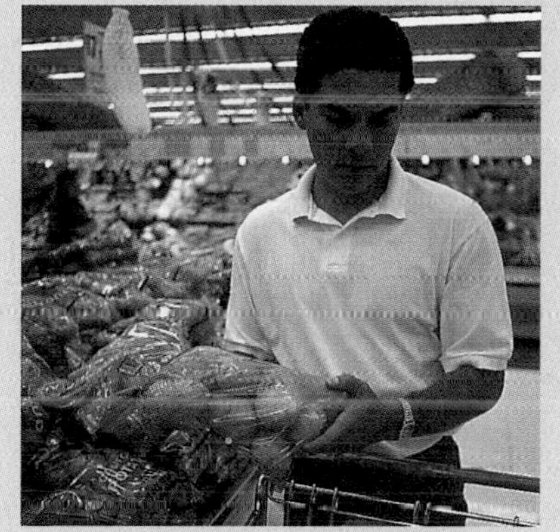
A 5-pound bag of potatoes weighs about 2 kilograms and a 176-pound person weighs 80 kilograms.

- **Height: Meters (m)**

1 m = 100 centimeters (cm).
2.54 cm = 1 inch.
1 mm = 0.04 inches.

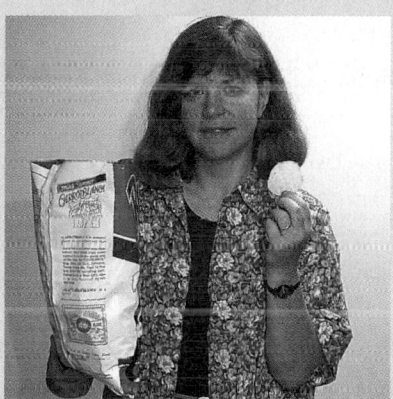
A person 5 feet 5 inches tall measures about 165 centimeters, and a rippled potato chip is about 1 millimeter thick.

book uses the term *kcalorie* and its abbreviation *kcal* throughout, as do other scientific books and journals. The accompanying box provides a few tips on how to "think metric."

A kcalorie is not a constituent of foods; it is a measure of the potential energy in foods. Thus to speak of the "kcalories" in a cookie is technically incorrect, just as to speak of the inches in a person is incorrect. It is correct to speak of the *energy* available from a food (and of the *height* of a person).

calorie: a unit by which energy is measured. Food energy is measured in **kilocalories** (1000 calories equal 1 kilocalorie), abbreviated **kcalories** or **kcal**. A capitalized version is also sometimes used: **Calories**. One kcalorie is the amount of heat necessary to raise the temperature of 1 kilogram (kg) of water 1°C.

Energy in Foods The energy content of a food depends on how much carbohydrate, fat, and protein it contains. When completely broken down in the body, a gram of carbohydrate yields about 4 kcalories of energy; a gram of protein

How to Calculate the Energy Available from Foods

To calculate the energy available from a food, multiply the number of grams of carbohydrate, protein, and fat by 4, 4, and 9, respectively. Then add the results together. For example, 1 slice of bread with 1 tablespoon of peanut butter on it contains 16 grams carbohydrate, 7 grams protein, and 9 grams fat:

$$\begin{aligned} 16 \text{ g carbohydrate} \times 4 \text{ kcal/g} &= 64 \text{ kcal.} \\ 7 \text{ g protein} \times 4 \text{ kcal/g} &= 28 \text{ kcal.} \\ 9 \text{ g fat} \times 9 \text{ kcal/g} &= 81 \text{ kcal.} \\ \text{Total} &= 173 \text{ kcal.} \end{aligned}$$

From this information, you can calculate the percentage of kcalories each of the energy nutrients contributes to the total. To determine the percentage of kcalories from fat, for example, divide the 81 fat kcalories by the total 173 kcalories:

$$81 \div 173 = 0.468 \text{ (rounded to 0.47).}$$

Then multiply by 100 to get the percentage:

$$0.47 \times 100 = 47\%.$$

Health recommendations that urge people to limit fat intake to 30 percent of kcalories refer to the day's total energy intake, not to individual foods. Still, if the proportion of fat in each food choice throughout a day exceeds 30 percent of kcalories, then the day's total surely will too. Knowing that this snack provides 47 percent of its kcalories from fat alerts a person to the need to make lower-fat selections at other times that day.

1 g carbohydrate = 4 kcal.
1 g protein = 4 kcal.
1 g fat = 9 kcal.
1 g alcohol = 7 kcal.

also yields 4 kcalories; and a gram of fat yields 9 kcalories.* The accompanying box explains how to calculate the energy available from foods.

One other substance contributes food energy: alcohol. Alcohol is not considered a nutrient because it interferes with the growth, maintenance, and repair of the body, but it does yield energy when metabolized in the body.†

Most foods contain all three energy-yielding nutrients, as well as water, vitamins, minerals, and other substances. Thus it is inaccurate to identify foods with their predominant nutrients—for example, to speak of meat as a protein or of bread as a carbohydrate. Meat and bread are *foods* rich in these nutrients. Meat contains water, fat, vitamins, and minerals as well as protein. Bread contains water, a trace of fat, a little protein, and some vitamins and minerals in addition to its carbohydrate. Only a few foods are exceptions to this rule, the common ones being sugar (pure carbohydrate) and oil (essentially pure fat).

Energy in the Body The body uses the energy-yielding nutrients to fuel its metabolic and physical activities. All the energy used to keep the heart beating, the brain thinking, and the legs walking comes from energy-yielding nutrients.

*For those using kilojoules: 1 g carbohydrate = 17 kJ; 1 g protein = 17 kJ; 1 g fat = 37 kJ.

†For those using kilojoules: 1 g alcohol = 29 kJ. For those using milliliters: 1 mL alcohol = 5.6 kcal.

When the body metabolizes the energy-yielding nutrients, the bonds between their atoms break. As the bonds break, they release energy in a controlled version of the process by which wood burns in a fire. When wood burns, it releases heat (energy), steam (water), some carbon and minerals as carbon dioxide and other oxides, and some carbon and minerals as ash. During the body's metabolism of nutrients, some of the energy from food is released as heat just as in the burning of wood, but some is used to send electrical impulses through the brain and nerves, to synthesize body compounds, and to move muscles. Thus the energy from food supports every activity from quiet thought to vigorous sports. To support this metabolism, you continually inhale oxygen and exhale carbon dioxide made by combining oxygen with the carbons of the foods you have eaten. You also excrete the hydrogens of foods, combined with oxygen, as water in your urine and vapor as you breathe. Thus food fuels all of life's activities.

The processes by which nutrients are broken down to yield energy or rearranged into body structures are known as *metabolism* (defined and described further in Chapter 7).

During energy metabolism, the carbon atoms combine with oxygen to yield carbon dioxide; the hydrogen atoms combine with oxygen to yield water.

If the body has an excess of any of the three energy-yielding nutrients, it rearranges them (and the energy they contain) into carbohydrate and fat storage compounds, to be drawn upon between meals and overnight when fresh energy supplies run low. If you take in more energy than you expend, especially when the excess energy is from foods rich in fat, you gain weight as body fat.

When taken in excess of energy need, alcohol, too, can be converted to body fat and stored. However, when alcohol contributes a substantial portion of the energy in a person's diet, the harm it does extends far beyond the problems of adding fat to the body. (Highlight 7 is devoted to alcohol and nutrition.)

The body's use (metabolism) of the energy-yielding nutrients can be summarized as follows. Carbohydrate, fat, and protein from foods are broken down to simpler compounds. The process yields energy and smaller molecules. The energy may:

- Escape as heat.
- Help build new compounds (and some energy may be stored in them).
- Help move the body (do work).

The smaller molecules may:

- Serve as building blocks for new compounds (fat, muscle, or other tissues).
- Be excreted as waste materials.

Other Roles of Energy-Yielding Nutrients In addition to providing energy, carbohydrate, fat, and protein provide the raw materials for building the body's tissues and regulating its many activities. In fact, protein's role as a fuel source is relatively minor compared with both the other two nutrients and its other roles. Proteins are found in structures such as the muscles and skin and help to regulate activities such as digestion and energy production.

Chapters 4, 5, and 6 provide more details about carbohydrate, fat, and protein. Chapter 4 includes the fibers in its discussion of the carbohydrates. Most fibers are carbohydrates, but unlike the carbohydrates, the fibers yield little or no energy. In fact, fibers pass through the body largely undigested. Fibers are important to health because they exercise the digestive tract muscles and carry potentially harmful substances out of the body, helping to lower the risks of heart disease and cancer. Fibers also provide bulk, which makes them filling, a characteristic that benefits weight control. Chapter 7 presents an introductory lesson on metabolism and sets

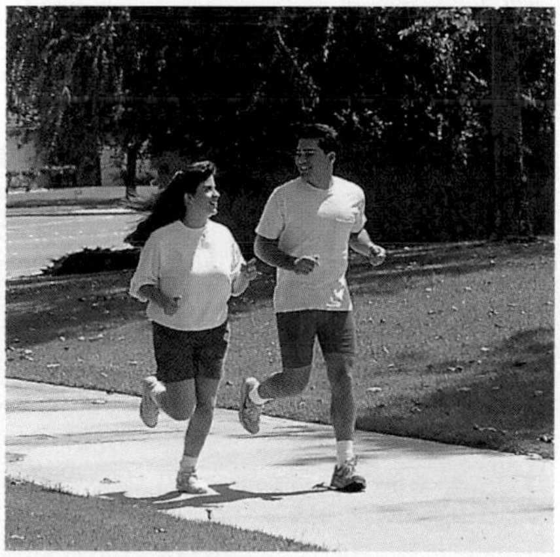

The energy to run a mile or read a book comes from the carbohydrate, fat, and protein in foods.

the stage for understanding energy balance and weight control (Chapters 8 and 9) and nutrition's role in exercise (Chapter 14).

THE VITAMINS

vitamins: organic, essential nutrients required in small amounts by the body for health. The water-soluble vitamins are vitamin C and the eight B vitamins: thiamin, riboflavin, niacin, vitamins B_6 and B_{12}, folate, biotin, and pantothenic acid. The fat-soluble vitamins are vitamins A, D, E, and K. The water-soluble vitamins are the subject of Chapter 10 and the fat-soluble vitamins, of Chapter 11.

Like the first three classes of nutrients (carbohydrate, fat, and protein), the vitamins are vital to life, organic, and available in food. They differ, however, in that the body does not extract usable energy from vitamins; rather, it uses them as helpers in metabolic processes.

Vitamins can function only if they are intact, but because they are complex organic molecules, they are vulnerable to destruction by heat, light, and chemical agents. This is why the body handles them carefully, and why nutrition-wise cooks do too. The strategies of cooking foods at moderate temperatures, in or over small amounts of water, and for short times all help to preserve the vitamins.

There are 13 different vitamins, each with its own special roles to play. One vitamin enables the eyes to see in dim light, another helps protect the lungs from air pollution, and still another helps make the sex hormones—among other things. When you cut yourself, one vitamin helps stop the bleeding and another helps repair the skin. Vitamins busily help replace old red blood cells and the lining of the digestive tract. Almost every action in the body requires the assistance of vitamins.

THE MINERALS

minerals: inorganic elements; some minerals are essential nutrients required in small amounts. The major minerals are calcium, phosphorus, potassium, sodium, chloride, magnesium, and sulfur. The trace minerals are iron, iodine, zinc, chromium, selenium, fluoride, molybdenum, copper, and manganese. Chapters 12 and 13 are devoted to the major and trace minerals, respectively.

The problems caused by one of the contaminant minerals, lead, are detailed in Highlight 19.

In contrast to the vitamins, which are organic compounds, the minerals are pure inorganic elements. That means the minerals occur in the simplest of chemical forms, as atoms of a single element. Some minerals may be put together into orderly arrays in such structures as bones and teeth. Some minerals are found in the fluids of the body and influence the properties of those fluids. Whatever their roles, minerals are not metabolized, nor do they yield energy.

Some 16 minerals are known to be essential in human nutrition; others are still being studied to determine whether they play significant roles in the human body. Still other minerals are important because they are *not* nutrients, but toxic environmental contaminants, which may displace nutrient minerals from their workplaces in the body, disrupting body functions.

Because they are indestructible, minerals in foods need not be handled with the special care that vitamins need. They can, however, be bound by substances that make it hard for the body to absorb them. They can also be lost during food refining processes or dissolve into water during cooking and then be discarded.

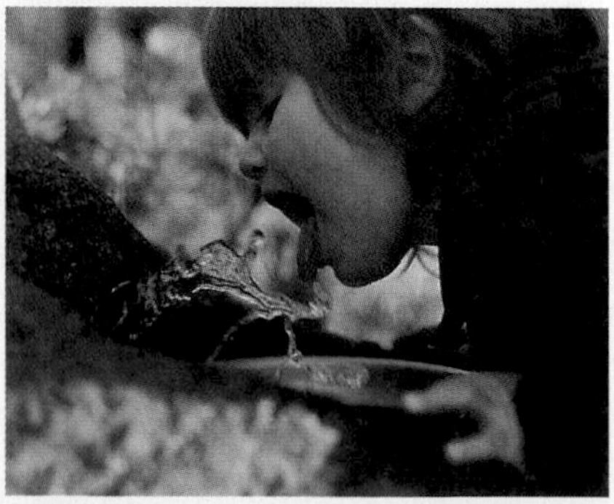

Water itself is an essential nutrient and naturally contains many minerals, which give it flavor.

WATER

Water, indispensable and abundant, provides the environment in which nearly all the body's activities are conducted. It participates in many metabolic reactions and supplies the medium for transporting vital materials to cells and waste products away from them. Water is discussed fully in Chapter 12, but it is mentioned in every chapter. If you watch for it, you cannot help but be impressed by water's participation in all life processes.

To sum up, foods provide energy and nutrients—substances that support the growth, maintenance, and repair of the body's tissue. Three nutrients (carbohydrate, fat, and protein) provide the major materials for building the body's tissues and yield energy for the body's use or storage. Energy is measured in kcalories. The other three (vitamins, minerals, and water) facilitate a variety of activities in the body. Without exaggeration, nutrients provide the physical basis for nearly all that we are and all that we do.

The Science of Nutrition

The science of nutrition is the study of the nutrients in foods and the body's handling of those nutrients. As sciences go, nutrition is a young one. To put its age in perspective, if the 3-million-year history of the human race were compressed into 24 hours, then scientific discoveries began about 12 seconds ago, and nutrition as an organized science emerged only during the last 3 to 6 seconds.[3] As you can see from the size of this book, though, much has happened in nutrition's short life. This section introduces the research methods scientists have used in uncovering the wonders of the nutrients.

science of nutrition: the study of the nutrients in foods and of the body's handling of them (including ingestion, digestion, absorption, transport, metabolism, interaction, storage, and excretion). A broader definition includes the study of the environment and of human behavior as it relates to food.

NUTRITION RESEARCH

Research always begins with a question. For example, "what foods or nutrients might protect against the common cold?" In search of an answer, scientists make educated guesses (hypotheses) and then systematically conduct research studies to test each hypothesis. Examples of some types of research studies follow:

- *Epidemiological studies* observe how much and what kinds of foods a group of people eat and how healthy those people are. Such findings bring to light factors that might influence the incidence of a disease in various populations.
- *Case-control studies* compare people who do and do not have a given condition such as a disease, closely matching them in age, occupation, and other key variables so that differences in other factors will stand out. Differences then appear that may account for the condition in the group that has it.
- *Animal studies* might feed specific nutrients or diets to animals and then observe any changes in health. Such studies test possible disease causes and treatments in a laboratory where all conditions can be controlled.
- *Human intervention (or clinical) trials* ask people to adopt a new behavior (for example, eat a citrus fruit, take a vitamin C supplement, or exercise daily). These trials help determine the effects such measures have on the development or prevention of disease. Each type of study has advantages and disadvantages. Findings must be interpreted with an awareness of the study's limitations. (See Highlight 1 for a discussion on evaluating research findings.)

In attempting to discover whether a nutrient relieves symptoms or cures a disease, all research tries to answer the same kinds of questions. Research on vitamin C and the common cold illustrates particularly well what those questions are.

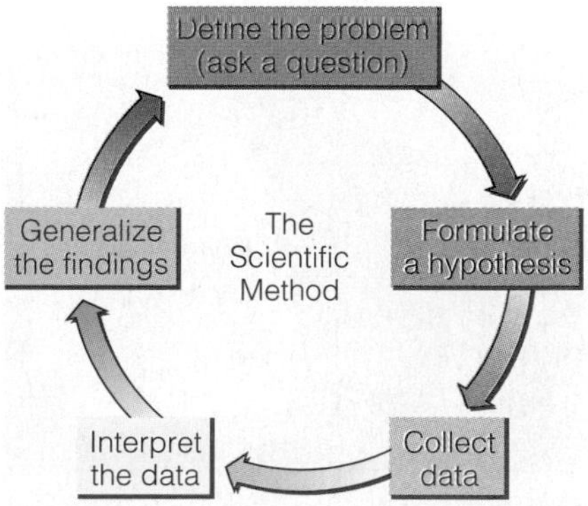

In conducting research, scientists follow these steps, which define the scientific method.

Controls In most studies on the efficacy of vitamin C, researchers divide people into two groups. One group (the experimental group) receives a vitamin C supplement, and the other (the control group) does not. Researchers follow both groups to determine whether the vitamin C group has fewer or shorter colds

Glossary of Research Terms

blind experiment: an experiment in which the subjects do not know whether they are members of the experimental group or the control group.

control group: a group of individuals similar in all possible respects to the experimental group except for the treatment. Ideally, the control group receives a placebo while the experimental group receives a real treatment.

correlation (CORE-ee-LAY-shun): the simultaneous increase, decrease, or change of two variables. If A increases as B increases, or if A decreases as B decreases, the correlation is positive. (This does not mean that A causes B or vice versa.) If A increases as B decreases, or if A decreases as B increases, the correlation is negative. (This does not mean that A prevents B or vice versa.) Some third factor may account for both A and B.

double-blind experiment: an experiment in which neither the subjects nor the researchers know which subjects are members of the experimental group and which are serving as control subjects, until after the experiment is over.

experimental group: a group of individuals similar in all possible respects to the control group except for the treatment. The experimental group receives the real treatment.

peer review: a process in which a panel of scientists rigorously evaluates a research study to assure that the scientific method was followed.

placebo (pla-SEE-bo): an inert, harmless medication given to provide comfort and hope; a sham treatment used in controlled research studies.

placebo effect: the healing effect that faith in medicine, even inert medicine, often has.

randomization (RAN-dom-ih-ZAY-shun): a process of choosing the members of the experimental and control groups without bias.

replication (REP-lee-KAY-shun): repeating an experiment and getting the same results. The skeptical scientist, on hearing of a new, exciting finding, will ask, "Has it been replicated yet?" If it hasn't, the scientist will withhold judgment regarding the finding's validity.

validity (va-LID-ih-tee): having the quality of being founded on fact or evidence.

variable: a factor that changes. A variable may depend on another variable (for example, a child's height depends on his age), or it may be independent (for example, a child's height does not depend on the color of her eyes). Sometimes both variables correlate with a third variable (a child's height and eye color both depend on genetics).

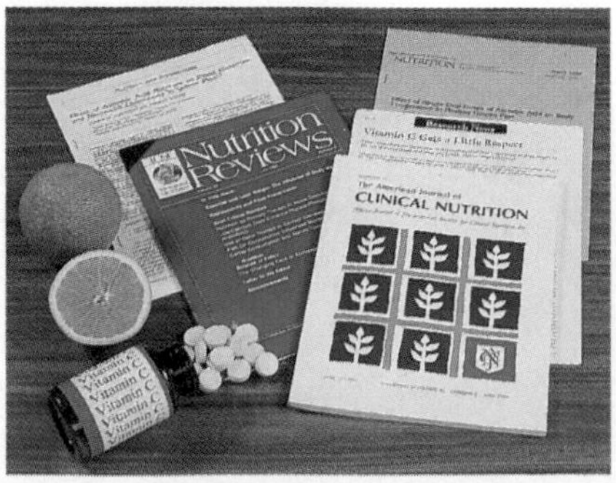

Knowledge about the nutrients and their effects on health comes from scientific study.

than the control group. A number of pitfalls are inherent in an experiment of this kind and must be avoided.

First, the two groups of people must be similar in all respects (except that one group receives vitamin C). Similarity of the experimental and control groups is accomplished by randomization, a process of choosing the members from the same population by throws of the dice or some other method involving chance.

Importantly, both groups must have the same track record with respect to colds to rule out the possibility that an observed difference might have occurred anyway. If group A would have caught twice as many colds as group B anyway, then the fact that group B happened to receive the treatment proves nothing.

In experiments involving a nutrient, the diets of both groups must also be similar, especially with respect to that nutrient. If those in group B were receiving less vitamin C from their diet, this might cancel the effects of the supplement.

Sample Size To ensure that chance variation between the two groups does not influence the results, the groups must be large. If one member of a group of five people catches a bad cold by chance, he will pull the whole group's average toward bad colds; but if one member of a group of 500 catches a bad cold, she will not unduly affect the group average. Statistical methods are used to determine whether differences between groups of various sizes support a hypothesis or are insignificant.

Placebos If people take vitamin C for colds and *believe* it will cure them, their chances of recovery are improved. Taking anything believed to be beneficial hastens recovery in about half of all cases. This phenomenon, the effect of faith on healing, is known as the placebo effect. In experiments designed to determine vitamin C's effect on colds, this mind-body effect must be rigorously controlled. Severity of symptoms is often a subjective measure, and people who believe they are being treated may report less severe symptoms.

One way experimenters control for the placebo effect is to give pills to all participants; some pills contain vitamin C, and others of similar appearance and taste contain an inactive ingredient (placebos). This way, the effects of faith will work equally in both groups. It is not necessary to convince all subjects that they are receiving vitamin C, but the extent of belief or unbelief must be the same in both groups. A study conducted under these conditions is called a blind experiment—that is, the subjects do not know (are blind to) whether they are members of the experimental group (receiving treatment) or the control group (receiving the placebo).

Double Blind The experimenters, too, must not know which subjects are in which group. Being fallible human beings and having an emotional investment in a successful outcome, researchers might interpret and record results with a bias in the expected direction. To prevent such distortions, the pills given to the subjects are coded by a third party, who does not reveal to the experimenters which subjects were which until all results have been recorded quantitatively.

Correlations and Causes Research often examines the relationships between two or more variables—for example, daily vitamin C intake and the number of colds. Findings sometimes suggest no correlation between the two variables (regardless of the amount of vitamin C eaten, the number of colds remains the same). Other times, studies find either a positive correlation (the more vitamin C, the more colds) or a negative correlation (the more vitamin C, the fewer colds). Correlational evidence proves only that two variables are associated, not that one is the cause of the other. People often jump to conclusions when they learn of correlations, but the conclusions are often wrong. To prove that A causes B, scientists have to find evidence of the *mechanism*—that is, to catch A in the act of causing B, so to speak. Furthermore, other scientists must confirm or disprove the findings through replication before the results are accepted into the body of nutrition knowledge. Before the findings are published, they are subjected to peer review—a process whereby a panel of scientists evaluates the study to confirm that it followed standard scientific methods.

RESEARCH VERSUS RUMORS

In discussing these subtleties of experimental design, our intent is to show you what a far cry scientific validity is from the experience of your neighbor Mary (sample size, one; no control group), who says she takes vitamin C when she feels a cold coming on and "it works every time." She knows what she is taking, she has faith in its efficacy, and she tends not to notice when it doesn't work. Before concluding that an experiment has shown that a nutrient cures a disease or alleviates a symptom, ask these questions:

- Was there similarity between the control group and the experimental group?
- Was the sample size large enough to rule out chance variation?
- Was a placebo effectively administered (blind)?
- Was the experiment double blind?

In summary, scientists learn about nutrition by conducting experiments that follow the protocol of scientific research. Researchers take care to establish similar control and experimental groups, large sample sizes, placebos, and blind treatments. Their findings must be reviewed and replicated by other scientists before being accepted as valid. These are a few of the characteristics of research that is well designed to study the actions of nutrients in the body. Such research has laid the foundation for quantifying how much of each nutrient the body needs.

Recommended Nutrient Intakes

If nutrition experts could define all the dietary factors a person needs to support good health, they ideally would:

1. Estimate the amount of food energy the person needs to consume and the amount of physical activity the person needs to engage in to balance that energy intake.
2. Distribute the three energy-yielding nutrients so that the person receives:
   a. enough protein to meet protein needs, and
   b. sufficient carbohydrate and fat to fill the remainder of the energy allowance, balanced in the way that supports health best.
3. Estimate how much water and fiber will support health optimally.
4. Estimate the minimum and maximum amounts of each vitamin and mineral consistent with health.
5. Set upper limits for intakes of dietary constituents that are harmful in large amounts (salt, fat, and alcohol are familiar examples).

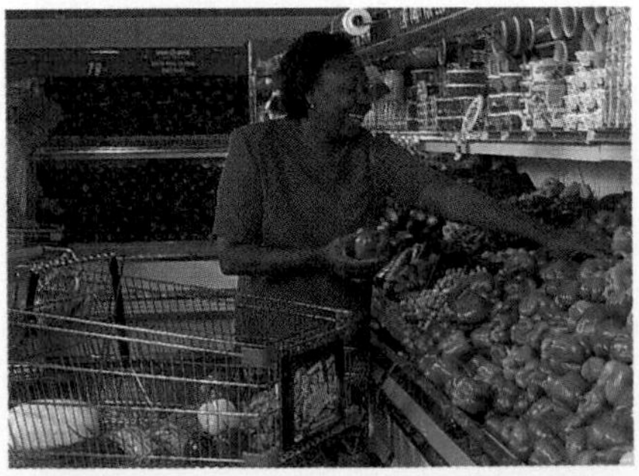

When people shop for foods, they are buying nutrients.

That is what the experts have done, and their dietary recommendations are presented in this section.

Two national committees take responsibility for defining the amounts of dietary factors that best support health. These committees are selected by the National Academy of Sciences and subject to approval by the National Research Council. The Committee on Dietary Allowances concerns itself primarily with maintaining health and focuses on energy and nutrient needs; the Committee on Diet and Health pays particular attention to reducing the risks of chronic diseases and focuses on dietary inadequacies and excesses.

RECOMMENDED DIETARY ALLOWANCES (RDA)

Recommended Dietary Allowances (RDA): the amounts of selected nutrients considered adequate to meet the known nutrient needs of practically all healthy people.

The RDA are based on scientific knowledge and are prepared by a committee of the Food and Nutrition Board (FNB) of the National Academy of Sciences (NAS).

The Canadian equivalent of the RDA is the Recommended Nutrient Intakes (RNI); see Appendix I.

The Committee on Dietary Allowances produces the set of nutrient standards known as the Recommended Dietary Allowances (RDA). A summary table of the RDA appears on the inside front cover (left) of this book; Appendix G presents additional RDA tables. At least 40 different nations and international organizations have published standards similar to the RDA.

The Committee on Dietary Allowances consists of highly qualified scientists. They base their estimates of nutrient needs on careful examination and interpretation of scientific evidence. Every few years, the committee reviews and revises the RDA as needed. For each new edition, committee members reexamine the data, concepts, and assumptions that underlie the RDA; restudy their own prior reasoning; and record how they have arrived at their recommendations.[4]

Developing the RDA is a huge task. Parts of it have occupied the committee's attention since the early 1940s. RDA have been established for energy and for nutrients for which deficiencies are known to occur. These recommendations change only a little from one revision to the next. For nutrients that are abundant in the diet, estimated minimum requirements have been set. For other nutrients that are less-well studied, Estimated Safe and Adequate Dietary Intakes (ESADDI) are given. The next paragraphs discuss specific aspects of the RDA.

RDA set for :
- Energy.
- Protein.
- Vitamins (A, D, E, K, C, thiamin, riboflavin, niacin, B_6, folate, B_{12}).
- Minerals (calcium, phosphorus, magnesium, iron, zinc, iodine, selenium)

Estimated minimum requirements set for:
- Sodium, potassium, chloride.

ESADDI set for:
- Vitamins (biotin, pantothenic acid).
- Minerals (copper, manganese, fluoride, chromium, molybdenum).

See inside front cover and Appendix G for details.

Energy RDA Each person's food energy *intake* must equal the energy *expended,* if the person is to maintain body weight. In recommending energy intakes, the Committee on Dietary Allowances reviewed research on thousands of individuals and derived *averages* for each of several age-sex groups. The committee finally arrived at a *single average number of kcalories* spent per day for each group—2900 kcalories, for example, for males 19 to 24 years of age.

Of course, tremendous variation surrounds this number. Males aged 19 to 24 come in all shapes and sizes and participate in all kinds of activities. The average energy recommendation is directly applicable to only a few individuals, but it serves as a ballpark figure; it gives a sense of how many kcalories are reasonable for this group.

The committee has not established an RDA for the output side of the energy balance equation—that is, how much energy people should expend. In deriving an RDA for energy intake, the Committee on Dietary Allowances assumes most people engage in light-to-moderate activity. The committee does say that people should balance energy intake with expenditure and that those who need to lose weight should increase energy expenditure rather than reduce energy intake. The more physical activity a person engages in, the more fit the person becomes, and the more food the person can eat without gaining weight. A person who can eat more food can obtain more nutrients, and this also supports health.

Chapters 8 and 9 revisit the energy RDA and show how to estimate your individual energy requirements and how to control your energy intake to meet your needs.

Protein RDA For protein, recommendations are based on body weight. The protein RDA is high, unlike the energy RDA, so it covers most people's needs.*

*The *average* daily requirement for protein is 0.6 grams per kilogram of body weight; the RDA is set at 0.8 grams per kilogram to meet the needs of 97.5 percent of the population—see Chapter 6.

No RDA for Carbohydrate and Fat The amount of protein recommended represents a relatively small percentage of a person's energy allowance; the remainder comes from carbohydrate and fat. No RDA for carbohydrate and fat is given, but the general guideline is that more than half of daily energy should come from carbohydrate, and no more than one-third should come from fat.

Water Recommendation The bigger and more active a person is, the more water the person needs. Water recommendations are tied directly to energy expenditures as described in Chapter 12. Generally, most people need at least six to eight 8-ounce glasses of water or liquids a day.

Fiber Recommendation There is no RDA for fiber. Instead, the Committee on Dietary Allowances recommends that people obtain sufficient fiber from fruits, vegetables, legumes, and whole-grain products, which provide vitamins, minerals, and water as well as fiber.

SETTING THE RDA FOR VITAMINS AND MINERALS

In contrast to some of the foregoing dietary constituents, many of the vitamins and minerals have specific recommended allowances in the main RDA table (inside front cover, left). They have been well studied and restudied for decades.

Estimating a Minimal Requirement To set vitamin and mineral recommendations, the Committee on Dietary Allowances reviews and selects the most valid studies of deficiency states, of the body's nutrient stores and their depletion, of nutrient intakes of apparently healthy people, and of findings from animal research. From this information, the committee estimates an *average requirement* for each nutrient—an amount that appears sufficient to maintain body processes *for a population*. When people consistently obtain a *deficient* intake (one that is less than the requirement), their nutrient stores decline, which over time leads to deficiency symptoms.

requirement: the amount of a nutrient that will maintain normal biochemical and physiological functions and prevent the development of specific deficiency signs; distinguished from the RDA, which is a recommended and generous allowance that provides for variability among individuals.

deficient: the amount of a nutrient below which *almost all healthy people* can be expected, over time, to experience deficiency symptoms.

Examining all the available data, the committee finds that each person's body is unique and has its own set of requirements. For example, Mr. A might need 40 units of the nutrient each day to prevent deficiency; Ms. B might need 35; Mr. C, 57. A look at enough individuals might reveal that their requirements fall into a symmetrical distribution (as shown in Figure 1–2), with most near the midpoint and only a few at the extremes.

Establishing a Generous Recommendation Then, to set the RDA, the committee must decide what intake to recommend for everybody. Should the RDA reflect the average requirement (shown in Figure 1–2 as 45 units)? The average requirement for each nutrient is probably closest to everyone's need, assuming the distribution shown in Figure 1–2. (Actually, the data for most nutrients other than protein have a distribution that is much less symmetrical.) But if people consumed exactly the average requirement of a given nutrient each day, half of the population would develop deficiencies of that nutrient; in Figure 1–2, Mr. C would be among them.

In this example, a reasonable choice for an RDA for everybody might be 63 units a day (see Figure 1–2). Such a point can be calculated mathematically so that it covers about 98 percent of a population. Even those whose needs were

Each of the 120 squares shown here represents a person. Some people require only a small amount of the nutrient, and some require a lot, but most fall somewhere near the middle. The text discusses three of these people: Mr. A, Ms. B, and Mr. C.

The RDA for nutrients is set well above the average requirement. It covers about 98% of the population.

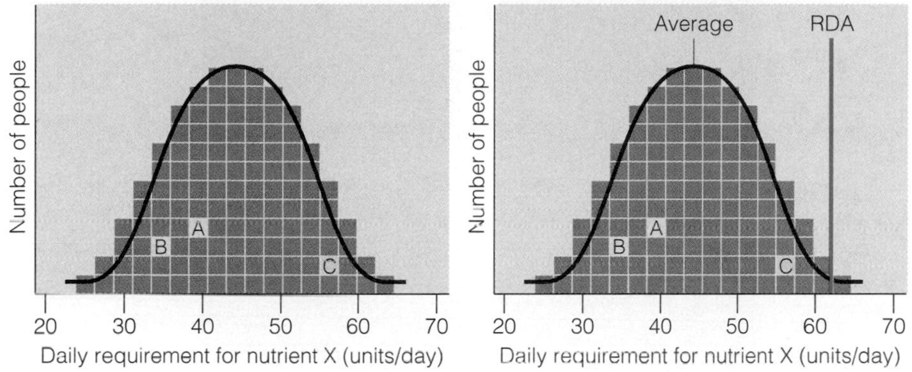

Figure 1–2

Setting the RDA for a Nutrient

higher than the average would be covered. Relatively few people's requirements would exceed the RDA, and even then, they wouldn't exceed by much.

Committee members make this kind of judgment in setting the RDA for each vitamin and mineral. They set it well above the average requirement determined from the best available information. For these reasons, people cannot use the RDA as their own individual requirements, but they can be reasonably sure that the RDA probably cover their needs adequately.

The RDA for protein, vitamins, and minerals are generous, and although the recommendations do not necessarily cover every individual for every nutrient, people's intakes should not exceed the RDA by much. People's tolerances for high doses of nutrients vary, and somewhere above the RDA there is an *upper safe* level beyond which some nutrients can be toxic. It is naive to think of the RDA as minimum amounts. A more accurate view is to see a person's nutrient needs as falling within a range, with marginal and danger zones both below and above it (see Figure 1–3). This consideration can be seen especially clearly in the RDA tables that state recommended intakes in terms of "safe and adequate" ranges, "safe" meaning "not too high" and "adequate" meaning "not too low."

upper safe: the amount of a nutrient that appears safe for *most healthy people* and beyond which there is concern that some people will experience toxicity symptoms.

Energy and Nutrient RDA Compared Figure 1–4 illustrates a contrast between the RDA for energy and the RDA for nutrients. The RDA for energy are set at the mean of the population's known requirements. In the case of energy, more than the need is as bad for health as less because excess energy leads to obesity, and deficient energy causes undernutrition. In contrast, in the case of vitamins and minerals, small amounts above the daily requirement do no harm, whereas amounts below the requirement lead to deficiencies. Their RDA are set near the top end of the range of the population's known requirements, so that as many people as possible will meet their needs given the RDA.

The preceding discussion has covered most of the goals listed at the start (p. 14)—setting recommended intakes for energy, energy-yielding nutrients, water, fiber,

Figure 1–3

Naive versus Accurate View of Nutrient Needs

The RDA for a given nutrient represents a point within a range of appropriate and reasonable intakes that lies between toxicity and deficiency. The recommendation is high enough to provide reserves in times of short-term dietary inadequacies, but not so high as to approach toxicity. Nutrient intakes above or below this range might be equally harmful.

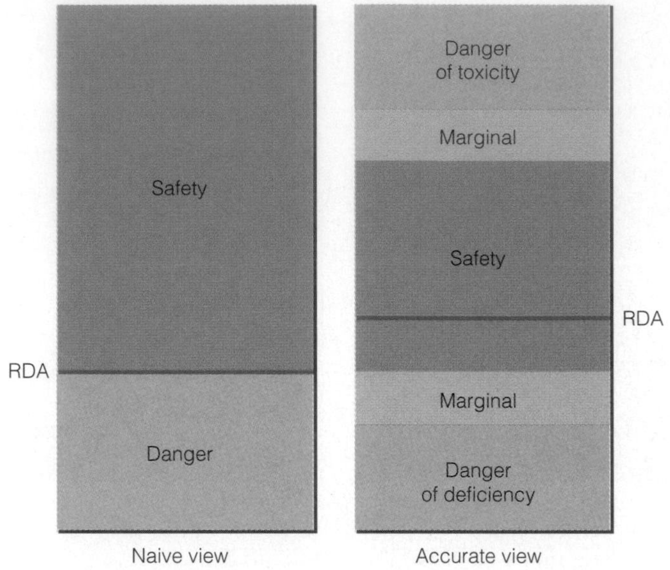

and vitamins and minerals. Energy and these nutrients represent the primary focus of the Committee on Dietary Allowances. The remaining dietary constituents (salt, fat, alcohol, and others) differ from these, in that deficiencies are not a risk, but excesses threaten health. This aspect of diet is the province of the Committee on Diet and Health and other agencies and is discussed further at the end of this chapter.

USING THE RDA

Although the intent of the RDA may seem simple enough, they are the subject of much misunderstanding and controversy. Perhaps the following facts will help

Figure 1–4

The Nutrient RDA and the Energy RDA Compared

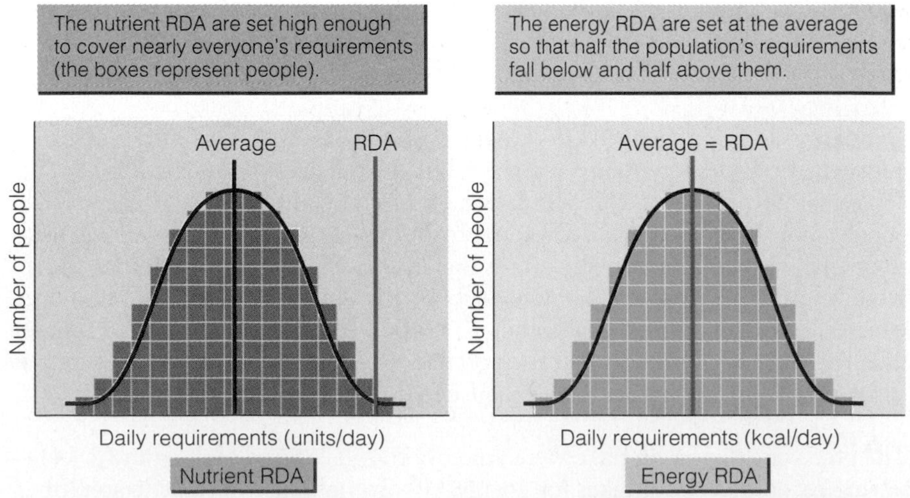

put the RDA in perspective. First, the RDA serve as estimates of adequate energy and nutrient intakes for *healthy* people. They do not apply to people with health problems who may require supplemented or restricted intakes.

Second, the RDA are safe and adequate *recommendations* that include a generous margin of safety. They are not minimum requirements, nor are they necessarily optimal intakes for all individuals.

Third, the RDA are intended to be met through diets composed of a variety of *foods*. Because foods contain mixtures of nutrients, they deliver more than just those nutrients named in the RDA table. Excess intakes of vitamins and minerals are unlikely when their sources are foods rather than supplements.

Fourth, the RDA apply to *average daily intakes*. To try to meet the RDA for every nutrient every day is difficult and unnecessary. The length of time over which a person's intake can deviate from the average without risk of deficiency or overdose varies; for most nutrients, it is best to try to achieve the average intakes recommended by the RDA within three days or so.

Fifth, the RDA are most appropriately used to develop and evaluate nutrition programs for *populations* such as schoolchildren or military personnel. The RDA can be used to estimate the risks of deficiencies for an individual only if the person's intakes are determined and averaged over a sufficient length of time.[5] After all, the recommended intakes do meet the needs of essentially all members of a healthy population, so by definition, they apply to individuals within that population. To use the RDA this way, though, an individual must compare the RDA with the *typical* intake, and not just with an arbitrary day's intake.

With these understandings, researchers use the RDA as a yardstick to assess the adequacy of diets—for example, in nutrition surveys. Diet planners use them as guidelines in planning and evaluating diets for groups of people—for example, the children in school districts. Dietitians working in social service programs use the RDA to establish criteria for foods delivered by food assistance programs. The Food and Drug Administration (FDA) uses the RDA as guidelines for the labeling of foods, and the food industry uses them to develop new food products.

Revising the RDA The RDA are not etched on stone tablets. They are revised periodically as convincing new evidence becomes available. Since the first edition in 1943, the RDA have been the authoritative standard for the nutrient needs of people in the United States.[6] In general, the current edition shares many similarities with previous editions. The RDA have served their purpose of protecting against nutrient deficiencies. Over the past several decades, deficiencies have not been reported in groups of people who were receiving the RDA. Clearly, the safety margins used in setting the nutrient RDA do indeed cover practically all people, just as they claim to do.

The Food and Nutrition Board now faces the challenge of redefining the RDA's goal beyond preventing nutrient deficiencies to include supporting optimal health and preventing chronic diseases.[7] Plans for the next edition of the RDA call for it to address "the potential roles of nutrients and other food constituents in reducing chronic disease risk."[8] Suggestions being considered for the next revision include:[9]

- Providing several sets of RDA (one for health, one for disease prevention, another for disease treatment).
- Providing a range of values to accommodate people's diverse needs.

- Using the most current RDA for food labels (labels now use the 1968 edition).
- Establishing RDA for nutrients and nonnutrients such as fiber, cholesterol, and beta-carotene (a relative of vitamin A) that influence health.
- Addressing the needs of elderly people and other nutritionally vulnerable subgroups such as minority populations and smokers.
- Changing the name from *dietary* to *nutrient* allowances in recognition that in some circumstances, desired intakes may not be possible from foods alone.

Unlike past revisions, the next edition of the RDA is likely to exhibit more differences from previous editions than similarities. It is appropriate that the RDA continue to evolve.

Comparing the RDA with Other Recommendations Other recommendations work similarly to the RDA. For example, like the RDA, recommendations of the international agencies FAO and WHO are considered sufficient for the maintenance of health in nearly all people. These recommendations differ from the RDA, however, in that they serve populations worldwide and are based on different judgment factors. For example, the FAO/WHO recommendations consider that people worldwide are generally smaller and more active than people in the United States. Nevertheless, the recommendations of all nations and agencies fall within the same range.

FAO: the Food and Agriculture Organization (of the United Nations).

WHO: the World Health Organization.

Nutrient recommendations from FAO/WHO are provided in Appendix G.

To recap, the RDA represent intakes of selected nutrients considered adequate to meet the needs of practically all healthy people. The energy RDA is set at the average of people's needs so as to discourage overconsumption of food energy. The RDA for protein, vitamins, and minerals, on the other hand, are set well above the average so as to cover the needs of most healthy people. The RDA are commonly used to assess the adequacy of diets.

Nutrition Assessment

What happens when a person doesn't get enough of a nutrient or energy or gets too much? If the deficiency or excess is significant over time, the person exhibits signs of malnutrition. With a deficiency of energy, the person may display the symptoms of undernutrition by becoming extremely thin, losing muscle tissue, and becoming prone to infection and disease. With a deficiency of a nutrient, the person may experience skin rashes, depression, hair loss, bleeding gums, muscle spasms, night blindness, or other symptoms. With an excess of energy, the person may become obese and vulnerable to diseases associated with overnutrition such as diabetes, heart disease, and cancer. With a sudden nutrient overdose, the person may experience hot flashes, yellowing skin, paralysis, a rapid heart rate, low blood pressure, or other symptoms.

malnutrition: any condition caused by excess or deficient food energy or nutrient intake or by an imbalance of nutrients.
mal = bad

undernutrition: deficiency of energy or nutrients.

overnutrition: excess energy or nutrients.

Malnutrition symptoms are easy to miss. They resemble the symptoms of other diseases: diarrhea, skin rashes, pain, and the like. But a person who has learned how to read the signs can tell when these conditions are caused by malnutrition and can take steps to correct it. Dietitians have developed assessment techniques to detect malnutrition. This discussion presents the basics of nutrition assessment; many more details are offered in later chapters and in Appendix E.

NUTRITION ASSESSMENT OF INDIVIDUALS

To prepare a nutrition assessment, the assessor, usually a registered dietitian or a physician trained in clinical nutrition, uses:

- Historical information.
- Anthropometric data.
- Physical examinations.
- Laboratory tests.

Each of these methods involves collecting data in various ways and interpreting each finding in relation to the others in order to create a total picture.

nutrition assessment: a comprehensive approach, completed by a registered dietitian, to defining nutrition status that uses health, socioeconomic, drug, and diet histories; anthropometric measurements; physical examinations; and laboratory tests.

A *registered dietitian* is a college-educated food and nutrition specialist who is qualified to evaluate people's nutritional health and needs. See Highlight 1 for more on what constitutes a nutrition expert.

Historical Information One step in evaluating nutrition status is to obtain information about a person's history with respect to health status, socioeconomic status, drug use, and diet. The health history may reveal a disease that interferes with the person's ability to eat or the body's use of nutrients. Socioeconomic circumstances may show a financial inability to buy foods or inadequate kitchen facilities in which to prepare them. A drug history may highlight possible drug-nutrient interactions that lead to nutrient deficiencies. A diet history can indicate whether the diet may be under- or oversupplying nutrients or energy.

To take a diet history, the assessor collects and analyzes data about the foods a person eats. The data may be collected by recording the foods the person has eaten over a period of 24 hours, three days, or a week or more or by asking what foods the person typically eats and how much of each. The days in a record have to be fairly typical of the person's diet, and the record has to pay special attention to portion sizes. To determine the amounts of nutrients consumed, the assessor usually enters the foods and their portion sizes into a computer using a diet analysis program. Alternatively, this step can be done manually by looking up each food in a table of food composition such as Appendix H in this book. Then the assessor compares the calculated nutrient intakes with recommended intakes such as the RDA.

Appendix E describes the tools used to obtain food intake data: the 24-hour recall, usual intake record, food frequency checklist, and food record.

An estimate of energy and nutrient intakes from a diet history, combined with other sources of information, can help confirm or rule out the *possibility* of suspected nutrition problems. A sufficient intake of a nutrient does not guarantee adequate nutrition status for an individual, and an insufficient intake does not always indicate a deficiency, but such findings warn of possible problems.

Anthropometric Data A second technique that may help reveal nutrition problems is the taking of measures such as height and weight. The assessor compares measurements taken on an individual with standards specific for sex and age or with previous measures on the same individual.

Measurements taken periodically and compared with previous measurements reveal patterns and indicate trends in a person's overall nutrition status; they provide little information about the status of specific nutrients. Measurements out of line with expectations may reveal such problems as growth failure in children, wasting or swelling of body tissue in adults, and obesity—conditions that may reflect nutrient deficiencies or excesses.

anthropometric (AN-throw-poe-MET-rick): relating to measurement of the physical characteristics of the body, such as height and weight.
anthropos = human
metric = measuring

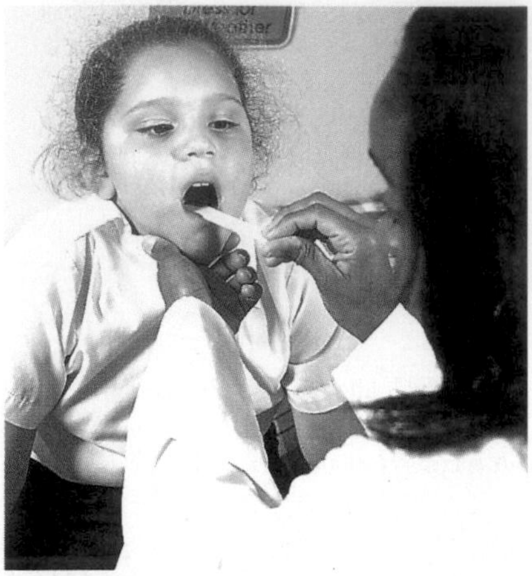

A peek inside the mouth provides clues to a person's nutrition status.

overt (oh-VERT): out in the open and easy to observe.
ouvrir = to open

primary deficiency: a nutrient deficiency caused by inadequate dietary intake of a nutrient.

secondary deficiency: a nutrient deficiency caused by something other than diet, such as a disease condition that reduces absorption, accelerates use, hastens excretion, or destroys the nutrient.

Physical Examinations A third nutrition assessment technique is a physical examination that looks for clues to poor nutrition status. Every part of the body that can be inspected can offer such clues: the hair, eyes, skin, posture, tongue, fingernails, and others. The examination requires skill, for many physical signs can reflect more than one nutrient deficiency or toxicity or even nonnutrition conditions. Like the other assessment techniques, a physical examination does not by itself point to firm conclusions. Instead, it reveals possible nutrient imbalances for other assessment techniques to confirm or confirms data collected from other assessment measures.

Laboratory Tests A fourth way to detect a developing deficiency, imbalance, or toxicity state is to take samples of body tissues or fluids (blood or urine), analyze them in the laboratory, and compare the results with normal values for a similar population. A goal of nutrition assessment is to uncover early signs of malnutrition before symptoms appear. Laboratory tests are useful this way and can also confirm suspicions raised by other assessment methods.

Iron, for Example The mineral iron can be used to illustrate the stages in the development of a nutrient deficiency and the assessment techniques useful in detecting them. The overt, or outward, signs of an iron deficiency appear at the end of a long sequence of events. Figure 1–5 describes what happens in the body as a nutrient deficiency progresses and shows how assessment methods can reveal those changes.

First, too little iron gets into the body—either because iron is lacking in the person's food (a primary deficiency) or because the person's body doesn't absorb or use iron normally (a secondary deficiency). A diet history provides clues to primary deficiencies; a health history provides clues to secondary deficiencies.

Figure 1–5

Stages in the Development of a Nutrient Deficiency

Internal changes precede outward signs of deficiencies. As a corollary, signs of sickness need not appear before a person takes corrective measures. Tests can either reveal the presence of problems in the early stages or confirm that nutrient stores are adequate.

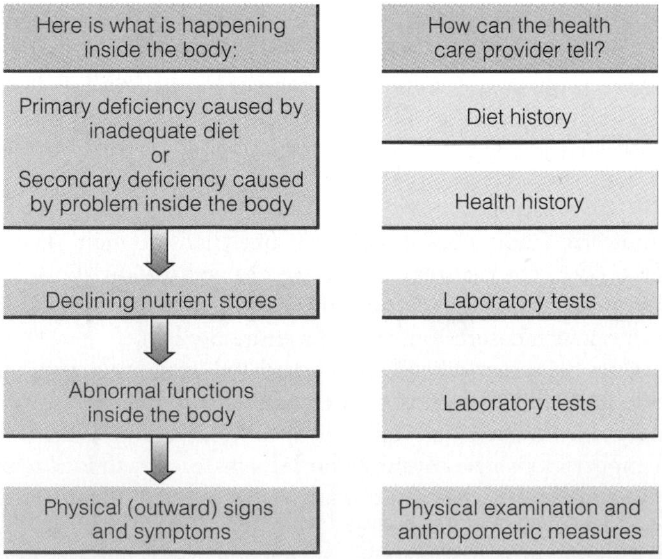

Then the body begins to use up its stores of iron. At this stage, the deficiency might be described as subclinical. It exists as a covert condition and might be detected by laboratory tests, but outward signs have not yet appeared.

Finally, iron stores are exhausted. Now, the body cannot make enough iron-containing red blood cells to replace those that are aging and dying. The red blood cells normally carry oxygen to all the body's tissues. When iron is lacking, fewer red blood cells are made, the new ones are pale and small, and every part of the body feels the effects of an oxygen shortage. Now, the overt symptoms of deficiency appear—weakness, fatigue, pallor, and headaches, reflecting the iron-deficient state of the blood. Physical examination would reveal these symptoms.

Thus reviewing dietary data may suggest a nutrition problem in its earliest stages. Laboratory tests may detect it before it becomes overt, whereas physical examination picks up on the problem only after it is causing symptoms.

subclinical deficiency: a deficiency in the early stages, before the outward signs have appeared.

covert (KOH-vert): hidden, as if under covers.
couvrir = to cover

HEALTHY PEOPLE 2000: Increase to at least 75% the proportion of primary care providers who provide nutrition assessment and counseling and/or referral to qualified nutritionists or dietitians.

The **Healthy People 2000** report sets national objectives in health promotion and disease prevention for the year 2000.[10] The 21 nutrition-related priorities are listed in Appendix G and appear in the text where their subjects are discussed.

NUTRITION ASSESSMENT OF POPULATIONS

To assess a population's nutrition status, researchers conduct surveys using techniques similar to those used on individuals. One kind of survey—a food consumption survey—determines the kinds and amounts of foods people eat. Then researchers calculate the energy and nutrients in the foods and compare the amounts consumed with a standard such as the RDA. An example of this type of survey is the Nationwide Food Consumption Survey (NFCS). Information for the third NFCS (1994–1996) was gathered from 15,000 people using food intake records for two nonconsecutive days.

food consumption survey: a survey that measures the amounts and kinds of foods people consume (using diet histories), estimates the nutrient intakes, and compares them with a standard such as the RDA.

Another kind of survey—a nutrition status survey—examines the people themselves, using nutrition assessment methods. The National Health and Nutrition Examination Survey (NHANES) is an example of a nutrition status survey. The third NHANES (1988–1996) gathered information from between 40,000 and 70,000 people using diet histories, anthropometric measurements, physical examinations, and laboratory tests. The data provide information on several nutrition-related conditions, such as growth retardation, heart disease, and nutrient deficiencies. Both the NFCS and the NHANES oversample high-risk groups (low-income families, infants and children, and the elderly) in order to glean an accurate estimate of their health and nutrition status.

nutrition status survey: a survey that evaluates people's nutrition status using diet histories, anthropometric measures, physical examinations, and laboratory tests.

Until 1990, findings from the nation's many nutrition surveys, including these two largest ones, were almost impossible to compare and synthesize into a single cohesive report. Then the National Nutrition Monitoring and Related Research Act was enacted and coordinated the many nutrition-related activities that had been underway within 22 different federal agencies. The law mandated that the U.S. Department of Agriculture (USDA) and the Department of Health and Human Services (DHHS) establish and implement a Ten-Year Comprehensive Plan for nutrition monitoring and related research.[11]

The resulting wealth of information can be used for a variety of purposes. For example, Congress uses this information to establish public policy on nutrition education, food assistance programs, and the regulation of the food supply. Scientists use the information to establish research priorities. All major reports that examine the contribution of diet and nutrition status to the health of the people of the United States depend on information collected and coordinated by this national program.* This data provided the basis for the mid-decade report on Healthy People 2000 that shows we are not meeting many of our health goals; in fact, we are not even heading in the right direction for some goals, such as reducing the prevalence of overweight in this country.[12]

To review, people become malnourished when they get too little or too much energy or nutrients. To detect malnutrition in individuals, health care professionals use nutrition assessment techniques. Assessments gather data from historical information, anthropometric measures, physical examinations, and laboratory tests. Assessment methods are also used in surveys to measure people's food consumption and to evaluate the nutrition status of populations.

Diet and Health

Diet has always played a vital role in supporting health. Early nutrition research focused on identifying the nutrients in foods that would prevent such common diseases as rickets and scurvy, the vitamin D– and vitamin C–deficiency diseases. More recently, with nutrient deficiencies no longer a major threat, nutrition research has focused on diseases associated with energy and nutrient excesses. Today, overconsumption of foods—especially foods high in fats—is a major health concern for people in the United States.[13]

Figure 1–6 shows the ten leading causes of illness and death in the United States. These "causes" are stated as if single conditions such as heart disease caused death, but most chronic diseases arise from multiple factors over many years. A person who died of heart failure may have had preexisting conditions such as overweight and high blood pressure, may have been a cigarette smoker, and may have spent years eating a high-fat diet and getting too little exercise.

chronic diseases: degenerative diseases characterized by deterioration of the body organs; also called chronic, **noncommunicable diseases (NCD)**. Examples include heart disease, cancer, and diabetes.

Of course, not all people who die of heart disease fit this description, nor do all people with these characteristics die of heart disease. People who are overweight might die from the complications of diabetes instead, or those who smoke might die of cancer. They might even die from something totally unrelated to any of these factors, such as an automobile accident. Still, statistical studies have shown that certain conditions and behaviors are linked to certain diseases.

RISK FACTORS

risk factors: factors associated with an elevated frequency of a disease but not proven to be causal.

Factors that increase or reduce the *risk* of developing chronic diseases are identified by analyzing statistical data. A strong association between a risk factor and a disease means that when the factor is present, the *likelihood* of developing the

*Such reports include:
- *Recommended Dietary Allowances.*
- *Healthy People 2000: National Health Promotion and Disease Prevention Objectives.*
- *Diet and Health: Implications for Reducing Chronic Disease Risks.*
- *Surgeon General's Report on Nutrition and Health.*
- *Dietary Guidelines for Americans.*

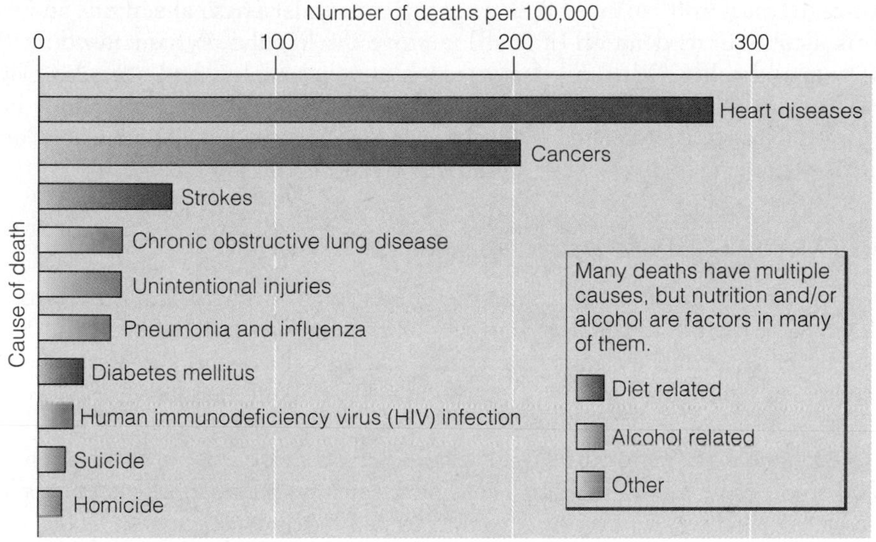

Figure 1–6

The Ten Leading Causes of Illness and Death in the United States

Diet influences the development of several chronic diseases—notably, heart disease, some types of cancer, stroke, and diabetes. Taken together, these four diseases account for about two-thirds of the nation's 2 million deaths each year.

Source: National Center for Health Statistics, *Monthly Vital Statistics Report,* October 1994.

disease is great. It does not mean that all people with the risk factor will develop the disease. Similarly, a lack of risk factors does not guarantee freedom from a given disease. On the average, though, the more risk factors in a person's life, the greater that person's chances of developing the disease. Conversely, the fewer risk factors in a person's life, the better the chances for good health.

Risk Factors Persist Risk factors tend to persist over time. Without intervention, a young adult with high blood pressure will most likely continue to have high blood pressure as an older adult, for example. To minimize the damage, then, early intervention is most effective.

Risk Factors Cluster Risk factors also tend to cluster. For example, a person who is overweight is likely to be physically inactive, to have high blood pressure, and to have high blood cholesterol—all risk factors associated with heart disease. Intervention that focuses on one risk factor often benefits the others as well. For example, physical activity can help reduce weight. Then both physical activity and weight loss will help to lower blood pressure and blood cholesterol.

Risk Factors in Perspective Many people live well into their later years. Today's average life expectancy is a record high of 75.5 years.[14] Whether those years are burdened by poor health depends, in part, on personal behaviors.

An estimated half of all deaths each year can be attributed to specific risk factors, many of which reflect personal behaviors.[15] The most prominent factor contributing to death in the United States is tobacco use, followed by diet and activity patterns, and alcohol use (see Table 1–1). The 1988 *Surgeon General's Report* concluded that for the two out of three Americans who do not smoke or drink alcohol excessively, the one choice that can influence long-term health prospects more than any other is diet.[16]

Some risk factors, such as smoking, dietary habits, physical activity, and alcohol consumption, are personal behaviors that can be changed. Decisions to not

Table 1–1

Actual Causes of Death in the United States (1990)

Cause	Percentage of Total Deaths
Tobacco	19
Diet/activity	14
Alcohol	5
Microbial agents	4
Toxic agents	3
Firearms	2
Sexual behavior	1
Motor vehicles	1
Illicit drugs	<1
Total	50

Source: J. M. McGinnis and W. H. Foege, Actual causes of death in the United States, *Journal of the American Medical Association* 270 (1993): 2207–2212

smoke, to eat a well-balanced diet, to engage in regular physical activity, and to drink alcohol in moderation (if at all) improve the likelihood that a person will enjoy good health. Other risk factors, such as genetics, sex, and age, also play important roles in the development of chronic diseases, but they cannot be changed. Health recommendations acknowledge the influence of such factors on the development of disease, but must focus on those that are changeable.

DIETARY RECOMMENDATIONS

Dietary recommendations represent the efforts of government and other agencies to meet the last of the five goals set out earlier (p. 14): to define upper limits for intakes of dietary constituents that harm health when eaten in excess. Recommendations are based on current knowledge about diet and disease.

Several agencies have published similar sets of recommendations, which differ only slightly in detail. The *Diet, Nutrition, and Prevention of Chronic Diseases* report from WHO is presented in Appendix G.

Recommendations for the Population After considering the results of over 7000 studies, the Committee on Diet and Health concluded that most people can gain some disease-prevention benefits by making dietary changes.[17] The *Diet and Health* recommendations are intended to be used together with the RDA in planning diets (see Table 1–2).[18] The RDA are aimed at maintaining health and provide guidelines for energy and nutrient intakes. The *Diet and Health* recommendations are aimed at reducing disease risks and describe the kinds of foods people should include, limit, or avoid. They also address weight maintenance and exercise and pinpoint trouble areas surrounding specific nutrients. Like the *Diet and Health* report, the *Nutrition Recommendations for Canadians* report makes recommendations that will supply enough nutrients, while reducing the risk of chronic disease (see Table 1–3).

Several of the *Diet and Health* recommendations are aimed at weight control: cut fat, add complex carbohydrates, and balance food intake with activity. Obesity is common in this country, and it is linked with most of the chronic diseases that threaten life. The problems of overweight people multiply when medical problems develop. For example, overweight people readily develop diabetes, which is often accompanied by high blood pressure and high blood cholesterol. Such a combination of problems may require only one treatment: lose the excess weight by adopting a healthful diet combined with regular exercise.

Recommendations that urge all people to make dietary changes believed to forestall or prevent diseases are taking a **preventive** or **population approach**. Alternatively, recommendations that urge dietary changes only for people who are known to need them are taking a **medical** or **individual approach**.

The *Diet and Health* recommendations are aimed at the general population in the hope that all people at all levels of risk may benefit. Such a strategy is similar to national efforts to vaccinate to prevent polio, fluoridate water to prevent dental caries, and fortify grains to prevent iron deficiency.

Recommendations for Individuals People's hereditary susceptibility to diseases and their responsiveness to dietary measures vary. Unlike nutrient-deficiency diseases, which develop when nutrients are lacking and disappear when the nutrients are provided, chronic diseases are neither caused nor prevented by diet alone. Many people have followed dietary advice and developed heart disease or cancer anyway; others have ignored all advice and lived long and healthy lives. For many people, though, diet does influence the time of onset and course of some chronic diseases, and many health care professionals urge dietary measures as part of a disease-prevention strategy. The recommendations were established for "the potential public health benefit, and the likelihood of minimal risk."[19]

Table 1–2

Diet and Health **Recommendations**

- Reduce total *fat* intake to 30 percent or less of kcalories. Reduce saturated fatty acid intake to less than 10 percent of kcalories and the intake of cholesterol to less than 300 milligrams daily.
- Increase intake of starches and other *complex carbohydrates*.
- Maintain *protein* intake at moderate levels.
- Balance food intake and physical activity to maintain appropriate *body weight*.
- For those who drink *alcoholic beverages*, limit consumption to the equivalent of less than 1 ounce of pure alcohol in a single day. Pregnant women should avoid alcoholic beverages.
- Limit total daily intake of *salt* (sodium chloride) to 6 grams or less.
- Maintain adequate *calcium* intake.
- Avoid taking dietary *supplements* in excess of the RDA in any one day.
- Maintain an optimal intake of *fluoride*, particularly during the years of primary and secondary tooth formation and growth.

Note: Italics added to highlight the areas of concern.
Source: Adapted from the Committee on Diet and Health, *Diet and Health: Implications for Reducing Chronic Disease Risk* (Washington, D.C.: National Academy Press, 1989).

Table 1–3

Nutrition Recommendations for Canadians

- The Canadian diet should provide energy consistent with the maintenance of *body weight* within the recommended range.
- The Canadian diet should include *essential nutrients* in amounts recommended.
- The Canadian diet should include no more than 30 percent of energy as *fat* (33 grams/1000 kcalories or 39 grams/5000 kilojoules) and no more than 10 percent as saturated fat (11 grams/1000 kcalories or 13 grams/5000 kilojoules).
- The Canadian diet should provide 55 percent of energy as *carbohydrate* (138 grams/1000 kcalories or 165 grams/5000 kilojoules) from a variety of sources.
- The *sodium* content of the Canadian diet should be reduced.
- The Canadian diet should include no more than 5 percent of total energy as *alcohol*, or two drinks daily, whichever is less.
- The Canadian diet should contain no more *caffeine* than the equivalent of four regular cups of coffee per day.
- Community water supplies containing less than 1 milligram per liter should be *fluoridated* to that level.

Note: Italics added to highlight areas of concern.
Source: Health and Welfare Canada, *Nutrition Recommendations: The Report of the Scientific Review Committee* (Ottawa: Canadian Government Publishing Centre, 1990).

To determine whether dietary recommendations are important to you personally, look at your family history to see which diseases are common to your relatives. In addition, examine your personal history, taking note of your blood pressure, blood test results, and lifestyle habits such as smoking.

In conclusion, diet is one of several factors that can influence the development of chronic diseases. To have the greatest impact possible, dietary recommendations are aimed at the entire population, and not just at the individuals who might benefit most. Recommendations focus on weight control and urge people to limit fat, increase complex carbohydrates, and balance food intake with activity.

The next several chapters will provide many more details about the nutrients and how they support health. Whenever appropriate, they will show how diet influences each of today's major diseases. The *Diet and Health* recommendations will appear again and again, as each nutrient's relationships with health are explored. Most people who follow the recommendations will benefit and can enjoy good health into their later years.

Study Questions

These questions will help you review the chapter.

1. Give several reasons (and examples) why people make the food choices that they do.
2. What is a nutrient? Name the six classes of nutrients found in foods. What is an essential nutrient?
3. Which nutrients are inorganic and which are organic? Discuss the significance of that distinction.
4. Which nutrients yield energy and how much energy do they yield per gram? How is energy measured?
5. Describe how alcohol resembles nutrients. Why is alcohol not considered a nutrient?
6. What is the science of nutrition? Describe the types of research studies and methods used in acquiring nutrition information.
7. Explain how variables might be correlational but not causal.
8. What factors must be included in the full definition of a healthy diet? Which are covered by the RDA?
9. What are the RDA? Who develops the RDA? To whom do they apply? How are they used? In your description, address the issues of whether the RDA represent minimum requirements, whether the RDA need to be met daily, and whether the RDA apply to individuals.
10. What judgment factors are involved in setting the energy and nutrient intake recommendations?
11. What balance of energy-yielding nutrients is recommended to meet energy needs?
12. What happens when people either get too little or too much energy or nutrients? Define malnutrition, undernutrition, and overnutrition. Describe the four methods used to detect energy and nutrient deficiencies and excesses.
13. What methods are used in nutrition surveys? What kinds of information can these surveys provide?
14. Describe the differences between the population approach and the individual approach to making dietary recommendations. Which approach do today's dietary recommendations take?
15. What recommendations are made in the *Diet and Health* report?

Notes

1. G. A. Falciglia and P. A. Norton, Evidence for a genetic influence on preference for some foods, *Journal of the American Dietetic Association* 94 (1994): 154–158.
2. I. M. Parraga, Determinants of food consumption, *Journal of the American Dietetic Association* 90 (1990): 661–663.
3. A. E. Harper, 1990 Atwater lecture—The science and the practice of nutrition: Reflections and directions, *American Journal of Clinical Nutrition* 53 (1991): 413–420.
4. Committee on Dietary Allowances, *Recommended Dietary Allowances*, 10th ed. (Washington, D.C.: National Academy Press, 1989).
5. Committee on Dietary Allowances, 1989, pp. 8–9.
6. P. Lachance and L. Langseth, The RDA concept: Time for a change? *Nutrition Reviews* 52 (1994): 266–270.
7. L. J. Machlin and H. E. Sauberlich, New views on the function and health effects of vitamins, *Nutrition Today*, January/February 1994, pp. 25–29.
8. How should the Recommended Dietary Allowances be revised? A concept paper from the Food and Nutrition Board, (Washington, D.C.: National Academy Press, 1994).
9. ADA testifies on need for revised RDAs, *Journal of the American Dietetic Association* 93 (1993): 864.
10. *Healthy People 2000: National Health Promotion and Disease Prevention Objectives* (Washington, D.C.: U.S. Department of Health and Human Services, 1990).
11. Ten-year comprehensive plan for the national nutrition monitoring and related research program, *Federal Register*, June 11, 1993.
12. J. M. McGinnis and P. R. Lee, *Healthy People 2000* at mid decade, *Journal of the American Medical Association* 273 (1995): 1123–1129.
13. *The Surgeon General's Report on Nutrition and Health: Summary and Recommendations*, DHHS (PHS) publication no. 88–50211 (Washington, D.C.: Government Printing Office, 1988).
14. National Center for Health Statistics, Monthly vital statistics report, August 1993.
15. J. M. McGinnis and W. H. Foege, Actual causes of death in the United States, *Journal of the American Medical Association* 270 (1993): 2207–2212.
16. *The Surgeon General's Report*, 1988.
17. Committee on Diet and Health, *Diet and Health: Implications for Reducing Chronic Disease Risk* (Washington, D.C.: National Academy Press, 1989).
18. Committee on Dietary Allowances, 1989, p. 9.
19. Committee on Diet and Health, 1989, pp. 665–710.

Problem Set

These problem sets have been created to provide you with practice in doing simple nutrition-related calculations. Answers appear in Appendix K. Once you have mastered these examples, you can, of course, create others of your own. Be sure to show your calculations for each problem.

1. Inspect some foods. Look up each of the following foods in Appendix H; enter the values in the following table:

Food	Item No.	Weight (g)	Water (%)	Protein (g)	Carbohydrate (g)	Fiber (g)	Fat (g)
Swiss cheese, 1 oz	______	______	______	______	______	______	______
Fried egg, 1	______	______	______	______	______	______	______
Cauliflower, cooked fresh, ½ c	______	______	______	______	______	______	______

a. How many grams of water are in each food?
1 oz swiss cheese: ______________________ = ______ g water.
1 fried egg: ______________________ = ______ g water.
½ c cooked cauliflower: ______________________ = ______ g water.

b. How many grams of solids must, therefore, be in each food?
1 oz swiss cheese: ______________________ = ______ g solids.
1 fried egg: ______________________ = ______ g solids.
½ c cooked cauliflower: ______________________ = ______ g solids.

c. How many grams of energy nutrients and fiber are in each food?
1 oz swiss cheese: ______________________ = ______ g energy nutrients and fiber.
1 fried egg: ______________________ = ______ g energy nutrients and fiber.
½ c cooked cauliflower: ______________________ = ______ g energy nutrients and fiber.

d. Compare your answers in (b) with those in (c) to determine how many grams remain unaccounted for. (These are vitamins, minerals, and incidental nonnutrient compounds.)
1 oz swiss cheese: ______________________ leaves ______ g unaccounted for.
1 fried egg: ______________________ leaves ______ g unaccounted for.
½ c cooked cauliflower: ______________________ leaves ______ g unaccounted for.

This inspection should satisfy you that most foods are, indeed, composed almost entirely of water, energy nutrients, and fiber.

2. Practice thinking in metric measures. Use the box on pp. 6–7 and Appendix D to help make the following conversions. A person is 5 ft 9 in tall and weighs 170 lb.

a. How tall is the person in centimeters? ______________________ = ______ cm

b. How much does the person weigh in kilograms? ______________________ = ______ kg

(continued on the next page)

Problem Set (continued)

c. Imagine you are following a soup recipe that is given in metric measures. Your measuring devices are all in cups, teaspoons, and tablespoons. The recipe's measures are only approximate, so *do not calculate*. Just pick the measure that is *about* equivalent to each of the following:

½ liter water: _____ 1 qt _____ 2 c _____ 1 c

100 g chopped onion: _____ ½ c _____ 1 tbs _____ 1 tsp

5 g minced garlic: _____ ½ cup _____ 1 tbs _____ 1 tsp

d. A Canadian and a U.S. citizen are sharing dessert. The Canadian gives the U.S. citizen a cookie and says it has about 400 kJ of energy. The American gives the Canadian a brownie and says it contains 80 kcal.

How many kcalories are in a kilojoule? 1 kJ = _____ kcal.

How many kilojoules are equal to 1 kcal? 1 kcal = _____ kJ.

Express the energy in the cookie in kcalories: ______________________ = _____ kcal.

Express the energy in the brownie in kilojoules: ______________________ = _____ kJ.

3. Calculate the energy in a food from its energy-nutrient contents. A cup of fried rice contains 5 g protein, 30 g carbohydrate, and 11 g fat.

a. How many kcalories does the rice provide from these energy nutrients?

______________________ = _____ kcal protein.

______________________ = _____ kcal carbohydrate.

______________________ = _____ kcal fat.

Total = _____ kcal.

b. What percentage of the energy in the fried rice comes from each of the energy-yielding nutrients? (Make sure that the percentages of energy add up to 100%. Sometimes they add to 99% or 101% due to rounding errors. These totals are acceptable.)

______________________ = _____ % kcalories from protein.

______________________ = _____ % kcalories from carbohydrate.

______________________ = _____ % kcalories from fat.

Total = _____ %

c. Even a little nutrition knowledge can help you identify some bogus claims. Consider an advertisement for a new "super supplement" that claims the product provides 15 g protein and 10 kcal per 100 g. Is this possible? _____. Why or why not? ______________________ = _____ kcal.

Who Speaks on Nutrition?

People are bombarded by nutrition news as they read newspapers, turn the pages of magazines, talk with friends, and watch television. Today, more than ever before, people want to know what nutrition news they can believe and safely use. They want to know how best to take care of themselves. Some people seek miracles: tricks to help them lose weight, foods to forestall aging, and supplements to prevent baldness. People's heightened interests in nutrition and health translate into billions of dollars spent on services and products peddled by both legitimate and fraudulent businesses. While consumers who obtain legitimate health care can improve their health, those enticed into scams may lose their health, their savings, or both. Unfortunately, fraudulent health care, most of it related to nutrition, rings cash registers to the tune of $25 billion annually.[1] Ironically, nutrition quackery prevents people from attaining the health they are searching for by giving them false hope and delaying effective strategies.

Science and quackery may be easy to tell apart at the extremes, but an abundance of nutrition information lies between the extremes. How can people distinguish valid nutrition information from misinformation? One excellent approach is to notice who is purveying the information. If an instructor at the gym praises a high-protein diet, or the author of a magazine article recommends eating three pineapples a day to lose weight, or a health-store clerk suggests an amino acid supplement, should you believe these people? What qualifies them to give nutrition advice? When you are confused or need sound dietary advice, whom should you ask?

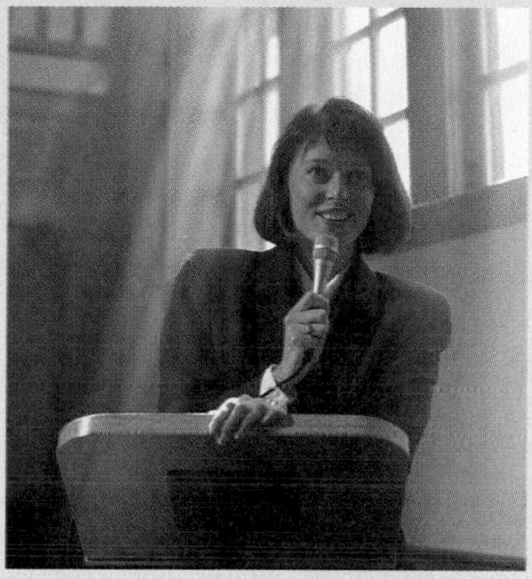

The quality of nutrition information depends on the provider's knowledge and credentials.

IDENTIFYING NUTRITION EXPERTS

Most people turn to their physicians for dietary advice. Physicians are expected to know all about health-related matters—but are they the best sources of accurate and current information on *nutrition?* Only about one-fourth of all medical schools in the United States require students to take even one nutrition course.[2] Students attending these classes receive an average of 20 hours of nutrition instruction—an amount they themselves consider inadequate.[3] (By comparison, most students reading this text are taking a nutrition class that provides an average of 45 hours of instruction.) Many experts call for nutrition to play a much larger role in the medical curriculum, but they acknowledge that the curriculum already carries a heavy burden. They prefer to integrate nutrition into already-existing courses such as biochemistry, microbiology, and physiology. Then clinical dietetics could be presented in the same way clinical pharmacology is taught, and community dietetics could be incorporated into public health courses.[4]

In 1990, Congress passed a law mandating that:

> Students enrolled in United States medical schools and physicians practicing in the United States [must] have access to adequate training in the field of nutrition and its relationship to human health.[5]

Plans are in the works to make nutrition education a standard course in medical schools. The American Dietetic Association (ADA) supports the inclusion of nutrition education as an essential component at all levels of medical education.[6] Furthermore, the ADA asserts that standardized nutrition education should be included in the curricula for all health care professionals: physician's assistants, dental hygienists, physical and occupational therapists, social workers, and all others who provide services directly to clients.[7] When these professionals have command of reliable nutrition information, then all the people they serve will also be better informed.

Most physicians appreciate the connections between health and nutrition. Those who have specialized in clinical nutrition are especially well qualified to speak on the subject. Membership in the American Society for Clinical Nutrition, whose journal is cited many times throughout this text, is another sign

Glossary

accredited: approved; in the case of medical centers or universities, certified by an agency recognized by the U.S. Department of Education.

American Dietetic Association (ADA): the professional organization of dietitians in the United States. The Canadian equivalent is the Canadian Dietetic Association (CDA), which operates similarly.

correspondence school: a school that offers courses and degrees by mail. Some correspondence schools are accredited; others are *diploma mills*.

dietetic technician registered (DTR): a person with an associate's degree and training in nutrition, food science, and diet planning who works under the guidance of an RD (registered dietitian).

dietitian: a person trained in nutrition, food science, and diet planning. See also *registered dietitian*.

DTR: see *dietetic technician registered*.

fraud or **quackery:** the promotion, for financial gain, of devices, treatments, services, plans, or products (including diets and supplements) that alter or claim to alter a human condition without proof of safety or effectiveness. (The word *quackery* comes from the term *quacksalver*, meaning a person who quacks loudly about a miracle product—a lotion or a salve.)

license to practice: permission under state or federal law, granted on meeting specified criteria, to use a certain title (such as dietitian) and offer certain services. Licensed dietitians may use the initials LD after their names.

misinformation: false or misleading information.

nutritionist: a person who specializes in the study of nutrition. Some nutritionists are registered dietitians, whereas others are self-described experts whose training is questionable. In states with responsible legislation, the term applies only to people who have MS or PhD degrees from properly accredited institutions.

public health nutritionist: a dietitian who specializes in public health nutrition.

RD: see *registered dietitian*.

registered dietitian (RD): a dietitian who has graduated from a university or college after completing a program of dietetics that has been accredited by the American Dietetic Association (or Canadian Dietetic Association), has served in an internship or coordinated program to practice the necessary skills, has passed the association's registration examination, and maintains competency through continuing education. Many states require licensing for practicing dietitians.

registration: listing; with respect to health professionals, listing with a professional organization that requires specific course work, experience, and passing of an examination.

---

of nutrition knowledge. Still, few physicians have the time or experience to develop diet plans and provide detailed diet instructions for clients. Often physicians wisely refer their clients to qualified nutrition experts—registered dietitians (RD).

A registered dietitian has the educational background necessary to deliver reliable nutrition advice and care. To become an RD, a person must earn an undergraduate degree requiring some 60 or so semester hours in nutrition and food science; complete a year's clinical internship or the equivalent; pass a national examination administered over five competency areas by the ADA;* and maintain up-to-date knowledge by participating in required continuing education activities: attending seminars, taking courses, or writing professional papers. Meeting these established criteria certifies that a dietitian is a true nutrition authority.

Dietitians perform a multitude of duties in many settings in most communities.† They work in the food industry, in pharmaceutical companies, in home health agencies, in long-term care institutions, in private practice, in public health departments, in research centers, in education settings, in fitness centers, and in hospitals.

Dietitians can assume a number of different job responsibilities depending on their work settings and positions.[8] In hospitals, administrative dietitians manage the foodservice system; clinical dietitians provide client care (see Table H1–1); and nutrition support team dietitians coordinate nutrition care with other health care professionals. In the food industry, dietitians conduct research, develop products, and market services.

Public health dietitians who work in government-funded agencies play a key role in delivering nutrition services to people in the community.[9] Among their many roles, public health nutritionists

*The five content areas included on the registration examination for dietitians are nutrition services, foodservice systems, management, education and communication, and evaluation and standards. L. C. Webb and J. O. Maillet, The development of test specifications for the registration examinations, *Journal of the American Dietetic Association* 90 (1990): 1134–1135.

†To find a registered dietitian in your area, call the American Dietetic Association hotline: (800) 366–1655.

Table H1–1

Responsibilities of a Clinical Dietitian

- Assesses clients' nutrition status.
- Determines clients' nutrient requirements.
- Monitors clients' nutrient intakes.
- Develops, implements, and evaluates clients' nutrition care plans.
- Counsels clients to cope with unique diet plans.
- Teaches clients and their families about nutrition and diet plans.
- Provides training for other dietitians, nurses, interns, and dietetics students.
- Serves as liaison between clients and the foodservice department.
- Communicates with physicians, nurses, pharmacists, and other health care professionals about clients' progress, needs, and treatments.
- Participates in professional activities to enhance knowledge and skill.

help plan, coordinate, and evaluate food-assistance programs; act as consultants to other agencies; manage finances; and much more.[10] Those with advanced degrees in public health are well placed for employment in this vast field.

In some facilities, dietetic technicians assist registered dietitians in both administrative and clinical responsibilities. A dietetic technician has been educated and trained to work under the guidance of a registered dietitian.

Other dietary employees may include clerks, aides, cooks, porters, and other assistants. These dietary employees do not have extensive formal training in nutrition and their ability to provide accurate information may be limited.

IDENTIFYING FAKE CREDENTIALS

In contrast to registered dietitians, thousands of people possess fake nutrition degrees and claim to be nutrition counselors, nutritionists, or "dietists." These and other such titles may sound meaningful, but most of these people lack the established credentials and training of the ADA-sanctioned dietitian. If you look closely, you can see signs of their fake expertise.

Take, for example, a nutrition expert's educational background. The minimal standards of education for a dietitian specify a bachelor of science (BS) degree in food science and human nutrition or related fields from an accredited college or university. Such a degree generally requires four to five years of study. In contrast, a fake nutrition expert may display a degree from a six-month correspondence course. Such a degree simply falls short.* In some cases, schools posing as legitimate correspondence schools offer even less—they sell certificates to anyone who pays the fees. To obtain these "degrees," a candidate need not read any books or pass any examinations.†

To guard educational quality, an accrediting agency recognized by the U.S. Department of Education (DOE) certifies that certain schools meet criteria established to ensure that an institution provides complete and accurate schooling. Unfortunately, fake nutrition degrees are available from schools "accredited" by more than 30 phony accrediting agencies.**

To dramatize the ease with which anyone can obtain a fake nutrition degree, one writer enrolled in a correspondence course for a fee of $82. She made every attempt to fail, intentionally answering all examination questions incorrectly. Even so, she received a "nutritionist" certificate at the end of the course. The "school" explained that it was sure she must have just misread the test.

In a similar stunt, Ms. Sassafras Herbert was named a "professional member" of a professional association. For her efforts, Sassafras has received a wallet card and is listed in a sort of fake *Who's Who* in nutrition that is distributed at health fairs and trade shows nationwide. Sassafras is a poodle; her master,

*To find out whether a corresponding school is accredited, write the Distance Education and Training Council, Accrediting Commission, 1601 Eighteenth Street, N.W., Washington, D.C. 20009, or call (202) 234–5100.

†To find out whether a school is properly accredited for a dietetics degree, write the American Dietetic Association, Division of Education and Research, 216 West Jackson Boulevard, Chicago, IL 60606, or call (312) 899–4870.

**The American Council on Education publishes a directory of accredited institutions, professionally accredited programs, and candidates for accreditation in *Accredited Institutions of Postsecondary Education Programs Candidates* (available from many libraries). For additional information, write the Council on Postsecondary Accreditation, One Dupont Circle, Suite 305, Washington, D.C. 20036, or call (202) 452–1433.

Victor Herbert, MD, paid $50 to prove that she could be awarded these honors merely by sending in her name. Mr. Charlie Herbert, who is also a professional member of such an organization, is a cat.

Some states allow anyone to use the titles *dietitian* or *nutritionist*, but others have responded to the need for professional regulation. Some states allow only RDs or people with certain graduate degrees to call themselves dietitians. Many states now provide a further guarantee: the license to practice.[11] Licensing provides a way to identify people who have met minimal standards of education and experience.

By knowing what qualifies someone to speak on nutrition, consumers can determine whether that person's advice might be harmful or helpful. Don't be afraid to ask for credentials. Does the instructor at the spa have a degree in nutrition from an accredited university? Is the author of the magazine article an RD or otherwise qualified to write on nutrition? Have you seen the health-store clerk's license to practice as a dietitian? If not, seek a better-qualified source. After all, your health depends on it.

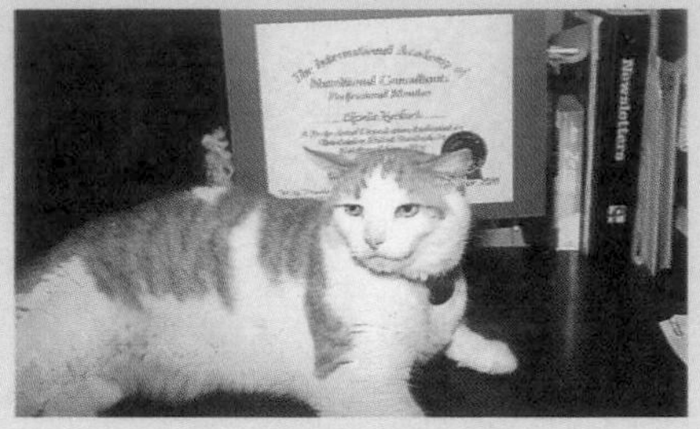

Charlie displays his professional credentials.

IDENTIFYING VALID INFORMATION

Where do nutrition experts get their information? As Chapter 1 explained, nutrition is a science; that is, it derives information from scientific research.

Researchers conduct experiments and then record and analyze their results, exercising caution in their interpretation of the findings. For example, in an epidemiological study, scientists may use a specific segment of the population—say, men 50 to 60 years old. When the scientists draw conclusions, they are careful not to generalize the findings to all people. Similarly, scientists performing research studies using animals are cautious in applying their findings to human beings. Conclusions from any one research study are always tentative and take into account findings from studies conducted by other scientists as well. As evidence accumulates, scientists gain confidence about making recommendations that affect people's health and lives. Still, their statements are worded cautiously, as in "A diet high in fruits and vegetables *may* protect against some cancers."

Quite often, as they approach an answer to one research question, scientists raise several more questions, so future research projects are never lacking. Further scientific investigation then seeks to answer questions such as "What substance or substances within fruits and vegetables provide protection?" If those substances turn out to be the vitamins A and C found so abundantly in fresh produce, then, "how much vitamin A and C is needed to offer protection?" "How do these vitamins protect against cancer?" "Is it their action as antioxidant nutrients?" "If not, might it be another action or even another substance that accounts for the protection fruits and vegetables provide against cancer?" (Highlight 11 explores the answers to these questions and reviews recent research on antioxidant nutrients and disease.)

The findings from a research study are submitted to a board of reviewers composed of other scientists who rigorously evaluate the study to assure that the scientific method was followed—a process known as peer review. The reviewers critique the study's hypothesis, methodology, statistical significance, and conclusions (Table H1–2 describes the parts of a research article). If the reviewers consider the conclusions to be well supported by the evidence, they endorse the work for publication in a scientific journal where others can read it. The readers can then evaluate the study and assess the findings in light of knowledge gleaned from other studies. Figure H1–1 (on p. 36) provides examples of reliable nutrition information.

Even when a new finding is published, it is still only preliminary, and not very meaningful by itself. Other scientists will need to confirm or disprove the findings through replication. To be accepted into the body of nutrition knowledge, a finding must stand up to rigorous, repeated testing in experiments performed by several different researchers. What we "know" in nutrition results from years of replicating study findings.

With each report from scientists, the field of nutrition changes a little—each finding contributes another piece to the whole body of knowledge. People who know how science works understand that single findings, like single frames in a movie, are just small parts of a larger story. Over years, the picture of what is "true" in nutrition gradually changes, and modifications in recommendations then follow.[12]

Table H1–2

Parts of a Research Article

- *Abstract*. The abstract provides a brief overview of the article.
- *Introduction*. The introduction clearly states the purpose of the current study by proposing a hypothesis and provides a comprehensive review of the literature.
- *Review of literature*. The review reveals all that science has uncovered on the subject to date.
- *Methodology*. The methodology section defines key terms and describes the instruments and procedures used in conducting the study.
- *Results*. The results report the findings and may include tables and figures that summarize the information.
- *Conclusions*. The conclusions drawn are those supported by the data and reflect the original purpose as stated in the introduction. Usually, they answer a few questions and raise several more.
- *References*. The references reflect the investigator's knowledge of the subject and should include an extensive list of relevant studies (including key studies several years old as well as current ones).

Instead of eating 4 servings of fruits and vegetables as recommended by the old Four Food Group plan, people are now encouraged to eat 2 to 4 servings of fruits and 3 to 5 servings of vegetables as suggested by the current Daily Food Guide (presented in Chapter 2).

There is much to learn about the effects of foods and nutrients on the body. The media, hungry for the latest news, often report scientific findings prematurely—without benefit of the careful interpretation, replication, and review that evaluate the findings. As a result, the public receives news quickly, but not always in perspective. Oftentimes findings from studies seem to contradict one another, and consumers feel frustrated and betrayed, when, in fact, this is simply the normal course of science at work. Science is constantly building on an already-existing foundation of knowledge.

People who do not understand how science operates may become distrustful as they try to learn nutrition from current news reports: "How am I supposed to know what to eat when the scientists themselves don't know?" General background knowledge about the science of nutrition is the best foundation a person can have in order to judge the validity of new nutrition information. (Congratulations on your decision to take this course.)

Because science is a step-by-step, information-gathering and testing process, old research still has value. A hypothesis first advanced in 1960 that stands up to decades of validation has real strength. When it comes to scientific information, "new" does not necessarily mean "improved." In fact, any science report based on all new references is suspect, for truly strong research is based on a body of work conducted over many years. This is why, even in books published just this year, you will see references to old reports. Some studies have become classics: they were exciting when they first appeared, and they have stood up to the test of time.

IDENTIFYING QUACKS

Nutrition is a hot topic and scattered among the valid research findings are thousands of unfounded claims. How can a person identify nutrition quackery? Once upon a time, quacks rode into town in wooden wagons hawking snake oil for 50 cents a bottle to "cure what ails you," but those days are gone. Today's purveyors manipulate consumers in less obvious ways. Fraudulent claims may *sound* logical, but they lack the research support found in nutrition science. The following techniques can alert consumers to quackery and misinformation:[13]

- Quacks use anecdotes, case histories, testimonials, and subjective evidence to support their claims.
- Quacks promise quick, dramatic, miraculous cures.
- Quacks use pseudo-medical terms and jargon, which lends a false legitimacy to the claim, confuses the client, and camouflages the lack of substance.
- Quacks display fake credentials.
- Quacks contend that most health problems are caused by poor nutrition and therefore can be corrected with proper nutrition.
- Quacks claim that "natural" vitamins are better than synthetic ones.
- Quacks sometimes recommend eating products derived from animal tissues to rejuvenate the counterpart in a human being.
- Quacks belittle medicine, science, and government regulations, offering "alternatives" that have not been proven safe or effective.

Figure H1–1

Sources of Reliable Nutrition Information

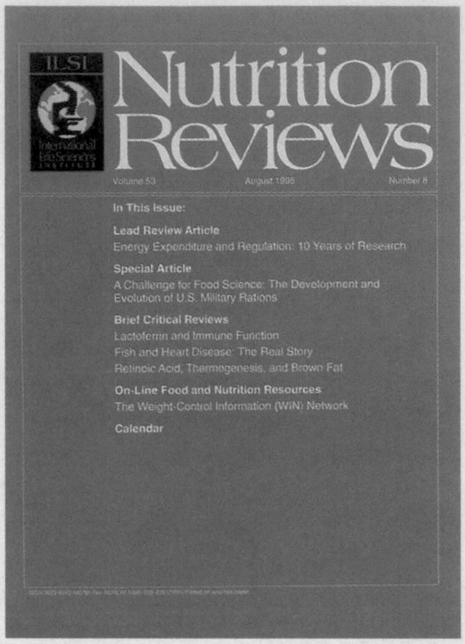

Reviews
Articles that examine all the major work on a subject are published in review journals like *Nutrition Reviews*. These articles provide references to all of the original work reviewed.

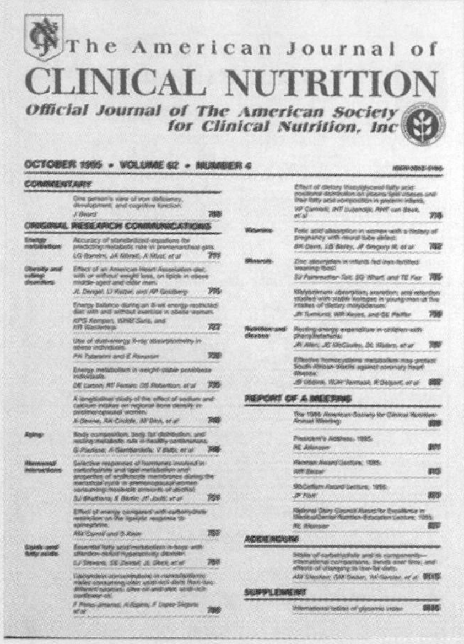

Journals
Articles that present all the details of the methods, results, and conclusions of a particular study are published in journals like the *American Journal of Clinical Nutrition*.

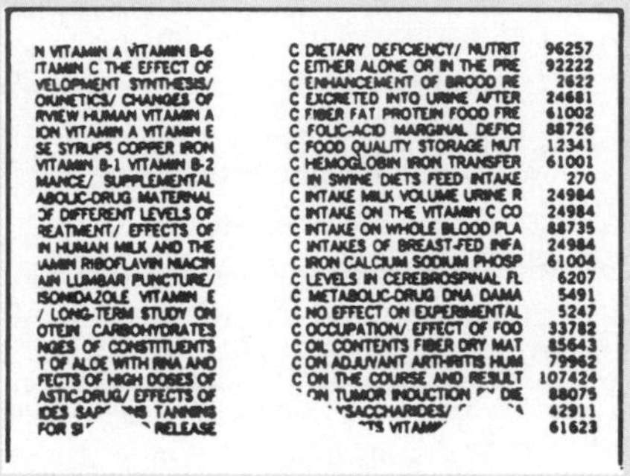

Indexes
An index of abstracts directs you to many research articles on a given subject. This index from *Biological Abstracts* lists recently published works on vitamin C.

- Quacks believe that products from health-food stores are better than those from regular grocery stores.
- Quacks oppose public health strategies such as fluoridating the water supply or vaccinating children against infectious diseases.
- Quacks claim that food processing and storage destroy all nutrients.
- Quacks depict food additives as poisons responsible for a variety of problems—from misbehavior to murder.
- Quacks insist that stress and other conditions raise nutrient needs higher than can be met by foods alone.
- Quacks make claims that people want to hear but that are too good to be true—such as that vitamin and mineral supplements will prevent cancer.
- Quacks use hair analysis and other unproven diagnostic tests to detect "alleged" nutrient deficiencies.
- Quacks profit from the sales of the products they are advocating.
- Quacks claim sugar is a poison.
- Quacks diagnose "nutrient deficiencies" by computerized questionnaires.
- Quacks advocate restrictive fad diets for a variety of health conditions.
- Quacks portray physicians as money-grabbing, incompetent misfits who are not to be trusted.

In short, quackery respects neither science nor honesty in its pursuit of ill-gotten gains.

In summary, when you hear nutrition news, consider its source. Ask yourself these two questions: Is the person purveying the information qualified to speak on nutrition? Is the information based on valid scientific research? To check an "expert's" qualifications, first look for the degrees and credentials listed by the person's name (such as MS, PhD, RD, or MD). Then find out

How to Find Credible Sources of Nutrition Information

Government health agencies, volunteer health agencies, consumer groups, and professional health organizations provide consumers with reliable health and nutrition information. Credible sources of nutrition information include:

- Government health agencies such as the Federal Trade Commission (FTC), the U.S. Department of Health and Human Services (DHHS), the Food and Drug Administration (FDA), and the U.S. Department of Agriculture (USDA).
- Local agencies such as the County Cooperative Extension Service.
- Nutrition and food science departments at a university or community college.
- Volunteer health agencies such as the American Cancer Society, the American Diabetes Association, and the American Heart Association.
- Reputable consumer groups such as the Better Business Bureau, the Consumers Union, the American Council on Science and Health, and the National Council Against Health Fraud.
- Professional health organizations such as the American Dietetic Association, the Society for Nutrition Education, and the American Medical Association.
- Journals such as the *American Journal of Clinical Nutrition*, *Journal of the American Dietetic Association*, and *Nutrition Reviews*.

Appendix F provides addresses for these and other organizations.

Source: Adapted from Position of The American Dietetic Association: Food and nutrition misinformation, *Journal of the American Dietetic Association* 95 (1995): 705–707.

about the reputation of the institution that awarded each degree. Call and ask your state's health-licensing agency if dietitians are licensed in your state and (if so) if the person giving you dietary advice has met licensing criteria. If not, find someone better qualified, for your health is your most precious asset.

NOTES

1. M. E. Shils, Separating food facts and myths, in *The Mount Sinai School of Medicine Complete Book of Nutrition*, eds. V. Herbert and G. J. Subak-Sharpe (New York: St. Martin's Press, 1990), pp. 21–29.
2. M. E. Shils, National Dairy Council award for excellence in medical and dental nutrition education lecture, 1994: Nutrition education in medical schools—The prospect before us, *American Journal of Clinical Nutrition* 60 (1994): 631–638.
3. A. G. Swanson, 1990 ASCN Nutrition educators' symposium and information exchange: Nutrition sciences in medical-student education, *American Journal of Clinical Nutrition* 53 (1991): 587–588.
4. D. S. McLaren, Nutrition in medical schools: A case of mistaken identity, *American Journal of Clinical Nutrition* 59 (1994): 960–963.
5. National Nutrition Monitoring and Related Research Act of 1990, public law 101–445, as quoted in C. H. Halstead, Toward standardized training of physicians in clinical nutrition, *American Journal of Clinical Nutrition* 56 (1992): 1–3.
6. Position of The American Dietetic Association: Nutrition—An essential component of medical education, *Journal of the American Dietetic Association* 94 (1994): 555–557.
7. Position of The American Dietetic Association: Nutrition education of health professionals, *Journal of the American Dietetic Association* 91 (1991): 611–613.
8. M. T. Kane and coauthors, Role delineation for dietetic practitioners: Empirical results, *Journal of the American Dietetic Association* 90 (1990): 1124–1133.
9. M. C. Egan, Public health nutrition: A historical perspective, *Journal of the American Dietetic Association* 94 (1994): 298–302.
10. B. Haughton and J. Shaw, Functional roles of today's public health nutritionist, *Journal of the American Dietetic Association* 92 (1992): 1218–1222.
11. Licensure of dietitians and nutritionists: Update on state laws, *Journal of the American Dietetic Association* 94 (1994): 974.
12. K. McNutt, Where truth comes from, *Nutrition Today*, March/April 1994, pp. 43–48.
13. Adapted with permission from Thirty ways to spot quacks and pushers, in S. Barrett and V. Herbert, *The Vitamin Pushers: How the "Health Food" Industry Is Selling America a Bill of Goods* (Amherst, NY: Prometheus Books, 1994), pp. 15–35.

Chapter 2

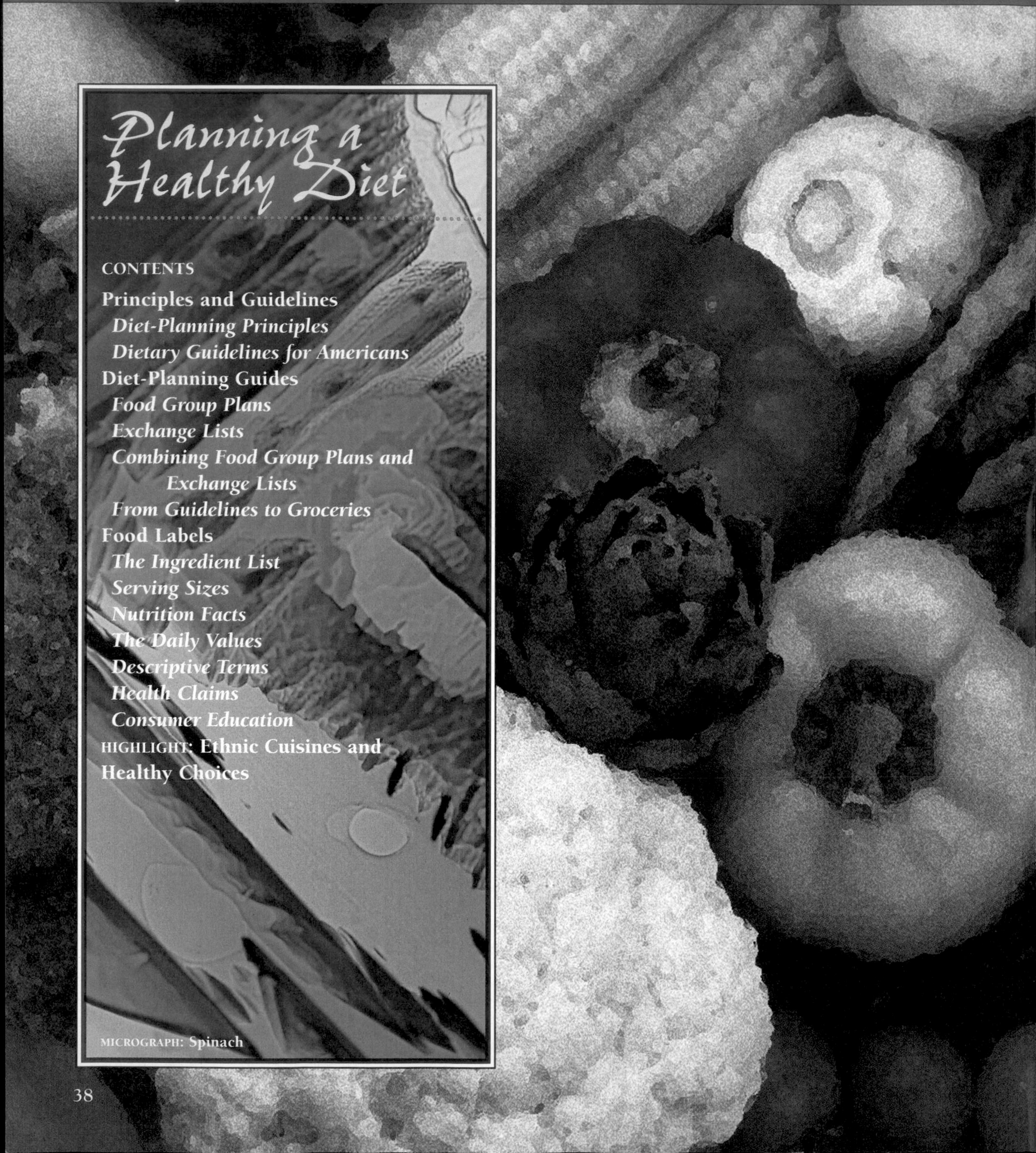

Planning a Healthy Diet

CONTENTS

MICROGRAPH: Spinach

Chapter 1 explained that the body's many activities are supported by the array of nutrients delivered by the foods people eat. Food choices made over years influence the body's health, and consistently poor choices increase the risks of developing chronic diseases. This chapter attempts to show how a person can select from the tens of thousands of foods available to create a diet that supports health. In a way, the task sounds simple: just select foods that will provide all the needed nutrients. On learning that an adult needs 800 milligrams of calcium a day, an enthusiastic novice might buy a quart of milk. To get the needed milligram of thiamin, the person might add ten slices of bread. This approach quickly runs into trouble, though. Faced with the need for 40-odd nutrients, a person who selected one type of food for each nutrient would soon have a basket of 40 different foods, and thousands too many kcalories to eat in a day. Fortunately, most foods provide several nutrients, so one trick for wise diet planning is to select a combination of foods that deliver a full array of nutrients. This chapter begins with an introduction of the diet-planning principles and dietary guidelines that assist people in selecting foods that will deliver nutrients without excess energy.

Principles and Guidelines

How well you nourish yourself does not depend on the selection of any one food. Instead it depends on the selection of many different foods at numerous meals, over days, months, and years. Diet-planning principles and dietary guidelines are key concepts to keep in mind whenever you are selecting foods—whether shopping at the grocery store, choosing from a restaurant menu, or preparing a home-cooked meal.

DIET-PLANNING PRINCIPLES

Diet planners have developed several ways to select foods. Whatever plan or combination of plans they use, though, they keep in mind the six basic diet-planning principles listed in the margin.

Diet-planning principles:

- Adequacy.
- Balance.
- kCalorie (energy) control.
- Nutrient Density.
- Moderation.
- Variety.

Adequacy The RDA discussion in Chapter 1 was all about dietary adequacy. An adequate diet provides sufficient energy and enough of all the nutrients to meet the needs of healthy people. Take the essential nutrient iron, for example. Each day the body loses some iron, so people have to replace it by eating foods that contain iron. A person whose diet fails to provide enough iron-rich foods may develop the symptoms of iron-deficiency anemia: the person may feel weak, tired, and listless; have frequent headaches; and find that even the smallest amount of muscular work brings disabling fatigue. To prevent these deficiency symptoms, diet planners include foods that supply adequate iron. The same is true for all the other essential nutrients introduced in Chapter 1.

adequacy (dietary): providing all the essential nutrients, fiber, and energy in amounts sufficient to maintain health.

Balance The essential minerals calcium and iron, taken together, illustrate the importance of dietary balance. Meats, fish, and poultry are rich in iron but poor in calcium. Similarly, milk and milk products are rich in calcium but poor in iron. In fact, milk (except breast milk) and milk products are so low in iron that overuse of these foods can actually lead to iron-deficiency anemia by

balance (dietary): providing foods of a number of types in proportion to each other, such that foods rich in some nutrients do not crowd out of the diet foods that are rich in other nutrients.

displacing iron-rich foods from the diet. Yet milk is the single most nutritious food for infants and can be an important source of calcium for people of all ages.

The art of balancing the diet involves using enough—but not too much—of each type of food. Use some meat or meat alternates for iron; use some milk and milk products for calcium; and save some space for other foods, too, since a diet consisting of milk and meat alone would not be adequate. For the other nutrients, people need vegetables, fruits, and grains.

Balance in the diet helps to ensure adequacy.

kCalorie (Energy) Control Clearly, the task of designing an adequate, balanced diet requires some thought and skillful planning. Even more thought and skill are required to create an adequate, balanced diet without overeating. The discussion of weight control in Chapter 9 examines this issue in more detail, but the key to controlling energy intake is to select foods of high nutrient density.

kcalorie (energy) control: management of food energy intake.

nutrient density: a measure of the nutrients a food provides relative to the energy it provides. The more nutrients and the fewer kcalories, the higher the nutrient density.

Nutrient density promotes adequacy and kcalorie control.

moderation: in relation to dietary intake, providing enough but not too much of a substance.

Moderation contributes to adequacy, balance, and kcalorie control.

variety (dietary): eating a wide selection of foods within and among the major food groups (the opposite of monotony).

Nutrient Density To eat well without overeating, select foods that deliver the most nutrients for the least food energy. Consider foods containing calcium, for example. You can get about 300 milligrams of calcium from either 1½ ounces of cheddar cheese or 8 ounces of nonfat milk, but the cheese contributes about twice as much food energy as the milk. The nonfat milk, then, is twice as calcium dense as the cheddar cheese; it offers the same amount of calcium for half the energy intake. Both foods are excellent choices for adequacy's sake alone, but to achieve adequacy while controlling kcalories, the nonfat milk is the better choice.

Just like a person who has to pay for rent, food, clothes, and tuition on a tight budget, a person whose energy allowance is limited has to obtain iron, calcium, and all the other essential nutrients on a tight energy budget. To succeed, the person has to get many nutrients for each kcalorie "dollar." In the cola and watermelon example in the margin, both provide about the same number of kcalories, but the watermelon delivers many more nutrients. A person who makes nutrient-dense choices such as fruit over cola can meet daily nutrient needs on a lower energy budget.

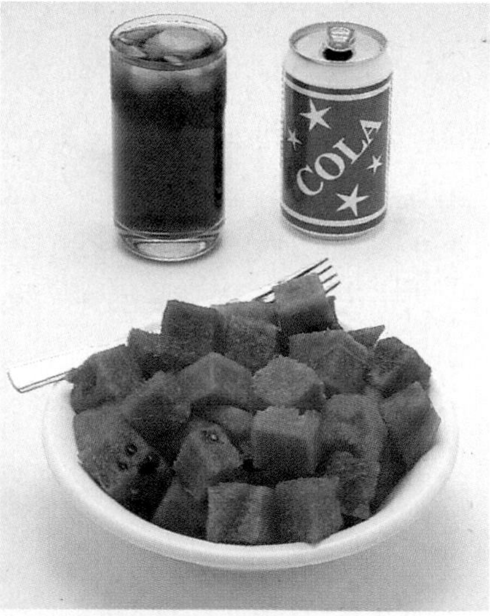

This cola and bowl of watermelon illustrate nutrient density. Each provides about 150 kcalories, but the watermelon offers a little protein, some vitamins, minerals, and fiber along with the energy; the cola beverage offers only "empty" kcalories. Watermelon, or any fruit for that matter, is more nutrient dense than cola beverages.

Moderation Foods rich in fat and sugar provide enjoyment and energy, but relatively few nutrients. In addition, they promote weight gain when eaten in excess. A person practicing moderation would eat such foods only on occasion and would regularly select foods low in fat and sugar, a practice that automatically improves nutrient density. Returning to the example of cheddar cheese and nonfat milk, the nonfat milk not only offers the same amount of calcium for less energy, but it contains far less fat than the cheese.

Variety A diet may have all of the virtues just described and still lack variety, if a person eats the same foods day after day. People should select foods from each of the food groups daily. Diets that omit several food groups are associated with an increased risk of mortality.[1] Furthermore, people should vary their choices within each food group from day to day for several reasons. First, different foods within the same group contain different arrays of nutrients. Among the fruits, for example, strawberries are especially rich in vitamin C while cantaloupes are rich in vitamin A. Second, no food is guaranteed entirely free of substances that, in excess, could be harmful. The strawberries might contain trace amounts of one contaminant, the cantaloupes another. By alternating fruit choices, a person will ingest very little of either contaminant. (Contamination of foods is the subject of Chapter 19.) Stated another way, variety within the diet helps ensure dilution of contaminants. Third, as the adage goes, variety is the spice of life. Even if a person eats beans frequently, the person can choose pinto beans in Mexican chili today, garbanzo beans in Greek salad tomorrow, and baked beans with barbecued chicken on the weekend. Eating nutritious meals need never be boring.

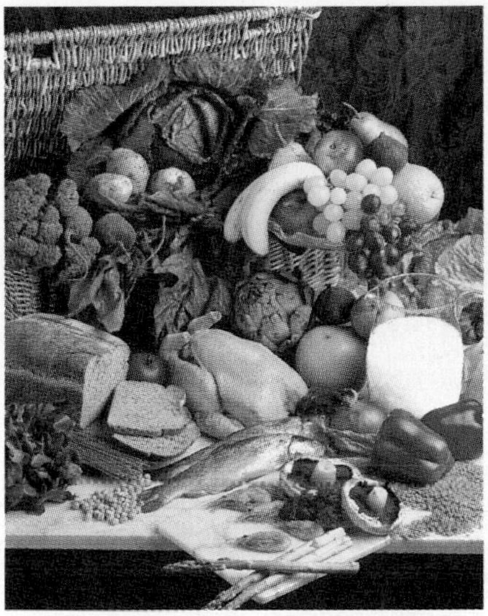

To ensure an adequate and balanced diet, eat a variety of foods daily, choosing different foods from each group.

DIETARY GUIDELINES FOR AMERICANS

The *Dietary Guidelines for Americans* coordinate the health recommendations introduced in Chapter 1 with the diet-planning principles just presented. For example, they combine the recommendation to "increase intake of starches and complex carbohydrates" with the principle of variety, offering the practical advice to "choose a diet with plenty of grain products, vegetables, and fruits." In general, the *Dietary Guidelines* answer the question, What should an individual eat to stay healthy?

Table 2–1 presents the 1990 and proposed 1995 *Dietary Guidelines*. The first two guidelines encourage people to eat a variety of foods to get the nutrients needed to support good health and to balance food intake with physical activity in order to maintain or improve body weight. The next two guidelines urge a shift in the balance of energy nutrients: they encourage people to increase their carbohydrate intakes and reduce their fat intakes by choosing a diet that is abundant in grains, vegetables, and fruits and low in fat, saturated fat, and cholesterol. The last three guidelines recommend a diet moderate in sugars, salt and sodium, and alcoholic beverages for those who partake. Together, these seven guidelines point the way toward better health. Table 2–2 presents *Canada's Guidelines for Healthy Eating*.

Table 2–1

Dietary Guidelines for Americans

1990 Guidelines	1995 Guidelines (proposed)
• Eat a variety of foods.	• Eat a variety of foods.
• Maintain healthy weight.	• Balance the food you eat with physical activity; maintain or improve your weight.
• Choose a diet low in fat, saturated fat, and cholesterol.	• Choose a diet with plenty of grain products, vegetables, and fruits.
• Choose a diet with plenty of vegetables, fruits, and grain products.	• Choose a diet low in fat, saturated fat, and cholesterol.
• Use sugars only in moderation.	• Choose a diet moderate in sugars.
• Use salt and sodium in moderation.	• Choose a diet moderate in salt and sodium.
• If you drink alcoholic beverages, do so in moderation.	• If you drink alcoholic beverages, do so in moderation.

Note: These guidelines are designed for healthy people over two years old.
Source: The *Dietary Guidelines for Americans* are developed by the U.S. Department of Agriculture and U.S. Department of Health and Human Services: the 1995 guidelines are based on the *Report of the Dietary Guidelines Advisory Committee, 1995*.

Table 2–2

Canada's Guidelines for Healthy Eating

- Enjoy a variety of foods.
- Emphasize cereals, breads, other grain products, vegetables, and fruits.
- Choose lower-fat dairy products, leaner meats, and foods prepared with little or no fat.
- Achieve and maintain a healthy body weight by enjoying regular physical activity and healthy eating.
- Limit salt, alcohol, and caffeine.

Source: These guidelines derive from *Action Towards Healthy Eating: The Report of the Communications/Implementation Committee* and *Nutrition Recommendations . . . . A Call for Action: Summary Report of the Scientific Review Committee and the Communications/ Implementation Committee*, which are available from Branch Publications Unit, Health Services and Promotion Branch, Department of Health and Welfare, 5th Floor, Jeanne Mance Building, Ottawa, Ontario K1A 1B4.

> HEALTHY PEOPLE 2000: Increase to at least 90% the proportion of restaurants and institutional foodservice operations that offer identifiable low-fat, low-kcalorie food choices, consistent with the *Dietary Guidelines for Americans*.

To sum up, a well-planned diet delivers adequate nutrients, a balanced array of nutrients, and an appropriate amount of energy. It is based on nutrient-dense foods, moderate in substances that can be detrimental to health, and varied in its selections. The *Dietary Guidelines* apply these principles, offering practical advice on how to eat for good health.

Diet-Planning Guides

To plan a diet that achieves all of the dietary ideals just outlined, a planner needs not only knowledge but tools. Two of the most widely used tools for diet planning are food group plans and exchange lists.

food group plans: diet-planning tools that sort foods of similar origin and nutrient content into groups and then specify that people should eat certain numbers of servings from each group.

The Daily Food Guide replaced the old Four Food Group Plan and is illustrated as the Food Guide Pyramid.

Five food groups:

- Breads, cereals, and other grain products.
- Vegetables.
- Fruits.
- Meat, poultry, fish, and alternates.
- Milk, cheese, and yogurt.

FOOD GROUP PLANS

Food group plans build a diet from clusters of foods that are similar in origin and nutrient content. One such cluster is the milk group, which includes milk, cheese, and yogurt. Another cluster is the grains: breads, cereals, rice, and pasta. Each food group may include dozens of different items. No two items are identical, but they can be arranged into families of foods with similar nutrient compositions. Thus each group represents a set of nutrients that differs from the nutrients supplied by the other groups. Selecting foods from each of the groups eases the task of creating a balanced diet.

Daily Food Guide Figure 2–1 (pp. 44–45) presents the USDA's Daily Food Guide, a food group plan that assigns foods to five major food groups. The figure lists the most notable nutrients of each group, the foods within each group categorized by nutrient density, the number of servings recommended, and the serving sizes. It also includes an illustration of the USDA's Food Guide Pyramid, a pictorial description of the Daily Food Guide.

Notable Nutrients The beauty of the Daily Food Guide lies in its simplicity and flexibility. For example, a person can substitute cheese for milk because both supply the key nutrients for the milk group. A person following a food group plan receives not only the nutrients each group is noted for, but small amounts of other nutrients as well. For example, milk, cheese, and yogurt are notable for their calcium, protein, and riboflavin, but they also provide other nutrients. In contrast, a drink concocted from sugar, water, calcium, protein, and riboflavin lacks this nutrient richness, although a label featuring these ingredients might make the drink appear to resemble milk. Milk, cheese, and yogurt are foundation foods; synthetic drinks are not.

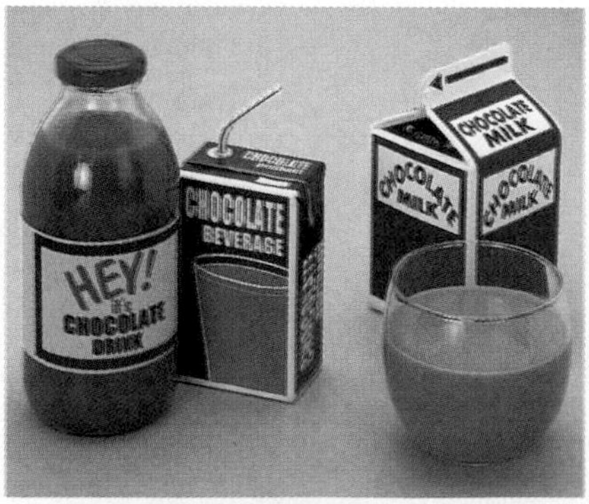

Milk "beverages" or "drinks" may taste delicious, but they lack the nutrient richness of real milk products.

Miscellaneous Foods Some foods—such as the synthetic drink just mentioned—do not fit into any of the food groups. Foods that are high in fat, sugar, or alcohol provide energy, but too few nutrients to hold a significant place in the diet. Such foods should be used sparingly and only after basic nutrient needs have been met by the foundation foods. Examples of "miscellaneous" foods include salad dressings, jams, and alcoholic beverages.

Nutrient Density The Daily Food Guide provides a strong foundation for a healthy diet, but it fails to specify food energy intakes. Large fat and energy differences exist within a single food group—for example, between nonfat milk and ice cream, fish and hot dogs, green beans and french fries, apples and avocados, or bread and biscuits—yet according to the Daily Food Guide, any of these substitutions would be acceptable. People who have low energy allowances are advised to select the most nutrient-dense foods within each group, whereas people with high energy needs may select some of the less nutrient-dense, higher-kcalorie foods. Notice that Figure 2–1 provides a key indicating which foods *within each group* are high, moderate, or low nutrient density choices.

Recommended Servings As mentioned earlier, all food groups are important, and people should make selections from each group daily. The recommended numbers of daily servings are:

- 6 to 11 servings of breads and cereals.
- 3 to 5 servings of vegetables.
- 2 to 4 servings of fruits.
- 2 to 3 servings of meats and meat alternates.
- 2 servings of milk and milk products. (Women who are pregnant or breastfeeding and teenagers are advised to have 3 servings, and teenagers who are pregnant or breastfeeding should have 4.)

The lower number of servings from each group provides about the right amount of food energy for sedentary women and older adults. The middle of the range is appropriate for most children, teenage girls, active women, and sedentary men. The upper end meets the needs of teenage boys, active men, and very active women. Table 2–3 provides estimated kcalorie amounts for each of these three levels. Physical activity raises a person's energy allowance and permits the person to eat more foods, or higher-kcalorie foods, to supply needed nutrients without gaining unwanted weight.

Table 2–3

Sample Diet Plans for Different Levels of Energy Intake

Food Group	Servings		
Bread	6	9	11
Vegetable	3	4	5
Fruit	2	3	4
Milk[a]	2–3[a]	2–3[a]	2–3[a]
Meat[b]	5	6	7
kCalories	1600	2200	2800

Note: The 1600-kcalorie plan assumes a total of 53 grams of fat and allows 6 teaspoons of added sugar. The 2200 kcalorie plan assumes a total of 73 grams of fat and allows 12 teaspoons of added sugar. The 2800-kcalorie plan assumes a total of 93 grams of fat and allows 18 teaspoons of added sugar.

[a]Women who are pregnant or breastfeeding, teenagers, and young adults to age 24 need 3 servings.

[b]Meat group amounts are in total ounces.

Serving Sizes What counts as a serving? The answer differs for each food group and for various foods within a group. Furthermore, serving sizes may not represent the amounts people actually put on their plates. Figure 2–1 provides the serving sizes for standard foods within each group. For example, ½ cup of cooked rice is considered one serving. So, 1 cup of rice counts as 2 of the recommended 6 to 11 daily servings from the bread group. Similarly, ¼ cup counts as ½ serving.

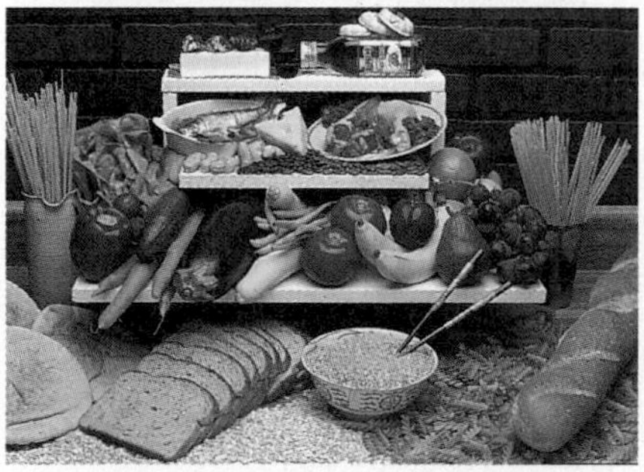

Each of the five major food groups appears in the Pyramid in proportion to the number of daily servings recommended.

Food Guide Pyramid The Food Guide Pyramid is a graphic depiction of the Daily Food Guide (see Figure 2–1 again). The illustration was designed to depict variety, moderation, and also proportions: the size of each section represents the number of daily servings recommended. The broad base at the bottom conveys the message that grains should be abundant and form the foundation of a healthy diet. Fruits and vegetables appear at the next level, showing that they have a less prominent, but still important, place in the diet. Meats and milks appear in a

Figure 2–1

The Daily Food Guide

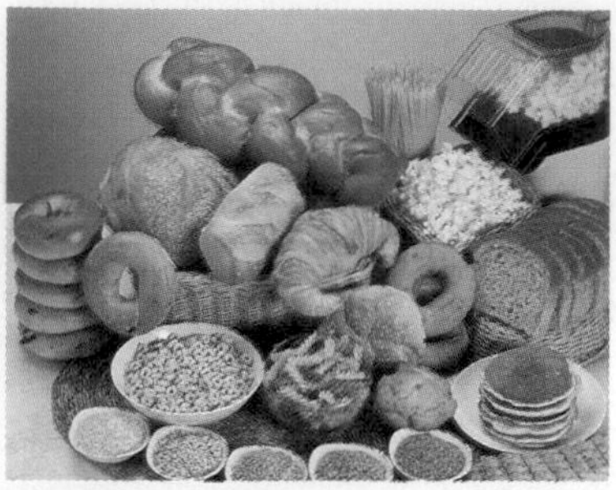

Breads, Cereals, and Other Grain Products

These foods are notable for their contributions of complex carbohydrates, riboflavin, thiamin, niacin, iron, protein, magnesium, and fiber.

6 to 11 servings per day.

Serving = 1 slice bread; ½ c cooked cereal, rice, or pasta; 1 oz ready-to-eat cereal; ½ bun, bagel, or English muffin; 1 small roll, biscuit, or muffin; 3 to 4 small or 2 large crackers.

- ♦ Whole grains (wheat, oats, barley, millet, rye, bulgur), enriched breads, rolls, tortillas, cereals, bagels, rice, pastas (macaroni, spaghetti), air-popped corn.
- ♦ Pancakes, muffins, cornbread, crackers, cookies, biscuits, presweetened cereals, granola, taco shells, waffles.
- ♦ Croissants, fried rice, doughnuts, pastries, cakes, pies.

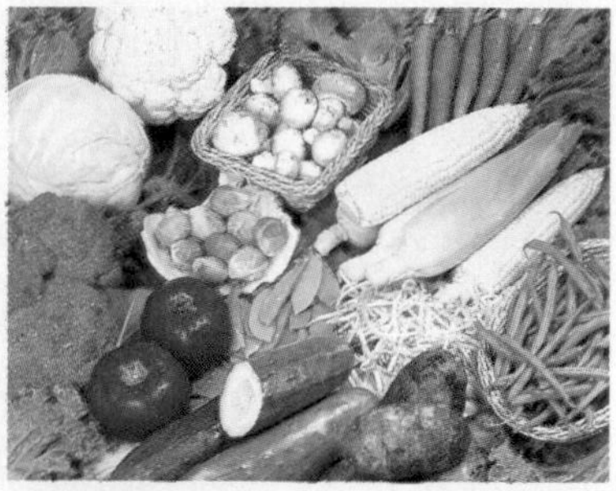

Vegetables

These foods are notable for their contributions of vitamin A, vitamin C, folate, potassium, magnesium, and fiber, and for their lack of fat and cholesterol.

3 to 5 servings per day (use dark green, leafy vegetables and legumes several times a week).

Serving = ½ c cooked or raw vegetables; 1 c leafy raw vegetables; ½ c cooked legumes; ¾ c vegetable juice.

- ♦ Bean sprouts, broccoli, brussels sprouts, cabbage, carrots, cauliflower, corn, cucumbers, green beans, green peas, leafy greens (spinach, mustard, and collard greens), legumes, lettuce, mushrooms, potatoes, tomatoes, winter squash.
- ♦ Candied sweet potatoes.
- ♦ French fries, tempura vegetables, scalloped potatoes, potato salad.

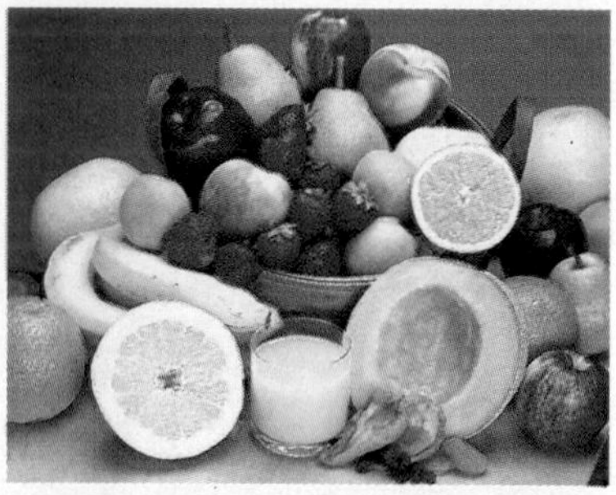

Fruits

These foods are notable for their contributions of vitamin A, vitamin C, potassium, and fiber, and for their lack of sodium, fat, and cholesterol.

2 to 4 servings per day.

Serving = typical portion (such as 1 medium apple, banana, or orange, ½ grapefruit, 1 melon wedge); ¾ c juice; ½ c berries; ½ c diced, cooked, or canned fruit; ¼ c dried fruit.

- ♦ Apricots, cantaloupe, grapefruit, oranges, orange juice, peaches, strawberries, apples, bananas, pears; unsweetened juices.
- ♦ Canned or frozen fruit (in syrup); sweetened juices.
- ♦ Dried fruit, coconut, avocados.

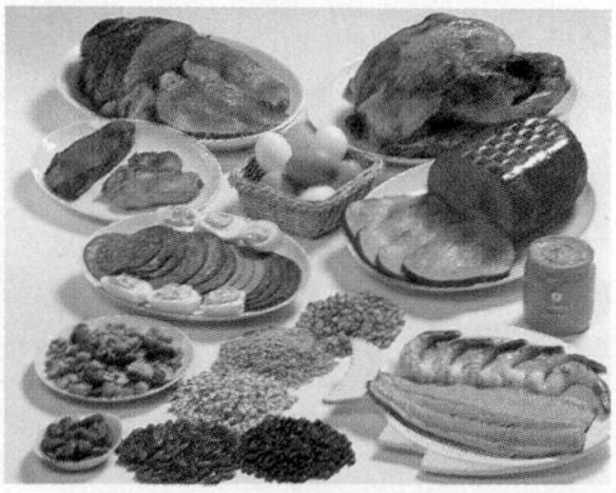

Meat, Poultry, Fish, and Alternates

These foods are notable for their contributions of protein, phosphorus, vitamin B_6, vitamin B_{12}, zinc, magnesium, iron, niacin, and thiamin.

2 to 3 servings per day.

Servings = 2 to 3 oz lean, cooked meat, poultry, or fish (total 5 to 7 oz per day); count 1 egg, ½ c cooked legumes, 4 oz tofu, or 2 tbs nuts, seeds, or peanut butter as 1 oz meat (or about ⅓ serving).

- ♦ Poultry (light meat, no skin), fish, shellfish, legumes, egg whites.
- ♦ Lean meat (fat-trimmed beef, lamb, pork); poultry (dark meat, no skin); ham; refried beans; whole eggs, tofu, tempeh.
- ♦ Hot dogs, luncheon meats, ground beef, peanut butter, nuts, sausage, bacon, fried fish or poultry, duck.

Key:

- ♦ Foods generally highest in nutrient density (good first choice).
- ♦ Foods moderate in nutrient density (reasonable second choice).
- ♦ Foods lowest in nutrient density (limit selections).

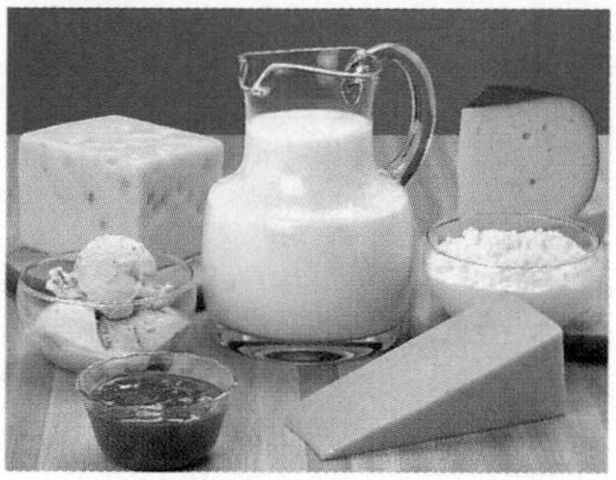

Milk, Cheese, and Yogurt

These foods are notable for their contributions of calcium, riboflavin, protein, vitamin B_{12}, and, when fortified, vitamin D and vitamin A.

2 servings per day.

3 servings per day for teenagers and young adults, pregnant/lactating women, women past menopause.

4 servings per day for pregnant/lactating teenagers.

Serving = 1 c milk or yogurt; 2 oz process cheese food; 1½ oz cheese.

- ♦ Nonfat and 1% low-fat milk (and nonfat products such as buttermilk, cottage cheese, cheese, yogurt); fortified soy milk.
- ♦ 2% low-fat milk (and low-fat products such as yogurt, cheese, cottage cheese); chocolate milk; sherbet; ice milk.
- ♦ Whole milk (and whole-milk products such as cheese, yogurt); custard; milk shakes; ice cream.

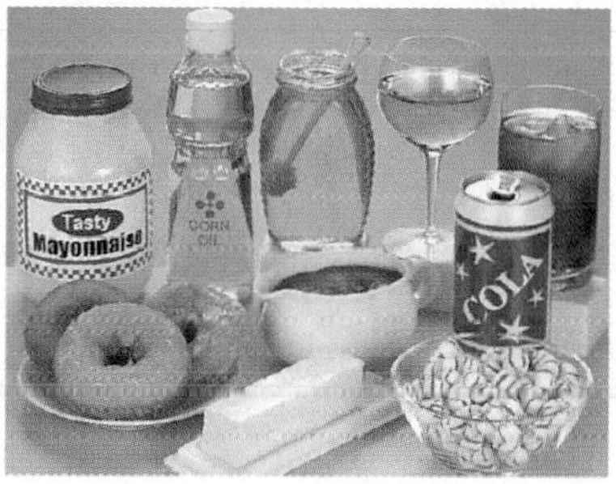

Fats, Sweets, and Alcoholic Beverages

These foods are notable for their contributions of sugar, fat, alcohol, and food energy. No servings are suggested because these foods provide few nutrients. Note that some of the following items, for example, doughnuts, are high in both sugar and fat. Alcoholic beverages are not classed as foods; they contribute few nutrients, but do provide food energy and so are included in this miscellaneous group. Miscellaneous foods not high in kcalories, such as spices, herbs, coffee, tea, and diet soft drinks, can be used freely.

- ♦ Foods high in fat include margarine, salad dressing, oils, mayonnaise, sour cream, cream cheese, butter, gravy, sauces, potato chips, chocolate bars.
- ♦ Foods high in sugar include cakes, pies, cookies, doughnuts, sweet rolls, candy, soft drinks, fruit drinks, jelly, syrup, gelatin, desserts, sugar, and honey.
- ♦ Alcoholic beverages include wine, beer, and liquor.

Note: Serve children at least the lower number of servings from each group, but in smaller amounts (for example, ¼ to ⅓ cup rice). Children should receive the equivalent of 2 cups of milk each day, but again in smaller quantities per serving (for example, 4 half-cup portions). Pregnant women may require additional servings of fruits, vegetables, meats, and breads to meet their higher needs for energy, vitamins, and minerals.

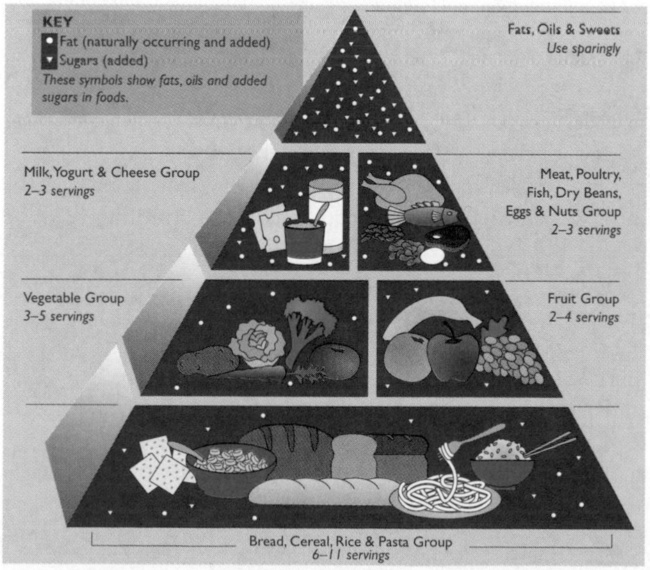

Food Guide Pyramid

A Guide to Daily Food Choices

The breadth of the base shows that grains (breads, cereals, rice, and pasta) deserve most emphasis in the diet. The tip is smallest: use fats, oils, and sweets sparingly.

smaller band near the top. A few servings of each can contribute valuable nutrients, such as protein, vitamins, and minerals, without too much fat and cholesterol. Fats, oils, and sweets occupy the tiny apex, indicating that they should be used sparingly.

Alcoholic beverages do not appear in the pyramid, but they too should be limited. Items such as spices, coffee, tea, and diet soft drinks provide few, if any, nutrients, but can add flavor and pleasure to meals when used judiciously.

Icons of tiny dots and triangles are sprinkled over the food groups, representing naturally occurring and added fats and added sugars, respectively. These icons are meant to remind users that specific foods within the various groups are high in fats, sugars, or both, and so should be eaten in moderation.

The Daily Food Guide plan and Food Guide Pyramid emphasize grains, fruits, and vegetables—all plant foods. Some 75 percent of a day's servings should come from these three groups. This strategy helps all people obtain complex carbohydrates, fiber, vitamins, and minerals with little fat. It also eases diet planning for vegetarians.

Highlight 6 defines vegetarian terms and provides more information on vegetarian diets.

legumes (lay-GYOOMS, LEG-yooms): plants of the bean and pea family. Bacteria in the root nodules of legumes "fix" nitrogen by trapping nitrogen from the air into the soil and then making it a part of the protein in the beans. Thus legumes are rich in high-quality protein compared with other plant-derived foods. Ultimately, the plant leaves more nitrogen in the soil than it takes out (sparing the land). Farmers sometimes plow under legume plants to fertilize the soil.

Vegetarian Food Guide Vegetarian diets rely mainly on plant foods: grains, vegetables, legumes, fruits, seeds, and nuts. Some vegetarian diets include eggs, milk products, or both. People who do not eat meats or milk products can still use the Daily Food Guide to create an adequate diet.[2] The food groups are similar, and the number of servings remain the same. Vegetarians select *meat alternates* from the meat group—foods such as legumes, seeds, nuts, tofu, and for those who eat them, eggs. Legumes help to supply the iron that meats usually provide, and vegetable selections need to include at least one cup of dark leafy greens for additional iron. Vegetarians who do not drink cow's milk can use soy "milk"—a product made from soybeans that provides similar nutrients if it has been fortified with calcium, vitamin D, and vitamin B_{12}.

Ethnic Food Guides The Daily Food Guide and Food Guide Pyramid can easily be adapted to include foods from different cultures.[3] For example, a Mexican-American guide would include tortillas in the bread group, jicama in the vegetable group, and guava in the fruit group.

Perceptions and Actual Intakes The Daily Food Guide and Food Guide Pyramid were developed to help people choose a balanced and healthful diet. Are we selecting foods that reflect the recommendations of the pyramid? According to one survey, many adults *think* they are, when, in fact, they are eating too many fats, sweets, and oils and too little from most of the other food groups.[4] In a sense, our pyramids are top heavy and "tumbling." They need more support from the bread, vegetable, fruit, milk, and meat groups to build a balanced diet.

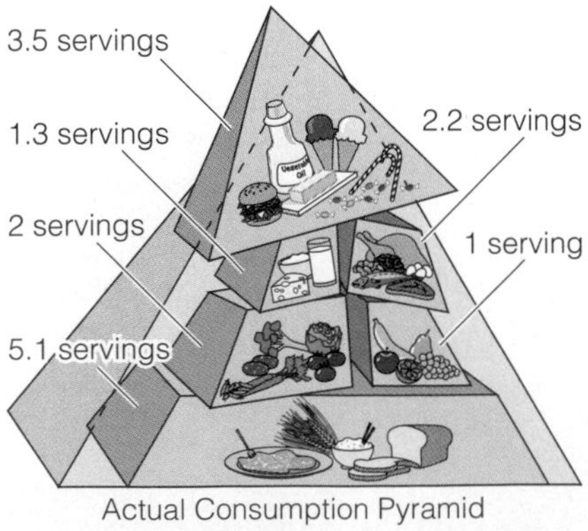

Compared with recommendations, actual consumption resembles a precariously built or "tumbling" pyramid.

Canada's Food Guide Canada's Food Guide to Healthy Eating, shown in Figure 2–2 (pp. 48–49), gives detailed information for selecting foods to meet the nutritional needs of all Canadians four years of age and older. Like the U.S. Daily Food Guide, Canada's Food Guide takes a total diet approach, rather than emphasizing a single food, meal, or day's meals and snacks.

The rainbow side of the Food Guide shows the four food groups with pictorial examples of foods in each group. Key statements advise consumers about selecting foods generally from all the groups, and more specifically within each group. The bar side shows the number of servings recommended for each group and the serving sizes for some foods.

EXCHANGE LISTS

Food group plans are particularly well suited to help the diet planner to achieve dietary adequacy, balance, and variety. Exchange lists provide additional help in achieving kcalorie control and moderation. Originally developed for people with diabetes, exchange systems have proved useful for general diet planning as well.

exchange lists: diet-planning tools that organize foods by their proportions of carbohydrate, fat, and protein. Foods on any single list can be used interchangeably.

Appendix G gives complete details of the major exchange system used in the United States, and Appendix I provides details of the exchange system used in Canada.

An exchange system:

- Names the foods on each list.
- Specifies portion sizes.
- States the amounts of carbohydrate, protein, fat, and kcalories each portion contributes.

Unlike the Daily Food Guide, which sorts foods primarily by their protein, vitamin, and mineral contents, the exchange system sorts foods into three main groups by their proportions of carbohydrate, fat, and protein. These three groups—the carbohydrate group, the fat group, and the meat and meat substitute group (protein)—organize foods into several exchange lists. The carbohydrate group covers these exchange lists:

- Starch (cereals, grains, pasta, breads, crackers, snacks, starchy vegetables, and dried beans, peas, and lentils).
- Fruit.
- Milk (nonfat, low-fat, and whole).
- Other carbohydrates (desserts and snacks with added sugars and fats).
- Vegetables.

The fat group covers this exchange list:

- Fats.

The meat and meat substitute group (protein) covers these exhange lists:

- Meat and meat substitutes (very lean, lean, medium-fat, and high-fat).

Portion Sizes All of the food portions in a given list provide approximately the same amounts of energy nutrients (carbohydrate, fat, and protein) and the same number of kcalories. Portion sizes are strictly defined so that every item on a given list provides roughly the same amount of energy. Any food on a list can then be exchanged, or traded, for any other food on that same list without affecting a plan's balance or total kcalories.

To apply the system successfully, users must become familiar with portion sizes. A convenient way to remember the portion sizes and energy values is to keep in mind a typical item from each list (see Table 2–4 on p. 50). Figure 2–3 (on pp. 52–53) shows the foods on each of the exchange lists and their accurate portion sizes.

The Foods on the Lists Foods are not always on the exchange list where you might first expect them to be because they are grouped according to their energy-nutrient contents rather than by their source (such as milks), their outward appearance, or their vitamin and mineral contents. For example, cheeses are grouped with meats in the exchange system because, like meats, cheeses contribute energy from protein and fat but provide negligible carbohydrate. (In the food group plans presented earlier, cheeses are classed with milk because they are milk products with a similar calcium content.)

Figure 2–2 Canada's Food Guide to Healthy Eating

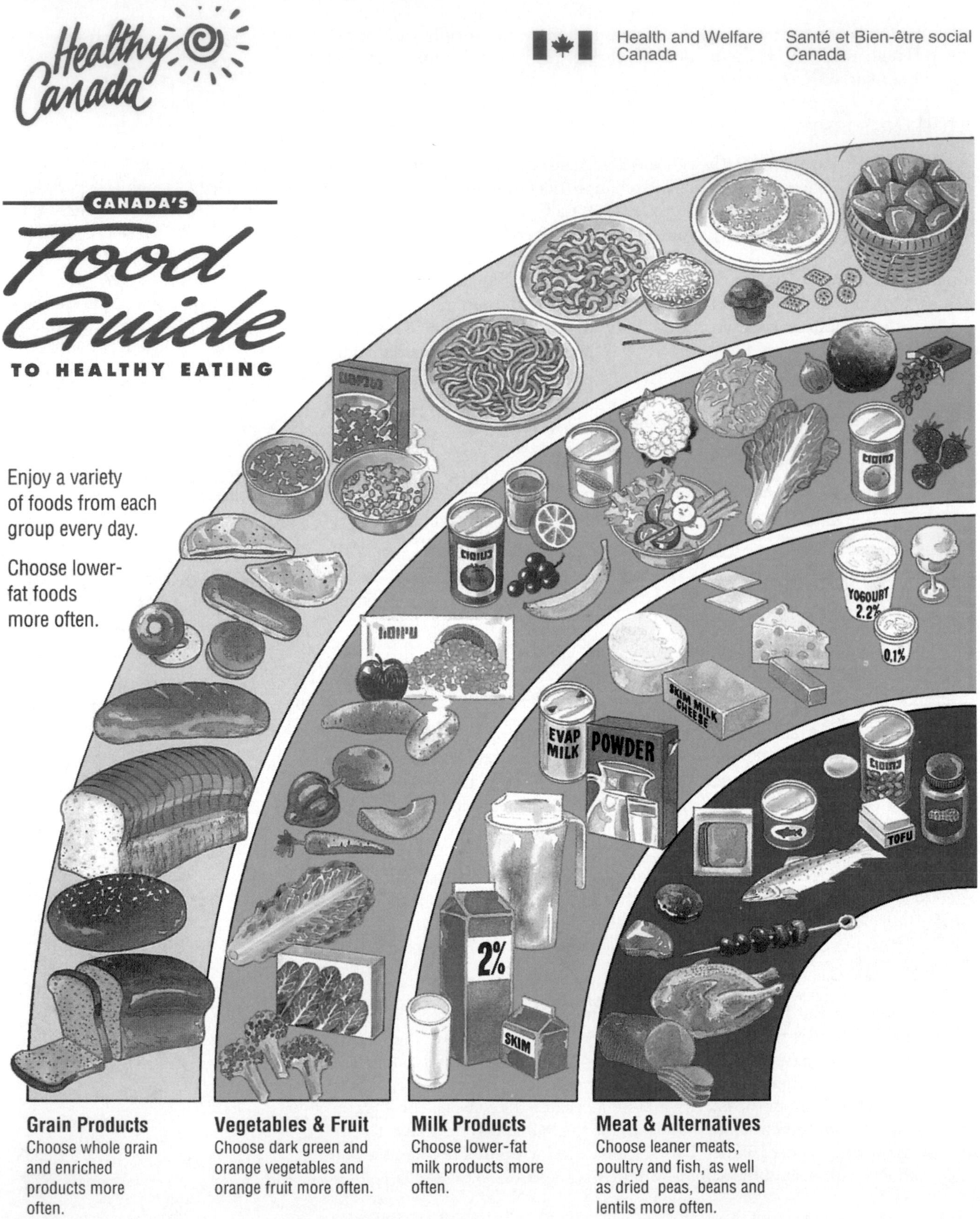
Healthy Canada
Health and Welfare Canada
Santé et Bien-être social Canada
CANADA'S
Food Guide
TO HEALTHY EATING
Enjoy a variety of foods from each group every day.
Choose lower-fat foods more often.
YOGOURT 2.2%
0.1%
SKIM MILK CHEESE
EVAP MILK
POWDER
TOFU
2%
SKIM
Grain Products
Choose whole grain and enriched products more often.
Vegetables & Fruit
Choose dark green and orange vegetables and orange fruit more often.
Milk Products
Choose lower-fat milk products more often.
Meat & Alternatives
Choose leaner meats, poultry and fish, as well as dried peas, beans and lentils more often.

CANADA'S

Food Guide

TO HEALTHY EATING

FOR PEOPLE FOUR YEARS AND OVER

Different People Need Different Amounts of Food

The amount of food you need every day from the 4 food groups and other foods depends on your age, body size, activity level, whether you are male or female and if you are pregnant or breast-feeding. That's why the Food Guide gives a lower and higher number of servings for each food group. For example, young children can choose the lower number of servings, while male teenagers can go to the higher number. Most other people can choose servings somewhere in between.

Grain Products

5–12

SERVINGS PER DAY

1 Serving | **2 Servings**

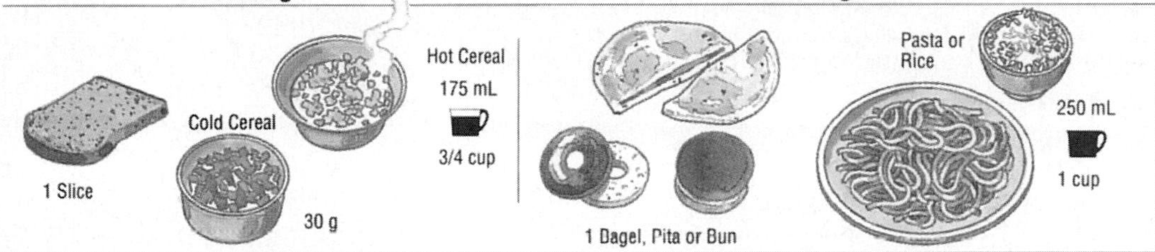

Vegetables & Fruit

5–10

SERVINGS PER DAY

1 Serving

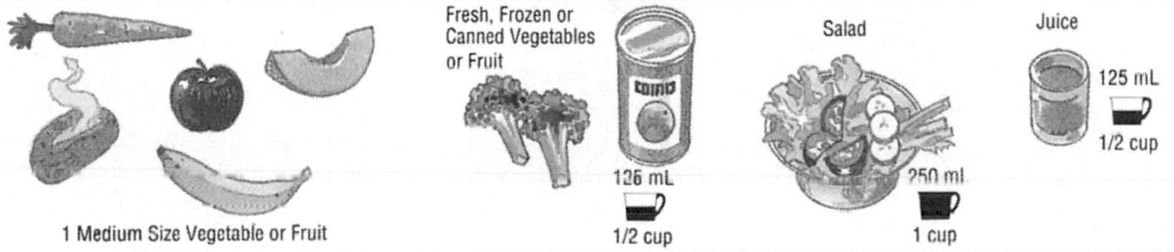

Milk Products

SERVINGS PER DAY

Children 4–9 years: 2–3
Youth 10–16 years: 3–4
Adults: 2–4
Pregnant & Breast-feeding Women: 3–4

1 Serving

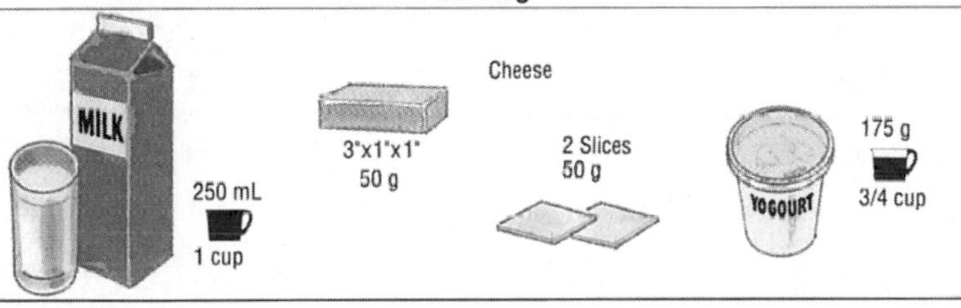

Meat & Alternatives

2–3

SERVINGS PER DAY

1 Serving

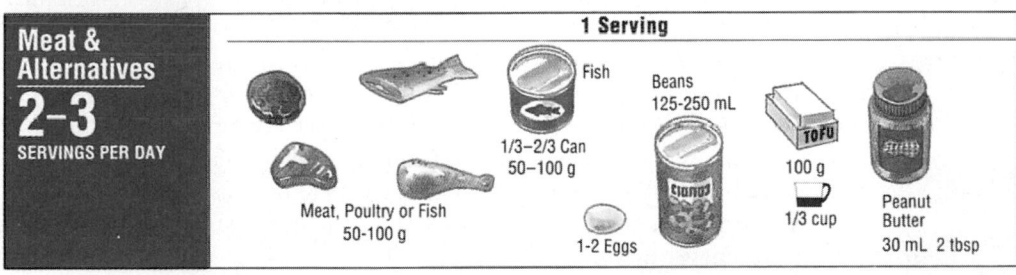

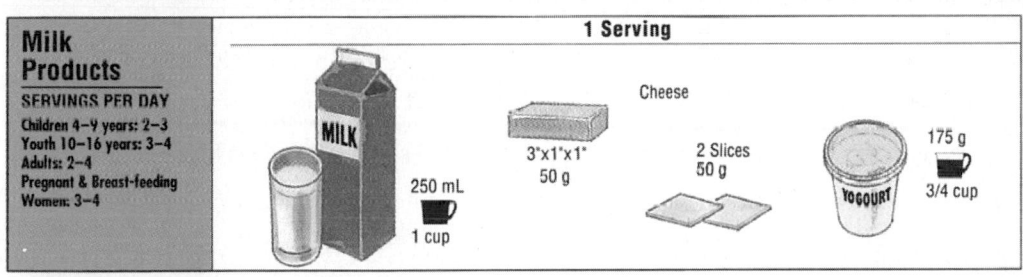

Other Foods

Taste and enjoyment can also come from other foods and beverages that are not part of the 4 food groups. Some of these foods are higher in fat or Calories, so use these foods in moderation.

Enjoy eating well, being active and feeling good about yourself. That's VITALITÉ

Table 2–4

The Exchange Lists

Group/Lists	Typical Item/Portion Size	Carbohydrate (g)	Protein (g)	Fat (g)	Energy[a] (kcal)
CARBOHYDRATE GROUP					
Starch[b]	1 slice bread	15	3	1 or less	80
Fruit	1 small apple	15	—	—	60
Milk					
Nonfat	1 c nonfat milk	12	8	0–3	90
Low-fat	1 c low-fat milk	12	8	5	120
Whole	1 c whole milk	12	8	8	150
Other carbohydrates[c]	2 small cookies	15	varies	varies	varies
Vegetable	½ c cooked carrots	5	2	—	25
MEAT AND MEAT SUBSTITUTE GROUP[d]					
Meat					
Very Lean	1 oz chicken (white meat, no skin)	—	7	0–1	35
Lean	1 oz lean beef	—	7	3	55
Medium-fat	1 oz ground beef	—	7	5	75
High-fat	1 oz pork sausage	—	7	8	100
FAT GROUP					
Fat	1 tsp butter	—	—	5	45

Note: The complete details of the U.S. exchange system are provided in Appendix G. Those of the Canadian system are shown in Appendix I.

[a]The energy value for each exchange list represents an approximate average for the group and does not reflect the precise number of grams of carbohydrate, protein, and fat. For example, a slice of bread contains 15 grams carbohydrate (that's 60 kcalories), 3 grams protein (that's another 12 kcalories), and a little fat—rounded up to 80 kcalories for ease in calculating. A half cup of vegetables (not including starchy vegetables) contains 5 grams carbohydrate (20 kcalories) and 2 grams protein (8 more), which has been rounded down to 25 kcalories.

[b]The starch list includes cereals, grains, breads, crackers, snacks, starchy vegetables (such as corn, peas, and potatoes), and legumes (dried beans, peas and lentils).

[c]The other carbohydrates list includes foods that contain added sugars and fats such as cakes, cookies, doughnuts, ice cream, potato chips, pudding, syrup, and frozen yogurt.

[d]The meat and meat substitutes list includes legumes, cheeses, and peanut butter.

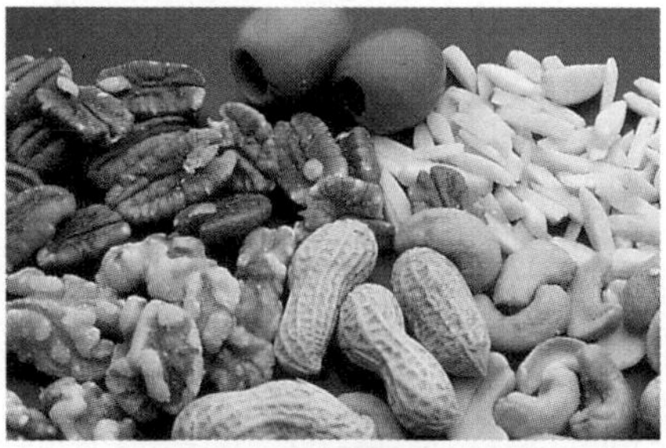

Nuts and olives are so high in fat that they are listed with butter, mayonnaise, and bacon in the fat exchange list.

For similar reasons, starchy vegetables such as corn, green peas, and potatoes are listed on the starch list in the exchange system, rather than with the vegetables. Likewise, olives are not classed as a "fruit" as a botanist would claim; they are classified as a "fat" because their fat content makes them more similar to butter than to berries. Bacon is also on the fat list to remind users of its high fat content. These groupings permit you to see the characteristics of foods that are significant to energy intake.

Users of the exchange lists learn to view mixtures of foods, such as casseroles and soups, as combinations of foods from different exchange lists. They also learn to interpret food labels with the exchange system in mind (see margin on the next page). Knowing that foods on the starch list provide 15 grams of carbohydrate and those on the vegetable list provide 5, you can count a lasagna dinner that provides 37 grams of carbohydrate as "2 starches and 1 vegetable;" knowing that foods on the meat list provide 7 grams of protein, you might count it as "3 meats;" the grams of fat suggest that the meat (and cheese) is probably medium-fat.

Controlling Energy and Fat The exchange system helps people control their energy intakes by paying close attention to portion sizes. A portion of any food on a given list provides roughly the same amount of energy nutrients and total kcalories. The portion sizes have been adjusted so that all portions have the same energy value. For example, 17 grapes count as one fruit portion, as does ½ grapefruit. A whole grapefruit counts as two portions.

A *portion* in the exchange system is not the same as a *serving* in the Daily Food Guide, especially when it comes to meats. The exchange system lists meats and most cheeses in single ounces; that is, 1 *portion* (or *exchange*) of meat is 1 ounce, whereas one *serving* is 2 to 3 ounces. Calculating meat by the ounce encourages the planner to keep close track of the exact amounts eaten. This in turn helps control energy and fat intakes. Be aware, too, that most people do not serve foods in carefully measured portions, nor do the portion sizes reflect the exchange system or Daily Food Guide serving sizes. Many restaurants, for example, offer steaks that are equivalent to four or five servings of meat. Similarly, a bakery may sell muffins that are twice the size of a typical bread serving. Taking actual serving sizes into account is an important part of diet planning.

By allocating items like bacon and avocados to the fat list, the exchange system alerts consumers to foods that are unexpectedly high in fat. Even the starch list specifies which grain products contain added fat (such as biscuits, muffins, and waffles). In addition, the exchange system encourages users to think of nonfat milk as milk and of whole milk as milk with added fat; and to think of very lean meats as meats and of lean, medium- and high-fat meats as meats with added fat. To that end, foods on the milk and meat lists are separated into categories based on their fat contents. The milk group is classed as nonfat, low-fat, and whole; the meat group as very lean, lean, medium-fat, and high-fat.

Control of food energy and fat intake can be highly successful with the exchange system. Exchange plans do not, however, guarantee adequate intakes of vitamins and minerals. Food group plans work better from that standpoint because the food groupings are based on similarities in vitamin-mineral content. In the exchange system, for example, meats are grouped with cheeses, yet the meats are iron-rich and calcium-poor, whereas the cheeses are iron-poor and calcium-rich. To take advantage of the strengths of both food group plans and exchange patterns, and to compensate for their weaknesses, diet planners often combine these two diet-planning tools.

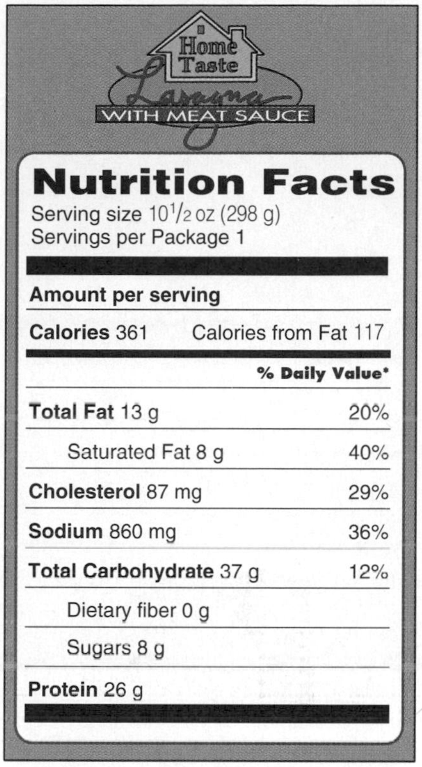

Can you "see" these exchanges in the label above?

Exchange	Carbohydrate	Protein	Fat
2 starches	**30 g**	**6 g**	—
1 vegetable	**5 g**	**2 g**	—
3 medium-fat meats	—	**21 g**	**15 g**
Total	**35 g**	**29 g**	**15 g**

COMBINING FOOD GROUP PLANS AND EXCHANGE LISTS

A diet planner may find that using a food group plan together with the exchange lists eases the task of choosing foods that will provide all the nutrients. The food group plan ensures that all classes of nutritious foods are included, thus promoting adequacy, balance, and variety. The exchange system classifies the food selections by their energy-yielding nutrients, thus controlling energy and fat intakes.

Table 2–5 (on p. 54) shows how to use the Daily Food Guide plan together with the exchange lists to plan a diet. The Daily Food Guide ensures that a certain number of servings is chosen from each of the five food groups (see the first column of the table). The second column translates the number of servings (using the midpoint) into exchanges. With the addition of a small amount of fat, this sample diet plan provides about 1750 kcalories. Most people can meet their

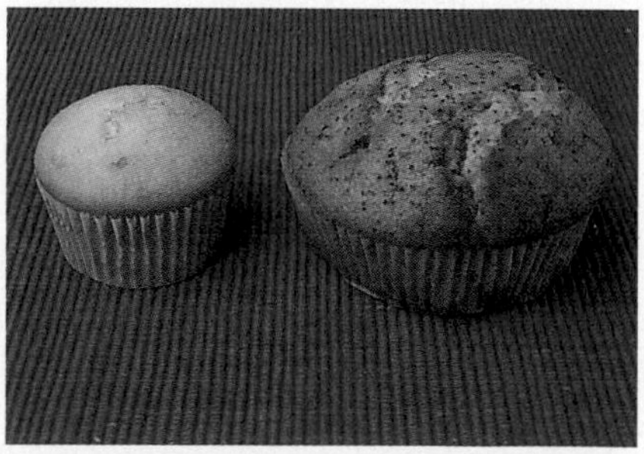

It may look like *one*, but the large muffin counts as *two* servings.

Figure 2–3 The Exchange System: Example Foods, Portion Sizes, and Energy-Nutrient Contributions

THE CARBOHYDRATE GROUP

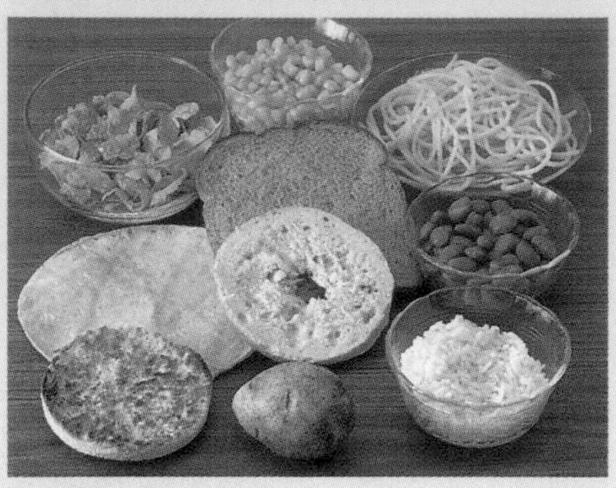

Starch
1 starch exchange is like:
1 slice bread.
¾ c ready-to-eat cereal.
½ c cooked pasta.
⅓ c cooked rice.
½ c cooked beans.[a]
½ c corn, peas, or yams.
1 small (3 oz) potato.
½ bagel, English muffin, or bun.
1 tortilla, waffle, or roll.
(1 starch = 15 g carbohydrate, 3 g protein, 0–1 g fat, and 80 kcal.)

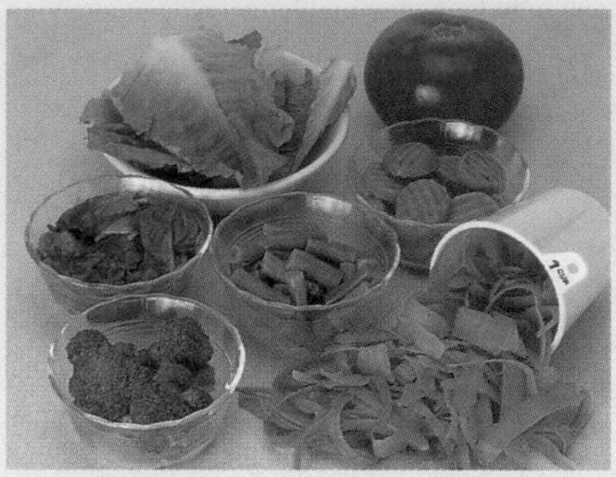

Vegetables
1 vegetable exchange is like:
½ c cooked carrots, greens, green beans, brussels sprouts, beets, broccoli, cauliflower, or spinach.
1 c raw carrots, radishes, or salad greens.
1 lg tomato.
(1 vegetable = 5 g carbohydrate, 2 g protein, and 25 kcal.)

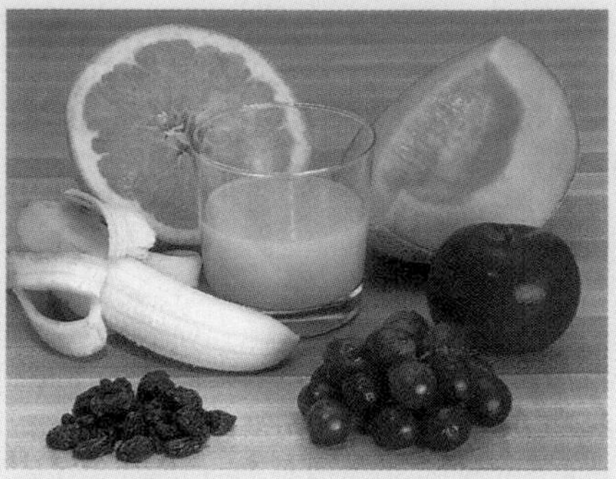

Fruits
1 fruit exchange is like:
1 small banana, nectarine, apple, or orange.
½ large grapefruit or pear.
½ c orange, apple, or grapefruit juice.
17 small grapes.
⅓ cantaloupe (or 1 c cubes).
2 tbs raisins.
(1 fruit = 15 g carbohydrate and 60 kcal.)

[a] ½ c cooked beans = 1 very lean meat exchange *plus* 1 starch exchange.

THE MEAT AND MEAT SUBSTITUTES GROUP (PROTEIN)

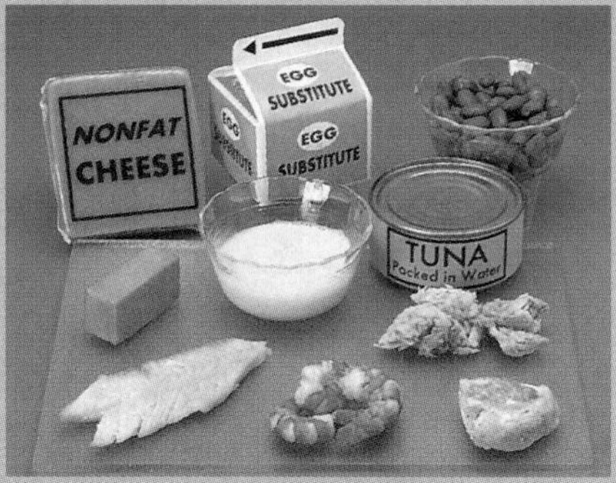

Meat and substitutes (very lean)
1 very lean meat exchange is like:
1 oz chicken (white meat, no skin).
1 oz cod, flounder, or trout.
1 oz tuna (canned in water).
1 oz clams, crab, lobster, scallops, shrimp, or imitation seafood.
1 oz fat-free cheese.
½ c cooked beans, peas, or lentils.
¼ c nonfat or low-fat cream cheese.
2 egg whites (or ¼ c egg substitute).
(1 very lean meat = 7 g protein, 0–1 g fat, and 35 kcal).

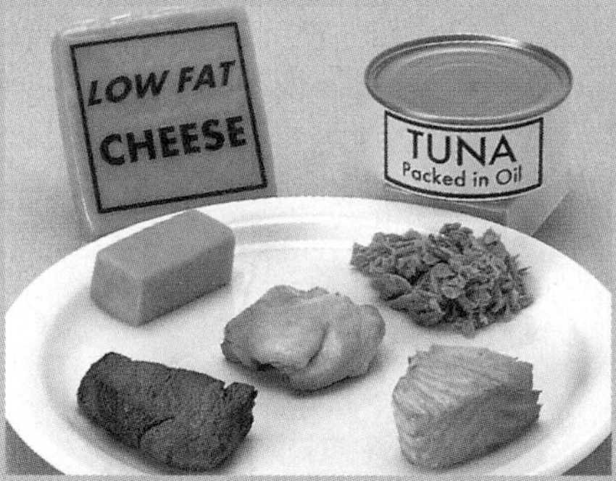

Meats and substitutes (lean)
1 lean meat exchange is like:
1 oz beef or pork tenderloin.
1 oz chicken (dark meat, no skin).
1 oz herring or salmon.
1 oz tuna (canned in oil, drained).
1 oz low-fat cheese or luncheon meats.
(1 lean meat = 7 g protein, 3 g fat, and 55 kcal.)

[b]A beef or pork hot dog counts as 1 high-fat meat exchange *plus* 1 fat exchange.

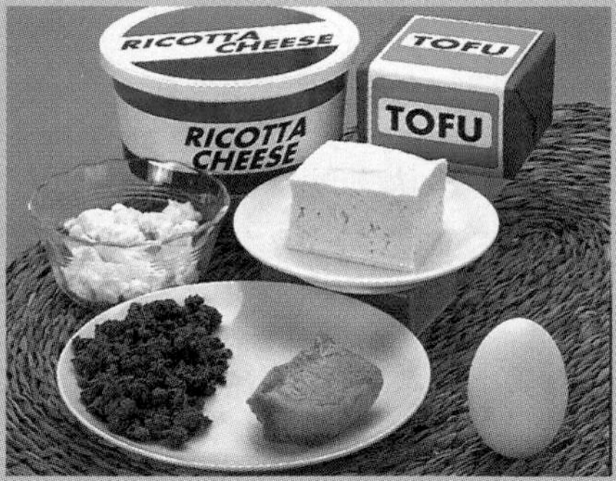

Meats and substitutes (medium-fat)
1 medium-fat meat exchange is like:
1 oz ground beef.
1 oz pork chop.
1 egg.
¼ c ricotta.
4 oz tofu.
(1 medium-fat meat = 7 g protein, 5 g fat, and 75 kcal.)

[c]Peanut butter counts as 1 high-fat meat exchange *plus* 1 fat exchange.

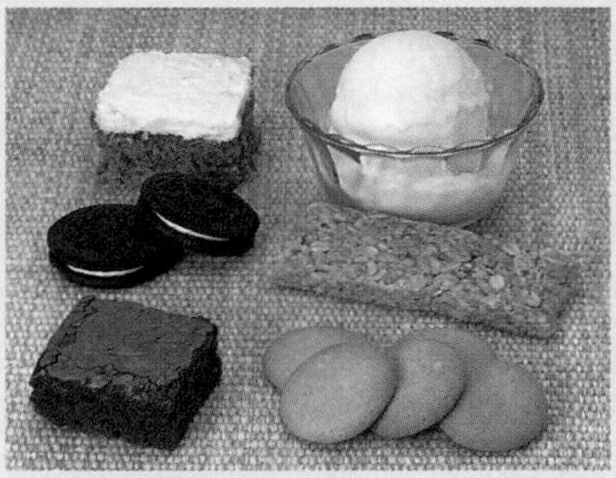

Other carbohydrates
1 other carbohydrates exchange is like:
2 small cookies.
1 small brownie or cake.
5 vanilla wafers.
1 granola bar.
½ c ice cream.
(1 other carbohydrate = 15 g carbohydrate and may be exchanged for 1 starch, 1 fruit, or 1 milk. Because many items on this list contain added sugar and fat, their fat and kcalorie values vary and their portion sizes are small.)

Milks (nonfat and very-low fat)
1 nonfat milk exchange is like:
1 c nonfat milk.
¾ c nonfat yogurt, plain.
1 c nonfat or lowfat buttermilk.
½ c evaporated nonfat milk.
⅓ c dry nonfat milk.
(1 nonfat milk = 12 g carbohydrate, 8 g protein, 0–3 g fat, and 90 kcal.)

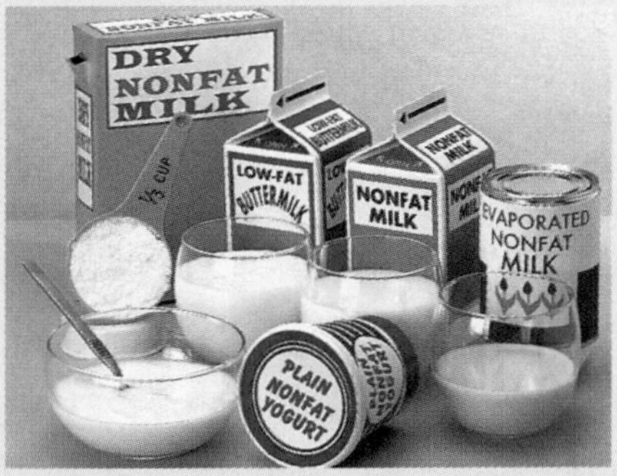

Milks (low-fat)
1 low-fat milk exchange is like:
1 c 2% milk.
¾ c low-fat yogurt, plain.
(1 low-fat milk = 12 g carbohydrate, 8 g protein, 5 g fat, and 120 kcal.)

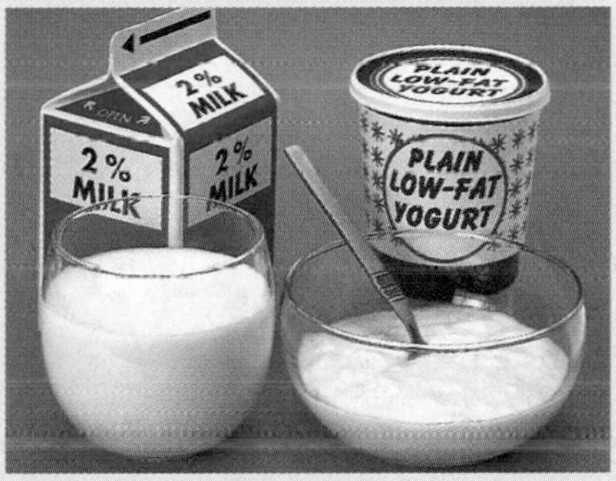

Milks (whole)
1 whole milk exchange is like:
1 c whole milk.
½ c evaporated whole milk.
(1 whole milk = 12 g carbohydrate, 8 g protein, 8 g fat, and 150 kcal.)

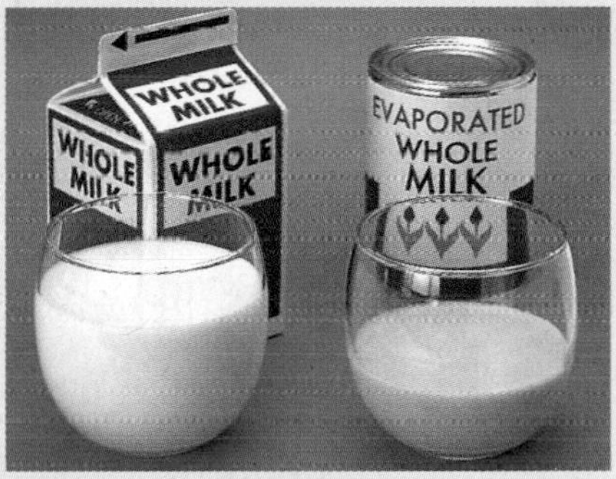

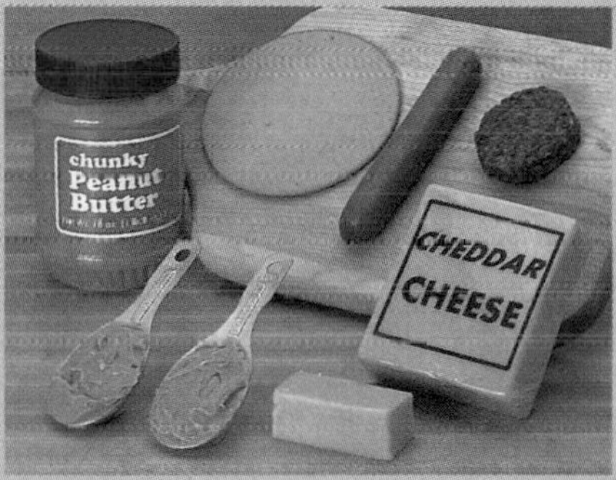

Meats and substitutes (high-fat)
1 high-fat meat exchange is like:
1 oz pork sausage.
1 oz luncheon meat (such as bologna).
1 oz regular cheese (such as cheddar or swiss).
1 small hot dog (turkey or chicken).[b]
2 tbs peanut butter.[c]
(1 high-fat meat = 7 g protein, 8 g fat, and 100 kcal.)

THE FAT GROUP

Fats
1 fat exchange is like:
1 tsp butter.
1 tsp margarine or mayonnaise (1 tbs reduced fat).
1 tsp any oil.
1 tbs salad dressing (2 tbs reduced fat).
8 large black olives.
10 large peanuts.
⅛ medium avocado.
1 slice bacon.
2 tbs shredded coconut.
1 tbs cream cheese (2 tbs reduced fat).
(1 fat = 5 g fat and 45 kcal.)

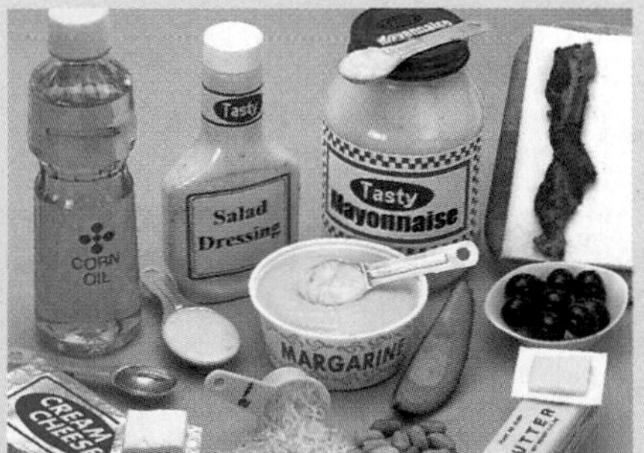

Note: Health recommendations urge people to limit their intakes of saturated fats; butter, bacon, coconut, and cream cheese contain saturated fats.

Table 2–5

Diet Planning with the Exchange System Using the Daily Food Guide Pattern

Pattern from Daily Food Guide Plan	Selections Made Using the Exchange System	Energy Cost (kcal)
Grains (breads and cereals)—6 to 11 servings	Starch list—select 9 exchanges	720
Vegetables—3 to 5 servings	Vegetable list—select 4 exchanges	100
Fruits—2 to 4 servings	Fruit list—select 3 exchanges	180
Meat—2 to 3 servings[a]	Meat list—select 6 lean exchanges	330
Milk—2 servings	Milk list—select 2 nonfat exchanges	180
	Fat list—select 5 exchanges	225
Total		1735

[a]In the food group plan, 1 serving is 2 to 3 ounces; in the exchange system, 1 exchange is 1 ounce. The Daily Food Guide suggests that amounts should total 5 to 7 ounces of meat daily.

needs for all the nutrients within this reasonable energy allowance. (Table 9–4 in Chapter 9 shows patterns for other energy intakes.) The next step in diet planning is to assign the exchanges to meals and snacks. The final plan might look like the one in Table 2–6.

Next, a person could begin to fill in the plan with real foods to create a menu (use Figure 2–3 and Appendix G). For example, the breakfast plan calls for 2 starches, 1 fruit, and 1 nonfat milk. A person might select a bowl of shredded wheat with banana slices and milk (1 cup shredded wheat = 2 starches, 1 small banana = 1 fruit, and 1 cup nonfat milk = 1 milk); or a bagel and a bowl of can-

Table 2–6

A Sample Diet Plan

Exchange	Breakfast	Lunch	Snack	Dinner	Evening Snack
9 starch	2	2	1	3	1
4 vegetable				4	
3 fruit	1	1	1		
6 lean meat		2		4	
2 nonfat milk	1	1			1
5 fat		1		4	

Note: This diet plan is one of many possibilities. It follows the number of servings suggested by the Daily Food Guide and meets dietary recommendations to provide 55 to 60% of its kcalories from carbohydrate, 15 to 20% from protein, and less than 30% from fat.

taloupe pieces topped with yogurt (1 bagel = 2 starches, ⅓ cantaloupe melon = 1 fruit, and ¾ cup nonfat plain yogurt = 1 milk). A person who wanted butter on the bagel could move a fat exchange or two from dinner to breakfast. If willing to use two fat exchanges at breakfast, the person could have pancakes with strawberries and milk (4 small pancakes = 2 starches plus 2 fats, 1¼ cup strawberries = 1 fruit, and a cup of nonfat milk = 1 milk). Then the person could move on to complete the menu for lunch, dinner, and snacks. As you can see, we all make countless food-related decisions daily—whether we have a plan or not. Following a plan, like the Daily Food Guide, that incorporates health recommendations and diet-planning principles helps anyone to make wise decisions.

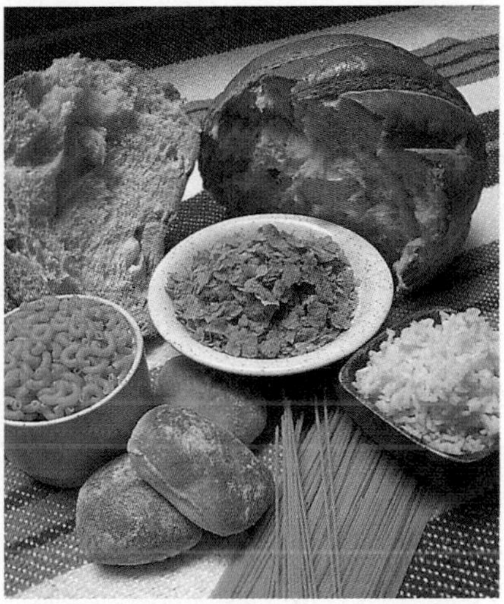

With its many grains (including wheat, rye, oats, corn, and rice) and types of foods (such as pastas, breads, and cereals), this group does more than its share for variety.

FROM GUIDELINES TO GROCERIES

Dietary recommendations emphasize foods low in fat such as grains, fruits, vegetables, lean meats, fish, poultry, and low-fat milk products. Only you can design such a diet for yourself, but how do you begin? Start with the foods you enjoy eating. Then try to make improvements, little by little. When shopping, think of the food groups, and choose nutrient-dense foods within each group.

Breads, Cereals, and Other Grain Products When shopping for grain products, you will find them described as *refined*, *enriched*, or *whole grain* (see the accompanying glossary). These terms refer to the milling process and the making

Glossary of Grain Terms

bran: the protective coating around the kernel similar in function to the shell of a nut; rich in nutrients and fiber.

endosperm (EN-doe-sperm): the bulk of the edible part of the kernel containing starch and proteins.

enriched: the addition of nutrients to a food to meet a specified standard; often used interchangeably with *fortified*. In the case of refined bread or cereal, four nutrients have been added: thiamin, niacin, and riboflavin in amounts approximately equivalent to, or higher than, those originally present and iron in amounts to alleviate the prevalence of iron-deficiency anemia.

germ: the nutrient-rich inner part of a grain. The germ is the seed that grows into a wheat plant, so it is especially rich in vitamins and minerals to support new life.

gluten (GLOO-ten): an elastic protein found in wheat and other grains that gives dough its structure and cohesiveness.

husk: the outer, inedible part of a grain; also called the *chaff*.

refined: the process by which the coarse parts of a food are removed. With respect to refining wheat into flour, the bran, germ, and husk have been removed, leaving only the endosperm.

unbleached flour: a tan-colored endosperm flour with texture and nutritive qualities that approximate those of regular white flour.

wheat flour: any flour made from wheat, including white flour; wheat flour has been refined whereas *whole-wheat flour* has not.

white flour: an endosperm flour that has been refined and bleached for maximum softness and whiteness.

whole grain: a grain milled in its entirety (all but the husk), not refined.

whole-wheat flour: flour made from whole-wheat kernels; a whole-grain flour.

of products, and they have different nutrition implications. Refined foods may have lost many nutrients during processing; enriched products may have had some nutrients added back; and whole-grain products may be rich in all nutrients found in the original grain (see Figure 2–4).

When it became a common practice to refine the wheat flour used for bread by milling it and throwing away the bran and the germ, consumers suffered a tragic loss of many nutrients. As a consequence, legislation was passed in the

Figure 2–4

A Wheat Plant

The milling process breaks wheat kernels into their parts, shown here.

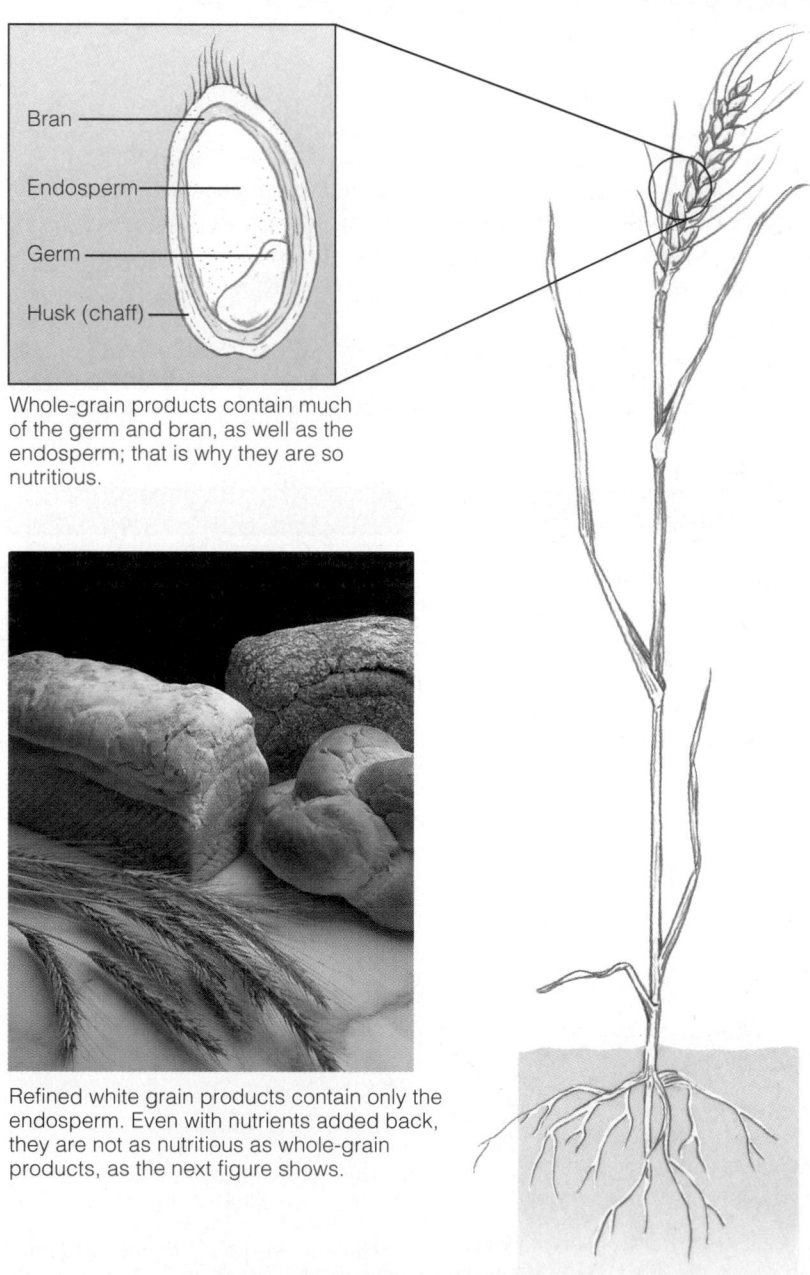

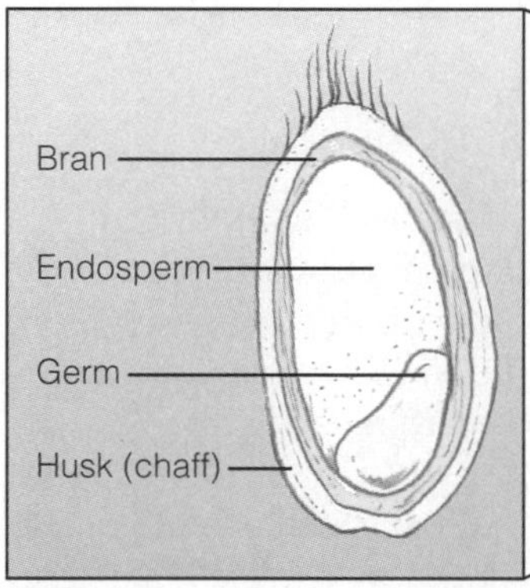

Whole-grain products contain much of the germ and bran, as well as the endosperm; that is why they are so nutritious.

Refined white grain products contain only the endosperm. Even with nutrients added back, they are not as nutritious as whole-grain products, as the next figure shows.

early 1940s requiring that all grain products that cross state lines be enriched with iron, thiamin, riboflavin, and niacin.[5] Enrichment restores these nutrients to the levels present in the original whole wheat and actually raises thiamin and especially riboflavin to higher levels. Most grain products that have been refined, such as rice, wheat pastas like macaroni and spaghetti, and cereals (both cooked and ready-to-eat types), have subsequently been enriched, and their labels say so.

Enrichment doesn't make a slice of bread rich in these added nutrients, but people who eat several slices a day obtain significantly more of these nutrients than they would from unenriched white bread. To a great extent, the enrichment of white flour helps to prevent deficiencies of these four nutrients, but it fails to compensate for losses of many other nutrients and fiber. As Figure 2–5 shows, whole-grain items still outshine the enriched ones. Only *whole-grain* flour contains all of the nutritive portions of the grain.

Whole-grain products, such as brown rice or oatmeal, not only provide more nutrients and fiber, but do not contain the added salt and sugar of flavored, processed rice or sweetened cereals. So, when grocery shopping, choose whole-grain breads and cereals often.

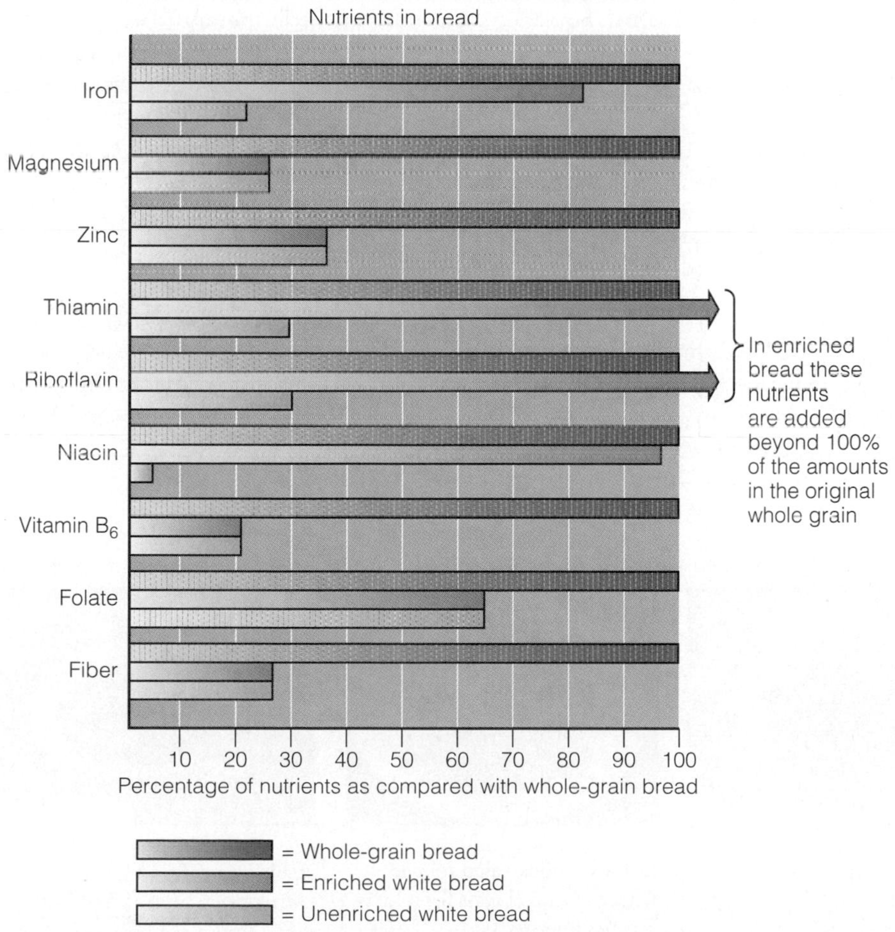

Figure 2–5

Nutrients in Bread

Whole-grain bread is more nutritious than other breads, even enriched bread. For iron, thiamin, riboflavin, and niacin, enriched bread provides about the same quantities as whole-grain bread and significantly more than unenriched bread. For fiber and the other nutrients (both those shown here and those not shown), enriched bread provides less than whole-grain bread.

fortified: the addition of nutrients that were either not originally present or present in insignificant amounts to a food. Fortification can be used to correct or prevent a widespread nutrient deficiency, to balance the total nutrient profile of a food, or to restore nutrients lost in processing.

Speaking of cereals, ready-to-eat breakfast cereals lead the list of the most highly fortified foods on the market. Like an enriched food, a *fortified* food has had nutrients added during processing, but in a fortified food, the added nutrients may not have been present in the original product. Some breakfast cereals made from refined flour and fortified with high doses of vitamins and minerals are actually more like supplements disguised as cereals than they are like whole grains. They may be nutritious—with respect to the nutrients added—but they still may fail to convey the full spectrum of nutrients that a whole-grain food or a mixture of such foods might provide.

Vegetables Choose fresh vegetables, especially green and yellow-orange vegetables like spinach, broccoli, and sweet potatoes. Cooked or raw, vegetables are good sources of vitamins, minerals, and fiber. Frozen and canned vegetables without added salt are acceptable alternatives to fresh. To control fat, energy, and sodium intakes, limit butter, salad dressings, and salt on vegetables.

Fruit Choose fresh fruits often, especially citrus fruits and yellow-orange fruits like cantaloupes and apricots. Fruits supply valuable vitamins, minerals, and fibers. They add flavors, colors, and textures to meals, and their natural sweetness makes them enjoyable as snacks or desserts.

Fruit juices are healthy beverages, but contain little dietary fiber compared with whole fruits. Whole fruits satisfy the appetite better than juices and are a better selection for people who need to limit food energy intakes. Juices, on the other hand, are a good choice for people who need extra food energy. Frozen, dried, and canned fruits without added sugar are acceptable alternatives to fresh. Be aware that sweetened fruit "drinks" or "ades" contain mostly water, sugar, and a little juice for flavor. Some may have been fortified with vitamin C, but lack any other significant nutritional value.

Legumes include:

- Black beans.
- Black-eyed peas.
- Garbanzo beans.
- Great northern beans.
- Kidney beans.
- Lentils.
- Navy beans.
- Peanuts.
- Pinto beans.
- Soybeans.
- Split peas.

Legumes Choose often from the legumes (beans and peas such as pinto beans, split peas, lima beans, and black beans). They are available fresh, frozen, dried, or canned. Whether you buy legumes ready to eat or incorporate them into a recipe, use them often as they are an economical, low-fat, nutrient- and fiber-rich food choice.

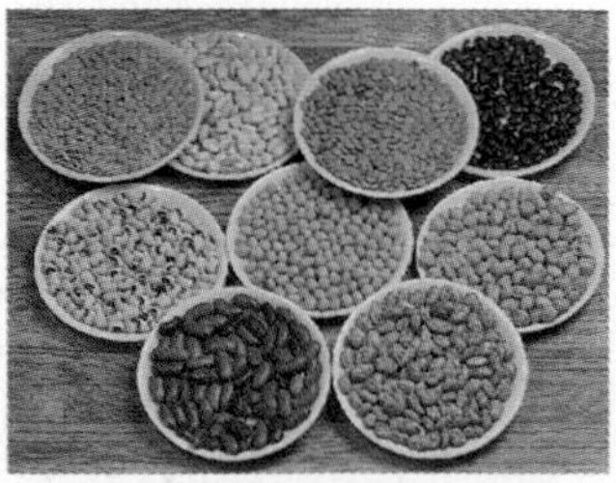

Combining legumes with foods from other food groups creates delicious meals.

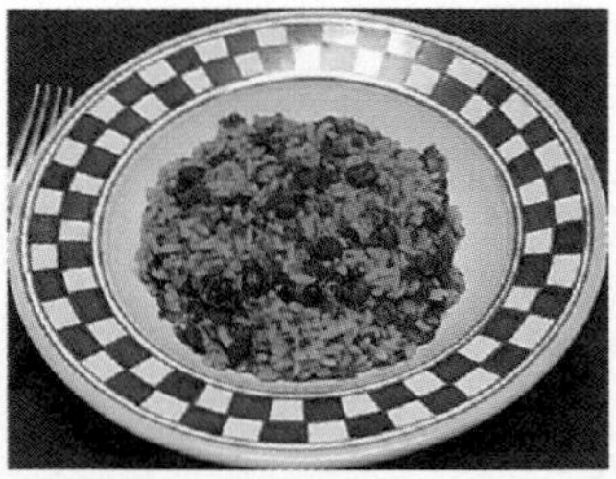

Add rice to red beans for a hardy meal.

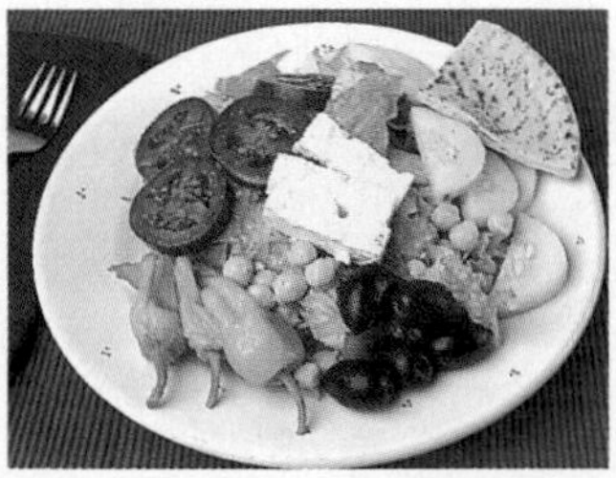

Enjoy a Greek salad topped with garbanzo beans for a little ethnic diversity.

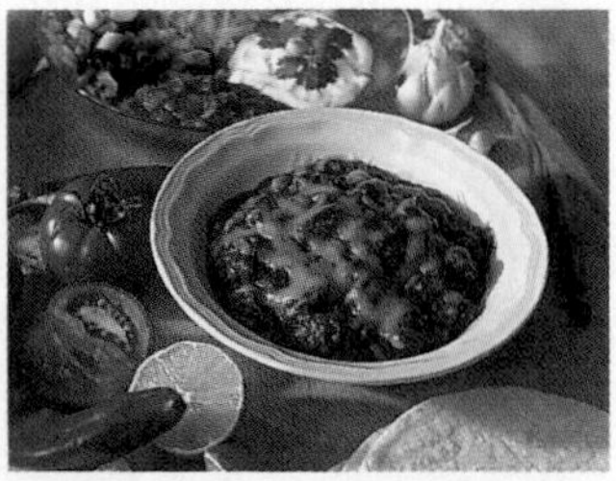

A bit of meat and lots of spices turn kidney beans into chile con carne.

Meat, Fish, and Poultry Meat, fish, and poultry provide essential minerals, such as iron and zinc, and abundant B vitamins as well as protein. To buy and prepare these foods without excess energy, fat, and sodium takes skill. Choose fish, poultry, and lean meats when shopping in the meat department. Lean cuts of beef and pork are named "round" or "loin" (as in top round or pork tenderloin). As a guide, "prime" and "choice" cuts generally have more fat than "select" cuts. Restaurants usually serve prime cuts. Ground beef, even "lean" ground beef, derives most of its food energy from fat as the accompanying table shows. Have the butcher trim and grind a lean round steak instead.

Weigh meat after it is cooked and the bones and fat are removed. In general, 4 ounces of raw meat is equal to about 3 ounces of cooked meat. Some examples of 3-ounce portions of meat include 1 medium pork chop, ½ chicken breast, or 1 steak or hamburger about the size of a deck of cards. To keep fat intake down, bake, roast, broil, grill, or braise meats (but do not fry them in fat); remove the skin from poultry; trim visible fat before cooking; and drain fat after cooking.

Milk Shoppers will find fortified foods in the dairy case. Examples are milk, to which vitamins A and D have been added, and soy milk, to which calcium, vitamin D, and vitamin B_{12} have been added. In addition, shoppers may find imitation foods (such as cheeses) and food substitutes. As food technology advances, many such foods offer low-fat alternatives. For example, egg substitutes help people who want to reduce their fat and cholesterol intakes. Highlight 5 gives other examples.

When shopping, choose low-fat or nonfat milk, yogurt, and cheeses. They are important sources of calcium, but can provide too much sodium and fat if selections aren't made with care.

In summary, food group plans select from different families of similar foods to provide adequacy, balance, and variety in the diet. Exchange lists define portion sizes so that foods within a given group supply similar amounts of energy nutrients, thus helping to attain kcalorie control and moderation. Together, they make it easier to plan a diet that includes abundant grains, vegetables, legumes, and fruits, and moderate amounts of meats and milk products. In making any food choice, remember to view the food in the context of your total diet. It is the combination of many different foods that provides the abundance of nutrients so essential to a healthy diet.

Food Labels

Many consumers want to eat less fat, saturated fat, cholesterol, and sodium and more complex carbohydrates and dietary fiber. Until recently, however, grocery shoppers found foods without nutrition labels or labels without enough useful information. The Nutrition Labeling and Education Act of 1990 brought sweeping changes to the regulations that define what is required on a food label.[6] The Food and Drug Administration (FDA) and the U.S. Department of Agriculture (USDA) designed the new requirements so that labels would provide consumers with useful information about the foods they eat, and especially about how individual foods fit into their daily diets. (Chapter 19 provides more information on how federal agencies monitor our food system.)

Percent kCalories Fat in Selected Meats

• Ground beef	
Regular	66%
Lean	57%
Extra lean	54%
• Ground turkey	51%
• Ground round (lean and trimmed)	27%

Quick and easy estimate:

- 3 oz meat is about the size of a deck of cards.
- ¼ lb (4 oz) hamburger patty, uncooked, is about 3 oz, cooked.

Chapter 5 offers many additional strategies for lowering fat intake.

imitation food: a food that substitutes for and resembles another food and is nutritionally inferior to it with respect to vitamin, mineral, or protein content. If the substitute is not inferior to the food it resembles and it provides an accurate name for itself, it need not be labeled "imitation."

substitute food: a food that is designed to replace another.

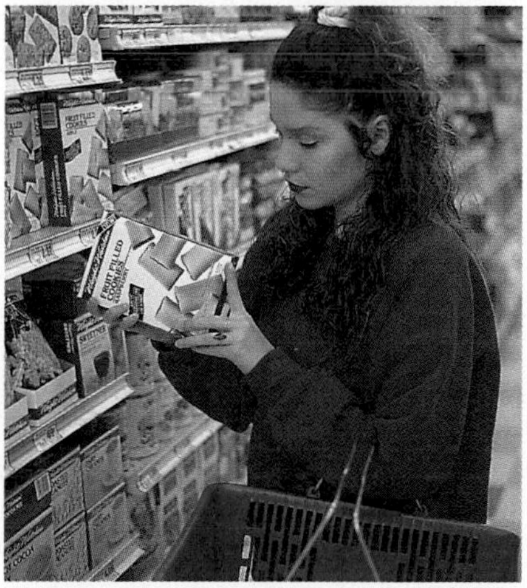

Consumers read food labels to learn about nutrition and its possible connections with health.

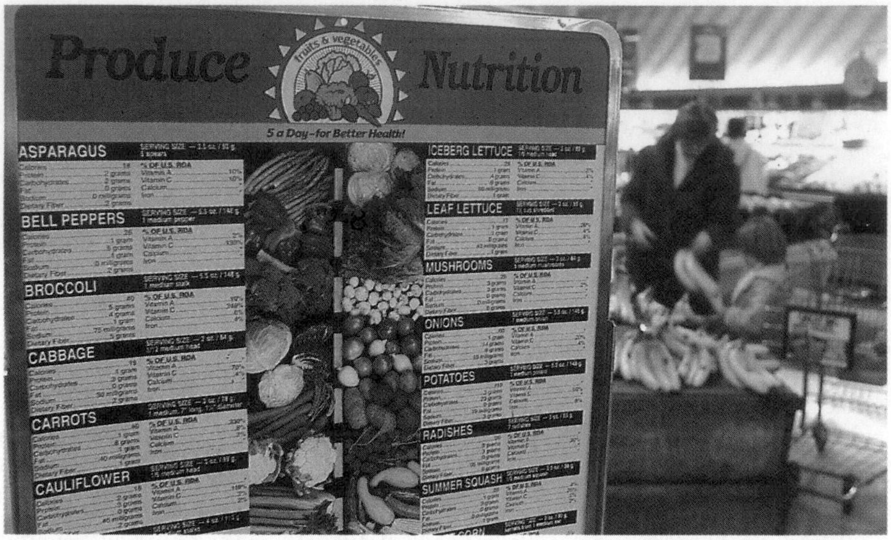

Posters in the produce department present nutrition information for nonpackaged items such as raw fruits and vegetables.

A major objective of the changes was to ensure that labels would appear on virtually all foods and would provide consistent nutrition information. A few foods need not carry nutrition labels: those contributing few nutrients, such as plain coffee, tea, and spices; those produced by small businesses; and those prepared and sold in the same establishment. Some of these items, however, are voluntarily using labels. Even nonpackaged items are encouraged to voluntarily present nutrient information, either in brochures or on signs posted at the point of purchase. The FDA provides guidelines and oversees this voluntary nutrition information program for the 20 most frequently eaten fresh fruits, vegetables, and seafoods (see Table 2–7). The USDA monitors a similar program for 45 major cuts of meat and poultry. Thus essentially all foods are now covered, and as a result, consumers can garner much more useful information in the grocery store than ever before.

HEALTHY PEOPLE 2000: Achieve useful and informative nutrition labeling for virtually all processed foods and at least 40% of fresh meats, poultry, fish, fruits, vegetables, baked goods, and ready-to-eat carry-away foods.

According to law, every food label must prominently display and express in ordinary words:

- The common or usual name of the product.
- The name and address of the manufacturer, packer, or distributor.
- The net contents in terms of weight, measure, or count.
- The ingredients in descending order of predominance by weight.
- The serving size and number of servings per container.
- The quantities of specified nutrients and food constituents.

The information in the first three items is useful, of course, but it is the last three items that tell consumers about the nutritional value of a product. Many manufacturers supply additional nutrition information upon request. Appendix F lists addresses for several food corporations.

Table 2–7

Most Frequently Eaten Raw Fruits, Vegetables, and Seafood

The FDA's voluntary nutrition labeling program applies to the 20 most frequently consumed members of each category: raw fruits, vegetables, and seafood. They are listed here in descending order of consumption.

Fruits	Vegetables	Seafood
Bananas	Potatoes	Shrimp
Apples	Iceberg lettuce	Cod
Watermelons	Tomatoes	Pollock
Oranges	Onions	Catfish
Cantaloupes	Carrots	Scallops
Grapes	Celery	Salmon
Grapefruits	Corn	Flounder
Strawberries	Broccoli	Sole
Peaches	Cabbage	Oysters
Pears	Cucumbers	Orange roughy
Nectarines	Bell peppers	Mackerel
Honeydew melons	Cauliflower	Ocean perch
Plums	Leaf lettuce	Rockfish
Avocados	Sweet potatoes	Whiting
Lemons	Mushrooms	Clams
Pineapples	Green onions	Haddock
Tangerines	Green beans	Blue crabs
Cherries	Radishes	Rainbow trout
Kiwi fruit	Summer squash	Halibut
Limes	Asparagus	Lobster

THE INGREDIENT LIST

In the past, a few foods, such as mayonnaise and bread, were exempt from listing ingredients. Instead, manufacturers were required simply to comply with standards of identity that specified the exact ingredients allowed in the products. Now all foods must list all ingredients on the label. Ingredients are listed in descending order of predominance by weight.

By knowing that the first ingredient named is the one that predominates by weight, consumers who read ingredient lists can glean much information. Compare these products, for example:

- An orange powder that contains "sugar, citric acid, orange flavor . . ." versus a juice that contains "water, tomato concentrate, concentrated juices of carrots, celery . . . ."
- A cereal that contains "puffed milled corn, sugar, corn syrup, molasses, salt . . ." versus one that contains "100 percent rolled oats."
- A canned fruit that contains "sugar, apples, water" versus one that contains simply "apples, water."

In each comparison, consumers can tell that the second product is the more nutrient dense.

The FDA considered—and rejected—a proposal to group sweeteners together in the ingredient list and declare them in the order of predominance appropriate for their *sum*. The agency reasoned that consumers can find the quantity of total sugars on the "nutrition facts" panel of a label and that this information is more valuable than determining from the ingredient list whether the combined weight of the sugar, corn syrup, and molasses exceeds that of puffed milled corn, for example.

The mandate to list *all* ingredients means that manufacturers must now list all the additives they have used. Such information is particularly useful to people who suffer adverse reactions to specific ingredients such as the milk protein casein or the flavor enhancer MSG (monosodium glutamate).

SERVING SIZES

Table 2–8

Household and Metric Measures

- 1 teaspoon (tsp) = 5 milliliters (ml)
- 1 tablespoon (tbs) = 15 ml
- 1 cup (c) = 240 ml
- 1 fluid ounce (fl oz) = 30 ml
- 1 ounce (oz) = 28 grams (g)

Because labels present nutrient information per serving, they must identify the size of a serving. The FDA has established specific serving sizes that reflect amounts that people customarily consume and requires that all labels for a given product use the same serving size. For example, the serving size for all ice creams is a half cup and for all beverages, 8 fluid ounces. This facilitates comparison shopping. Consumers can see at a glance whether one brand or another has more or fewer kcalories or grams of fat. Standard serving sizes are expressed in both common household measures, such as cups, and metric measures, such as milliliters, to accommodate users of both types of measures (see Table 2–8).

NUTRITION FACTS

An easy way to recognize a new label is to look for the words "Nutrition Facts" (old labels read "Nutrition Information"). In addition to the serving size and the servings per container, the "Nutrition Facts" panel on a label shows quantities of energy (in kcalories), of fat (in both kcalories and grams), and of certain other nutrients (in grams or milligrams) in a serving:

- Total food energy (kcalories).
- Food energy from fat (kcalories).
- Total fat (grams).
- Saturated fat (grams).
- Cholesterol (milligrams).
- Sodium (milligrams).
- Total carbohydrate, including starch, sugar, and fiber (grams).
- Dietary fiber (grams).
- Sugars (grams).
- Protein (grams).

In addition, labels must present nutrient content information as compared with a standard for the following vitamins and minerals:

- Vitamin A.
- Vitamin C.

- Iron.
- Calcium.

Comparing nutrient amounts against a standard helps make them meaningful to label readers. A label reader might wonder, for example, whether 1 milligram of iron or calcium is a little or a lot. Well, the standard value for iron is 18 milligrams, so 1 milligram of iron is enough to take notice of: it is over 5 percent. But the standard value for calcium is 1000 milligrams, so 1 milligram of calcium is essentially nothing.

It would be nice for consumers if food labels could express each food's nutrient contents as a percentage of each individual's recommended intakes. Unfortunately, though, recommended intakes, such as the RDA, are not the same for everybody; they depend on age and sex. Manufacturers can't know who will be reading the label—an 8-year-old boy, a 70-year-old woman, or a pregnant teenage girl. Label makers do the best they can with this variability, though: they use one set of standard values to represent the needs of a "typical consumer." These standard values, developed by the FDA for use on food labels, are called the Daily Values.

Table 2–9

Reference Daily Intakes (RDI)

Nutrient	Amount
Protein[a]	50g
Thiamin	1.5 mg
Riboflavin	1.7 mg
Niacin	20 mg NE
Biotin	300 μg
Pantothenic acid	10 mg
Vitamin B_6	2 mg
Folate	400 μg
Vitamin B_{12}	6 μg
Vitamin C	60 mg
Vitamin A[b]	5000 IU
Vitamin D[b]	400 IU
Vitamin E[b]	30 IU
Calcium	1000 mg
Iron	18 mg
Zinc	15 mg
Iodine	150 μg
Copper	2 mg

[a]The RDI for protein varies for different groups of people: pregnant women, 60 g; nursing mothers, 65 g; infants under 1 year, 14 g; children 1 to 4 years, 16 g.

[b]The RDI for fat-soluble vitamins are expressed in International Units (IU), an old system of measurement. The current RDA and tables of food composition use a more accurate system of measurement. Equivalent values are as follows: for vitamin A, 875 μg RE; for vitamin D, 6.5 μg; for vitamin E, 9 mg α-TE.

THE DAILY VALUES

In creating the Daily Values, the FDA first established two sets of reference values: Reference Daily Intakes (RDI) and Daily Reference Values (DRV). These two sets of standards are "behind the scenes" characters only; they do not appear as such on labels but are used to determine the Daily Values. The following paragraphs explain each set individually before describing the Daily Values information found on labels.

Reference Daily Intakes (RDI) The first set of standards, the Reference Daily Intakes (RDI), are for protein, some vitamins, and some minerals. They are based on the RDA and represent intakes to achieve. For example, the RDI for calcium is 1000 milligrams—an amount to aim for daily. (The RDI replace an earlier set of label standards, the U.S. RDA, in name only: except for protein, the RDI values are the same as the old U.S. RDA, which were based on the 1968 edition of the RDA.) Most labels use the RDI developed for adults and children four years old and older (see Table 2–9); foods designed for certain groups (such as cereals for infants) must use the RDI developed specifically for that group.

Daily Reference Values (DRV) The second set of standard values, the Daily Reference Values (DRV), are for nutrients and food components, such as fat and fiber, that have important relationships with health, but no RDA. The DRV are based on scientific evidence and reflect current dietary recommendations. For example, several agencies have consistently recommended that fat intake be limited to 30 percent of total energy intake. The DRV represent some intakes to achieve, as for complex carbohydrates, and some to limit, as for cholesterol (see Table 2–10).

The FDA decided to use 2000 kcalories as a standard for energy intake in calculating the DRV for energy-yielding nutrients. A 2000-kcalorie diet is considered about right for moderately active women, teenage girls, and sedentary men. Older adults, children, and sedentary women may need fewer kcalories. Large

Daily Values (DV): reference values developed by the FDA specifically for use on food labels. The Daily Values represent two sets of standards: Reference Daily Intakes (RDI) and Daily Reference Values (DRV).

Reference Daily Intakes (RDI): a set of standards for protein, vitamins, and minerals used on food labels as part of the Daily Values; previously known as the U.S. RDA.

Daily Reference Values (DRV): a set of standards for nutrients and food components (such as fat and fiber) that have important relationships with health; used on food labels as part of the Daily Values.

Table 2–10

Daily Reference Values (DRV)

Food Component	DRV	Calculation
Fat	65 g	30% of kcalories
Saturated fat	20 g	10% of kcalories
Cholesterol	300 mg	Same regardless of kcalories
Carbohydrate (total)	300 g	60% of kcalories
Fiber	25 g	11.5 g per 1000 kcalories
Protein	50 g	10% of kcalories
Sodium	2400 mg	Same regardless of kcalories
Potassium	3500 mg	Same regardless of kcalories

Note: The DRV were established for adults and children over four years old. The values for energy-yielding nutrients are based on 2000 kcalories a day.

labels list, at the bottom, Daily Values for both a 2000-kcalorie and a 2500-kcalorie diet, but the "% Daily Value" column on all labels applies only to a 2000-kcalorie diet. A 2500-kcalorie diet is considered about right for many men, teenage boys, and active women. People who are exceptionally active may need still higher kcalorie intakes. Labels may also provide a reminder of the kcalories in a gram of carbohydrate, fat, and protein below the Daily Value information.

The Two Combined: Daily Values The FDA strongly believes that the RDI and DRV serve different purposes and prefers to treat them separately. For example, the RDI serve as standards for federal food assistance programs, whereas the DRV do not. But the FDA also recognizes the need to use only one set of values on labels to limit consumer confusion. Hence the Daily Values, which include both the RDI and the DRV and cover all the nutrients that labels list.

Percent Daily Values Labels present nutrient information in two ways—in quantities (such as grams) and as percentages of Daily Values. The "% Daily Value" column provides a ballpark estimate of how individual foods contribute to the total diet. It compares key nutrients in a serving of food with the daily goals of a person consuming 2000 kcalories. A person who consumes 2000 kcalories a day can simply add up all the "% Daily Values" for a particular nutrient to see if the day's diet fits with recommendations. If the "% Daily Values" total 100 percent, then recommendations are met.

People who require more or less than 2000 kcalories daily must do some calculations to see how foods compare with their personal nutrition goals. They can use the last column in the DRV table shown in Table 2–10 or the suggestions described in the accompanying box.

Consumers can use Daily Values to evaluate the contributions of individual foods to their daily diets and health goals. Such information helps consumers see easily whether a food contributes "a little" or "a lot" of a nutrient. For example, the "% Daily Value" column on a label of macaroni and cheese may say 20 percent for fat. This tells the consumer that each serving of this food contains about

How to Calculate Personal Daily Values

The Daily Values on food labels are designed for a 2000 kcalorie intake, but you can calculate a personal set of Daily Values based on your energy allowance. Consider a person with a 1500-kcalorie intake, for example. To calculate a daily goal for fat, multiply energy intake by 30 percent:

$$1500 \text{ kcal} \times 0.30 \text{ kcal from fat} = 450 \text{ kcal from fat.}$$

The "kcalories from fat" are listed on food labels, so a person could then add all the "kcalories from fat" values for a day, using 450 as a goal. A person who preferred to count grams of fat could divide this 450 kcalories from fat by 9 kcalories per gram to determine the goal in grams:

$$450 \text{ kcal from fat} \div 9 \text{ kcal/g} = 50 \text{ g fat.}$$

Alternatively, a person could calculate that 1500 kcalories is 75 percent of 2000 kcalories.

$$1500 \text{ kcal} \div 2000 \text{ kcal} = 0.75.$$

$$0.75 \times 100 = 75\%.$$

Then, instead of trying to achieve 100 percent of the Daily Value, a person consuming 1500 kcalories would aim for 75 percent. Similarly, a person consuming 2800 kcalories would aim for 140 percent:

$$2800 \text{ kcal} \div 2000 \text{ kcal} = 1.40 \text{ or } 140\%.$$

20 percent of the day's allotted 65 grams of fat. That leaves about 80 percent available for other foods to contribute. A person consuming 2000 kcalories a day could simply keep track of the percentages of Daily Values from foods eaten in a day and try not to exceed 100 percent. To determine whether a particular food was a wise choice, a consumer would need to consider the other foods to be eaten during the day.

Daily Values make it easy to compare foods. For example, a consumer might discover that frozen macaroni and cheese has a Daily Value for fat of 20 percent, whereas macaroni and cheese prepared from a boxed mix has a Daily Value of 15 percent. By comparing labels, consumers who are concerned about their fat intakes will be able to make informed decisions.

With an understanding of the Daily Values, consumers can extract a lot of information from a nutrition label. Labels provide different amounts of information based on their package size. Figure 2–6 highlights key information areas on a large food label; Figure 2–7 presents the abbreviated versions that small packages can use.

DESCRIPTIVE TERMS

The FDA specifies what words a label may use to describe a product and what those words mean. See Table 2–11 (on p. 68) for definitions of such terms as

Figure 2–6

An Example of a Large Food Label

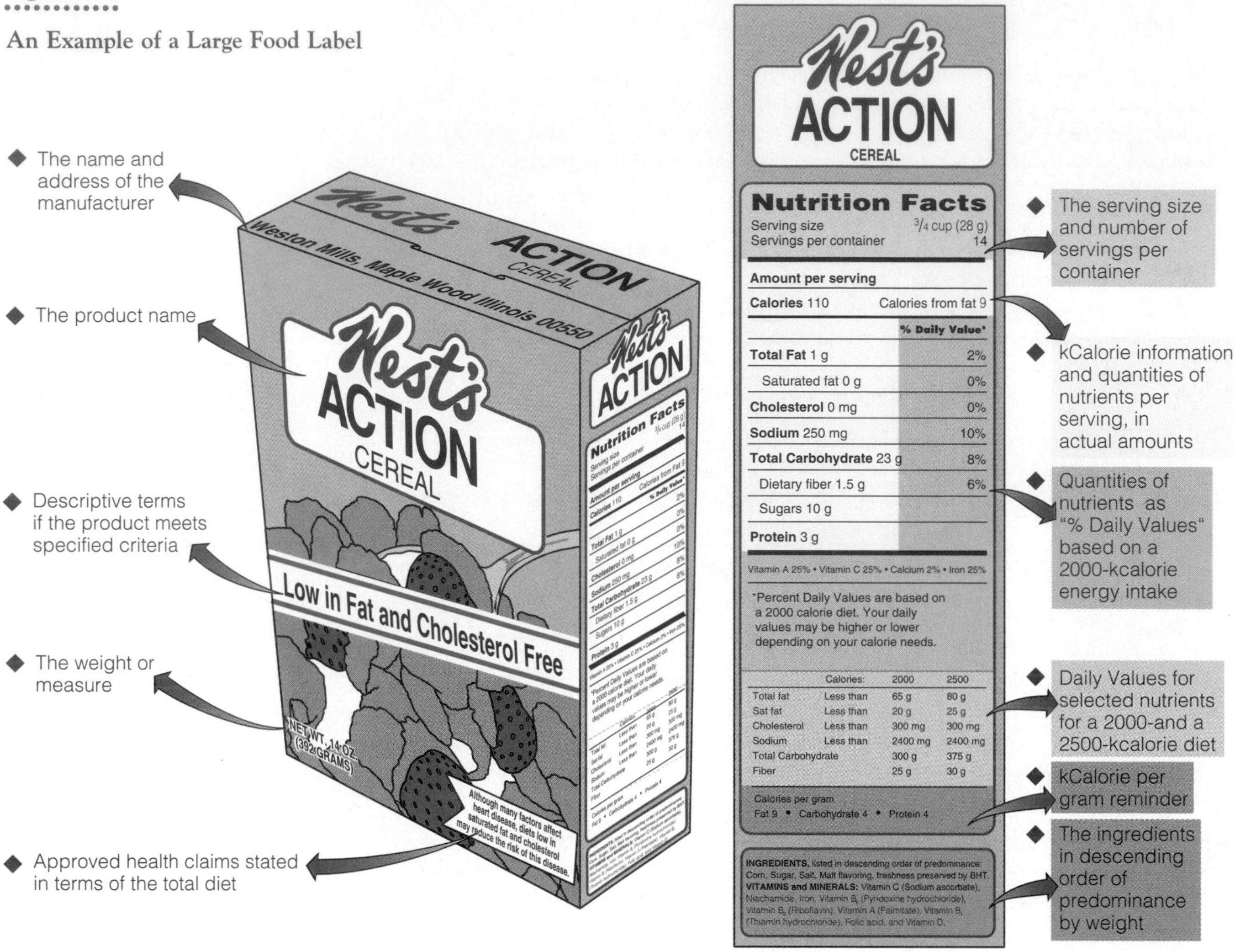

"free" (as in fat-free), "low" (as in low-sodium), "high" (as in high-fiber), "light" or "lite," and "more" and "less."

The FDA's definitions also state the conditions under which each term can be used. For example, in addition to having less than 2 milligrams of cholesterol, a "cholesterol-free" product may not contain more than 2 grams of saturated fat per serving. The term "fresh" can be used only for raw food; the descriptive term "freshly" (baked or prepared) can be used only if the food has been recently made and has not been frozen, heated, processed, or chemically preserved.

Some descriptions *imply* that a food contains, or does not contain, a nutrient. Implied claims are prohibited unless they meet specified criteria. For example, a claim that a product "contains no oil" *implies* that the food contains no fat. If the product is truly fat-free, then it may make the no-oil claim, but if it contains another source of fat, such as butter, it may not.

Figure 2–7

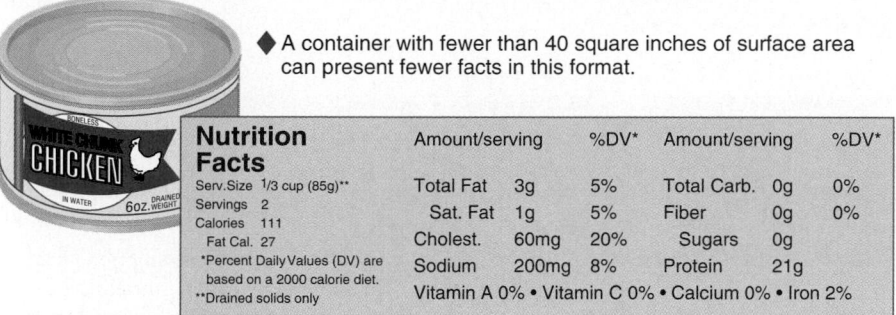

Examples of Small Food Labels

◆ A container with fewer than 40 square inches of surface area can present fewer facts in this format.

Nutrition Facts	Amount/serving		%DV*	Amount/serving		%DV*
Serv.Size 1/3 cup (85g)**	Total Fat	3g	5%	Total Carb.	0g	0%
Servings 2	Sat. Fat	1g	5%	Fiber	0g	0%
Calories 111	Cholest.	60mg	20%	Sugars	0g	
Fat Cal. 27	Sodium	200mg	8%	Protein	21g	
*Percent Daily Values (DV) are based on a 2000 calorie diet. **Drained solids only	Vitamin A 0% • Vitamin C 0% • Calcium 0% • Iron 2%					

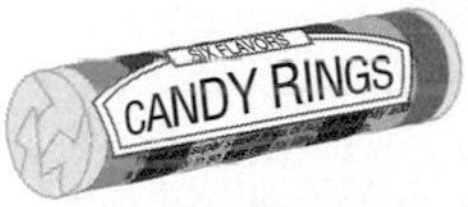

◆ Packages with fewer than 12 square inches of surface area need not carry nutrition information, but they must provide an address or telephone number for obtaining information.

HEALTH CLAIMS

Health claims describe an association between a specific nutrient or food substance and a specific health problem. They are permitted only in cases where scientifically valid links between diet and health have been clearly established. The FDA has approved several health claims based on specified criteria, including:

health claim: any statement that characterizes the relationship between any nutrient or other substance in a food and a disease or health-related condition.

- The nutrient or food substance must be related to a disease or health condition for which most people or a specific group of people, such as the elderly, are at risk.
- The claim is supported by scientific evidence from well-designed studies conducted with recognized scientific procedures and principles.

Health claims on products must emphasize the importance of the total diet and not exaggerate the role of a particular food or diet in disease prevention. No one food possesses magical healing powers, and manufacturers must take care not to distort the roles of their products in promoting health.

Claims must be honest and balanced. For example, health claims can say that foods high in calcium "may" or "might" reduce the risk of osteoporosis. Claims must also explain that diseases develop in response to many factors. They may even mention beneficial factors, such as exercise. For example, a health claim may state that "Development of cancer depends on many factors. A diet low in total fat may reduce the risk of some cancers." The health claim is true, it acknowledges that diet is among many factors influencing disease development, and it is phrased in terms of total diet, not in terms of the particular product. The following relationships for health claims on labels have been authorized:

Health claims on supplement labels are presented in Highlight 10.

- *Calcium and osteoporosis*. Foods or supplements must be high in calcium (at least 20 percent of the RDI) and contain no more phosphorus than calcium.
- *Sodium and hypertension (high blood pressure)*. Foods must qualify as "low sodium" (see Table 2–11)."
- *Dietary saturated fat and cholesterol and risk of coronary heart disease*. Foods must qualify as "low saturated fat," "low cholesterol," and "low fat" or, in the case of meat and poultry, as "extra lean" (see Table 2–11).

Table 2–11

Terms on Food Labels

General Terms

Free: "nutritionally trivial" and unlikely to have a physiological consequence; synonyms include "without," "no," and "zero." A food that does not contain a nutrient naturally may make such a claim, but only as it applies to all similar foods (for example, "applesauce, a fat-free food").

Healthy: a food that is low in fat, saturated fat, cholesterol, and sodium and that contains at least 10% of the Daily Values for vitamin A, vitamin C, iron, calcium, protein, or fiber.

High: 20% or more of the Daily Value for a given nutrient per serving; synonyms include "rich in" or "excellent source."

Less: at least 25% less of a given nutrient or kcalories than the comparison food (see individual nutrients below); synonyms include "fewer" and "reduced."

Light or lite: any use of the term other than as defined below must specify what it is referring to (for example, "light in color" or "light in texture").

Low: an amount that would allow frequent consumption of a food without exceeding the Daily Value for the nutrient. A food that is naturally low in a nutrient may make such a claim, but only as it applies to all similar foods (for example, "fresh cauliflower, a low-sodium food"); synonyms include "little," "few," and "low source of."

More: at least 10% more of the Daily Value for a given nutrient than the comparison food; synonyms include "added."

Good source of: product provides between 10 and 19% of the Daily Value for a given nutrient per serving.

Energy

kCalorie-free: fewer than 5 kcal per serving.

Light: one-third fewer kcalories than the comparison food.

Low kcalorie: 40 kcal or less per serving.

Reduced kcalorie: at least 25% fewer kcalories per serving than the comparison food.

Fat and Cholesterol

Percent fat-free: may be used only if the product meets the definition of *low fat* or *fat-free* and must reflect the amount of fat in 100 g (for example, a food that contains 2.5 g of fat per 50 g can claim to be "95 percent fat free").

Fat-free: less than 0.5 g of fat per serving (and no added fat or oil).

Low fat: 3 g or less fat per serving.

Less fat: 25% or less fat than the comparison food.

Saturated fat-free: less than 0.5 g of saturated fat and 0.5 grams of *trans*-fatty acids per serving.

Low saturated fat: 1 g or less saturated fat per serving.

Less saturated fat: 25% or less saturated fat than the comparison food.

Cholesterol-free: less than 2 mg cholesterol per serving and 2 g or less saturated fat per serving.

Low cholesterol: 20 mg or less cholesterol per serving and 2 g or less saturated fat per serving.

Less cholesterol: 25% or less cholesterol than the comparison food (reflecting a reduction of at least 20 mg per serving), and 2 g or less saturated fat per serving.

Extra lean: less than 5 g of fat, 2 g of saturated fat, and 95 mg of cholesterol per serving and per 100 g of meat, poultry, and seafood.

Lean: less than 10 g of fat, 4.5 g of saturated fat, and 95 mg of cholesterol per serving and per 100 g of meat, poultry, and seafood.

Light: 50% or less of the fat than in the comparison food (for example, 50% less fat than our regular cookies).

Note: Foods containing more than 13 g total fat per serving or per 50 g of food must indicate those contents immediately after a cholesterol claim. As you can see, all cholesterol claims are prohibited when the food contains more than 2 g saturated fat per serving.

Carbohydrates: Fiber and Sugar

High fiber: 5 g or more fiber per serving; a high-fiber claim made on a food that contains more than 3 g fat per serving and per 100 g of food must also declare total fat.

Sugar-free: less than 0.5 g of sugar per serving.

Sodium

Sodium-free and **salt-free:** less than 5 mg of sodium per serving.

Low sodium: 140 mg or less per serving.

Light: a low-kcalorie, low-fat food with a 50% reduction in sodium.

Light in sodium: no more than 50% of the sodium of the comparison food.

Very low sodium: 35 mg or less per serving.

- *Dietary fat and cancer.* Foods must qualify as "low fat" or, in the case of meat and poultry, as "extra lean." Claims may not specify types of fat and must speak in terms of "some types of cancers" or "some cancers."
- *Fiber-containing grain products, fruits, and vegetables and cancer.* Grain products, fruits, or vegetables must qualify both as "low fat" and as "good sources" (without fortification) of dietary fiber (see Table 2–11). Claims may not specify types of fiber and must speak in terms of "some types of cancer" or "some cancers."
- *Fruits, vegetables, and grain products that contain fiber, particularly soluble fiber, and risk of coronary heart disease.* Fruits, vegetables, or grain products must qualify as "low saturated fat," "low cholesterol," and "low fat" and provide (without fortification) at least 0.6 grams of soluble fiber per serving.
- *Fruits and vegetables and cancer.* Fruits or vegetables must qualify as "low fat" and as "good sources" (without fortification) of vitamin A, vitamin C, or dietary fiber.

Two additional criteria must also be met. First, a food making a health claim must be a *naturally* good source (containing at least 10 percent of the Daily Value) of at least one of the following nutrients: vitamin A, vitamin C, iron, calcium, protein, or fiber. Second, foods are disqualified from making health claims if a standard serving contains more than 20 percent of the Daily Value for total fat, saturated fat, cholesterol, or sodium. Thus milk, which is high in calcium, may make a calcium and osteoporosis claim if it is nonfat or low-fat milk, but not if it is whole milk. Excess fat increases the risks of some cancers and heart disease.

CONSUMER EDUCATION

Labels are valuable only if people know how to use them, and so the labeling law contains an education component. Consumers who understand how to read labels will be best able to apply the information to achieve and maintain healthful dietary practices. The FDA has designed several programs to educate consumers about the nutrition information on food labels and the benefits of using that information to maintain healthful dietary habits.

HEALTHY PEOPLE 2000: Increase to at least 85% the proportion of people aged 18 and older who use food labels to make nutritious food selections.

In conclusion, food labels provide consumers with information they need to select foods that will help them meet their nutrition and health goals.[7] Given labels with relevant information presented in a standardized, easy-to-read format, consumers are well prepared to plan and create healthful diets.*

*The National Center for Nutrition and Dietetics hotline (800–366–1655) offers messages and answers consumers' questions about food labeling.

Study Questions

1. Name the diet-planning principles and briefly describe how each principle helps in diet planning.
2. What recommendations appear in the *Dietary Guidelines for Americans?* How do they compare with the *Diet and Health* recommendations introduced in Chapter 1?
3. Name the five food groups in the Daily Food Guide and identify several foods typical of each group. Explain how such plans group foods and what diet-planning principles the plans best accommodate. How are food group plans used, and what are some of their strengths and weaknesses?
4. Name the exchange lists and identify a food typical of each list. Explain how the exchange system groups foods and what diet-planning principles the system best accommodates. How are exchange systems used, and what are some of their strengths and weaknesses?
5. Review the *Dietary Guidelines*. What types of grocery selections would you make to achieve those recommendations?
6. What information can you expect to find on a food label? How can this information help you choose between two similar products?
7. What are the Daily Values? How can they help you meet health recommendations?
8. What health claims have been approved by the FDA for use on labels? What criteria must all health claims meet?

Notes

1. A. K. Kant and coauthors, Dietary diversity and subsequent mortality in the First National Health and Nutrition Examination Survey Epidemiological Follow-up Study, *American Journal of Clinical Nutrition* 57 (1993): 434–440.
2. Position of The American Dietetic Association: Vegetarian diets, *Journal of the American Dietetic Association* 93 (1993): 1317–1319.
3. C. Achterberg, E. McDonnell, and R. Bagby, How to put the Food Guide Pyramid into practice, *Journal of the American Dietetic Association* 94 (1994): 1030–1035.
4. National Live Stock and Meat Board, *Eating in America Today: A Dietary Pattern and Intake Report*, 1994.
5. W. H. Sebrell, A fiftieth anniversary—Cereal enrichment, *Nutrition Today*, January/February 1992, pp. 20–21.
6. The information on food labels reflects the final regulations as published in the *Federal Register*, January 6, 1993, subsequent amendments, and a special report published in *FDA Consumer*, May 1993.
7. Position of The American Dietetic Association: Nutrition and health information on nutrition labels, *Journal of the American Dietetic Association* 90 (1990): 583–585.

Problem Set

1. *Nutrient density*. Recall that nutrient density is a measure of the nutrients in a food compared with the energy provided. A food can be nutrient dense in one nutrient, but not in another.

   a. This exercise asks you to calculate the calcium density, iron density, and vitamin C density for each of several foods. First look up these foods in Appendix H and record their energy, calcium, iron, and vitamin C values.

Item No./Food		Energy (kcal)	Calcium (mg)	Iron (mg)	Vitamin C (mg)
#93	Whole milk, 1 c	149	290	_____	_____
#98	Nonfat milk, 1 c	_____	_____	_____	_____
#41	Cottage cheese, 1 c	_____	_____	_____	_____
#598	Ground beef patty, 4 oz	_____	_____	_____	_____
#876	Navy beans, cooked, 1 c	_____	_____	_____	_____
#269	Fresh orange juice, 1 c	_____	_____	_____	_____

   b. *Calcium density*. Now calculate the calcium density of each food (milligrams of calcium per 100 kcal, rounded off to the nearest whole number). Appendix D offers help with this type of calculation, which involves using ratios, and the first example has been done for you. For whole milk with 290 mg calcium and 149 kcal, the question is, how many milligrams of calcium are in 100 kcal? Let "x" stand for the unknown quantity: x = number of milligrams of calcium in 100 kcal of the food. Next, set up a ratio: 290 mg calcium is to 149 kcal as x mg calcium is to 100 kcal:

$$\frac{290 \text{ mg}}{149 \text{ kcal}} = \frac{x \text{ mg}}{100 \text{ kcal}}.$$

Now multiply the "top" of each side of the equation by the "bottom" of the other side:

$$290 \text{ mg} \times 100 \text{ kcal} = x \text{ mg} \times 149 \text{ kcal}.$$
$$29{,}000 = 149x$$

Now, solve for x: $29{,}000 \div 149 = x$, so $x = 194.6$ or 195 mg. A food with 149 kcal and 290 mg calcium has a calcium density of 195 mg/100 kcal.

Item No./Food	Calcium Density (mg/100 kcal)
#93 Whole milk, 1 c	195
#98 Nonfat milk, 1 c	________
#41 Cottage cheese, 1 c	________
#598 Ground beef patty, 4 oz	________
#876 Navy beans, cooked, 1 c	________
#269 Fresh orange juice, 1 c	________

c. Which of these foods is the best calcium "buy" per 100 kcal? ____________________

d. *Iron density*. Now calculate the iron densities the same way (milligrams of iron per 100 kcal).

e. Which food is the best iron "buy" per 100 kcal?

f. Which food is the least iron dense? __________

g. How does milk's calcium density compare with its iron density? ____________________

Item No./Food	Iron Density (mg/100 kcal)
#93 Whole milk, 1 c	________
#98 Nonfat milk, 1 c	________
#41 Cottage cheese, 1 c	________
#598 Ground beef patty, 4 oz	________
#876 Navy beans, cooked, 1 c	________
#269 Fresh orange juice, 1 c	________

h. *Vitamin C density*. No doubt you can guess which food offers the best "buy" for vitamin C, but prove yourself correct by doing the calculation.

i. Which food is the most vitamin C dense? ______

Item No./Food	Vitamin C Density (mg/100 kcal)
#93 Whole milk, 1 c	________
#98 Nonfat milk, 1 c	________
#41 Cottage cheese, 1 c	________
#598 Ground beef patty, 4 oz	________
#876 Navy beans, cooked, 1 c	________
#269 Fresh orange juice, 1 c	________

These comparisons should make it clear that some foods may be more dense in one particular nutrient than in another. It is for reasons like this that varied food choices are recommended.

2. *Meal planning*. Improve a meal's nutrient density by making successive changes. Start with one meal, check its energy and nutrient contributions, and then substitute some items to see how the balances change.

a. Start with the "A" meal shown below and calculate the energy and nutrients in the meal:

"A" Meal Item No./Food	Energy (kcal)	Iron (mg)	Vitamin A (μg RE)	Vitamin C (mg)
# 637 Fried, batter-dipped chicken thigh, 1	________	________	________	________
# 715 Potato salad with mayonnaise and eggs, ½ c	________	________	________	________
# 800 Snap beans cooked from fresh, 1 c[a]	________	________	________	________
# 211 Unsweetened applesauce, ½ c[a]	________	________	________	________
Totals:	________	________	________	________

[a]Be careful: The serving size for green beans in Appendix H is ½ c, so double all values; for applesauce, it is 1 c, so cut all values in half.

(continued on the next page)

b. Now replace the fried chicken with 4 oz of dark-meat turkey; take the totals, subtract the chicken values, and add the turkey values. Recalculate the totals to create the "B" meal:

"B" Meal Item No./Food	Energy (kcal)	Iron (mg)	Vitamin A (μg RE)	Vitamin C (mg)
Previous totals from "A" meal				
Minus chicken from "A" meal				
Plus #652 Dark-meat turkey, 4 oz				
New totals:				

c. Looking just at the energy and the iron, how did this substitution improve the meal? ______

d. By how many milligrams did the iron values in this meal change? ______

e. What percentage of an 18-year-old woman's iron RDA (15 mg) does this change represent? ______

f. Assuming that any increase of more than 5% in an essential nutrient intake is beneficial, would it be beneficial for a woman to make such a change in her meal plan? ______

g. By the same standard, a loss of more than 5% in an essential nutrient is significant. How much vitamin A was lost by making this substitution? ______

h. What percentage of the woman's vitamin A RDA (800 μg RE) was this? ______

i. Comparing the gain of iron with the loss of vitamin A, was the substitution worth making? ______

j. Now replace the ½ c of potato salad with ½ c of lima beans:

"C" Meal Item No./Food	Energy (kcal)	Iron (mg)	Vitamin A (μg RE)	Vitamin C (mg)
Previous totals from "B" meal				
Minus potato salad from "A" meal				
Plus #797 lima beans, thick seeded ½ c				
New totals:				

k. How did this substitution improve the "B" meal? ______

l. Were losses significant? (The RDA for vitamin C is 60 mg.) ______

m. Keep going. Alter the "C" meal by trading the cup of snap beans for a cup of chopped broccoli:

"D" Meal Item No./Food	Energy (kcal)	Iron (mg)	Vitamin A (μg RE)	Vitamin C (mg)
Previous totals from "C" meal				
Minus snap beans from "A" meal				
Plus #822 chopped broccoli, cooked from frozen, 1 c				
New totals:				

n. Which nutrients changed most significantly?

o. Finally, compare the totals from meal "A" and meal "D." For the energy and each nutrient, indicate whether the amount in meal "D" is "significantly more," "not significantly changed," or "significantly less" (use 2200 kcalorie RDA for energy):

	Energy (kcal)	Iron (mg)	Vitamin A (μg RE)	Vitamin C (mg)
Meal "A"				
Meal "D"				
Change				

This exercise shows how simple changes in food choices can improve the nutrient density of meals.

Ethnic Cuisines and Healthy Choices

Do some foodways support health better than others? This highlight presents a few of the many ethnic foodways to show how basic diet-planning principles can apply to many different cuisines (the glossary on p. 74 defines foodways, cuisines, and related terms). A look at the traditional foods of other countries is a delightful way to learn about the world's people and is especially useful to those who advise others on nutrition. A counselor who is familiar with the cultural and religious traditions that influence a person's food choices is better able to make suggestions that fit into the person's life.[1]

Every country, and in fact every region of a country, has its own typical foods and ways of combining them into meals. Ethnic foods have become an integral part of the "American diet," expanding the number of foods available and thus helping people to achieve variety in their diets. While variety helps to ensure nutrient adequacy, only moderation can control energy and fat intakes, and these are the keys to reducing the risks of chronic diseases. How can people enjoy ethnic meals and still limit their energy and fat intakes? Keep this question in mind as you read the following sections.

NORTHERN EUROPEAN INFLUENCE

An evening meal of hearty roast beef, mashed potatoes, boiled cabbage, and bread, with fruit pie for dessert, is typical of cuisines of Germany, England, and Ireland. Such

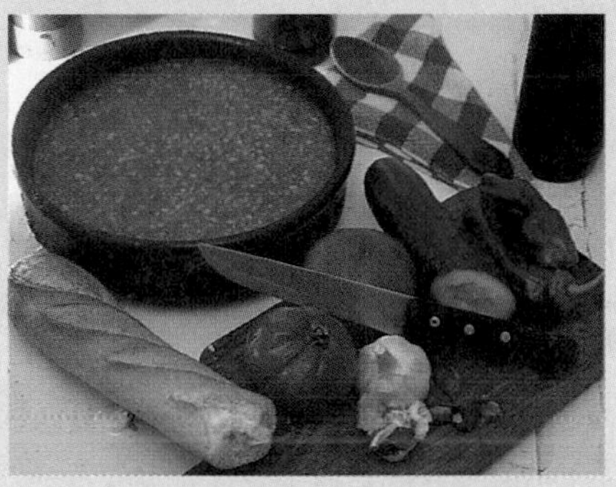

Low-fat ethnic foods, such as gazpacho, have become such common restaurant fare that we often forget their origins.

meals are served for countless diners across the United States, too, and variations on this plan are numerous. Even a Thanksgiving turkey dinner with all the trimmings follows this pattern.

Traditionally, people have filled their plates with meat and served starches and vegetables on the side. Today's health advice, however, encourages people to load their plates with tasty grains and vegetables and to limit meat to 2- to 3-ounce portions. This way, the meal provides plenty of carbohydrate and fiber, adequate protein, and not too much fat.

Another familiar meal that derives from northern Europe is the bacon and eggs breakfast. The English serve it with baked beans; in the United States, northerners select potatoes and southerners choose grits. The legumes offer a fiber advantage. More fruit and a lower-fat meat choice would improve the breakfast further.

Every eating style has advantages and drawbacks. The northern European style ensures adequate protein and all the other nutrients associated with meat. It delivers a lot of fat, though, and is short on fiber and the vitamins and minerals associated with fruits and vegetables. For better health, people who eat this way need to reduce portions of meats and added fats and choose more whole grains, fruits, and vegetables.

French cuisine is among the world's most popular foodways. The French expertly combine butter, cream, eggs, herbs, and wine into classic sauces. They prepare pastries filled with seafood, cheese, or meats and covered with rich sauces for a main dish or wrapped around sweetened fruits and creams for dessert. These choices are extraordinarily high in fat, but typical serving sizes are small. Eating French food can be healthful when a person follows the suggestion to "keep it simple." The country cuisine of southern France along the Mediterranean Sea offers equally wonderful options: elegant clear soups; steamed and poached seafood; lean meats, legumes, and vegetables seasoned with lemon, herbs, or wine; fruit; and huge loaves of french bread.

The notion that red wine protects the French and others of the Mediterranean region against heart disease, while not proved, may have some validity. Studies do show low rates of heart disease in populations that drink moderate amounts of wine (red or white) with meals. Other correlations have not been ruled out, though, and correlations are not causes. Furthermore, any advantage of cardiovascular protection may be offset by other health problems. French people have a higher incidence of stomach and

Glossary

cuisine (kwi-ZEEN): style of cooking or preparing food.

ethnic diets: foodways and cuisines typical of national origins, cultural heritages, or geographic locations.

foodways: the sum of the food habits, customs, beliefs, and preferences of a culture.

kosher (KOE-sure): foods prepared according to Jewish dietary laws.

esophagus cancer than people in the United States, and they suffer high rates of liver disease as a direct result of high alcohol intakes. Still, the French have heart disease rates lower than U.S. rates despite a similar fat intake.

The French have clearly influenced the bayou regions of Louisiana, and so have the African-American ancestors of the present population there. The settlers in southern Louisiana adapted their heritages to the local food supply, creating the Cajun style of cooking that is now popular across the nation. Many Cajun dishes are based on a roux made by browning flour and salt with oil. Cajun dishes include spicy stews (gumbo, jambalaya), sausages, hot pepper sauce, red beans and rice, seafood, and dirty rice (rice made brown with chopped chicken livers and seasonings). Many people enjoy Cajun coffee brewed with chicory root and a sugared doughnut known as a beignet (pronounced ben-YAY).

Nutritionists agree with enthusiastic diners that red beans and rice is a classic dish—full of flavor from expert use of spices and abundant in carbohydrate, protein, and fiber, while low in fat. A jambalaya (stew) of seafood (crawfish, shrimp, and fish), tomatoes, vegetables, and rice seasoned with a little strong-flavored sausage is packed with vitamins and minerals, adequate in protein, rich in carbohydrate, and usually low in fat. With a careful eye on the fat during food preparation and a limit on the beignets, people eating Cajun style can easily achieve the goals embodied in the *Dietary Guidelines*.

MEDITERRANEAN DIETS AND HEART HEALTH

Coastal populations that share the bounty of the Mediterranean waters may also share some important health advantages. Mediterranean people die less frequently of heart disease and certain cancers than do people of northern Europe and North America.[2] While popular sources report the marvels of "the Mediterranean diet," scientists who have attempted to define that diet or its health benefits have run into problems.[3] One problem is that many countries border the Mediterranean Sea: Italy, Spain, Portugal, France, Greece, Syria, Lebanon, Israel, Turkey, Egypt, Algeria, and more. Consequently, there is no single "Mediterranean diet." Also, some of the data backing claims about causes of death in Mediterranean countries were collected in the 1960s, when the majority of people still consumed traditional diets. Even with these limitations, the links between Mediterranean diets and health are worth pondering, and Highlight 6 reviews some of the findings of recent research.

Today's Greek and Italian cuisines stem from some of the world's most ancient foodways.[4] Ancient Greeks and Romans ate mostly grain foods such as breads and cakes, along with seeds including lentils and beans, fish and other seafoods, goat cheese, vegetables, and fruits (especially grapes and figs). They ate meat on special occasions only and drank wine diluted half-and-half with water. Their favored cooking fat was oil pressed from olives; butter was shunned as a "food of barbarians." In modern U.S. terms, the ancient Greek and Roman diets fit fairly well into the Daily Food Guide pattern. Unfortunately, no one knows much about the causes of death in those days, but the average life span was only about 40 years or so. So many people died of childhood diseases, in war, in childbirth, or from infectious diseases that few lived long enough to develop heart disease or cancer.

Today, Greeks are known for a robust cuisine that includes whole broiled fish and other seafoods; roasts and stews of vegetables such as eggplant with lamb, chicken, or beef; and the flavors of fresh lemons, garlic, and herbs (dill, mint, and parsley); and, always, olives and their oil, which lavishly season many dishes.[5] Traditional Greek salads contain no lettuce but combine chunks of tomato, peppers, cucumbers, onions, a salty cheese (feta), anchovies, and cured ripe olives with a tangy olive oil and lemon dressing. Stuffed grape leaves may be topped by a famous Greek soup of eggs and lemon juice. Gyros (pronounced YEE-roce, meaning "a circle" in Greek) is a high-fat, highly seasoned meat that is roasted over open flames as it slowly turns on a spit. When cooked, the gyros is thinly sliced, dressed with yogurt and cucumber, and served in a pita (pocket) bread. As for Greek desserts, pastries (baklava) soaked with butter and honey and layered with nuts are traditional at celebrations. Because of their intense sweetness, small servings of these desserts are usually satisfying.

The Greek diet provides a startling 42 percent of its kcalories from fat, mostly from olive oil and olives.[6] Yet people living in Greece have a lower incidence of cardiovascular disease than northern Europeans and North Americans and enjoy one of the longest life expectancies worldwide (1986 data), despite the tendency of many Greeks to carry excess body fat.[7] These facts have led some to suggest that a diet similar to that of Greece might be healthier and easier to follow than the limited fat diet recommended in the United States for heart health (Highlight 6 revisits this topic).[8]

Like Greece, Italy relies on the Mediterranean Sea for seafoods, but its cuisine is perhaps best known for its pastas. Italian cuisines—and pastas—differ from north to south. Generally, northern pastas are egg based and usually ribbon shaped or stuffed like dumplings (tortellini). Northern Italians eat their pasta with plenty of meat, butter, cheese, eggs, and cream. In the southern regions, the diet is more "Mediterranean" in character; wheat pastas are made without eggs, shaped more like macaroni, and served with vegetables such as artichokes, eggplants, peppers, and tomatoes. Beans appear on the table more often than meat, and all dishes are seasoned with olive oil, not butter. Unlike the Greeks, southern Italians keep total fat intakes relatively low.[9] Death rates from heart disease are low among natives of Italy (and neighboring Spain), so health experts are reluctant to suggest "improvements" for their diets.[10]

While heart disease rates may be low in Mediterranean countries, no one can explain why the incidence of stroke is almost double that of the United States. If diet is credited for heart health, shouldn't it also be blamed for stroke?

Also, while the link between diet and heart disease is strong, no one knows what part of the diet might be beneficial. Some think using olive oil instead of butter or shortening is the key factor, while others point to the protective effects of both nutrients and nonnutrients found in vegetables, seafoods, or seasonings.[11] They say that while fat may play a role, an antioxidant effect from constituents of plant foods is probably more important in defending the heart. (More about antioxidants appears in Highlight 11.)

A valid question is whether Mediterranean people may be naturally resistant to heart disease, but this seems not to be the case. People who move from one place to another and adopt the dietary habits of the new locale have heart disease rates typical of people native to that area.[12] Mediterranean populations are, however, more physically active than those in the United States and Canada. They also consume more fruits and vegetables, less meat and animal fat, more olive oil, and more of each day's kcalories early in the day. The effects of meal timing on heart disease risk may be important. A small but significant improvement in blood lipids has been observed in people who eat frequent small meals each day, rather than the standard larger meals.[13] Many aspects of life affect heart health.

WEST AFRICAN FOODS IN THE DEEP SOUTH

Peanut *butter* is considered an American food, invented by the agricultural scientist George Washington Carver, but peanuts are native to South America. They were spread by Portuguese explorers to Africa, where peanuts and peanut paste became staple foods and were brought to U.S. soil by African slaves. Many southern specialties, such as boiled peanuts, okra, and black-eyed (cow) peas, are of African origin. Today's rural southern cuisine varies little between African Americans and people of European descent.

Southern cuisine provides ample vitamins and minerals from a variety of vegetables: sweet potatoes, collards and other leafy greens, okra, tomatoes, meats, and corn. Unfortunately, many of these traditional vegetable dishes are flavored with salted pork, smoked bacon and its fat, or lard, or they are fried in shortening. Fried green tomatoes, a southern specialty, have been dredged in spicy cornmeal and then deep-fried. Many southerners enjoy large servings of high-fat, high-salt meats, such as fried chicken, fatty pork cuts or sausages, and spareribs, greatly overemphasizing protein and fat in the diet while slighting whole grains, fruits, and vegetables. Biscuits, a favored bread, are made with almost as much shortening as flour and are often served with butter or fat-rich gravy. Southern families take pride in their recipes for pecan pie, a pastry shell filled with butter, syrup, and nuts.

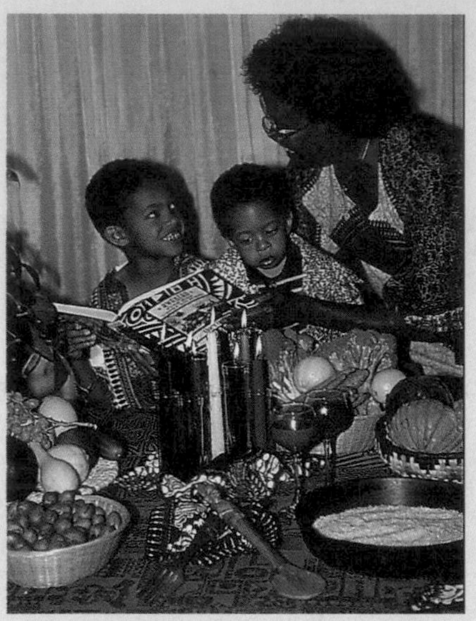

Ethnic meals and family gatherings nourish the spirit as well as the body.

Such a high-fat diet is associated with many health problems, including obesity, heart disease, and stroke. The southeastern United States has the dubious distinction of being the nation's Stroke Belt because of its high incidence of cardiovascular disease. People indulging in traditional southern cuisine need to keep moderation in mind if they are to maintain their health. The trick to choosing health-promoting rural southern food is to limit the fatty, salty meats and vegetables, biscuits, and gravies. Instead select low-fat meats; prepare sweet potatoes, greens, and other vegetables without fat and salt; and eat beans, rice, and cornbread with nonfat seasonings and spreads.

NATIVE AMERICAN DIETS

Over the last 200 years, Native Americans have seen unprecedented changes in their foodways. Hunter-gatherer and agricultural lifestyles have given way to a modern culture relying on fast foods, alcohol, abundant high-fat meats, and dairy products. For Native Americans, the effects of these changes on health have been overwhelmingly negative.

The Pima Indians of central Arizona are a well-studied example of a group that has experienced the effects of a "modernized" diet. Until the 1930s, the Pima diet consisted of wild and cultivated desert legumes, cactus leaves and fruit, fish, venison (deer meat), small seeds, mesquite pods, acorns, and corn.[14] Then, a change began. The Pima largely replaced their traditional wild foods, which had become scarce, with modern ones such as wheat flour, lard, sugar, coffee, and ready-to-eat cereals that were easily obtained. The result has been tragic: the Pima now suffer the highest per capita rate of diabetes known among any people in the world.[15] Likewise, the Sioux Indians rarely suffered heart disease when consuming their traditional diets, but now suffer one of the highest known rates of heart and artery disease.

Both the Pima and the Sioux changed not only their diets, but also their highly active lifestyles. Modern-day Pima and Sioux no longer hunt game on the windswept plains, toil in the fields, or cook over stone fireplaces as their ancestors did. Like others in the United States, they now drive to supermarkets to purchase convenience foods and cook them in microwave ovens. The Sioux also traded their traditional ceremonial pipes for daily cigarette smoking, a habit that is especially damaging to the heart.

While changed diets and lifestyles have almost certainly contributed to the declines in health, disease rates and risk factors differ greatly among tribes, despite a universal adoption of modern foods and television watching.[16] Genetic, as well as environmental, factors must account for these differences.

Native diets are not perfect. They may not provide adequate amounts of some nutrients, and availability of foods depends on such unpredictable factors as weather changes and herd movements. While modern foods are usually safe and sanitary, Native Alaskans eating traditional foods suffer more botulism (a deadly food poisoning described in Chapter 19) than any other group worldwide. Modern descendants changed the ancient methods of preserving meat, fish, and blubber (fat) in slight but critical ways that encourage the growth of the bacteria that cause botulism.[17] The point is that all diets, even those that have supported human beings through many centuries, have drawbacks. Still, by studying them, scientists are beginning to believe that when Native Americans consumed their original high-fiber, low-fat native foods, their hearts and bodies benefited.

MEXICAN ETHNIC FOODS

Mexican restaurants in the United States typically offer beautiful plates of complex food mixtures—tortillas filled with meats and cheeses, some fried and crisp and others baked and soft, along with flavored rice, refried beans, sour cream, guacamole (avocado sauce), and salsa (tomato sauce). These foods are of Mexican origin, but Mexican families typically eat them only on special occasions, not as daily fare. A typical Mexican lunch or dinner is rather simple, consisting of a stew of beans, meat, rice, and potatoes served with tortillas or bread, tomato salsa, and lettuce salad or

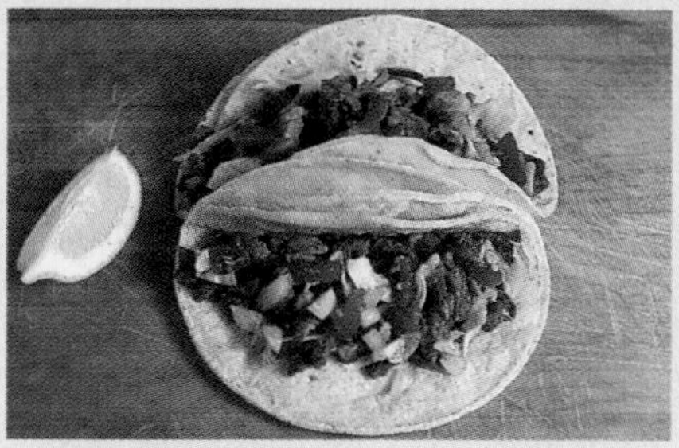
Tortillas filled with lean beef and fresh vegetables are a welcome alternative to sandwiches.

cooked vegetables.[18] A Mexican breakfast might include tortillas and eggs with a beverage.

If carefully chosen, the foods from both taco stands and fancier Mexican restaurants can make valuable contributions to the diet. Many traditional Mexican dishes, even the fast-food type, provide beans in abundance. Beans are high in nutrient density and fiber while low in fat (although some restaurants prepare the refried variety with lard). Soft corn tortillas filled with beans, lettuce, and salsa with a side order of rice are high in nutrient density. Without careful selection, though, Mexican foods can be extraordinarily high in fat, such as a fried tortilla shell filled with high-fat ground beef and topped with cheese and sour cream.

For a healthy special-occasion Mexican meal, use sour cream lightly, and skip the fried varieties of stuffed tortillas. Try instead a low-fat dish called fajita—lean meats, marinated and sizzled on a grill, wrapped in soft tortillas with chili salsa toppings. Salsa (made of chopped tomatoes, onions, and hot peppers) is rich in vitamins and zest but adds no fat to a meal. As for guacamole, even though avocados are high in fat, they add interest and flavor to a meal, and the type of fat avocados contain is not implicated in disease causation. Their high fat content does mean that people who tend to gain weight easily should eat avocados in small quantities on infrequent occasions.

THE CHINESE ADVANTAGE

Tried and true, the diet of China has supported the health of its people for thousands of years. China's foodways reflect the efficiency that is essential in a country where the population density is more than 1000 people per acre, yet only 10 percent of the land can be used to grow food. China has over a billion people, and 75 percent of them are involved in agriculture. Contrast these figures with the United States: population density, 113 per acre; land in farms, about 50 percent; population, 250 million; farmers, 1 to 2 percent.

There seems to be little malnutrition or obesity in China, even though the people consume 20 percent more food energy each day than we do.[19] On the whole, Chinese people eating traditional foods consume three times the fiber of people eating the American way, take in about half the fat, and have blood cholesterol values about half of what they are in the United States.[20] Only 4 out of every 100,000 men in China dies of heart disease each year compared with 67 in the United States. Chinese living in China also suffer much less cancer of the colon and rectum than do Chinese Americans who have adopted a Western diet.[21] It seems worthwhile to study the fine points of a diet so conservative of resources yet so superbly supportive of health—not to convince everyone to eat Chinese meals three times a day, but to illustrate the governing principles that can be applied to foods of all origins.

Typical Chinese meals do not follow the meat-vegetable-starch pattern of northern Europe that is common in much of the United States today. Instead, the vegetables and meats are cooked together. The total amount of meat (or fish or egg) in a Chinese dish is small by Western standards; meals center on a staple starch food—every diner has a dish of rice and chooses other foods from serving dishes according to appetite. The Chinese also usually drink soup or tea throughout each meal, which slows dining to a relaxing pace.

Vegetables and fruits provide tremendous variety, and subtle flavors in main dishes come largely from fat-free seasonings and sauces such as ginger root, scallions, rice wine, garlic, soy, hoisin, oyster, bean, and plum. Most sauces add tasty flavors but little fat unlike our gravies, butter, or sour cream. The Chinese mode of cooking in a wok requires just a tablespoon or two of oil for an entire dish. Chinese dishes do, however, tend to be high in sodium. Diners can enjoy low-sodium meals if they are prepared without salt or monosodium glutamate (MSG) and with judicious use of soy sauce.

Cooking foods the Chinese way tends to preserve nutrients. All food is cut into bite-sized pieces before cooking, so cooking is quick and destroys few nutrients. No cooking water is thrown away, so nutrients are not lost that way either. The water in which the rice is cooked soaks back into the rice, so the rice retains its nutrients.

The Chinese diet and cooking techniques are also land-efficient, as they must be in view of the scarcity of agricultural land and fuels. Nearly all of the food energy comes from plants rather than animals. A million kcalories in wheat or rice can be produced on less than 1 acre of land; a million kcalories in beef require 17 acres. In a world that is often wasteful of fuel and land, the Chinese way of eating offers a model to all nations.

Some Chinese dishes do have nutrition drawbacks, though. In China, deep-fried foods are eaten only seldom, but Chinese restaurants in this country often feature these and other high-fat items. Another drawback is the inclusion of salted, fermented pickles, which have been linked to a high incidence of digestive tract cancers. Chinese restaurants in the United States rarely serve these fermented items because they are not suited to Western tastes.

THE CHANGING JAPANESE DIET

Traditional Japanese cuisine bears similarities to the Chinese diet. Grains such as rice or millet form the bulk of most traditional Japanese meals. Vegetables and fruits are next in prominence, and seafood, eggs, poultry, and meats play a supporting role. For a favored traditional snack, a Japanese commuter might stop by a "noodle house" for a bowl of noodles (somen) in a clear, seasoned broth—a dish of Chinese origin. A Japanese delicacy popular in the United States is sushi—vinegar-flavored rice holding bits of colorful vegetables and seafood, wrapped in seaweed and served with horseradish or seasoned soy sauce. In the United States, the word *sushi* has come to mean "raw fish," which may be an ingredient, but sushi actually refers to vinegared rice, and many types of sushi are made with

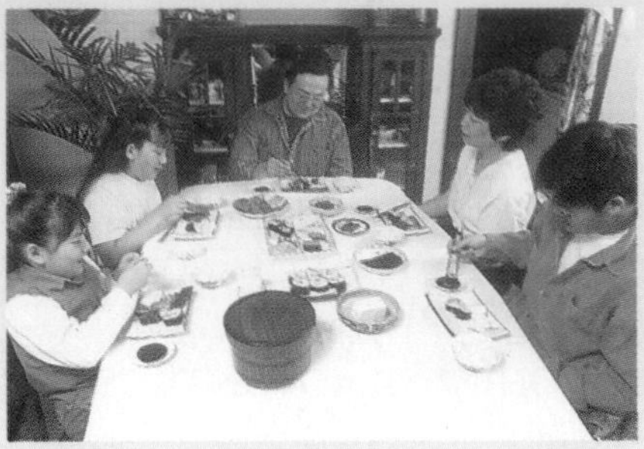

Foodways and cuisines of all cultures can support heart health when dietary fat is limited.

cooked ingredients. Sushi delights diners visually, as do most traditional Japanese foods. In Japan, the visual imagery created on the plate is at least as important as the taste of the food.

Since the 1950s, Japan has transformed itself from a wartorn, still largely traditional country struggling to feed its population to an industrial and economic world leader. Today, Japan's cuisine reflects the "hurry-up" lifestyle of a nation buzzing with mass communications media, high incomes, and high expenses. Time-consuming, home-cooked traditional dishes, though still favored in restaurants, have proved impractical for the two-income family of the 1990s.

In a land where rice once occupied center stage at every meal, meats, breads, and milk products now dominate. Meat consumption in Japan has jumped more than tenfold since the 1940s.[22] Egg intakes rose more than sixfold in the same period. Vegetable intakes have fallen precipitously, and margarine intakes have more than doubled. Japanese families choose microwavable frozen entrees; instant noodle and curry mixes; precooked hamburgers and fried shrimp. Ice cream has replaced fruit as the preferred dessert, and instant coffee is replacing tea. High-fat snacks from hamburger places, southern fried chicken restaurants, and doughnut shops have shoved low-fat noodle houses into the background.

The health implications of such changes are turning out to be two-sided. Deaths in Japan have declined as modern sanitation and immunizations have brought infectious diseases under control, but a steady increase in heart attacks and strokes is now reversing this trend. Japanese men who grew up consuming a "Western" diet are more likely to suffer from diabetes than are men who grew up on a traditional Japanese diet, and diabetes is a risk factor for heart disease.[23] On the other side, the new diet provides much more protein than a traditional rice-based diet, and extra protein during the growing years has enabled the younger generation to grow taller and stronger than any generation before them.[24] In general, Japan still enjoys a lower overall rate of heart disease than many other nations, but new choices present new risks.

People in the United States who wish to dine in the Japanese style can freely choose from traditional dishes, being wary only of a few battered and deep-fried meats and vegetables (tempuras). A traditional Japanese chef may toss together a mixture of mushrooms, carrots, and bamboo shoots with bits of seafood or meat; season it with fat-free (but salty) soy sauce; add sesame seeds; and serve it with a large portion of rice. Shrimp in rice-cake soup features a clear broth, mushrooms, shrimp, and spinach and is served with rice cakes (mochi). A fish-and-noodle casserole might combine a lean fish fillet and broth seasoned with sugar, soy sauce, and mirin (a syrupy rice wine) with a big bowl of thick noodles. Beware of any restaurant that claims to serve traditional Japanese meals but centers the meals around large portions of meat. Today's Japanese diners may consume such meals, but they are not traditional cuisine, and they incur the same warnings that accompany northern European foodways.

RELIGIOUS DIETARY TRADITIONS

A discussion of ethnic foodways would be incomplete without mentioning foodways practiced by religious groups. According to many religions, ritual and ceremony surrounding food can provide nourishment for the spirit as well as for the body. Like national groups, religious groups derive their distinct identity in part from special foodways.

The Jewish laws set forth an extensive set of dietary rules. Many people, on hearing the word *kosher,* think of foods such as pickles, bagels and lox, corned beef, or matzoh crackers. Kosher is not a cuisine, however, but rather a set of restrictions that Orthodox Jews place on the selection and preparation of animal-derived foods. Jews from Eastern Europe, Germany, the former Soviet Union, the Middle East, or India eat different foods, but the kosher rules apply to all.[25]

Religious commitment is the sole intent of those who keep kosher. Occasionally, someone suggests that the laws of kosher originated for reasons of health—that kosher food was "clean" and therefore kept people safe from food-borne illnesses, but the rules of kosher offer no special benefits to health. These rules permit Orthodox Jews to eat beef but not pork, fish but not shellfish, and they dictate special handling methods for permitted foods. Because blood is forbidden as food, kosher rules govern methods of animal slaughter, cuts that may be eaten, and preparation rituals.

Kosher law prohibits Jews from consuming milk and meat in the same meal. This law leads some kosher cooks to replace milk with nondairy creamer in meals that include meat. Nutritionally, however, creams do not resemble milk, and they are high in saturated fat. A better choice is to use soy "milk" products formulated to resemble the nutrient and cooking qualities of milk products.

Like other cuisines, Jewish cuisines and kosher foods can be evaluated according to dietary standards. A meal might be improved by reducing the schmaltz (chicken fat) used in cooking or by frying latke (potato pancakes) in nonstick pans rather than in oil. Bagels with lox (a form of salmon) and nonfat cream cheese are an excellent breakfast choice—bagels are naturally low in fat, and lox is rich in fish oils thought to be protective against the development of heart disease. A person dining on European Jewish cuisine might limit meat to the 2- to 3-ounce serving sizes recommended by the Daily Food Guide and fill in with grains, legumes, fruits, and vegetables.

Food symbolism abounds in most other religions as well. During certain days of Lent, the period prior to Easter, many Christians eat only vegetarian dishes, giving up meat until Easter dinner. Eastern Orthodox Christians observe many fast days on which they consume no animal products at all. The Mormon faith allows no alcohol, coffee, or tea. Many Seventh-Day Adventists consume no meat, but eat eggs and milk products; they also shun alcohol, coffee, and tea. Their doctrine advises them to avoid strong spices such as mustard or pepper and discourages between-meal snacks. Other faiths, such as Islam, Hinduism, and Buddhism, prohibit some dietary practices while promoting others.

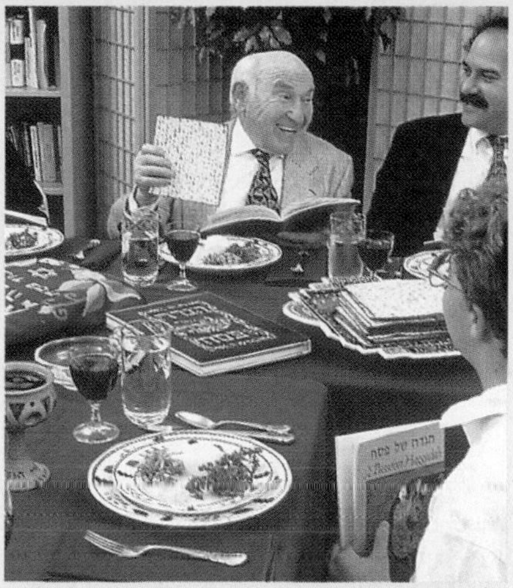

Many religions include foods in their ceremonies.

As you can see by now, consumers can apply the diet-planning principles introduced in Chapter 2 to any ethnic foodway. It is not the ethnic cuisine itself, but the diner's habitual selections from the many traditional choices that determine whether a diet will benefit health. Whatever the cuisine, consumers must learn to balance all foods in a way that provides adequate nourishment without excess.*

*The American Diabetes Association and the American Dietetic Association offer a series of booklets on the ethnic and regional food practices of dozens of foodways. These booklets describe food practices, customs, and holidays; present meals modified according to nutrition recommendations; provide exchange lists, food composition values, and glossaries for ethnic foods; and list additional resources. See Appendix F for addresses.

NOTES

1. K. P. Sucher and P. G. Kittler, Nutrition isn't color blind, *Journal of the American Dietetic Association* 91 (1991): 297–299.

2. F. Berrino and P. Muti, Mediterranean diet and cancer, *European Journal of Clinical Nutrition* 43 (1989): 49–55.

3. A. Ferro-Luzzi and S. Sette, The Mediterranean diet: An attempt to define its present and past composition, *European Journal of Clinical Nutrition* 43 (1989): 13–29.

4. J. C. Waterlow, Diet of the classical period of Greece and Rome, *European Journal of Clinical Nutrition* 43 (1989): 3–12.

5. D. Kromhout and coauthors, Food consumption patterns in the 1960s in seven countries, *American Journal of Clinical Nutrition* 49 (1989): 889–894.

6. A. Trichopoulou, Correspondence, *New England Journal of Medicine* 327 (1992): 53.

7. World Health Organization, Life expectancy, number of survivors, and chances per 1000 of eventually dying from specified causes, at selected ages, by sex, latest available year, in *World Health Statistics Annual* (Geneva: World Health Organization, 1989), pp. 158–163.

8. F. M. Sacks and W. W. Willet, More on chewing the fat, *New England Journal of Medicine* 325 (1991): 1740–1742.

9. Ferro-Luzzi and Sette, 1989.

10. L. Masana and coauthors, The Mediterranean-type diet: Is there a need for further modification? *American Journal of Clinical Nutrition* 53 (1991): 886–889.

11. W. P. T. James, G. G. Duthie, and K. W. J. Whale, The Mediterranean diet: Protective or simply nontoxic? *European Journal of Clinical Nutrition* 43 (1989): 31–41.

12. National Research Council, *Diet and Health: Implications for Reducing Chronic Disease Risk* (Washington, D.C.: U.S. Government Printing Office, 1991), pp. 177–178.

13. L. M. Arnold and coauthors, Effect of isoenergetic intake of three or nine meals on plasma lipoproteins and glucose metabolism, *American Journal of Clinical Nutrition* 57 (1993): 446–451.

14. J. C. Brand and coauthors, Plasma glucose and insulin responses to traditional Pima Indian meals, *American Journal of Clinical Nutrition* 51 (1990): 416–420.

15. B. A. Swinburn, Deterioration in carbohydrate metabolism and lipoprotein changes induced by modern, high-fat diet in Pima Indians and Caucasians, *Journal of Clinical Endocrinology and Metabolism* 73 (1991): 156–165.

16. R. Fabsitz, Administrator of the Strong Heart Study, as quoted by K. A. Fackelmann, *Science News* 142 (1992): 168–170.

17. M. Segal, Native food preparation fosters botulism, *FDA Consumer*, January/February 1992, pp. 23–26.

18. S. J. Algert and T. H. Ellison, Mexican American food practices, customs, and holidays, *Ethnic and Regional Food Practices* (series) (Chicago and Alexandria, Va.: American Dietetic Association and American Diabetes Association, 1989).

19. L. Roberts, Diet and health in China, *Science* 240 (1988): 27.

20. Roberts, 1988.

21. A. S. Whittemore and coauthors, Diet, physical activity, and colorectal cancer among Chinese in North America and China, *Journal of the National Cancer Institute* 82 (1990): 915–926.

22. M. Motoko, Eating is a solitary pastime, *Japan Quarterly* 36 (1989): 207–210.

23. E. H. Tsunehara, D. L. Leonetti, and W. Y. Fujimoto, Diet of second-generation Japanese-American men with and without noninsulin-dependent diabetes, *American Journal of Clinical Nutrition* 52 (1990): 731–738.

24. E. A. Martin and V. A. Beal, *Roberts' Nutrition Work with Children*, 4th ed. (Chicago: University of Chicago Press, 1978) presents details of these classic findings.

25. C. Higgins and H. S. Warshaw, Jewish food practices, customs, and holidays, *Ethnic and Regional Food Practices* (series) (Chicago and Alexandria, Va.: American Dietetic Association and American Diabetes Association, 1989).

Chapter 3

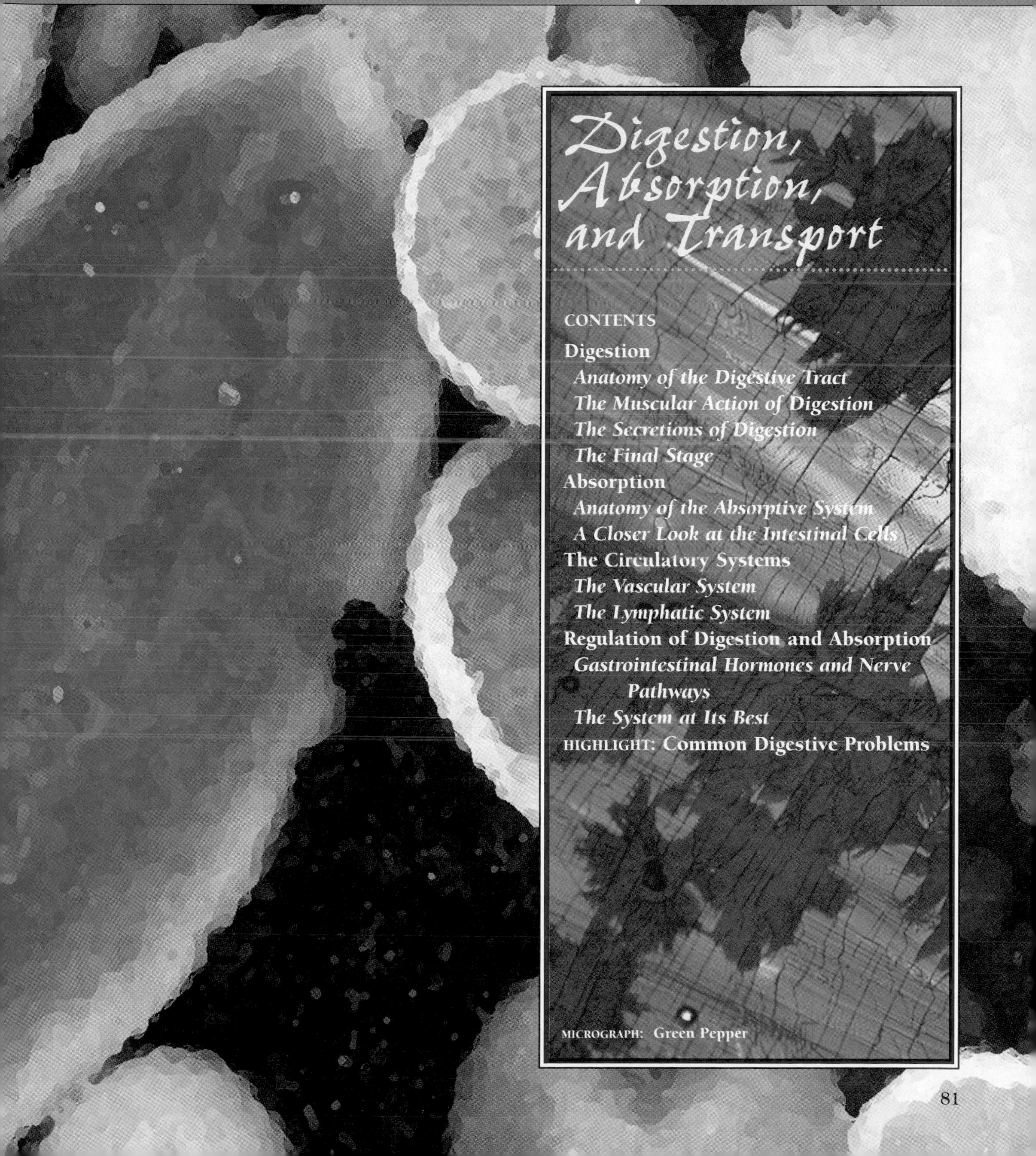

Digestion, Absorption, and Transport

CONTENTS

MICROGRAPH: Green Pepper

Have you ever wondered what happens to the food you eat after you swallow it? Or how your body extracts nutrients from food? Have you ever marveled how it all just seems to happen? This chapter takes you on the journey that transforms the foods you eat into the nutrients featured in the later chapters. Then it follows the nutrients as they travel through the intestinal cells and into the body to do their work. This introduction presents a general overview of the processes common to all nutrients; later chapters discuss the specifics of digesting and absorbing individual nutrients.

digestion: the process by which food is broken down into absorbable units.

Digestion

The digestive tract is the body's ingenious way of getting the nutrients ready for absorption, and it solves many problems for you without any conscious effort on your part. Consider these problems:

1. Human beings breathe, eat, and drink through their mouths. Air taken in through the mouth must go to the lungs; food and liquid must go to the stomach. The throat must be arranged so that swallowing and breathing don't interfere with each other.
2. Below the lungs lies the diaphragm, a dome of muscle that separates the upper half of the major body cavity from the lower half. Food must pass through this wall to reach the stomach.
3. To move through the system, food must be lubricated with water. Too much water would form a liquid that would flow too rapidly; too little water would form a paste too dry and compact to move at all. The amount of water must be regulated to keep the intestinal contents at the right consistency to move smoothly along.
4. When the digestive enzymes are breaking food down, they need it in finely divided form, suspended in enough water so that every particle is accessible. Once digestion is complete and the needed nutrients have been absorbed out of the tract into the body, the system must excrete the residue that remains, but excreting all the water along with the solid residue would be both wasteful and messy. Some water should be withdrawn, leaving a paste just solid enough to be smooth and easy to pass.
5. The materials within the tract should be kept moving, slowly but steadily, at a pace that permits all reactions to reach completion.
6. The enzymes of the digestive tract are designed to digest carbohydrate, fat, and protein. The walls of the tract, composed of living cells, are also made of carbohydrate, fat, and protein. These cells need protection against the action of the powerful digestive juices that they secrete.
7. Once waste matter has reached the end of the tract, it must be excreted, but it would be inconvenient and embarrassing if this function occurred continuously. Provision must be made for periodic, voluntary evacuation.

The following sections show how the body elegantly and efficiently handles these problems.

GI tract: the gastrointestinal tract or digestive tract; the principal organs are the stomach and intestines.
gastro = stomach

ANATOMY OF THE DIGESTIVE TRACT

The gastrointestinal (GI) tract is a flexible muscular tube from the mouth, through the esophagus, stomach, small intestine, large intestine, and rectum to the anus. Figure 3–1 (on p. 84) traces the path followed by food from one end to the other, and the glossary (on p. 85) defines GI anatomy terms. In a sense, the human body surrounds the GI tract. Only when a nutrient or other substance penetrates the GI tract's wall does it enter the body proper; many nonnutritive materials pass through the GI tract without being digested or absorbed.

Mouth The process of digestion begins in the mouth. As you chew, your teeth crush large pieces of food into smaller ones, and fluids blend with these pieces to ease swallowing. Fluids also help dissolve the food so that you can taste it; only particles in solution can react with taste buds. The tongue not only allows you to taste food, but to move food around the mouth, facilitating chewing and swallowing. When you swallow a mouthful of food, it first slides across your epiglottis, bypassing the entrance to your lungs. This is the body's solution to problem 1: the epiglottis closes off your air passages so that you don't choke when you swallow. After a mouthful of food has been swallowed, it is called a bolus.

Choking is discussed on p. 104.

bolus (BOH-lus): a portion; with respect to food, the amount swallowed at one time.

Esophagus to the Stomach Next, the bolus slides down the esophagus, which conducts it through the diaphragm (problem 2) to the stomach. The stomach cells produce secretions both to break down food particles and to protect themselves from being broken down (problem 6). The cardiac sphincter at the entrance to the stomach closes behind the bolus so that it can't slip back into the esophagus (problem 5). The stomach retains the bolus for a while in its upper portion. Little by little, the stomach transfers the food to its lower portion, adds juices to it, and grinds it to a semiliquid mass called chyme. Then, bit by bit, the stomach releases the chyme through the pyloric sphincter, which opens into the small intestine and then closes behind the chyme.

chyme (KIME): the semiliquid mass of partly digested food expelled by the stomach into the duodenum.
chymos = juice

Small Intestine At the top of the small intestine, the chyme bypasses the opening from the common bile duct, which is dripping fluids (problem 3) into the small intestine from two organs outside the GI tract—the gallbladder and the pancreas. The chyme travels on down the small intestine through its three segments—the duodenum, the jejunum, and the ileum—almost 10 feet of tubing coiled within the abdomen.[1]

Large Intestine (Colon) Having traveled the length of the small intestine, the chyme arrives at another sphincter (problem 5 again): the ileocecal valve, at the beginning of the large intestine (colon) in the lower right-hand side of the abdomen. As the chyme enters the colon, it passes another opening. Had it slipped into this opening, it would have ended up in the appendix, a blind sac about the size of your little finger. The chyme bypasses this opening, however, and travels along the large intestine up the right-hand side of the abdomen, across the front to the left-hand side, down to the lower left-hand side, and finally below the other folds of the intestines to the back side of the body, above the rectum.

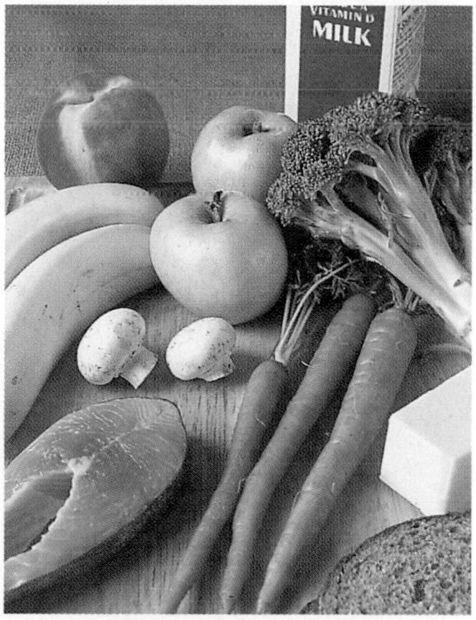

The process of digestion transforms all kinds of *foods* into *nutrients*.

Rectum During the chyme's passage to the rectum, the colon withdraws water from it, leaving semisolid waste (problem 4). The strong muscles of the rectum hold back this waste until it is time to defecate. Then the rectal muscles relax (problem 7), and the last sphincter in the system, the anus, opens to allow passage of the waste.

Figure 3–1

The Gastrointestinal Tract

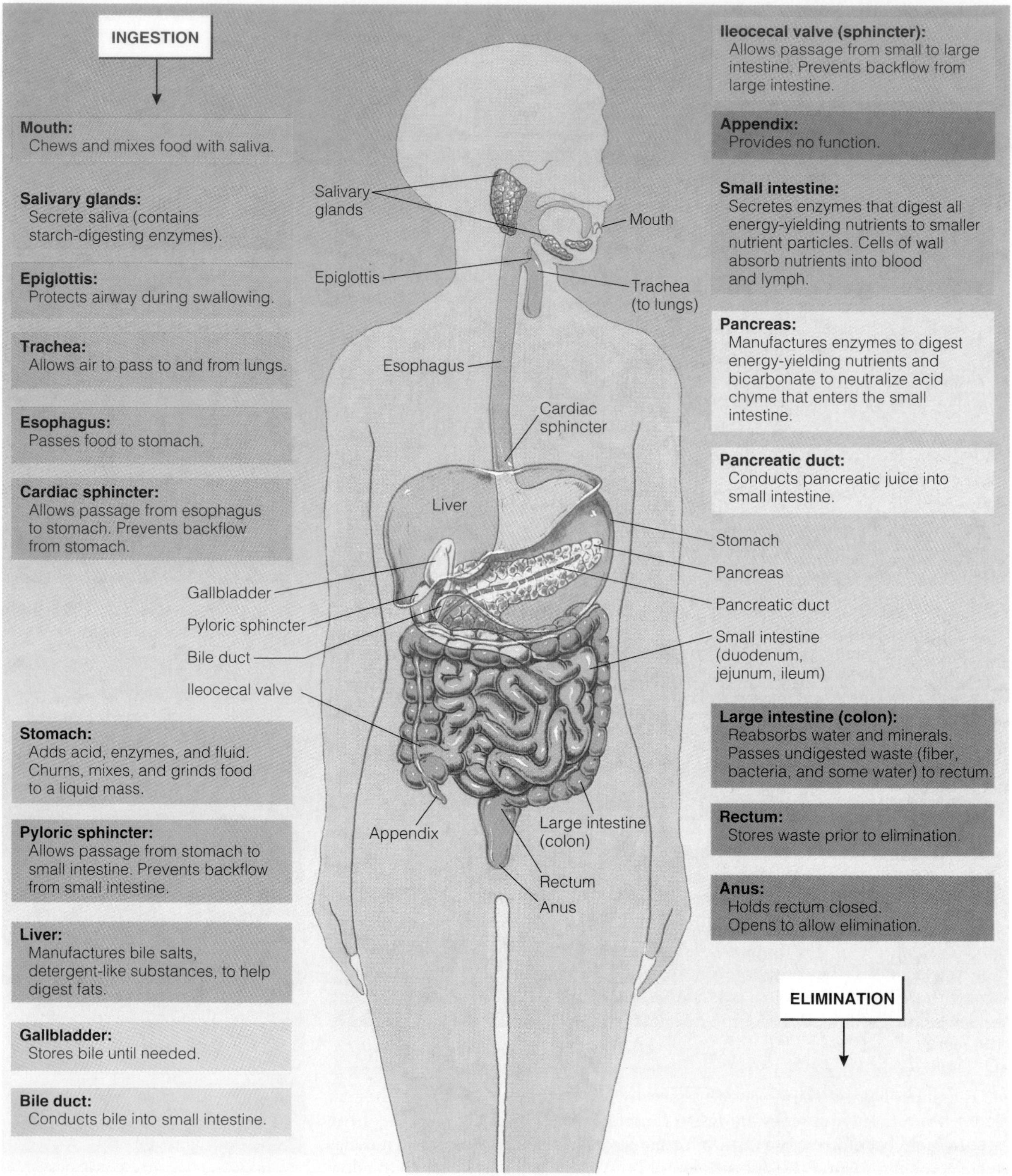

INGESTION
Mouth: Chews and mixes food with saliva.
Salivary glands: Secrete saliva (contains starch-digesting enzymes).
Epiglottis: Protects airway during swallowing.
Trachea: Allows air to pass to and from lungs.
Esophagus: Passes food to stomach.
Cardiac sphincter: Allows passage from esophagus to stomach. Prevents backflow from stomach.
Stomach: Adds acid, enzymes, and fluid. Churns, mixes, and grinds food to a liquid mass.
Pyloric sphincter: Allows passage from stomach to small intestine. Prevents backflow from small intestine.
Liver: Manufactures bile salts, detergent-like substances, to help digest fats.
Gallbladder: Stores bile until needed.
Bile duct: Conducts bile into small intestine.
Salivary glands
Epiglottis
Esophagus
Mouth
Trachea (to lungs)
Cardiac sphincter
Liver
Stomach
Pancreas
Pancreatic duct
Gallbladder
Pyloric sphincter
Bile duct
Ileocecal valve
Small intestine (duodenum, jejunum, ileum)
Appendix
Large intestine (colon)
Rectum
Anus
Ileocecal valve (sphincter): Allows passage from small to large intestine. Prevents backflow from large intestine.
Appendix: Provides no function.
Small intestine: Secretes enzymes that digest all energy-yielding nutrients to smaller nutrient particles. Cells of wall absorb nutrients into blood and lymph.
Pancreas: Manufactures enzymes to digest energy-yielding nutrients and bicarbonate to neutralize acid chyme that enters the small intestine.
Pancreatic duct: Conducts pancreatic juice into small intestine.
Large intestine (colon): Reabsorbs water and minerals. Passes undigested waste (fiber, bacteria, and some water) to rectum.
Rectum: Stores waste prior to elimination.
Anus: Holds rectum closed. Opens to allow elimination.
ELIMINATION

Glossary of GI Anatomy Terms

These terms are listed in order from start to end of the digestive tract.

epiglottis (epp-ee-GLOTT-iss): cartilage in the throat that guards the entrance to the trachea and prevents fluid or food from entering it when a person swallows.
epi = upon (over)
glottis = back of tongue

trachea (TRAKE-ee-uh): the windpipe; the passageway from the mouth and nose to the lungs.

esophagus (e-SOFF-uh-gus): the food pipe; the conduit from the mouth to the stomach.

cardiac sphincter (CARD-ee-ack SFINK-ter): the sphincter muscle at the junction between the esophagus and the stomach; also called the *lower esophageal sphincter* or the *gastroesophageal sphincter*.
cardiac = the heart

sphincter: a circular muscle surrounding, and able to close, a body opening.
sphincter = band (binder)

stomach: a muscular, elastic, saclike portion of the digestive tract that grinds and churns swallowed food, mixing it with acid and enzymes to form chyme.

pyloric (pie-LORE-ic) **sphincter:** the circular muscle that separates the stomach from the small intestine and regulates the flow of partially digested food into the small intestine (also called **pylorus** or **pyloric valve**).
pylorus = gatekeeper

liver: the organ that manufactures bile and is the first to receive nutrients from the intestines. The liver's many other functions are described in Chapter 7.

gallbladder: the organ that stores and concentrates bile. When it receives the signal that fat is present in the duodenum, the gallbladder contracts and squirts bile through the bile duct into the duodenum.

pancreas: a gland that secretes digestive enzymes and juices into the duodenum.

small intestine: a 10-foot length of small-diameter intestine that is the major site of digestion of food and absorption of nutrients; its segments are the duodenum, jejunum, and ileum.

duodenum (doo-oh-DEEN-um, doo-ODD-num): the top portion of the small intestine (about "12 fingers' breadth" long in ancient terminology).
duodecim = twelve

jejunum (je-JOON-um): the first two-fifths of the small intestine beyond the duodenum.

ileum (ILL-ee-um): the last segment of the small intestine.

ileocecal (ill-ee-oh-SEEK-ul) **valve:** the sphincter separating the small and large intestines.

large intestine or **colon** (COAL-un): the lower portion of intestine that completes the digestive process; its segments are the ascending colon, the transverse colon, the descending colon, and the sigmoid colon.
sigmoid = shaped like an S (sigma in Greek)

appendix: a narrow blind sac extending from the beginning of the colon; a vestigial organ with no known function.

rectum: the muscular terminal part of the intestine, extending from the sigmoid colon to the anus.

anus (AY-nus): the terminal sphincter of the GI tract.

To sum up, food follows the path shown in Figure 3–1. Food enters the mouth and travels past the epiglottis, down the esophagus and through the cardiac sphincter to the stomach, then through the pyloric sphincter to the small intestine (duodenum, with entrance from the gallbladder and pancreas; then jejunum; then ileum), on through the ileocecal valve to the large intestine, past the appendix to the rectum, ending at the anus. Considering all that happens on the way, the route is remarkably simple.

THE MUSCULAR ACTION OF DIGESTION

The first step in the reduction of food to a liquid takes place in the mouth, where chewing, the addition of saliva, and the action of the tongue reduce the food to a coarse mash. Then you swallow, and thereafter, you are generally unaware of all the activity that follows. As is the case with so much else that happens in the body, the muscles of the digestive tract meet internal needs without your having to exert any conscious effort. They keep things moving at just the right pace, slow enough to get the job done and fast enough to make progress.

The ability of the GI tract muscles to move is called their **motility**.

peristalsis (peri-STALL-sis): wavelike muscular contractions of the GI tract that push its contents along.
peri = around
stellein = wrap

Peristalsis Peristalsis begins when the bolus enters the esophagus. The entire GI tract is ringed with circular muscles that can squeeze it tightly. Surrounding these rings of muscle are longitudinal muscles. When the rings tighten and the long muscles relax, the tube is constricted. When the rings relax and the long muscles tighten, the tube bulges. These actions follow each other continuously and push the intestinal contents along (problem 5). (If you have ever watched a lump of food pass along the body of a snake, you have a good picture of how these muscles work.)

The waves of contraction ripple along the GI tract at varying rates and intensities depending on the part of the GI tract and on whether food is present. For example, waves occur three times per minute in the stomach, but speed up to ten times per minute when chyme reaches the small intestine. When you have just eaten a meal, the waves are slow and continuous; when the GI tract is empty, the intestine is quiet except for periodic bursts of powerful rhythmic waves. Peristalsis, along with the sphincter muscles that surround the tract at key places, keeps things moving along (Figure 3–2).

Stomach Action The stomach has the thickest walls and strongest muscles of all the GI tract organs. In addition to the circular and longitudinal muscles, it has a third layer of diagonal muscles that also alternately contract and relax. These three sets of muscles work to force the chyme downward, but the pyloric sphincter usually remains tightly closed, preventing the chyme from passing into the duodenum. As a result, the chyme is churned and forced down, hits the pyloric sphincter, and remains in the stomach. Meanwhile, the stomach wall releases juices. When the chyme is completely liquefied, the pyloric sphincter opens briefly, about three times a minute, to allow small portions of chyme through. At this point, the chyme no longer resembles food in the least.

segmentation (SEG-men-TAY-shun): a periodic squeezing or partitioning of the intestine at intervals along its length by its circular muscles.

Segmentation The intestines not only push, but also periodically squeeze, their contents—as if a string tied around the intestines were being pulled gently. This motion, called segmentation, momentarily forces the intestinal contents back a few inches, mixing them and promoting close contact with the digestive juices and the absorbing cells of the intestinal walls before letting the contents move slowly along (see Figure 3–2).

Figure 3–2

Peristalsis and Segmentation

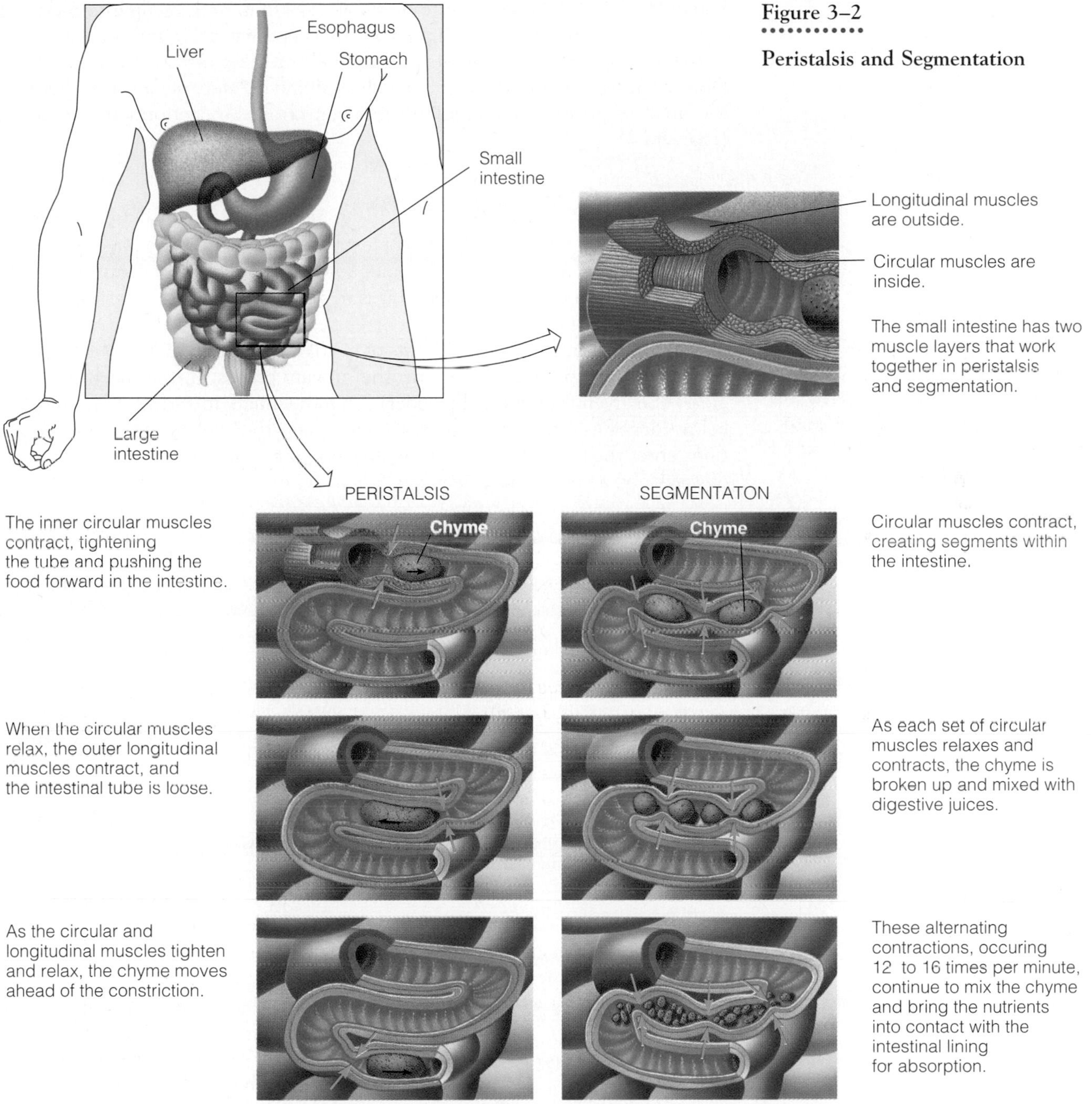
Esophagus
Liver
Stomach
Small intestine
Large intestine
Longitudinal muscles are outside.
Circular muscles are inside.
The small intestine has two muscle layers that work together in peristalsis and segmentation.
PERISTALSIS
SEGMENTATON
The inner circular muscles contract, tightening the tube and pushing the food forward in the intestine.
Chyme
Chyme
Circular muscles contract, creating segments within the intestine.
When the circular muscles relax, the outer longitudinal muscles contract, and the intestinal tube is loose.
As each set of circular muscles relaxes and contracts, the chyme is broken up and mixed with digestive juices.
As the circular and longitudinal muscles tighten and relax, the chyme moves ahead of the constriction.
These alternating contractions, occuring 12 to 16 times per minute, continue to mix the chyme and bring the nutrients into contact with the intestinal lining for absorption.

Sphincter Contractions Four major sphincter muscles divide the GI tract into its principal divisions. At the bottom of the esophagus, the cardiac sphincter prevents reflux of the stomach contents. At the bottom of the stomach, the pyloric sphincter, which stays closed most of the time, holds the bolus in the stomach long enough so that it can be thoroughly mixed with gastric juice and

reflux: a backward flow.
re = back
flux = flow

liquefied. It also prevents the intestinal contents from backing up into the stomach. At the end of the small intestine, the ileocecal valve performs a similar function, emptying the contents of the small intestine into the large intestine. Finally, the tightness of the rectal muscle is a kind of safety device; together with the anus, it prevents elimination until you choose to perform it voluntarily (problem 7).

THE SECRETIONS OF DIGESTION

Remember from Chapter 1 how people can eat differently yet have essentially the same body composition? It all comes down to the process of digestion, of rendering food—whatever kind of food it is to start with—into the basic units that make up the nutrients.

To break down food to small units of nutrients that the body can absorb, five different organs produce secretions: the salivary glands, the stomach, the pancreas, the liver (via the gallbladder), and the small intestine. (The glossary below identifies some of the digestive glands and their secretions.) These secretions enter the GI tract at various points along the way, bringing an abundance of water and a variety of enzymes.

gland: a cell or group of cells that secretes materials for special uses in the body. Glands may be **exocrine** (EKS-oh-crin) **glands**, secreting their materials "out" (into the digestive tract or onto the surface of the skin), or **endocrine** (EN-doe-crin) **glands**, secreting their materials "in" (into the blood).
exo = outside
endo = inside
krine = to separate

Glossary of Digestive Glands and Their Secretions

These terms are listed in order from start to end of the digestive tract.

salivary glands: exocrine glands that secrete saliva into the mouth.

saliva: the secretion of the salivary glands; its principal enzyme begins carbohydrate digestion.

gastric glands: exocrine glands in the stomach wall that secrete gastric juice into the stomach.
gastro = stomach

gastric juice: the digestive secretion of the gastric glands of the stomach.

hydrochloric acid: an acid composed of hydrogen and chloride atoms (HCl). The gastric glands normally produce this acid.

mucus (MYOO-cuss): a slippery substance secreted by goblet cells of the GI lining (and other body linings) that protects the cells from exposure to digestive juices (and other destructive agents). The lining of the GI tract with its coat of mucus is a **mucous membrane**. (The noun is **mucus**; the adjective is **mucous**.)

bile: an emulsifier that prepares fats and oils for digestion; an exocrine secretion made by the liver, stored in the gallbladder, and released into the small intestine when needed.

emulsifier (ee-MUL-sih-fire): a substance with both water-soluble and fat-soluble portions that promotes the mixing of oils and fats in a watery solution.

pancreatic (pank-ree-AT-ic) **juice:** the exocrine secretion of the pancreas, containing enzymes for the digestion of carbohydrate, fat, and protein as well as bicarbonate, a neutralizing agent. The juice flows from the pancreas into the small intestine through the pancreatic duct. (The pancreas also has an endocrine function, the secretion of insulin and other hormones.)

bicarbonate: an alkaline secretion of the pancreas, part of the pancreatic juice. (Bicarbonate also occurs widely in all cell fluids.)

Glossary of Digestive Enzymes

digestive enzymes: proteins found in digestive juices that act on food substances, causing them to break down into simpler compounds.

-ase (ACE): a word ending denoting an enzyme. Enzymes are often identified by the place they come from and the compounds they work on; *gastric lipase*, for example is a stomach enzyme that acts on lipids, whereas *pancreatic lipase* come from the pancreas (and also works on lipids).

carbohydrase (KAR-boe-HIGH-drase): an enzyme that hydrolyzes carbohydrates.

hydrolysis (high-DROL-ih-sis): a chemical reaction in which a major reactant is split into two products, with the addition of a hydrogen atom (H) to one and a hydroxyl group (OH) to the other (from water, H_2O).
hydro = water
lysis = breaking

lipase (LYE-pase): an enzyme that hydrolyzes lipids (fats).

protease (PRO-tee-ase): an enzyme that hydrolyzes proteins.

All enzymes and some hormones are proteins, but an enzyme is not a hormone. Enzymes facilitate the making and breaking of bonds in chemical reactions; hormones act as chemical messengers, sometimes regulating enzyme action.

Enzymes are formally introduced in Chapter 6, but for now, a simple definition will suffice. An enzyme is a giant protein molecule that facilitates a chemical reaction—making a molecule from smaller parts, breaking a molecule into smaller parts, changing the arrangement of a molecule, or exchanging parts of molecules. As a catalyst, the enzyme itself remains unchanged. The enzymes involved in digestion facilitate a chemical reaction known as hydrolysis—the addition of water (hydro) to break (lysis) a molecule into smaller pieces. The glossary above identifies some of the digestive enzymes and defines related terms.

catalyst (CAT-uh-list): a compound that facilitates chemical reactions without itself being changed in the process.

Saliva The salivary glands squirt just enough saliva to moisten each mouthful of food so that it can pass easily down the esophagus (problem 3). The saliva contains water, salts, and enzymes that initiate the digestion of carbohydrates. In fact, you can taste the change if you hold a piece of starchy food like a cracker in your mouth for a few minutes without swallowing it—the cracker begins tasting sweeter as the enzyme acts on it. Saliva also protects the tooth surfaces and the linings of the mouth, esophagus, and stomach from attack by substances that might harm them.

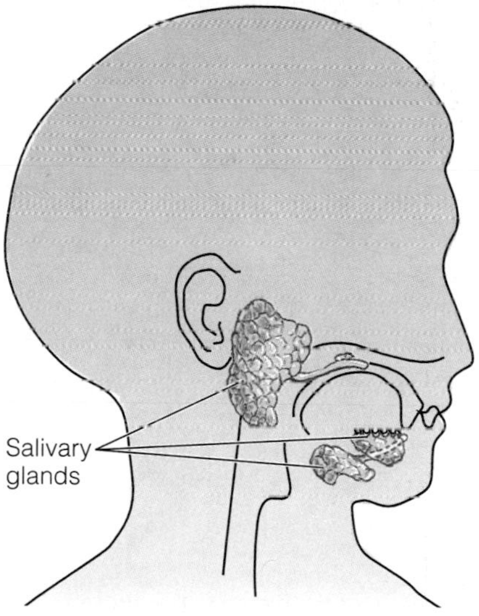

The salivary glands secrete saliva into the mouth and begin the digestive process. Given the short time food is in the mouth, salivary enzymes contribute little to digestion.

Gastric Juice Cells in the stomach secrete gastric juice, a mixture of water, enzymes, and hydrocholoric acid. The acid is so strong that it causes the sensation of heartburn if it chances to reflux into the esophagus. Highlight 3, following this chapter, discusses heartburn and other common digestive problems.

The strong acidity of the stomach prevents bacterial growth and kills most bacteria that enter the body with food. It would destroy the cells of the stomach as well, but for their natural defenses. To protect themselves from gastric juice, the goblet cells of the stomach wall secrete mucus, a thick, slippery, white substance that coats the cells, protecting them from the acid and enzymes that might otherwise harm them.

goblet cells: cells of the GI tract (and lungs) that secrete mucus.

Figure 3–3 shows how the strength of acids is measured—in pH units. Note that the acidity of gastric juice registers below "2" on the pH scale—stronger than vinegar. The stomach enzymes work most efficiently in the stomach's strong acid, but

Figure 3–3

The pH Scale

A substance's acidity or alkalinity is measured in pH units. The pH is the negative logarithm of the hydrogen ion concentration. Each increment presents a tenfold increase in concentration of hydrogen particles. For example, a pH of 2 is 1000 times stronger than a pH of 5.

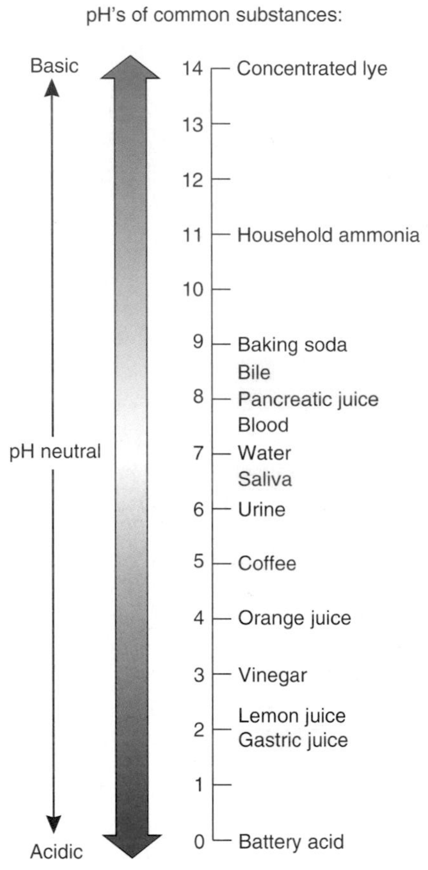

pH: the unit of measure expressing a substance's acidity or alkalinity (Chapter 12 and Appendix B provide a more detailed definition).

The bacterial inhabitants of the GI tract are known as the **intestinal flora**
flora = plant growth

the salivary enzymes, which are swallowed with food, do not work in acid this strong. Consequently, the salivary digestion of carbohydrate gradually ceases as the stomach acid penetrates each newly swallowed bolus of food. In fact, salivary enzymes become just other proteins to be digested, and carbohydrate digestion waits to resume in the next digestive organ, the small intestine.

The major digestive event in the stomach is the partial breakdown (hydrolysis) of proteins. There, the acid helps to uncoil proteins, making them available for digestion. Both an enzyme and the stomach acid itself act as catalysts for this reaction. Minor events are the digestion of a very little fat by a gastric lipase; the breakdown of some carbohydrate by gastric acid; and the attachment of a protein carrier to vitamin B_{12}.

Pancreatic Juice and Intestinal Enzymes By the time food leaves the stomach, digestion of all three energy nutrients has begun, and the action gains momentum in the small intestine. There, the pancreas and liver contribute additional digestive juices by way of ducts leading into the duodenum. The pancreatic juice contains enzymes that act on all three energy nutrients, and the cells of the intestinal wall also possess digestive enzymes on their surfaces.

In addition to enzymes, the pancreatic juice contains sodium bicarbonate, which is basic or alkaline—the opposite of the stomach's acid (review Figure 3–3). The pancreatic juice thus neutralizes the acid chyme arriving in the small intestine from the stomach. From this point on, the chyme remains at a neutral or slightly alkaline pH. The enzymes of both the intestine and the pancreas work best in this environment.

Bile Bile also flows into the duodenum. Bile is secreted by the liver continuously, and it is concentrated and stored in the gallbladder, which squirts it into the duodenum when fat arrives there. Bile is not an enzyme, but an emulsifier that brings fats into suspension in water so that enzymes can break them down into their component parts. Thanks to all these secretions, the three energy-yielding nutrients are digested in the small intestine (see Table 3–1 for a summary of digestive secretions and their actions).

Protective Factors Both the small and large intestine, being neutral in pH, permit the growth of bacteria. In fact, a healthy intestinal tract supports a thriving bacterial population that normally does the body no harm and may actually do some good. Bacteria in the GI tract produce a couple of vitamins, including a significant amount of vitamin K, although the amount is insufficient to meet the body's total need for that vitamin.[2]

Provided that the normal intestinal flora are thriving, infectious bacteria have a hard time getting established and launching an attack on the system. Diet is one of several factors that influence the bacterial population and its environment.[3] In addition, secretions from the GI tract—saliva, mucus, gastric acid, and digestive enzymes—not only help with digestion, but also defend against foreign invaders. The GI tract also maintains several different kinds of defending cells that confer specific immunity against intestinal diseases.

THE FINAL STAGE

The story of how digestion prepares food for absorption is now nearly complete. The three energy-yielding nutrients—carbohydrate, fat, and protein—have been

Table 3–1

Summary of Digestive Secretions

Organ or Gland	Target Organ	Secretion	Action
Salivary glands	Mouth	Saliva	Fluid eases swallowing; salivary enzyme breaks down carbohydrate.
Gastric glands	Stomach	Gastric juice	Fluid mixes with bolus; hydrochloric acid uncoils proteins; enzymes break down proteins; mucus protects stomach cells.
Pancreas	Small intestine	Pancreatic juice	Bicarbonate neutralizes acidic gastric juices; pancreatic enzymes break down carbohydrates, fats, and proteins.
Liver	Gallbladder	Bile	Bile stored until needed.
Gallbladder	Small intestine	Bile	Bile emulsifies fat into small particles that enzymes can attack.
Intestinal glands	Small intestine	Intestinal juice	Intestinal enzymes break down carbohydrate and protein fragments; mucus protects the intestinal wall.

disassembled to basic building blocks and are ready to be absorbed. Most of the other nutrients—vitamins, minerals, and water—need no such disassembly; they are absorbed as they are. Undigested residues, such as some fibers, are not absorbed, but continue through the digestive tract, providing a semisolid mass that helps exercise the muscles and keep them strong enough to perform peristalsis efficiently. Fiber also retains water, accounting for the stools' pasty consistency, and carries some bile acids, some minerals, and some additives and contaminants with it out of the body.

Some vitamins and minerals are slightly altered during digestion as later chapters explain.

Chapter 4 discusses fiber in more detail.

stools: waste matter discharged from the colon; also called **feces** (FEE-seez).

The process of absorbing the nutrients into the body presents its own problems, to be discussed in the next section. For the moment, assume that the digested nutrients simply are absorbed from the GI tract as soon as they are ready. Most are gone by the time the contents of the GI tract reach the end of the small intestine. Little remains but water, a few dissolved salts and body secretions, and undigested materials such as fiber. These enter the large intestine (colon).

In the colon, intestinal bacteria degrade some of the fiber to simpler compounds, while the colon itself retrieves all materials that the body is designed to recycle—water and dissolved salts. The waste that is finally excreted has little or nothing of value left in it. The body has extracted all that it can use from the food. Figure 3–4 (on p. 92) summarizes digestion by following a sandwich through the GI tract and into the body.

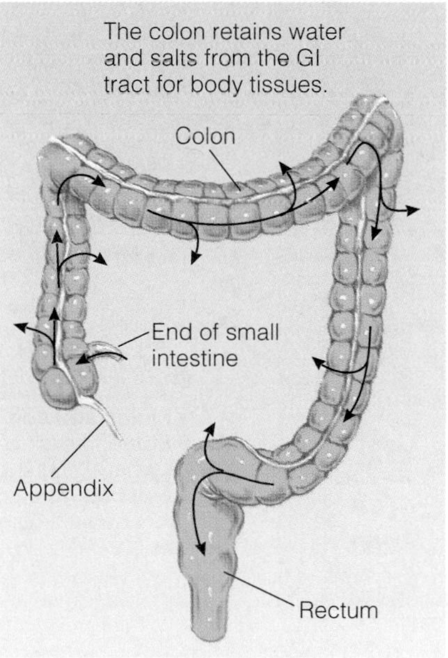

The colon reabsorbs water and salts.

Absorption

Problem: Given an elaborate production in which 1000 actors are on stage at once, provide a means by which all can exit simultaneously. This is the problem of absorption. Within three or four hours after you have eaten a dinner of beans and rice (or spinach lasagna, or steak and potatoes) with vegetable, salad, beverage, and dessert, your body must find a way to absorb—one by one—some two

Figure 3–4

The Digestive Fate of a Sandwich

To review the digestive processes and enzymes, follow a peanut butter and banana sandwich on whole-wheat, sesame seed bread through the GI tract.

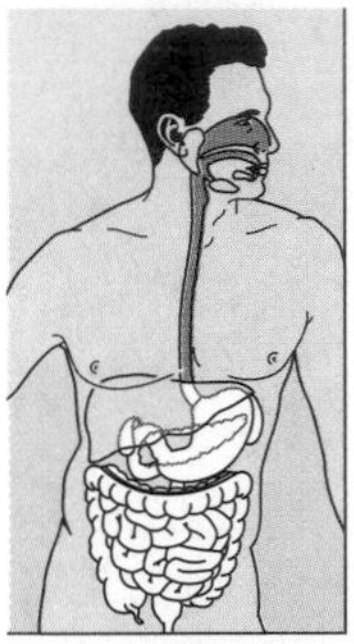

MOUTH: CHEWING AND SWALLOWING, WITH LITTLE DIGESTION

- **Carbohydrate** digestion begins as the salivary enzyme starts to break down the starch from bread and peanut butter.
- **Fiber** covering on the sesame seeds is crushed by the teeth, which exposes the nutrients inside the seeds to the upcoming digestive enzymes.

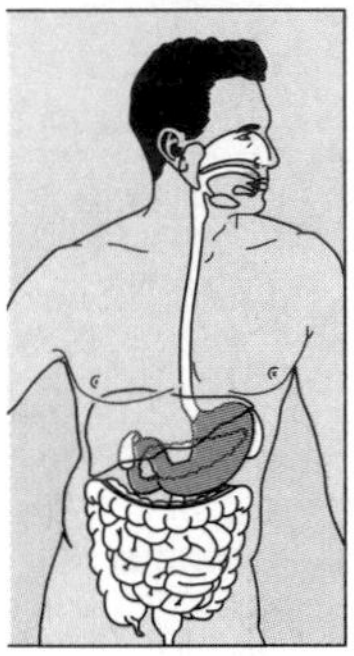

STOMACH: COLLECTING AND CHURNING, WITH SOME DIGESTION

- **Carbohydrate** digestion continues until the mashed sandwich has been mixed with the gastric juices; the stomach acid of the gastric juices inactivates the salivary enzyme.
- **Proteins** from the bread, seeds, and peanut butter begin to uncoil when they mix with the gastric acid, making them available to the gastric protease enzymes that begin to digest proteins.
- **Fat** from the peanut butter forms a separate layer on top of the watery mixture.

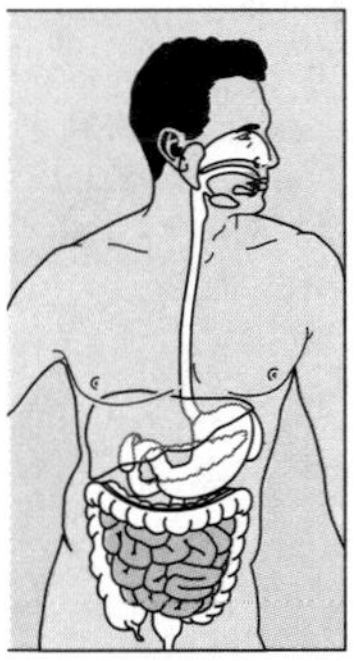

SMALL INTESTINE: DIGESTING AND ABSORBING

- **Sugars** from the banana require so little digestion that they begin to traverse the intestinal cells immediately on contact.
- **Starch** digestion picks up when the pancreas sends pancreatic enzymes to the small intestine via the pancreatic duct. Enzymes on the surfaces of the small intestinal cells complete the process of breaking down starch into small fragments that can be absorbed through the intestinal cell walls and into the blood.
- **Fat** from the peanut butter and seeds is emulsified with the watery digestive fluids by bile. Now the pancreatic and intestinal lipases can begin to break down the fat to smaller fragments that can be absorbed through the cells of the small intestinal wall and into the lymph.
- **Protein** digestion depends on the pancreatic and intestinal proteases. Small fragments of protein are liberated and absorbed through the cells of the small intestinal wall and into the blood.
- **Vitamins and minerals** are absorbed.

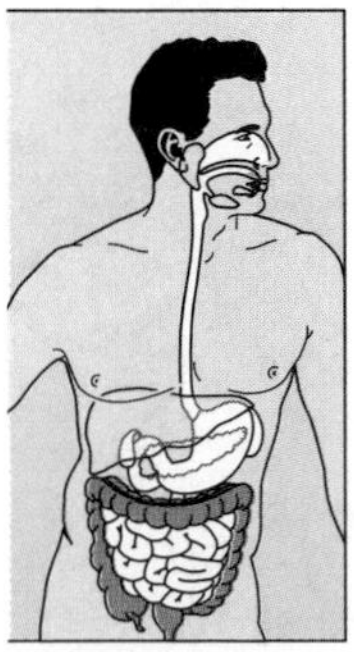

LARGE INTESTINE: REABSORBING AND ELIMINATING

- **Fluids and some minerals** are absorbed.
- **Some fibers** from the seeds, whole-wheat bread, peanut butter, and banana are partly digested by the bacteria living there, and some of these products are absorbed.
- **Most fibers** pass through the large intestine and are excreted as feces; some fat, cholesterol, and minerals bind to fiber and are also excreted.

hundred thousand million, million, million molecules derived from carbohydrate digestion; a comparable number of molecules derived from protein and fat digestion; and many vitamin and mineral molecules as well.

For the stage production, the manager might design multiple wings that the actors could crowd into, a dozen at a time. A mechanical genius might somehow design conveyor-belt wings that would actively sweep up the actors as they approached. The absorptive system is no such fantasy; the lowly "gut" is actually one of the most elegantly designed organ systems in the body. In 10 feet of small intestine, it provides a surface area equivalent to a quarter of a football field, which engulfs and absorbs the nutrient molecules. To remove the molecules rapidly and provide room for more to be absorbed, a rush of circulating blood continuously washes the underside of this surface, carrying the absorbed nutrients away to the liver and other parts of the body.

absorption: the taking up of nutrients into the intestinal cells.

ANATOMY OF THE ABSORPTIVE SYSTEM

The inner surface of the small intestine looks smooth and slippery, but viewed through a microscope, it turns out to be wrinkled into hundreds of folds. Each fold, in turn, is contoured into thousands of nipplelike projections, as numerous as the hairs on velvet fabric. These small intestinal projections are the villi. A single villus, magnified still more, turns out to be composed of hundreds of cells, each covered with its own microscopic hairs, the microvilli (see Figure 3–5 on p. 94). In the crevices between the villi lie the crypts—tubular glands that secrete the intestinal juices into the small intestine.

The villi are in constant motion. Each villus is lined by a thin sheet of muscle, so it can wave, squirm, and wriggle like the tentacles of a sea anemone. Any nutrient molecule small enough to be absorbed is trapped among the microvilli that coat the cells and then drawn into the cells. Some partially digested nutrients are caught in the microvilli, digested further by enzymes there, and then absorbed into the cells. Figure 3–6 (on p. 95) describes how nutrients are absorbed by diffusion, facilitated diffusion, or active transport.

The body's two transport systems—the bloodstream and the lymphatic system—supply vessels to each villus, as shown in Figure 3–5. When a nutrient molecule has crossed the cell of a villus, it may enter either the lymph or the blood, but before following nutrients through the body, we must look more closely at the digestive cells themselves.

villi (VILL-ee, VILL-eye): fingerlike projections from the folds of the small intestine; singular **villus**.

microvilli (MY-cro-VILL-ee, MY-cro-VILL-eye): tiny, hairlike projections on each cell of every villus that can trap nutrient particles and transport them into the cells; singular **microvillus**.

crypts: tubular glands that lie between the intestinal villi and secrete intestinal juices into the small intestine.

A CLOSER LOOK AT THE INTESTINAL CELLS

One of the beauties of the digestive tract is that it is selective. Materials that are nutritive for the body are broken down into particles that can be assimilated into the bloodstream. Most of the materials that are not nutritive are left undigested and pass out the other end of the digestive tract. The cells of the villi are among the most amazing in the body, for they recognize and select the nutrients the body needs and regulate their absorption. A close look at these cells is worthwhile, because it will help to explode a common misconception about nutrition: that you have to do anything to ensure that your digestive tract does its job. Nothing could be further from the truth.

The problem of food contaminants, which may be absorbed defenselessly by the body, is the subject of Chapter 19.

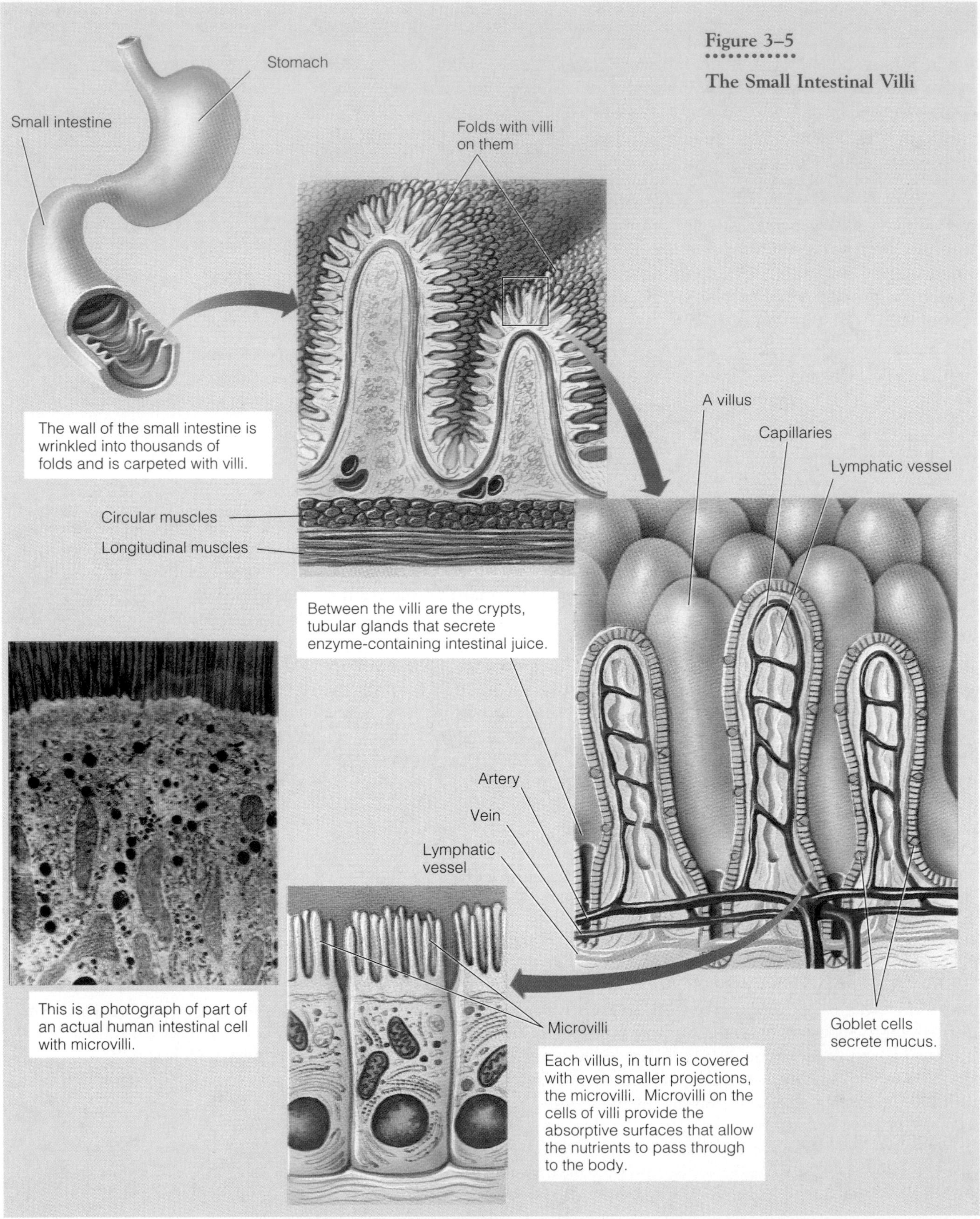

Stomach
Small intestine
Folds with villi on them
The wall of the small intestine is wrinkled into thousands of folds and is carpeted with villi.
Circular muscles
Longitudinal muscles
A villus
Capillaries
Lymphatic vessel
Between the villi are the crypts, tubular glands that secrete enzyme-containing intestinal juice.
Artery
Vein
Lymphatic vessel
This is a photograph of part of an actual human intestinal cell with microvilli.
Microvilli
Each villus, in turn is covered with even smaller projections, the microvilli. Microvilli on the cells of villi provide the absorptive surfaces that allow the nutrients to pass through to the body.
Goblet cells secrete mucus.

Figure 3–5

The Small Intestinal Villi

Figure 3–6

Absorption of Nutrients

Absorption of nutrients into intestinal cells typically occurs by diffusion, facilitated diffusion, or active transport.

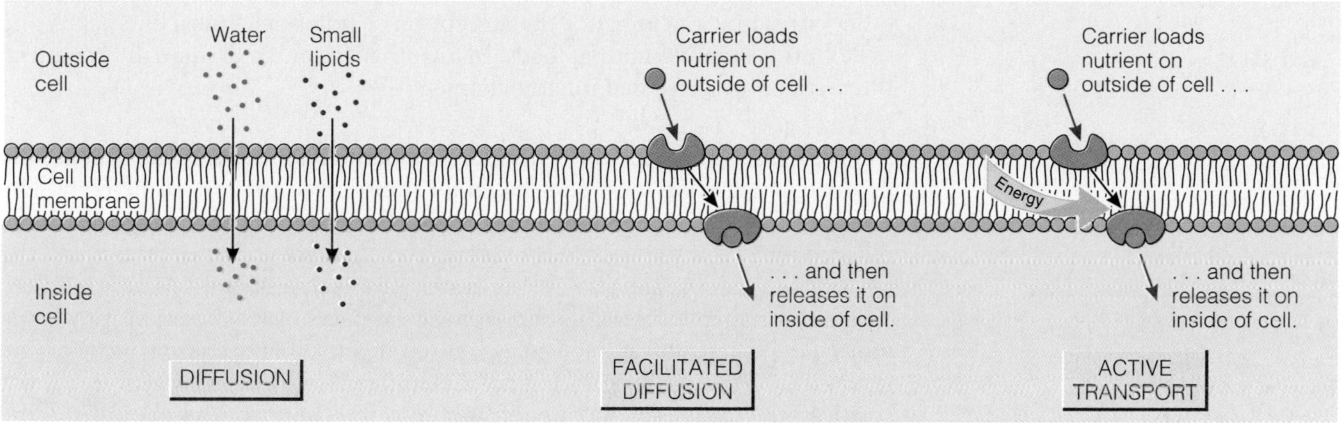

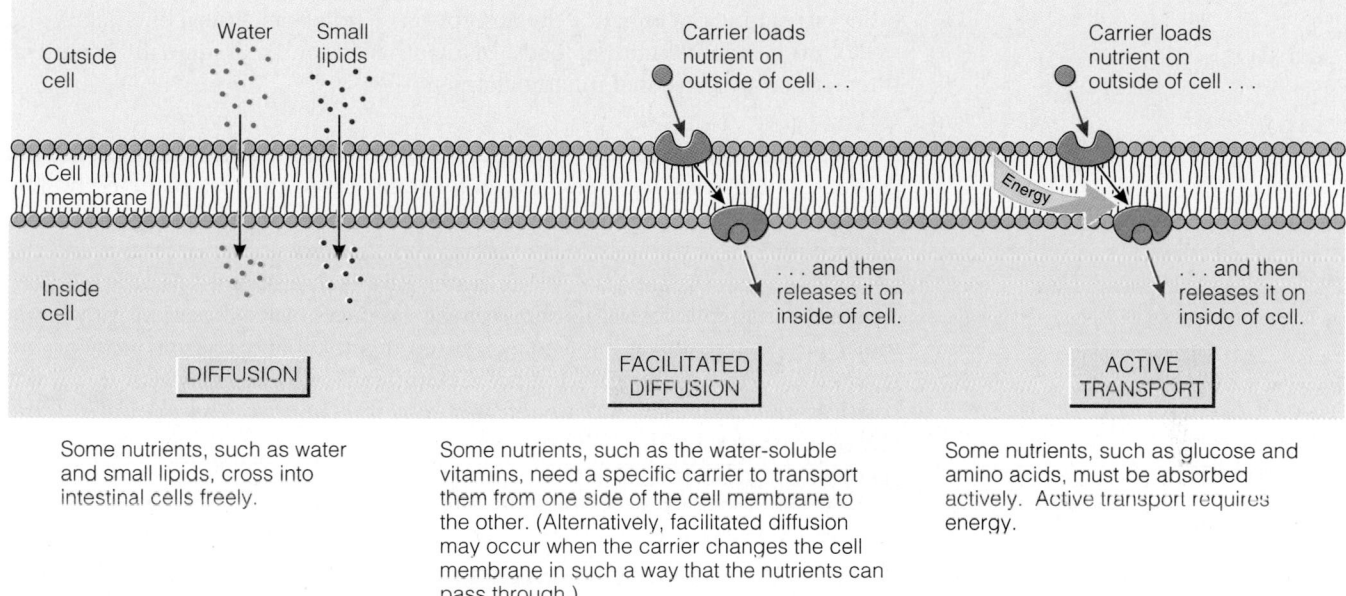

Some nutrients, such as water and small lipids, cross into intestinal cells freely.

Some nutrients, such as the water-soluble vitamins, need a specific carrier to transport them from one side of the cell membrane to the other. (Alternatively, facilitated diffusion may occur when the carrier changes the cell membrane in such a way that the nutrients can pass through.)

Some nutrients, such as glucose and amino acids, must be absorbed actively. Active transport requires energy.

The Cells' Capabilities As already described, each cell of a villus is coated with thousands of microvilli, which project from the cell's membrane (review Figure 3–5). In these microvilli and in the membrane lie hundreds of different kinds of enzymes and "pumps," which recognize and act on different nutrients. Descriptions of specific enzymes and "pumps" for each nutrient are presented in the following chapters where appropriate, but the point here is that the cells are equipped to handle all kinds and combinations of foods and nutrients.

Specialization in the GI Tract A further refinement of the system is that the cells of successive portions of the intestinal tract are specialized to absorb different nutrients. The nutrients that are ready for absorption early are absorbed near the top of the tract; those that take longer to be digested are absorbed farther down. The rate at which digested nutrients travel through the GI tract is finely adjusted to maximize their availability to the appropriate absorptive segments of the tract. Medical and health professionals who deal with digestion learn the specialized absorptive functions of different parts of the GI tract so that if one part becomes dysfunctional, the diet can be adjusted accordingly.

The Myth of "Food Combining" The idea that people should not eat certain food combinations (for example, fruit and meat) at the same meal, because the digestive system cannot handle more than one task at a time, is a myth. The art of "food combining" (which actually emphasizes "food separating") is based on this idea, and it represents faulty logic and a gross underestimation of the body's capabilities. If a person ate only fruit, the carbohydrate enzymes for digestion and carriers for absorption would be extremely busy while those for protein and fat sat idle. In fact, the contrary is often true; foods eaten together can enhance each other's use by the body. For example, vitamin C in a pineapple or other citrus fruit can enhance the absorption of iron from a meal of chicken and rice or other iron-containing foods. Many other instances of mutually beneficial interactions are presented in later chapters.

Preparing Nutrients for Transport Once inside the intestinal cells, the products of digestion must be released for transport to the rest of the body. The water-soluble nutrients (including the smaller products of fat digestion) are released directly into the bloodstream via the capillaries. The larger fats and the fat-soluble vitamins are insoluble in water, however, and blood is mostly water. The intestinal cells assemble many of the products of fat digestion into larger molecules. These larger molecules cluster together, and special proteins are inserted into their surfaces, forming chylomicrons. These chylomicrons cannot pass into the capillaries and are released into the lymphatic system instead; the chylomicrons move through the lymph and later enter the bloodstream at a point near the heart.

Chylomicrons (kye-lo-MY-cronz) are described in Chapter 5.

The Circulatory Systems

Once a nutrient has entered the bloodstream, it may be transported to any part of the body and thus become available to any of the cells, from the tips of the toes to the roots of the hair. The circulatory systems are arranged to deliver nutrients wherever they are needed.

THE VASCULAR SYSTEM

The vascular, or blood circulatory, system is a closed system of vessels through which blood flows continuously in a figure eight, with the heart serving as a pump at the crossover point (see Figure 3–7). As the blood circulates through this system, it picks up and delivers materials as needed.

All the body tissues derive oxygen and nutrients from the blood and deposit carbon dioxide and other wastes into it. The lungs exchange carbon dioxide (which leaves the blood to be exhaled) and oxygen (which enters the blood to be delivered to all cells). The digestive system supplies the nutrients to be picked up. In the kidneys, wastes other than carbon dioxide are filtered out of the blood to be excreted in the urine (see Figure 3–8 on p. 98).

Blood leaving the right side of the heart circulates by way of arteries into the lung capillaries and then back through veins to the left side of the heart. The left side of the heart then pumps the blood out through arteries to all systems of the body. The blood circulates in the capillaries, where it exchanges material with the cells, and then collects into veins, which return it again to the right side of the heart. In short, blood travels this simple route:

- Heart to arteries to capillaries to veins to heart.

artery: a vessel that carries blood away from the heart.

capillary (CAP-ill-ary): a small vessel that branches from an artery. Capillaries connect arteries to veins. Exchange of oxygen, nutrients, and waste materials takes place across capillary walls.

vein: a vessel that carries blood back to the heart.

Figure 3–7

The Vascular System

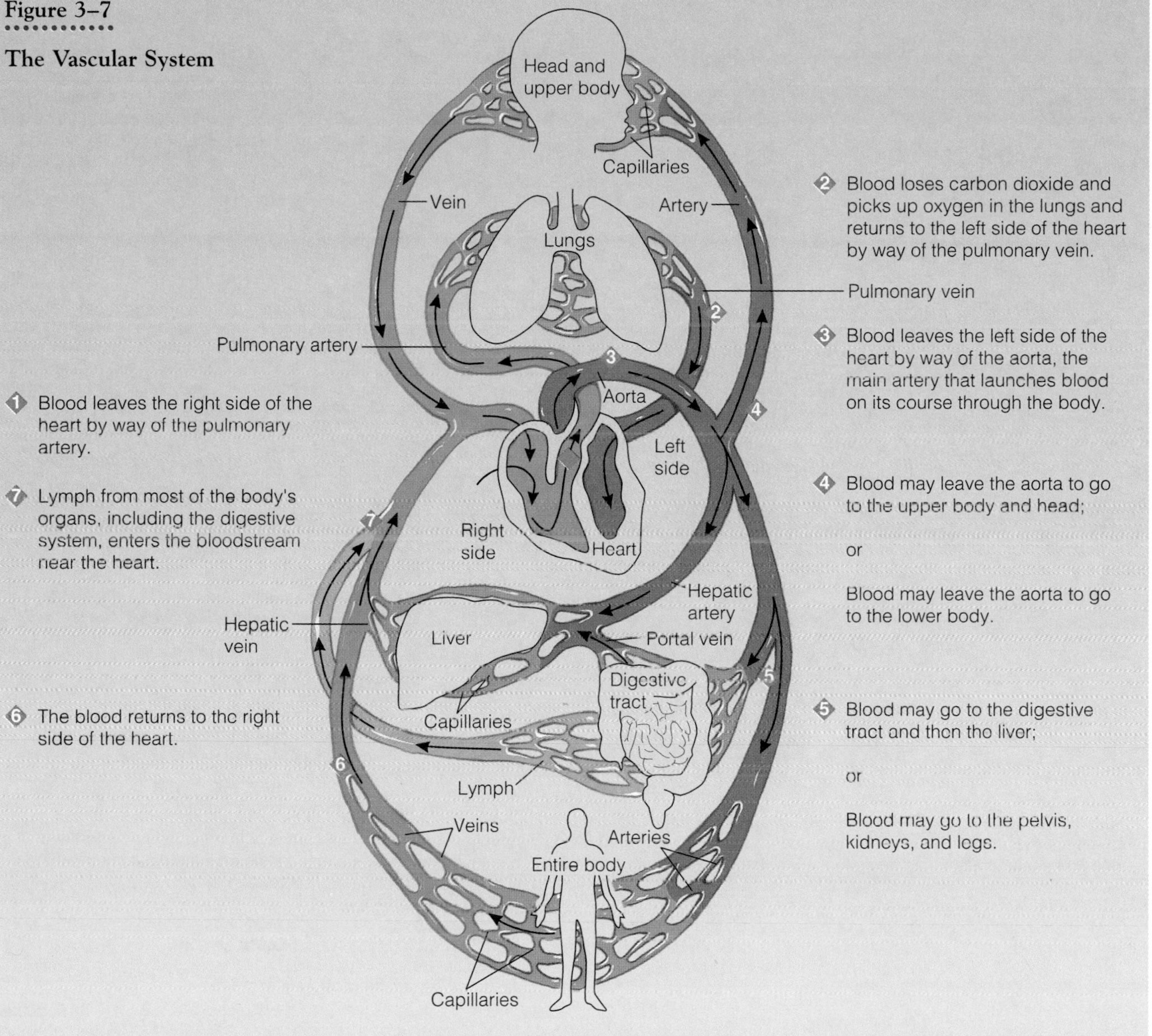
Head and upper body
Capillaries
Vein
Artery
Lungs
Pulmonary vein
Pulmonary artery
Aorta
Left side
Right side
Heart
Hepatic artery
Hepatic vein
Liver
Portal vein
Digestive tract
Capillaries
Lymph
Veins
Arteries
Entire body
Capillaries
1 Blood leaves the right side of the heart by way of the pulmonary artery.
2 Blood loses carbon dioxide and picks up oxygen in the lungs and returns to the left side of the heart by way of the pulmonary vein.
3 Blood leaves the left side of the heart by way of the aorta, the main artery that launches blood on its course through the body.
4 Blood may leave the aorta to go to the upper body and head;
or
Blood may leave the aorta to go to the lower body.
5 Blood may go to the digestive tract and then the liver;
or
Blood may go to the pelvis, kidneys, and legs.
6 The blood returns to the right side of the heart.
7 Lymph from most of the body's organs, including the digestive system, enters the bloodstream near the heart.

The routing of the blood past the digestive system has a special feature. The blood is carried to the digestive system (as to all organs) by way of an artery, which (as in all organs) branches into capillaries to reach every cell. Blood leaving the digestive system, however, goes by way of a vein, not back to the heart, but to another organ—the liver. This vein *again* branches into *capillaries,* so that every cell of the liver also has access to the blood carried by the vein. Blood leaving the liver then *again* collects into a vein, which returns to the heart.

The vein that collects blood from the GI tract and conducts it to capillaries in the liver is the portal vein.
portal = gateway

The vein that collects blood from the liver capillaries and returns it to the heart is the hepatic vein.
hepatic = liver

Figure 3–8

A Nephron, One of the Kidney's Many Functioning Units

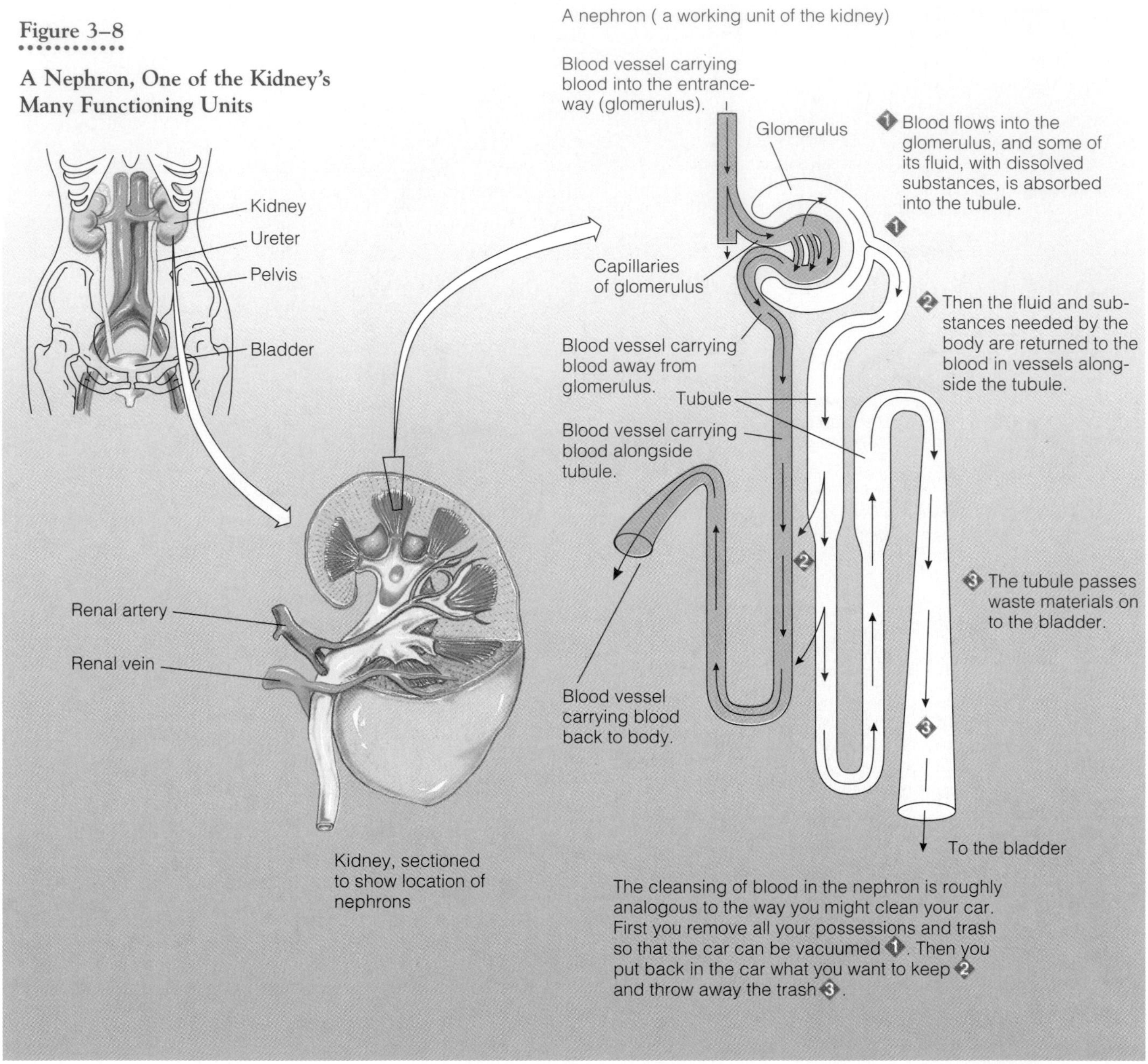
Kidney
Ureter
Pelvis
Bladder
Renal artery
Renal vein
Kidney, sectioned to show location of nephrons
A nephron (a working unit of the kidney)
Blood vessel carrying blood into the entrance-way (glomerulus).
Glomerulus
1 Blood flows into the glomerulus, and some of its fluid, with dissolved substances, is absorbed into the tubule.
Capillaries of glomerulus
2 Then the fluid and substances needed by the body are returned to the blood in vessels alongside the tubule.
Blood vessel carrying blood away from glomerulus.
Tubule
Blood vessel carrying blood alongside tubule.
3 The tubule passes waste materials on to the bladder.
Blood vessel carrying blood back to body.
To the bladder
The cleansing of blood in the nephron is roughly analogous to the way you might clean your car. First you remove all your possessions and trash so that the car can be vacuumed 1. Then you put back in the car what you want to keep 2 and throw away the trash 3.

The route is:

- Heart to arteries to capillaries (in intestines) to vein to capillaries (in liver) to vein to heart.

An anatomist studying this system knows there must be a reason for this special arrangement. The liver is placed in the circulation at this point so that it will have the first chance at the materials absorbed from the GI tract. In fact, the

Figure 3–9

The Liver

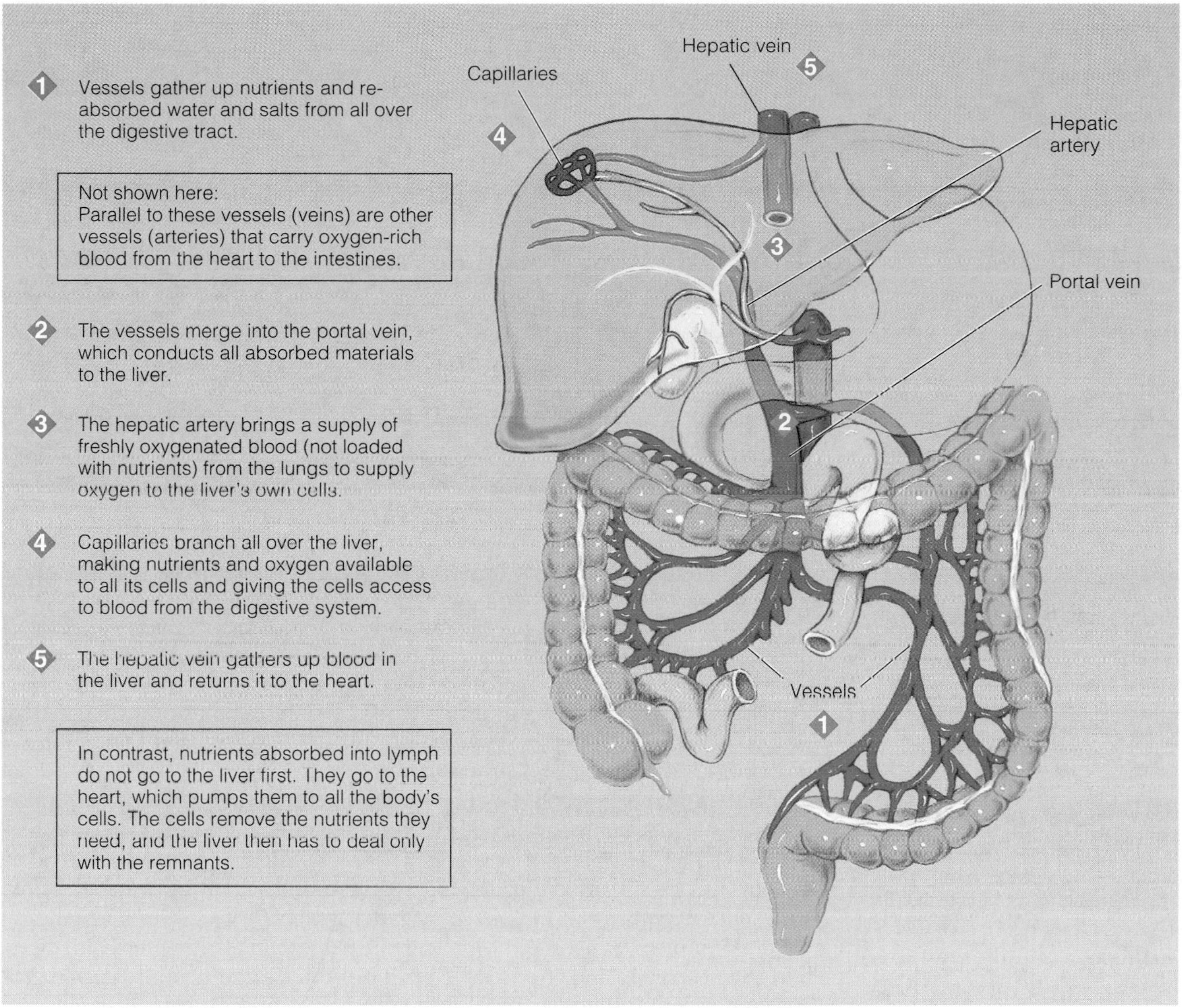
1 Vessels gather up nutrients and reabsorbed water and salts from all over the digestive tract.
Not shown here:
Parallel to these vessels (veins) are other vessels (arteries) that carry oxygen-rich blood from the heart to the intestines.
2 The vessels merge into the portal vein, which conducts all absorbed materials to the liver.
3 The hepatic artery brings a supply of freshly oxygenated blood (not loaded with nutrients) from the lungs to supply oxygen to the liver's own cells.
4 Capillaries branch all over the liver, making nutrients and oxygen available to all its cells and giving the cells access to blood from the digestive system.
5 The hepatic vein gathers up blood in the liver and returns it to the heart.
In contrast, nutrients absorbed into lymph do not go to the liver first. They go to the heart, which pumps them to all the body's cells. The cells remove the nutrients they need, and the liver then has to deal only with the remnants.
Hepatic vein
5
Capillaries
4
Hepatic artery
3
Portal vein
2
Vessels
1

liver has many jobs to do in preparing the absorbed nutrients for use by the body. It is the body's major metabolic organ.

You might guess that, in addition, the liver stands as gatekeeper to waylay intruders that might otherwise harm the heart or brain. Perhaps this is why, when people ingest poisons that succeed in passing the first barrier (the intestinal cells), the liver quite often suffers the damage—from the hepatitis virus, from drugs such as barbiturates or alcohol, from poisons, and from contaminants such as mercury. Perhaps, in fact, you have been undervaluing your liver, not knowing what heroic tasks it quietly performs for you. Figure 3–9 shows the liver's key position in nutrient transport.

lymphatic (lim-FAT-ic) system: a loosely organized system of vessels and ducts that convey fluids toward the heart; the GI part of the lymphatic system carries the products of digestion into the bloodstream.

lymph (LIMF): a clear yellowish fluid that resembles blood without the red blood cells; lymph from the GI tract transports fat and fat-soluble vitamins to the bloodstream via lymphatic vessels.

The duct that conveys lymph toward the heart is the thoracic (thor-ASS-ic) duct. The subclavian vein connects this duct with the right upper chamber of the heart, providing a passageway by which lymph can be returned to the vascular system.

THE LYMPHATIC SYSTEM

The lymphatic system provides a one-way route for fluid from the tissue spaces to enter the blood. Lymph fluid circulates between the cells of the body and collects into tiny vessels. Lymph is almost identical to blood except that it contains no red blood cells or platelets, because they cannot escape through the blood vessel walls.

The lymphatic system has no pump; instead, lymph is squeezed from one portion of the body to another like water in a sponge, as muscles contract and create pressure here and there. Ultimately, much of the lymph collects in a large duct behind the heart. This duct terminates in a vein that conducts the lymph toward the heart. Thus materials from the GI tract that enter lymphatic vessels (large fats and fat-soluble vitamins) ultimately enter the blood circulatory system, circulating through arteries, capillaries, and veins like the other nutrients, with a notable exception—they bypass the liver at first.

Once inside the vascular system, the nutrients can travel freely to any destination and can be taken into cells and used as needed. What becomes of them is described in later chapters.

Regulation of Digestion and Absorption

homeostasis (HOME-ee-oh-STAY-sis): the maintenance of constant internal conditions (such as blood chemistry, temperature, and blood pressure) by the body's control systems. A homeostatic system is constantly reacting to external forces so as to maintain limits set by the body's needs.
homeo = the same
stasis = staying

Factors influencing GI function:
- Physical immaturity.
- Aging.
- Illness.
- Nutrition.

There is nothing random about digestion and absorption; they are coordinated in every detail. The ability of the digestive tract to handle its ever-changing contents routinely illustrates an important physiological principle that governs the way all living things function—the principle of homeostasis. Simply stated, conditions have to stay about the same for an organism to survive; if they deviate too far from the norm, the organism must "do something" to bring them back to normal. The body's regulation of digestion is one example of homeostatic regulation. The body also regulates its temperature, its blood pressure, and all other aspects of its blood chemistry in similar ways.

The following paragraphs describe the regulation of digestion and absorption in healthy adults, but many factors can influence normal GI function. For example, peristalsis and sphincter action are poorly coordinated in newborns, and so infants tend to "spit up" during the first several months of life. Older adults often experience constipation, in part because the intestinal wall loses strength and elasticity with age, which slows GI motility. Diseases can also interfere with digestion and absorption and often lead to malnutrition. Lack of nourishment, in general, and lack of certain dietary constituents such as fiber, in particular, alter the structure and function of GI cells. Quite simply, GI tract health depends on food.

hormones: chemical messengers. Hormones are secreted by a variety of glands in response to altered conditions in the body. Each hormone travels to one or more specific target tissues or organs, where it elicits a specific response to restore normal conditions. In general, a gastrointestinal hormone is called an enterogastrone (EN-ter-oh-GAS-trone).*

GASTROINTESTINAL HORMONES AND NERVE PATHWAYS

Two intricate and sensitive systems coordinate all the digestive and absorptive processes: the hormonal (or endocrine) system and the nervous system. The contents of the GI tract either stimulate or inhibit digestive secretions by way of

*The term *enterogastrone* refers specifically to any hormone that inhibits gastric secretions, including secretin, cholecystokinin (CCK), and gastric-inhibitory peptide; more broadly, the term refers to any hormone released from the intestine.

messages that are carried from one section of the GI tract to another by both hormones and nerve pathways.

Appendix A presents a brief summary of the body's hormonal system and nervous system.

Notice that the kinds of regulation that will be described are all examples of *feedback* mechanisms. A certain condition demands a response. The response changes that condition, and the change then cuts off the response. Thus the system is self-corrective. Examples follow.

The stomach normally maintains a pH between 1.5 and 1.7. How does it stay that way? One of the regulators of the stomach pH is the hormone gastrin, secreted by cells in the stomach wall. The entrance of food into the stomach stimulates these cells to release gastrin, which, in turn, stimulates other stomach glands to secrete the components of hydrocholoric acid. When pH 1.5 is reached, the acid itself turns off the gastrin-producing cells, so that they stop releasing the hormone. Once the hormone stimulus has ceased, the glands stop producing hydrochloric acid. Thus the system adjusts itself.

gastrin: a hormone secreted by cells in the stomach wall. Target organ: the stomach. Response: secretion of gastric juice.

Another regulator consists of nerve receptors in the stomach wall. These receptors respond to the presence of food and stimulate both the gastric glands to secrete juices and the muscles to contract. As the stomach empties, the receptors are no longer stimulated, the flow of juices slows, and the stomach quiets down.

The pyloric sphincter opens to let out a little chyme, then closes again. How does it know when to open and close? When the pyloric sphincter relaxes, acidic chyme slips through. The cells of the pyloric muscle on the intestinal side sense the acid, causing the pyloric sphincter to close tightly. Only after the chyme has been neutralized by pancreatic bicarbonate and the medium surrounding the pyloric sphincter has become alkaline can the muscle relax again. This process ensures that the chyme will be released slowly enough to be neutralized as it flows through the small intestine. This is important, because the small intestine has less of a mucous coating than the stomach does and so is not as well protected from acid.

As the chyme enters the intestine, the pancreas adds bicarbonate to it, so that the intestinal contents always remain at a slightly alkaline pH. How does the pancreas know how much to add? The presence of chyme stimulates the cells of the duodenum wall to release the hormone secretin into the blood. As this hormone circulates through the pancreas, it stimulates the pancreas to release its bicarbonate-rich juices. Thus, whenever the duodenum signals that acidic chyme is present, the pancreas responds by sending bicarbonate to neutralize it. When the need has been met, the secretin cells of the duodenal wall are no longer stimulated to release the hormone, the hormone no longer flows through the blood, the pancreas no longer receives the message, and it stops sending pancreatic juice. Nerves also regulate pancreatic secretions.

secretin (see-CREET-in): a hormone produced by cells in the duodenum wall. Target organ: the pancreas. Response: secretion of bicarbonate-rich pancreatic juice.

Pancreatic secretions contain a mixture of enzymes to digest carbohydrate, fat, and protein. How does the pancreas know how much of each type of enzyme to provide? This is one of the most interesting questions physiologists have asked. The question awaits final answer, but clearly the pancreas does know, somehow, what its owner has been eating, and it secretes enzyme mixtures tailored to deal with the food mixtures that have been arriving lately (over the last several days). Enzyme activity changes proportionately in response to the amounts of carbohydrate, fat, and protein in the diet.[4] If a person has been eating mostly carbohydrates, the pancreas makes and secretes mostly carbohydrases; if the person's diet has been high in fat, the pancreas produces more lipases; and so forth. Presumably, hormones from the GI tract, secreted in response to meals, keep the pancreas informed as to its digestive tasks. The day or two lag between the time a person's diet changes and the time digestion of the new diet becomes efficient explains why dietary changes can "upset digestion" and should be made gradually.

When fat is present in the intestine, the gallbladder contracts to squirt bile into the intestine to emulsify the fat. How does the gallbladder get the message that fat is present? Fat in the intestine stimulates cells of the intestinal wall to release the hormone cholecystokinin (CCK). This hormone, traveling by way of the blood to the gallbladder, stimulates it to contract, releasing bile into the small intestine. Once the fat in the intestine is emulsified and enzymes have begun to work on it, the fat no longer provokes release of the hormone, and the message to contract is canceled.

cholecystokinin (coal-ee-sis-toe-KINE-in), or CCK: a hormone produced by cells of the intestinal wall. Target organ: the gallbladder. Response: release of bile and slowing of GI motility.

Fat takes longer to digest than carbohydrate does. When fat is present, intestinal motility slows to allow time for its digestion. How does the intestine know when to slow down? Cholecystokinin and gastric-inhibitory peptide slow GI tract motility. By slowing the digestive process, fat helps to maintain a pace that will allow all reactions to reach completion. Gastric-inhibitory peptide also inhibits gastric acid secretion. Hormonal and nervous mechanisms like these account for much of the body's ability to adapt to changing conditions.

gastric-inhibitory peptide: a hormone produced by the intestine. Target organ: the stomach. Response: slowing of the secretion of gastric juices and of GI motility.

Once a person has started to learn the answers to questions like these, it may be hard to stop. Some people devote their whole lives to the study of physiology. For now, however, these few examples will be enough to illustrate how all the processes throughout the digestive system are precisely and automatically regulated without any conscious effort.

THE SYSTEM AT ITS BEST

This chapter has described the anatomy of the digestive tract on several levels: the sequence of digestive organs, the cells and structures of the villi, and the selective machinery of the cell membranes. The intricate architecture of the GI tract makes it sensitive and responsive to conditions in its environment. Knowing what the optimal conditions are will help you to promote the best functioning of the system.

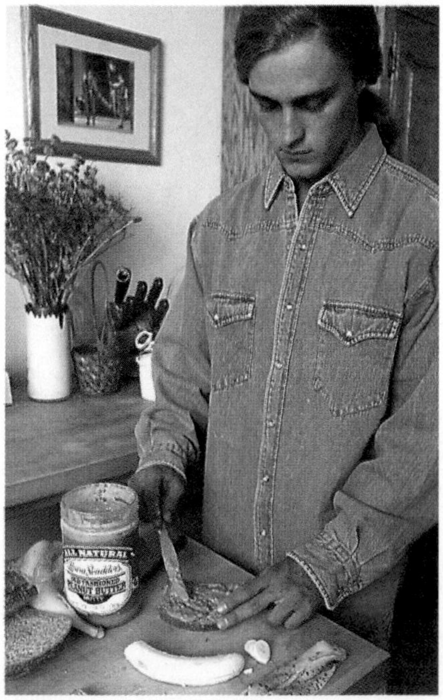

To become part of your body, food must first be digested and absorbed.

One indispensable condition is good health of the digestive tract itself. This health is affected by such lifestyle factors as sleep, physical activity, and state of mind. Adequate sleep allows for repair, maintenance of tissue, and removal of wastes that might impair efficient functioning. Activity promotes healthy muscle tone. Mental state profoundly affects digestion and absorption through the activity of regulatory nerves and hormones; for healthy digestion, you should be relaxed and tranquil at mealtimes.

Another factor is the kind of meals you eat. Among the characteristics of meals that promote optimal absorption of nutrients are those mentioned in Chapter 2: balance, moderation, variety, and adequacy. Balance and moderation require having neither too much nor too little of anything. For example, too much fat is harmful, but some fat is needed to slow down intestinal motility, permitting time for absorption of some of the nutrients that are slow to be absorbed.

Variety is important for many reasons, but partly because some food constituents interfere with nutrient absorption. For example, some compounds that occur in whole-grain cereals, certain leafy green vegetables, and legumes bind with minerals, so, to some extent, the minerals in those foods may become "unavailable." This does not mean that these high-fiber foods are undesirable;

they are rightly prized for their nutrient contributions. It does mean, though, that people who use cereals, leafy greens, and legumes to the exclusion of other foods may be obtaining fewer minerals from their diets than they would if they were to vary their choices. They might want to exercise moderation in their use of these high-fiber foods.

As for adequacy—in a sense, this entire book is about dietary adequacy. But here, at the end of this chapter, is a good place to underline the interdependence of the nutrients. It could almost be said that every nutrient depends on every other. All the nutrients work together and are all present in the cells of a healthy digestive tract. To maintain health and promote the functions of the GI tract, you should make balance, moderation, variety, and adequacy features of every day's menus.

Study Questions

1. Describe the problems involved with digesting food and the solutions offered by the human body.
2. Describe the path food follows as it travels through the digestive system. Summarize the muscular actions that take place along the way.
3. Name five organs that secrete digestive juices. How do the juices and enzymes facilitate digestion?
4. Describe the problems involved with absorbing nutrients and the solutions offered by the small intestine.
5. How is blood routed through the digestive system? Which nutrients enter the bloodstream directly? Which are first absorbed into the lymph?
6. Describe how the body coordinates and regulates the processes of digestion and absorption.
7. How does the composition of the diet influence the functioning of the GI tract?
8. What steps can you take to help your GI tract function at its best?

Notes

1. The length of the small intestine in living adults is almost 2½ times shorter than at death, when muscles are relaxed and elongated. W. F. Ganong, *Review of Medical Physiology*, (Norwalk, Conn.: Appleton & Lange, 1993), pp. 438–465; E. A. Shaffer, Disgestive system, physiology, and biochemistry, in *Encyclopedia of Human Biology* (San Diego: Academic Press, 1991), p. 76.
2. Committee on Dietary Allowances, *Recommended Dietary Allowances*, 10th ed. (Washington, D.C.: National Academy of Sciences, 1989), pp. 108–109.
3. M. B. Roberfroid and coauthors, Colonic microflora: Nutrition and health, *Nutrition Reviews* 53 (1995): 127–130; D. Kelly, R. Begbie, and T. P. King, Nutritional influences on interactions between bacteria and the small intestinal musoca, *Nutrition Research Reviews* 7 (1994): 233–257.
4. P. M. Brannon, Adaptation of the exocrine pancreas to diet, *Annual Review of Nutrition* 10 (1990): 85–105.

Common Digestive Problems

The facts of anatomy and physiology presented in Chapter 3 permit easy understanding of some common situations. Everyone, at one time or another, has to deal with choking on food, vomiting, diarrhea, constipation, belching, gas, and heartburn; and everyone is familiar with ulcers (the glossary on p. 106 defines these terms).

CHOKING ON FOOD

When someone chokes on food, it is because the food has slipped into the air passage and cut off breathing (see Figure H3–1). Food can lodge so securely in the trachea that it cuts off all air. No sound can be made, because the larynx is in the trachea and makes sounds only when air is pushed across it.

The choking scenario might read like this. A person is dining in a restaurant with friends. A chunk of food, usually meat, becomes lodged in his trachea so firmly that he cannot make a sound. Often he chooses to suffer alone rather than "make a scene in public." If he tries to communicate distress to his friends, he must depend on pantomime. The friends are bewildered by his antics and become terribly worried when the victim "faints" after a few minutes without air. They call for an ambulance. By the time the victim arrives at the hospital, however, he is dead from suffocation.

To help a person who is choking, first ask this critical question: "Can you make any sound at all?" If the victim makes a sound, relax. You have time to continue with your questioning to see what you can do to help; you are not going to have to make a quick decision. But whatever you do, don't hit him on the back—the particle may become lodged more firmly in his air passage. If the victim cannot make a sound, follow the procedures described in Figure H3–2. You would do well to take a life-saving course and practice these techniques, for you will have no time for hesitation once you are called on to perform this death-defying act.

Almost any food can cause choking, although some are cited more often than others: tough meats, hot dogs, nuts, grapes, carrots, hard candies, popcorn, and peanut butter. These foods are particularly difficult for young children to safely chew and swallow. Each year, more than 300 children in the United States choke to death. Always remain alert to the dangers of choking whenever young children are eating. To prevent choking, cut food into small pieces, chew thoroughly before swallowing, don't talk or laugh with food in your mouth, and don't eat when breathing hard.

VOMITING

Another common digestive mishap is vomiting. Vomiting can be a symptom of many different diseases or may arise in any situation that upsets the body's equilibrium, such as air or sea travel. For whatever reason, the waves of peristalsis reverse direction, and the contents of the stomach are propelled up through the esophagus to the mouth and expelled.

Figure H3–1

Normal Swallowing and Choking

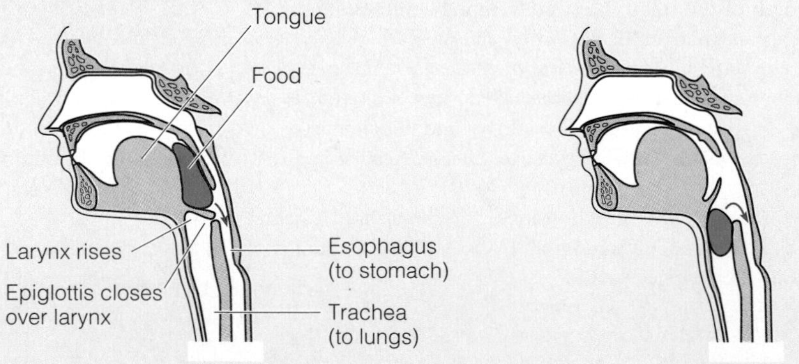

Swallowing. The epiglottis closes over the larynx, blocking entrance to the lungs via the trachea. The red arrow shows that food is heading down the esophagus normally.

Choking. A choking person cannot speak or gasp because food lodged in the trachea blocks the passage of air. The red arrow points to where the food should have gone to prevent choking.

- If the choking victim is an infant, lay her face down on your lap with her head firmly supported and held lower than her body.

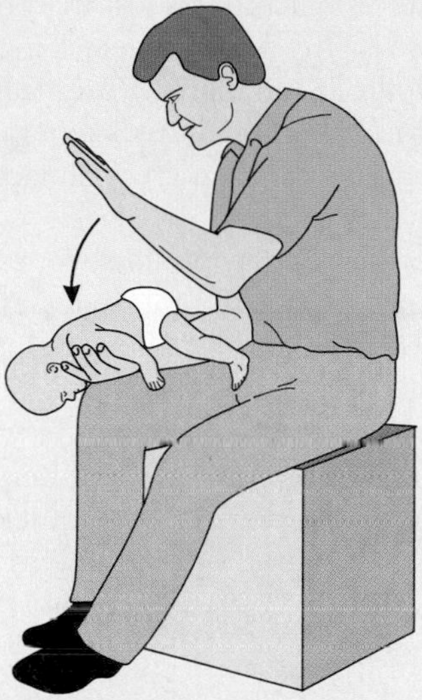

Administer five blows rapidly with the heel of your hand high between her shoulder blades.

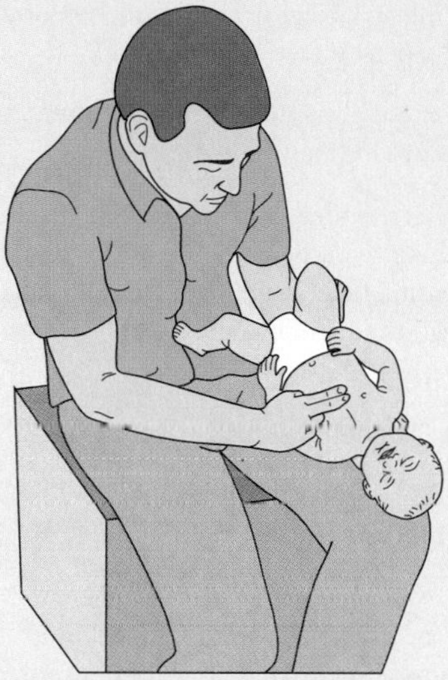

If that doesn't work, turn her over and deliver five quick downward thrusts over her sternum using two fingers.

- If the choking victim is an older child or adult, the strategy most likely to succeed is abdominal thrusts, sometimes called the Heimlich maneuver.

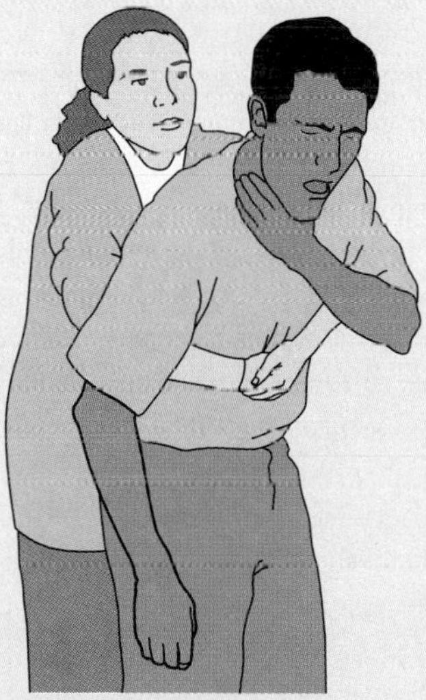

Stand behind the victim, and wrap your arms around him. Place the thumb side of one fist snugly against his body, slightly above the navel and below the rib cage. Grasp your fist with your other hand and give him a sudden strong hug inward and upward. Repeat thrusts as necessary.

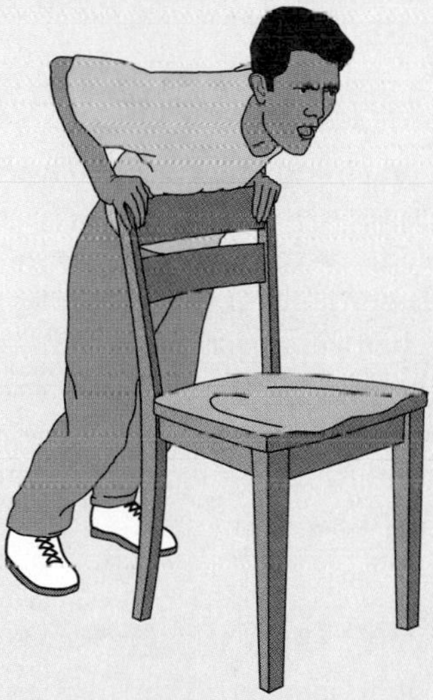

To self–administer first aid, place the thumb side of one fist slightly above the navel and below the rib cage, grasp the fist with your other hand, and then press inward and upward with a quick motion. If this is unsuccessful, quickly press your upper abdomen over any firm surface such as the back of a chair, a countertop, or a railing.

- If all else fails, open the mouth by grasping both the tongue and lower jaw and lifting. Then, and only if you can see the object, use your finger to sweep it out and begin rescue breathing.

Figure H3–2

First Aid for Choking

Source: Adapted from Committee on Pediatric Emergency Medicine, First aid for the choking child, *Pediatrics* 92 (1993): 477–479; H. J. Heimlich and M. H. Uhley, The Heimlich maneuver, *Clinical Symposia* 31 (1979): 1–32; H. J. Heimlich, Self-application of the Heimlich maneuver, *New England Journal of Medicine* 318 (1988): 714–715.

If vomiting continues long enough or is severe enough, the reverse peristalsis will extend beyond the stomach and carry the contents of the duodenum, with its green bile salts, into the stomach and then up the esophagus. Although certainly unpleasant and wearying for the nauseated person, vomiting such as this is no cause for alarm. Vomiting is one of the body's adaptive mechanisms to rid itself of something irritating. The best advice is to rest and drink small amounts of fluids as tolerated until the nausea subsides.

Vomiting can be serious, however, when large quantities of fluid are lost from the GI tract, causing dehydration. A physician's care may be needed in those cases. With massive fluid loss from the GI tract, all of the body's other fluids redistribute themselves so that, eventually, fluid is taken from every cell of the body. Leaving the cells with the fluid are salts that are absolutely essential to the life of the cells, and they must be replaced, which is difficult while the vomiting continues. Intravenous feedings of saline and glucose are frequently necessary while the physician is diagnosing the cause of the vomiting and instituting corrective therapy.

In an infant, vomiting is likely to become serious early in its course, and a physician should be contacted

Glossary

belch: the expulsion of gas from the stomach through the mouth.

colonic irrigation: the popular, but potentially harmful practice of "washing" the large intestine with a powerful enema machine.

constipation: the condition of having painful or difficult bowel movements (elapsed time between movements is not relevant).

defecate (DEF-uh-cate)**:** to move the bowels and eliminate waste.
defaecare = to remove dregs

diarrhea: the frequent passage of watery bowel movements.

heartburn: a burning sensation in the chest area caused by backflow of stomach acid into the esophagus.

Heimlich maneuver: a technique for removing an object from the trachea of a choking person (see Figure H3–2).

hemorrhoids: painful swelling of the veins surrounding the rectum.

hiccups: repeated cough-like sounds and jerks that are produced when an involuntary spasm of the diaphragm muscle sucks air down the windpipe; also spelled *hiccoughs*.

larynx: the voice box (see Figure H3–1).

peptic ulcer: an erosion in the mucous membrane of either the stomach (a gastric ulcer) or duodenum (a duodenal ulcer).

ulcer: an erosion in the topmost, and sometimes underlying, layers of cells in an area. See also *peptic ulcer*.

vomiting: expulsion of the contents of the stomach up through the esophagus to the mouth.

---

soon after onset. Infants have more fluid between their body cells than adults do, so more fluid can move readily into the digestive tract and be lost from the body. Consequently, the body water of infants becomes depleted and their body salt balance upset faster than in adults.

Self-induced vomiting, such as occurs in bulimia, also has serious consequences. (Bulimia nervosa is the subject of Highlight 9.) In addition to fluid and salt imbalances, repeated vomiting can cause irritation and infection of the pharynx, esophagus, and salivary glands; erosion of the teeth; and dental caries. The esophagus may rupture or tear, as may the stomach. Sometimes the eyes become red from pressure during vomiting. Bulimic behavior reflects underlying problems that require intervention.

Projectile vomiting is also serious. The contents of the stomach are expelled with such force that they leave the mouth in a wide arc like a bullet leaving a gun. This type of vomiting requires immediate medical attention.

DIARRHEA

Diarrhea is characterized by frequent, loose, watery stools. This sort of stool indicates that the intestinal contents have moved too quickly through the intestines for fluid absorption to take place, or that water has been drawn from the cells lining the intestinal tract and added to the food residue. Like vomiting, diarrhea can lead to considerable fluid and salt losses, but the composition of the fluids is different. Stomach fluids lost in vomiting are highly acidic, whereas intestinal fluids lost in diarrhea are nearly neutral. When fluid losses require medical attention, correct replacement is crucial.

For short bouts of diarrhea, rest and drink fluids to replace losses. If diarrhea continues, call for help. A medical evaluation is needed to identify and correct the underlying problem.[1] For an infant, get help promptly, for diarrhea may quickly lead to dehydration so severe as to require emergency medical treatment.

CONSTIPATION

Unlike diarrhea, constipation is generally not a cause for immediate concern. Each person's GI tract responds to food in its own way, with its own rhythm. Food is digested and the waste becomes ready for excretion in a predictable number of hours. Each GI tract thus has its own cycle, which depends on its owner's physical makeup and such environmental considerations as the type of food eaten, when it was eaten, and when the person's schedule allows time to defecate. Even when several days pass between movements, a person is not constipated, as long as these movements take place without discomfort. But if a movement is passed with difficulty, discomfort, or pain, then the person is constipated. The time that has elapsed since the previous bowel movement is irrelevant.

Often a person's lifestyle may cause constipation. If a person receives the signal to defecate and ignores it, the signal may not return for several hours. In the meantime, water continues to be withdrawn from the fecal matter, so that when the person does defecate, the bowel movement is dry and hard.

Careful review of daily habits may reveal the causes of the constipation. Being too busy to respond to the defecation signal is a common complaint. In that case, a person's daily regimen may need to be revised to allow time to have a bowel movement when the body sends its signal. One possibility is to go to bed earlier in order to rise earlier, allowing ample time for a leisurely breakfast and a movement.

Another cause of constipation is lack of physical activity.[2] In today's society many people drive cars or ride buses to work, stand at assembly lines or sit behind desks, and then sit in front of television sets in the evening. Increasing physical activity may require some rearrangement of one's lifestyle. People can work out in spas or health clubs; more simply, they can just park their cars a distance from the office and walk the extra blocks, or they can walk up several flights of stairs a day rather than taking the elevator. Such activity will improve the muscle tone, not just of the outer body, but also of the digestive tract.

Although constipation usually reflects lifestyle habits, in some cases it may be a side effect of medication or may reflect a medical problem such as tumors that are obstructing the passage of waste. If discomfort is associated with passing fecal matter, a physician's help should be sought to rule out disease. Once this has been done, dietary or other measures for correction can be considered.

One dietary measure that may be appropriate is to increase dietary fiber. Some fibers—those found in cereal products—help to prevent constipation by increasing fecal mass. In the GI tract, fiber attracts water, creating soft, bulky stools that stimulate bowel contractions to push the contents along. These contractions strengthen the intestinal muscles. The improved muscle tone, together with the water content of the stools, eases elimination, reducing the pressure in the rectal veins and helping to prevent hemorrhoids. Although the major impact of dietary fiber is on the colon, fiber acts as a bulking agent all along the intestine. Chapter 4 provides more information on fiber's role in maintaining a healthy colon and reducing the risks of colon cancer and diverticulosis.

Drinking plenty of water in conjunction with eating high-fiber foods also helps with constipation. The increased bulk physically stimulates the upper GI tract, promoting peristalsis throughout.

Eating prunes can also be helpful. Prunes are high in fiber and also contain a laxative substance.* If a morning defecation is desired, a person can drink prune juice at bedtime; if the evening is preferred, the person can drink prune juice with breakfast.

Adding fat to the diet can relieve some constipation by stimulating the hormone cholecystokinin, which summons bile into the duodenum. Bile's high salt content draws water from the intestinal wall, which stimulates peristalsis and softens the fecal matter.

These suggested changes in lifestyle or diet should correct chronic constipation without the use of laxatives, enemas, or mineral oil, although television commercials often try to persuade people otherwise. One of the fallacies often perpetrated by television commercials is that one person's successful use of a product is a good recommendation for others to use that product.

As a matter of fact, even diet changes that relieve constipation for one person may increase the constipation of another. For instance, increasing fiber intake stimulates peristalsis and helps the person with a sluggish colon. Some people, though, have a spastic type of constipation, in which peristalsis promotes strong contractions that close off a segment of the colon and prevent passage; for these people, increasing fiber intake would be exactly the wrong thing to do.

A person who seems to need products such as laxatives should seek a physician's opinion. Advice from friends or alternative medicine practitioners may cause more harm than good. One potentially harmful but currently popular practice that is being promoted by some alternative medicine practitioners is colonic irrigation—the internal washing of the large intestine with a powerful enema machine. Such an extreme cleansing is not only unnecessary, but the force of the machine can rupture the intestine. Less extreme practices can cause problems, too. Frequent use of laxatives and enemas can lead to dependency; can upset the body's fluid, salt, and mineral balances; and, in the case of mineral oil, can interfere with the absorption of fat-soluble vitamins. (Mineral oil dissolves the vitamins, but is not itself absorbed; instead, it leaves the body, carrying the vitamins with it.)

*This substance is dihydroxyphenyl isatin.

BELCHING AND GAS

Many people complain of problems that they attribute to excessive gas. For some, belching is the complaint. Others blame intestinal gas for abdominal discomforts and embarrassment. Most people believe that the problems occur after they eat certain foods. This may be the case with intestinal gas, but belching results from swallowing air. The best advice for belching seems to be to eat slowly, chew thoroughly, and relax while eating.

Everyone swallows a little bit of air with each mouthful of food, but people who eat too fast may swallow too much air and then have to belch. Ill-fitting dentures, carbonated beverages, and chewing gum can also contribute to the swallowing of air with resultant belching. Occasionally, belching can be a sign of a more serious disorder, such as gallbladder pain, colonic distress, or an impending obstruction of a coronary blood vessel.

People who eat or drink too fast may also trigger hiccups, the repeated spasms that produce a cough-like sound and jerky movement. Normally, hiccups soon subside and are of no medical significance, but they can be bothersome. The most effective cure is to hold the breath for as long as possible, which helps to relieve the spasms of the diaphragm.

Little is known about intestinal gas, but techniques for collecting gas directly from the abdomen have allowed researchers to gain some knowledge. While expelling gas can be a humiliating experience, it is quite normal. (People experiencing painful bloating from malabsorption diseases, however, require medical treatment.) Healthy people expel several hundred milliliters of gas several times a day. Almost all (99 percent) of the gases expelled—nitrogen, oxygen, hydrogen, methane, and carbon dioxide—are odorless. The remaining "volatile" gases are the infamous ones.

Foods that produce gas usually must be determined individually. The most common offenders are foods rich in the carbohydrates—sugars, starches, and fibers. When partially digested carbohydrates reach the large intestine, bacteria digest them, giving off gas as a by-product. People can test foods suspected of forming gas by omitting them individually for a trial period and seeing if there is any improvement.

One aspect of gas may offer an important medical opportunity. An association observed in methane-producing people may help in the early diagnosis of colon cancer. Twice as many people with colon cancer produce methane as members of the general population. Methane-producing people may have a high risk of cancer because the changes in acid balance associated with methane production may favor cancer formation.[3] In addition, researchers believe that methane production increases in response to the presence of the tumor.[4]

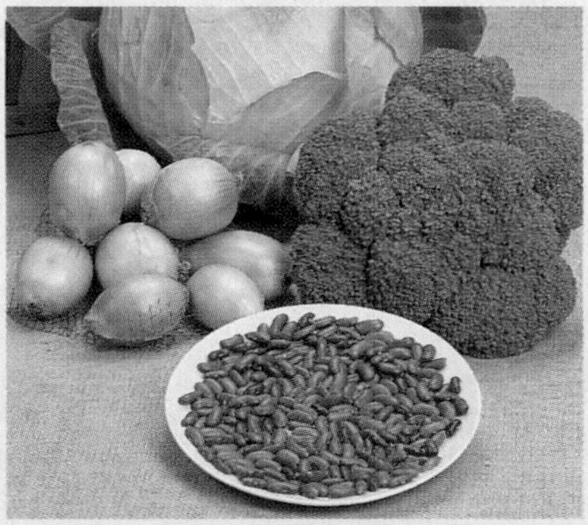

Beans, broccoli, cabbage, and onions produce gas in many people. People troubled by gas need to determine which foods bother them and then eat those foods in moderation.

HEARTBURN AND "ACID INDIGESTION"

Almost everyone has experienced heartburn at one time or another, usually after a meal. Heartburn is the painful sensation a person feels when the cardiac sphincter fails to prevent the stomach contents from refluxing into the esophagus. This may happen if a person eats or drinks too much (or both): back-pressure from the stomach forces food up into the esophagus. Tight clothing and even changes of position (lying down, bending over) can cause it, too, as can some medications and smoking. A defect of the cardiac sphincter itself is a possible, but less likely cause.

If the heartburn is not caused by an anatomical defect, treatment is fairly simple. Tips for people suffering from heartburn include the following:

- Eat small meals.
- Drink liquids one hour before or one hour after meals.
- Refrain from lying down or bending over and from wearing tight-fitting clothing, particularly after a meal.
- Lose weight, if overweight.
- Elevate the head of the bed by 4 to 6 inches.
- Avoid food, beverages, and medicines that seem to aggravate the heartburn.
- Refrain from smoking cigarettes.

Use antacids infrequently for occasional heartburn; they may mask or cause problems if used regularly. Chewing gum may bring relief of symptoms by increasing the flow of saliva, which helps in re-swallowing the esophageal contents.

As far as "acid indigestion" is concerned, recall from Chapter 3 that the strong acidity of the stomach is a desirable condition—television commercials for antacids notwithstanding. People who overeat or eat too quickly are likely to suffer from indigestion. The muscular reaction of the stomach to unchewed lumps or to being overfilled may be so violent that it causes regurgitation (reverse peristalsis). When this happens, overeaters may taste the stomach acid and feel pain. Responding to television commercials, they may take antacids to neutralize the "acid indigestion."

Antacids will provide quick relief, but they are not appropriate therapy for the stomach's discomfort. An antacid places a demand on the stomach to secrete more acid to counteract the neutralizer and enable the digestive enzymes to do their work. So the person still ends up with acid in the stomach, but the stomach has had to work against the antacid to produce it.

Antacids are designed to help relieve the acute symptoms from abnormal conditions, such as the pain felt by an ulcer patient whose stomach or duodenal lining has been attacked by acid. The person who overeats or swallows unchewed food needs to sit upright until the unhappy stomach has had a chance to cope with the problem it faces. Then, to avoid such misery in the future, the person needs to learn to eat less at a sitting, chew food more thoroughly, and eat it more slowly.

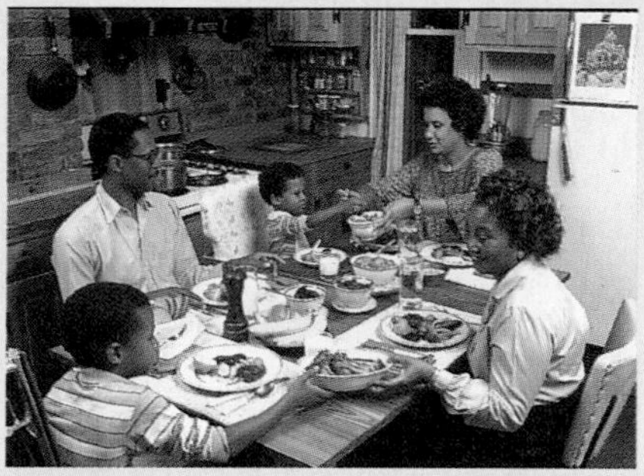

Taking the time to enjoy a meal can enhance people's physical and emotional health.

ULCERS

Ulcers of the stomach (gastric ulcers) or duodenum (duodenal ulcers) are another common digestive problem. (The term *peptic ulcer* includes both types.) An ulcer is an erosion of the top layer of cells from an area, such as the wall of the stomach or duodenum. This erosion leaves the underlying layers of cells unprotected and exposed to gastric juices. The erosion may proceed until the gastric juices reach the capillaries that feed the area, leading to bleeding, and reach the nerves, causing pain. If the erosion penetrates all the way through the GI lining, a life-threatening infection can develop.

Some people naively believe that an ulcer is caused by the secretion of stomach acid, but this is not the case—at least not at first. The stomach lining in a healthy person is well protected by its mucous coat. What, then, causes ulcers to form?

Three major causes of ulcers have been identified: bacterial infection, the use of certain anti-inflammatory drugs, and disorders that cause excessive gastric acid secretion.[5]* The treatment of ulcers aims at relieving pain, healing the ulcer, and minimizing the likelihood of recurrence. Drug therapy plays the primary role in the treatment; the specific type of drug depends on the cause of the ulcer. The most widely used treatment regimen includes the mineral bismuth and two other antimicrobial drugs.[6] Other drugs may be used to neutralize gastric acidity, reduce gastric acid secretion, or otherwise protect the stomach and duodenal wall from the eroding effect of gastric acid. The same treatment regimen is used for both gastric and duodenal ulcers.

Diet therapy once played a major role in ulcer treatment, but it no longer does. Current practice is simply to treat for infection, eliminate any food that routinely causes indigestion or pain, and avoid coffee and caffeine- and alcohol-containing beverages. Both regular and decaffeinated coffee stimulate stomach acid secretion and so aggravate *existing* ulcers.

Many of the common GI problems presented here reflect hurried lifestyles. For this reason, many of their remedies require that people slow down: take the time to eat slowly; chew food thoroughly to prevent choking, heartburn, and acid indigestion; take the time to rest until vomiting and diarrhea subside; and take the time to heed the urge to defecate. In addition,

*The bacterial infection frequently associated with ulcers is caused by *Helicobacter pylori*. The drugs associated with ulcers are nonsteroidal anti-inflammatory agents such as ibuprofen and naproxen.

learn how to handle life's day-to-day problems and challenges without overreacting and becoming upset; learn how to relax, to get enough sleep, and to enjoy life. Remember, "what's eating you" may cause more GI distress than what you eat.

NOTES

1. M. Donowitz, F. T. Kokke, and R. Saidi, Evaluation of patients with chronic diarrhea, *New England Journal of Medicine* 332 (1995): 725–729.

2. R. S. Sandler, M. C. Jordan, and B. J. Shelton, Demographic and dietary determinants of constipation in the US population, *American Journal of Public Health* 80 (1990): 185–189.

3. J. A. Flick and J. A. Perman, Nonabsorbed carbohydrate: Effect on fecal pH in methane-excreting and nonexcreting individuals, *American Journal of Clinical Nutrition* 49 (1989): 1252–1257.

4. J. M. Pique, Methane production and colon cancer, *Gastroenterology* 87(1987): 601–605.

5. D. Y. Graham, *Helicobacter pylori:* Its epidemiology and its role in duodenal ulcer disease, *Journal of Gastroenterology and Hepatology* 6 (1991): 105–113.

6. D. Y. Graham, Treatment of peptic ulcers caused by *Helicobacter pylori*, *New England Journal of Medicine* 328 (1993): 349–350.

Chapter 4

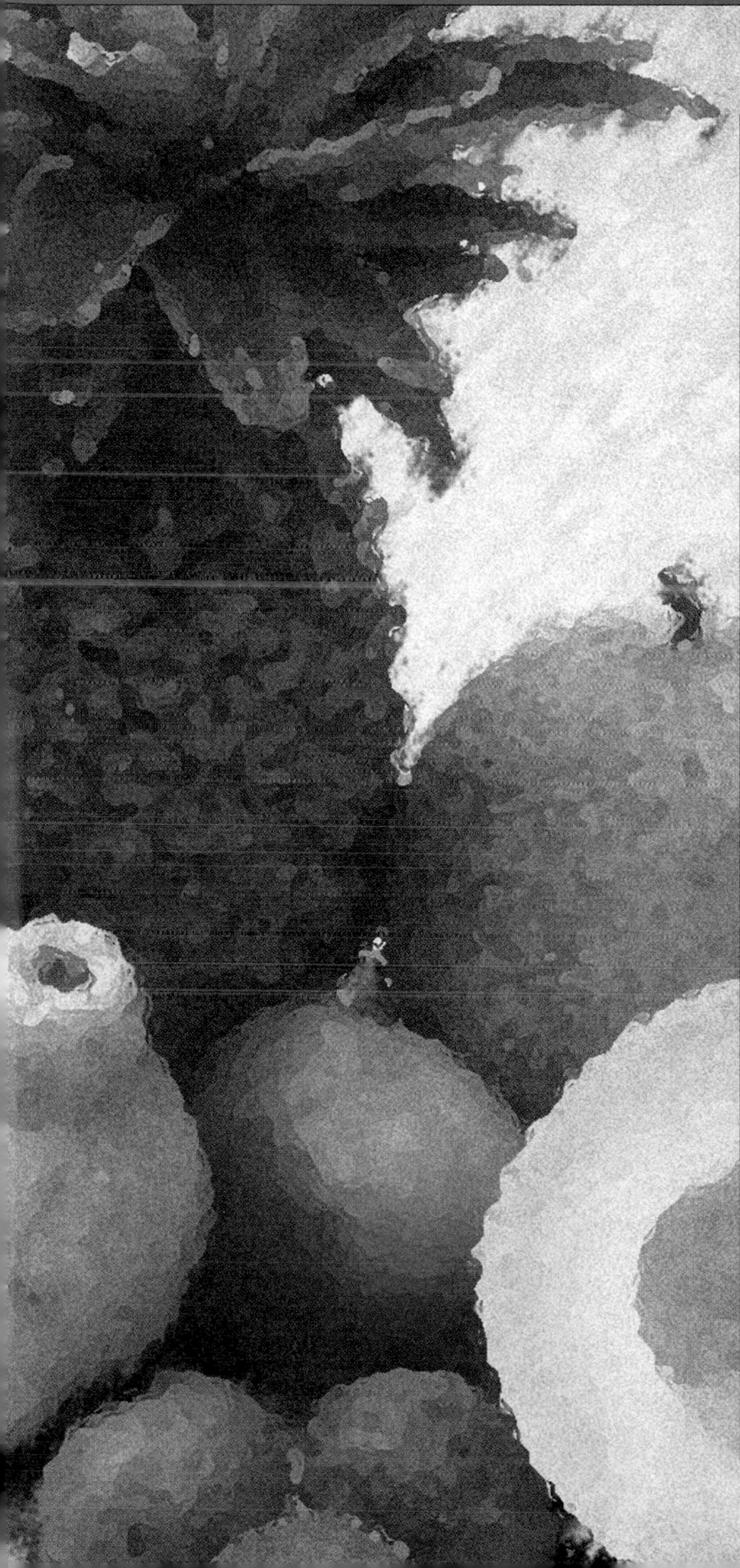

The Carbohydrates: Sugars, Starch, and Fibers

CONTENTS

MICROGRAPH: Fructose, the sugar of fruits

A student, quietly studying a textbook, is seldom aware that within his brain cells, billions of glucose molecules are splitting each second to provide the energy that permits him to learn. Yet glucose provides nearly all of the energy the human brain uses daily. Similarly, a marathon runner, bursting across the finish line in an explosion of sweat and triumph, seldom gives thanks to the glycogen fuel her muscles have devoured to help her finish the race. Yet, together, glucose and its storage form glycogen provide about half of all the energy human nerves, muscles, and other body tissues use. The other half of the body's energy comes mostly from fat.

People don't eat glucose and glycogen directly; they eat foods rich in carbohydrates. Then their bodies convert the carbohydrates mostly into glucose for immediate energy and into glycogen for reserve energy.

Carbohydrates contribute so much to the bulk of most foods that many people mistakenly think of them as "fattening" and avoid them when trying to lose weight. Actually, such a strategy may be counterproductive. People can better control body weight by selecting high-carbohydrate, high-fiber foods and limiting fat-rich foods. All unrefined plant foods—vegetables, fruits, legumes, and grains—provide ample carbohydrate and fiber with little or no fat. (Milk also contains carbohydrates. So do shellfish and organ meats such as liver, but only a little.)

Table 4–1 offers a preview of the dietary carbohydrate family, which includes the simple carbohydrates (the sugars) and the complex carbohydrates (the starches and fibers). All of the carbohydrates are made of simple sugars; they are *complex* when they have more than two simple sugars in a molecule. The simple carbohydrates are those that chemists describe as:

- Monosaccharides—single sugars.
- Disaccharides—sugars composed of pairs of monosaccharides.

The complex carbohydrates are:

- Polysaccharides—large molecules composed of chains of monosaccharides.

Table 4–1
The Carbohydrate Family

Simple Carbohydrates (sugars)
• Monosaccharides
Glucose
Fructose
Galactose
• Disaccharides
Sucrose
Lactose
Maltose
Complex Carbohydrates[a]
• Starch (polysaccharides)
• Fibers (nonstarch polysaccharides)
Soluble
Insoluble

[a]Glycogen is a complex carbohydrate (a polysaccharide), but not a *dietary* source of carbohydrate.

The Chemist's View of Carbohydrates

To understand the structure of carbohydrates, look at the units of which they are made. The sugars most important in nutrition are the monosaccharides known as 6-carbon sugars, or hexoses. Each contains 6 carbon atoms, 12 hydrogens, and 6 oxygens (written in shorthand as $C_6H_{12}O_6$).

Each atom can form a certain number of chemical bonds with other atoms:

- Carbon atoms can form four bonds.
- Nitrogen atoms, three.
- Oxygen atoms, two.
- Hydrogen atoms, only one.

Chemists represent the bonds as lines between the chemical symbols (such as C, N, O, and H) that stand for the atoms (see Figure 4–1).

Atoms form molecules in ways that satisfy the bonding requirements of each atom. Figure 4–1 shows the structure of ethyl alcohol, the active ingredient of alcoholic beverages, as an example. The two carbons each have four bonds represented by lines; the oxygen has two; and each hydrogen has one bond con-

carbohydrates: compounds composed of carbon, oxygen, and hydrogen arranged as monosaccharides or multiples of monosaccharides.
carbo = carbon (C)
hydrate = with water (H_2O)

simple carbohydrates (sugars): monosaccharides and disaccharides.

complex carbohydrates (starches and fibers): polysaccharides composed of straight or branched chains of monosaccharides.

Most of the monosaccharides important in nutrition are **hexoses**, simple sugars with six atoms of carbon and the formula $C_6H_{12}O_6$.
hex = six

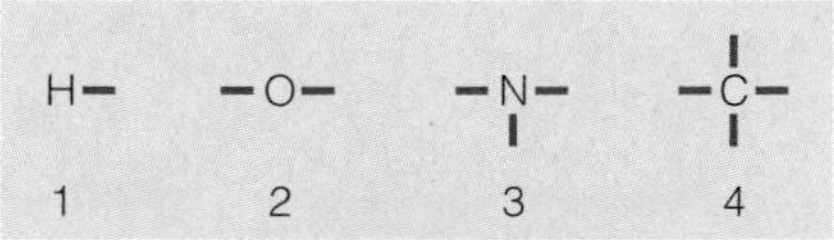

Each atom has a characteristic number of bonds it can form with other atoms.

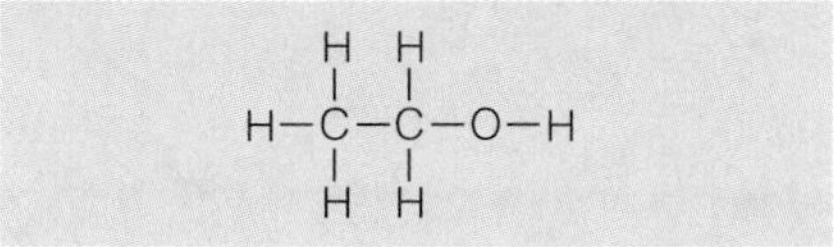

Ethyl alcohol, a simple molecule showing bonding.

Figure 4–1

Atoms and Their Bonds

The four main types of atoms found in nutrients are hydrogen, oxygen, nitrogen, and carbon. Appendix B presents basic chemistry terms and relationships.

necting it to other atoms. An accurate drawing of a chemical structure must obey these rules because the laws of nature demand it.

To quickly recap, the carbohydrates are made of carbon (C), oxygen (O), and hydrogen (H). Each of these atoms can form a specified number of chemical bonds: carbon forms four, oxygen forms two, and hydrogen forms one.

The Simple Carbohydrates

The following list of the six sugars most important in nutrition symbolizes them as hexagons and pentagons of different colors. The shapes reflect their chemical structures as drawn on paper. Three are single sugars or monosaccharides:

- Glucose. 
- Fructose.* 
- Galactose.† 

Three are double sugars or disaccharides:

- Maltose (glucose + glucose). 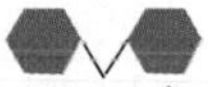
- Sucrose (glucose + fructose). 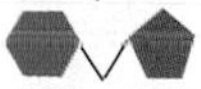
- Lactose (glucose + galactose). 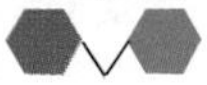

See Appendix C for the complete chemical structures of the sugars.

monosaccharide (mon-oh-SACK-uh-ride): a carbohydrate of the general formula $C_nH_{2n}O_n$ that consists of a single ring.
mono = one
saccharide = sugar

MONOSACCHARIDES

The three monosaccharides important in nutrition all have the same numbers and kinds of atoms, but in different arrangements. These chemical differences account for the differing sweetness of the monosaccharides. A pinch of purified glucose on the tongue gives only a mild sweet flavor and galactose hardly tastes sweet at all, but fructose is as intensely sweet as honey and, in fact, is the sugar primarily responsible for honey's sweetness.

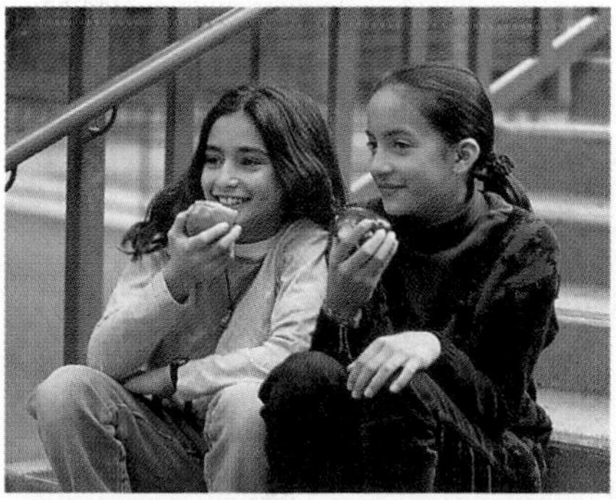

Fruits package their simple sugars with fibers, vitamins, and minerals, making them a sweet and healthy snack.

*Fructose is shown as a pentagon, but it does have 6 carbon atoms. The ring contains 4 carbons and an oxygen; 2 carbons stick out from the ring (see Figure 4–4).

†Galactose occurs only as a part of lactose.

Figure 4–2

Chemical Structure of Glucose
On paper, the structure of glucose has to be drawn flat, but in nature the five carbons and oxygen are roughly in a plane. The atoms attached to the ring carbons extend above and below the plane.

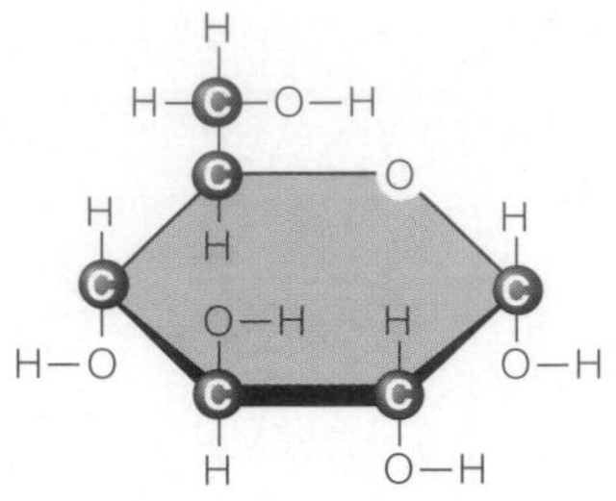

glucose: a monosaccharide; sometimes known as blood sugar or dextrose.
ose = carbohydrate
 = glucose

Glucose Chemically, glucose is a larger and more complicated molecule than ethyl alcohol, but it obeys the same rules of chemistry: each carbon atom has four bonds; each oxygen, two bonds; and each hydrogen, one bond. Figure 4–2 illustrates the chemical structure of a glucose molecule.

The diagram of a glucose molecule shows all the relationships between the parts and proves simple on examination, but chemists have adopted even simpler ways to depict chemical structures. Figure 4–3 shows that a chemical structure can combine or omit a number of letters without losing the information it conveys.

The significance of glucose to nutrition is tremendous. Glucose is one of the two sugars in every disaccharide and is the unit from which the polysaccharides are made almost exclusively. One of these polysaccharides, starch, is the chief energy food of the world's people; another, glycogen, is a major storage form of energy in the body. Glucose will therefore reappear frequently throughout this chapter and all those that follow.

Figure 4–3 Simplified Diagrams of Glucose

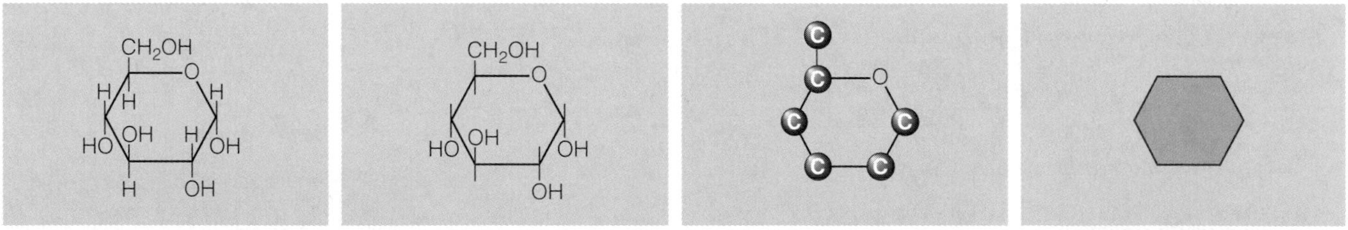

The carbons at the corners are not shown and the formula CH_2OH stands for the structure in Figure 4-2.

Now the single hydrogens are not shown, but lines still extend upward or downward from the ring to show where they belong. You can easily reconstruct the complete structure, with all its details, from such a diagram by putting a C for carbon at each corner of the hexagon and an H for hydrogen at the end of each single line. This is the traditional chemical shorthand used for glucose.

Another way to look at glucose is to notice that its six carbon atoms are all connected.

For convenience, in this and other illustrations throughout this book, glucose is represented as a blue hexagon.

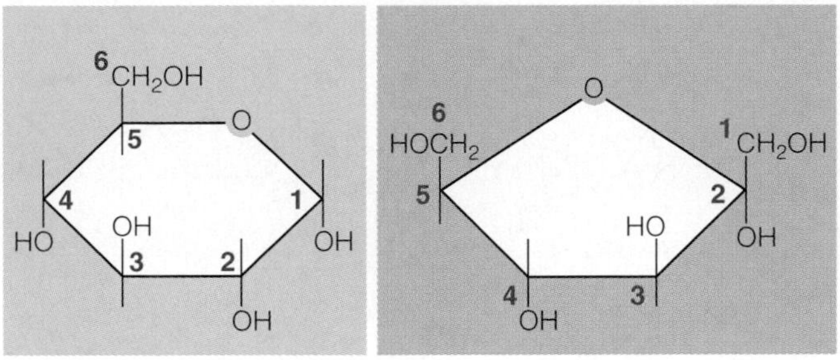

Glucose Fructose

Figure 4–4

Two Monosaccharides: Glucose and Fructose

Can you see the similarities? If you learned the rules in Figure 4–3, you will be able to "see" 6 carbons (numbered), 12 hydrogens, and 6 oxygens in both these compounds.

Fructose Fructose is the sweetest of the sugars. Curiously, fructose has exactly the same chemical *formula* as glucose—$C_6H_{12}O_6$—but its *structure* differs (see Figure 4–4). The arrangement of the atoms in fructose stimulates the taste buds on the tongue to produce the sweet sensation. Fructose occurs naturally in fruits and honey; food manufacturers also use it in products sweetened with high-fructose corn syrup (HFCS), a corn product used as an additive.

fructose: a monosaccharide; sometimes known as fruit sugar or levulose, fructose is found abundantly in fruits, honey, and saps.
fruct = fruit
⬟ = fructose

Galactose Seldom occurring free in nature, galactose binds with another monosaccharide to form the sugar in milk. Galactose has the same numbers and kinds of atoms as glucose and fructose, but in yet another arrangement. Figure 4–5 shows galactose beside a molecule of glucose for comparison.

galactose: a monosaccharide; part of the disaccharide lactose.
⬢ = galactose

DISSACCHARIDES

The disaccharides are pairs of the three sugars just discussed. Glucose occurs in all three; the second member of the pair is either fructose, galactose, or another glucose. These carbohydrates and all the other energy nutrients are put together and taken apart by similar chemical reactions.

disaccharide: a pair of monosaccharides linked together.
di = two

Condensation To make a disaccharide, a chemical reaction known as condensation links two monosaccharides together (see Figure 4–6). A hydroxyl (OH) group from one monosaccharide and a hydrogen atom (H) from the other combine to create a molecule of water (H_2O). The two originally separate monosaccharides link together with a single oxygen (O).

condensation: a chemical reaction in which two reactants combine to yield a larger product.

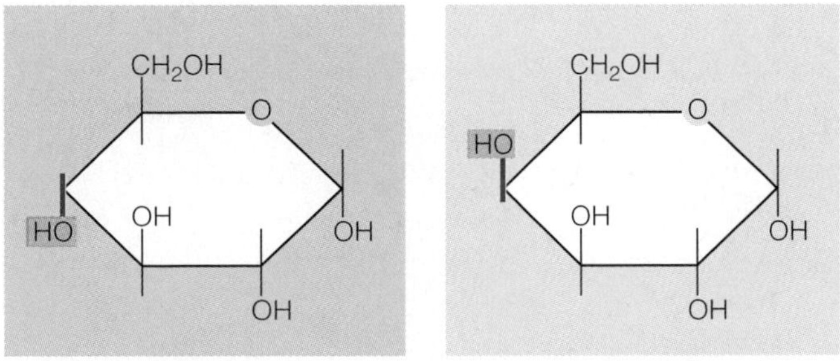

Glucose Galactose

Figure 4–5

Two Monosaccharides: Glucose and Galactose

Notice the similarities and the difference.

Figure 4–6

Condensation of Two Monosaccharides to Form a Disaccharide

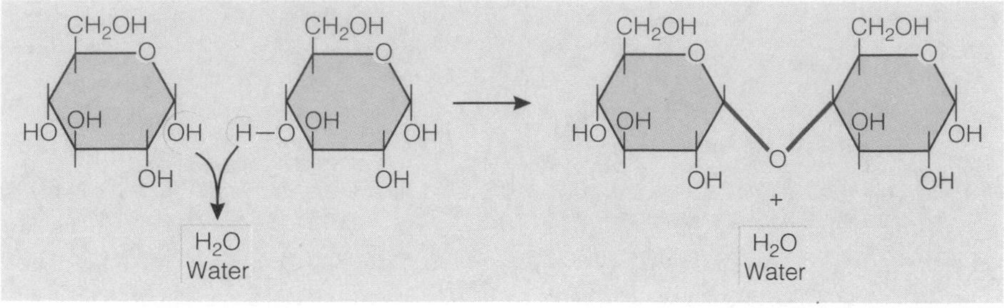

Glucose + glucose

An OH group from one glucose and an H atom from another glucose combine to create a molecule of H_2O.

Maltose

The two glucose molecules bond together with a single O atom to form the disaccharide maltose.

Reminder: A *hydrolysis* reaction splits a major reactant into two products, with H added to one and OH to the other (from water).

Hydrolysis To break a disaccharide in two, a chemical reaction known as hydrolysis occurs (Figure 4–7). A molecule of water splits to provide the H and OH needed to complete the resulting monosaccharides. Hydrolysis reactions commonly occur during digestion.

maltose: a disaccharide composed of two glucose units; sometimes known as malt sugar.

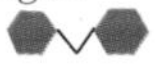 = maltose

Maltose The disaccharide maltose consists of two glucose units. Maltose is produced whenever starch breaks down—as happens in plants when seeds germinate and in human beings during carbohydrate digestion. It also occurs during the fermentation process that yields alcohol. Maltose is only a minor constituent of a few foods.

sucrose: a disaccharide composed of glucose and fructose; commonly known as table sugar, beet sugar, or cane sugar. Sucrose also occurs in many fruits and some vegetables and grains.

sucro = sugar

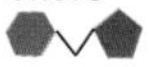 = sucrose

Sucrose Fructose and glucose together form sucrose, or table sugar, the most familiar of the sugars. Because the fructose is in a position accessible to the taste receptors, sucrose tastes sweet, accounting for some of the natural sweetness of fruits, vegetables, and grains. To make table sugar, sucrose is refined from the juices of sugar cane and sugar beets, then granulated. Depending on the extent to which it is refined, the product becomes the brown, white, and powdered sugars available at grocery stores.

Figure 4–7

Hydrolysis of a Disaccharide

Hydrolysis occurs during digestion.

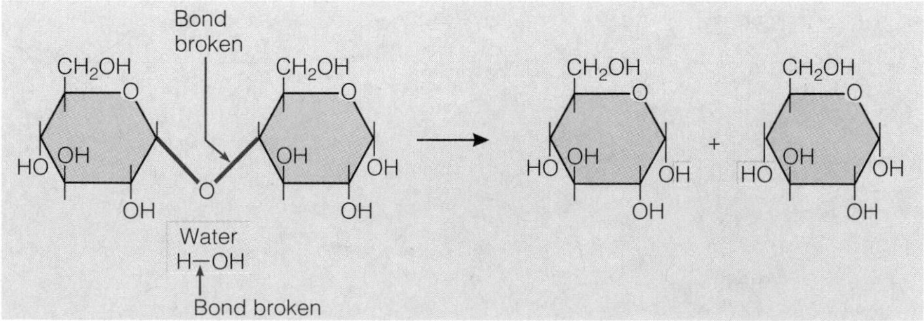

Maltose

Glucose + glucose

The disaccharide maltose splits into two glucose molecules with H added to one and OH to the other (from water).

Lactose The combination of galactose and glucose makes the disaccharide lactose, the principal carbohydrate of milk. Known as milk sugar, lactose contributes about 5 percent of milk's weight. Depending on the milk's fat content, lactose contributes 30 to 50 percent of milk's energy.

lactose: a disaccharide composed of glucose and galactose; commonly known as milk sugar.
lact = milk
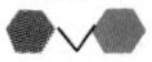 = lactose

In summary, then, six major simple carbohydrates, or sugars, are important in nutrition. The three monosaccharides (glucose, fructose, and galactose) all have the same chemical formula ($C_6H_{12}O_6$), but their structures differ. The three disaccharides (sucrose, lactose, and maltose) are pairs of monosaccharides. The sugars derive primarily from plants, except for lactose and its component galactose, which come from milk and milk products. Two monosaccharides can be linked together by a condensation reaction to form a disaccharide and water. A disaccharide, in turn, can be broken into its two monosaccharides by a hydrolysis reaction using water.

The Complex Carbohydrates

The simple carbohydrates are the sugars just mentioned: glucose, fructose, and galactose, either singly or paired with glucose. In contrast, the complex carbohydrates contain many glucose units and a few other monosaccharides strung together as polysaccharides. Three are important in nutrition: glycogen, starch, and the fibers.

polysaccharide: many monosaccharides linked together.
poly = many
saccharide = sugar

Glycogen is a storage form of energy in the animal body; starch plays that role in plants; and the fibers of plants serve as structural elements in stems, trunks, roots, leaves, and skins. Both glycogen and starch are built of glucose units, but they are linked together differently. The fibers are composed of a variety of monosaccharides and other carbohydrate derivatives.

GLYCOGEN

Glycogen is found only to a limited extent in meats and not at all in plants.* For this reason, glycogen is not a significant food source of carbohydrate, but it does perform an important role in the body. It is the form in which the human body stores much of its glucose. Glycogen consists of many glucose molecules linked together in highly branched chains (see the left side of Figure 4–8). This arrangement permits rapid hydrolysis. When the hormonal message "Release energy" arrives at the storage sites in a liver or muscle cell, enzymes respond by attacking all the many branches of each glycogen simultaneously, making a surge of fuel available.†

glycogen (GLY-co-gen): an animal polysaccharide composed of glucose; it is manufactured and stored in the liver and muscles as a storage form of glucose. Glycogen is not a significant food source of carbohydrate and is not counted as one of the complex carbohydrates in foods.
glyco = glucose
gen = gives rise to

*Glycogen in animal muscles rapidly hydrolyzes after slaughter.

†Normally, only the liver can return glucose *directly* from glycogen to the blood; muscle cells use glycogen internally to produce glucose. Muscle cells can restore the blood glucose level *indirectly*, however: when muscles oxidize glucose without oxygen for energy, they release a breakdown product (lactic acid) into the blood, which the liver can pick up and reconvert to glucose. The return of glucose via this pathway is called the Cori cycle, and it accounts for 15 percent or more of blood glucose. L. J. Hoffer, Cori cycle contribution to plasma glucose appearance in man, *Journal of Parenteral and Enteral Nutrition* 14 (1990): 646–648.

Figure 4–8

Glycogen and Starch Molecules Compared (Small Segments)

Notice that the more highly branched the structure, the greater the number of ends from which glucose can be released. (These units would have to be magnified millions of times to appear at the size shown in this figure. For details of the chemical structures, see Appendix C.)

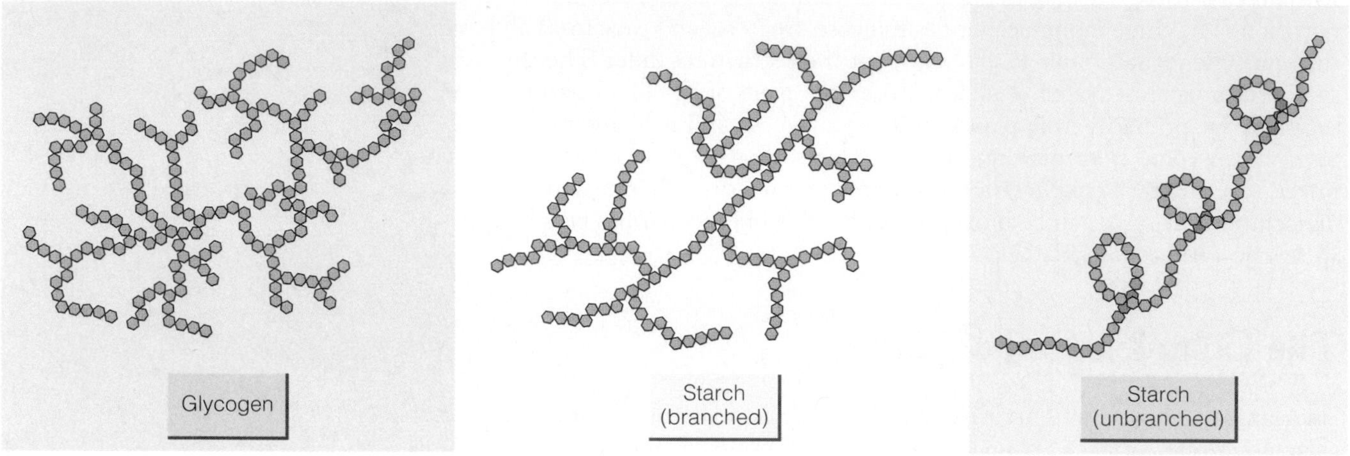

A glycogen molecule contains hundreds of glucose units in long highly branched chains.

A starch molecule contains hundreds of glucose molecules in either occasionally branched chains or unbranched chains.

STARCH

Just as the human body stores glucose as glycogen, plant cells store glucose as starch—long, unbranched or branched chains of hundreds or thousands of glucose molecules linked together (see the middle and right side of Figure 4–8). These giant molecules are packed side by side in grains such as wheat or rice, in tubers such as potatoes, and in legumes such as peas and beans. A cubic inch of food may contain as many as a million starch molecules.

In a plant such as a potato, starch stores the glucose needed to support the plant's first growth. When you eat the plant, your body hydrolyzes the starch to glucose and uses the glucose for its own energy purposes. Together with the sugars, then, starch is considered to be an available carbohydrate.

All starchy foods come from plants. Grains are the richest food source of starch, providing much of the food energy for people all over the world—rice in Asia; wheat in Canada, the United States, and Europe; corn in much of Central and South America; and millet, rye, barley, and oats elsewhere. The legumes are another important source of starch, as well as of dietary fibers and protein. Tubers, such as potatoes, yams, and the cassava of many non-Western societies, are another major source of starch.

starch: a plant polysaccharide composed of glucose that is digestible by human beings. For the structures of starch's two forms, amylose (straight chain) and amylopectin (branched chain), see Appendix C.

Starch and sugar are called **available carbohydrates** because human digestive enzymes make them available to the body. In contrast, fibers are called **unavailable carbohydrates** because human digestive enzymes cannot break their bonds.

fiber: a general term denoting in plant foods the *nonstarch polysaccharides* that are not digested by *human* digestive enzymes, although some are digested by GI tract bacteria; fibers include cellulose, hemicelluloses, pectins, gums, and mucilages and the nonpolysaccharides lignins, cutins, and tannins.

THE FIBERS

Fibers are the structural parts of plants and thus are found in all plant-derived foods—vegetables, fruits, grains, and legumes. Most are polysaccharides, but starch is not one of them; in fact, fibers are often described as nonstarch poly-

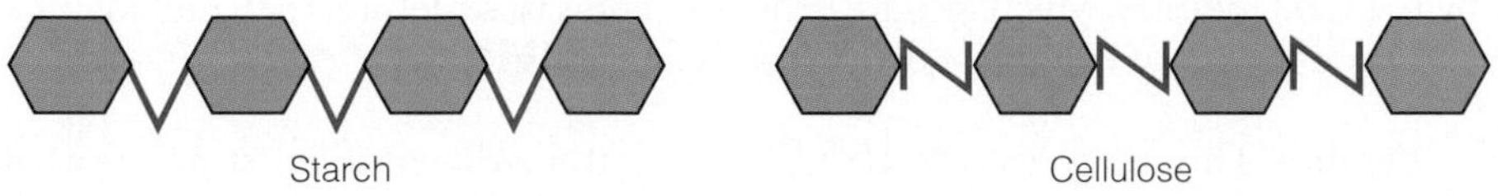

Figure 4–9

Starch and Cellulose Molecules Compared (Small Segments)
The bonds that link the glucose units together in cellulose are different from the bonds in starch (and glycogen). Human enzymes cannot digest cellulose. See Appendix C for chemical structures and descriptions of linkages.

saccharides. Nonstarch polysaccharides include cellulose, hemicelluloses, pectins, gums, and mucilages. Fibers also include some nonpolysaccharides such as lignins, cutins, and tannins.*

Even though most are polysaccharides, fibers differ from starch in that the bonds between their monosaccharide units cannot be broken down by human digestive enzymes. The bacteria of the GI tract can break some fibers down, however, and this is important to digestion and to health.

Each of the fibers has a different structure. Most contain monosaccharides, but differ in the types they contain and in the bonds that link the monosaccharides to each other. These differences produce diverse health effects.

Cellulose Cellulose is the primary constituent of plant cell walls and therefore occurs in all vegetables, fruits, and legumes. Like starch, cellulose is composed of glucose units connected in long chains. Unlike starch, however, the chains do not branch, and the bonds holding the glucose units together resist digestion by human enzymes (see Figure 4–9).

Hemicelluloses The hemicelluloses are the main constituent of cereal fibers. They are composed of various monosaccharide backbones with branching side chains of monosaccharides.† The many backbones and side chains make the hemicelluloses a diverse group; some are soluble, while others are insoluble.

Pectins All pectins consist of a backbone derived from carbohydrate with side chains of various monosaccharides. Commonly found in vegetables and fruits (especially citrus fruits and apples), pectins may be isolated and used by the food industry to thicken jelly, keep salad dressing from separating, and otherwise control texture and consistency. Pectins can perform these functions because they readily form gels in water.

---

*The terms *crude fiber, neutral-detergent fiber,* and *dietary fiber* reflect different methodologies used to estimate the fiber contents of foods; they do not identify different types of fiber. The structure of cellulose is shown in Appendix C; the other polysaccharide fibers are similar, but differ slightly in their bonding. Besides glucose, their component sugars may include rhamnose, arabinose, and others. As for the lignins, they are polymers of several dozen molecules of phenol (an organic alcohol), with strong internal bonds that make them impervious to digestive enzymes.

†In hemicelluloses, the most common backbone monosaccharides are xylose, mannose, and galactose; the common side chains are arabinose, glucuronic acid, and galactose (see Appendix C for structures).

Gums and Mucilages When cut, the branch of a plant secretes gums from the site of the injury. Like the other fibers, gums are composed of various monosaccharides and their derivatives. Gums such as *gum arabic* are used as additives by the food industry. Mucilages are similar to gums in structure; they include *guar* and *carrageenan*, which are added to foods as stabilizers.

Lignin This *nonpolysaccharide* fiber has a three-dimensional structure that gives it strength. Because of its toughness, few of the foods that people eat contain much lignin. It occurs in the woody parts of vegetables such as carrots or the small seeds of fruits such as strawberries.

Other Classifications of Fibers Scientists classify fibers in several ways. The previous paragraphs classified them according to their chemical properties. Fibers can also be classified according to their solubility. The effects of fibers on the body do not neatly divide along the lines of solubility, but some generalizations of significance to health can be made.

Soluble fibers:
- Gums.
- Pectins.
- Some hemicelluloses.
- Mucilages.

Insoluble fibers:
- Cellulose.
- Many hemicelluloses.
- Lignins.

In general, soluble fibers occur in higher concentrations in fruits, oats, barley, and legumes. In the body, soluble fibers:

- Delay the stomach's emptying and the transit of chyme through the intestines.
- Delay glucose absorption.
- Lower blood cholesterol.[1]

In general, insoluble fibers are found in higher concentrations in vegetables, wheat, and cereals. In the body, insoluble fibers:

- Accelerate the transit of chyme through the intestines.
- Increase fecal weight.
- Slow starch breakdown and delay glucose absorption into the blood.

In the body, *both* soluble and insoluble fibers:

- Influence transit time and nutrient absorption in the GI tract.
- Are partially fermented by microorganisms in the digestive tract to fragments that the body can use.*

Table 4–2 summarizes these fiber facts. Such generalizations are useful, but exceptions occur. For example, insoluble rice bran also lowers blood cholesterol, and the soluble fiber psyllium effectively promotes bowel movements.[2]

Some researchers classify fibers according to other physical properties that affect GI function and nutrient absorption. Physical properties of fibers include:

- *Water-holding capacity*—the capacity to capture water like a sponge, swelling and increasing the bulk of the intestines' contents.
- *Viscosity*—the capacity to form viscous, gel-like solutions.
- *Cation-exchange capacity*—the ability to bind minerals.
- *Bile-binding capacity*—the ability to bind bile.
- *Fermentability*—the extent to which bacteria can ferment them in the digestive tract.

---

*Dietary fibers are fermented by colon bacteria to short-chain fatty acids, which are absorbed and metabolized by the GI mucosa and liver.

Table 4–2

Fibers: Their Sources, Actions, and Structures

	Soluble Fibers	Insoluble Fibers
Food sources	Fruits (apples, citrus), oats, barley, legumes	Wheat bran, whole-grain breads and cereals, vegetables
Action in the body	Delay GI transit. Delay glucose absorption. Lower blood cholesterol.	Accelerate GI transit. Increase fecal weight. Slow starch hydrolysis. Delay glucose absorption.
Type of fiber	Gums, pectins, some hemicelluloses, mucilages	Cellulose, many hemicelluloses, lignins

Clearly, the fibers are a diverse group of compounds. Like a basket of threads of various colors and sizes, they can be used for many different projects depending on the interests of the craftsperson selecting them.[3]

A compound not classed as a fiber but often found with it in foods is phytic acid. Most dietary phytic acid comes from seeds such as the cereal grains. A person on a high-fiber diet may lose minerals that become bound to phytic acid and are excreted with it. (In plant seeds, phytic acid may store these minerals and hold them in plant tissue during germination.) The nutrition consequences of such mineral losses are described in Chapters 12 and 13.

phytic acid: a nonnutrient component of plant seeds; also called **phytate** (FYE-tate). Phytic acid occurs in the husks of grains, legumes, and seeds and is capable of binding minerals such as zinc, iron, calcium, magnesium, and copper in insoluble complexes in the intestine, which the body excretes unused.

In summary, the complex carbohydrates are the polysaccharides (chains of monosaccharides): glycogen, starch, and fibers. Both glycogen and starch are storage forms of glucose—glycogen in the body, and starch in plants—and both yield energy for human use. The fibers also contain glucose (and other monosaccharides), but their bonds cannot be broken by human digestive enzymes, so they yield little, if any, energy.

Digestion and Absorption of Carbohydrates

The ultimate goal of digestion and absorption of sugars and starch is to render all available carbohydrates into small compounds that the body can absorb and use—chiefly glucose. The large starch molecules require extensive breakdown; the disaccharides need only to be split once. The splitting of the larger carbohydrates begins in the mouth; the final splitting and absorption occur in the small intestine; and conversion to a common energy currency (glucose) is the task of the liver. The details follow.

THE PROCESSES OF DIGESTION AND ABSORPTION

Figure 4–10 traces the digestion of carbohydrates through the GI tract. When a person eats foods containing starch, enzymes hydrolyze the long chains to shorter chains, the short chains to disaccharides, and, finally, the disaccharides to monosaccharides. This process begins in the mouth.

The short chains of glucose units that result from the breakdown of starch are known as **dextrins**. The word sometimes appears on food labels because dextrins can be used as thickening agents in foods.

Figure 4–10

Carbohydrate Digestion in the GI Tract

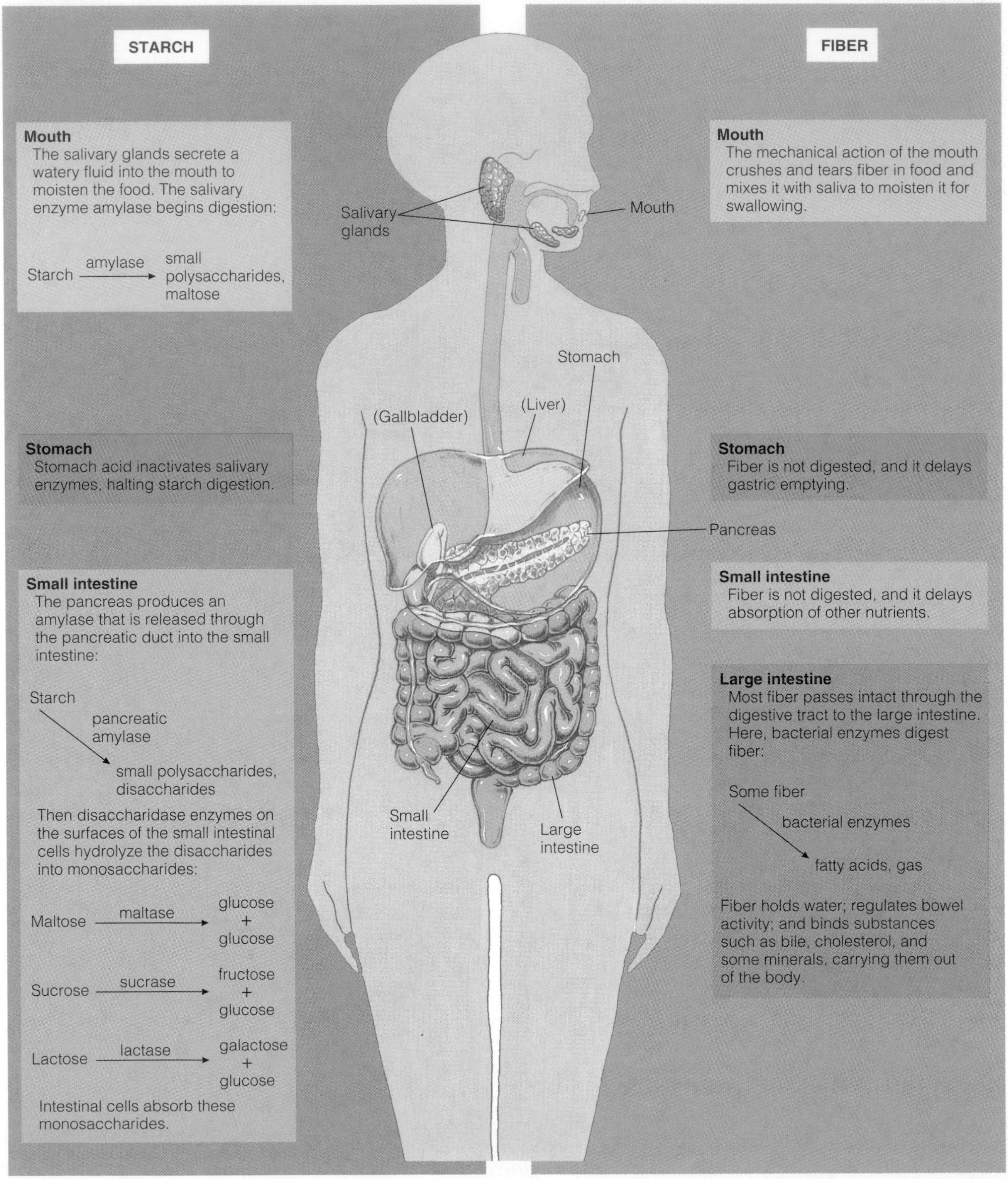
STARCH
FIBER
Mouth
The salivary glands secrete a watery fluid into the mouth to moisten the food. The salivary enzyme amylase begins digestion:
Starch —amylase→ small polysaccharides, maltose
Stomach
Stomach acid inactivates salivary enzymes, halting starch digestion.
Small intestine
The pancreas produces an amylase that is released through the pancreatic duct into the small intestine:
Starch —pancreatic amylase→ small polysaccharides, disaccharides
Then disaccharidase enzymes on the surfaces of the small intestinal cells hydrolyze the disaccharides into monosaccharides:
Maltose —maltase→ glucose + glucose
Sucrose —sucrase→ fructose + glucose
Lactose —lactase→ galactose + glucose
Intestinal cells absorb these monosaccharides.
Salivary glands
Mouth
Stomach
(Liver)
(Gallbladder)
Pancreas
Small intestine
Large intestine
Mouth
The mechanical action of the mouth crushes and tears fiber in food and mixes it with saliva to moisten it for swallowing.
Stomach
Fiber is not digested, and it delays gastric emptying.
Small intestine
Fiber is not digested, and it delays absorption of other nutrients.
Large intestine
Most fiber passes intact through the digestive tract to the large intestine. Here, bacterial enzymes digest fiber:
Some fiber —bacterial enzymes→ fatty acids, gas
Fiber holds water; regulates bowel activity; and binds substances such as bile, cholesterol, and some minerals, carrying them out of the body.

In the Mouth In the mouth, vigorous chewing of high-fiber foods slows eating and stimulates the flow of saliva. The salivary enzyme amylase starts to work, hydrolyzing starch to shorter polysaccharides and to maltose. Because food is in the mouth for only a short time, very little digestion takes place there.

amylase (AM-ih-lace): an enzyme that hydrolyzes amylose (a form of starch). Amylase is a carbohydrase, an enzyme that breaks down carbohydrates.

Reminder: A *bolus* is a portion of food swallowed at one time.

In the Stomach The swallowed bolus mixes with the stomach's acid and protein-digesting enzymes, and these digest the salivary enzyme amylase. Thus amylase is removed from the scene before its job of starch digestion is completed. To a small extent, the stomach's acid continues breaking starch down, but its juices contain no enzymes to digest carbohydrate. Fibers tend to linger in the stomach, delaying gastric emptying. This provides a feeling of fullness and satiety. Carbohydrate digestion speeds up again in the small intestine.

In the Small Intestine The small intestine carries out most of the work of carbohydrate digestion. A major carbohydrate-digesting enzyme, pancreatic amylase, enters the intestine via the pancreatic duct and continues breaking down the polysaccharides to shorter glucose chains and disaccharides. The final step takes place on the outer membranes of the intestinal cells. There, specific enzymes dismantle specific disaccharides:

- Maltase breaks maltose into 2 glucose molecules.
- Sucrase breaks sucrose into 1 glucose and 1 fructose molecule.
- Lactase breaks lactose into 1 glucose and 1 galactose molecule.

maltase: an enzyme that hydrolyzes maltose.

sucrase: an enzyme that hydrolyzes sucrose.

lactase: an enzyme that hydrolyzes lactose.

At this point, all disaccharides contribute at least one glucose molecule to the body. Other monosaccharides can eventually become glucose after being processed in the liver, as explained later.

Fibers delay the absorption of carbohydrates and fats in the small intestine, conferring benefits on health that a later section describes further. In addition, fibers in the intestines can bind with minerals there. This prevents the minerals' absorption and presents a risk of deficiency, but the risk is minimal when fiber intake is reasonable and mineral intake adequate.

In the Large Intestine Within one to four hours after a meal, all the sugars and most of the starches have been digested. Only a small fraction of the starches and the indigestible fibers remain in the digestive tract.[4]

Starch that is not absorbed in the small intestine of healthy people is known as **resistant starch**.

Most of the fibers' actions occur in the large intestine. There, fibers attract water, which softens the stools for passage without straining. Also, bacteria in the human digestive tract ferment fibers—that is, they digest fibers in the absence of oxygen. This process generates water, gas, and short-chain fatty acids (described in Chapter 5).* The short-chain fatty acids are absorbed in the colon and yield energy when metabolized. Metabolism of short-chain fatty acids occurs in both the intestinal mucosa and the liver.[5] Food fibers, therefore, do contribute some energy, depending on the extent to which they are broken down and absorbed. The energy contribution can rise to as much as 15 percent of daily food energy intake on a high-fiber diet.

*The short-chain fatty acids produced by GI bacteria are primarily acetic acid, propionic acid, and butyric acid.

Figure 4–11

Absorption of Monosaccharides

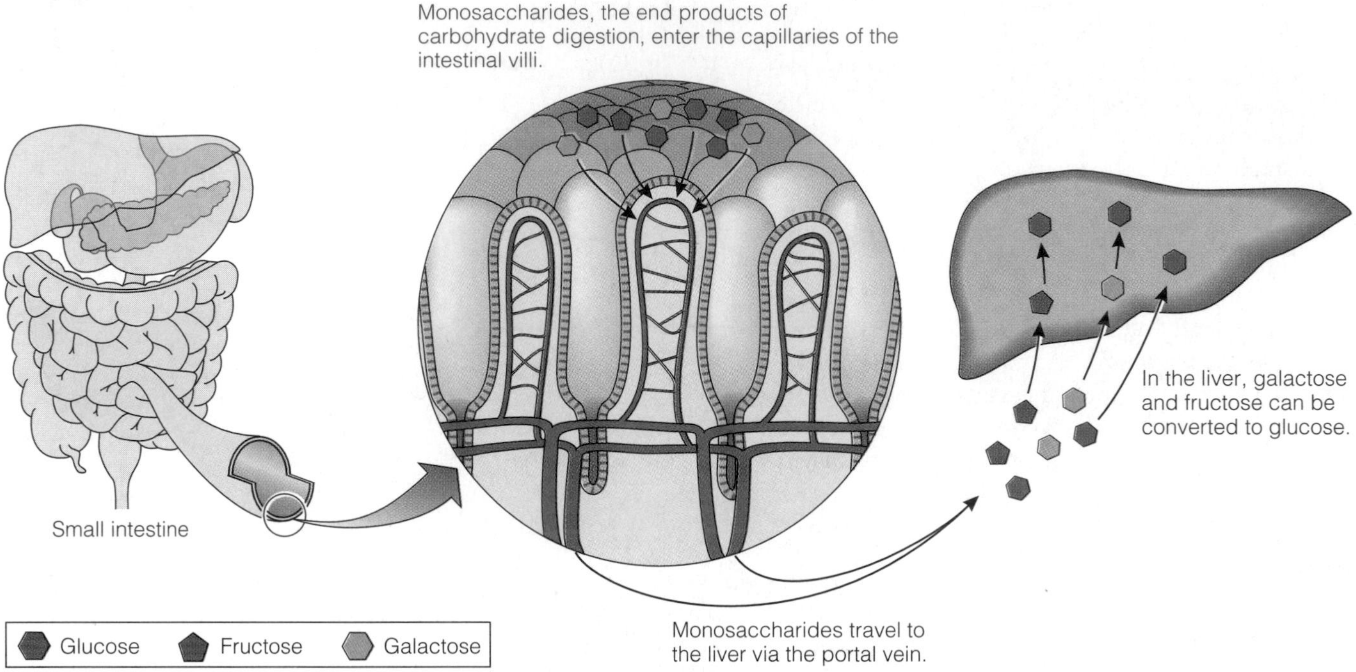

Monosaccharides, the end products of carbohydrate digestion, enter the capillaries of the intestinal villi.
Small intestine
In the liver, galactose and fructose can be converted to glucose.
Glucose
Fructose
Galactose
Monosaccharides travel to the liver via the portal vein.

Absorption into the Bloodstream Glucose is unique in that it can be absorbed to some extent through the lining of the mouth, but for the most part, all nutrient absorption takes place in the small intestine. The monosaccharides traverse the cells lining the small intestine by active transport and are washed away in the circulating blood.*

The blood then circulates through the liver, whose cells take up fructose and galactose and convert them to other compounds, most often to glucose, as shown in Figure 4–11. Thus all disaccharides not only provide at least one glucose molecule directly, but they also can provide another one indirectly—through the conversion of fructose and galactose to glucose. (The body does not use fructose and glucose in exactly the same ways, but for purposes of this book, they are treated as being metabolically identical.)

This description of the way the body receives carbohydrate should help explode a myth perpetrated by advertisers of high-sugar foods and beverages. They describe sugar as "quick energy" and imply that when you need quick energy, you should reach for a candy bar and a cola beverage. Clearly, though, the best pick-me-ups are not concentrated sugars. Sugars do offer energy, but so does any other food containing carbohydrate. Why not have a delicious peanut butter and banana sandwich, a tall, cool glass of milk, and a fresh, juicy orange as a pick-me-up?

---

*Fructose is absorbed by facilitated diffusion (see Figure 3–6 on p. 95).

LACTOSE INTOLERANCE

Normally, the enzyme lactase ensures that the disaccharide lactose found in milk is both digested and absorbed efficiently. Lactase levels are highest immediately after birth, as befits an infant whose first and only food for a while will be milk.[6] In the great majority of the world's populations, lactase activity declines dramatically during childhood and adolescence to about 5 to 10 percent of the activity at birth.[7] Only a relatively small percentage (about 30 percent) of the people in the world retain enough lactase to digest and absorb lactose efficiently throughout adult life.

Symptoms When more lactose is consumed than the available lactase can handle, lactose molecules remain in the intestine undigested, attracting water and causing bloating, abdominal discomfort, and diarrhea—the symptoms of lactose intolerance. The undigested lactose becomes food for intestinal bacteria, which multiply and produce irritating acid and gas, further contributing to the discomfort and diarrhea.

lactose intolerance: a condition that results from inability to digest the milk sugar lactose; characterized by bloating, gas, abdominal discomfort, and diarrhea. Lactose intolerance differs from milk allergy, which is caused by an immune reaction to the protein in milk.

lactase deficiency: a lack of the enzyme required to digest the disaccharide lactose into its component monosaccharides (glucose and galactose).

Causes As mentioned, lactase activity commonly declines with age. Lactase deficiency may also develop when the intestinal villi are damaged by disease, certain medicines, prolonged diarrhea, or malnutrition; this can lead to temporary or permanent lactose malabsorption, depending on the extent of the intestinal damage. In extremely rare cases, an infant is simply born with a lactase deficiency.

Prevalence The prevalence of lactose intolerance varies widely among ethnic groups, indicating that the trait is genetically determined.[8] The prevalence of lactose intolerance is lowest among Scandinavians and other Northern Europeans and highest among native North Americans and Southeast Asians.

Estimated prevalence of lactose intolerance:

- >80% Asian Americans.
- 80% Native Americans.
- 75% African Americans.
- 70% Mediterranean peoples.
- 60% Inuits.
- 50% Hispanics.
- 20% Caucasians.
- <10% Northern Europeans.

Dietary Changes Managing lactose intolerance requires some dietary changes, although total elimination of milk products is usually not necessary. Excluding all milk products from the diet can lead to nutrient deficiencies, for milk is a major source of several nutrients, notably the mineral calcium and the B vitamin riboflavin. Fortunately, many people with lactose intolerance can consume small amounts of milk products, especially if they take them with other foods in meals. In some cases, people can increase their tolerance by gradually increasing the amounts of milk products they consume; they may become able to tolerate as much as a cup of milk a day.[9] A change in the GI bacteria, not the reappearance of the missing enzyme, accounts for the ability to adapt to milk products.

In many cases, lactose-intolerant people can tolerate fermented milk products such as yogurt and acidophilus milk. The bacteria in these products digest lactose for their own use, leaving these foods relatively low in lactose. Hard cheeses and cottage cheese are often well tolerated because most of the lactose is removed with the whey during manufacturing. Lactose continues to diminish as the cheese ages.

Many lactose-intolerant people use commercially prepared milk products that have been treated with an enzyme that breaks down the lactose. Alternatively, they take enzyme tablets with meals or add enzyme drops to their milk. The

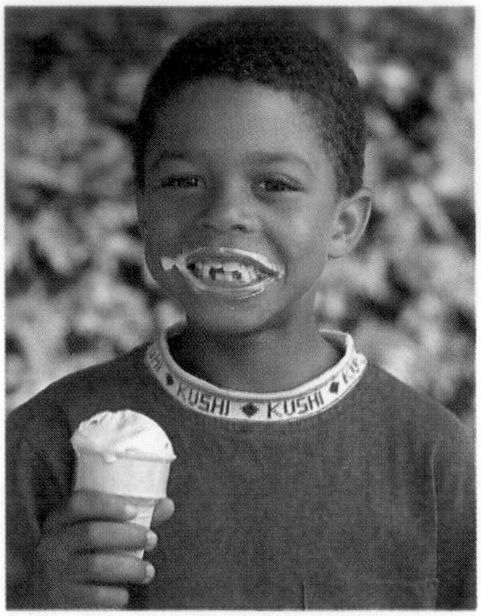

Many people who are lactose intolerant cannot enjoy ice cream without GI distress.

enzyme hydrolyzes much of the lactose in milk to glucose and galactose, which lactose-intolerant people can absorb without ill effects. Most healthy adults with lactose intolerance can drink milk when the lactose content has been reduced by 50 percent.[10]

Because people's tolerance to lactose varies widely, lactose-restricted diets must be highly individualized. Each case differs. A completely lactose-free diet can be difficult because lactose appears not only in milk and milk products but as an ingredient in many nondairy foods such as breads, cereals, breakfast drinks, salad dressings, and cake mixes. People on strict lactose-free diets need to read labels and avoid foods that include milk, milk solids, whey (milk liquid), and casein (milk protein, which may contain traces of lactose). They also need to check all drugs with the pharmacist because 20 percent of prescription drugs and 5 percent of over-the-counter drugs contain lactose as a filler.

People who consume few or no milk products must take care to meet riboflavin and calcium needs. Later chapters on the vitamins and minerals offer help with finding good nonmilk sources of these nutrients.

To summarize the digestion and absorption of carbohydrates, the body breaks down starches into disaccharides and disaccharides into monosaccharides, and then converts monosaccharides mostly to glucose to fuel the cells' work. The fibers help to regulate the passage of food through the GI system, but contribute only a little energy. Lactose intolerance is a common condition that occurs when there is insufficient lactase to digest the disaccharide lactose found in milk and milk products. Symptoms include GI distress. Because treatment requires limiting milk intake, other calcium-rich substitutes must be included in the diet.

Glucose in the Body

The primary role of the available carbohydrates in human nutrition is to supply the body's cells with glucose to deliver the indispensable commodity, energy. Starch contributes most to the body's glucose supply, but as explained earlier, any of the sugars can also be converted to glucose.

Glucose plays the central role in carbohydrate metabolism. The next two sections provide an overview first of the pathways glucose can follow in the body and then of the ways the body regulates those pathways.

A PREVIEW OF CARBOHYDRATE METABOLISM

This brief discussion provides just enough information about carbohydrate metabolism to illustrate that the body needs and uses glucose as a chief energy nutrient. Chapter 7 provides a full description of how all of the energy-yielding nutrients—carbohydrate, fat, and protein—contain energy and how the body metabolizes these molecules to free that energy for its use.

Storing Glucose as Glycogen The liver stores and releases glucose as needed. During times of plenty, liver cells combine excess glucose molecules into long, branching chains of glycogen. The liver stores one-third of the body's total glycogen. When blood glucose falls, the liver cells dismantle the glycogen into single molecules of glucose and release them into the bloodstream. Thus glucose can supply energy to the central nervous system and other organs regardless of whether the person has eaten recently. Muscle cells can also store glucose as glycogen (the other two-thirds), but they hoard most of their own supply, using it just for themselves during exercise.

Glycogen holds water and therefore is rather bulky. The body can store only enough glycogen to provide energy for relatively short periods of time—during exercise, a few hours' worth at most. For its long-term energy reserves, for use over days or weeks of food deprivation, the body employs its unlimited, water-free fuel, fat, as Chapter 5 describes.

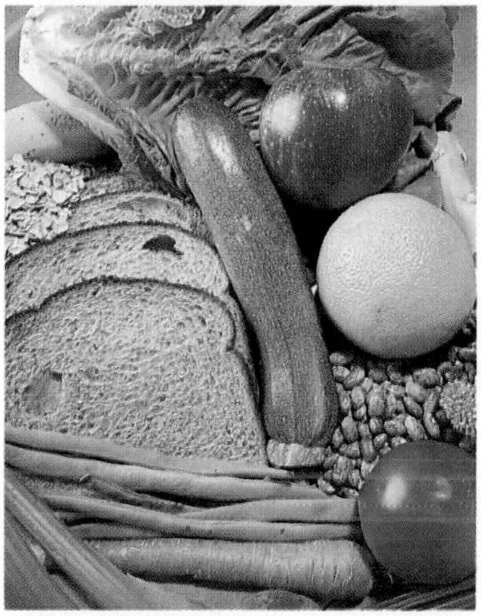

The carbohydrates of grains, vegetables, fruits, and legumes supply most of the energy in a healthful diet.

Using Glucose for Energy Glucose fuels the work of most of the body's cells. Inside a cell, enzymes break glucose in half. These halves can be put back together to make glucose, or they can be further broken down into smaller fragments (never again to be reassembled to form glucose). The small fragments can yield energy when broken down completely to carbon dioxide and water, or they can be reassembled, but only into units of body fat.

To keep providing glucose to meet the body's energy needs, a person has to eat dietary carbohydrate frequently, for as mentioned, glycogen stores last only for hours, not for days. People do not always attend faithfully to their bodies' carbohydrate needs, yet they survive. How do they manage without glucose from dietary carbohydrate? Do they simply draw energy from the other two energy-yielding nutrients, fat and protein? They do draw energy, but not simply.

Making Glucose from Protein Body protein can be converted to glucose to some extent, but protein has jobs of its own that no other nutrient can do. Body fat cannot be converted to glucose to any significant extent, and although fat breakdown can yield energy for many of the body's cells "as is," glucose does some jobs that fat cannot normally do—for example, glucose provides energy for brain cells, other nerve cells, and developing red blood cells.

Thus, when a person does not replenish depleted glycogen stores by eating carbohydrate, body proteins are dismantled to make glucose to fuel these special cells. The conversion of protein to glucose is called gluconeogenesis—literally, the making of new glucose. Only adequate dietary carbohydrate can prevent this use of protein for energy, and this role of carbohydrate is known as its protein-sparing action.

Making Ketone Bodies from Fat Fragments Without sufficient glucose, the body also changes its way of using fat. Normally, when fat breaks down to provide energy, glucose is also present, and the two fuels are metabolized together. Fat fragments combine with glucose fragments, and the combined molecules then break down completely. Without glucose, fat fragments do not break down completely but combine with each other, forming ketone bodies. Muscles and other tissues can use ketone bodies for energy, but when their production exceeds their use, they accumulate in the blood, causing ketosis, a condition that disturbs the body's normal acid-base balance, as described in Chapter 7.

To ensure complete sparing of body protein and prevent ketosis requires 50 to 100 grams of carbohydrate a day.[11] Dietary recommendations urge people to select abundantly from carbohydrate-rich foods to provide for this allowance and considerably more.

gluconeogenesis (gloo-co-nee-oh-GEN-ih-sis): the making of glucose from a noncarbohydrate source (described in more detail in Chapter 7).
gluco = glucose
neo = new
genesis = making

protein-sparing action: the action of carbohydrate (and fat) in providing energy that allows protein to be used for other purposes.

ketone (KEE-tone) **bodies:** the product of the incomplete breakdown of fat when glucose is not available in the cells.

ketosis (kee-TOE-sis): an undesirably high concentration of ketone bodies in the blood and urine.

acid-base balance: the equilibrium in the body between acid and base concentrations; see Chapter 12.

Converting Glucose to Fat Given more carbohydrate than it needs, the body uses glucose to meet its energy needs, fills its glycogen stores to capacity, and may still have some left over. To store the extra glucose, the liver breaks it (and energy-containing fragments from protein or fat, too) into smaller molecules and puts them together into the more permanent energy-storage compound—fat. Then the fat travels to the fatty tissues of the body for storage. Unlike the liver cells, which can store only about half a day's worth of glycogen, fat cells can store unlimited quantities of fat.

Even though excess carbohydrate can be converted to fat and stored, this is a minor pathway.[12] The amount of fat being made from carbohydrate at any given time is less than the amount of fat being used for energy. Body fat comes mainly from dietary fat.[13] A balanced diet high in complex carbohydrates actually helps control body weight. Most carbohydrate-rich foods are so bulky and naturally so low in fat that when large quantities are eaten, they tend to crowd fat out of the diet. Since carbohydrate is less energy dense than fat (with only 4 kcalories to the gram compared with fat's 9), eating a diet high in carbohydrate usually tends to *reduce* energy intake. Thus abundant dietary carbohydrate combined with little dietary fat supports weight control.

THE CONSTANCY OF BLOOD GLUCOSE

Every body cell depends on glucose for its fuel to some extent, and ordinarily, the cells of the brain and the rest of the nervous system depend *primarily* on glucose for their energy. The activities of these cells never cease, and they do not have the ability to store glucose. Day and night they continually draw on the supply of glucose in the fluid surrounding them. To maintain the supply, a steady stream of blood moves past these cells bringing more glucose from either the intestines (food) or the liver (glycogen).

Reminder: *Homeostasis* is the maintenance of constant internal conditions by the body's control systems.

Normal blood glucose: 80 to 120 mg/dL.

Maintaining Glucose Homeostasis To function optimally, the body must maintain blood glucose within limits that permit the cells to nourish themselves. If blood glucose falls below normal, the person may become dizzy and weak; if it rises above normal, the person may become confused and have difficulty breathing. Left untreated, fluctuations to the extremes—either high or low—can be fatal.

insulin (IN-suh-lin): a hormone secreted by special cells in the pancreas in response to (among other things) increased blood glucose concentration. The primary role of insulin is to control the transport of glucose from the bloodstream into the cells.

glucagon (GLOO-ka-gon): a hormone secreted by special cells in the pancreas in response to low blood glucose concentration that elicits release of glucose from storage.

The Regulating Hormones Blood glucose homeostasis is regulated primarily by two hormones: insulin, which moves glucose from the blood into the cells, and glucagon, which brings glucose out of storage when necessary. Figure 4–12 depicts these hormonal regulators at work.

After a meal, as blood glucose rises, special cells of the pancreas respond by secreting insulin into the blood.* As the circulating insulin contacts the receptors on the body's other cells, the receptors respond by ushering glucose from the blood into the cells. Most of the cells take only the glucose they can use for energy right away, but the liver and muscle cells can assemble the small glucose units into long, branching chains of glycogen for storage. The liver cells can also convert glucose to fat for export to other cells. Thus high blood glucose returns

*The *beta* (BAY-tuh) *cells*, one of several types of cells in the pancreas, secrete insulin in response to elevated blood glucose concentration.

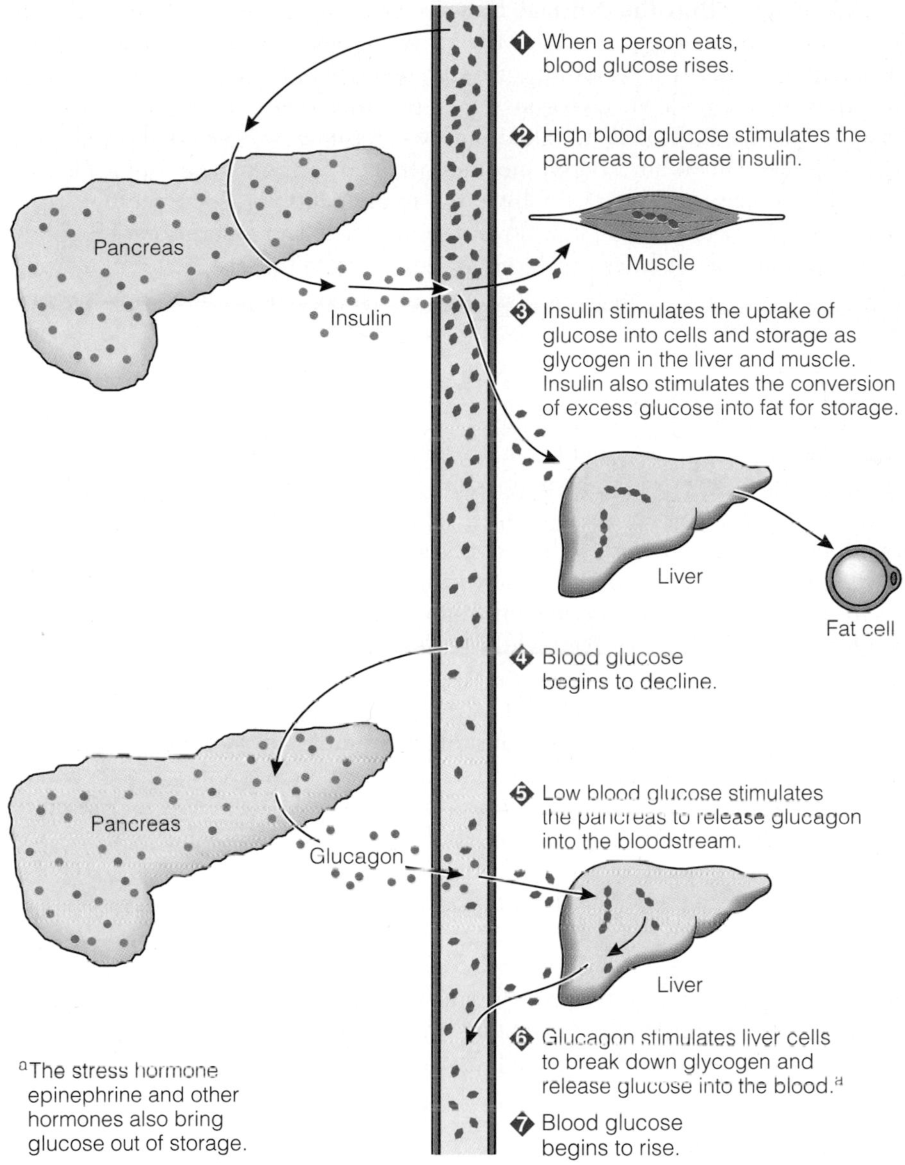

1 When a person eats, blood glucose rises.
2 High blood glucose stimulates the pancreas to release insulin.
Pancreas
Insulin
Muscle
3 Insulin stimulates the uptake of glucose into cells and storage as glycogen in the liver and muscle. Insulin also stimulates the conversion of excess glucose into fat for storage.
Liver
Fat cell
4 Blood glucose begins to decline.
5 Low blood glucose stimulates the pancreas to release glucagon into the bloodstream.
Pancreas
Glucagon
Liver
6 Glucagon stimulates liver cells to break down glycogen and release glucose into the blood.[a]
7 Blood glucose begins to rise.
[a]The stress hormone epinephrine and other hormones also bring glucose out of storage.

Figure 4–12

Maintaining Blood Glucose Homeostasis

to normal as excess glucose is stored as glycogen (which can be converted back to glucose) and fat (which cannot be).

When blood glucose falls (as occurs between meals), other special cells of the pancreas respond by secreting glucagon into the blood.* Glucagon raises blood glucose by signaling the liver to dismantle its glycogen stores and release glucose into the blood for use by all the other body cells.

Another hormone that calls glucose from the liver cells is the "fight-or-flight" hormone, epinephrine. Epinephrine acts quickly when a person experiences stress, ensuring that all the body cells have energy fuel in emergencies. Like glucagon, epinephrine works to return glucose to the blood from liver glycogen.

epinephrine (EP-ih-NEFF-rin): a hormone of the adrenal gland that modulates the stress response; formerly called *adrenaline*.

*Glucagon is produced by the *alpha cells* of the pancreas.

Balancing within the Normal Range The maintenance of normal blood glucose thus ordinarily depends on two processes. When blood glucose falls too low, food can readily replenish it, or in the absence of food, glucagon can signal the liver to break down glycogen stores. When blood glucose rises too high, insulin can signal the cells to take in glucose for energy. Eating balanced meals helps the body maintain a happy medium between the extremes. Balanced meals provide abundant complex carbohydrates, including fibers, some protein, and a little fat. The fibers and fat slow down the digestion and absorption of carbohydrate, so that glucose enters the blood gradually, providing a steady, ongoing supply. Dietary protein elicits the secretion of glucagon, whose effects oppose those of insulin, helping maintain blood glucose within the normal range.[14]

Falling outside the Normal Range This influence of foods on blood glucose has given rise to the oversimplification that foods *govern* blood glucose concentrations. Foods do not; the body does. In some people, however, blood glucose regulation fails. When this happens, either of two conditions can result: diabetes or hypoglycemia. People with these conditions can often use special diet patterns to help maintain their blood glucose within a normal range.

hypoglycemia: an abnormally low blood glucose concentration.

In diabetes, blood glucose remains high after a meal because insulin is either inadequate or ineffective. Thus while *blood* glucose is central to diabetes, *dietary* carbohydrates do not cause diabetes.

In insulin-dependent diabetes (IDDM), which is the less common type of diabetes, the pancreas fails to make insulin; researchers hold genetics, toxins, a virus, and a disordered immune system responsible. In noninsulin-dependent diabetes (NIDDM), which is the more common type of diabetes, the cells fail to respond to insulin; this condition tends to occur as a consequence of obesity. Because obesity can precipitate NIDDM, the best preventive measure is to maintain a healthy body weight. Recommendations for those who have diabetes encourage a diet low in fat and rich in complex carbohydrates and fibers. Concentrated sweets are not strictly excluded from the diabetic diet as they once were, but can be eaten in limited amounts with meals as part of a healthy diet.[15] The many environmental, genetic, and metabolic factors surrounding diabetes and its associated problems receive full attention in Chapter 18.

insulin-dependent diabetes mellitus (IDDM): the less common type of diabetes in which the person produces no insulin at all; also known as type I diabetes or juvenile-onset diabetes (because it frequently develops in childhood), although some cases arise in adulthood.

noninsulin-dependent diabetes mellitus (NIDDM): the more common type of diabetes in which the fat cells resist insulin; also called type II diabetes or adult-onset diabetes. NIDDM is usually milder than IDDM and progresses more slowly.

The Glycemic Effect The term *glycemic effect* describes the effect of food on blood glucose: how quickly glucose is absorbed after a person eats, how high blood glucose rises, and how quickly it returns to normal. Slow absorption, a modest rise in blood glucose, and a smooth return to normal are considered desirable; fast absorption, a surge in blood glucose, and an overreaction that forces glucose below normal are undesirable. Different foods have different effects on blood glucose depending on a number of factors working together, and the effect is not always what a person might expect.[16] Ice cream, for example, is a high-sugar food, but it produces less of a response than potatoes, a high-starch food.

glycemic (gligh-SEEM-ic) effect: a measure of the extent to which a food, as compared with pure glucose, raises the blood glucose concentration and elicits an insulin response.

Most relevant to real life, a food's glycemic effect differs depending on whether it is eaten alone or as part of a mixed meal. In addition, eating small meals frequently spreads glucose absorption across the day and thus offers the same metabolic advantages as do foods with a low glycemic effect.[17]

Popular articles sometimes describe eating many small meals and snacks throughout the day as grazing.

The rate of glucose absorption is particularly important to people with diabetes, who may benefit from avoiding foods that produce too great a rise, or too sudden a fall, in blood glucose. Indeed, some studies have shown that taking the glycemic effect into account in meal planning is a practical way to improve glucose control.[18] Overall, though, meal planning should focus on total carbohydrate intake rather than the source of carbohydrate.[19]

To sum up, dietary carbohydrates provide glucose that can be used by the cells for energy, stored by the liver and muscle as glycogen, or converted into fat if intakes exceed needs. All of the body's cells depend on glucose; those of the central nervous system are especially dependent on it. Without glucose, the body is forced to break down its protein tissues to make glucose and alter its metabolism to make ketone bodies from fats. Blood glucose regulation depends primarily on two pancreatic hormones: insulin to remove glucose from the blood into the cells when levels are high and glucagon to free glucose from glycogen stores and release it into the blood when levels are low.

Health Effects and Recommended Intakes of Sugars

Ever since people first discovered honey and dates, they have enjoyed the sweetness of sugars. In the United States, the natural sugars of milk, fruits, vegetables, and grains account for about half of the sugar intake; the other half consists of sugars that have been refined and added to foods for a variety of purposes. Added sugars assume various names: sucrose, invert sugar, corn sugar, corn syrups and solids, high-fructose corn syrup, and honey (see the glossary on p. 132).

The use of sweeteners in food manufacturing has risen steadily over the past two decades, reaching a record high of 139 pounds per person per year (see Figure 4–13). This estimate represents all sweeteners used in the marketing

As an additive, sugar:

- Enhances flavor.
- Supplies texture and color to baked goods.
- Provides fuel for fermentation, causing bread to rise or producing alcohol.
- Acts as a bulking agent in ice cream and baked goods.
- Acts as a preservative in jams.
- Balances the acidity of tomato- and vinegar-based products.

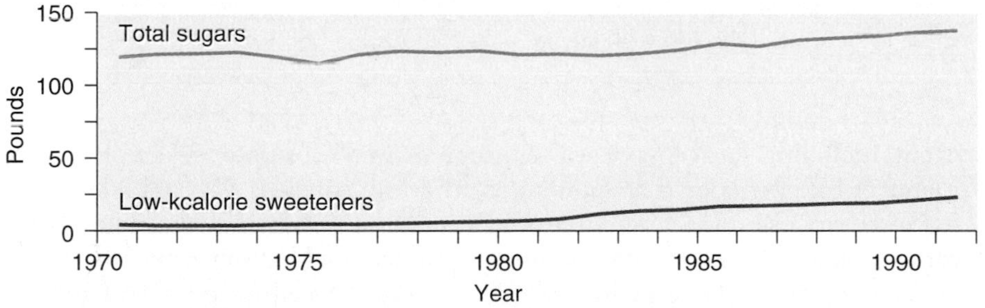

Figure 4–13

Use of Sweeteners

Source: U.S. Department of Agriculture, Economic Research Service, Commodity Economics Division.

Total per capita use of sugars increased 15 percent from 1971 to 1991. In that same time, use of low-kcalorie sweeteners increased approximately 10 percent.

These data do not represent the amount of sugars actually consumed; instead, they represent the total disappearance of sweeteners into the marketing system divided by the total U.S. population. Estimates based on dietary intake indicate that the average consumption of refined sugar is less than half of the per capita estimate.

Glossary of Sugars

brown sugar: refined white sugar crystals to which manufacturers have added molasses syrup with natural flavor and color; 91 to 96 percent pure sucrose.

confectioners' sugar: finely powdered sucrose; 99.9 percent pure.

corn sweeteners: corn syrup and sugars derived from corn.

corn syrup: a syrup produced by the action of enzymes on cornstarch; contains mostly glucose. See also *high-fructose corn syrup (HFCS)*.

dextrose: an older name for glucose.

granulated sugar: crystalline sucrose; 99.9 percent pure.

high-fructose corn syrup (HFCS): a corn-syrup sweetener made especially for use in processed foods and beverages, where it is the predominant sweetener. HFCS is mostly fructose; glucose makes up the balance.

honey: sugar (mostly sucrose) formed from nectar gathered by bees. An enzyme splits the sucrose into glucose and fructose. Composition and flavor vary, but honey always contains a mixture of sucrose, fructose, and glucose.

invert sugar: a mixture of glucose and fructose formed by the hydrolysis of sucrose in a chemical process; sold only in liquid form and sweeter than sucrose. Invert sugar is used as a food additive to help preserve freshness and prevent shrinkage.

levulose: an older name for fructose.

maple sugar: a sugar (mostly sucrose) purified from the concentrated sap of the sugar maple tree.

molasses: the thick brown syrup produced during sugar refining. Molasses retains residual sugar and other by-products and a few minerals; blackstrap molasses contains significant amounts of calcium and iron—the iron comes from the *machinery* used to process the sugar.

raw sugar: the first crop of crystals harvested during sugar processing. Raw sugar cannot be sold in the United States because it contains too much filth (dirt, insect fragments, and the like). Sugar sold as "raw sugar" domestically has actually gone through over half of the refining steps.

turbinado (ter-bih-NOD-oh) sugar: sugar produced using the same refining process as white sugar, but without the bleaching and anti-caking treatment; traces of molasses give turbinado its sandy color.

white sugar: pure sucrose or "table sugar," produced by dissolving, concentrating, and recrystallizing raw sugar.

---

system, including sugar lost or wasted, such as in the brine of sweet pickles or in jams or bakery goods that spoil before they are eaten. It also includes sugar used in pet foods and in fermentation. Estimates of *intake* indicate that on the average, each person consumes about 45 pounds of added sugar per year.[20] As a percentage of daily energy intake, this amount is roughly equivalent to current recommendations that sugar contribute no more than about 10 percent of energy intake.

HEALTH EFFECTS OF SUGARS

In moderate amounts (similar to current consumption levels), sugars add pleasure to meals without harming health. In excess, however, they can be detrimental in two ways. One, sugars can contribute to nutrient deficiencies by supplying energy (kcalories) without providing nutrients, and so dietary guidelines caution people against eating large quantities. Two, sugars contribute to tooth decay, and so dietary guidelines caution people against eating frequent snacks containing sugars and starches.

empty-kcalorie food: a popular term used to denote foods that contribute energy but lack protein, vitamins, and minerals. Empty-kcalorie foods are *low-nutrient density foods*. The most notorious empty-kcalorie foods are sugar, fat, and alcohol.

Nutrient Deficiencies Foods that contain lots of added sugar deliver energy without other nutrients—they are empty-kcalorie foods. By comparison, starch comes packaged in foods with protein, vitamins, and minerals.

A person spending 200 kcalories of a day's energy allowance on a 16-ounce cola gets nothing of value for those kcaloric "dollars." In contrast, a person using 200 kcalories on three slices of whole-wheat bread gets 9 grams of protein plus several of the B vitamins with those kcalories. For the person who wants something sweet, perhaps a reasonable compromise would be to have two slices of bread with a teaspoon of jam on each. The amount of sugar a person can afford depends on how many kcalories are available beyond those needed to deliver indispensable vitamins and minerals.

With careful food selections, a person can obtain all the needed nutrients within an allowance of about 1500 kcalories. Some people have more generous energy allowances with which to "purchase" nutrients. For example, an active teenage boy may need as many as 4000 kcalories to get all the energy he needs. If he eats mostly nutritious foods, then the "empty kcalories" of cola beverages are probably an acceptable addition to his diet. On the other hand, an inactive older woman who can use fewer than 1500 kcalories a day cannot afford any but the most nutrient-dense foods.

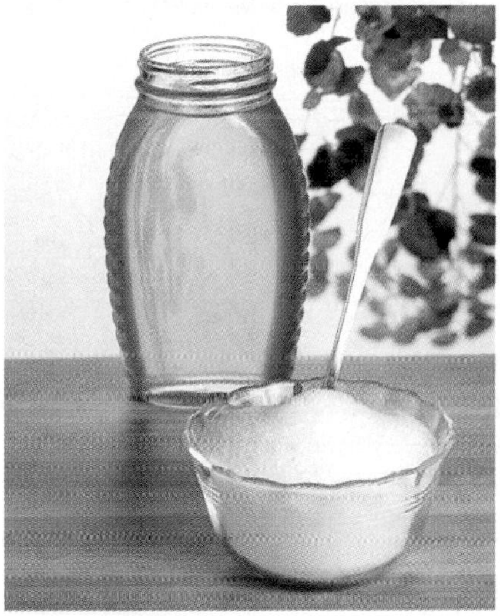

1 tsp honey = 22 kcal.
1 tsp sugar = 16 kcal.

Some people believe that because honey is a natural food, it is nutritious—or, at least, more nutritious than sugar. A look at their chemical structures reveals the truth. Honey, like table sugar, contains glucose and fructose. The primary difference is that in table sugar the two monosaccharides are bonded together, whereas in honey some of them are free. Whether a person eats monosaccharides individually, as in honey, or linked together, as in table sugar, they end up the same way in the body: as glucose and fructose.

Honey does contain a few vitamins and minerals, but not many, as Table 4–3 (on p. 134) shows. Honey is denser than crystalline sugar, too, so it provides more energy per spoon.

This is not to say that all sugar sources are alike, for some are more nutritious than others. Consider a fruit, say, an orange. The fruit may give you the same amounts of fructose and glucose and the same number of kcalories as a dose of sugar or honey, but the packaging is more valuable nutritionally. The fruit's sugars arrive in the body diluted in a large volume of water, packaged in fiber, and mixed with valuable minerals and vitamins.

As these comparisons illustrate, the really significant difference between sugar sources is not between "natural" honey and "purified" sugar but between concentrated sweets and the dilute, naturally occurring sugars that sweeten foods. You can suspect an exaggerated nutrition claim when you hear the assertion that one product is more nutritious than another because it contains honey.

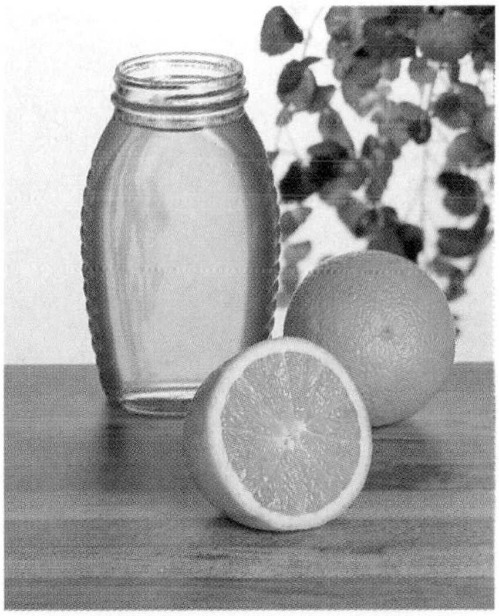

You receive the same sugars from an orange as from honey, but the packaging makes a big nutrition difference.

Sugar can contribute to nutrient deficiencies only by displacing nutrients. The appropriate attitude to take is not that sugar is "bad" and must be avoided, but that nutritious foods must come first. If the nutritious foods end up crowding

Table 4–3

Sample Nutrients in Sugars and Other Foods

The indicated portion of any of these foods provides approximately 100 kcalories. Notice that for a similar number of kcalories and grams of carbohydrates, milk, legumes, fruits, vegetables, and grains offer more of the other nutrients than do the sugars.

	Size of 100 kcal Portion	Carbohydrate (g)	Protein (g)	Calcium (mg)	Iron (mg)	Vitamin A (μg RE)	Vitamin C (mg)
Foods							
Milk, 1% low-fat	1 c	12	8	300	0.1	144	2
Kidney beans	½ c	20	7	30	1.6	0	2
Apricots	6	24	2	30	1.1	554	22
Bread, whole wheat	1½ slices	20	4	30	1.9	0	0
Broccoli, cooked	2 c	20	12	188	2.2	696	148
Sugars							
Sugar, white	2 tbs	24	0	trace	trace	0	0
Molasses, blackstrap	2½ tbs	28	0	343	12.6	0	0.1
Cola beverage	1 c	26	0	6	trace	0	0
Honey	1½ tbs	26	trace	2	0.2	0	trace

sugar out of the diet, that is fine—but not the other way around. As always, the goals to seek are balance, variety, and moderation.

dental caries: decay of teeth.
caries = rottenness

Dental Caries Both sugars and starches begin breaking down to sugars in the mouth and so can contribute to tooth decay. Bacteria in the mouth ferment the sugars and in the process produce an acid that dissolves tooth enamel. People can eat sugar without this happening, though, for much depends on how long acid-yielding foods stay in the mouth. Sticky foods stay on tooth surfaces longer and keep yielding acid longer than foods that are readily cleared from the mouth. For that reason, sugar consumed quickly in a soft drink, for example, is less likely to cause dental caries than sugar in a pastry. By the same token, the sugar in sticky foods such as dried fruits is more detrimental than its quantity alone would suggest.

To prevent dental caries:

- Eat sugary foods with meals.
- Limit between-meal snacks containing sugars and starches.
- Brush and floss teeth regularly.
- If brushing and flossing are not possible, at least rinse with water.

Another concern is how often people eat sugar. Bacteria produce acid for 20 to 30 minutes after each exposure. If a person ate three pieces of candy at one time, the teeth would be exposed to approximately 30 minutes of acid destruction. But, if the person ate three pieces at half-hour intervals, the time of exposure would increase to 90 minutes. Likewise, slowly sipping a sugary soft drink may be more harmful than drinking quickly and clearing the mouth of sugar. Nonsugary foods can help remove sugar from tooth surfaces; hence, it is better to eat sugar with meals than between meals.

plaque, dental: a gummy mass of bacteria that grows on teeth and can lead to dental caries and gum disease.

The development of caries depends on several factors: the bacteria that reside in the plaque, the saliva that cleanses the mouth, the minerals that form the teeth, and the foods that remain after swallowing.[21] For most people, good oral hygiene and a well-balanced diet will prevent dental caries. In short, sugars cause dental caries, but they require a cooperating victim to do so.

ACCUSATIONS AGAINST SUGARS

Sugars have been blamed for a variety of other problems. The following paragraphs evaluate some of these accusations.

Accusation: Sugar Causes Obesity Population studies show that obesity rises as sugar consumption increases, but sugar is not the sole cause. Foods high in added sugars are usually high in fat, too, so that whenever sugar intake increases, total energy and fat intakes do, too. Simultaneously, physical activity often declines. Obesity also occurs where sugar intakes are low. In some instances, obese people eat less sugar than thin people.[22] Thus sugar can contribute to obesity but does not cause obesity by itself—and obesity can occur without it.

Accusation: Sugar Causes Heart Diseases Researchers agree that unusually high doses of refined sugar can alter blood lipids to promote heart disease. This effect is most dramatic in "carbohydrate-sensitive" individuals—people who respond to sucrose with abnormally high insulin secretion, which promotes the making of excess fat. For most people, though, moderate sugar intakes do *not* influence the risk of heart disease. To keep these findings in perspective, consider that heart disease correlates most closely with factors that have nothing to do with nutrition, such as smoking and genetics. Among dietary risk factors, several—such as total fats, saturated fats, cholesterol, and obesity have much stronger associations with heart disease than sugar intakes.

Accusation: Sugar Causes Misbehavior in Children and Criminal Behavior in Adults Sugar has been blamed for the misbehaviors of hyperactive children, delinquent adolescents, and lawbreaking adults. Such speculations have been based on personal stories and have not been confirmed by scientific research.[23] No scientific evidence supports a relationship between sugar and hyperactivity or other misbehaviors. Chapter 16 provides accurate information on diet and children's behavior.

RECOMMENDED INTAKES OF SUGARS

The *Dietary Guidelines* urge people to use sugars only in moderation. Other recommendations specify that sugars should occupy only 10 percent or less of the day's total energy intake. A person consuming 2000 kcalories a day, then, should receive no more than 200 kcalories (that is, 50 grams or less) from concentrated sugars.

Food labels list the total grams of sugar a food provides. This total reflects both added sugars and those occurring naturally in foods. A food is likely to be high in sugars if its ingredient list starts with any of the sugars named in the glossary on p. 132 or if it includes several of them.

In summary, as currently consumed, sugars pose no major health threat except for an increased risk of dental caries. Excessive intakes may displace needed nutri-

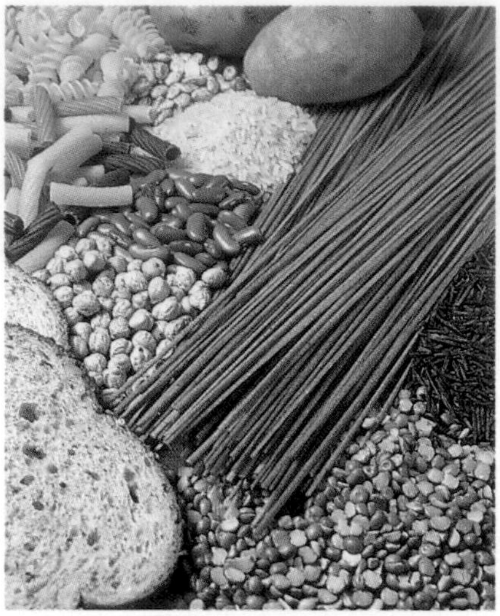

Foods rich in starch and fiber offer many health benefits.

ents and fiber; when accompanied by fat, sugars may be associated with obesity. If on these grounds a person decides to limit daily sugar intake, it is important to recognize that not all sugars need to be restricted, just *concentrated* sweets, which are relatively empty of other nutrients and high in kcalories. Sugars that occur naturally in fruits, vegetables, and milk are acceptable.

Health Effects and Recommended Intakes of Starch and Fibers

Carbohydrates and fats are the two major sources of energy in the diet. When one is high, the other is usually low—and vice versa. The average fat intake in the United States is high compared with health recommendations. To lower fat intake and improve the balance between these two energy nutrients, people need to replace fatty foods with vegetables, legumes, fruits, and grain products—foods noted for their complex carbohydrates.

HEALTH EFFECTS OF STARCH AND FIBERS

In addition to starch and dietary fibers, vegetables, legumes, fruits, and grains supply valuable vitamins and minerals and little or no fat. The following paragraphs describe some of the health benefits of diets rich in complex carbohydrates.

Weight Control Foods rich in complex carbohydrates tend to be low in fat and simple sugars and can therefore promote weight loss by providing less food energy per bite. They also provide satiety and delay hunger. In addition, fiber-rich foods slow the rate at which food leaves the stomach and draw water into the GI tract, prolonging the satiety enjoyed from carbohydrate-rich meals. Several studies have found that people who eat a high-carbohydrate breakfast take in fewer kcalories at later meals and snacks than people who eat low-fiber or high-fat breakfasts.[24]

Many weight-loss products on the market today contain bulk-inducing fibers such as methylcellulose, but buying pure fiber compounds like this is neither necessary nor advisable. To use fiber in a weight-loss plan, select fresh fruits, vegetables, legumes, and whole-grain foods. High-fiber foods not only add bulk to the diet, but are economical and nutritious. (A note of caution, though: on baked goods, read the label—those popular large bran muffins are high in fat, and many items, of course, contain added sugar.)

The role of animal fat and cholesterol in heart disease is discussed in Chapter 5. The role of vegetable proteins in heart disease is discussed in Chapter 6.

Heart Disease High-carbohydrate diets are associated with low blood cholesterol and a low risk of heart disease.[25] Sorting out the exact reasons why can be difficult. Such diets are low in animal fat and cholesterol and high in soluble fibers and vegetable proteins—all factors associated with a lower risk of heart disease.

Foods rich in soluble fibers (such as oat bran, barley, and legumes) lower blood cholesterol by binding with bile, the emulsifier that otherwise would assist with fat and cholesterol absorption.[26] With less bile available, less fat and cholesterol are absorbed and blood cholesterol declines. Then the liver makes more bile from cholesterol to compensate for the bile bound to fiber and excreted in the

GI tract.[27] This reduces blood cholesterol further. The products of fiber digestion, once absorbed, also inhibit cholesterol synthesis.

Several researchers have speculated that fiber also exerts an indirect cholesterol-lowering effect by displacing fats in the diet.[28] Even when dietary fat is low, however, research shows high intakes of soluble fibers exert a separate and significant cholesterol-lowering effect.[29]

Cancer A high-carbohydrate diet, especially one that includes plenty of green and yellow vegetables and citrus fruits, protects against some types of cancer. Again, it is unclear whether the protection derives from the fiber or the vitamins.

The role antioxidant vitamins and nutrients play in cancer prevention is discussed in Highlight 11.

Populations consuming high-fiber diets generally have lower rates of colon cancer than similar populations consuming low-fiber diets. Fiber may help prevent colon cancer by diluting, binding, and rapidly removing potentially cancer-causing agents from the colon. Alternatively, the protective effect may be due to the fermentation of resistant starch and fiber in the colon, which lowers the pH. A decreased pH in the colon is associated with decreased colon cancer risks.[30]

Diabetes Populations eating high-carbohydrate diets often have low rates of diabetes, most likely because such diets are low in fat. High-carbohydrate, low-fat diets help control weight, and this is the most effective way to prevent the most common type of diabetes (NIDDM). Furthermore, when soluble fibers trap nutrients and delay their exit from the stomach, glucose absorption is slowed, and this helps to prevent the glucose surge and rebound that seem to be associated with diabetes onset.

GI Health Dietary fibers enhance the health of the large intestine. Their short-chain fatty acid products promote salt absorption and help maintain mucosal integrity. The healthier the intestinal walls, the better they can block absorption of unwanted constituents, such as bacteria. Fibers enlarge the stools, easing passage, and they speed up transit time; up to a point, transit time depends on stool weight. Insoluble fibers such as cellulose (as in cereal brans, fruits, and vegetables) are most important in this regard. Their undigested residue, together with the microbial growth they stimulate, enlarges the stools, helping to alleviate or prevent constipation. Fibers also stimulate microbial digestion of absorbable products.

Taken with ample fluids, fibers help to prevent several GI disorders. Large, soft stools ease elimination for the rectal muscles and reduce the pressure in the lower bowel, making it less likely that rectal veins will swell (hemorrhoids). Fiber prevents compaction of the intestinal contents, which could obstruct the appendix and permit bacteria to invade and infect it (appendicitis). In addition, fiber stimulates the GI tract muscles so that they retain their strength and resist bulging out into pouches known as diverticula (illustrated in Figure 4–14 on p. 138).

diverticula (dye-ver-TIC-you-la): a sac or pouch that develops in the weakened areas of the intestinal wall (like bulges in an inner tube where the tire wall is weak). The term **diverticulosis** (DYE-ver-tic-you-LOH-sis) describes the condition of having diverticula. The danger of diverticulosis is that it can give rise to **diverticulitis** (DYE-ver-tic-you-LYE-tis), in which the pockets become infected or inflamed and may rupture. About one in every six people in Western countries develops diverticulosis in middle or later life.

- *divertir* = to turn aside
- *osis* = condition
- *itis* = infection or inflammation

Harmful Effects of Excessive Fiber Intake Despite fiber's benefits to health, research indicates that a diet high in fiber also has a few drawbacks. A person who has a small capacity and eats mostly high-fiber foods may not be able to take in enough food energy or nutrients. The malnourished, the elderly, and children adhering to all-plant diets are especially vulnerable to this problem.

Figure 4–14

Diverticula

Outpocketings of intestinal linings that balloon through weakened intestinal wall muscles are known as diverticula. Diverticula may develop anywhere along the GI tract, but most commonly in the colon.

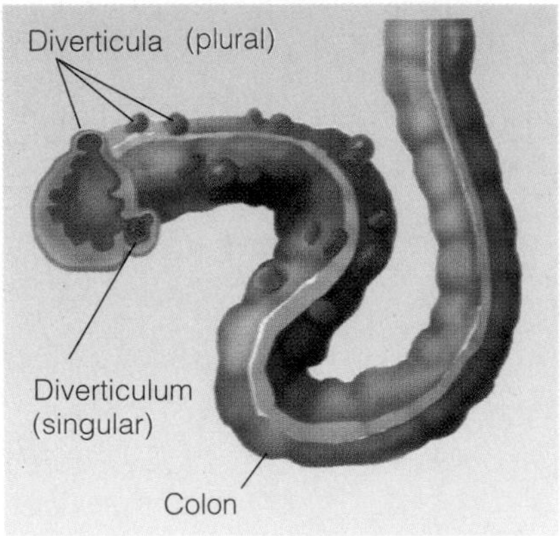

Launching suddenly into a high-fiber diet can cause temporary bouts of abdominal discomfort, gas, and diarrhea and, more seriously, can obstruct the GI tract. To prevent such complications, a person adopting a high-fiber diet is advised to:

- Increase fiber intake gradually over several weeks to give the GI tract time to adapt.
- Drink lots of fluids to soften the fiber as it moves through the GI tract.
- Select fiber-rich foods from a variety of sources—fruits, vegetables, legumes, and whole-grain breads and cereals.

By speeding the transit of foods through the GI tract, excess fiber can limit the absorption of some nutrients. Also, insoluble fibers can bind to minerals and interfere with their absorption. When mineral intake is adequate, however, a reasonable intake of high-fiber foods does not seem to compromise mineral balance.

Clearly, fiber is like all the nutrients in that "more" is only "better" up to a point. Too much is no better than too little. Again, the key words are balance, moderation, and variety.

RECOMMENDED INTAKES OF STARCH AND FIBER

Quick and easy estimate: To attain 55 to 60% of energy from carbohydrate, look for 14 to 15 g of carbohydrate for each 100 kcal of food.

The Committee on Dietary Allowances has not established a specific RDA for carbohydrates, but it does suggest that carbohydrates provide more than half the energy requirement.[31] Most nutrition experts suggest that 55 to 60 percent of total energy should be from carbohydrate to support long-term health. A person consuming 2000 kcalories a day should therefore have 1100 to 1200 kcalories of carbohydrate, or about 275 to 300 grams. The FDA used this guideline in establishing a Daily Value for carbohydrate of 300 grams per day or 60 percent of kcalories. For most people, this means increasing total carbohydrate intake. To this end, the *Dietary Guidelines* and the *Diet and Health* report both suggest a diet with plenty of vegetables, fruits, and grain products.

HEALTHY PEOPLE 2000: Increase complex carbohydrate and fiber-containing foods in the diets of adults to five or more daily servings for vegetables (including legumes) and fruits and to six or more daily servings for grain products.

Chapter 2 described how whole-grain products retain many nutrients that are commonly lost during processing (see Figure 2–5 on p. 57).

The Committee on Dietary Allowances has not established a fiber RDA; instead, the committee suggests the same foods just mentioned: fruits, vegetables, legumes, and whole-grain cereals, which also provide minerals and vitamins.[32] The *Dietary Guidelines* and the *Diet and Health* report make similar suggestions. The FDA set a Daily Value for fiber at 25 milligrams or 11.5 grams per kcalorie energy intake. The American Dietetic Association suggests 20 to 35 grams of dietary fiber daily, which is about two times higher than the average intake in the United States.[33] An effective way to add fiber while cutting fat is to substitute plant sources of proteins (legumes) for animal sources (meats). Table 4–4 presents a listing of fiber sources.

Choose Wisely In selecting high-fiber foods, keep in mind the principle of variety. The fibers in some foods lower cholesterol, those in other foods help pro-

Table 4–4

Fiber in Selected Foods

Bread, Cereal, Rice, and Pasta Group

Whole-grain products provide about 2 grams of fiber per serving:

- 1 slice whole-wheat, pumpernickel, rye bread.
- 1 oz ready-to-eat bran cereal.
- ½ c cooked barley, bulgur, grits, oatmeal.

Vegetable Group

Most vegetables contain 2 to 3 grams of fiber per serving:

- 1 c raw bean sprouts.
- ½ c cooked broccoli, brussels sprouts, cabbage, carrots, cauliflower, collards, corn, eggplant, green beans, green peas, kale, mushrooms, okra, parsnips, potatoes, pumpkin, spinach, sweet potatoes, swiss chard, winter squash.
- ½ c chopped raw carrots, peppers.

Fruit Group

Fresh, frozen, and dried fruits have about 2 grams of fiber per serving:

- 1 medium apple, banana, kiwi, nectarine, orange, pear.
- ½ c applesauce, blackberries, blueberries, raspberries, strawberries.
- Fruit juices contain very little fiber.

Legumes

Many legumes provide about 8 grams of fiber per serving:

- ½ c cooked baked beans, black beans, black-eyed peas, kidney beans, navy beans, pinto beans.

Some legumes provide about 5 grams of fiber per serving:

- ½ c cooked garbanzo beans, great northern beans, lentils, lima beans, split peas.

Note: Appendix H provides fiber grams for over 2000 foods.

Adequate fiber:
- Fosters weight control.
- Lowers blood cholesterol.
- Helps prevent colon cancer.
- Helps prevent and control diabetes.
- Helps prevent and alleviate hemorrhoids.
- Helps prevent appendicitis.
- Helps prevent diverticulosis.

Excess fiber:
- Displaces energy- and nutrient-dense foods.
- Causes intestinal discomfort and distention.
- Interferes with mineral absorption.

mote GI tract health. The FDA authorizes two health claims on food labels concerning fiber: one is for "fruits, vegetables, and grain products that contain fiber, particularly soluble fiber, and risk of coronary heart disease," and the other is for "fiber-containing grain products, fruits, and vegetables and cancer." Another more general health claim addresses "fruits and vegetables and cancer." Chapter 2 describes the criteria foods must meet to bear these health claims.

A diet following the Daily Food Guide plan, which includes 3 to 5 vegetable servings, 2 to 4 fruit servings, and 6 to 11 bread servings daily, can easily supply the recommended amount of carbohydrates and fiber. The box (on pp. 140–141) describes an easy way to estimate the carbohydrate content of a meal. Notice that the exchange system has no sugar list, but sugars do contribute to carbohydrate and energy intake. To help estimate carbohydrate and energy intakes accurately, the list in the margin shows what concentrated sweets are equivalent to 1

1 tsp white sugar =
- 1 tsp brown sugar.
- 1 tsp candy.
- 1 tsp corn sweetener or corn syrup.
- 1 tsp honey.
- 1 tsp jam or jelly.
- 1 tsp maple sugar or maple syrup.
- 1 tsp molasses.
- 1½ oz carbonated soda.
- 1 tbs catsup.

How to Use the Exchange System to Estimate Carbohydrate

One Exchange	Carbohydrate (g)
Starch	15
Fruits	15
Milks	12
Other carbohydrates	15
Vegetables	5
Meats	—
Fats	—
Sugars (1 tsp)[a]	5

[a]Sugars are not officially part of the exchange system, but do have to be counted.

The exchange system described in Chapter 2 provides a convenient way to estimate carbohydrate intake because the foods within each list have a similar carbohydrate content. To use the system, you need to know the carbohydrate value for each list (see the accompanying table) and the foods on that list with their portion sizes (review Figure 2–3).

Familiarity with portion sizes makes estimations easier. For example, it helps to recognize that this lunch contains a sandwich with 2 slices of bread and 2 ounces of turkey, 1 cup of milk, and 1 small bunch of grapes. Then you can translate these portions into exchanges: 2 starches, 2 meats, 1 milk, and 1 fruit. Finally, you can calculate 15 grams of carbohydrate for each starch, 0 grams for the meats, 12 grams for the milk, and 15 grams for the fruit.

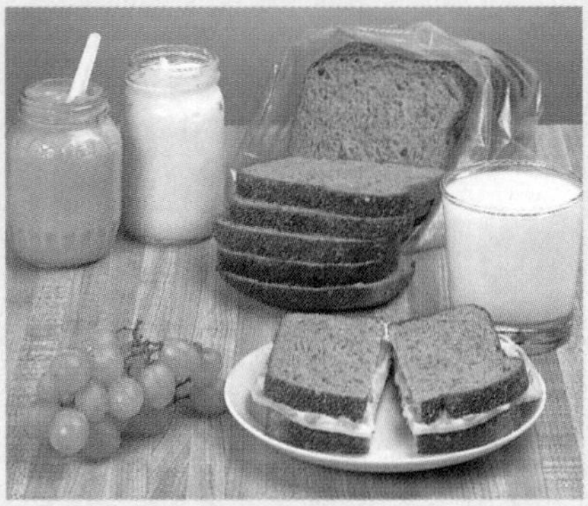

Lunch		Exchange	Carbohydrate (g) Estimate	Actual
2 slices bread	=	2 starches	30	32 (bread and turkey)
2 oz turkey	=	2 meats	0	
1 c 1% low-fat milk	=	1 milk	12	12
1 small bunch of grapes	=	1 fruit	15	15
			57	59

Using the exchange system to estimate, this lunch provides about 57 grams of carbohydrate. A computer diet analysis program came to a similar conclusion (59 grams), as would a diet analysis using the values in Appendix

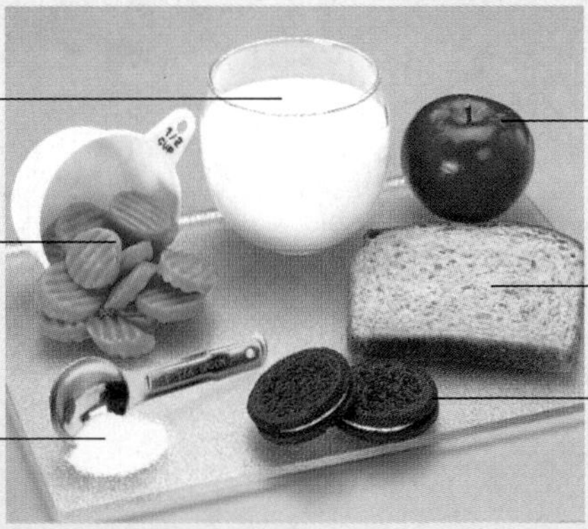
12 g in 1 c milk (lactose)
5 g in ½ c vegetables (starch/sugars)
5 g in 1 tsp sugar (sugars)
15 g in 1 fruit portion (sugars)
15 g in 1 slice bread (starch)
15 g in 1 small dessert or snack (starch/sugars)

Carbohydrate-containing foods appear in several exchange lists: starch, vegetable, fruit, milk, and "others" such as desserts and snacks. Sugars also contribute carbohydrate.

H. Small variations between values arrived at differently may seem disconcerting, but remember that all are only estimates. Estimates save time; often only a ballpark figure is needed anyway. In this example, the values are essentially the same, and the differences between them are insignificant.

Most estimates of the nutrient contents of foods are rough but serviceable approximations. A "90-kcalorie potato" actually means a "90-kcalorie plus or minus about 20 percent potato," which makes it not significantly different from a 100-kcalorie potato. In general, for most purposes, a variation of about 20 percent is considered reasonable.

Fiber appears in only the starch, vegetable, and fruit lists. To estimate fiber, remember that most items on these lists provide at least 2 grams of fiber per serving; some provide 3 or more. Knowing this, a reasonable fiber estimate for this lunch would be 6 to 9 grams—and a diet analysis report of 8 grams would agree.

Just a few calculations of this kind will give you a feel for the carbohydrate content of a diet. Once you are aware of the major carbohydrate contributing foods you eat, you can return to thinking simply in terms of foods, developing a sense of how much of each is enough.

teaspoon of white sugar. These sugars all provide *about* 5 grams of carbohydrate and *about* 20 kcalories per teaspoon. Some are lower (16 kcalories for table sugar), while others are higher (22 kcalories for honey), but a 20-kcalorie average is an acceptable approximation. For a person who uses catsup liberally, it may help to remember that 1 tablespoon of catsup supplies about 1 teaspoon of sugar.

Read Food Labels Food labels list the amount, in grams, of total carbohydrate—including starch, fibers, and sugars—per serving. Fiber grams are also listed separately, as are the grams of sugars. (With this information, you can calculate starch grams by subtracting the grams of fibers and sugars from the total carbohydrate.) Sugars reflect both added sugars and those that occur naturally in foods. Total carbohydrate and dietary fiber are also expressed as "% Daily Values" for a person consuming 2000 kcalories; there is no Daily Value for sugars.

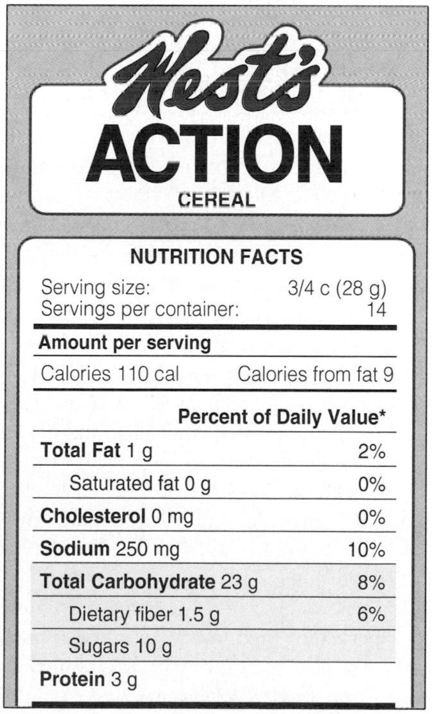
West's
ACTION
CEREAL
NUTRITION FACTS
Serving size: 3/4 c (28 g)
Servings per container: 14
Amount per serving
Calories 110 cal Calories from fat 9
Percent of Daily Value*
Total Fat 1 g 2%
Saturated fat 0 g 0%
Cholesterol 0 mg 0%
Sodium 250 mg 10%
Total Carbohydrate 23 g 8%
Dietary fiber 1.5 g 6%
Sugars 10 g
Protein 3 g

Clearly, a diet rich in complex carbohydrates—starches and fibers—supports efforts to control body weight and prevent heart disease, cancer, diabetes, and GI disorders.[34] For these reasons, recommendations urge people to eat plenty of grains, vegetables, legumes, and fruits—enough to provide 55 to 60 percent of the daily energy intake from carbohydrate.

In today's world, there is one other reason why plant foods high in starch and natural sugars are a better choice than animal foods or foods high in concentrated sweets: in general, the energy and resources required to grow and process plant foods are less, and the health benefits greater. Chapter 20 takes a closer look at the environmental impacts of food production and use.

Study Questions

1. Which carbohydrates are described as simple and which are complex?
2. Describe the structure of a monosaccharide and name the three monosaccharides important in nutrition. Name the three disaccharides commonly found in foods and their component monosaccharides. In what foods are these sugars found?
3. What happens in a condensation reaction? In a hydrolysis reaction?
4. Describe the structure of polysaccharides and name the ones important in nutrition. How are starch and glycogen similar, and how do they differ? How do the fibers differ from the other polysaccharides?
5. Describe carbohydrate digestion and absorption. What role does fiber play in the process?
6. What are the possible fates of glucose in the body? What is the protein-sparing action of carbohydrate?
7. How does the body maintain blood glucose concentrations? What happens when it rises too high or falls too low?
8. What are the health effects of sugars? What are the dietary recommendations regarding concentrated sugar intakes?
9. What are the health effects of starches and fibers? What are the dietary recommendations regarding these complex carbohydrates?
10. What foods provide starches and fibers?

Notes

1. S. R. Glore and coauthors, Soluble fiber and serum lipids: A literature review, *Journal of the American Dietetic Association* 94 (1994): 425–436.
2. M. Kestin and coauthors, Comparative effects of three cereal brans on plasma lipids, blood pressure, and glucose metabolism in mildly hypercholesterolemic men, *American Journal of Clinical Nutrition* 52 (1990): 661–666; J. K. C. Chan and V. Wypyszyk, A forgotten natural dietary fiber: Psyllium mucilloid, *Cereal Foods World* 33 (1988): 921–922.
3. J. L. Slavin, Dietary fiber: Mechanisms or magic on disease prevention? *Nutrition Today*, November/December 1990, pp. 6–10.
4. G. Annison and D. L. Topping, Nutritional role of resistant starch: Chemical structure vs physiological function, *Annual Review of Nutrition* 14 (1994): 297–320; N. Asp, Nutritional classification and analysis of food carbohydrates, *American Journal of Clinical Nutrition* 59 (1994): 679S–681S.
5. M. I. McBurney and P. J. van Soest, Structure-function relationships: Lessons from other species, in *The Large Intestine: Physiology, Pathophysiology, and Diseases*, eds. S. F. Phillips, J. H. Pemberton, and R. G. Shorter (New York: Raven Press, 1991), pp. 37–50.
6. J. M. Saavedra and J. A. Perman, Current concepts in lactose malabsorption and intolerance, *Annual Review of Nutrition* 9 (1989): 475–502.
7. S. Auriechio and G. Semenza, Late-onset hypolactasia and persistent high lactose activity in humans, in *Sugars in Nutrition*, eds. M. Gracey, N. Kretchmer, and E. Rossi (New York: Raven Press, 1991).
8. G. Flatz, Genetics of lactose digestion in humans, in *Advances in Human Genetics*, eds., H. Harris and K. Hirschhorn (New York: Plenum Press, 1987), pp. 1–77; Committee on Nutrition, Practical significance of lactose intolerance in children: Supplement, *Pediatrics* 86 (1990): 643–644.
9. Committee on Nutrition, 1990; A. O. Johnson and coauthors, Adaptation of lactose maldigesters to continued milk intakes, *American Journal of Clinical Nutrition* 58 (1993): 879–881; F. L. Suarez, D. A. Savaiano, and M. D. Levitt, A comparison of symptoms after the consumption of milk or lactose-hydrolyzed milk by people with self-reported severe lactose intolerance, *New England Journal of Medicine* 333 (1995): 1–4.
10. J. C. Brand and S. Holt, Relative effectiveness of milks with reduced amounts of lactose in alleviating milk intolerance, *American Journal of Clinical Nutrition* 54 (1991): 148–151.
11. Committee on Dietary Allowances, *Recommended Dietary Allowances*, 10th ed. (Washington, D.C.: National Academy Press, 1989), p. 41.
12. E. Jéquier, Carbohydrates as a source of energy, *American Journal of Clinical Nutrition* (supplement) 59 (1994): 682S–685S.
13. J. Hirsch, Role and benefits of carbohydrate in the diet: Key issues for future dietary guidelines, *American Journal of Clinical Nutrition* 61 (1995): 996S–1000S.
14. S. A. Westphal, M. C. Gannon, and F. Q. Nuttall, Metabolic response to glucose ingested with various amounts of protein, *American Journal of Clinical Nutrition* 52 (1990): 267–272.
15. B. Vessby, Dietary carbohydrates in diabetes, *American Journal of Clinical Nutrition* (supplement) 59 (1994): 742S–746S.
16. T. M. S. Wolever and J. B. Miller, Sugars and blood glucose control, *American Journal of Clinical Nutrition* 62 (1995): 212S–227S; I. Björck and coauthors, Food properties affecting the digestion and absorption of carbohydrates, *American Journal of Clinical Nutrition* (supplement) 59 (1994): 699S–705S.

17. D. J. A. Jenkins and coauthors, Low glycemic index: Lente carbohydrates and physiological effects of altered food frequency, *American Journal of Clinical Nutrition* (supplement) 59 (1994): 706S–709S.
18. J. C. B. Miller, Importance of glycemic index in diabetes, *American Journal of Clinical Nutrition* (supplement) 59 (1994): 747S–752S.
19. Position statement: Nutrition recommendations and principles for people with diabetes mellitus, *Diabetes Care* 17 (1994): 519–522.
20. W. H. Glinsmann and Y. K. Park, Perspective on the 1986 Food and Drug Administration Assessment of Carbohydrate Sweeteners: Uniform definitions and recommendations for future assessments, *American Journal of Clinical Nutrition* 62 (1995): 161S–169S.
21. J. M. Navia, Carbohydrates and dental health, *American Journal of Clinical Nutrition* (supplement) 59 (1994): 719S–727S.
22. C. J. Lewis and coauthors, Nutrient intakes and body weights of persons consuming high and moderate levels of added sugars, *Journal of the American Dietetic Association* 92 (1992): 708–713.
23. M. L. Wolraich and coauthors, Effects of diets high in sucrose or aspartame on the behavior and cognitive performance of children, *New England Journal of Medicine* 330 (1994): 301–307; D. A. Gans, Sucrose and unusual childhood behavior, *Nutrition Today*, May/June 1991, pp. 8–14; J. A. Bachorowski and coauthors, Sucrose and delinquency: Behavioral assessment, *Pediatrics* 86 (1990): 244–253.
24. J. E. Blundell, S. Green, and V. Burley, Carbohydrates and human appetite, *American Journal of Clinical Nutrition* 59 (1994): 728S–734S; A. S. Levine and coauthors, Effect of breakfast cereals on short-term food intake, *American Journal of Clinical Nutrition* 50 (1989): 1303–1307; L. Lissner and coauthors, Dietary fat and the regulation of energy intake in human subjects, *American Journal of Clinical Nutrition* 46 (1987): 886–892.
25. A. S. Truswell, Food carbohydrates and plasma lipids—An update, *American Journal of Clinical Nutrition* 59 (1994): 710S–718S.
26. G. H. McIntosh and coauthors, Barley and wheat foods: Influence on plasma cholesterol concentrations in hypercholesterolemic men, *American Journal of Clinical Nutrition* 53 (1991): 1205–1209; Kestin and coauthors, 1990; J. W. Anderson and coauthors, Serum lipid response of hypercholesterolemic men to single and divided doses of canned beans, *American Journal of Clinical Nutrition* 51 (1990): 1013–1019; L. P. Bell and coauthors, Cholesterol-lowering effects of soluble-fiber cereals as part of a prudent diet for patients with mild to moderate hypercholesterolemia, *American Journal of Clinical Nutrition* 52 (1990): 1020–1026; J. W. Anderson and N. J. Gustafson, Hypocholesterolemic effects of oat and bean products, *American Journal of Clinical Nutrition* 48 (1988): 749–753.
27. Y. A. Kesaniemi, S. Tarpila, and T. A. Miettinen, Low vs high dietary fiber and serum, biliary, and fecal lipids in middle-aged men, *American Journal of Clinical Nutrition* 51 (1990): 1007–1112.
28. J. F. Swain and coauthors, Comparison of the effects of oat bran and low-fiber wheat on serum lipoprotein levels and blood pressure, *New England Journal of Medicine* 322 (1990): 147–152; W. Denmark-Wahnefried, J. Bowering, and P. S. Cohen, Reduced serum cholesterol with dietary change using fat-modified and oat bran supplemented diets, *Journal of the American Dietetic Association* 90 (1990): 223–229.
29. D. J. A. Jenkins and coauthors, Effect on blood lipids of very high intakes of fiber in diets low in saturated fat and cholesterol, *New England Journal of Medicine* 329 (1993): 21–26.
30. I. P. Munster and coauthors, Effect of resistant starch on breath-hydrogen and methane excretion in healthy volunteers, *American Journal of Clinical Nutrition* 59 (1994): 626–630.
31. Committee on Dietary Allowances, 1989, p. 41.
32. Committee on Dietary Allowances, 1989, p. 42.
33. Position of The American Dietetic Association: Health implications of dietary fiber, *Journal of the American Dietetic Association* 93 (1993): 1446–1447.
34. J. W. Anderson, B. M. Smith, and N. J. Gustafson, Health benefits and practical aspects of high-fiber diets, *American Journal of Clinical Nutrition* 59 (1994): 1242S–1247S.

Problem Set appears on the next page

Problem Set

1. Seek a perspective on sugary foods. Suppose you are so sensitive to your own energy needs that you know you can afford a snack of about 450 kcal.

   a. How many packages of M&M candy (item #1134 in Appendix H) could you eat? Show your calculations.

   ____

   b. In place of the candy, how many peaches (item #277) could you eat? Show your calculations.

   ____

   c. How many pieces of melba toast (item #420) could you eat? Show your calculations.

   ____

   d. How many frozen fruit juice bars (item #1482) could you eat? Show your calculations.

   ____

   e. How many cups of ice cream (the rich, hard type, item #128) could you eat? Show your calculations.

   ____

Look up some other possibilities if you like.

2. Use a quick and easy method to estimate the carbohydrate in foods. Recall from the chapter that if a food contains more than 14 to 15 g of carbohydrate per 100 kcal, then over half of its energy comes from carbohydrate. The calculation is:

   14 to 15 g carbohydrate × 4 kcal per g carbohydrate = 56 to 60 kcal of carbohydrate and therefore 56 to 60% of 100 kcal.

Example: A label says that a serving of food contains 400 kcal and 20 g of carbohydrate. Is more than half of the energy from carbohydrate? No, because 20 g of carbohydrate deliver only 80 kcal (20 g carbohydrate × 4 kcal/g), much less than half of 400 kcal.

   a. First, try a packaged food. The label says the food contains 33 g of carbohydrate in each 200-kcalorie serving. Are half the kcalories from carbohydrate?

   b. Now try a food such as Asian bean curd or tofu (item #927 under "Vegetables and Legumes—Soybean products" in Appendix H). How big is a serving? _______ How many kcalories are in a serving? _______ How much carbohydrate? _______ How many kcalories from carbohydrate? _______ Is that more than half of the total kcalories? _______ Is tofu, therefore, a good source of carbohydrate? _______

   c. Try another food. Look up cooked wild rice (item #548 in Appendix H). How big is a serving? _______ How many kcalories are in a serving? _______ How much carbohydrate? _______ How many kcalories from carbohydrate? _______ Is that more than half of the total kcalories? _______ Is cooked wild rice, therefore, a good source of carbohydrate? _______

3. Check the portion sizes a person would have to eat to meet the Healthy People 2000 goal that suggests a person should eat 5 or more servings of vegetables and fruits, and 6 or more servings of grains, each day. To discover what "a serving" is, first look up each of the following foods in Figure 2–1 on pp. 44–45, and record the

Problem Set (continued)

serving size given there. Then look up each food in Appendix H and see how much carbohydrate that serving size delivers.

5 Servings of Vegetables and Fruits	Serving Size (from Figure 2–1)	Carbohydrate per Serving (g)
a. Banana (whole)	____________	____________
b. Fresh orange juice	____________	____________
c. Black-eyed peas (cooked from frozen)	____________	____________
d. Corn (cooked from frozen)	____________	____________
e. Mashed potatoes (home-cooked with milk)	____________	____________
6 Servings of Grains		
f. English muffin (plain)	____________	____________
g. Cooked oatmeal (regular)	____________	____________
h. Sliced wheat bread	____________	____________
i. Bagel (plain)	____________	____________
j. Brown rice (cooked)	____________	____________
k. Macaroni (enriched)	____________	____________
l. Now, total the carbohydrate grams:	Total:	____________

m. Do these foods, taken together, meet recommendations for a person eating 1500 kcal per day? Show your calculations.

____

____

Alternatives to Sugar

People who want to limit their use of sugar may encounter two sets of alternative sweeteners. One set, the artificial sweeteners, provide virtually no energy and are sometimes referred to as nonnutritive sweeteners. The other set, the sugar alcohols, yield energy and are sometimes referred to as nutritive sweeteners. The artificial sweeteners are sugar substitutes; the sugar alcohols are sugar relatives. The glossary on p. 148 presents the most common members of both groups.

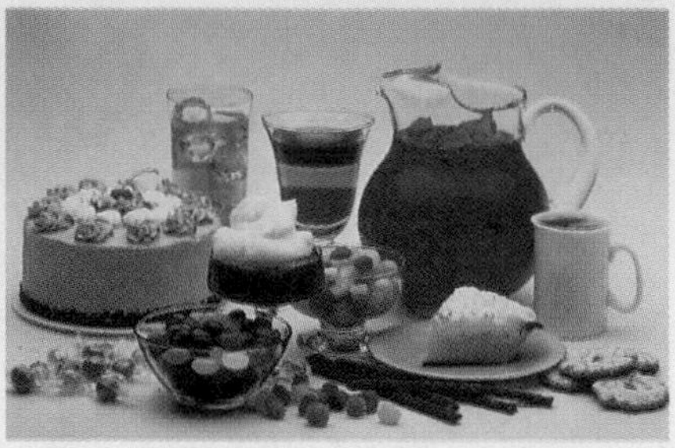

People wanting to limit their sugar intake can find a variety of foods and beverages made with artificial sweeteners.

ARTIFICIAL SWEETENERS

Artificial sweeteners permit people to keep their sugar and energy intakes down, yet still enjoy the delicious sweet tastes of their favorite foods and beverages. The Food and Drug Administration (FDA) has approved the use of three artificial sweeteners—saccharin, aspartame, and acesulfame potassium (acesulfame-K). Saccharin holds the honor of being the oldest artificial sweetener, having been around since before 1900. Aspartame was approved by the FDA in 1981 and currently dominates the world market for artificial sweeteners. Acesulfame-K is the "new kid on the block," having received FDA approval in 1988. Three others have petitioned the FDA and are awaiting approval—alitame, cyclamate, and sucralose. Table H4–1 provides general details about each of these sweeteners.

Both saccharin and acesulfame-K present the body with no chemical compounds to deal with and pass through the digestive system unchanged. In contrast, the body does digest aspartame, receiving tiny quantities of nutrients and other compounds. Aspartame is, in fact, *technically* classified as a nutritive sweetener because it yields tiny amounts of energy, but for all practical purposes, that energy is negligible.

Some consumers have challenged the safety of using artificial sweeteners. Considering that all compounds are toxic at some dose, it is little surprise that large doses of artificial sweeteners (or their components or metabolic by-products) have toxic effects. The question to ask is whether their ingestion is safe for human beings in quantities people normally use (and potentially abuse). The answer is yes, except in the special case described for aspartame later.

The Safety of Saccharin

Saccharin, used for over 100 years in the United States, is currently used by some 50 million people—primarily in soft drinks, secondarily as a tabletop sweetener. Saccharin is rapidly excreted in the urine and does not accumulate in the body.

Questions about saccharin's safety surfaced in 1977, when experiments suggested that large doses of saccharin increased the risk of bladder cancer in rats. The FDA proposed banning saccharin as a result. Public outcry in favor of saccharin was so loud, however, that Congress imposed a moratorium on the ban—a moratorium that was repeatedly extended until 1991, when the FDA withdrew its proposal to ban saccharin.[1] Products containing saccharin must still carry the warning label, "use of this product may be hazardous to your health. This product contains saccharin, which has been determined to cause cancer in laboratory animals."

Does saccharin cause cancer? The largest population study to date, involving 9000 men and women, showed overall that saccharin use did not raise the risk of cancer. Among certain small groups of the population, however, such as those who both smoked heavily and used saccharin, the risk of bladder cancer was slightly greater. Other studies involving more than 5000 people with bladder cancer showed no association between bladder cancer and saccharin use.[2] Common sense dictates that consuming large amounts of any substance is probably not wise, but at current, moderate intake levels, saccharin is assumed to be safe for most people. It has been approved for use in more than 90 countries.

The Safety of Aspartame

Aspartame is one of the most studied of all food additives; extensive animal and human studies docu-

Table H4–1

Artificial Sweeteners

Artificial Sweeteners	Properties	Allowable Intakes	Uses
APPROVED SWEETENERS			
• Saccharin (an organic compound) 300–400 times as sweet as sugar 0 kcal/g	Heat stable, long shelf life, water soluble, colorless, odorless; bitter, metallic aftertaste	GRAS[a]: 500 mg/day in children 1000 mg/day in adults	Cakes, cookies, jams, beverages, vitamin supplements and medicines
• Aspartame (aspartic acid + phenylalanine) 180–200 times as sweet as sugar 4 kcal/g[b]	Loses sweetness with heat, no aftertaste	ADI[c]: 50 mg/kg body weight[d] Warning to people with PKU: Contains phenylalanine	Presweetened cold cereals, soft drinks, chewing gum, hot chocolate, yogurt, wine coolers, fruit juice beverages, gelatins, puddings, frozen dairy and nondairy desserts, tabletop sweeteners
• Acesulfame-K (an organic salt) 150–200 times as sweet as sugar 0 kcal/g	Heat stable, long shelf life, water soluble, synergistic sweetening effect when used with other sweeteners, no aftertaste	ADI[c]: 15 mg/kg body weight[e]	Tabletop sweeteners, dry beverage mixes, instant coffee and tea, gelatins, puddings, chewing gum, candies, baked goods, soft drinks, desserts
SWEETENERS WITH APPROVAL PENDING			
• Alitame (aspartic acid + alanine) 2000 times as sweet as sugar 4 kcal/g[b]	Heat stable, water soluble, no aftertaste except in acidic foods at high temperatures, synergistic sweetening effect when used with other sweeteners		Beverages, baked goods, tabletop sweeteners, frozen desserts
• Cyclamate (cyclamic acid, calcium cyclamate, sodium cyclamate) 30–60 times as sweet as sugar 0 kcal/g	Heat stable, water soluble, no aftertaste		Tabletop sweeteners, baked goods
• Sucralose (a chlorinated sugar derivative) 400–800 times as sweet as sugar 0 kcal/g	Extremely stable, water soluble		Carbonated beverages, dairy products, baked goods, coffee and tea, fruit spreads, syrups, tabletop sweeteners, chewing gum, frozen desserts, salad dressing

[a]GRAS is the FDA's designation of generally recognized as safe.
[b]Aspartame and alitame yield 4 kcal/g, but such small amounts are needed to achieve desired sweetness that energy contribution is negligible.
[c]ADI is the FDA's designation of an Acceptable Daily Intake.
[d]Recommendations from the World Health Organization and in Europe and Canada limit aspartame intake to 40 mg/kg body weight.
[e]Recommendations from the World Health Organization limit acesulfame-K intake to 9 mg/kg body weight.

Source: S. A. Schlicker and C. Regan, Innovations in reduced-calorie foods: A review of fat and sugar replacement technologies, *Topics in Clinical Nutrition* 6 (1990): 50–60; A. M. Bertorelli and J. V. Czarnowski, Review of present and future use of nonnutritive sweeteners, *The Diabetes Educator* 16 (1990): 415–420.

Glossary

acesulfame (AY-see-sul-fame) **potassium:** a low-kcalorie sweetener recently approved by the FDA; also known as acesulfame-K, because K is the chemical symbol for potassium; approved in Canada.

ADI (Acceptable Daily Intake): the amount of a sweetener that individuals can safely consume each day over the course of a lifetime without adverse effect. It includes a 100-fold safety factor.

alitame (AL-ih-tame): a compound of two amino acids (alanine and aspartic acid) that is 2000 times sweeter than sucrose; FDA approval pending.

artificial sweeteners: sugar substitutes that provide no energy; sometimes called **nonnutritive sweeteners**.

aspartame (ah-SPAR-tame or ASS-par-tame): a compound of two amino acids (phenylalanine and aspartic acid) that tastes like the sugar sucrose but is much sweeter. It provides 4 kcalories per gram, as does protein, but because so little is used, it is virtually kcalorie-free. In powdered form it is sometimes mixed with lactose, however, so a 1-gram packet may provide 4 kcalories. It is used in both the United States and Canada.

cyclamate (SIGH-klo-mate): a 0-kcalorie sweetener; FDA approval pending in the United States; available in Canada on grocery-store shelves but only as a table-top sweetener, not as an additive.

diketopiperazine (dye-KEY-toe-pie-PER-a-zeen), or **DKP:** a product to which aspartame breaks down during metabolism.

nutritive sweeteners: sweeteners that yield energy, including both sugars and sugar alcohols.

saccharin (SAK-ah-ren): a 0-kcalorie sweetener used in the United States but available in Canada only in pharmacies and only as a sweetener, not as an additive.

sucralose (SUE-kra-lose): a 0-kcalorie sweetener that is 600 times sweeter than sucrose; FDA approval pending in the United States; approved in Canada.

sugar alcohols: sugarlike compounds that can be derived from fruits or commercially produced from dextrose; also called **polyols**. Like sugars, sugar alcohols are sweet to taste and yield 4 kcalories per gram, but they are absorbed more slowly and metabolized differently than other sugars in the human body, and are not readily utilized by ordinary mouth bacteria. Examples are **maltitol**, **mannitol**, **sorbitol**, and **xylitol**.

---

ment its safety. Long-term consumption of aspartame is not associated with any adverse health effects.[3]

The nutrients in aspartame may present a problem for certain people, however, and for this reason, aspartame also carries a warning on its label. Aspartame is a simple chemical compound made of components common to many foods: two amino acids (phenylalanine and aspartic acid) and a methyl group (CH_3). Figure H4–1 shows its chemical structure. The flavors of the components give no clue to the combined effect; one of them tastes bitter, and the other is tasteless, but the combination creates a product that is 200 times sweeter than sucrose.

In the digestive tract, enzymes split aspartame into its three component parts. The body absorbs the two amino acids and uses them just as if they had come from food protein, which is made entirely of amino acids including these two.

Because this sweetener contributes phenylalanine, products containing aspartame must bear a warning label for people with the inherited disease phenylketonuria (PKU). People with PKU are unable to dispose of any excess phenylalanine. The accumulation of phenylalanine and its by-products is toxic to the developing nervous system, causing irreversible brain damage. For this reason, all newborns in the United States are screened for PKU. The treatment for PKU is a special diet that must strike a balance, providing enough phenylalanine to support normal growth and health but not enough to cause harm. The question then is does aspartame raise blood phenylalanine high enough to be toxic to people with PKU? Apparently not. The little extra phenylalanine from aspartame, even in heavy users, poses only a small risk.[4]

Still, there is a compelling reason why children with PKU need to get all their phenylalanine from foods, and not from an artificial sweetener. The PKU diet excludes such protein-rich and nutrient-rich foods as milk, meat, fish, poultry, cheese, eggs, nuts, legumes, and many bread products. Only with difficulty can these children obtain the many essential nutrients—such as calcium, iron, and the B vitamins—found along with phenylalanine in these foods. To suggest that children with PKU squander any of their limited phenylalanine allowance on the purified phenylalanine of aspartame, which contributes none of the associated vitamins or minerals essential for good health and normal growth, would open the way for poor nutrition.

Setting aside the special case of PKU, how do people ordinarily metabolize aspartame? Is there any

Figure H4–1

Structure of Aspartame

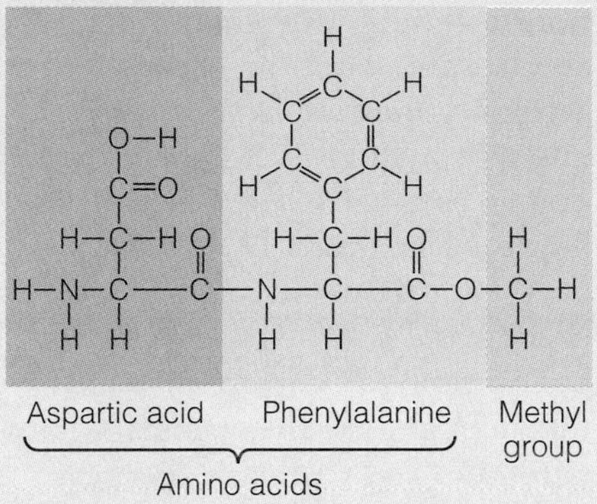

reason to be concerned about the products it yields in the body? During metabolism, the methyl group momentarily becomes methyl alcohol (methanol)—a potentially toxic compound (see Figure H4–2). Then enzymes convert methanol to formaldehyde, another toxic compound. Finally, formaldehyde is broken down to carbon dioxide. Before aspartame could be approved for public use, the quantities of these products generated during metabolism had to be determined; they were found to fall below the threshold at which they would cause harm. In fact, ounce for ounce, tomato juice yields six times as much methanol as a diet soda.[5]

Finally, aspartame breaks down to diketopiperazine, or DKP for short. Long-term studies using animals have directly tested this product and eliminated it as a source of concern.

Still another concern was over the effect aspartame use might have on the brain. Experiments with rats, monkeys, and human beings were performed, and none showed any cause for concern. In the monkey study, infant monkeys were given up to 3000 milligrams of aspartame per kilogram of body weight for nine months, and the researchers found no ill effects on growth, development, health, or behavior either during the test or on the withdrawal of aspartame. The conclusion reached was that aspartame is safe except for people with PKU. Some 500 individual complaints received after its approval were reviewed by the Centers for Disease Control, which concluded that some individuals may exhibit vague, but not dangerous, symptoms due to unusual sensitivity to aspartame, but that the product is generally safe. Like saccharin, aspartame has been approved for use in more than 90 countries.

The Safety of Acesulfame-K

The FDA approved acesulfame-K in 1988 after reviewing more than 90 safety studies conducted over 15 years. Some consumer groups believe that acesulfame-K causes tumors in rats and should not have been approved by the FDA. The FDA counters that the tumors were not caused by the sweetener, but were typical of those commonly found in rat studies.

The Safety of Alitame, Cyclamate, and Sucralose

FDA approval for alitame, cyclamate, and sucralose is still pending. To date, no safety issues have been raised for alitame or sucralose. Cyclamate, on the other hand, has been battling safety issues for 50 years. Approved by the FDA in 1949, cyclamate was banned in 1969 principally on the basis of one study indicating that it caused bladder cancer in rats.

Figure H4–2

Metabolism of Aspartame

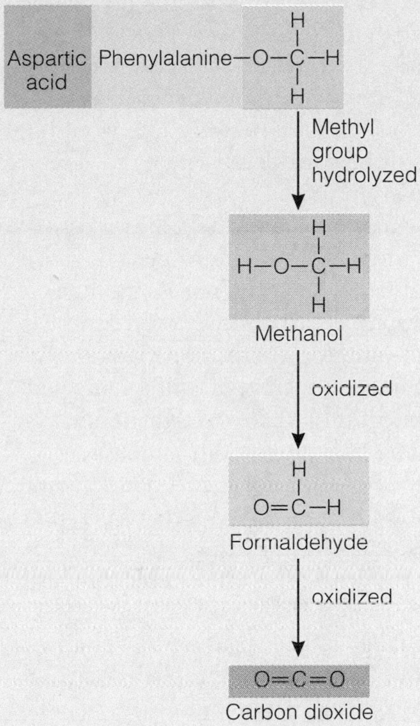

The National Research Council has reviewed dozens of studies on cyclamate and concluded that neither cyclamate nor its metabolites cause cancer. They did, however, recommend further research to determine the risks for heavy or long-term use. Although cyclamate does not initiate cancer, it may promote cancer development once started. The FDA has no policy on substances that enhance the cancer-causing activities of other substances. Consequently, the FDA is unlikely to approve cyclamate soon, if at all. Agencies in more than 50 other countries have approved cyclamate, however. In fact, Canada has approved cyclamate and banned saccharin.

Acceptable Daily Intake

The FDA has established an Acceptable Daily Intake (ADI) for artificial sweeteners. The ADI represents the level of consumption that, if maintained every day throughout a person's life, would still be considered safe by a wide margin.

For example, the ADI for aspartame is 50 milligrams per kilogram of body weight. That is, the FDA approved aspartame based on the assumption that no one would consume more than 50 milligrams per kilogram of body weight in a day. This maximum daily intake is indeed a lot: for a 150-pound adult, it adds up to 97 packets of Equal or 20 cans of soft drinks sweetened only with aspartame. The company that produces aspartame estimates that if all the sugar and saccharin in the U.S. diet were replaced with aspartame, 1 percent of the population would be consuming the FDA maximum. Most people who use aspartame consume less than 5 milligrams per kilogram of body weight per day.[6] A five-year-old child who drinks four glasses of aspartame-sweetened beverages on a hot day and has five servings of other products with aspartame that day (such as pudding, chewing gum, cereal, gelatin, and frozen desserts) takes in the FDA maximum level. Although this presents no proven hazard, it seems wise to offer children other foods so as not to exceed the limit. Table H4–2 lists the average amounts of aspartame in some common foods.

For persons choosing to use artificial sweeteners, the American Dietetic Association wisely advises that they be used in moderation and only as part of a well-balanced nutritious diet.[7] The dietary principles of both moderation and variety are useful in reducing the possible risks associated with any food.

Artificial Sweeteners and Weight Control

Many people eat and drink products sweetened with artificial sweeteners to help them control weight. Does this work? Ironically, a few studies have reported that intense sweeteners, such as aspartame, may stimulate appetite, which could lead to weight gain. Contradicting these reports, most studies find either no change or a decline in feelings of hunger and conclude that most people using the sweeteners don't seem to increase their food intakes.[8] Adding to the confusion, some studies report reduced food intakes and weight losses when people eat or drink artificially sweetened products.[9]

In studying the effects of artificial sweeteners on food intake and body weight, different researchers ask different questions and take different approaches in searching for the answers. It matters, for example, whether the people used in the study were of a healthy weight or obese, and whether they were on weight-loss diets or not. Motivations for using sweeteners differ, too, and this influences a person's actions. For example, a person might drink a low-kcalorie beverage now so as to be able to eat a high-kcalorie food later. This person's energy intake might stay the same or increase. On the other hand, a person trying to control food energy intake might use the artificial sweetener and then still choose a low-kcalorie food in place of the high-kcalorie option. This would reduce the person's energy intake.

In designing experiments on artificial sweeteners, researchers have to distinguish between the effects of sweetness and the effects of a particular substance. If a person wants to eat again shortly after eating an artificially sweetened snack, is that because the sweet taste (of all sweeteners, including sugars) stimulates appetite? Or is it because the artificial sweetener itself stimulates appetite? Research must also distinguish between the effects of food energy and the effects of the substance. If a person is hungrier after eating an artificially sweetened food than after a sugar-sweetened product, is that because less food energy was available to satisfy hunger? Or is it because the artificial sweetener itself triggers hunger? Furthermore, if appetite is stimulated and a person feels hungry, does that actually lead to increased food intake?

One recent study tried to answer these questions by feeding normal-weight people one of four cheese samples for breakfast and then measuring their food intake at later meals throughout the day.[10] Two of the samples provided 700 kcalories:

Table H4–2

Aspartame Contents of Selected Foods

Food	Aspartame (mg)
12 oz diet soft drink	170
8 oz powdered drink	100
8 oz sugar-free fruit yogurt	124
4 oz gelatin dessert	80
1 packet sweetener	35

one contained sucrose, and the other aspartame with enough starch to equalize the kcalories. The other two samples provided 300 kcalories: one was plain and the other contained aspartame. Those who ate the lower-kcalorie breakfast, regardless of sweetness, were hungrier later. They also ate more at lunch (100 kcalories on average), although not enough to fully compensate for the 400-kcalorie difference between the breakfasts. Because energy intake at later meals was similar, those who ate the 700-kcalorie breakfasts had higher total energy intakes.

Overall it seems that artificial sweeteners alone do not stimulate appetite but that low-kcalorie intakes may leave people hungry, so that they compensate at later meals. Whether a person compensates for the energy reduction either partially or fully depends on several factors, including the person's characteristics. Using artificial sweeteners will not automatically lower energy intake; to control energy intake successfully, a person will need to make informed diet and activity decisions throughout the day (as Chapter 9 explains).

SUGAR ALCOHOLS

Some "sugar-free" dietary products such as hard candies, sugarless gums, jams, and jellies contain the sugar alcohols—mannitol, sorbitol, xylitol, and maltitol. They claim to be "sugar-free" on their labels, but in this case, "sugar-free" does not mean they are free of kcalories. Sugar alcohols occur naturally in fruits and vegetables; they are also used by manufacturers as a low-energy bulk ingredient in many products.[11] Sugar alcohols provide energy, although the exact kcalorie value has not been determined.[12] The FDA uses 4 kcalories per gram as a standard, but some research indicates that the value may be only 2.5 to 3.5 kcalories per gram. Table H4–3 presents a general description of each of the sugar alcohols.

Sugar alcohols evoke a low glycemic response. The body absorbs sugar alcohols slowly; consequently, they are slower to enter the bloodstream than other sugars. Side effects such as gas, abdominal discomfort, and diarrhea, however, make them less attractive than the artificial sweeteners. For this reason, labeling regulations require foods to state that "Excess consumption may have a laxative effect" if reasonable consumption could result in the daily ingestion of 50 grams of a sugar alcohol.

The real benefit of using sugar alcohols is that they do not contribute as much to dental caries as sugar does. Bacteria in the mouth cannot metabolize sugar alcohols as rapidly as sugar. They are therefore valuable in chewing gums, breath mints, and other products that people keep in their mouths for a while.

The sugar alcohols, like the artificial sweeteners, can occupy a place in the diet, and provided they are used in moderation, they will do no harm. In fact, they can help, both by providing an alternative to sugar for people with diabetes and by inhibiting caries-causing bacteria. People may find it appropriate to use all three sweeteners at times: the artificial kind, the sugar alcohols, and sugar itself.

Table H4–3
Sugar Alcohols

Sugar Alcohols	Sweetness Compared with Sucrose	Advantages	Disadvantages
Sorbitol	One-half as sweet	Opposes dental caries; controls browning, stability, and moisture loss in foods	Abdominal cramps, gas, diarrhea
Mannitol	Three-fourths as sweet		Abdominal cramps, gas, diarrhea
Maltitol	Three-fourths as sweet	Opposes dental caries	Expensive
Xylitol	Equivalent	Opposes dental caries; may assist in weight control	Diarrhea

NOTES

1. Withdrawal of certain pre-1986 proposed rules: Final actions, *Federal Register* 56 (1991): 67422.
2. Position of The American Dietetic Association: Use of nutritive and nonnutritive sweeteners, *Journal of the American Dietetic Association* 93 (1993): 816–821.
3. Position of The American Dietetic Association, 1993.
4. Position of The American Dietetic Association, 1993.
5. H. H. Butchko and F. N. Kotsonis, Acceptable intake vs actual intake: The aspartame example, *Journal of American College of Nutrition* 10 (1991): 258–266.
6. Butchko and Kotsonis, 1991.
7. Position of The American Dietetic Association, 1993.
8. D. J. Canty and M. M. Chan, Effects of consumption of caloric vs noncaloric sweet drinks on indices of hunger and food consumption in normal adults, *American Journal of Clinical Nutrition* 53 (1991): 1159–1164; B. J. Rolls, Effects of intense sweeteners on hunger, food intake, and body weight: A review, *American Journal of Clinical Nutrition* 53 (1991): 872–878; L. A. Chen and E. S. Parham, College students' use of high-intensity sweeteners is not consistently associated with sugar consumption, *Journal of the American Dietetic Association* 91 (1991): 686–690.
9. M. G. Tordoff and A. M. Alleva, Effect of drinking soda sweetened with aspartame or high-fructose corn syrup on food intake and body weight, *American Journal of Clinical Nutrition* 51 (1990): 963–969.
10. A. Drewnowski and coauthors, Comparing the effects of aspartame and sucrose on motivational ratings, taste preferences, and energy intake in humans, *American Journal of Clinical Nutrition* 59 (1994): 338–345.
11. F. R. J. Bonet, Undigestible sugars in food products, *American Journal of Clinical Nutrition* 59 (1994): 763S–769S.
12. Position of The American Dietetic Association, 1993.

Chapter 5

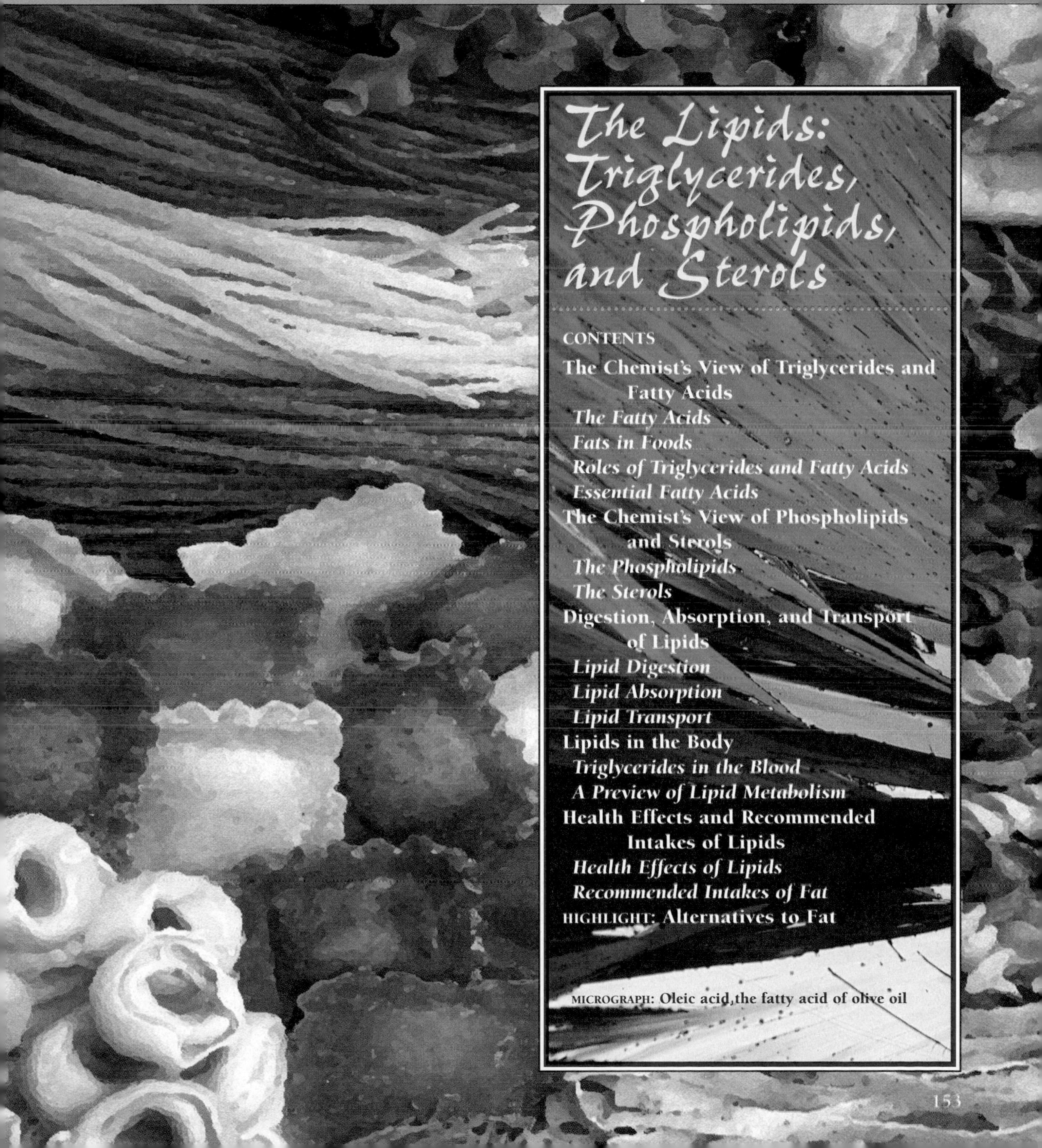

The Lipids: Triglycerides, Phospholipids, and Sterols

CONTENTS

MICROGRAPH: Oleic acid, the fatty acid of olive oil

Most people are surprised to learn that fat has some virtues. It is only when people consume either too much or too little of it that ill health follows. It is true, though, that in our society of abundance, people are likely to encounter too much fat.

Fat is actually a subset of the class of nutrients known as lipids, but the term *fat* is often used to refer to all the lipids. Table 5–1 offers a preview of the lipid family, which includes triglycerides (fats and oils), phospholipids, and sterols, all important to nutrition. The triglycerides provide the body with a continuous fuel supply, keep it warm, and protect it from mechanical shock; their component fatty acids serve as starting materials for important hormonal regulators. The phospholipids and sterols contribute to the cells' structures, and the sterol cholesterol serves as the raw material for some hormones, vitamin D, and bile.

In foods, triglycerides carry with them the four fat-soluble vitamins—A, D, E, and K—together with many of the compounds that give foods their flavor, tenderness, and palatability. Fat is responsible for the delicious aromas associated with sizzling bacon and hamburgers on the grill, onions being sautéed, or vegetables in a stir-fry. Of course, these wonderful aromas lure people into eating too much from time to time. Studies have found that obese people have a strong preference for fat, but have not revealed whether the preference or the obesity comes first.[1]

When people speak of fats and oils, they are usually speaking of triglycerides. The triglycerides predominate, both in foods and in the body.

Table 5–1

The Lipid Family

Triglycerides (fats and oils)
• Glycerol (1 per triglyceride)
• Fatty acids (3 per triglyceride)
Saturated
Monounsaturated
Polyunsaturated
Omega-6
Omega-3
Phospholipids (such as lecithin)
Sterols (such as cholesterol)

fat: the lipids in foods or body fat, both of which are composed mostly of triglycerides.

lipids: a family of compounds that includes triglycerides (fats and oils), phospholipids, and sterols.

Of the lipids in foods, 95% are fats and oils (triglycerides), and 5% are other lipids (phospholipids and sterols). Of the lipids stored in the body, 99% are triglycerides.

triglycerides (try-GLISS-er-rides): the chief form of fat in the diet and the major storage form of fat in the body; composed of a molecule of glycerol with three fatty acids attached; also called **triacylglycerols** (try-ay-seel-GLISS-er-ols).
tri = three
glyceride = a compound of glycerol
acyl = a carbon chain

glycerol (GLISS-er-ol): an alcohol composed of a three-carbon chain, which can serve as the backbone for a triglyceride.
ol = alcohol

Figure 5–1

Glycerol

Notice that glycerol has three OH groups to which three fatty acids can attach to form a triglyceride.

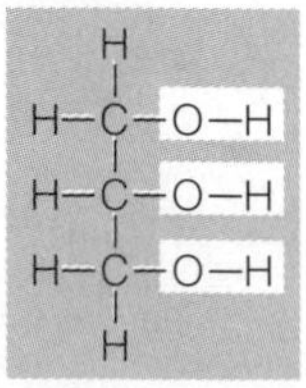

The Chemist's View of Triglycerides and Fatty Acids

Like carbohydrates, triglycerides are composed of carbon, hydrogen, and oxygen. However, triglycerides have many more carbons and hydrogens in proportion to their oxygens, and so can supply more energy per gram (Chapter 7 provides details).

For people who think more easily in words than in chemical symbols, this *preview* of the upcoming chemistry may be helpful. The following paragraphs and diagrams demonstrate that:

1. Every triglyceride contains one molecule of glycerol (see Figure 5–1) and three fatty acids (basically chains of carbon atoms).
2. Fatty acids may be 4 to 24 (even numbers of) carbons long, the 18-carbon ones being the most common in foods and especially noteworthy in nutrition.
3. Fatty acids may also be saturated or unsaturated. The latter may have one or more points of unsaturation (may be mono- or polyunsaturated).
4. Polyunsaturated fatty acids of special importance in nutrition are the ones whose *first* point of unsaturation is next to the third carbon (known as omega-3 fatty acids) or next to the sixth carbon (omega-6), when counting from the methyl end (CH_3) of the carbon chain.
5. The 18-carbon fatty acids that fit this description are linolenic acid (omega-3) and linoleic acid (omega-6). Each is the primary member of a "family" of longer-chain fatty acids that regulate blood pressure, clotting, and other body functions important to health.

THE FATTY ACIDS

A fatty acid is an organic acid—a chain of carbon atoms with hydrogens attached—that has an acid group (COOH) at one end and a methyl group (CH_3) at the other end. The organic acid shown in Figure 5–2 is acetic acid, the compound that gives vinegar its sour taste. Acetic acid is the simplest such acid, with a "chain" only two carbon atoms long.

fatty acid: an organic compound composed of a carbon chain with hydrogens attached and an acid group (COOH) at one end. The COOH group of an organic acid can be represented this way:

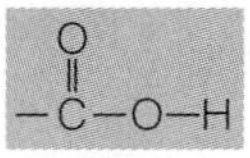

Notice that this structure meets the requirement that C must have four bonds and O two. To accomplish this, O and C form a double bond.

The Carbon Chain Most naturally occurring fatty acids contain even numbers of carbons in their chains—up to 24 carbons in length. This discussion begins with the 18-carbon fatty acids, which are abundant in our food supply. Stearic acid is the simplest of the 18-carbon fatty acids; the bonds between its carbons are all alike:

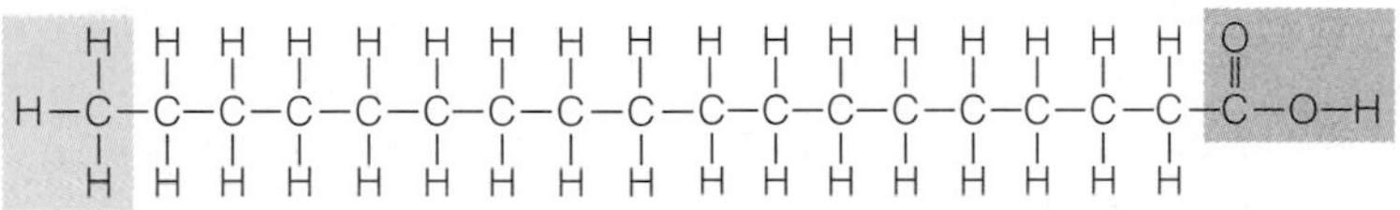

Stearic acid, an 18-carbon saturated fatty acid.

(As you can see, stearic acid is 18 carbons long and each atom meets the rules of chemical bonding described in Chapter 4.) A fatty acid like stearic acid that contains only single bonds between its carbon atoms is a saturated fatty acid. The following structure also depicts stearic acid, but in a simpler way, with each "corner" on the zigzag line representing a carbon atom with two attached hydrogens:

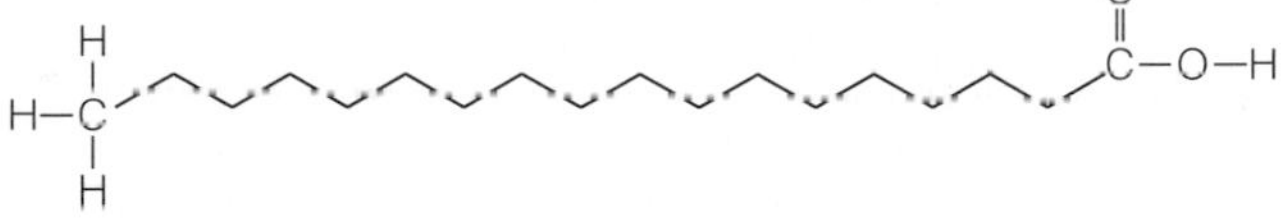

Stearic acid (simplified structure).

Figure 5–2

Acetic Acid

Acetic acid is a two-carbon organic acid.

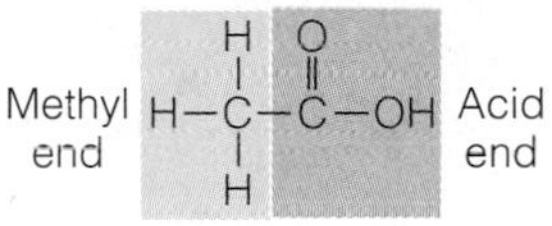

Triglyceride Formation Few fatty acids occur free in foods or in the body. Most often, they are incorporated into triglycerides. To make a triglyceride, three fatty acids are attached to a glycerol molecule by condensation reactions (see Figure 5–3 on p. 156). Each condensation reaction combines a hydrogen atom (H) from the glycerol and a hydroxyl (OH) group from a fatty acid, forming a molecule of water (H_2O) and leaving a bond between the other two molecules.

Degree of Saturation The glossary on p. 157 defines the terms that describe fatty acids. The triglyceride shown in Figure 5–3 is a saturated fat because all three fatty acids are saturated fatty acids—that is, fully loaded with hydrogen atoms. If hydrogens were missing, there would be points of unsaturation where the carbons would have to form double bonds with one another. The result would be an unsaturated, or even a polyunsaturated, fat. Consider stearic acid once more. If two hydrogens were missing from the middle of the carbon chain, the structure that remained might be:

point of unsaturation: the double bond of a fatty acid, where hydrogen atoms can easily be added to the structure.

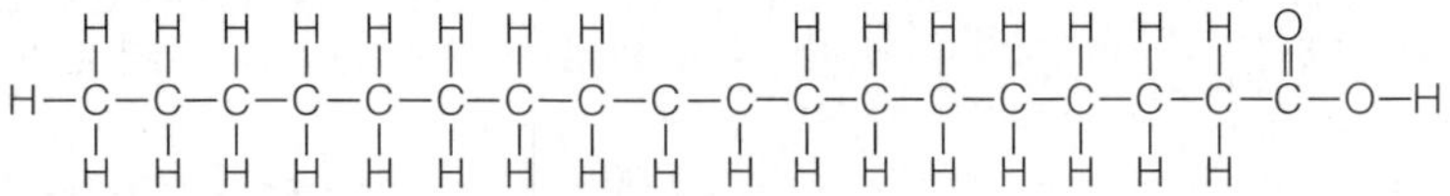

An impossible chemical structure.

Such a compound cannot exist, however, because two of the carbons have only three bonds each, and nature requires that every carbon have four bonds.

Figure 5–3

Condensation of Glycerol and Fatty Acids to Form a Triglyceride

To make a fat (triglyceride), three fatty acids attach to glycerol in condensation reactions:

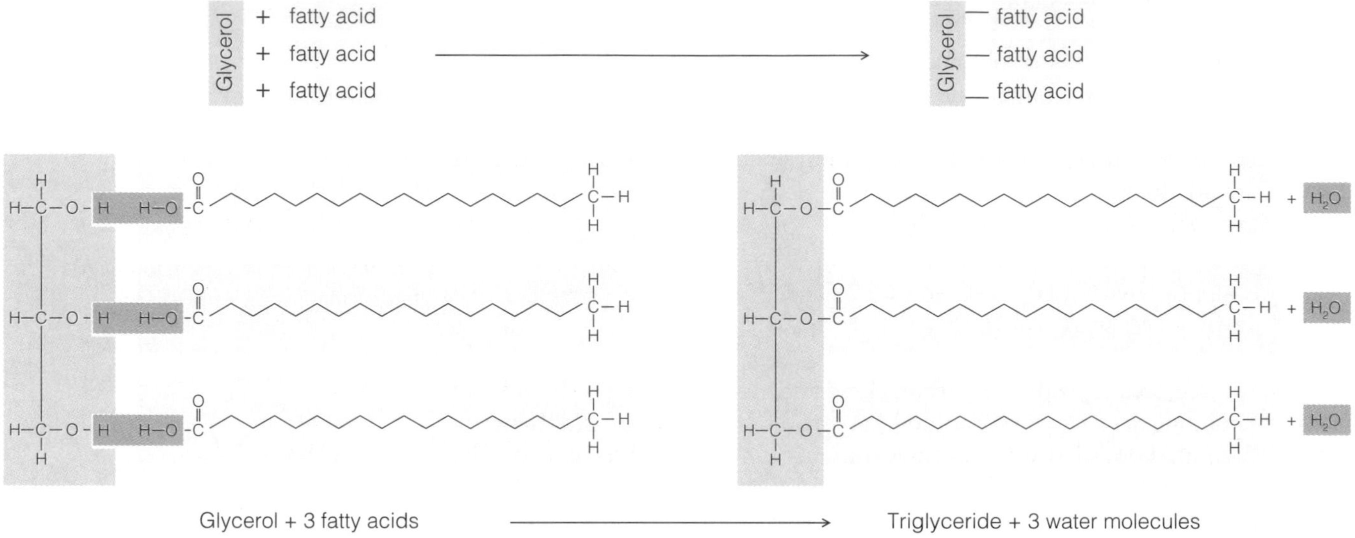

Water is removed from the glycerol and the fatty acids, forming a bond between the O on the glycerol and the C at the acid end of each fatty acid.

Three fatty acids attached to a glycerol form a triglyceride and yield water. In this example, all three fatty acids are stearic acid, but most often triglycerides contain mixtures of fatty acids.

The two carbons therefore form a double bond:

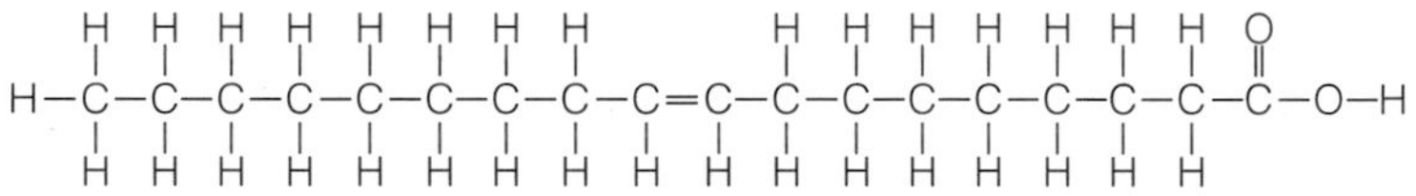

Oleic acid, an 18-carbon monounsaturated fatty acid.

The same structure drawn more simply looks like this:*

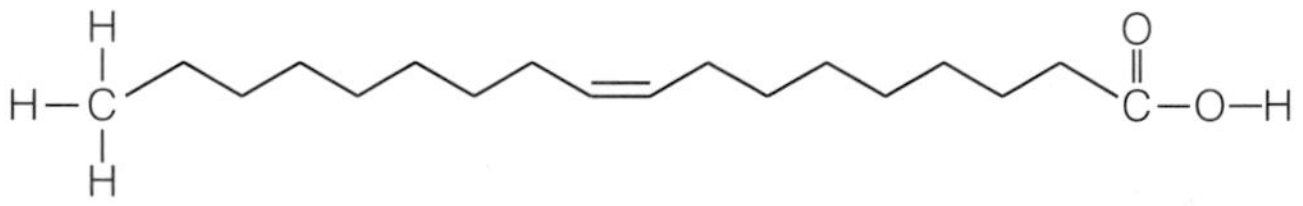

Oleic acid (simplified structure).

A fatty acid like this—with two hydrogens missing and a double bond—is an *un*saturated fatty acid. This one is the 18-carbon *mono*unsaturated fatty acid oleic acid, which is abundant in the triglycerides of olive oil.

A *poly*unsaturated fat contains triglycerides whose fatty acids have two or more carbon-to-carbon double bonds. The best known of these is linoleic acid,

linoleic acid (lin-oh-LAY-ick): an essential fatty acid with 18 carbons and two double bonds (18:2).

*Remember that each "corner" on the zigzag line represents a carbon atom with two attached hydrogens. In addition, the actual shape bends at the double bonds and rotates around single bonds. These molecules, although drawn straight on paper, are constantly twisting and bending. At any given moment, they may be coiled, horseshoe shaped, or straight.

Glossary of Fatty Acids

These terms are listed in order from the most saturated to the most unsaturated.

saturated fatty acid: a fatty acid carrying the maximum possible number of hydrogen atoms—for example, stearic acid. A **saturated fat** is composed of triglycerides in which all or virtually all of the fatty acids are saturated.

unsaturated fatty acid: a fatty acid that lacks hydrogen atoms and has at least one double bond between carbons (includes monounsaturated and polyunsaturated fatty acids). An **unsaturated fat** is composed of triglycerides in which some of the fatty acids are unsaturated.

monounsaturated fatty acid: a fatty acid that lacks two hydrogen atoms and has one double bond between carbons—for example, oleic acid.
mono = one

polyunsaturated fatty acid (PUFA): a fatty acid that lacks four or more hydrogen atoms and has two or more double bonds between carbons—for example, linoleic acid (two double bonds) and linolenic acid (three double bonds). A **polyunsaturated fat** is composed of triglycerides containing a high percentage of PUFA.
poly = many

---

the 18-carbon fatty acid common in vegetable oils. Linoleic acid lacks four hydrogens and has two double bonds:

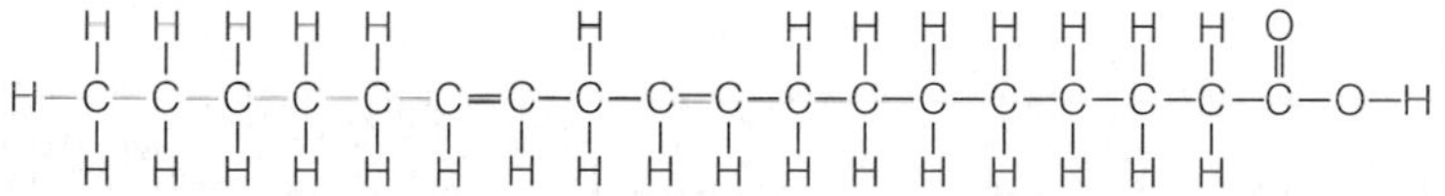

Linoleic acid, an 18-carbon polyunsaturated fatty acid.

Drawn more simply, linoleic acid looks like this:

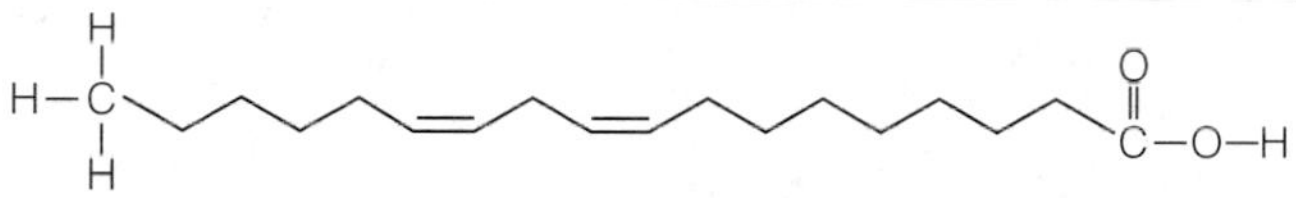

Linoleic acid (simplified structure).

A fourth 18-carbon fatty acid is linolenic acid, which has three double bonds (see Table 5–2).

linolenic acid (lin-oh-LEN-ick): an essential fatty acid with 18 carbons and three double bonds (18:3).

Having looked at four of the most common fatty acids in foods, one can predict what the others will look like. They vary only in their degrees of unsaturation

Table 5–2

18-Carbon Fatty Acids

Name	Notation[a]	Number of Double Bonds	Saturation
Stearic acid	18:0	0	Saturated
Oleic acid	18:1	1	Monounsaturated
Linoleic acid	18:2	2	Polyunsaturated
Linolenic acid	18:3	3	Polyunsaturated

[a]Chemists use a shorthand notation to describe fatty acids. The first number indicates the number of carbon atoms; the second, the number of double bonds.

Figure 5–4

A Mixed Triglyceride

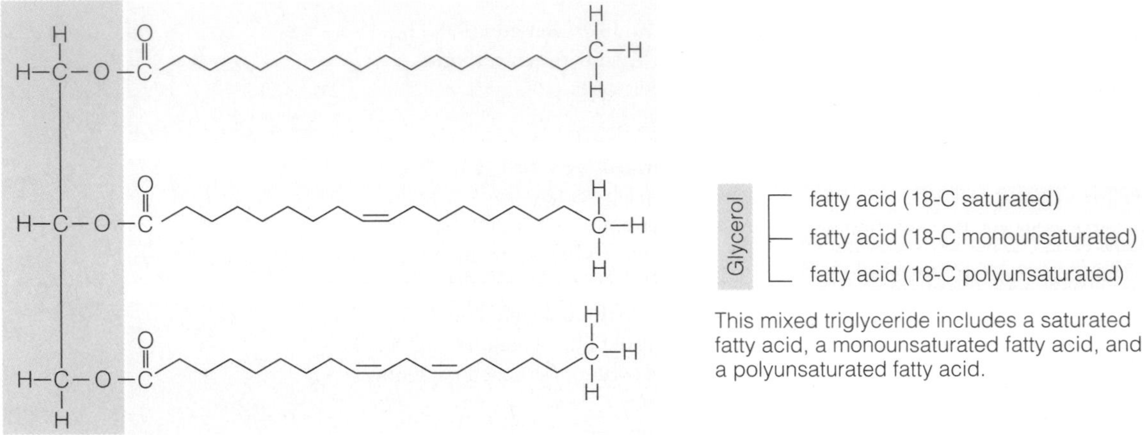

This mixed triglyceride includes a saturated fatty acid, a monounsaturated fatty acid, and a polyunsaturated fatty acid.

Another way to show the chemical structure of a triglyceride is to draw the second fatty acid to the left of the glycerol.

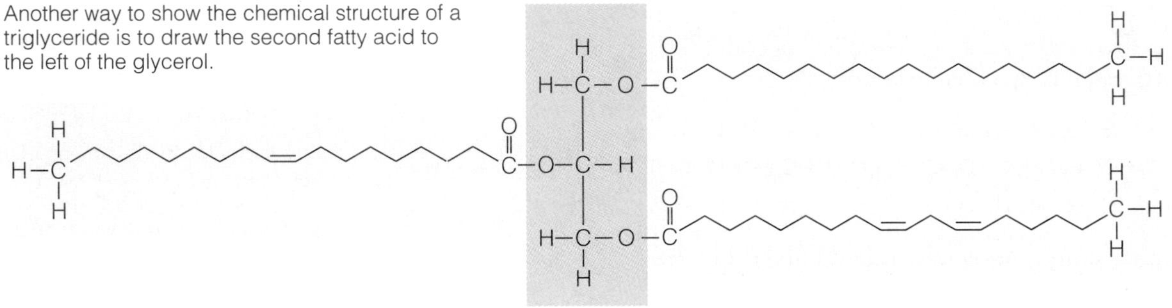

Tables C–1 and C–2 in Appendix C provide the names, chain length, and sources of fatty acids commonly found in foods.

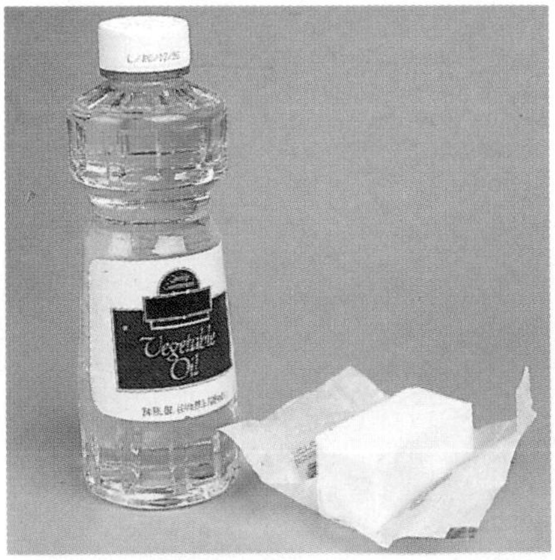

At room temperature, unsaturated fats (such as those found in vegetable oils) are usually liquid, whereas saturated fats (such as those found in butter) are solid.

and the lengths of their chains. The long-chain fatty acids (12- to 24-carbon) of meats and fish are most common in the diet. Smaller amounts of medium-chain (6- to 10-carbon) and short-chain (less than 6 carbon) fatty acids also occur, primarily in dairy products.

To sum up to this point, dietary fats and oils are mostly (95 percent) triglycerides: glycerol backbones with three fatty acids attached. Fats that are fully loaded with hydrogens are saturated; fats that are missing hydrogens and therefore have double bonds are unsaturated (monounsaturated and polyunsaturated). The degree of unsaturation of fats affects health, as a later section in this chapter explains. The vast majority of triglycerides contain mixtures of more than one type of fatty acid. Figure 5–4 provides an example. The fatty acid compositions of some typical dietary fats are shown in Figure 5–5, and Appendix H provides the fat and fatty acid contents of many other foods.

FATS IN FOODS

The degree of saturation influences the firmness of fats at room temperature. Generally speaking, the polyunsaturated vegetable oils are liquid and the more

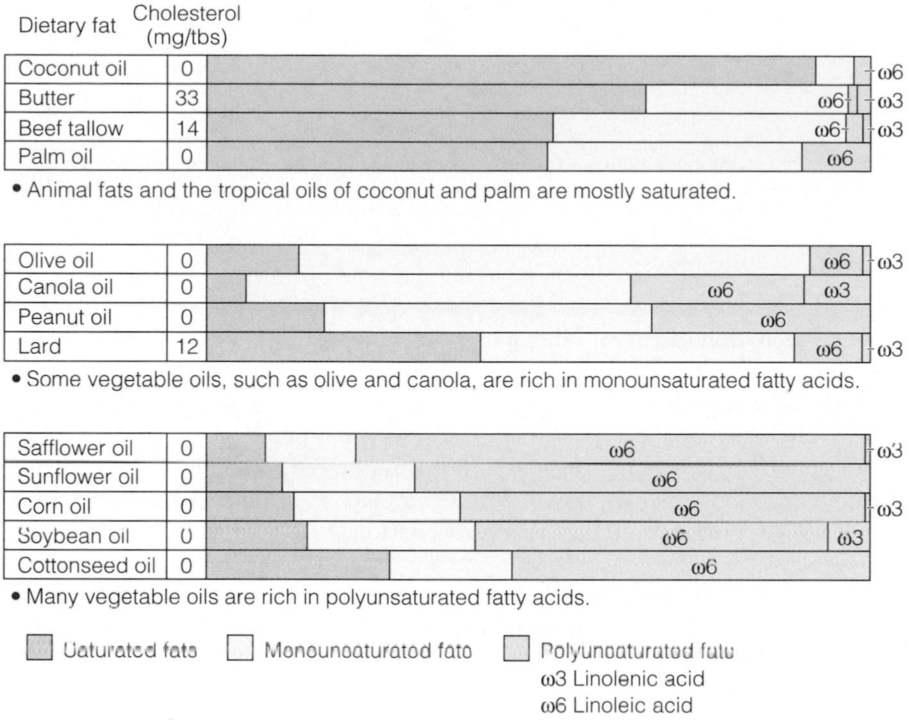

Figure 5–5

Comparison of Dietary Fats

Most fats are a mixture of saturated, monounsaturated, and polyunsaturated fatty acids. See pp. 161–163 for information on omega-6 (ω6) and omega-3 (ω3) fatty acids.

Source: The Lipid Handbook, ed. F. D. Gunstone (London: Chapman and Hall, 1986) and USDA data, as cited by the Malaysian Palm Oil Promotion Council in material distributed by Edelman Public Relations, 1420 K Street, NW, Washington, D.C. 20005 in undated materials received in 1991; J. B. Reeves and J. L. Weihrauch, *Composition of Foods, Agriculture Handbook No. 8–1* (Washington, D.C.: USDA, 1979) as cited by Procter & Gamble in copyrighted material provided as a professional service, 1992.

saturated animal fats are harder at room temperature (review Figure 5–5). Butter is harder than margarine because butter is more saturated than margarine; this is why people limiting their intakes of saturated fats use margarine. Not all vegetable oils are polyunsaturated, however. Palm and coconut oils are saturated even though they are of vegetable origin; they are firmer than most vegetable oils because of their saturation, but softer than most animal fats because of their short carbon chains (only 10 and 12 carbons long, respectively). Generally, the longer the carbon chain, the more liquid the fat is at room temperature.

The food industry often refers to palm and coconut oils as the "tropical oils."

Processed Fat Saturation also influences stability. All fats can become rancid when exposed to oxygen. Polyunsaturated fatty acids spoil most readily because their double bonds are unstable. The oxidation of unsaturated fats yields a variety of products that smell and taste rancid; saturated fats are more resistant to oxidation and thus less likely to become rancid. Other types of spoilage can occur due to microbial growth.

oxidation (OK-see-day-shun): the process of a substance combining with oxygen.

Manufacturers can protect fat-containing products against rancidity in three ways—none of them perfect. First, products may be sealed air-tight and refrigerated—an expensive and inconvenient storage system. Second, manufacturers may add antioxidants to compete for the oxygen and thus protect the oil (examples are the additives BHA and BHT and vitamins C and E); the advantages and disadvantages of antioxidants in food processing are presented in Chapter 19. Third, manufacturers may saturate some or all of the points of unsaturation by adding hydrogen molecules—a process known as partial or complete hydrogenation.

antioxidant: a compound that protects others from oxidation by being oxidized itself; Chapter 10 provides more details.

Figure 5–6

Hydrogenation

Hydrogenation yields a product that is more saturated, more spreadable, and more resistant to oxidation.

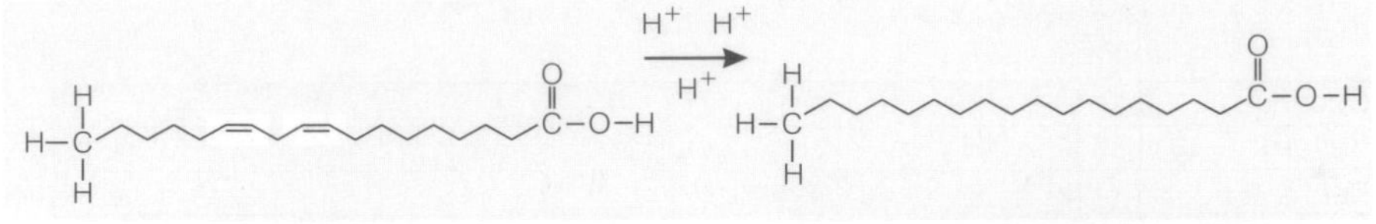

Double bonds carry a slightly negative charge and readily accept positively charged hydrogen atoms, creating a saturated fatty acid.

---

hydrogenation (high-dro-gen-AY-shun): a chemical process by which hydrogens are added to monounsaturated or polyunsaturated fats to reduce the number of double bonds, making the fats more saturated (solid) and more resistant to oxidation (protecting against rancidity). Hydrogenation produces *trans*-fatty acids.

trans-fatty acids: fatty acids with an unusual configuration around the double bond.

Hydrogenation of Fats The process of hydrogenation offers two advantages: it protects against oxidation (thereby prolonging shelf life) and alters the texture of foods. When partially hydrogenated, vegetable oils become spreadable margarine. Hydrogenated fats make pie crusts flaky and puddings creamy. A disadvantage is that hydrogenation makes polyunsaturated fats more saturated (see Figure 5–6). Consequently, any health advantages of using polyunsaturated fats instead of saturated fats are lost in hydrogenation.

Formation of *Trans*-Fatty Acids Another disadvantage of hydrogenation has to do with some of the molecules that remain unsaturated after processing. Some of these molecules change shape from *cis* to *trans*. In nature, most unsaturated fatty acids are *cis*-fatty acids—meaning that the hydrogens next to the double bonds are on the same side of the carbon chain. Only a few (notably those found in milk and butter) are *trans*-fatty acids—meaning that the hydrogens next to the double bonds are on opposite sides of the carbon chain (see Figure 5–7). These arrangements result in different configurations for the fatty acids, and the differences affect function.

Major sources of *trans*-fatty acids:

- Margarine (the hard stick type).
- Cakes, cookies, doughnuts, crackers.
- Snack chips.
- Meat and dairy products.
- Peanut butter.
- Fried foods.

People's intakes of *trans*-fatty acids from food products have risen in recent years as manufacturers have increased their use of partially hydrogenated vegetable oils.[2] A food that lists partially hydrogenated oils among its first three ingredients usually contains substantial amounts of *trans*-fatty acids, as well as some saturated fat. The relationship between *trans*-fatty acids and heart disease has been the subject of much recent research, as a later section describes.

Figure 5–7

***Cis*- and *Trans*-Fatty Acids Compared**

Manufacturers rarely use total hydrogenation; most often a fat is partially hydrogenated, yielding a *trans*-monounsaturated fatty acid. This example shows the *cis* configuration for oleic acid and its corresponding *trans* configuration (elaidic acid).

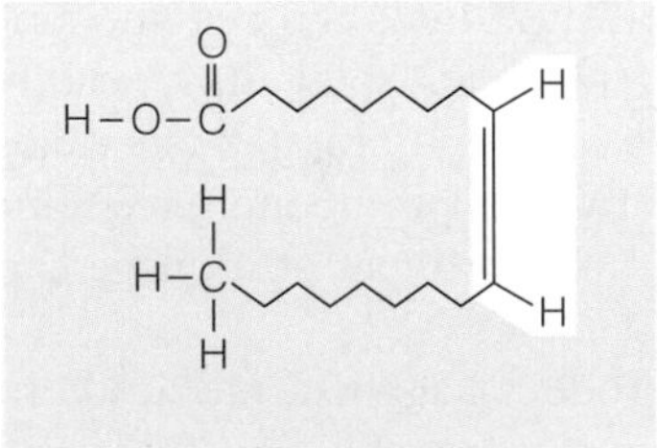

Cis-fatty acid

A *cis*-fatty acid has its hydrogens on the same side of the double bond; *cis* molecules fold back into a U-like formation. Most unsaturated fatty acids in foods are *cis*.

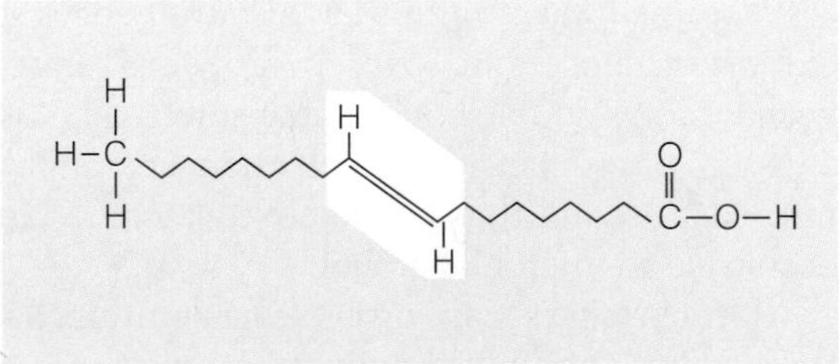

Trans-fatty acid

A *trans*-fatty acid has its hydrogens on the opposite sides of the double bond; *trans* molecules are more linear. The *trans* form typically occurs in partially hydrogenated foods when hydrogen atoms shift around some double bonds and change the configuration from *cis* to *trans*.

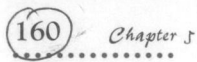

ROLES OF TRIGLYCERIDES AND FATTY ACIDS

First and foremost, the triglycerides provide the body with energy. When a person dances all night, her stored triglycerides provide the fuel to keep her moving; when a person loses his appetite, his stored triglycerides fuel much of his body's work until he can eat again. Stored fat supports many of life's activities.

Stored fat also insulates the body. Fat is a poor conductor of heat; the layer of fat beneath the skin helps keep the body warm. Fat pads also serve as shock absorbers, supporting and cushioning the vital organs.

Fat also helps the body use its two other energy nutrients—carbohydrate and protein—efficiently. Fat fragments combine with glucose fragments in the release of energy, and fat helps spare protein, providing energy so that protein can be used for other important tasks.

ESSENTIAL FATTY ACIDS

The human body can make all but two fatty acids—linoleic acid and linolenic acid. Because these two fatty acids are indispensable to body function, they must be supplied by the diet. They are therefore called essential fatty acids. The body uses these essential fatty acids to maintain the structural parts of cell membranes and to make many hormonelike substances known as eicosanoids. Eicosanoids help regulate blood pressure, blood clot formation, blood lipids, and the immune response to injury and infection.[3]

Linoleic acid and linolenic acid are the 18-carbon members of the two omega families mentioned in the introductory remarks.* Figure 5–8 (on p. 162) shows the structures of these two omega families.

Linoleic Acid, an Omega-6 Fatty Acid Linoleic acid is the primary member of the omega-6 family. Given linoleic acid, the body can make other members of the omega-6 family—such as the 20-carbon polyunsaturated fatty acid, arachidonic acid. Should a linoleic acid deficiency develop, arachidonic acid, and all the other fatty acids that derive from linoleic acid, would also become essential and would have to be obtained from the diet. Normally, vegetable oils and meats supply enough omega-6 fatty acids to meet the body's needs.

Linolenic Acid, an Omega-3 Fatty Acid Linolenic acid is the primary member of the omega-3 family.† Like linoleic acid, this 18-carbon acid cannot be made in the body and must be supplied by foods. Given dietary linolenic acid, the body can make the 20- and 22-carbon members of the omega-3 series, eicosapentaenoic acid (EPA) and docosahexaenoic acid (DHA). Many body tissues

---

*A fatty acid has two ends, designated the methyl (CH_3) end and the acid (COOH) end. Chemists usually number the carbons beginning at the acid end, but make an exception for polyunsaturated fatty acids. Because the body lengthens fatty acid chains by adding carbons at the acid end of the chain, these numbers would change as the chains grew longer. Chemists therefore number the carbons beginning at the methyl end, which eases the task of keeping track of fatty acids: when an omega-3 fatty acid is lengthened, the derivative is also an omega-3 fatty acid.

†This omega-3 linolenic acid is known as alpha-linolenic acid and is the fatty acid referred to in this discussion. Another fatty acid, also with 18 carbons and three double bonds, belongs to the omega-6 family and is known as gamma-linolenic acid.

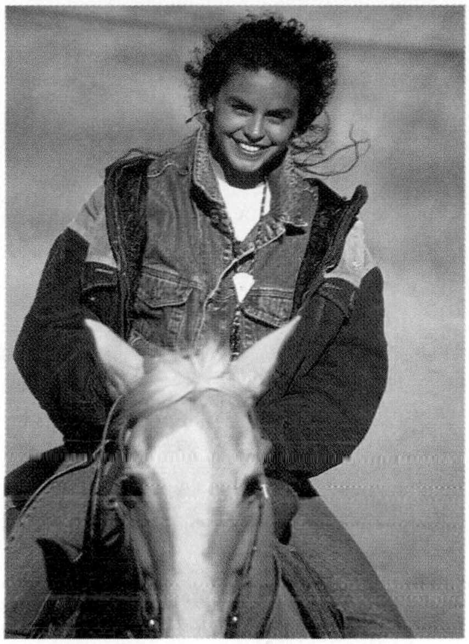

Thanks to the body's fat pads, a horseback ride causes no serious damage to internal organs.

Triglycerides in the body:

- Provide energy.
- Insulate against temperature extremes.
- Protect organs against shock.
- Help the body use carbohydrate and protein efficiently.

essential fatty acids: fatty acids needed by the body, but not made by the body in amounts sufficient to meet physiological needs.

eicosanoids (eye-COSS-uh-noyds): derivatives of fatty acids; hormonelike compounds that regulate blood pressure, clotting, and other body functions. They include *prostaglandins*, *thromboxanes*, and *leukotrienes*.

omega: the last letter of the Greek alphabet (ω), used by chemists to refer to the position of the endmost double bond in a fatty acid.

omega-6 fatty acid: a polyunsaturated fatty acid in which the first double bond is six carbons from the methyl (CH_3) end of the carbon chain.

arachidonic (a-RACK-ih-DON-ic) **acid:** an omega-6 polyunsaturated fatty acid with 20 carbons and four double bonds (20:4); synthesized from linoleic acid.

Figure 5–8

Structural Formulas for Omega-3 and Omega-6 Fatty Acids

The omega number indicates the position of the first double bond in a fatty acid, counting from the methyl (CH_3) end. Thus an omega-3 fatty acid's first double bond occurs three carbons from the methyl end, and an omega-6 fatty acid's first double bond occurs six carbons from the methyl end. The members of a given family may have different lengths and different numbers of double bonds, but the first double bond occurs at the same point in all of them.

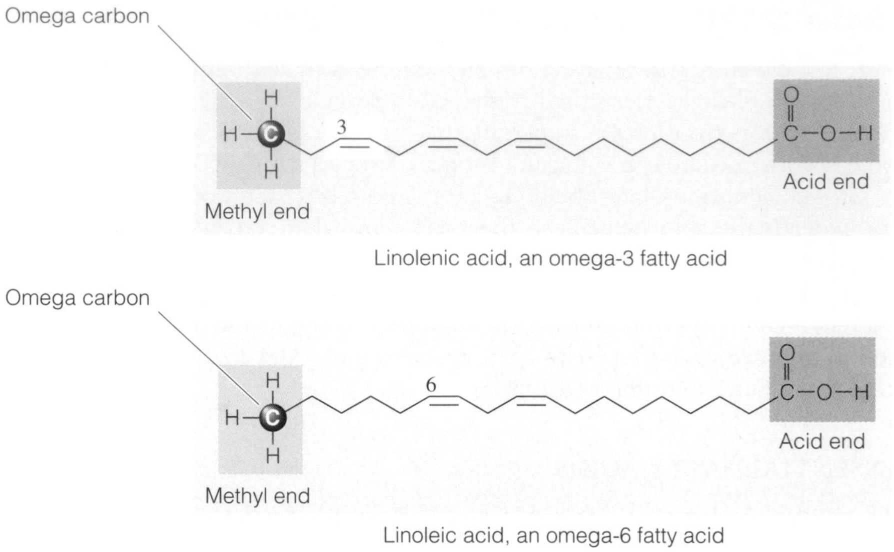

---

omega-3 fatty acid: a polyunsaturated fatty acid in which the first double bond is three carbons away from the methyl (CH_3) end of the carbon chain.

eicosapentaenoic (EYE-cossa-PENTA-ee-NO-ic) **acid (EPA):** an omega-3 polyunsaturated fatty acid with 20 carbons and five double bonds (20:5); synthesized from linolenic acid.

docosahexaenoic (DOE-cossa-HEXA-ee-NO-ic) **acid (DHA):** an omega-3 polyunsaturated fatty acid with 22 carbons and six double bonds (22:6); synthesized from linolenic acid.

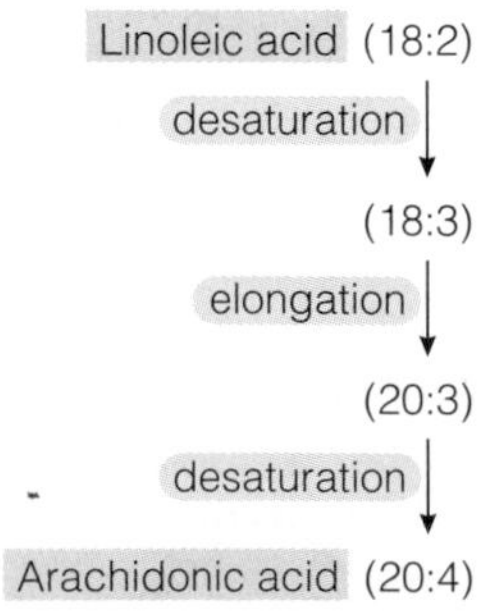

Note: The first number indicates the number of carbons and the second, the number of double bonds. Similar reactions occur when the body makes EPA and DHA from linolenic acid.

contain EPA and DHA; they make up a large proportion of the communicating membranes of the brain, and so their availability is necessary for normal brain development.[4] EPA and DHA are also active in the retina of the eye.[5] These omega-3 fatty acids are essential for normal growth and development, and they may play an important role in the prevention and treatment of heart disease, hypertension, arthritis, and cancer.[6]

A Comment on Essentiality A simple definition of an essential nutrient has already been given: a nutrient that the body cannot make, or cannot make in sufficient quantities to meet its physiological needs. In the case of fatty acids, though, the body can make some fatty acids only if others are available. Also, some may be essential only for growth or for disease prevention.

The cells do not possess the enzymes to make any of the omega-6 or omega-3 fatty acids from scratch; nor can they convert an omega-6 fatty acid to an omega-3 fatty acid or vice versa. They *can* start with the 18-carbon member of a series and make the longer fatty acids of that series by forming double bonds (desaturation) and lengthening the chain two carbons at a time (elongation). This is a slow process because the two families compete for the same enzymes. Therefore the most effective way to maintain body supplies of these polyunsaturated fatty acids is to obtain them directly from foods.

Polyunsaturated Fats in Foods A balanced diet that includes grains, seeds, nuts, leafy vegetables (or small amounts of vegetable oils), and fish supplies all the omega-6 and omega-3 fatty acids in abundance. Table 5–3 lists the chief dietary sources of the omega fatty acids.

When dietary intakes exceed the body's immediate needs, the body stores the omega-3 fatty acids EPA and DHA.[7] Most North Americans, however, do not eat enough fish to store any extra EPA and DHA. (Optimal omega-3 intake is estimated to be about 1 to 1.5 grams a day; current intake in the United States is about one-tenth of that.) They do, however, receive plenty of the omega-6

Table 5–3

Sources of Omega Fatty Acids

Omega-6	
Linoleic acid	Leafy vegetables, seeds, nuts, grains, vegetable oils (corn, safflower, soybean, cottonseed, sesame, sunflower)
Arachidonic acid	Meats (or can be made from linoleic acid)
Omega-3	
Linolenic acid	Fats and oils (canola, soybean, walnut, wheat germ, margarine and shortening made from canola and soybean oil)
	Nuts and seeds (butternuts, walnuts, soybean kernels)
	Vegetables (soybeans)
EPA and DHA	Human milk
	Shellfish and fish[a] (mackerel, tuna, salmon, bluefish, mullet, sturgeon, menhaden, anchovy, herring, trout, sardines)
	(or can be made from linolenic acid)

[a]These fish provide at least 1 gram of omega-3 fatty acids in 100 grams of fish (3.5 ounces); the fish oil content of each species varies with the season and site of harvest.

fatty acids. A comparison with the fish-eating people of Greenland is illuminating. Greenlanders have higher energy intakes and a higher percentage of kcalories from omega-3 fatty acids. North Americans have lower energy intakes and a higher percentage of kcalories from omega-6 fatty acids; indeed, they eat about twice as many omega-6 and half as many omega-3 fatty acids as Greenlanders do. Researchers have speculated that this difference may explain why the heart attack rate in North America is so much higher than in Greenland. It also explains why the people in Greenland have prolonged bleeding times and a high incidence of stroke. Such findings highlight the importance of dietary balance. Ideally, the ratio between these two lipid families in the diet is 4 to 10 grams of omega-6 fatty acids to 1 gram of omega-3 fatty acids.[8]

Fatty Acid Deficiencies Essential fatty acids should make up at least 3 percent of the day's energy intake. Deficiencies of these polyunsaturated fatty acids cause growth retardation, reproductive failure, skin lesions, kidney and liver disorders, and subtle neurological and visual problems. There is no need to panic, though; most diets meet minimum requirements more than adequately.[9] Deficiencies have historically developed only in infants and young children fed nonfat milk and low-fat diets or in hospital clients fed formulas that provided no polyunsaturated fatty acids for long times.

In summary, the lipids important in nutrition, commonly called simply *fat,* are of three classes: triglycerides, phospholipids, and sterols. The triglycerides are by far the predominant class both in foods and in the body. They are energy-dense, important energy-storage compounds. Each triglyceride contains three fatty acids, which may be long, medium, or short chain; may be saturated, monounsaturated, or polyunsaturated; and if the latter, may be members of the omega-3 or omega-6 families of fatty acids. Linoleic acid (18 carbons, omega-6) and linolenic acid (18 carbons, omega-3) are essential nutrients; the essentiality of other polyunsaturated fatty acids is debated.

Fatty acid saturation affects fats' cooking qualities, their storage properties, and their contributions to people's susceptibility to heart disease and cancer. Hydrogenation, which makes polyunsaturates more saturated, gives rise to some *trans*-fatty acids, altered fatty acids that may exert adverse health effects. Small amounts of fats are necessary to support health, carry fat-soluble vitamins, and spare protein; deficiencies are unlikely.

The Chemist's View of Phospholipids and Sterols

phospholipid: a compound similar to a triglyceride but having choline (or another nitrogen-containing compound) and a phosphate group (a phosphorus-containing salt) in place of one of the fatty acids.

lecithin (LESS-uh-thin): one of the phospholipids; a compound of glycerol to which are attached two fatty acids, a phosphate group, and a choline molecule. Both nature and the food industry use lecithin as an emulsifier to combine two ingredients that do not ordinarily mix, such as water and oil.

Reminder: An *emulsifier* promotes the mixing of two substances, such as oil and water, that are not mutually soluble.

The preceding pages have been devoted to one of the three classes of lipids, the triglycerides, and their component parts, the fatty acids. The other two classes of lipids, the phospholipids and sterols, make up only 5 percent of the lipids in the diet, but they are nevertheless interesting and important.

THE PHOSPHOLIPIDS

The best-known phospholipids are the lecithins. Each lecithin has a backbone of glycerol with two of its three attachment sites occupied by fatty acids like those in triglycerides. The third site is occupied by a phosphate group and a molecule of choline. The fatty acids make phospholipids soluble in fat; the phosphate-containing group enables them to dissolve in water. Such versatility enables the food industry to use phospholipids as emulsifiers, mixing fats with water in such products as mayonnaise and candy bars. A diagram of a lecithin molecule is shown in Figure 5–9.

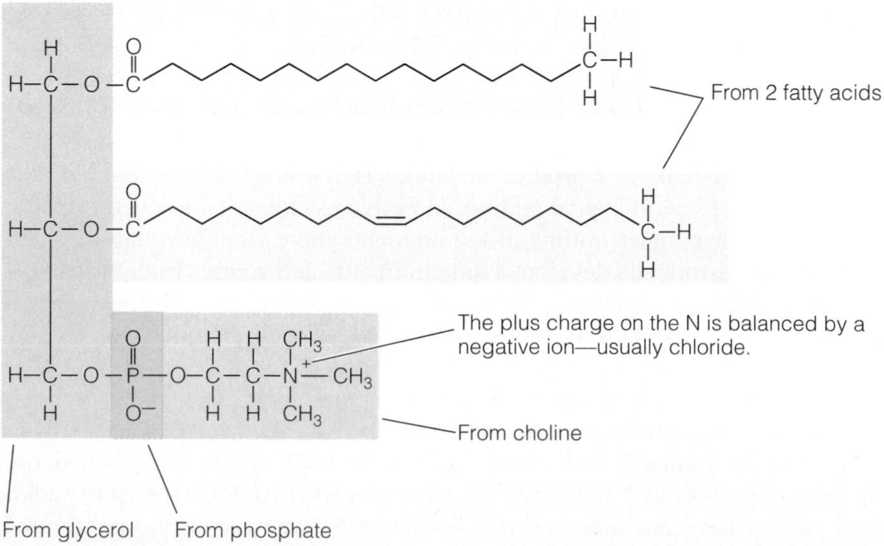

Figure 5–9

A Lecithin

This is one of the lecithins. Other lecithins have different fatty acids at the upper two positions. Notice that a molecule of lecithin is similar to a triglyceride but contains only two fatty acids. The third position is occupied by a phosphate group and a molecule of choline.

choline (KOH-leen): a nitrogen-containing compound found in plant and animal tissues as part of lecithin and other phospholipids.

Phospholipids in Foods In addition to the phospholipids used by the food industry as emulsifiers, phospholipids are also found in foods naturally. The richest food sources of lecithin are eggs, liver, soybeans, wheat germ, and peanuts.

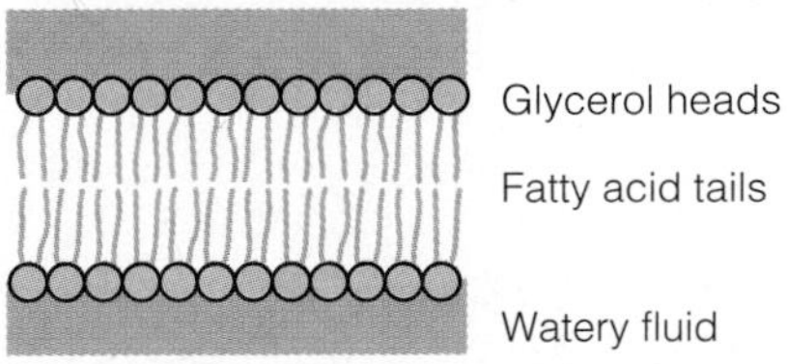

A cell membrane is made of phospholipids assembled into an orderly formation called a bilayer. The fatty acid "tails" orient themselves away from the watery fluid inside and outside of the cell. The glycerol and phosphate "heads" are attracted to the watery fluid.

Roles of Phospholipids The lecithins and other phospholipids are important constituents of cell membranes. Because phospholipids can dissolve in both water and fat, they can help lipids move back and forth across the lipid-containing cell membranes into the watery fluids on both sides. They thus allow fat-soluble substances, including vitamins and hormones, to pass easily in and out of cells. The phospholipids also act as emulsifiers in the body, helping to keep fats suspended in the blood and body fluids.

Lecithin periodically receives attention in the popular press. Its fans claim that it is a major constituent of cell membranes (true), that all cells depend on the integrity of their membranes (true), and that consumers must therefore take lecithin supplements (false). The liver makes from scratch all the lecithin a person needs. As for lecithin taken as a supplement, the digestive enzyme lecithinase in the intestine hydrolyzes most of it before it passes into the body fluids, so little lecithin reaches the body tissues intact. In other words, the lecithins are *not essential nutrients*; they are just another lipid. Like all the other lipids, they contribute 9 kcalories per gram to the body's energy economy—an unexpected "bonus" many people taking lecithin supplements fail to realize. Labels on lecithin supplements suggest a 7-gram daily dosage, which can add 6½ pounds a year to body weight. Furthermore, large doses of lecithin may cause GI distress, sweating, salivation, and loss of appetite. Perhaps these symptoms are beneficial because they may warn people to stop self-dosing with lecithin.

Reminder: The word ending *-ase* denotes an enzyme. Hence, lecithinase is an enzyme that works on lecithin.

THE STEROLS

The sterols are lipid compounds with a multiple-ring structure. The most famous sterol is cholesterol; Figure 5–10 shows its chemical structure. All sterols have the same multiple-ring structure, but each has different side groups attached.

sterol: a compound composed of C, H, and O atoms arranged in rings, like those of cholesterol, with any of a variety of side chains attached.

cholesterol: one of the sterols.

Sterols in Foods Both plant and animal foods contain sterols, but only animal foods contain cholesterol: meats, eggs, fish, poultry, and dairy products. Organ meats, such as liver and kidneys, and eggs, are richest in cholesterol; cheeses and meats have less. Shellfish contain many sterols, but much less cholesterol than has been thought in the past. Table 5–4 lists the cholesterol contents of selected foods. Many more foods, with their cholesterol contents, appear in Appendix H.

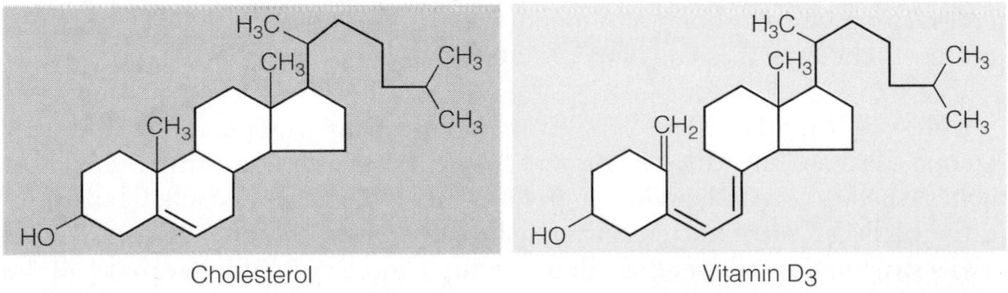

Figure 5–10

Cholesterol

The fat-soluble vitamin D is synthesized from cholesterol; notice the similarities. Notice, too, how different cholesterol is from the triglycerides and phospholipids.

Table 5–4

Approximate Amounts of Cholesterol in Common Foods

Foods	Cholesterol (mg)
Grains, vegetables, fruits	0
Milks (1 c serving)	
Whole milk and yogurt	30–35
Low-fat milk and yogurt	15–20
Nonfat milk and buttermilk	5–10
Cheeses (1 oz serving)	25–30
Ice cream (½ c serving)	30
Pudding (½ c serving)	15
Butter (1 tsp)	10
Margarine, all vegetable (1 tsp)	0
Creams (1 tsp)	10–20
Meats (3 oz serving)	
Veal cutlet	100
Beef steak, chicken, lamb chop, pork chop	70–85
Hot dog	45
Organ meats (3 oz serving)	
Brains	1696
Liver	410
Kidneys	329
Egg yolk	213
Egg white	0
Seafood (3 oz serving)	
Shrimp	165
Lobster, clams, fish fillets, oysters	50–60

Note: Only foods of animal origin contain cholesterol.
Source: Food Processor computer diet analysis program, ESHA, Salem, OR 97302.

Eggs contain just over 200 milligrams of cholesterol each, all of it in the yolks. A person on a strict low-cholesterol diet must curtail the use of egg yolks, and food manufacturers have produced several nonfat, no-cholesterol egg substitutes. For most people trying to lower blood cholesterol, however, limiting saturated fat is more effective than limiting cholesterol intake. Eggs are a valuable part of the diet because they are inexpensive, useful in cooking, and a source of high-quality protein. The American Heart Association approves an intake of up to four eggs a week.

Some people, confused about the distinction between dietary and blood cholesterol, have asked which foods contain the "good" cholesterol. "Good" cholesterol is not a type of cholesterol found in foods, but refers to the way the body transports cholesterol in the blood, as explained later (pp. 172–173).

Roles of Sterols Many vitally important body compounds are sterols. Among them are bile, the sex hormones (such as testosterone), the adrenal hormones (such as cortisol), and vitamin D, as well as cholesterol itself. Cholesterol in the body can serve as the starting material for synthesis of these compounds or as a structural component of cell membranes; more than nine-tenths of all the body's cholesterol resides in the cells. Despite popular impressions to the contrary, therefore, cholesterol is not a villain lurking in some evil foods—it is a compound the body makes and uses. Your liver is manufacturing cholesterol now, as you read. At the rate of perhaps 5×10^{16} (50,000,000,000,000,000) molecules per second (800 to 1500 milligrams per day), the liver contributes much more cholesterol to the body's total than does the diet. The liver can use fragments derived from carbohydrate, protein, or fat as the starting material from which to make cholesterol.

Cholesterol that is made in the body is **endogenous** (en-DODGE-eh-nus), whereas cholesterol from outside the body (from foods) is **exogenous** (eks-ODGE-eh-nus).
- *endo*= within
- *gen* = arising
- *exo* = outside (the body)

Cholesterol synthesis depends on the availability of the raw materials, the extent of bile production, and the presence of regulating hormones such as insulin. When insulin concentrations remain low, as occurs when people eat many small meals, cholesterol synthesis slows. Spreading total food intake over many meals and snacks a day without an increase in energy intake is a relatively easy and effective way to lower blood cholesterol.[10]

Reminder: Eating many small meals and snacks throughout the day is sometimes called *grazing*.

Cholesterol's harmful effects in the body occur when it forms deposits in the artery walls. These deposits lead to atherosclerosis, a disease that causes heart attacks and strokes.

atherosclerosis (ath-er-oh-scler-OH-sis): a type of artery disease characterized by accumulations of lipid-containing material on the inner walls of the arteries (see Chapter 18).
- *athero* = porridge or soft
- *scleros* = hard
- *osis* = condition

In summary, phospholipids, including lecithin, have a unique chemical structure that allows them to be soluble in both water and fat. In the body, phospholipids are part of cell membranes; the food industry uses phospholipids as emulsifiers. Sterols, including cholesterol, have a multiple-ring structure that differs from the other lipids. Sterols in the body include bile, vitamin D, and the sex hormones. Only animal-derived foods contain cholesterol.

Digestion, Absorption, and Transport of Lipids

Each day, the GI tract receives, on the average, 50 to 100 grams of triglycerides, 4 to 8 grams of phospholipids, and 300 to 450 milligrams of cholesterol. The body faces a challenge in digesting and absorbing these lipids: getting at them.

Fats carry no net charge and are neutral. They are hydrophobic—that is, they tend to separate from water—whereas the enzymes for digesting fats are hydrophilic. Since the watery fluids of the GI tract tend to settle at the bottom of the stomach while the dietary fats tend to float on top, the fats start out separated from their enzymes. The following paragraphs describe how the body mixes the fats into the watery fluids and then digests them.

hydrophobic: a term referring to water-fearing, or non-water-soluble, substances; also known as **lipophilic** (fat loving).
- *hydro* = water
- *phobia* = fear
- *lipo* = lipid
- *phile* = friend

hydrophilic: a term referring to water-loving, or water-soluble, substances.

LIPID DIGESTION

The goal of fat digestion is to dismantle triglycerides into small molecules that the body can absorb and use—namely, monoglycerides, fatty acids, and glycerol. Figure 5–11 traces the digestion of triglycerides through the GI tract.

monoglyceride: a molecule of glycerol with one fatty acid attached. A molecule of glycerol with two fatty acids attached is a **diglyceride**.

In the Mouth Fat digestion starts off slowly in the mouth, with some hard fats beginning to melt when they reach body temperature. The salivary glands at the base of the tongue release a lipase enzyme that plays a small role in fat digestion in adults and an active role in infants. In infants, this enzyme efficiently digests the short- and medium-chain fatty acids found in milk.[11]

Reminder: An enzyme that hydrolyzes lipids is called a *lipase*.

In the Stomach In the stomach, fat floats as a layer above the other components of swallowed food. As a result, little fat digestion takes place.

Figure 5–11

Triglyceride Digestion in the GI Tract

FAT

Salivary glands and mouth
Sublingual salivary gland in the base of the tongue secretes a lipase known as lingual lipase. Some hard fats begin to melt as they reach body temperature.

Stomach
The acid-stable lingual lipase initiates lipid digestion by hydrolyzing one bond of triglycerides to produce diglycerides and fatty acids. The degree of hydrolysis by lingual lipase is slight for most fats but may be appreciable for milk fats. The stomach's churning action mixes fat with water and acid. A gastric lipase accesses and hydrolyzes (only a very small amount of) fat.

Small intestine
Bile flows in from the gallbladder (via the common bile duct):

$$\text{Fat} \xrightarrow{\text{bile}} \text{emulsified fat}$$

Pancreatic lipase flows in from the pancreas (via the pancreatic duct):

Emulsified fat (triglycerides) → [Pancreatic (and intestinal) lipase] → monoglycerides, glycerol, fatty acids (absorbed)

Large intestine
Some fat and cholesterol, trapped in fiber, exit in feces.

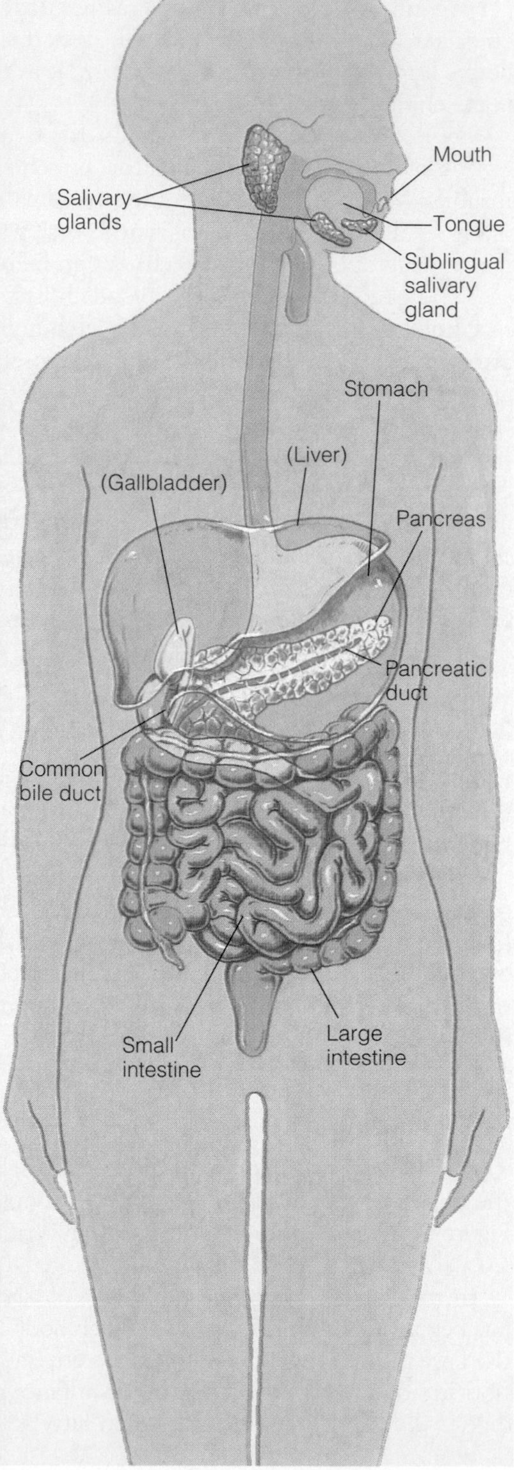

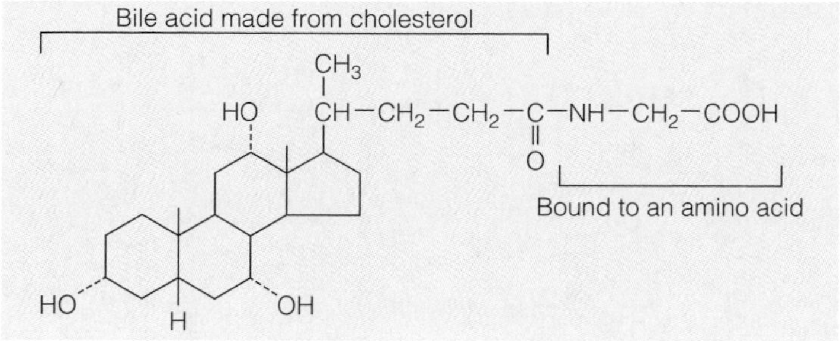

Figure 5–12

A Bile Acid

This is one of several bile acids the liver makes from cholesterol. It is then bound to an amino acid to improve its ability to form micelles, spherical complexes that carry fatty acids into the intestinal cells during digestion. Most bile acids occur as bile salts, usually in association with sodium, but sometimes with potassium or calcium. In addition to bile acids and bile salts, bile contains cholesterol, phospholipids (especially lecithin), antibodies, water, electrolytes, and bilirubin (a pigment resulting from the breakdown of heme).

In the Small Intestine When fat enters the small intestine, the hormone cholecystokinin (CCK) signals the gallbladder to release its stores of bile, an emulsifier. (The liver manufactures bile acids from cholesterol, and the gallbladder stores the bile until it is needed.)

At one end of each bile acid are side chains of amino acids (units of protein) that are attracted to water, and at the other end is a sterol portion that is attracted to fat (see Figure 5–12). Bile draws fat molecules into the surrounding watery fluids. There, the fats meet lipase enzymes from the pancreas and small intestine and are fully digested. The process of emulsification is diagrammed in Figure 5–13.

Reminder: Fat in the intestine triggers the release of the hormone *cholecystokinin* (CCK), which signals the gallbladder to send bile.

Reminder: *Bile* is an emulsifier, as are lecithins and other phospholipids. An *emulsifier* promotes the mixing of oils and fats in a watery solution.

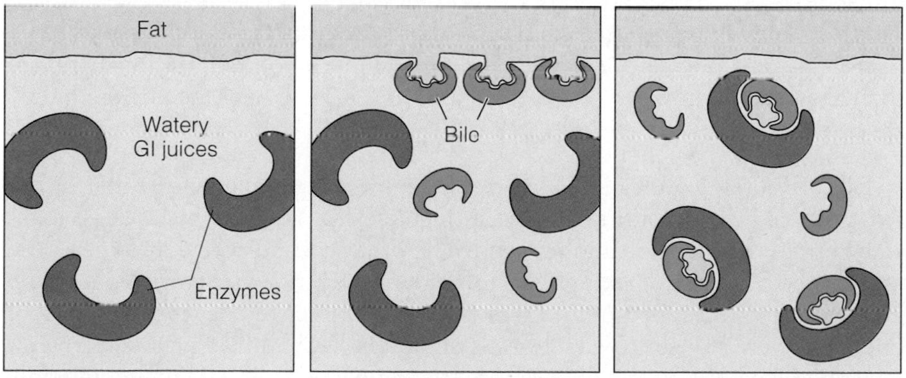

In the stomach, the fat and watery GI juices tend to separate. The enzymes are in the water and can't get at the fat.

When fat enters the small intestine, the gallbladder secretes bile. Bile has an affinity for both fat and water, so it can bring the fat into solution in the water.

After emulsification, the fat is mixed in the water solution, so the enzymes have access to it.

Figure 5–13

Emulsification of Fat by Bile

Detergents are emulsifiers and work the same way, which is why they are effective in removing grease spots from clothes. Molecule by molecule, the grease is dissolved out of the spot and suspended in the water, where it can be rinsed away.

Figure 5–14

Digestion (Hydrolysis) of a Triglyceride

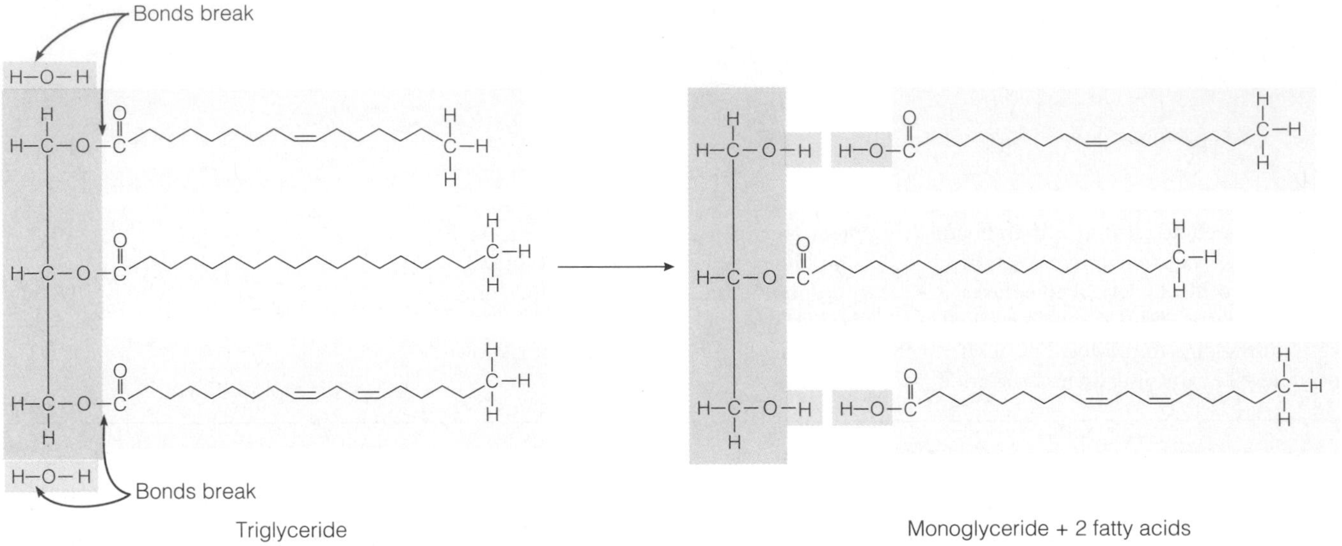

The triglyceride and two molecules of water are split, and the pieces combine to give two fatty acids and a monoglyceride.

These products may pass into the intestinal cells, but sometimes the monoglyceride is split with another molecule of water to give a third fatty acid and glycerol. Fatty acids, monoglycerides, and glycerol are absorbed into intestinal cells.

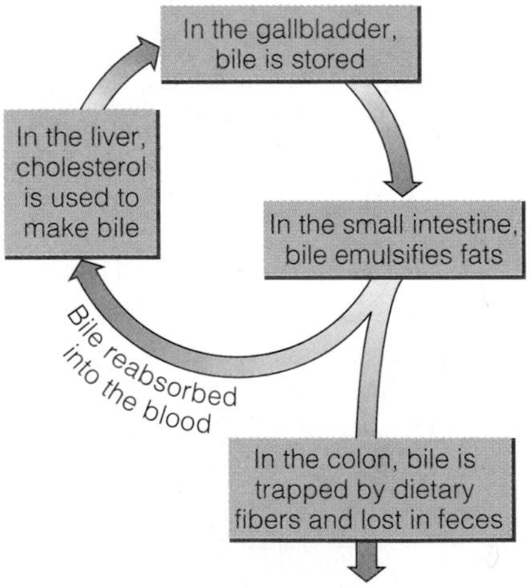

Figure 5–15

Enterohepatic Circulation

The recycling of cholesterol and bile through the intestine and liver is known as the enterohepatic circulation of bile.

enteron = intestine
hepat = liver

Most of the hydrolysis of triglycerides occurs in the small intestine. The major fat-digesting enzymes are pancreatic lipases; some intestinal lipases are also active. These enzymes remove one, then the other, of each tryglyceride's outer fatty acids, leaving a monoglyceride. Occasionally, enzymes remove all three fatty acids, leaving a free molecule of glycerol. The process of hydrolysis is shown in Figure 5–14.

Phospholipids are digested similarly—that is, their fatty acids are removed by hydrolysis. The two fatty acids and the remaining phospholipid fragment are then absorbed. Sterols can be absorbed as is; if any fatty acids are attached, they are first hydrolyzed off.

Bile's Routes After bile has entered the intestine and emulsified fat, it has two possible destinations, illustrated in Figure 5–15. For one, bile can be reabsorbed from the intestine and recycled. The other possibility is that some of the bile can be trapped by dietary fibers in the large intestine and carried out of the body with the feces. Because it takes cholesterol to make bile, the excretion of bile effectively reduces elevated blood cholesterol. The fibers most effective at lowering blood cholesterol this way are the soluble pectins and gums commonly found in fruits, oats, and legumes.

LIPID ABSORPTION

Figure 5–16 illustrates the absorption of lipids. Small units of digested fats (glycerol and short- and medium-chain fatty acids) can diffuse easily into the intesti-

Figure 5–16

Absorption and Transport of Lipids

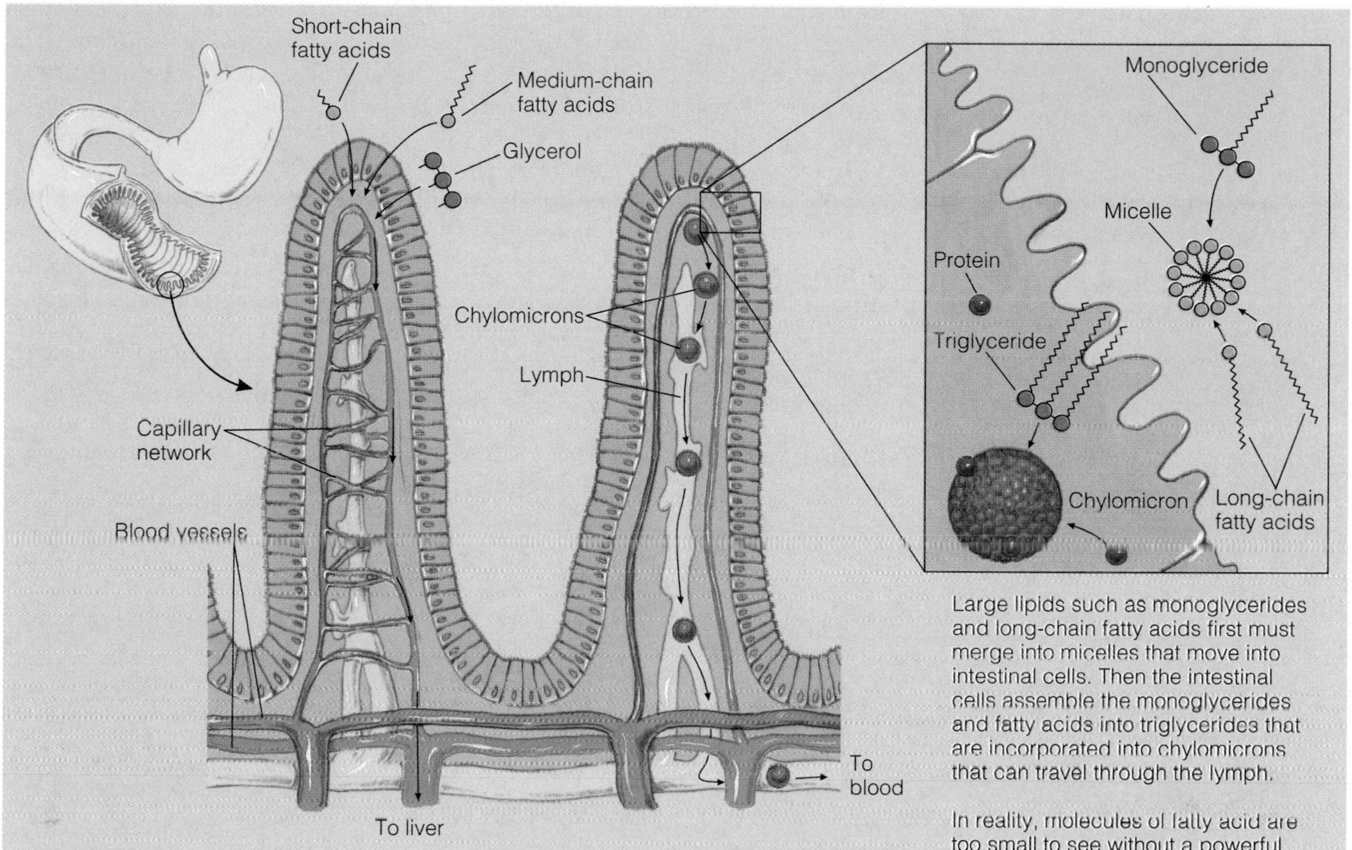

The end products of fat digestion are mostly monoglycerides, some fatty acids, and very little glycerol. Glycerol and short- and medium-chain fatty acids can move directly into the bloodstream.

Large lipids such as monoglycerides and long-chain fatty acids first must merge into micelles that move into intestinal cells. Then the intestinal cells assemble the monoglycerides and fatty acids into triglycerides that are incorporated into chylomicrons that can travel through the lymph.

In reality, molecules of fatty acid are too small to see without a powerful microscope, while villi are visible to the naked eye.

nal cells; they are absorbed directly into the bloodstream. Larger units (the monoglycerides and long-chain fatty acids) merge into spherical complexes, known as micelles, which are so small that they can fit between the tiny, hair-like microvilli of a single intestinal cell. (Emulsified fat particles are 100 times larger in diameter and contain tens of thousands of molecules.) The micelles easily diffuse into the intestinal cells. Once inside, the monoglycerides and long-chain fatty acids are reassembled into new triglycerides.

Within the intestinal cells, the newly made triglycerides and the other large lipids (cholesterol and phospholipids) are packed into transport vehicles known as chylomicrons. The intestinal cells then release the chylomicrons into the lymphatic system. The chylomicrons glide through the lymph until they reach a point of entry into the bloodstream at the thoracic duct near the heart. The blood can then carry these lipids to the rest of the body. The margin summarizes the absorption of lipids.

micelles (MY-cells): tiny spherical complexes that arise during fat digestion; each carries about 20 fatty acids and/or monoglycerides into intestinal cells.

Absorbed directly into blood:
- Glycerol.
- Short-chain fatty acids.
- Medium-chain fatty acids.

Merge into micelles, move into the intestinal cells, and made into triglycerides:
- Long-chain fatty acids.
- Monoglycerides.

Assembled into chylomicrons, absorbed into lymph, then into blood:
- Triglycerides.
- Phospholipids.
- Cholesterol.

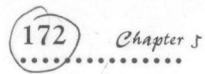

LIPID TRANSPORT

The chylomicrons are only one of several clusters of lipids and proteins that are used as transport vehicles for fats. As a group, these vehicles are known as lipoproteins, and they solve the body's problem of transporting fatty materials through the watery medium of the bloodstream. The body makes four main types of lipoproteins, distinguished by their size and density.* Each type contains different kinds of special proteins and carries different amounts of the various lipids.

lipoproteins (LIP-oh-PRO-teenz): clusters of lipids associated with proteins that serve as transport vehicles for lipids in the lymph and blood.

chylomicrons (kye-lo-MY-cronz): the class of lipoproteins that transport lipids from the intestinal cells into the body.

Chylomicrons The chylomicrons are the largest and least dense of the lipoproteins. They transport *diet*-derived lipids (mostly triglycerides) from the intestine to the rest of the body. Cells all over the body remove lipids from the chylomicrons as they pass by, so the chylomicrons get smaller and smaller. Within 14 hours after absorption, little is left of them but protein remnants and a few odds and ends of lipid. Special protein receptors on the membranes of the liver cells recognize and remove these remnants from the blood.[12] Once the liver cells have collected the chylomicron remnants, they dismantle them.

VLDL (very-low-density lipoprotein): the type of lipoprotein made primarily by liver cells to transport lipids to various tissues in the body; composed primarily of triglycerides.

VLDL Meanwhile, the liver cells are synthesizing other lipids to be shipped out to other parts of the body. The liver cells pick up fatty acids arriving in the blood and use them to make cholesterol, other fatty acids, and other compounds. At the same time, the liver cells may be making lipids from carbohydrates, proteins, or alcohol. The liver is the most active site of lipid synthesis. Ultimately, the lipids made in the liver are shipped to other parts of the body and packaged with proteins as very-low-density lipoproteins (VLDL).

As the VLDL travel through the body, cells remove triglycerides, causing the VLDL to shrink. As they lose triglycerides, the VLDL gather cholesterol from other lipoproteins circulating through the bloodstream and eventually become low-density lipoproteins (LDL).† This exchange explains why LDL contain few triglycerides but are loaded with cholesterol.

LDL (low-density lipoprotein): the type of lipoprotein derived from very-low-density lipoproteins (VLDL) as cells remove triglycerides from them; composed primarily of cholesterol.

LDL The LDL circulate throughout the body, making their contents available to the cells of all tissues—muscle, including the heart muscle; fat stores; the mammary glands; and others. The cells take triglycerides from the LDL; they also collect cholesterol and phospholipids to build new membranes, to make hormones or other compounds, or to store for later use. Special LDL receptors on the liver cells play a crucial role in the control of blood cholesterol concentrations by removing LDL from circulation.

HDL (high-density lipoprotein): the type of lipoprotein that transports cholesterol back to the liver from peripheral cells; composed primarily of protein.

HDL Fat cells may release glycerol, fatty acids, cholesterol, and phospholipids to the blood. The liver makes high-density lipoprotein (HDL) packages to

*The lipoproteins are distinguished by density because the chemist uses this feature to separate them in the laboratory. The chemist layers a blood sample below a thick fluid in a test tube and spins the tube in a centrifuge. The most buoyant particles (highest in lipids) rise to the top, and the densest particles (highest in proteins) remain at the bottom. Lipoproteins with a low protein-to-lipid ratio have a low density; those with a high protein-to-lipid ratio have a high density.

†Before becoming LDL, the VLDL are first transformed into intermediate-density lipoproteins (IDL), sometimes called VLDL remnants. Some IDL may be picked up by the liver and rapidly broken down; those IDL that remain in circulation pick up cholesterol and become LDL. Researchers debate whether IDL are simply transitional particles or a separate class of lipoproteins.

carry cholesterol and phospholipids from the cells back to the liver for recycling or disposal.

In summary, all four types of lipoproteins carry all classes of lipids (triglycerides, phospholipids, and cholesterol), but the chylomicrons are the largest and the highest in triglycerides; VLDL are smaller and are about half triglycerides; LDL are smaller still and are high in cholesterol; and HDL are the smallest and are rich in protein. Figure 5–17 (on p. 174) shows the relative sizes and compositions of the lipoproteins.

The distinction between LDL and HDL has implications for the health of the heart and blood vessels. The blood cholesterol linked to heart disease is LDL cholesterol. HDL also carry cholesterol, but elevated HDL represent cholesterol returning from the arteries to the liver for breakdown and excretion. High LDL cholesterol is associated with a high risk of heart attack, whereas high HDL cholesterol seems to have a protective effect.[13] This is why some people refer to LDL as "bad," and HDL as "good," cholesterol. Keep in mind, though, that there is only *one* kind of cholesterol, and that the differences between LDL and HDL reflect the *proportions* of lipids and proteins within them—not the type of cholesterol. The margin lists factors that influence LDL and HDL, and Chapter 18 provides many more details.

To help you remember, think of elevated **H**DL as **H**ealthy and elevated **L**DL as **L**ess healthy.

Factors that improve the LDL-to-HDL ratio:

- Weight control.
- Monounsaturated or polyunsaturated, instead of saturated, fatty acids in the diet.
- Soluble fibers (see Chapter 4).
- Antioxidants (see Highlight 11).
- Moderate alcohol consumption.
- Physical activity.

Lipids in the Body

The blood carries lipids to various sites around the body. Once they arrive at their destinations, the lipids can get to work providing energy, insulating against temperature extremes, protecting against shock, and building cell structures. This section provides an overview first of the triglycerides in the blood and then of the metabolic pathways triglycerides can follow within the body's cells.

TRIGLYCERIDES IN THE BLOOD

The body's cells use both glucose and fat to fuel their activities. The energy to make a muscle contract, including the heart muscle, is supplied mostly from fat, so the blood must continuously deliver a supply of triglycerides—either from the intestines where foods have provided fat or from the adipose tissue where fat has been stored. Either way, triglycerides are always circulating in the blood.

adipose (ADD-ih-poce) **tissue:** the body's fat tissue, which consists of masses of fat-storing cells.

A PREVIEW OF LIPID METABOLISM

The blood delivers its cargo of triglycerides to the cells for their use. This discussion provides a preview of how the cells store and release energy from fat; Chapter 7 provides many more details.

Storing Fat as Fat The triglycerides, familiar as the fat in foods and as body fat, serve the body primarily as a source of fuel. Fat provides more than twice the energy of carbohydrate and protein, making it an extremely efficient storage form of energy. The body's storage space for energy is virtually unlimited, thanks to the special cells of the adipose tissue. Unlike most body cells, which can store

Figure 5–17

Sizes and Compositions of the Lipoproteins

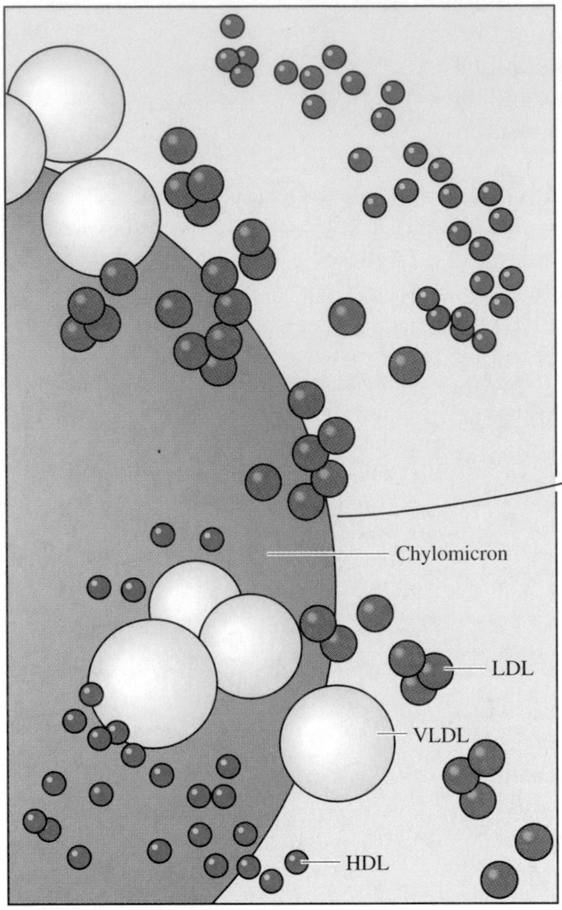

This solar system of lipoproteins shows their relative sizes. Notice how large the fat-filled chylomicron is compared with the others and how the others get progressively smaller as their proportion of fat declines and protein increases.

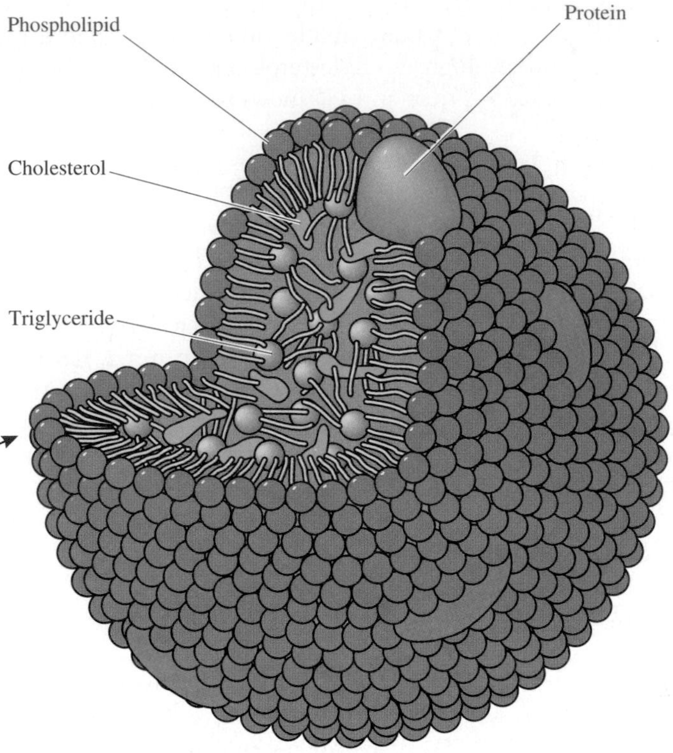

A typical lipoprotein contains an interior of triglycerides and cholesterol surrounded by phospholipids. The phospholipids' fatty acid "tails" point toward the interior, where the lipids are. Proteins near the outer ends of the phospholipids cover the structure. This arrangement of hydrophobic molecules on the inside and hydrophilic molecules on the outside allows lipids to travel through the watery fluids of the blood.

Chylomicrons contain so little protein and so much triglyceride that they are the lowest in density.

Very-low-density lipoproteins (VLDL) are half triglycerides, accounting for their low density.

Low-density lipoproteins (LDL) are half cholesterol, accounting for their implication in heart disease.

High-density lipoproteins (HDL) are half protein, accounting for their high density.

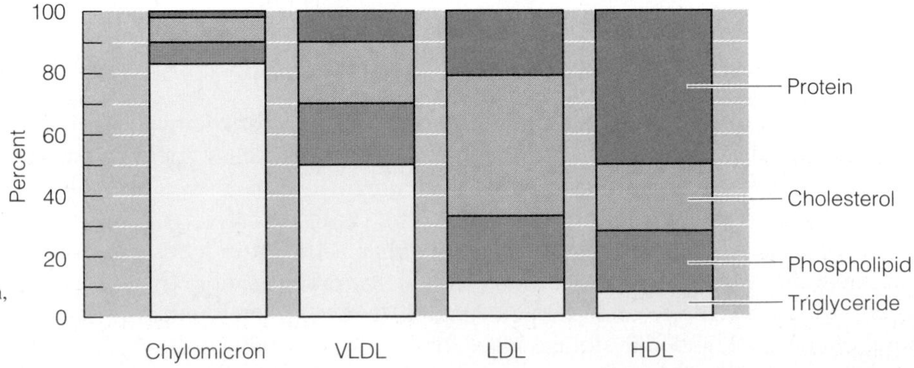

only limited amounts of fat, the fat cells of the adipose tissue readily take up and store fat. An adipose cell is depicted in Figure 5–18.

Adipose cells have a special enzyme on their surfaces—lipoprotein lipase (LPL)—that captures circulating triglycerides from lipoproteins passing by after meals. This enzyme hydrolyzes the triglycerides to fatty acids and monoglycerides and passes these products into the cells' interiors. Inside the cells, other enzymes reassemble the pieces into triglycerides again for storage. Triglycerides pack tightly together within adipose cells, storing a lot of energy in a relatively small space. Adipose cells always store fat after meals, when a heavy traffic of chylomicrons and VLDL loaded with triglycerides passes by; they release it later when the blood cargo needs replenishing.

Figure 5–18

An Adipose Cell

An adipose, or fat, cell seems to expand almost indefinitely. The more fat it stores, the larger it grows.

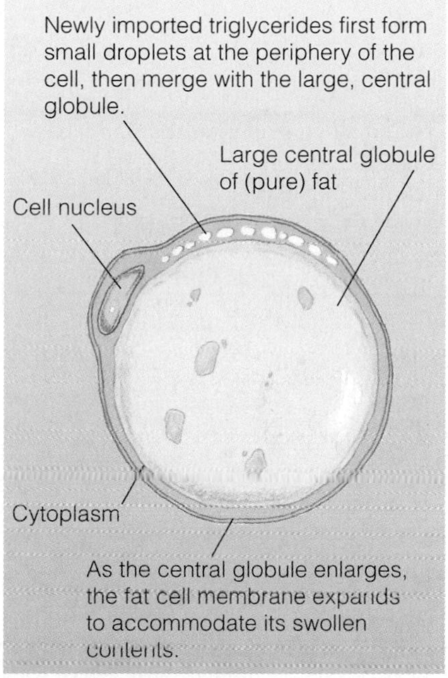

Newly imported triglycerides first form small droplets at the periphery of the cell, then merge with the large, central globule.
Large central globule of (pure) fat
Cell nucleus
Cytoplasm
As the central globule enlarges, the fat cell membrane expands to accommodate its swollen contents.

lipoprotein lipase (LPL): an enzyme mounted on the surface of fat cells (and other cells) that hydrolyzes triglycerides passing by in the bloodstream and directs their parts into the cells, where they can be metabolized or reassembled for storage.

Making Fat from Carbohydrate or Protein Earlier, Figure 5–3 showed how the body can make triglycerides from glycerol and fatty acids. Fatty acids, in turn, can be made from 2-carbon fragments derived from any nutrient. (This is why most fatty acid carbon chains come in even numbers.) Thus glucose can be converted to body fat: enzymes break glucose into 2-carbon fragments and then combine them to make long-chain fatty acids. Enzymes can also convert some of the components of protein (certain amino acids) to fatty acids. The food source from which the body most easily makes fat for storage, though, is fat itself.

Efficiency of Making Fat from Fat To convert food fats to body fat, the body simply absorbs the parts and puts them (or others) together again in storage. It requires very little energy to do this. By comparison, to convert dietary carbohydrate to body fat, the body must first break starches into disaccharides and then into monosaccharides, absorb the monosaccharides, then dismantle glucose, and reassemble many of the fragments into fatty acid chains. Each conversion requires energy. Thus it costs less (energetically) to store dietary fat as body fat than to convert and store dietary carbohydrate as body fat. Whether fat is stored at all depends more on total energy intake and on how much fat is eaten than on how much carbohydrate is eaten. The message is clear: to limit fat storage in the body, limit fat intake from foods. Chapter 8 discusses energy balance in more detail.

Using Fat for Energy Unlike the liver's glycogen stores, the body's fat stores have virtually unlimited capacity, and fat supplies 60 percent of the body's ongoing energy needs during rest.[14] During exercise or prolonged periods of food deprivation, fat stores may make an even greater contribution to energy needs.

When cells demand energy, an enzyme (hormone-sensitive lipase) inside the adipose cells responds by dismantling stored triglycerides and releasing the glycerol and fatty acids directly into the blood. Energy-hungry cells anywhere in the body can then break down these components into small fragments and take them through a series of chemical reactions to yield energy, carbon dioxide, and water.

In the last stages before being completely oxidized to carbon dioxide and water, each fat fragment combines with a fragment from the breakdown of glucose. Body fat cannot break down completely unless carbohydrate is simultaneously present. Without carbohydrate, ketosis will develop, as mentioned in Chapter 4.

hormone-sensitive lipase: an enzyme inside adipose cells that responds to the body's need for fuel by hydrolyzing triglycerides so that their parts (glycerol and fatty acids) escape into the general circulation and thus become available to other cells as fuel. The signals to which this enzyme responds include epinephrine and glucagon, which oppose insulin (see Chapter 4).

Reminder: When fat is metabolized in the absence of carbohydrate, *ketone bodies* are formed.

1 lb body fat = 3500 kcal.

A person who fasts (drinking only water) will rapidly metabolize body fat. A pound of body fat provides 3500 kcalories, so you might think a fasting person who expends 2000 kcalories a day could lose more than half a pound of body fat each day.* Actually, the person has to obtain some energy from lean tissue because the brain, nervous system, and red blood cells need glucose, which fat cannot supply. Also, as mentioned, fat itself needs glucose to break down completely. Even on a total fast, a person cannot lose more than half a pound of pure fat per day. Still, in conditions of enforced starvation—say, during a siege or a famine—a fatter person can survive longer than a thinner person thanks to this energy reserve.

The small contribution that fat can make to the body's glucose supply is detailed in Chapter 7.

Although fat provides energy during a fast, it can provide only very little glucose to give energy to the brain and nerves. Only the small glycerol molecule can be converted to glucose; fatty acids cannot be. After prolonged glucose deprivation, brain and nerve cells develop the ability to derive about two-thirds of their energy from the ketone bodies that the body makes from fat without carbohydrate. Ketone bodies cannot sustain life by themselves, however. As Chapter 7 explains, fasting for too long will cause death, even if the person still has ample body fat.

In summary, the body makes special arrangements to digest, absorb, transport, store, and use lipids. It provides the emulsifier bile to make them accessible to the fat-digesting lipases that dismantle triglycerides, mostly to monoglycerides, for absorption by the intestinal cells. The intestinal cells assemble freshly absorbed lipids into chylomicrons, lipid packages with protein escorts, for transport so that cells all over the body may select needed lipids from them. The liver also packages lipids and proteins into other lipoproteins—VLDL, LDL, and HDL—for transport around the body. Cells, especially fat cells, select and store triglycerides from these lipoproteins for later use as an energy fuel and assimilate other lipids such as cholesterol into their membranes. Unneeded lipids are returned to the liver for disposal. High LDL (which are high in cholesterol) portend a high risk of heart disease; high HDL (which are returning lipids for disposal) signify a low risk.

The body can easily store unlimited amounts of fat if excesses are available, and this body fat is used for energy when needed. The liver can also convert excess carbohydrate and protein into fat. Fat breakdown requires simultaneous carbohydrate breakdown for maximum efficiency; without carbohydrate, fats break down to ketone bodies producing ketosis.

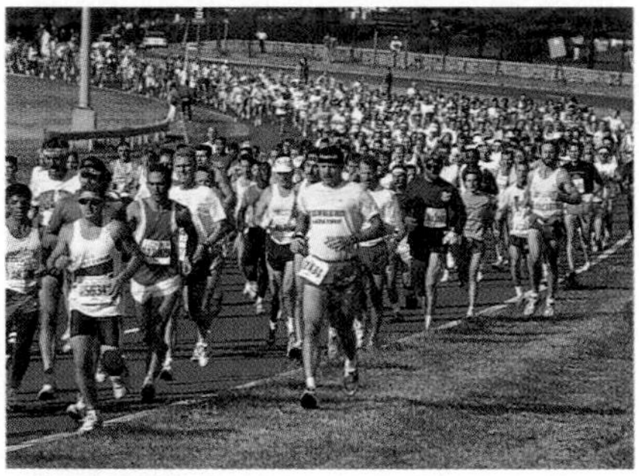

Fat supplies most of the energy in a long-distance run.

Health Effects and Recommended Intakes of Lipids

Of all the nutrients, fat is most often linked with chronic diseases. A high-fat diet raises the risks of heart disease, some types of cancer, and obesity. Fortunately, the same recommendation can help with all of these health problems: eat less fat.

*The reader who knows that 1 pound = 454 grams and that 1 gram fat = 9 kcalories may wonder why a pound of body fat does not equal 9 × 454 kcalories. The reason is that body fat contains some cell water and other materials; it is not quite pure fat.

HEALTH EFFECTS OF LIPIDS

Hearing a physician say, "Your blood lipid profile looks fine," is reassuring. The blood lipid profile reveals the concentrations of various lipids in the blood, notably triglycerides and cholesterol, and their lipoprotein carriers (VLDL, LDL, and HDL). This information alerts people to their disease risks and their need to change eating habits.

blood lipid profile: results of blood tests that reveal a person's total cholesterol, triglycerides, and various lipoproteins.

Desirable blood lipid profile:

- Total cholesterol: <200 mg/dL.
- LDL cholesterol: <130 mg/dL.
- HDL cholesterol: >35 mg/dL.
- Triglycerides: <200 mg/dL.

Heart Disease Most people realize that elevated blood cholesterol is a major risk factor for cardiovascular disease*. Cholesterol accumulates in the arteries, restricting blood flow and raising blood pressure. The consequences are deadly; in fact, heart disease is the nation's number one killer of adults. Blood cholesterol is often used to predict the likelihood of a person's suffering a heart attack or stroke; the higher the cholesterol, the earlier and more likely the tragedy.

Commercials advertise products that are low in cholesterol, and magazine articles tell readers how to cut the cholesterol in their favorite recipes. What most people don't realize, though, is that *food* cholesterol does not raise *blood* cholesterol as dramatically as *saturated fat* does.

cardiovascular disease (CVD): a general term for all diseases of the heart and blood vessels. Atherosclerosis is the main cause of CVD. When the arteries that carry blood to the heart muscle become occluded, the heart suffers damage known as **coronary heart disease (CHD)**.

cardio = heart
vascular = blood vessels

Other risk factors for heart disease include smoking, high blood pressure, diabetes, family history, sex, race, and obesity. Chapter 18 provides many more details about these risk factors, the development of heart disease, and dietary recommendations.

Risks from Saturated Fats Recall that LDL cholesterol raises the risk of heart disease. LDL concentrations respond to both the total amount and the type of fat in the diet. Most often implicated in raising LDL cholesterol are the saturated fats, although not all saturated fats have the same cholesterol-raising effect.[15] Most notable among the saturated fatty acids that raise blood cholesterol are lauric, myristic, and palmitic acids (12, 14, and 16 carbons, respectively). In contrast, stearic acid (18 carbons) does not seem to raise blood cholesterol.[16] Common sources of stearic acid are beef (tallow) and milk chocolate (cocoa butter).

Effects of Polyunsaturated and Monounsaturated Fats In general, polyunsaturated fatty acids lower LDL cholesterol, and monounsaturated fatty acids have little or no independent effect.[17] Dietary cholesterol's influence on blood cholesterol is relatively minor.

Also of interest are the effects these fats have on the "good" HDL cholesterol. Some research suggests that polyunsaturated fats tend to lower both HDL and LDL, whereas monounsaturated fats raise HDL, thus improving the blood lipid profile.[18] Other research finds that both polyunsaturated and monounsaturated fatty acids lower both LDL and HDL.[19]

Risks from *Trans*-Fatty Acids In the body, *trans*-fatty acids—even the monounsaturated ones—alter blood cholesterol the same way as some saturated fats do: they raise LDL and lower HDL cholesterol, although not to the same extent.[20] Recent epidemiological studies have linked dietary *trans*-fatty acids to heart disease risk,[21] but a study examining *trans*-fatty acids in adipose tissue found no correlation.[22] Clearly, this is an area of active research that is not yet ready for the evening news.

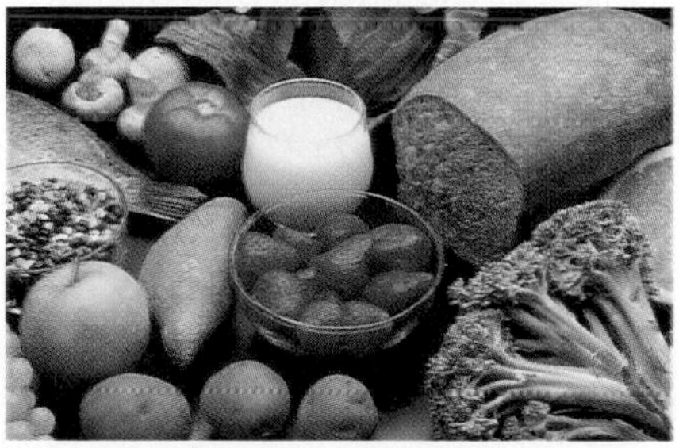

Enjoy low-fat foods for good heart health.

*The concentration of cholesterol is similar in *blood*, *plasma*, and *serum*; this book uses the term *blood* cholesterol. Plasma is blood with the cells removed; serum is plasma with the clotting factors also removed.

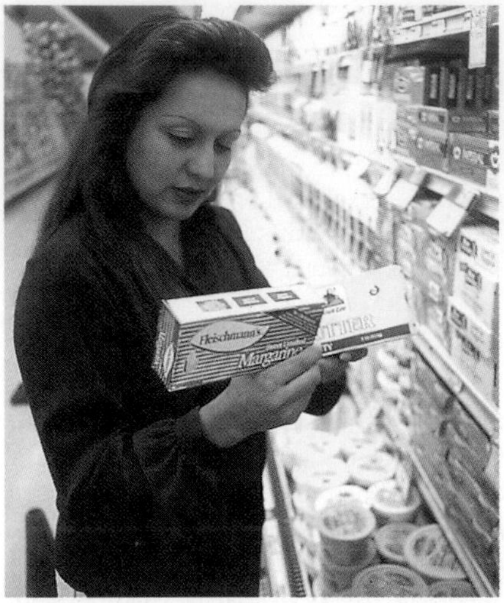

Whether you decide to use butter or margarine, remember to use them sparingly.

Reports on *trans*-fatty acids have raised consumer doubts about whether margarine is, after all, a better choice than butter for heart health. The American Heart Association has stated that because butter is rich in both saturated fat and cholesterol and because margarine is made from vegetable fat with no dietary cholesterol, margarine is still preferable to butter.[23] Others disagree, claiming the occasional use of butter is preferable to the use of products containing *trans*-fatty acids.[24] In addition to strict limits on *trans*-fatty acid use, some experts are calling for food labels to state the *trans*-fatty acid amounts in foods.[25]

The exact amount of *trans*-fatty acids in the diet is unknown, but it is lower than saturated fat intake.[26] If consumers limit their consumption of all types of fat, their *trans*-fatty acid intakes will most likely remain the same or decline.[27] The American Dietetic Association considers that current intakes are not harmful and that health risks from saturated fatty acids far outweigh those from *trans*-fatty acids.[28]

Benefits from Omega-3 Fatty Acids Research on the omega-3 polyunsaturated fatty acids has spotlighted the unique effects of different types of fat on blood cholesterol and heart disease. Inuit peoples of Alaska and Greenland enjoy relative freedom from heart disease despite high-energy, high-fat, high-cholesterol diets. Why? Their foods derive primarily from marine animals and are rich in omega-3 fatty acids, particularly EPA and DHA. Research reveals that a diet rich in fish oils can lower blood cholesterol, just as a low-fat, low-saturated fat diet can.[29] (The research compared a diet with 2 percent of daily intake from fish oils with a diet of 25 percent total fat, 5 percent saturated.) A diet with both attributes produces an optimal lipid profile. In addition to improving blood lipids, fish oils prevent blood clots and may also lower blood pressure, especially in people with hypertension or atherosclerosis.[30]

Chapter 18 presents many more details on the action of omega-3 fatty acids in preventing heart disease.

hypertension: high blood pressure; defined further in Chapter 18.

Data from Japan seem to confirm that a diet low in fat and high in fish benefits health. The Japanese diet today has become westernized with few Japanese people eating the large quantities of rice and fish their ancestors ate. These dietary changes have been accompanied by health consequences: higher rates of cardiovascular disease and cancer.[31]

Other risk factors for cancer include smoking, alcohol, and environmental contaminants. Chapter 18 provides many more details about these risk factors and the development of cancer.

Cancer The evidence linking dietary fats with cancer is less conclusive than for heart disease, but it does suggest an association between total fat and some types of cancers. Dietary fat seems not to *initiate* cancer development but to *promote* cancer once it has arisen. Some epidemiological studies suggest a relationship between specific cancers and saturated fats or dietary fat from animal sources (which is mostly saturated). Thus health advice to reduce cancer risks parallels that given to reduce heart disease risks: reduce total fat, especially saturated fat, intake.

Animal studies confirm that high-fat diets promote cancer development.[32] The data, however, are not fully consistent with evidence from epidemiological studies, most likely because the animals are fed extremely large amounts of specific fats—much higher than people typically eat. Animal studies suggest that *polyunsaturated fats* from vegetable oils (mostly omega-6 fatty acids) are more likely to promote cancer than are saturated fats. On the other hand, polyunsaturated fats from fish oils (mostly omega-3 fatty acids) are likely to delay cancer development and reduce the rate of growth and the size and number of tumors.[33] Research indicates that the omega-6 linoleic acid promotes tumor activity through the synthesis of prostaglandins derived from arachidonic acid and that omega-3 fatty acids inhibit that metabolism.[34]

The relationship between dietary fat and the risk of cancer differs for various types of cancers. In the case of breast cancer, some studies suggest little or no association between dietary fat and cancer.[35] Others find that total *energy* intake is a better predictor than percentage of kcalories from fat.[36] In the case of prostate cancer, there does appear to be a strong association with fat.[37] Research suggests that this association is due primarily to the saturated fat from meats; fat from milk or fish is not implicated in cancer risk.

Obesity As the photos in Figure 5–19 show, fat accounts for a lot of the energy in foods, and removing the fat from foods cuts energy intake dramatically. Fat contributes twice as many kcalories per gram as either carbohydrate or protein. Consequently, people who eat high-fat diets tend to exceed their energy needs and gain weight.

Furthermore, people who eat high-fat diets tend to store body fat efficiently.[38] Some studies suggest that dietary fat influences body fat independently of total

Remember, fat is a more concentrated energy source than the other energy nutrients: 1 g carbohydrate or protein = 4 kcal, but 1 g fat = 9 kcal.

Figure 5–19

Cutting Fat Cuts kCalories

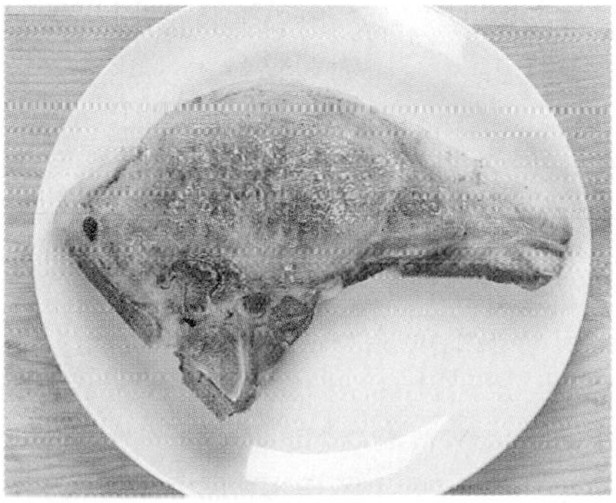

Pork chop with a half-inch of fat (275 kcal and 19 g fat).

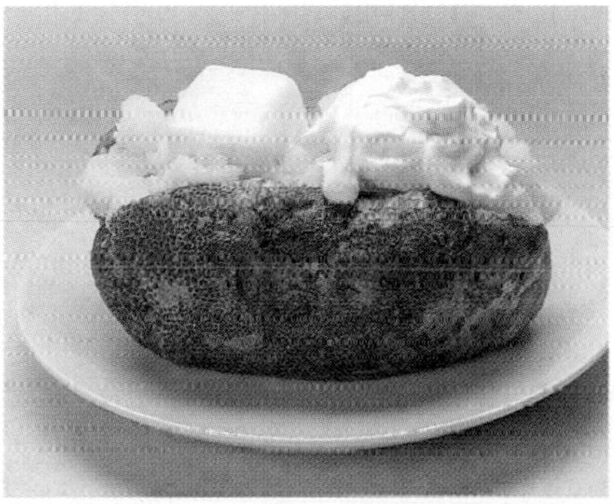

Potato with 1 tbs butter and 1 tbs sour cream (350 kcal and 14 g fat).

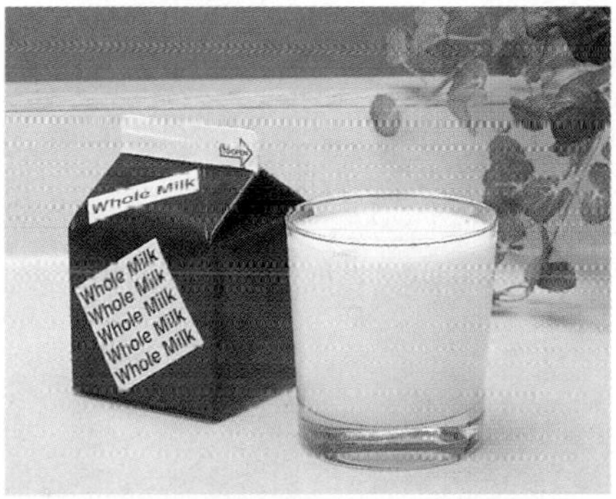

Whole milk, 1 c (150 kcal and 8 g fat).

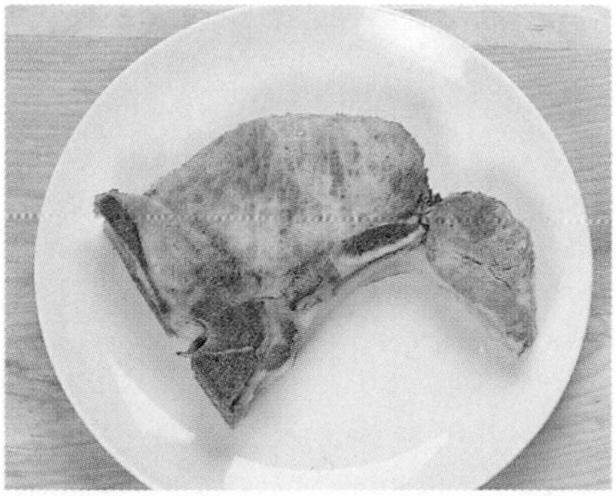

Pork chop with fat trimmed off (165 kcal and 8 g fat).

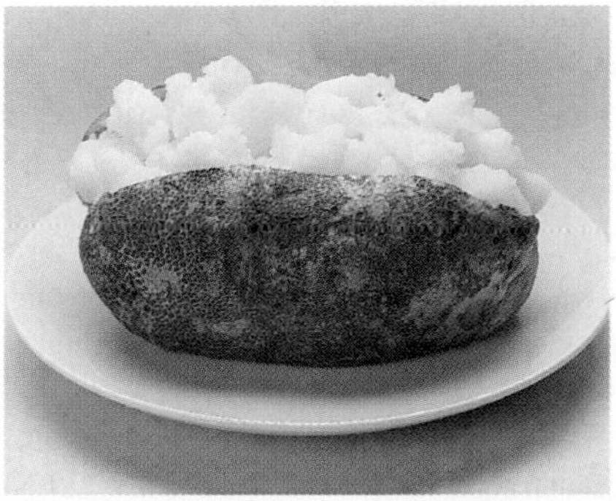

Plain potato (220 kcal and <1 g fat).

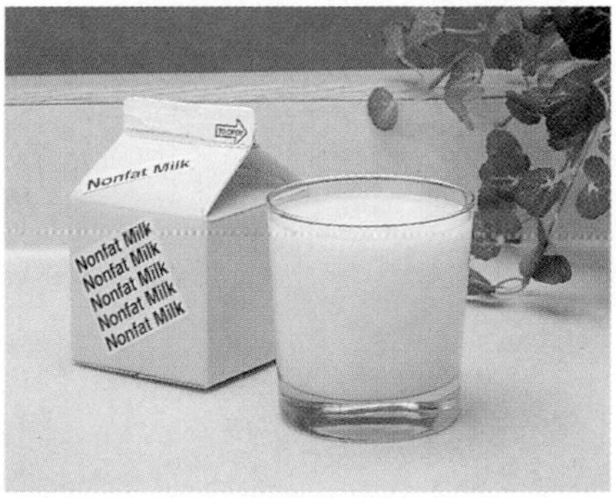

Nonfat milk, 1 c (90 kcal and 1 g fat).

energy intake; that is, people who eat high-fat diets have more body fat than their energy intakes would predict.[39] Highlight 8 revisits the issue of the fattening power of fat and concludes that low-fat, high-carbohydrate foods are most appropriate for satisfying hunger and controlling appetite.[40]

Don't Overdo Fat Restriction Although it is very difficult to do, some people actually manage to eat too little fat—to their detriment. Among them are people with eating disorders, described in Highlight 9. As a practical guideline, it is wise to include the equivalent of at least a teaspoon of fat in every meal—a little peanut butter on toast or mayonnaise on tuna, for example. Parents should not restrict the fat intakes of their infants and young children; dietary recommendations that limit fat were developed for healthy people over age two.

RECOMMENDED INTAKES OF FAT

The Committee on Dietary Allowances has not established an RDA for fat, but the Committee on Diet and Health makes the following recommendations:

- Reduce total fat intake to 30 percent or less of energy intake.
- Reduce saturated fat intake to less than 10 percent of energy intake.
- Reduce cholesterol intake to less than 300 milligrams daily.

A person consuming 2000 kcalories a day should therefore have 600 kcalories or less from fat (roughly 65 grams). Of those fat kcalories, only 200 should come from saturated fats (roughly 22 grams).

HEALTHY PEOPLE 2000: Reduce dietary fat intake to an average of 30% of energy or less and average saturated fat intake to less than 10% of energy among people aged two years and older.

To meet dietary fat recommendations, many people have reduced their fat intakes. Fat intake peaked at 42 percent of daily kcalories in the late 1950s and has fallen steadily ever since.[41] The most recent surveys report that adults in the United States receive about 34 percent of their total energy from fat, with saturated fat contributing about 12 percent of the total.[42] The average cholesterol intake in the United States is 300 to 450 milligrams a day.[43]

Reduce Total Fat Intake Triglycerides are abundant in all fats and oils. They also accompany protein in foods derived from animals, such as meat, fish, poultry, and eggs, and carbohydrate in foods derived from plants, such as avocados and coconuts.

To reduce dietary fat, eliminate fat as a seasoning and in cooking; remove the fat from high-fat foods; replace high-fat foods with low-fat alternatives; and emphasize grains, fruits, and vegetables. The accompanying box provides additional tips for reducing fat in the diet, food group by food group.

Reduce Saturated Fat Intake Fats from animal sources are the main sources of saturated fats in most people's diets. Some vegetable fats (coconut and palm) and hydrogenated fats provide smaller amounts of saturated fats. Selecting lean meats and nonfat milk products helps to lower saturated fat intake.

How to Lower Fat Intake—by Food Group

Meat, Fish, and Poultry

- Fat adds up quickly, even with lean meat; limit intake to about 6 ounces (cooked weight) daily.
- Choose fish, poultry, or lean cuts of pork or beef; look for unmarbled cuts named *round* or *loin* (eye of round, top round, round tip, tenderloin, sirloin, and top loin).
- Trim the fat from pork and beef; remove the skin from poultry.
- Grill, roast, broil, bake, stir-fry, stew, or braise meats; don't fry. When possible, place meat on a rack so that fat can drain.
- Use lean ground turkey or lean ground beef in recipes; brown ground meats without added fat, then drain off fat.
- Refrigerate meat pan drippings and broth; when it solidifies, remove the fat and use the defatted broth in recipes.
- Select tuna and other canned meats packed in water; rinse oil-packed items with hot water to remove much of the fat.
- Fill kabob skewers with lots of vegetables and slivers of meat; create main dishes and casseroles by combining a little meat, fish, or poultry with a lot of pasta, rice, or vegetables.
- Make meatless spaghetti sauces and casseroles; use legumes often.
- Eat a meatless meal or two daily.

Milk and Cheeses

- Drink nonfat and low-fat milk instead of whole milk.
- Use nonfat and low-fat cheeses (such as part-skim ricotta and low-fat mozzarella) instead of regular cheeses.
- Use nonfat or low-fat yogurt or fat-free sour cream instead of regular sour cream.
- Use evaporated nonfat milk instead of cream.
- Enjoy nonfat frozen yogurt, sherbet, or ice milk instead of ice cream.

Fruits and Vegetables

- Enjoy the natural flavor of steamed vegetables for dinner and fruits for dessert.
- Use butter-flavored granules on vegetables instead of butter or margarine.
- Use nonfat yogurt or nonfat salad dressing instead of sour cream, cheese, mayonnaise, or other sauces on vegetables and in casseroles.
- Select nonfat or low-fat salad dressings, or use herbs, lemon juice, and spices instead of regular salad dressing.
- Add a little water to thick, bottled salad dressing to dilute the amount of fat each serving provides.
- Eat at least two vegetables (in addition to a salad) with dinner.
- Snack on raw vegetables or fruits instead of high-fat items like potato chips.

Breads and Cereals

- Use fruit butters or jellies on bread instead of butter or margarine.
- Select breads, cereals, and crackers that are low in fat (for example, bagels instead of croissants).

Other Foods and Cooking Tips

- Use a nonstick pan or coat the pan lightly with vegetable oil.
- Use egg substitutes in recipes instead of whole eggs or use 2 egg whites in place of each whole egg.
- Use half the margarine, butter, or oil called for in a recipe. (The minimum amount of fat for muffins, quick breads, and biscuits is 1 to 2 tablespoons per cup of flour; for cakes and cookies, 2 tablespoons per cup.)
- Use less butter or margarine. Select the whipped types of butter, margarine, or cream cheese for use at the table; they contain half the kcalories of the regular types.
- Use butter replacers instead of butter.
- For sandwiches and salads, use spicy mustard, nonfat salad dressing, lemon juice, flavored vinegar, salsa or the nonfat versions instead of regular mayonnaise, salad dressing, or sour cream.
- Use wine; lemon, orange, or tomato juice; herbs; spices; fruits; or broth instead of butter, margarine, or oil when cooking.
- Stir-fry in a small amount of oil; add moisture and flavor with broth, tomato juice, or wine.
- Use variety to enhance enjoyment of the meal: vary colors, textures, and temperatures—hot cooked versus cool raw foods—and use garnishes to complement food.

Reduce Cholesterol Intake Recall that cholesterol is found only in animal products. Consequently, eating less fat from meat, eggs, and milk products will also help lower dietary cholesterol intake (as well as total and saturated fat intakes).

Balance Omega-3 and Omega-6 Intakes The Committee on Dietary Allowances has not established an RDA for omega-3 and omega-6 fatty acids, but recommends that future committees consider the possibility.[44] The 1990 Canadian RNI include specific amounts for both omega-3 and omega-6 fatty acids.* Many researchers believe the body's requirements depend on an optimal ratio; that is, not necessarily that more omega-3 fatty acids are better, but that an appropriate balance between the two omega families may be crucial.[45] A ratio of about 1 to 4 (omega-3 to omega-6 fatty acids) has been suggested as appropriate.

To obtain the right balance between omega-3 and omega-6 fatty acids, most people need to eat more fish and less vegetable oil. Eating fish instead of meat two or three meals a week supports heart health, especially when combined with physical activity.[46] Even one fish meal a week may be enough to make a difference.[47] The fish may not even need to be rich in omega-3 fatty acids; one study found that farm-raised catfish (which is relatively low in omega-3 fatty acids) improves lipid profiles similarly to wild Alaskan salmon.[48] Fish provides many minerals (except iron) and vitamins and is leaner than most other animal-protein sources. In an effort to improve health, people are well advised to eat fish periodically.

Fish oil should come from fish, not from supplements. Fish oil supplements are not recommended for a number of reasons.† Perhaps most importantly, the scientific evidence on their safety and effectiveness is not conclusive.[49] Also, high intakes of fish oil increase bleeding time, interfere with wound healing, worsen diabetes, and impair immune function.[50] Fish oil supplements are made from fish skins and livers, which may contain other environmental contaminants. Fish oils also naturally contain high levels of the two most potentially toxic vitamins, A and D. Lastly, supplements are expensive; money is better spent on foods that can provide a full array of nutrients.

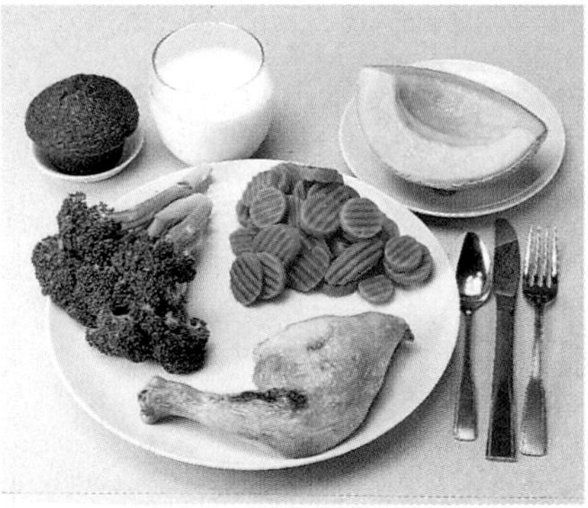

Even well-balanced, healthy meals provide some fat. In this meal, no butter is used and the beverage is nonfat milk, but 30 percent of the kcalories come from fat.

Select Lean Meats and Nonfat Milks Many foods that contain fat, saturated fat, and cholesterol—such as meats, milk, cheese, and eggs—also provide high-quality protein and valuable vitamins and minerals. They can be included in a healthy diet if a person selects lean and nonfat products and prepares them using the suggestions outlined in the box on p. 181. Figure 2–3 on pp. 52–53 shows examples of very lean, lean, medium-fat, and high-fat meats, and of nonfat, low-fat, and whole milk products.

Eat Plenty of Vegetables, Fruits, and Grains Choosing vegetables, fruits, cereals, and legumes also helps lower fat intake. Vegetables and fruits contain no fat, and most grains contain only trace amounts. Some grain *products* such as fried taco shells, croissants, and granola cereal are high in fat, though, so consumers need to read product labels.

*For omega-3 fatty acids, the RNI is 0.5 percent of total energy or 0.55 grams per 1000 kcalories; for omega-6 fatty acids, the RNI is 3 percent of total energy or 3.3 grams per 1000 kcalories.

†In Canada, fish oil supplements require a physician's prescription.

Because a low-fat diet is usually rich in vegetables, fruits, cereals, and legumes, it offers abundant vitamin C, folate, vitamin A, and dietary fiber—all important in supporting health. Consequently such a diet protects against disease in two ways, reducing fat and increasing nutrients.[51]

Use Fats and Oils Sparingly Practice moderation when using oils and fats such as butter, margarine, mayonnaise, and salad dressings. These foods offer much fat and little nourishment.

Look for Invisible Fat It can be surprising how much *invisible* fat some foods contain. Any *fried* food contains abundant fat: potato chips, french fries, fried wontons, fried fish. Many *baked* goods, too, are high in fat: pie crusts, pastries, biscuits, cornbread, doughnuts, sweet rolls, cookies, and cakes. Most chocolate bars contain more fat energy than sugar energy. Even cream-of-mushroom soup prepared with water derives 66 percent of its energy from fat. Abundant fat lurks on salad bars, too, not only in the dressings, but also in the potato salad, the macaroni salad, the coleslaw, and the marinated beans that are mixed with oil-based dressings. Keep invisible fats in mind when making food selections.

Some fat is easy to see: *visible fat,* such as butter, the oil in salad dressing, and the fat trimmed from meat. Other fat is less apparent: *invisible fat,* such as the fat that "marbles" a steak or is hidden in foods like nuts, cheese, crackers, avocados, olives, fried foods, bakery items, and chocolate.

Choose Wisely The *Dietary Guidelines* urge people to choose a diet low in fat, saturated fat, and cholesterol. A diet following the Daily Food Guide plan can support this goal if selections are made carefully. Only by following such a plan and making low-fat choices consistently can the goals of the *Diet and Health* recommendations be met. The accompanying box describes an easy way to estimate the fat content of a meal.

Consumers are finding more low-fat food choices available than ever before. In many cases, they are familiar foods presented now with less fat. Leaner animals are raised for meat, and cuts of meat are often trimmed of fat more closely than in the past. In the dairy case, nonfat and reduced-fat milk, yogurt, cheeses, and sour cream offer healthy alternatives to their higher-fat counterparts. Many processed foods such as salad dressings, crackers, chips, and cookies are now available with little or no fat. Such choices make low-fat eating easy. A simple switch to nonfat salad dressing can bring the average fat intake for women down from 37 to 34 percent of total kcalories.[52] Every little fat-saving step helps a person get closer to the 30 percent goal.

Many fat-free foods have been developed using familiar nutrients. Milk and egg proteins or carbohydrate derivatives, for example, are heated, acidified, or blended to simulate the properties of fat. Highlight 5 examines some of these new alternatives to fat.

HEALTHY PEOPLE 2000: Increase to at least 5000 brand items the number of processed food products that are reduced in fat and saturated fat.

Read Food Labels Labels list total fat, saturated fat, and cholesterol contents of foods in addition to fat kcalories per serving. (Labels do not provide information on *trans*-fatty acids; if the ingredients list includes hydrogenated oils, though, you know the food contains *trans*-fatty acids—you just don't know how much.) Because each package provides information for a single serving and serving sizes are standardized, consumers can easily compare similar products. Total

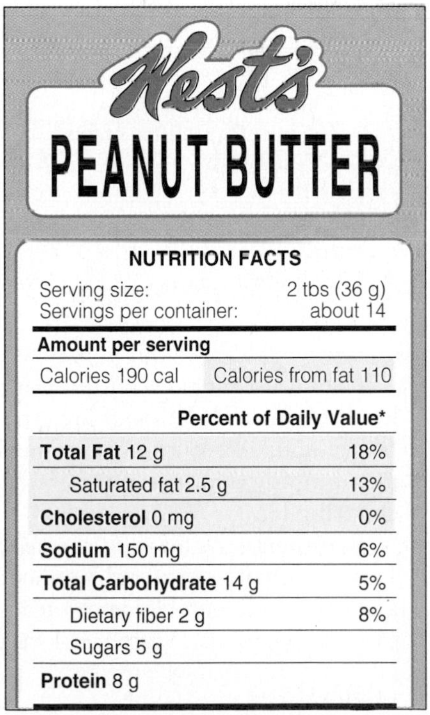

NUTRITION FACTS

Serving size:	2 tbs (36 g)
Servings per container:	about 14
Amount per serving	
Calories 190 cal	Calories from fat 110
	Percent of Daily Value*
Total Fat 12 g	18%
Saturated fat 2.5 g	13%
Cholesterol 0 mg	0%
Sodium 150 mg	6%
Total Carbohydrate 14 g	5%
Dietary fiber 2 g	8%
Sugars 5 g	
Protein 8 g	

How to Use the Exchange System to Estimate Fat

The exchange system is especially informative about the fats in foods. To use the exchange system, you need to know the fat value for each list (see the accompanying table) and the foods on that list with their portion sizes (review Figure 2–3 on pp. 52–53). Two of the lists—vegetables and fruits—contain no fat. A third list—starch—provides only a little. (Starch foods prepared with fat are counted as one starch exchange *plus* a fat exchange.) So you only need to learn the fat values for three lists: milks, meats, and fats.

The milk list offers three fat values for nonfat, low-fat, and whole milk. Think of nonfat milk as milk and of low-fat and whole milk as milk with added fat.

The meat list offers four fat values for very lean, lean, medium-fat, and high-fat products. People are often surprised to learn how much fat comes from meats and cheeses. An ounce of lean meat or low-fat cheese supplies about half of its energy from fat (28 protein kcalories and 27 fat kcalories). An ounce of high-fat meat or most cheeses supplies 72 percent of its energy from fat (28 protein kcalories and 72 fat kcalories). As for the meat alternate, peanut butter, 2 tablespoons supply 76 percent of their energy from fat (32 protein kcalories and 144 fat kcalories). Note that one meat exchange is a single ounce; to use the exchange system, learn to recognize the number of ounces in a serving.

One Exchange	Fat (g)
Milks	
Nonfat	0–3
Low-fat	5
Whole	8
Meats	
Very lean	0–1
Lean	3
Medium-fat	5
High-fat	8
Fats	
1 tsp butter, margarine, or oil (or any other serving of food on the fat list)	5
Starch	1 or less
Vegetables	—
Fruits	—
Other carbohydrates	varies

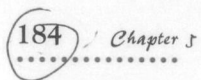

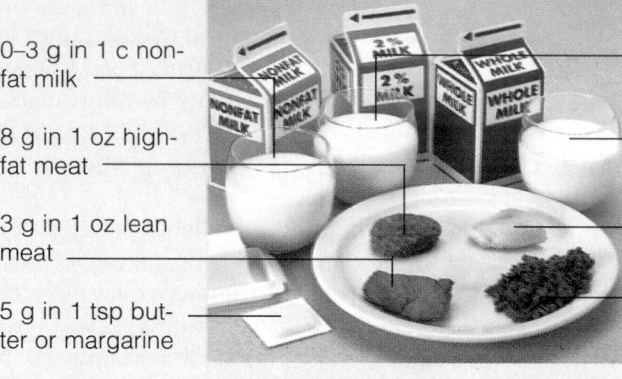

Fat-containing foods appear primarily in three of the exchanges lists: milks, meats, and fats.

The fat list includes butter, margarine, and oil, of course, but it also includes bacon, olives, avocados, and many kinds of nuts. These foods are grouped together because a portion of any of them contains as much fat as a pat of butter and, like butter, offers negligible protein and carbohydrate. In Appendix G, the fat list is sorted into monounsaturated, polyunsaturated, and saturated groups, which helps people make heart-wise selections when choosing fat.

To estimate the fat in this meal, you first need to recognize that this spaghetti dinner is really 1 cup of pasta, with 1 cup of tomato sauce and 3 ounces of lean ground beef. Then you need to translate these portions into exchanges: 2 starches, 1 vegetable, and 3 lean meats, respectively. Ignore the vegetables in the salad, but count the ½ cup of garbanzo beans as 1 starch + 1 very lean meat, and the sunflower seeds and ranch dressing as 1 fat each.

Dinner	Exchange	Fat (g) Estimate	Fat (g) Actual
Salad:			
1 c raw spinach leaves, shredded carrots, and sliced mushrooms	= free	0	0
½ c garbanzo beans	= 1 starch and 1 very lean meat	2	2
1 tbs sunflower seeds	= 1 fat	5	4
1 tbs ranch salad dressing	= 1 fat	5	6
Entree:			
Spaghetti with meat sauce			
1 c pasta (cooked)	= 2 starches	2	
1 c tomato sauce	= 1 vegetable	—	12
3 oz ground round	= 3 lean meats	9	
½ c green beans	= 1 vegetable	—	0
1 medium corn on the cob	= 1 starch	1	0
2 tsp butter	= 2 fats	10	8
Dessert:			
1/12 angel food cake	= 1 other carbohydrate	—	0
Beverage:			
1 c 1% low-fat milk	= 1 nonfat milk	3	3
		37	35

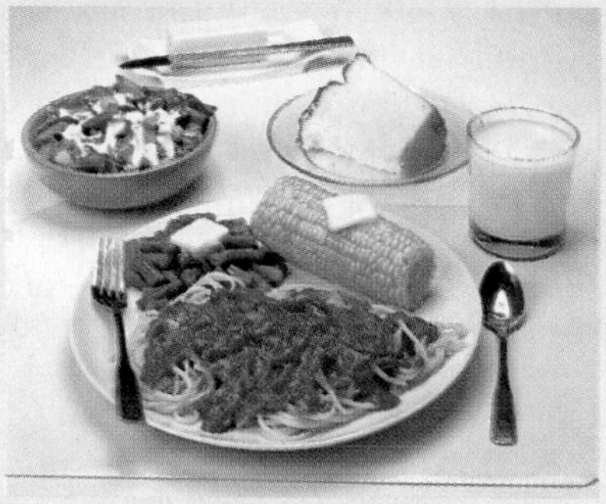

Using the exchange system to estimate, this dinner provides about 37 grams of fat. A computer diet analysis program came to a similar conclusion (35 grams), as would a diet analysis using the values in Appendix H. To keep from underestimating fat intake, count "1 or less" and "0–1" as "1 gram of fat" and count "0–3" as 3 grams of fat.

fat, saturated fat, and cholesterol are also expressed as "% Daily Values" for a person consuming 2000 kcalories. People who are consuming more or less than 2000 kcalories daily can calculate their personal Daily Value for fat as described in the box on p. 186.

Be aware that the "% Daily Value" for fat is not the same as "% kcalories from fat." Consider, for example, a piece of lemon meringue pie that provides 140 kcalories and 12 grams of fat. Because the Daily Value for fat is 65 grams for a 2000-kcalorie intake, 12 grams represents about 18 percent, or almost one-fifth, of the day's fat allowance (the pie's "% Daily Value" is 18). Uninformed consumers may mistakenly believe that this food meets the guideline to limit fat to "30 percent kcalories," but it doesn't—for two reasons. First, the pie's 12 grams of fat contribute 108 of the 140 kcalories, for a total of 77 percent kcalories from fat. Second, the "30 percent kcalories from fat" guideline applies to a day's total intake, not to an individual food. (Of course, if every selection throughout the day exceeds 30 percent kcalories from fat, you can be certain that the day's total intake does, too.)

Because recommendations apply to average daily intakes and not to individual food items, food labels do not provide the percent kcalories from fat. Still, you can get an idea of whether a particular food is high or low in fat. To quickly compare recommendations with the fat content of a food, use the rule of thumb that 3 grams of fat (27 kcalories of fat) represent about 30 percent of the kcalories in 100

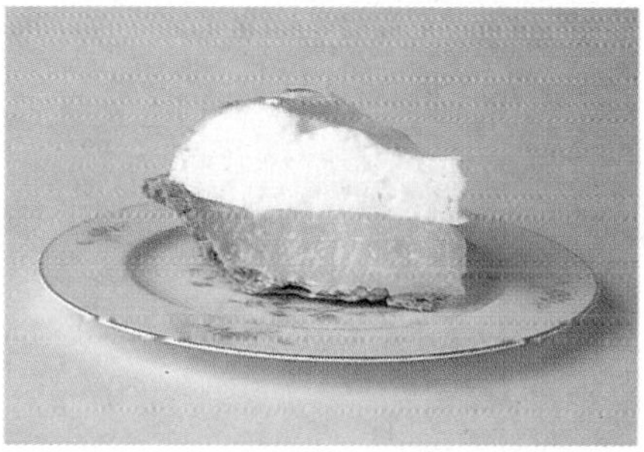

% Daily Value:

- $12\text{ g} \div 65\text{ g} = 0.18 \times 100 = 18\%$.

% kCalories from Fat:

- $12\text{ g} \times 9\text{ kcal/g} = 108\text{ kcal}$.
  $108\text{ kcal} \div 140\text{ kcal} = 77\%$.

How to Calculate a Personal Daily Value for Fat

The % Daily Value for fat on food labels is based on 65 grams. To know that you've met recommendations, you can either count grams until you reach 65, or add the "% Daily Values" until you reach 100%—if your energy intake is 2000 kcalories a day. If your energy intake is more or less, there are a couple of options.

You can calculate your personal daily fat allowance in grams. Multiply your total energy intake by 30 percent, then divide by 9. Suppose your energy intake is 1800 kcalories per day and your goal is 30 percent kcalories from fat:

$$1800 \text{ total kcal} \times 0.30 \text{ from fat} = 540 \text{ fat kcal.}$$

$$540 \text{ fat kcal} \div 9 \text{ kcal/g} = 60 \text{ g fat.}$$

Another way to calculate your personal fat allowance is to cross out the last digit of your energy intake and divide by 3.[a] For example, 1800 kcalories becomes 180; then you divide by 3:

$$\frac{180}{3} = 60 \text{ g fat/day.}$$

(In familiar measures, 60 grams of fat is about the same as ⅔ stick of butter or ¼ cup of oil.)

The accompanying table shows the numbers of grams of fat allowed per day for various energy intakes. With one of these numbers in mind, you can quickly evaluate the number of fat grams in foods you are considering eating.

Recommended Grams of Fat for Different Energy Intakes

Energy (kcal/day)	30 Percent kCalories	Fat (g/day)
1200	360	40
1500	450	50
1800	540	60
1900 (RDA for women 51 years and over)	570	63
2000 (Daily Value for food labels)	600	65
2200 (RDA for women 19 to 50 years old)	660	73
2300 (RDA for men 51 years and over)	690	77
2600	780	87
2900 (RDA for men 19 to 50 years old)	870	97
3000	900	100

[a]K. McNutt, Fat traps, tips, and tricks, *Nutrition Today*, May/June 1992, pp. 47–49.

Quick and easy estimates:
- A food is low in fat if it has: $\leq$ 3 g fat in 100 kcal food.
- A food is low in fat if: g fat $\times$ 30 < kcal.

kcalories of food. Alternatively, you can multiply the grams of fat in a serving by 30 and then compare that number to the kcalories.[53] If it is less, then the food has less than 30 percent kcalories from fat.

The FDA authorizes two health claims on labels concerning fat: one for "dietary saturated fat and cholesterol and risk of coronary heart disease" and one for "dietary fat and cancer." To make these claims, foods must meet specified criteria, as described in Chapter 2.

In summary, health authorities single out high fat intakes as a major flaw in the North American diet: excess fat contributes to heart disease, cancer, obesity, and other health problems. High blood LDL cholesterol, specifically, poses a risk of heart disease, and high intakes of saturated fat contribute most to high LDL. Cholesterol itself, in foods, presents much less of a risk; *trans*-fatty acids' effects are not yet clear from research. Omega-3 fatty acids appear to be protective, especially if consumed in a 1-to-4 ratio with omega-6 fatty acids. High fat diets also accelerate (but do not initiate) cancer development. Health authorities recommend limiting total fat to 30 percent or less of energy intake; saturated fat to one-third of total fat, or 10 percent of energy intake; and cholesterol to less than 300 milligrams a day. They also recommend consuming relatively more polyunsaturates, particularly omega-3 fatty acids, than in the past from foods such as fish, not from supplements. Many purchasing and cooking strategies can help bring these goals within reach, and the new food labels make it easier to select foods consistent with these guidelines.

If people were to make only one change in their diets, they would be wise to limit their intakes of total fat, which would control their energy intake as well. A second change might be to specifically limit saturated fat. Chances are good that if total fat and saturated fat meet recommendations, then cholesterol intake will, too. Many guidelines suggest these changes in that order of priority: low in fat, saturated fat, and cholesterol.

Lowering fat intake can be difficult, though, because fats make foods taste delicious. To maintain good health, must a person give up all high fat foods forever—never again to eat marbled steak, hollandaise sauce, or gooey chocolate cake? Not at all. These foods bring pleasure to a meal and can be enjoyed as part of a healthy diet when eaten in small quantities on occasion, but it is true that they are not everyday foods. The key word for fat is not deprivation, but moderation: appreciate the energy and enjoyment that fat provides, but take care not to exceed your needs.

Study Questions

1. Name the three classes of lipids found in the body and in foods. What features do fats bring to foods? What are some of their functions in the body?
2. Describe the structure of a triglyceride. What are the differences between saturated, unsaturated, monounsaturated, and polyunsaturated fats?
3. What two features distinguish fatty acids from each other?
4. What does hydrogenation do to fats? What are *trans*-fatty acids and how do they influence heart disease?
5. What does the term "omega" mean with respect to fatty acids? Describe the roles of the omega fatty acids in disease prevention.
6. Which of the fatty acids are essential? Name their chief dietary sources.
7. How do phospholipids differ from triglycerides in structure? How does cholesterol differ? How do these differences in structure affect function?
8. Trace the steps in fat digestion, absorption, and transport.
9. What do lipoproteins do? What are the differences among the chylomicrons, VLDL, LDL, and HDL?
10. What roles does cholesterol play in the body?
11. Describe the routes cholesterol takes in the body.
12. What roles do the triglycerides and phospholipids perform in the body?
13. How does excessive fat intake influence health? What factors influence LDL, HDL, and total blood cholesterol?
14. What are the dietary recommendations regarding fat and cholesterol intake? List ways to reduce intake.
15. Which food lists of the exchange system supply fat in abundance? In moderation? Not at all?
16. What is the Daily Value for fat (for a 2000-kcalorie diet)? What does this number represent?

Problem Set appears on pp. 190–192

Notes

1. D. J. Mela and D. A. Sacchetti, Sensory preferences for fat: Relationships with diet and body composition, *American Journal of Clinical Nutrition* 53 (1991): 908–915.
2. J. E. Hunter and T. H. Applewhite, Reassessment of *trans* fatty acid availability in the US diet, *American Journal of Clinical Nutrition* 54 (1991): 363–369; M. G. Enig and coauthors, Isomeric *trans* fatty acids in the U.S. diet, *Journal of the American College of Nutrition* 9 (1990): 471–486.
3. C. A. Drevon, Marine oils and their effects, *Nutrition Reviews* 50 (1992): 38–45.
4. M. A. Crawford, The role of essential fatty acids in neural development: Implications for perinatal nutrition, *American Journal of Clinical Nutrition* 57 (1993): 703S–710S; J. A. Nettleton, Are n-3 fatty acids essential nutrients for fetal and infant development? *Journal of the American Dietetic Association* 93 (1993): 58–64.
5. W. E. Connor, M. Neuringer, and S. Reisbick, Essential fatty acids: The importance of n-3 fatty acids in the retina and brain, *Nutrition Reviews* 50 (1992): II21–II29.
6. A. P. Simopoulos, Omega-3 fatty acids in health and disease and in growth and development, *American Journal of Clinical Nutrition* 54 (1991): 438–463.
7. D. S. Lin and W. E. Connor, Are the n-3 fatty acids from dietary fish oil deposited in the triglyceride stores of adipose tissue? *American Journal of Clinical Nutrition* 51 (1990): 535–539.
8. Scientific Review Committee, *Nutrition Recommendations: The Report of the Scientific Review Committee, 1990* (Ottawa: Canadian Government Publishing Centre, 1990), p. 45; P. J. Nestel, Polyunsaturated fatty acids (n-3, n-6), *American Journal of Clinical Nutrition* 45 (1987): 1161–1167; M. Neuringer, G. J. Anderson, and W. E. Connor, The essentiality of N-3 fatty acids for the development and function of the retina and brain, *Annual Review of Nutrition* 8 (1988): 517–541.
9. J. A. Nettleton, ω-3 Fatty acids: Comparison of plant and seafood sources in human nutrition, *Journal of the American Dietetic Association* 91 (1991): 331–337; J. E. Hunter, n-3 Fatty acids from vegetable oils, *American Journal of Clinical Nutrition* 51 (1990) 809–814; Committee on Dietary Allowances, *Recommended Dietary Allowances*, 10th ed. (Washington, D.C.: National Academy Press, 1989), pp. 47–48.
10. L. M. Arnold and coauthors, Effect of isoenergetic intake of three or nine meals on plasma lipoproteins and glucose metabolism, *American Journal of Clinical Nutrition* 57 (1993): 446–451; P. J. H. Jones, C. A. Leitch, and R. A Pederson, Meal-frequency effects on plasma hormone concentrations and cholesterol synthesis in humans, *American Journal of Clinical Nutrition* 57 (1993): 868–874; D. J. A. Jenkins and coauthors, Nibbling versus gorging: Metabolic advantages of increased meal frequency, *New England Journal of Medicine* 321 (1989): 929–934.
11. M. Hamosh, *Lingual and Gastric Lipases: Their Role in Fat Digestion* (Boston: CRC Press, 1990).
12. R. Havel, McCollum Award Lecture, 1993: Triglyceride-rich lipoproteins and atherosclerosis—New perspectives, *American Journal of Clinical Nutrition* 59 (1994): 795–799.
13. NIH Consensus Conference, Triglyceride, high-density lipoprotein, and coronary heart disease, *Journal of the American Medical Association* 269 (1993): 505–510; M. J. Stampfer and coauthors, A prospective study of cholesterol, apolipoproteins, and the risk of myocardial infarction, *New England Journal of Medicine* 325 (1991): 373–381.
14. J. L. Groff, S. S. Gropper, and S. M. Hunt, *Advanced Nutrition and Human Metabolism* (St. Paul, Minn.: West, 1995), pp. 466–483.
15. R. P. Mensink, Effects of the individual saturated fatty acids on serum lipid and lipoprotein concentrations, *American Journal of Clinical Nutrition* (supplement) 57 (1993): 711S–714S.
16. S. M. Grundy, Influence of stearic acid on cholesterol metabolism relative to other long-chain fatty acids, *American Journal of Clinical Nutrition* 60 (1994): 986S–990S.
17. B. V. Howard and coauthors, Polyunsaturated fatty acids result in greater cholesterol lowering and less triacylglycerol elevation than do monounsaturated fatty acids in a dose-response comparison in a multiracial study group, *American Journal of Clinical Nutrition* 62 (1995): 392–402; M. B. Katan, P. L. Zock, and R. P. Mensink, Effects of fats and fatty acids on blood lipids in humans: An overview, *American Journal of Clinical Nutrition* 60 (1994): 1017S–1022S; D. M. Hegsted and coauthors, Dietary fat and serum lipids: An evaluation of the experimental data, *American Journal of Clinical Nutrition* 57 (1993): 875–883.
18. Katan, Zock, and Mensink, 1994; P. Mata and coauthors, Effects of long-term monounsaturated- vs polyunsaturated-enriched diets on lipoproteins in healthy men and women, *American Journal of Clinical Nutrition* 55 (1992): 846–850.
19. M. C. Nydahl, I. B. Gustafsson, and B. Vessby, Lipid-lowering diets enriched with monounsaturated or polyunsaturated fatty acids but low in saturated fatty acids have similar effects on serum lipid concentrations in hyperlipidemic patients, *American Journal of Clinical Nutrition* 59 (1994): 115–122.
20. M. B. Katan, and P. L. Zock, *Trans* fatty acids and their effects on lipoproteins in humans, *Annual Review of Nutrition* 15 (1995): 473–493; A. H. Lichtenstein, *Trans* fatty acids and hydrogenated fat—What do we know? *Nutrition Today*, 30 (1995): 102–107; J. T. Judd and coauthors, Dietary *trans* fatty acids: Effects on plasma lipids and lipoproteins of healthy men and women, *American Journal of Clinical Nutrition* 59 (1994):

861–868; R. Troisi, W. C. Willett, and S. T. Weiss, *Trans*-fatty acid intake in relation to serum lipid concentrations in adult men, *American Journal of Clinical Nutrition* 56 (1992): 1019–1024.

21. A. Ascherio and coauthors, *Trans*-fatty acids intake and risk of myocardial infarction, *Circulation* 89 (1994): 94–101; W. C. Willett and coauthors, Intake of *trans* fatty acids and risk of coronary heart disease among women, *Lancet* 341 (1993): 581–585.
22. L. C. Hudgins, J. Hirsch, and E. A. Emken, Correlation of isomeric fatty acids in human adipose tissue with clinical risk factors for cardiovascular disease, *American Journal of Clinical Nutrition* 53 (1991): 474–482.
23. American Heart Association, Nutrition Advisory Committee, *News Release*, Trans fatty acids, May 13, 1994.
24. W. C. Willett and A. Ascherio, *Trans* fatty acids: Are the effects only marginal? *American Journal of Public Health* 84 (1994): 722–724.
25. A. P. Simopoulos and coauthors, Conferences, symposia, and reports—The 1st Congress of the International Society for the Study of Fatty Acids and Lipids (ISSFAL): Fatty acids and lipids from cell biology to human disease, *Nutrition Today*, July/August 1994, pp. 24–27; Willett and Ascherio, 1994; M. B. Katan, European researcher calls for reconsideration of *trans* fatty acids, *Journal of the American Dietetic Association* 94 (1994): 1097–1098.
26. A. Lichtenstein, *Trans* fatty acids, blood lipids, and cardiovascular risk: Where do we stand? *Nutrition Reviews* 51 (1993): 340–343.
27. American Dietetic Association, *News Release*, Evidence inconclusive on trans fatty acids, May 16, 1994.
28. Editor's note (in response to Katan, 1994), *Journal of the American Dietetic Association* 94 (1994): 1097–1098.
29. A Nordöy and coauthors, Individual effects of dietary saturated fatty acids and fish oil on plasma lipids and lipoproteins in normal men, *American Journal of Clinical Nutrition* 57 (1993): 634–639.
30. M. C. Morris, F. Sacks, and B. Rosner, Does fish oil lower blood pressure? A meta-analysis of controlled trials, *Circulation* 88 (1993): 523–533; L. J. Appel and coauthors, Does supplementation of diet with 'fish oil' reduce blood pressure? A meta-analysis of controlled clinical trials, *Archives of Internal Medicine* 153 (1993): 1429–1438.
31. Y. Goto, Changing trends in dietary habits and cardiovascular disease in Japan: An overview, *Nutrition Reviews* 50 (1992): 398–401.
32. K. K. Carroll, Dietary fats and cancer, *American Journal of Clinical Nutrition* 53 (1991): 1064S–1067S.
33. M. Anti and coauthors, Effect of ω-3 fatty acids on rectal mucosal cell proliferation in subjects at risk for colon cancer, *Gastroenterology* 103 (1992): 883–891; Simopoulos, 1991; L. A. Sauer, R. T. Dauchy, and A. S. Hurtubise, Effects of omega-6 and omega-3 fatty acids on rate of ^{3}H-thymidine incorporation in hepatoma, *FASEB Journal* 4 (1990): A508; D. Magrane and M. Philley, Effects of dietary corn oil and menhaden oil on rat mammary tumorigenesis and PGE_2 levels, *FASEB Journal* 4 (1990): A1176.
34. R. A. Karmali, Fatty acid metabolism and biochemical mechanisms in cancer, in *Health Effects of Dietary Fatty Acids*, ed. G. J. Nelson (Champaign, Ill.: American Oil Chemists' Society, 1991), pp. 150–156.
35. L. H. Kushi and coauthors, Dietary fat and postmenopausal breast cancer, *Journal of the National Cancer Institute* 84 (1992): 1092–1099; W. C. Willett and coauthors, Dietary fat and fiber in relation to risk of breast cancer: An 8-year follow-up, *Journal of the American Medical Association* 628 (1992): 2037–2044.
36. E. Barrett-Connor and N. J. Friedlander, Dietary fat, calories, and the risk of breast cancer in postmenopausal women: A prospective population-based study, *Journal of the American College of Nutrition* 12 (1993): 390–399.
37. K. J. Pienta and P. S. Esper, Is dietary fat a risk factor for prostate cancer? *Journal of the National Cancer Institute* 85 (1993): 1538–1540; E. Giovannuci and coauthors, A prospective study of dietary fat and risk of prostate cancer, *Journal of the National Cancer Institute* 85 (1993): 1571–1579.
38. C. Bennett and coauthors, Short-term effects of dietary-fat ingestion on energy expenditure and nutrient balance, *American Journal of Clinical Nutrition* 55 (1992): 1071–1077.
39. T. E. Prewitt and coauthors, Changes in body weight, body composition, and energy intakes in women fed high- and low-fat diets, *American Journal of Clinical Nutrition* 54 (1991): 304–310.
40. B. J. Rolls, Carbohydrates, fats, and satiety, *American Journal of Clinical Nutrition* 61 (1995): 960S–967S.
41. A. M. Stephen and N. J. Wald, Trends in individual consumption of dietary fat in the United States, 1920–1984, *American Journal of Clinical Nutrition* 52 (1990): 457–469.
42. Daily dietary fat and total food-energy intakes—Third National Health and Nutrition Examination Survey, Phase 1, 1988–91, *Morbidity and Mortality Weekly Report* 43 (1994): 116–117, 123–125.
43. C. L. Johnson and coauthors, Declining serum total cholesterol levels among US adults, *Journal of the American Medical Association* 269 (1993): 3002–3008.
44. Committee on Dietary Allowances, 1989, p. 48.
45. M. D. Boudreau and coauthors, Lack of dose response by dietary n-3 fatty acids at a constant ratio of n-3 to n-6 fatty acids in suppressing eicosanoid biosynthesis from arachidonic acid, *American Journal of Clinical Nutrition* 54 (1991): 111–117.
46. Simopoulos, 1991; K. N. Seidelin, B. Myrup, and B. Fischer-Hansen, n-3 fatty acids in adipose tissue and coronary artery disease are inversely related, *American Journal of Clinical Nutrition* 55 (1992): 1117–1119.
47. A. Ascherio and coauthors, Dietary intake of marine n-3 fatty acids, fish intake, and the risk of coronary disease among men, *New England Journal of Medicine* 332 (1995): 977–982; K. H. Bönaa, K. S. Bjerve, and A. Nordöy, Habitual fish consumption, plasma phospholipid fatty acids, and serum lipids: The Tromsö Study, *American Journal of Clinical Nutrition* 55 (1992): 1126–1134.

48. D. K. Tidwell and coauthors, Comparison of the effects of adding fish high or low in n-3 fatty acids to a diet conforming to the Dietary Guidelines for Americans, *Journal of the American Dietetic Association* 93 (1993): 1124–1128.
49. Fish oil supplements, *FDA Consumer,* October 1990, p. 32.
50. S. J. Bhathena and coauthors, Effects of ω-3 fatty acids and vitamin E on hormones involved in carbohydrate and lipid metabolism in men, *American Journal of Clinical Nutrition* 54 (1991): 684–688; K. L. Fritsche, S. C. Huang, and M. Misfeldt, Fish oil and immune function (letter), *Nutrition Reviews* 51 (1993): 24; H. Flaten and coauthors, Fish-oil concentrate: Effects on variables related to cardiovascular disease, *American Journal of Clinical Nutrition* 52 (1990): 300–306.
51. A. F. Subar and coauthors, US dietary patterns associated with fat intake: The 1987 National Health Interview Survey, *American Journal of Public Health* 84 (1994): 359–366.
52. M. Hudnall, M. G. Hermann-Zaidins, and J. S. Stern, Fat replacements: Helpful or not? *Journal of the American Dietetic Association* 92 (1992): 1330–1331.
53. D. Green-Burgeson, Calculating fat the easy way, *Journal of the American Dietetic Association* 94 (1994): 256.

Problem Set

1. Learn how food choices can affect energy and fat contents of meals. Start with one meal, check its energy, fat, calcium, iron, and vitamin C contributions, then substitute an item to see how the balances change.

   a. Start with a fast-food, fried chicken dinner and record the analysis for energy and four nutrients here:

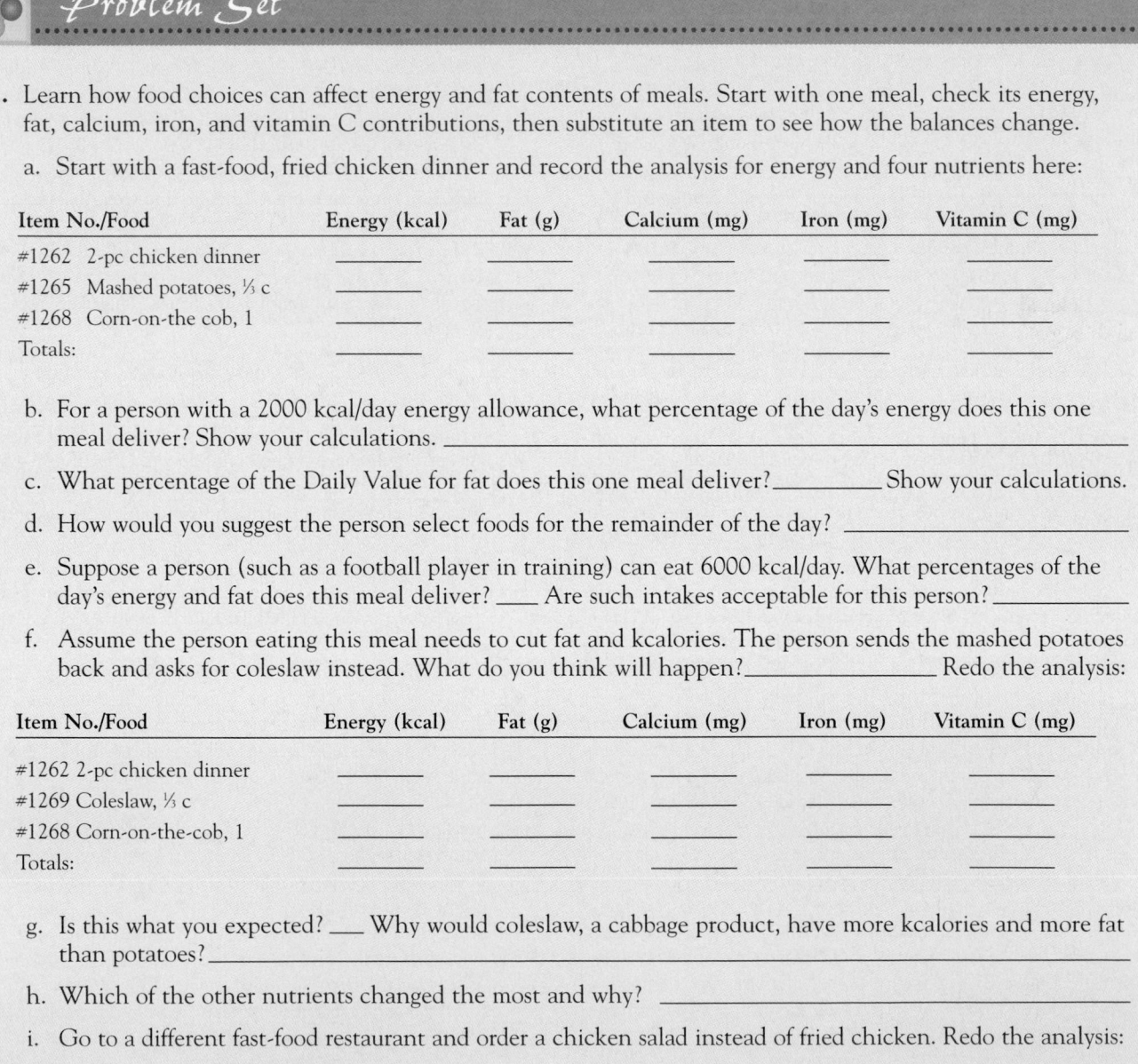

Item No./Food	Energy (kcal)	Fat (g)	Calcium (mg)	Iron (mg)	Vitamin C (mg)
#1262 2-pc chicken dinner	______	______	______	______	______
#1265 Mashed potatoes, ⅓ c	______	______	______	______	______
#1268 Corn-on-the cob, 1	______	______	______	______	______
Totals:	______	______	______	______	______

   b. For a person with a 2000 kcal/day energy allowance, what percentage of the day's energy does this one meal deliver? Show your calculations. ________________

   c. What percentage of the Daily Value for fat does this one meal deliver?________ Show your calculations.

   d. How would you suggest the person select foods for the remainder of the day? ________________

   e. Suppose a person (such as a football player in training) can eat 6000 kcal/day. What percentages of the day's energy and fat does this meal deliver? ____ Are such intakes acceptable for this person?__________

   f. Assume the person eating this meal needs to cut fat and kcalories. The person sends the mashed potatoes back and asks for coleslaw instead. What do you think will happen?______________ Redo the analysis:

Item No./Food	Energy (kcal)	Fat (g)	Calcium (mg)	Iron (mg)	Vitamin C (mg)
#1262 2-pc chicken dinner	______	______	______	______	______
#1269 Coleslaw, ⅓ c	______	______	______	______	______
#1268 Corn-on-the-cob, 1	______	______	______	______	______
Totals:	______	______	______	______	______

   g. Is this what you expected? ___ Why would coleslaw, a cabbage product, have more kcalories and more fat than potatoes?________________

   h. Which of the other nutrients changed the most and why? ________________

   i. Go to a different fast-food restaurant and order a chicken salad instead of fried chicken. Redo the analysis:

Item No./Food	Energy (kcal)	Fat (g)	Calcium (mg)	Iron (mg)	Vitamin C (mg)
#1401 Chunky chicken salad, 1	______	______	______	______	______
#1269 Coleslaw, ⅓ c	______	______	______	______	______
#1268 Corn-on-the-cob, 1	______	______	______	______	______
Totals:	______	______	______	______	______

This substitution makes a significant change in fat and kcalories, even though the salad is from a fast-food place. This goes to prove that people who try hard enough can eat a low-fat diet, even on the run.

2. Suppose one day a person eats 1700 kcal, including 60 g fat. Now the person wants to have dessert, but doesn't want to exceed 2000 kcal with 65 g fat for the day.

   a. Look up the following desserts in Appendix H and sort them into: (1) desserts that deliver less than 300 kcal and 5 g fat (acceptable), and (2) desserts that deliver more kcalories, more fat, or both (not acceptable).

Item No./Food		Energy (kcal)	Fat (g)	Acceptable?	
				YES	NO
#1724	Ice cream, ½ c	______	______	______	______
#133	Sherbet, ½ c	______	______	______	______
#147	Vanilla yogurt, 1 c	______	______	______	______
#1584	Yogurt, frozen, low-fat, ½ c	______	______	______	______
#318	Strawberries fresh, whole, 1 c	______	______	______	______
#372	Angel food cake, 1 piece	______	______	______	______
#384	Carrot cake, 1 piece	______	______	______	______
#404	Brownie homemade, 1	______	______	______	______
#407	Chocolate chip cookies, 4	______	______	______	______
#464	Pecan pie, 1 piece	______	______	______	______
#778	Popsicle, 1	______	______	______	______
#1131	Snickers candy bar, 1	______	______	______	______

   b. Suppose the person wanted to eat that piece of carrot cake but not exceed the 65-gram fat allowance for the day. What could the person have done earlier in the day to earn the cake? ______

3. Be aware of the fats in milks. Following are three categories of milk.

	Wt (g)	Fat (g)	Prot (g)	Carb (g)
Milk A (1 c)	244	8	8	12
Milk B (1 c)	244	5	8	12
Milk C (1 c)	244	0	8	12

	Milk A	Milk B	Milk C
a. Based on *weight,* what percentage of this milk is fat (round off to a whole number)?	______	______	______
b. A person who drinks a cup of this milk will receive how much energy from fat?	______	______	______
c. How much total energy will the person receive from 1 c of this milk?	______	______	______

(continued on the next page)

Problem Set (continued)

Problem 3 continued	Milk A	Milk B	Milk C
d. What percentage of the energy in the milk comes from fat?	______	______	______
e. In the grocery store, this milk is labeled:	______	______	______

4. Find the hidden fat in foods. Look up the following foods in Appendix H and record the total kcalories and fat. Then determine the percentage of the kcalories that comes from fat. The first one is done for you.

Item No./Food		Energy (kcal)	Fat (g)	Energy from Fat (g × 9 kcal/g)	% of kcal from Fat
#1414	Granola bar (soft), 1 ea	188	7	63	34%
#426	Croissant, 1 ea	______	______	______	______
#1271	Plain tortilla chips, 1 oz	______	______	______	______
#482	Waffle (home recipe), 1 ea	______	______	______	______
#1318	Oat bran cereal, 1 c	______	______	______	______
#537	Chow mein, dry, 1 c	______	______	______	______
#583	Salmon, broiled or baked, 4 oz	______	______	______	______
#661	Turkey patty, breaded, fried, 2 oz	______	______	______	______
#682	Chicken à la king, 1 c	______	______	______	______
#220	Avocado, 1 ea	______	______	______	______
#927	Tofu (regular), ½ c	______	______	______	______

a. Do any of these foods and their fat grams surprise you? Which ones? ______________________________

b. In all of these foods, fat contributes more than 30% of the kcalories. Is there any place in a healthy diet for these foods? (Think carefully.) ______________________________

5. Judge foods' fat contents by their labels.

a. A food label says that one serving of the food contains 6.5 g fat. What would the % Daily Value for fat be (show your calculations)? __________ What does the Daily Value you just calculated mean? ______

b. How many kcalories from fat does a serving contain? (Show your calculations and round off to the nearest whole number.) ______________________________

c. If a *serving* of the food contains 200 kcal, then what percentage of the energy is from fat (show your calculations and round off)? ______________________________

This example should show you how easy it is to evaluate foods' fat contents by reading labels and to see the difference between the % Daily Value and the percentage of kcalories from fat.

6. Now reconsider that carrot cake from problem 2. Remember that the Daily Value suggests 65 g of fat as acceptable within a 2000-kcalorie diet. A serving of carrot cake provides 30 g fat. What percentage of the Daily Value is that? __________ What does this mean? ______________________________

Alternatives to Fat

As people learn more and more about the health consequences of high-fat diets, they want to lower their fat intake, but they'd rather not give up their favorite foods. As the adage goes, they want to have their cake and eat it, too—both figuratively and literally. Fat replacements offer an easy way to lower fat intake, while enjoying many foods that were once high in fat. Skeptics say that people will use these artificial fats the same way they use artificial sweeteners: in *addition* to fats rather than *instead* of fats, but preliminary reports indicate that people who use fat substitutes do eat less fat. They compensate with more carbohydrate, however, so that their total energy intakes remain constant.[1] Still, even if energy intakes remain steady, eating carbohydrate in place of fat improves blood lipids and helps to shift body composition toward the lean.

Food chemists have been working for decades on ways to reduce the fat in foods. Juggling the needs of the human body, the taste perceptions of consumers, and the requirements of food preparation is a complex task. For the body, products must contribute little food energy, must be nontoxic and completely excreted, and must not rob the body of valuable fat-soluble nutrients. To satisfy consumers, products must be attractive, feel right in the mouth, and have the right flavor. Food manufacturers need a compound that remains stable while meeting a product's requirements for temperature, moisture, and texture. That's a tall order, but it looks as though food chemists are mastering the task. Today shoppers can select from thousands of new reduced-fat products. Many bakery goods, cheeses, frozen desserts, and other products are available that offer less than half a gram of fat in a serving.

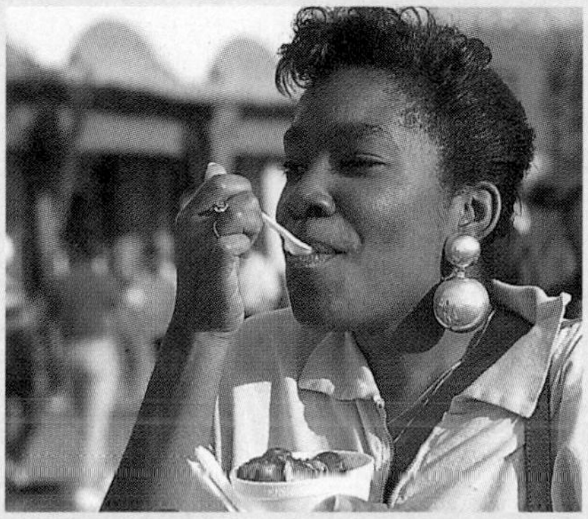

Low-fat and nonfat foods offer as much flavor and enjoyment as their high-fat counterparts—for less fat and fewer kcalories.

Some techniques for reducing food fat are quite simple. For example, manufacturers can lower fat by adding water or whipping in air. They use nonfat milk in creamy desserts and lean meats in frozen entrees. Sometimes they simply prepare the products differently. For example, fat-free potato chips are now baked instead of fried.

Some new products contain common food ingredients such as carbohydrates or proteins that replicate the texture of fat. Many of these products lack the sensation of richness provided by the fatty ingredients they replace. Innovative technologies are attempting to solve this problem by imitating the experience of eating fat—the creaminess as well as the taste—without the kcalories.[2] The many laboratories working to develop artificial fats are currently testing some 20 possible fat substitutes, most of them based on either carbohydrate, protein, or fat.

OATRIM AND OTHER CARBOHYDRATE-BASED FAT REPLACEMENTS

Several fat replacements are based on carbohydrate derivatives such as dextrins, modified food starches, and gums. One such product is maltodextrin, a carbohydrate derived from corn. When sprinkled on hot, moist foods such as baked potatoes, this product melts, providing a flavor similar to that of butter or margarine.

Another carbohydrate-based fat replacement is Oatrim, which is derived from oat fiber. Oatrim was developed by the U.S. Department of Agriculture to both reduce fat intake and lower blood cholesterol. An added advantage is that it provides satiety.

Most carbohydrate-based fat replacements are heat stable and can be used in baking, but not in frying. They mimic the texture and feel of fat by forming gels in foods such as margarines, frozen desserts, and salad dressings.

Because these carbohydrate derivatives are common dietary substances, companies can ask the FDA to approve them as generally recognized as safe (GRAS) substances. In fact, manufacturers have used these carbohydrate-based compounds for years as thickeners and stabilizers. The body digests and absorbs these substances, so they contribute some energy, although significantly less than fat's 9 kcalories per gram.

SIMPLESSE AND OTHER PROTEIN-BASED FAT REPLACEMENTS

Perhaps the best-known protein-based fat replacement, and the only one to receive FDA approval to date, is Simplesse. The FDA declared Simplesse safe for use in ice cream and frozen desserts in 1990. Simplesse is made from either egg white or milk proteins processed into mistlike particles that feel and taste like fat. Because the components of Simplesse are common in foods, safety studies have not been required.

Simplesse cannot be used for frying or baking because it gels when heated and loses its creaminess. It works fine on hot foods, though; for example, it makes a good imitation butter spread for toast or a sour cream–type topping for a baked potato. Simplesse is not available for home use.

Simplesse creates the *perception* of fat without all the kcalories. In the body, Simplesse is digested and absorbed, contributing 1 to 2 kcalories per gram—a substantial reduction from fat's 9 kcalories per gram. Substituting Simplesse for fat reduces the energy values of some foods dramatically. In some cases, though, such as fat-free ice cream, so much sugar is added that the kcalorie count of a fat-free product may be as high as in the original (see Table H5–1). Replacing both the fat and sugar in a product is difficult to do, because both contribute to flavor, texture, and stability. Substituting Simplesse for fat, however, does reduce a food's fat and cholesterol content appreciably.

Table H5–1

Fat Content of Regular Foods and Foods Prepared with Fat Replacements

Food	Fat (g)	Cholesterol (mg)	Energy (kcal)
Ice cream			
Super premium (½ c)	19	97	274
Regular (½ c)	7	30	135
Ice milk (½ c)	3	9	92
Frozen dessert			
Made with Simplesse (½ c)	<1	14	120
Made with Oatrim (½ c)	1	4	135
Butter (1 tsp)	4	11	36
Margarine (1 tsp)	4	0	34
Maltodextrin sprinkles (½ tsp)	<1	0	3
French fries			
Fried in vegetable oil	12.3	0	227
Fried in 75% olestra blend	3.1	0	144
Chicken			
Fried in vegetable oil	14.6	0	252
Fried in 75% olestra blend	8.6	0	198
Onion rings			
Fried in vegetable oil	19.5	0	315
Fried in 75% olestra blend	4.9	0	184

Note: Equivalent serving sizes were compared; in the case of butter and margarine, ½ teaspoon of sprinkles was compared with 1 teaspoon butter or margarine as per label directions.

Source: Oatrim: A potential fat substitute, *Nutrition Today*, July/August 1990, p. 4; M. Segal, Fat substitutes: A taste of the future? *FDA Consumer*, December 1990, pp. 25–27; J. E. Shields and E. Young, Fat in fast foods—Evolving changes, *Nutrition Today*, March/April 1990, pp. 32–35.

Some people, such as those who are allergic or sensitive to egg or milk proteins, may have to avoid Simplesse. (New regulations require a product's label to identify the source of its protein in the ingredient list.) People on protein-restricted diets may have to consult with their dietitians before including Simplesse in their diets, although its use is not expected to raise protein intake by more than 2 grams daily. Companies have developed other protein-derived products similar to Simplesse but have yet to petition the FDA for approval.

OLESTRA AND OTHER FAT-BASED FAT REPLACEMENTS

One product the FDA has had under consideration for several years is a kcalorie-free fat replacement formerly known as sucrose polyester; its generic name is now olestra. Olestra's chemical structure is similar to that of triglycerides, but olestra has a sucrose molecule instead of a glycerol molecule and six to eight fatty acids attached instead of three. Unlike sucrose or fatty acids, though, olestra is indigestible. It passes through the digestive tract unabsorbed. In the digestive tract, it interferes with the absorption of both dietary cholesterol and cholesterol being recycled through the enterohepatic pathway; as a result, it lowers blood cholesterol.

Olestra looks, feels, and tastes like dietary fat and can substitute for fats and oils in meals without diminishing flavor, adding energy, or raising blood lipids. It has the same properties as fats and oils when used in frying, cooking, and baking. Because olestra contains many of the fatty acids common to shortening and cooking oils, it shares many physical properties with them such as appearance, color, taste, heat stability, and shelf life. If approved, olestra can be used as a partial substitute for fats in shortenings and oils for home and restaurant use and in snack foods such as potato chips.

Most likely, olestra will be blended with other oils. Fats for home use may contain 35 percent olestra, while commercial fats may contain up to 75 percent. These mixtures will provide between 2 and 6 kcalories per gram instead of fat's typical 9.

Scientific research on animals and human beings seems to support the safety of olestra as a partial replacement for dietary fats and oils.[3] Studies on animals have reported no evidence of cancer or birth defects caused by olestra.

One action of olestra has both positive and negative consequences—it carries some fat-soluble substances out of the body. Olestra reduces cholesterol absorption, but on the negative side, it interferes with vitamin E absorption. The other fat-soluble vitamins are unaffected.[4] One proposed solution to this problem is to supplement olestra products with vitamin E. Studies suggest that people routinely using olestra might need to increase their intake of vitamin E to two times the RDA. Early formulations of olestra caused diarrhea in some people, but this seems to have been corrected by changing the composition.

To date, olestra is awaiting FDA approval. Other companies are expected to submit petitions to the FDA for approval of similar kcalorie-free fat substitutes.

Skeptics say that fat substitutes only encourage people to eat more food, that people will feel that they can afford to indulge if they've saved energy elsewhere. Of course, fat substitutes are not magic; they cannot make people eat healthy diets. What they can do, though, is offer a low-fat alternative to the high-fat foods that bring flavor and pleasure to meals and snacks. Used wisely, they can help consumers achieve their dietary goals.[5]

NOTES

1. L. L. Birch and coauthors, Effects of a nonenergy fat substitute on children's energy and macronutrient intake, *American Journal of Clinical Nutrition* 58 (1993): 326–333; R. W. Foltin and coauthors, Caloric, but not macronutrient, compensation by humans for required-eating occasions with meals and snack varying in fat and carbohydrate, *American Journal of Clinical Nutrition* 55 (1992): 331–342; B. J. Rolls and coauthors, Effects of olestra, a noncaloric fat substitute, on daily energy and fat intakes in lean men, *American Journal of Clinical Nutrition* 56 (1992): 84–92.

2. A. Drewnowski, Sensory properties of fats and fat replacements, *Nutrition Reviews* 50 (1992): II17–II20.

3. K. L. Skare, J. A. Skare, and E. O. Thompson, Evaluation of olestra in short-term genotoxic assays, *Food and Chemical Toxicology* 28 (1990): 69–73.

4. D. Y. Jones and coauthors, Vitamin K status of free-living subjects consuming olestra, *American Journal of Clinical Nutrition* 53 (1991): 943–946; D. Y. Jones and coauthors, Serum 25-hydroxyvitamin D concentrations of free-living subjects consuming olestra, *American Journal of Clinical Nutrition* 53 (1991): 1281–1287.

5. Position of The American Dietetic Association: Fat replacements, *Journal of the American Dietetic Association* 91 (1991): 1285–1288.

Chapter 6

Protein: Amino Acids

CONTENTS

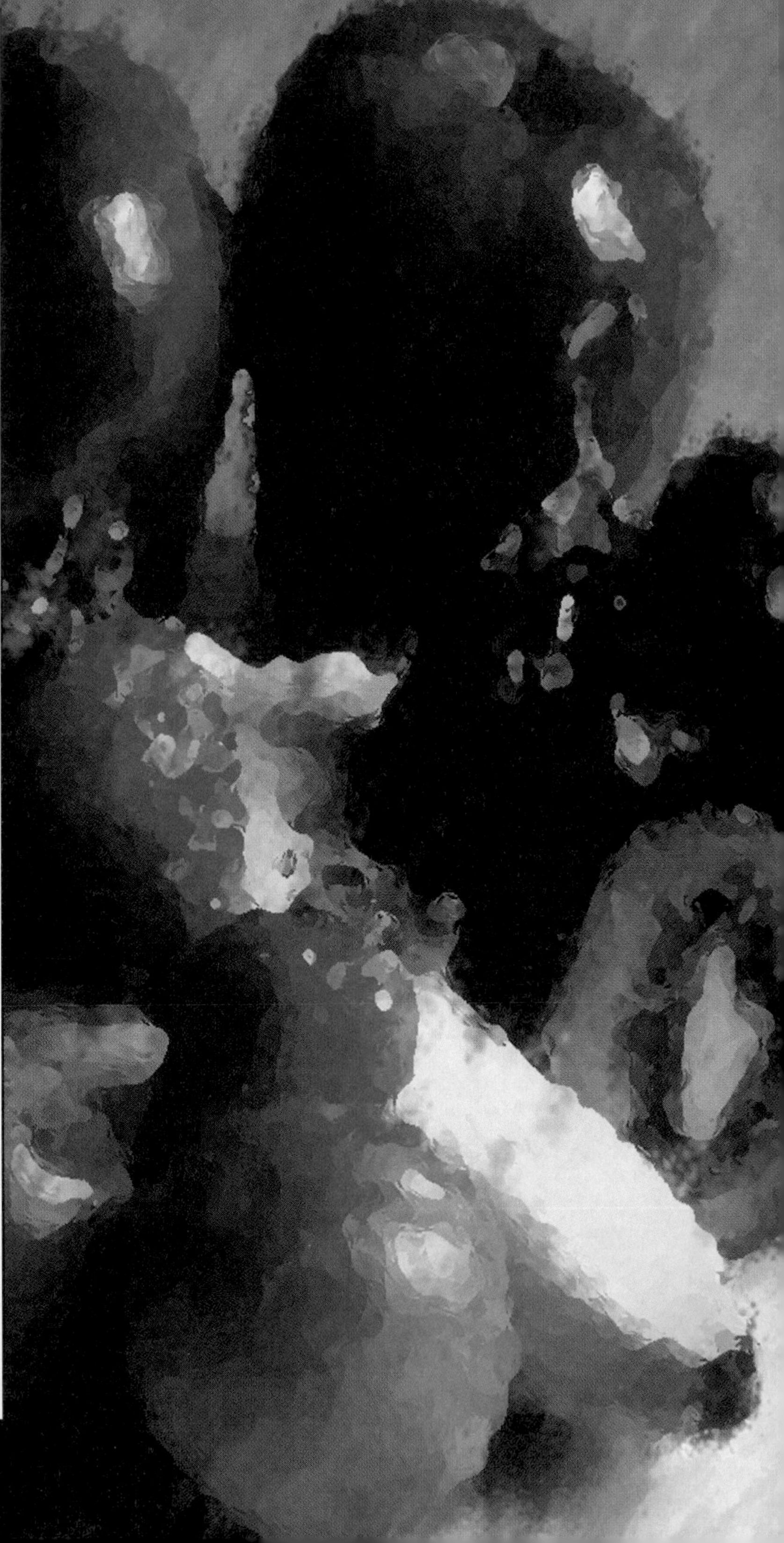

MICROGRAPH: Hemoglobin, the body's oxygen-carrying protein

People commonly associate protein with strength and meat with protein. Consequently, they eat steak to build their muscles, but their thinking is only partly correct. Protein is a vital structural and working substance in all cells, not just muscle cells. Meat is a good source of protein, but so are milk, eggs, legumes, and many grains and vegetables. People who overvalue protein may overemphasize meat in their diets, sometimes at the expense of other, equally important nutrients and foods. Protein is important, but it is only one of the nutrients needed to maintain the body's health.

The Chemist's View of Proteins

Chemically, proteins contain the same atoms as carbohydrates and lipids—carbon, hydrogen, and oxygen—but proteins also contain nitrogen atoms. These nitrogen atoms give the name *amino* (nitrogen containing) to the amino acids—the links in the chains of proteins. Also, proteins assume extraordinary and unique shapes, which enable them to play their vital roles in the body.

proteins: compounds composed of carbon, hydrogen, oxygen, and nitrogen atoms, arranged into amino acids linked in a chain. Some amino acids also contain sulfur atoms.

amino (a-MEEN-oh) **acids:** building blocks of proteins; each contains an amino group, an acid group, a hydrogen atom, and a distinctive side group attached to a central carbon atom.
amino = containing nitrogen

Reminder:
- H forms 1 bond.
- O forms 2 bonds.
- N forms 3 bonds.
- C forms 4 bonds.

AMINO ACIDS

All amino acids have the same basic structure—a central carbon atom with a hydrogen (H), an amino group (NH_2), and an acid group (COOH) attached to it. Carbon atoms need to form four bonds, though, so a fourth attachment is necessary, and it is this fourth site that distinguishes each amino acid from the others. Attached to the carbon atom at the fourth bond is a distinct atom, or group of atoms, known as the *side group* or *side chain* (see Figure 6–1).

Unique Side Groups The side groups on amino acids vary from one amino acid to the next, making proteins more complex than either carbohydrates or lipids. A polysaccharide (starch, for example) may be several thousand units long, but every unit is a glucose molecule just like all the others. A protein, on the other hand, is made up of about 20 different amino acids, each with a different side group. Table 6–1 lists the amino acids most common in proteins.*

The simplest amino acid, glycine, has a hydrogen atom as its side group. A slightly more complex amino acid, alanine, has an extra carbon with three hydrogen atoms. Other amino acids have more complex side groups (see Figure 6–2 for examples). Thus, although all amino acids share a common structure, they differ in size, shape, electrical charge, and other characteristics because of differences in these side groups.

Figure 6–1

Amino Acid Structure

All amino acids have a carbon (known as the alpha-carbon), with an amino group (NH_2), an acid group (COOH), a hydrogen (H), and a side group attached. The side group is a unique chemical structure that differentiates one amino acid from another.

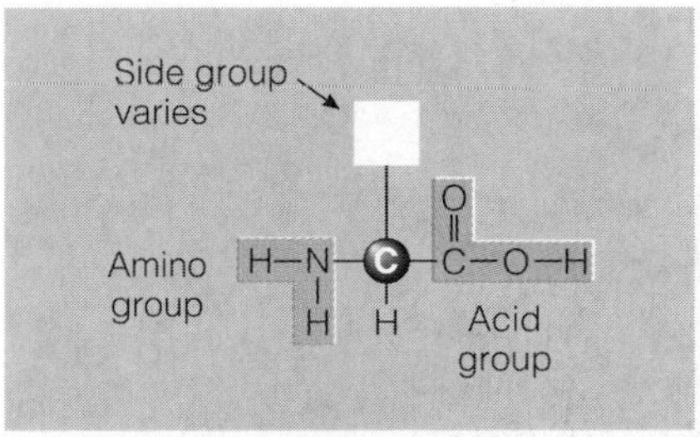

Nonessential Amino Acids The body can synthesize more than half of the amino acids for itself, if it is given nitrogen to form the amino group and fragments

*Amino acids sometimes occur in related forms (for example, proline can acquire an OH group to become hydroxyproline; two cysteines in a protein chain can bind to make cystine). Besides the 20 common amino acids, which can all be components of proteins, others occur individually (for example, taurine and ornithine). Chemists can make still others. This text presents (in Appendix C) the chemical structures of the 20 amino acids most common in proteins, as in Nomenclature policy: Abbreviated designations of amino acids, *Journal of Nutrition* 117 (1987): 15.

Table 6–1

Amino Acids

Proteins are made up of about 20 common amino acids. The first column lists the *essential* amino acids (those the body cannot make—that must be provided in the diet).

Essential Amino Acids		Nonessential Amino Acids	
Histidine	(HISS-tuh-deen)	Alanine	(AL-ah-neen)
Isoleucine	(eye-so-LOO-seen)	Arginine	(ARJ-ih-neen)
Leucine	(LOO-seen)	Asparagine	(ah-SPAR-ah-geen)
Lysine	(LYE-seen)	Aspartic acid	(ah-SPAR-tic acid)
Methionine	(meh-THIGH-oh-neen)	Cysteine	(SIS-teh-een)
Phenylalanine	(fen-il-AL-ah-neen)	Glutamic acid	(GLU-tam-ic acid)
Threonine	(THREE-oh-neen)	Glutamine	(GLU-tah-meen)
Tryptophan	(TRIP-toe-fan, TRIP-toe-fane)	Glycine	(GLY-seen)
		Proline	(PRO-leen)
Valine	(VAY-leen)	Serine	(SEER-een)
		Tyrosine	(TIE-roe-seen)

Note: In special cases, some nonessential amino acids may become conditionally essential (see the text).

from carbohydrate and fat to form the rest of the structure. Proteins in foods usually deliver these amino acids, but it is not essential that they do so.

essential amino acids: amino acids that the body cannot synthesize in amounts sufficient to meet physiological needs (see Table 6–1). Some researchers refer to essential amino acids as **indispensable** and to nonessential amino acids as **dispensable**.

conditionally essential amino acid: an amino acid that is normally nonessential, but must be supplied by the diet in special circumstances when the need for it exceeds the body's ability to produce it.

Essential Amino Acids There are nine amino acids that the body either cannot make at all or cannot make in sufficient quantity to meet its needs. These nine amino acids must be supplied by the diet; they are essential.

Conditionally Essential Amino Acids Sometimes a nonessential amino acid becomes essential under special circumstances. For example, the body normally makes tyrosine (a nonessential amino acid) from the essential amino acid phenylalanine. But if the diet fails to supply enough phenylalanine, or if the body cannot make the conversion for some reason (as happens in the inherited disease phenylketonuria), then tyrosine becomes *conditionally* essential.

Figure 6–2

Examples of Amino Acids

Note that all amino acids have a common chemical structure but that each has a different side chain.

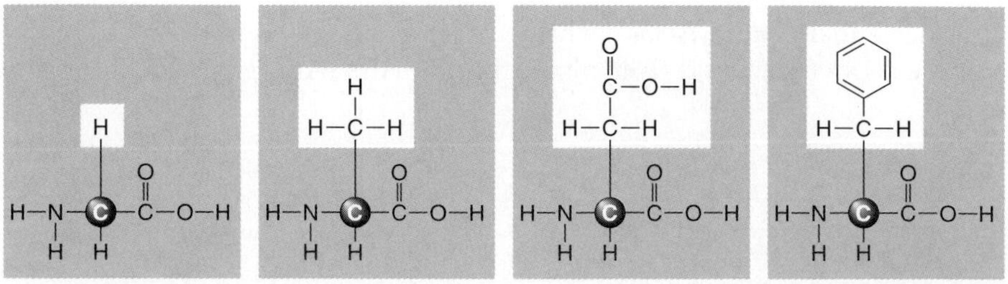

Glycine Alanine Aspartic acid Phenylalanine

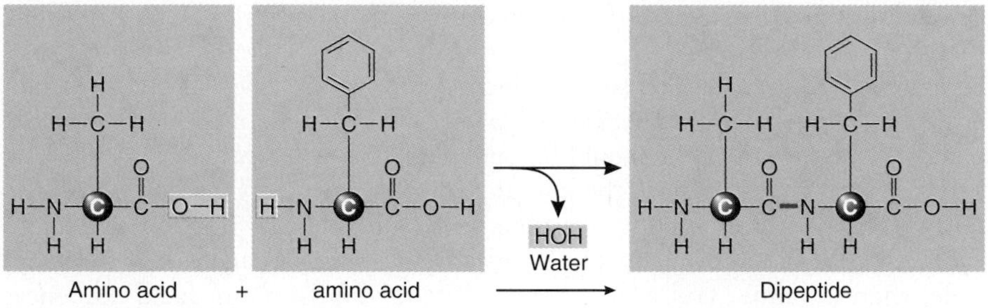

An OH group from the acid end of one amino acid and an H atom from the amino group of another join to form a molecule of water.

A peptide bond (highlighted in red) forms between the two amino acids, creating a dipeptide.

Figure 6–3

Condensation of Two Amino Acids to Form a Dipeptide

PROTEINS

Cells link amino acids end-to-end in a virtually infinite variety of sequences to form thousands of different proteins. Each link connecting one amino acid with another is a peptide bond.

Amino Acid Chains Condensation reactions create the bonds between amino acids, just as they combine monosaccharides to form disaccharides, and fatty acids with glycerol to form triglycerides.* Two amino acids bonded together form a dipeptide (see Figure 6–3). By another such reaction, a third amino acid can be added to the chain to form a tripeptide. As additional amino acids join the chain, a polypeptide is formed. Most proteins are a few dozen to several hundred amino acids long. Figure 6–4 provides an example—insulin.

*Later in this chapter, Figure 6–6 shows how each protein's sequence is dictated by the genetic code in DNA, and the text describes how the sequence shapes the protein.

peptide bond: a bond that connects the acid end of one amino acid with the amino end of another, forming a link in a protein chain.

dipeptide: two amino acids bonded together.
di = two
peptide = amino acid

tripeptide: three amino acids bonded together.
tri = three

polypeptide: many (ten or more) amino acids bonded together. An intermediate string of four to nine amino acids is an **oligopeptide**.
poly = many
oligo = few

Figure 6–4

Amino Acid Sequence of Human Insulin

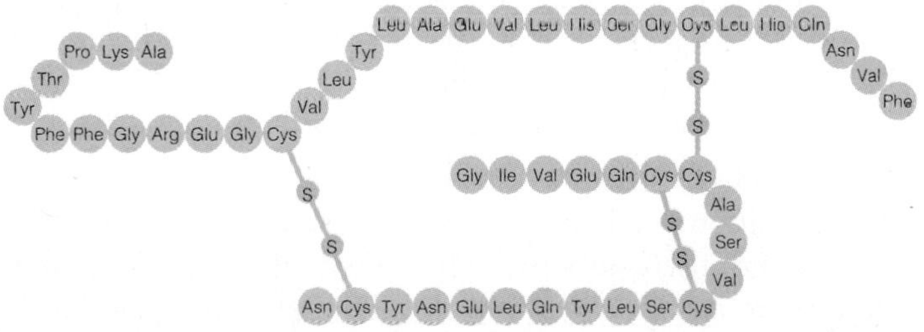

Human insulin is a relatively small protein that consists of 51 amino acids in two short polypeptide chains. (For amino acid abbreviations, see Appendix C.) Two bridges link the two chains. A third bridge spans a section within the short chain.

Known as disulfide bridges, these links always involve the amino acid cysteine (cys), whose side group contains sulfur. Cysteines connect to each other when bonds form between these side groups.

Amino Acid Sequences If a person could step onto a carbohydrate molecule like starch and walk along it, the first stepping stone would be a glucose. The next stepping stone would also be a glucose, and it would be followed by a glucose, and yet another glucose. But if a person were to walk along a polypeptide chain, each stepping stone would be one of 20-odd different amino acids. The first stepping stone might be the amino acid methionine. The second might be an alanine. The third might be a glycine, and the fourth a tryptophan, and so on. Walking along another polypeptide path, a person might step on a phenylalanine, then a valine, and a glutamine. In other words, amino acid sequences within proteins vary.

The amino acids can act somewhat like the letters in an alphabet. If you only had the letter G, you could write an unvarying string of Gs: G–G–G–G–G–G–G. But with 20 different letters available, you could create poems, songs, or novels. The 20 amino acids can be linked together in an even greater variety of sequences than are possible for letters in a word or words in a sentence. Thus the variety of possible sequences for polypeptide chains is tremendous.

Protein Shapes Polypeptide chains twist into complex, tangled shapes. Each amino acid has a unique chemical character that attracts it to, or repels it from, the surrounding fluids and other amino acids. Some amino acid side chains carry electrical charges that are attracted to water molecules (they are hydrophilic). Other side chains are neutral and are repelled by water (they are hydrophobic). As amino acids are strung together to make a polypeptide, the chain folds so that its charged hydrophilic side chains are on the outer surface near water; the neutral hydrophobic groups tuck themselves inside, away from water. The intricate, coiled shape the polypeptide finally assumes gives it maximum stability in the body's watery fluids.

Reminder: Substances that are attracted to water are *hydrophilic;* those that are repelled by water are *hydrophobic*.

Protein Functions The different shapes of proteins enable them to perform various tasks in the body. Some form hollow balls that can carry and store materials within them, and some, such as those of tendons, are more than ten times as long as they are wide, forming strong, rodlike structures. Some polypeptides may be functioning proteins as they are; others may need to associate with other polypeptides to form larger working complexes. Some proteins require minerals to activate them. One molecule of hemoglobin—the large, globular protein molecule that, by the billions, packs the red blood cells and carries oxygen—is made of four associated polypeptide chains, each holding the mineral iron.

hemoglobin: the globular protein of the red blood cells that carries oxygen from the lungs to the cells throughout the body.
hemo = blood
globin = globular protein

denaturation: the change in a protein's shape brought about by heat, acid, base, alcohol, heavy metals, or other agents.

Protein Denaturation When proteins are subjected to heat, acid, or other conditions that disturb their stability, they undergo denaturation—that is, they uncoil and lose their shapes and, consequently, their functions. Past a certain point, denaturation is irreversible. Familiar examples of denaturation include the hardening of an egg when it is cooked, the curdling of milk when acid is added, and the stiffening of egg whites when they are whipped.

In summary, proteins are made of some 20 different amino acids, 9 of which the body cannot make (they are essential). Cells synthesize each protein that they need by stringing together amino acids in a distinctive sequence.

Digestion and Absorption of Protein

Proteins in foods do not become body proteins, but supply the amino acids from which the body makes its own proteins. When a person eats foods containing protein, enzymes break the long polypeptide strands into shorter strands, the short strands into tripeptides and dipeptides, and finally, the tripeptides and dipeptides into amino acids.

THE PROCESS OF DIGESTION

Figure 6–5 illustrates the digestion of protein through the GI tract. Proteins are crushed and moistened in the mouth, but the real action begins in the stomach.

In the Stomach In the stomach, hydrochloric acid uncoils (denatures) each protein's tangled strands so that digestive enzymes can attack the peptide bonds. The hydrochloric acid also converts the inactive form of the enzyme pepsinogen to its active form pepsin. Pepsin cleaves proteins—large polypeptides—into smaller polypeptides and some amino acids.

Reminder: An enzyme that hydrolyzes protein is a *protease*.

The inactive form of an enzyme is called a **proenzyme**.

pro = before

pepsin: a gastric protease. Pepsin is secreted in an inactive form, **pepsinogen**, which is activated by stomach acid.

In the Small Intestine When polypeptides enter the small intestine, pancreatic and intestinal proteases hydrolyze them further into short peptide chains (oligopeptides), tripeptides, dipeptides, and amino acids. Figure 6–5 includes the details of digestive enzyme action for dietary protein. A number of distinct carriers transport these protein pieces into the intestinal cells.

THE PROCESS OF ABSORPTION

The cells of the small intestine absorb amino acids and have peptidase enzymes on their surfaces that split most of the dipeptides and tripeptides into single amino acids. A few dipeptides, tripeptides, and even larger molecules sometimes escape digestion and cross the digestive tract wall to enter the bloodstream.

peptidase: a digestive enzyme that hydrolyzes peptide bonds. *Tripeptidases* cleave tripeptides; *dipeptidases* cleave dipeptides. *Endopeptidases* cleave peptide bonds *within* the chain to create smaller fragments, whereas *exopeptidases* cleave bonds at the *ends* to release free amino acids.

Some nutrition faddists fail to realize that most proteins are broken down to amino acids before absorption. They urge consumers to "Eat enzyme A. It will help you digest your food." Or "Don't eat food B. It contains enzyme C, which will digest cells in your body." In reality, though, enzymes in foods are digested, just as all proteins are. Only the digestive enzymes, whose design prevents them from being denatured or digested, can work in such an environment.

Another misconception is that eating predigested proteins (amino acid supplements) saves the body from having to digest proteins and keeps the digestive system from "overworking." Such a belief grossly underestimates the body's abilities. As a matter of fact, the digestive system handles whole proteins *better* than predigested ones because it dismantles and absorbs the amino acids at rates that are optimal for the body's use.[1] (The last section of this chapter discusses amino acid supplements further.)

In short, via digestion facilitated mostly by the stomach's acid and enzymes, the body first denatures dietary proteins, then cleaves them into polypeptides, then oligo-, tri-, and dipeptides, and some amino acids. Intestinal enzymes split these

Figure 6–5

Protein Digestion in the GI Tract

Protein Digestive Enzymes

In the Stomach:

HCl
- Denatures protein structure.
- Activates pepsinogen to pepsin.

Pepsin
- Cleaves proteins to smaller polypeptides and some free amino acids.
- Inhibits pepsinogen synthesis.

In the Small Intestine:

Enteropeptidase[a]
- Converts pancreatic trypsinogen to trypsin.

Trypsin
- Converts pancreatic chymotrypsinogen to chymotrypsin.
- Converts pancreatic procarboxypeptidases to carboxypeptidases.
- Inhibits trypsinogen synthesis.
- Cleaves peptide bonds next to the amino acids lysine and arginine.

Chymotrypsin
- Cleaves peptide bonds next to the amino acids phenylalanine, tyrosine, tryptophan, methionine, asparagine, and histidine.

Elastase and collagenase
- Cleave polypeptides into smaller polypeptides and tripeptides.

Carboxypeptidases
- Cleave amino acids from the acid (carboxyl) ends of polypeptides.

Aminopeptidases
- Cleave amino acids from the amino ends of small polypeptides (oligopeptides).

Tripeptidases
- Cleave tripeptides to dipeptides and amino acids.

[a]Enteropeptidase was formerly known as *enterokinase*.

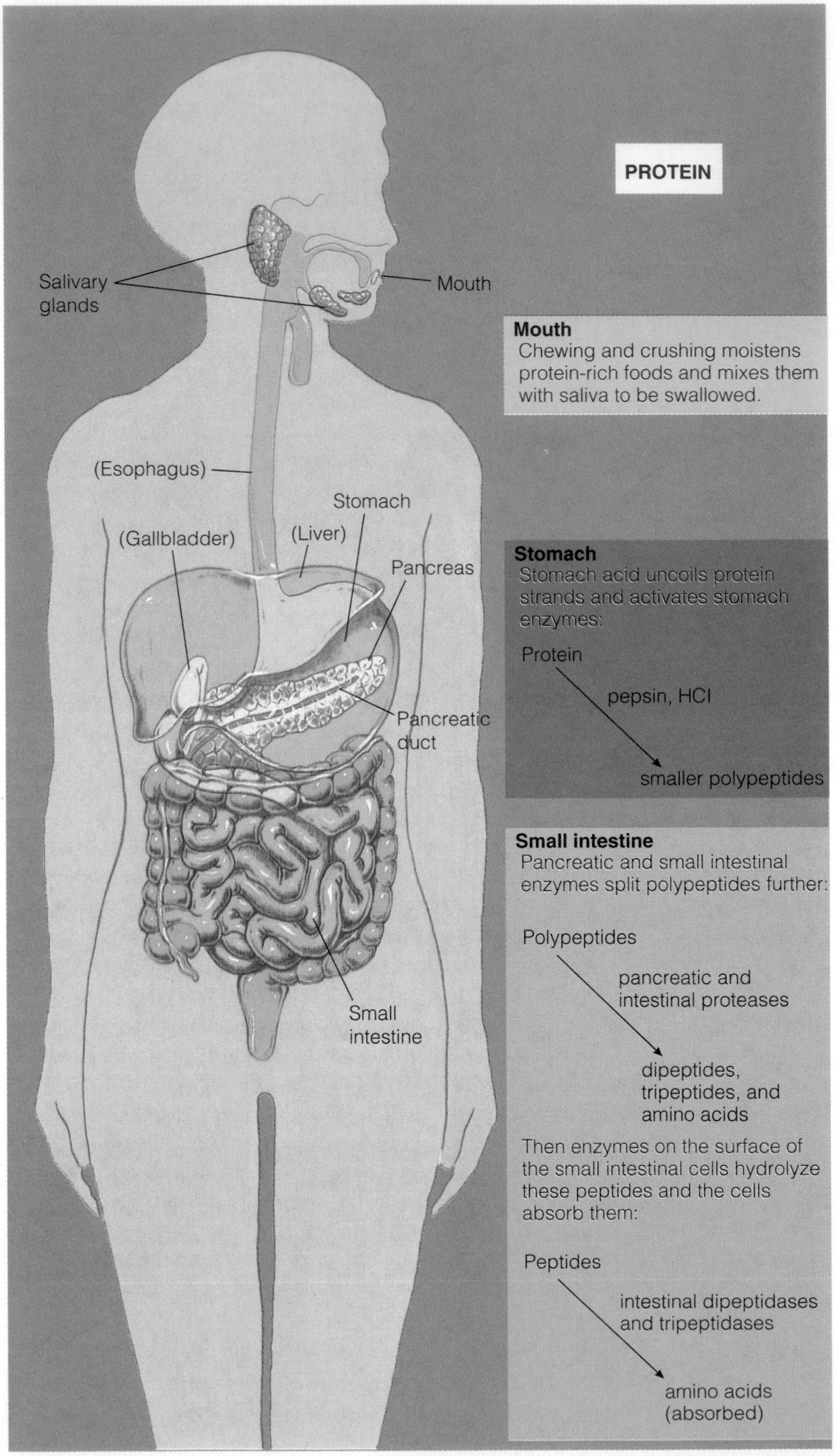
PROTEIN
Salivary glands
Mouth
(Esophagus)
Stomach
(Gallbladder)
(Liver)
Pancreas
Pancreatic duct
Small intestine
Mouth
Chewing and crushing moistens protein-rich foods and mixes them with saliva to be swallowed.
Stomach
Stomach acid uncoils protein strands and activates stomach enzymes:
Protein
pepsin, HCl
smaller polypeptides
Small intestine
Pancreatic and small intestinal enzymes split polypeptides further:
Polypeptides
pancreatic and intestinal proteases
dipeptides, tripeptides, and amino acids
Then enzymes on the surface of the small intestinal cells hydrolyze these peptides and the cells absorb them:
Peptides
intestinal dipeptidases and tripeptidases
amino acids (absorbed)

further, mostly to single amino acids. Then carriers in the membranes of intestinal cells transport the amino acids into the cells, where they are released into the bloodstream.

Proteins in the Body

The human body contains an estimated 10,000 to 50,000 different kinds of proteins. Of these, about 1000 have been studied. Only about 10 are described in this chapter—but these should be enough to illustrate proteins' versatility, uniqueness, and importance. As you will see, each protein has a specific function and that function is determined during protein synthesis.

PROTEIN SYNTHESIS

Each human being is unique because of minute differences in the body's proteins. These differences are determined by the amino acid sequences of proteins, which are in turn determined by genetics. The following paragraphs describe in words the ways cells synthesize proteins; Figure 6–6 provides a pictorial description.

The instructions for making every protein in a person's body are transmitted by way of the genetic information received at conception. This body of knowledge, which is filed in the DNA within the nucleus of every cell, never leaves the nucleus.

Delivering the Instructions To inform a cell of the sequence of amino acids for a needed protein, a stretch of DNA serves as a template for making a strand of RNA that carries a code, listing in order the amino acids that will be needed to make a given protein. Known as messenger RNA, this molecule escapes through the nuclear membrane. Messenger RNA seeks out and attaches itself to one of the ribosomes (a protein-making machine, which is itself composed of RNA and protein). Thus situated, messenger RNA presents its list, specifying the sequence in which the amino acids are to line up to make a strand of protein.

Lining Up the Amino Acids Other forms of RNA, called transfer RNA, collect amino acids from the cell fluid and bring them to the messenger. Each of the 20 amino acids has a specific transfer RNA. Thousands of transfer RNA, each carrying its amino acid, cluster around the ribosomes, awaiting their turn to unload. When the messenger's list calls for a specific amino acid, the transfer RNA carrying that amino acid moves into position. Then the next loaded transfer RNA moves into place and then the next and the next. Thus the amino acids line up in the sequence that is called for, and enzymes bind them together. Finally, the completed protein strand is released, the messenger is degraded, and the transfer RNA are freed to return for another load of amino acids.

Sequencing Errors The sequence of amino acids in each protein determines its configuration, which supports a specific function. If a genetic error alters the amino acid sequence of a protein, or if a mistake is made in copying the sequence, an altered protein will result, sometimes with dramatic consequences. The protein hemoglobin offers one example of such a genetic variation. In a person with sickle-cell anemia, two of hemoglobin's four polypeptide chains (described earlier

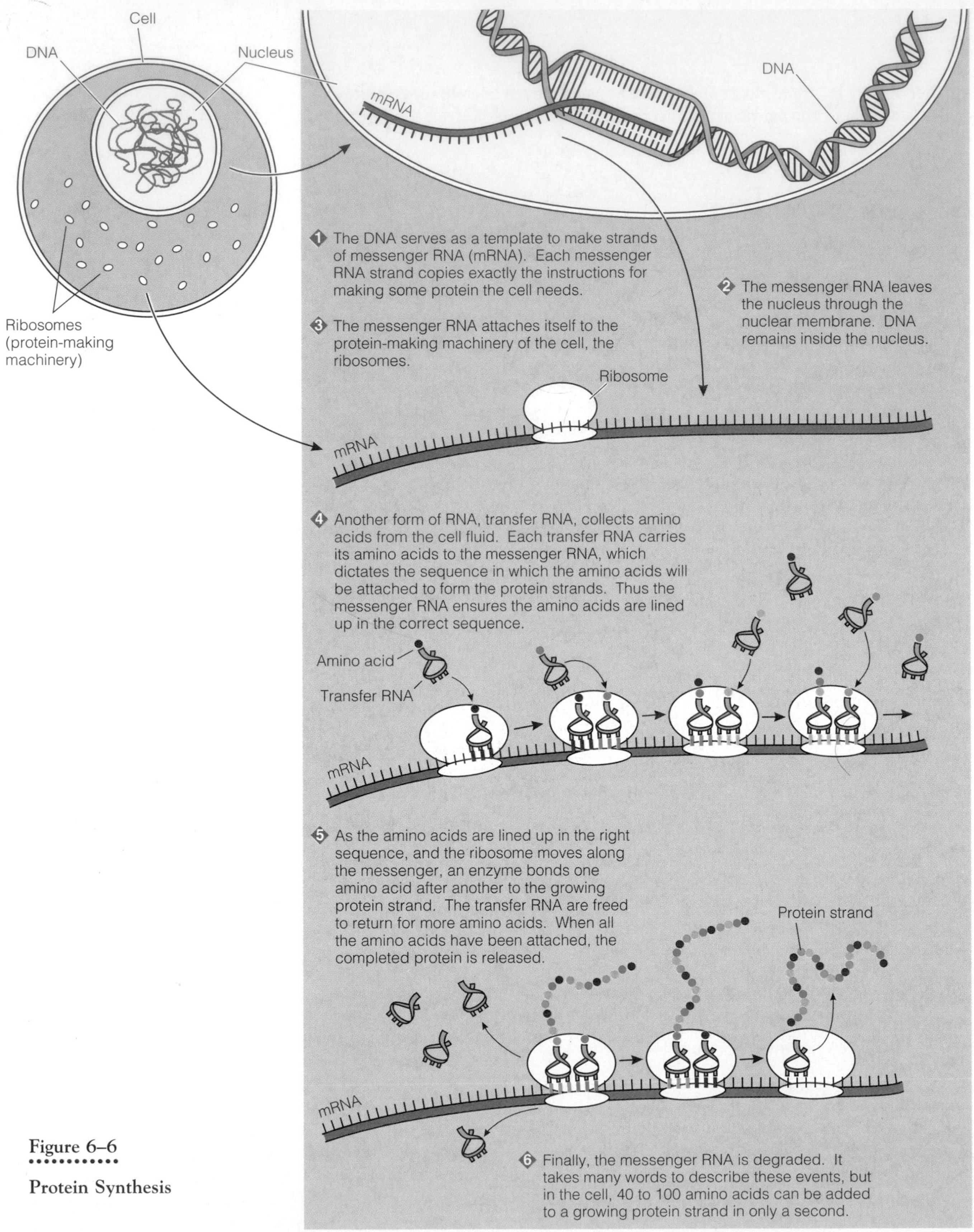
Cell
DNA
Nucleus
Ribosomes (protein-making machinery)
mRNA
DNA
1 The DNA serves as a template to make strands of messenger RNA (mRNA). Each messenger RNA strand copies exactly the instructions for making some protein the cell needs.
2 The messenger RNA leaves the nucleus through the nuclear membrane. DNA remains inside the nucleus.
3 The messenger RNA attaches itself to the protein-making machinery of the cell, the ribosomes.
Ribosome
mRNA
4 Another form of RNA, transfer RNA, collects amino acids from the cell fluid. Each transfer RNA carries its amino acids to the messenger RNA, which dictates the sequence in which the amino acids will be attached to form the protein strands. Thus the messenger RNA ensures the amino acids are lined up in the correct sequence.
Amino acid
Transfer RNA
mRNA
5 As the amino acids are lined up in the right sequence, and the ribosome moves along the messenger, an enzyme bonds one amino acid after another to the growing protein strand. The transfer RNA are freed to return for more amino acids. When all the amino acids have been attached, the completed protein is released.
Protein strand
mRNA
6 Finally, the messenger RNA is degraded. It takes many words to describe these events, but in the cell, 40 to 100 amino acids can be added to a growing protein strand in only a second.

Figure 6–6

Protein Synthesis

Figure 6–7

Normal Red Blood Cells Compared with Sickle-Cells

Normally, red blood cells are disc-shaped; in the inherited disorder sickle-cell anemia, red blood cells are sickle- or crescent-shaped. This alteration in shape occurs because valine replaces glutamic acid in the amino acid sequence of hemoglobin's polypeptide chain. As a result of this one amino acid's being in the wrong place, the hemoglobin has a diminished capacity to carry oxygen.

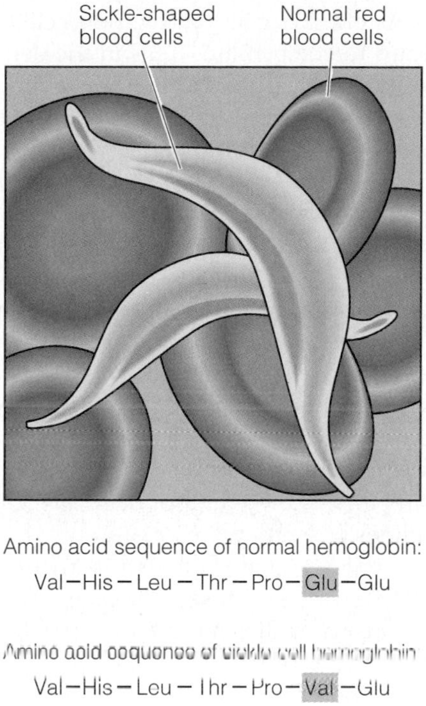

sickle-cell anemia: a hereditary form of anemia characterized by abnormal sickle- or crescent-shaped red blood cells. Sickled cells interfere with oxygen transport and blood flow. Symptoms include hemolytic anemia (red blood cells burst), fever, and severe pain in the joints and abdomen; they are precipitated by dehydration and insufficient oxygen (as may occur at high altitudes).

Note: Anemia is not a disease, but a symptom of various diseases. In the case of sickle-cell anemia, a defect in the hemoglobin molecule changes the shape of the red blood cells. Later chapters describe how vitamin and mineral deficiencies change the size and color of the red blood cells. In all cases, the abnormal blood cells are unable to meet the body's oxygen demands.

on p. 200) have the normal sequence of amino acids, but the other two chains do not—they have the amino acid valine in a position that is normally occupied by glutamic acid (see Figure 6–7). This single alteration in the amino acid sequence changes the character and shape of the protein so much that hemoglobin loses its ability to carry oxygen effectively. The red blood cells filled with this abnormal hemoglobin stiffen into elongated sickle, or crescent, shapes instead of maintaining their normal pliable disc shape—hence the name, sickle cell anemia. Sickle-cell anemia causes many medical problems and can be fatal.

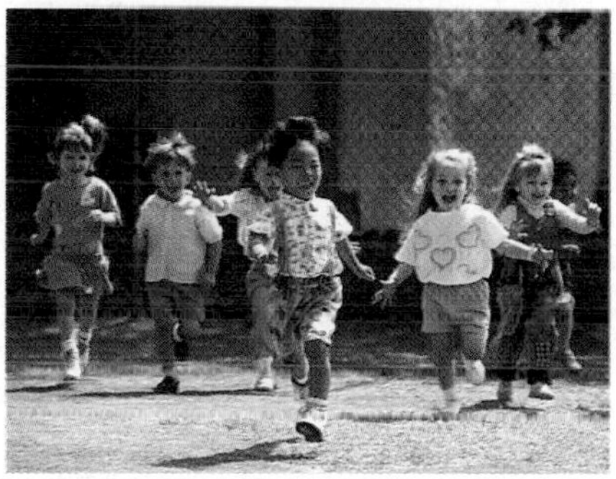

Growing children end each day with more bone, blood, muscle, and skin cells than they had at the beginning of the day.

ROLES OF PROTEINS

Whenever the body is growing, repairing, or replacing tissue, proteins are involved. Sometimes their role is to facilitate or to regulate; other times it is to become part of a structure. Yes, versatility is a key feature of proteins.

As Building Materials From the moment of conception, as the body grows, it uses proteins as building blocks. For example, to build a bone or a tooth, cells first lay down a matrix of the protein collagen and then fill it with crystals of calcium, phosphorus, fluoride, and other minerals.

The protein collagen is also the material of ligaments and tendons and the strengthening glue between the cells of the artery walls that enables the arteries to withstand the pressure of the blood surging through them with each heartbeat. Also made of collagen are scars that knit the separated parts of torn tissues together.

collagen: the protein material from which connective tissues such as scars, tendons, ligaments, and the foundations of bones and teeth are made.

matrix (MAY-tricks): the basic substance that gives form to a developing structure; in the body, the formative cells from which teeth and bones grow.

As old skin cells fall off, new cells made largely of protein grow from underneath to compensate. Cells in the deeper skin layers synthesize new proteins to go into hair and fingernails. GI tract cells are replaced every three days. Both inside and outside, then, the body constantly deposits protein into new cells that replace those that have been lost.

enzymes: proteins that facilitate chemical reactions without being changed in the process; protein catalysts.

The breakdown of large molecules into smaller ones is known as *catabolism;* the synthesis of small molecules into larger ones is known as *anabolism*. These two types of reactions receive further attention in Chapter 7.

synthetase (SIN-the-tase): an enzyme that enables two or more substances to form a more complex structure.

As Enzymes Digestive enzymes have appeared in every chapter since Chapter 3, but digestion is only one of the many processes enzymes facilitate. Enzymes not only break down substances, they also build substances and transform one substance into another. Figure 6–8 diagrams a synthesis reaction.

An analogy may help to clarify the role of enzymes. Enzymes are comparable to the clergy and judges who make and dissolve marriages. When a minister marries two people, they become a couple, with a new bond between them. They are joined together—but the minister remains unchanged. The minister represents synthetase enzymes that make large compounds from smaller ones. One minister can perform thousands of marriage ceremonies, just as one enzyme can perform billions of synthetic reactions.

Similarly, a judge who lets married couples separate may decree many divorces before retiring or dying. The judge represents enzymes that hydrolyze larger compounds to smaller ones; for example, the digestive enzymes. The point is that, like the minister and the judge, enzymes themselves are not altered by the reactions they facilitate. They are catalysts, permitting reactions to occur more quickly and efficiently than if substances depended on chance encounters alone.

The chemical structures in the margin and the paragraphs that follow provide an example of enzyme action. This single biochemical pathway illustrates how one compound encounters an enzyme, is converted to another compound that encounters another enzyme, and so forth until the final product is entirely different from the starting material. The details are offered only to give you insight into the kinds of processes that take place in the daily lives of the body's cells.

In the breakdown of glucose (a 6-carbon compound), enzymes add two phosphate groups, alter the arrangement of the atoms, and then split the molecule in half, leaving two 3-carbon compounds. One of these is compound A and the other is converted to compound A, so the two halves derived from glucose follow the same path from that point on.

Figure 6–8

Enzyme Action

Each enzyme facilitates a specific chemical reaction. In this diagram, an enzyme enables two compounds to make a more complex structure, but the enzyme itself remains unchanged.

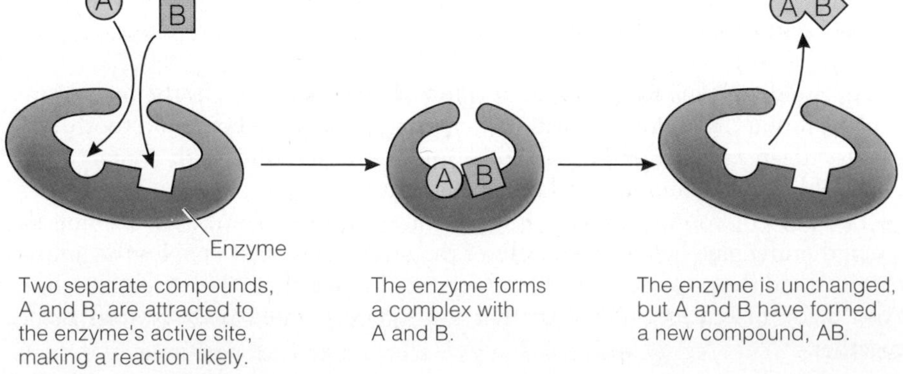

A
B
Enzyme
A B
A B
Two separate compounds, A and B, are attracted to the enzyme's active site, making a reaction likely.
The enzyme forms a complex with A and B.
The enzyme is unchanged, but A and B have formed a new compound, AB.

Compound A floats around until it encounters an enzyme that recognizes it. This enzyme removes hydrogens from molecules of compound A. Without hydrogens, carbon and oxygen must form a double-bond; thus compound B is created. Compound B is released from this enzyme and encounters another enzyme that removes an oxygen and substitutes an amino group in its place; the result is compound C. The next enzyme removes the phosphate group and replaces it with a hydrogen, leaving compound D.

The characteristics of compound D become apparent upon close examination and may not surprise some readers, but this example takes the process one step further before revealing the identity of compound D. Another enzyme, whose function is to remove CH_2OH groups from molecules, forms compound E.

Compound E appeared earlier in this chapter. It has an amino group at one end, an acid group at the other, and a central carbon carrying two hydrogen atoms. It is the amino acid glycine (introduced in Figure 6–2).

Amazing! The cellular machinery started with a molecule of glucose (a derivative of dietary carbohydrate), made one small change after another, and transformed it into an amino acid (a member of the protein family). The lesson of this sequence of events is that the body can use glucose and nitrogen-containing compounds to make many of the amino acids needed to build body proteins. The nonessential amino acid glycine is just one example. Compound D, which precedes glycine on the pathway, is another example: the nonessential amino acid serine. Thus, among the thousands of tasks that enzymes perform, they even manufacture many of the nonessential amino acids they themselves are made of.

Perhaps you have realized by now that the protein story is circular. To follow the circle in nutrition, start with a person eating food proteins. The proteins are broken down by proteins (digestive enzymes) into amino acids. The amino acids enter the body cells, where proteins (synthetases) link them into long chains whose sequences are specified by DNA. The chains twist and fold forming proteins, some of which are enzymes. Some enzymes break apart compounds; others put compounds together. Day by day, in billions of reactions, these processes repeat themselves, and life goes on. Only living systems work with such self-renewal. A car cannot make another car; a toaster cannot fix another toaster. Only living creatures and the parts they are composed of—the cells—can duplicate and repair themselves.

As Hormones Cells can switch their protein machinery on or off in response to the body's needs. Often hormones do the switching, with marvelous precision. The body's many hormones are messenger molecules, and some hormones are proteins. Various glands in the body release hormones in response to changes in the internal environment. The blood carries the hormones to their target tissues, where they elicit the appropriate responses to restore normal conditions.

The hormone insulin provides a familiar example. When blood glucose rises, the pancreas steps up its release of insulin. Insulin stimulates the cells' transport proteins to pump glucose into the cells faster than it can leak out. (After acting on the message, the cells destroy the insulin.) Then, as blood glucose falls the pancreas reduces its insulin output. Many other proteins act as hormones maintaining the distribution of hundreds of substances in the body (see Table 6–2).

As Regulators of Fluid and Electrolyte Balance Proteins help to maintain the body's fluid and electrolyte balance. As Figure 6–9 shows, the body's fluids

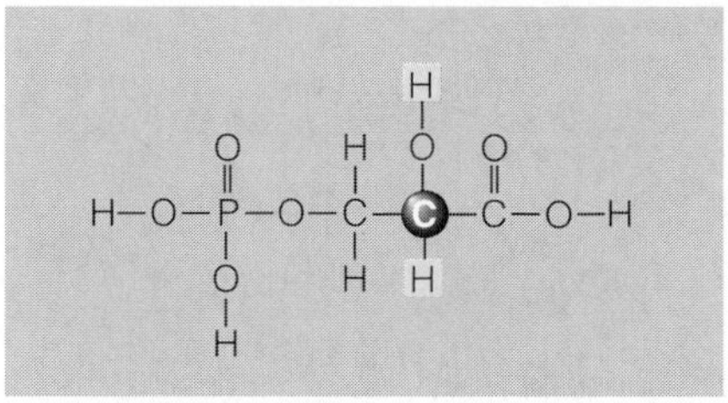

Compound A

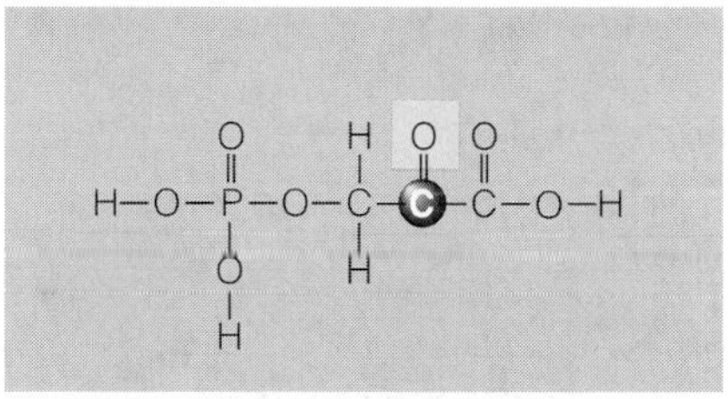

Compound B

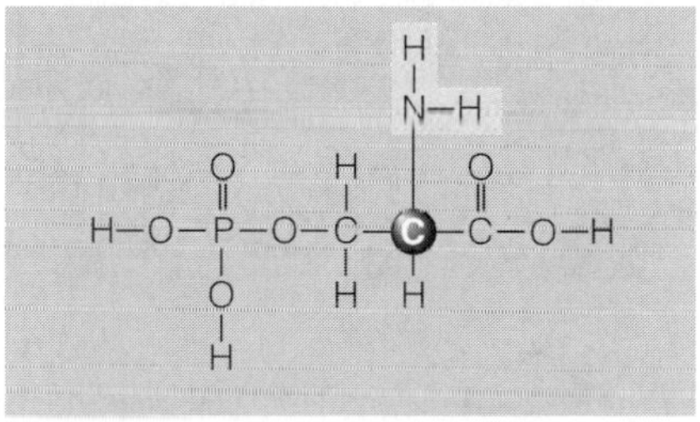

Compound C

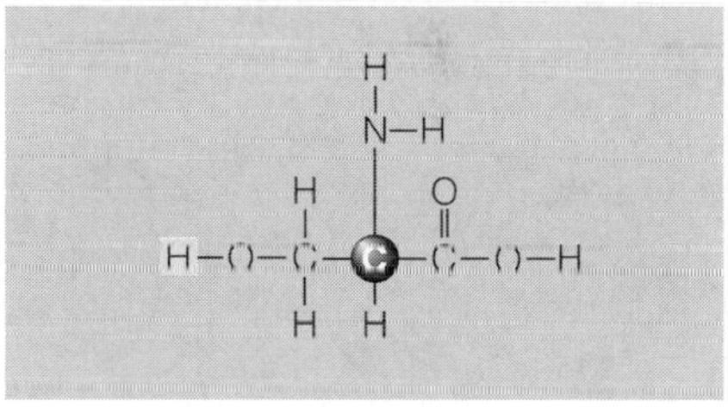

Compound D

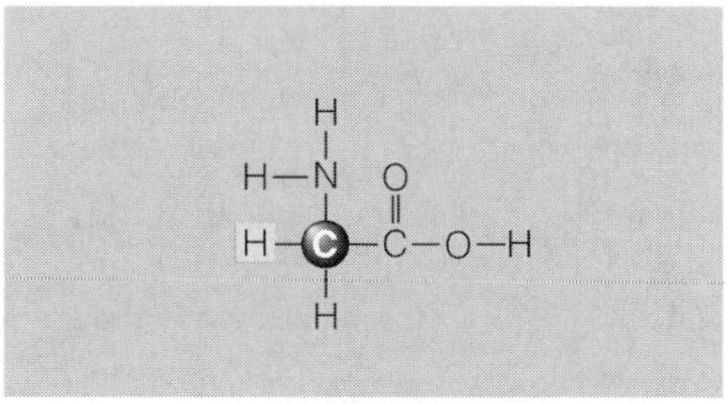

Compound E

fluid and electrolyte balance: maintenance of the proper types and amounts of fluid and minerals in each compartment of the body fluids (see also Chapter 12).

Figure 6–9

One Cell and Its Associated Fluids

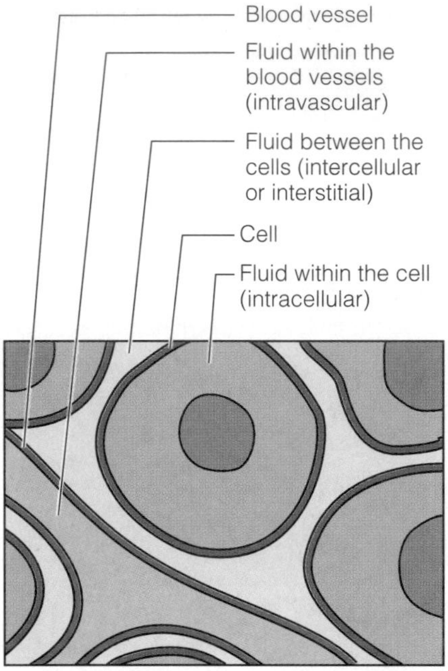

Minerals also help regulate fluid distribution; Chapter 12 provides more details.

edema (eh-DEEM-uh): the swelling of body tissue caused by excessive amounts of fluid in the interstitial spaces; seen in protein deficiency (among other conditions).

acids: compounds that release hydrogen ions in a solution.

bases: compounds that accept hydrogen ions in a solution.

Reminder: The *acid-base balance* is the equilibrium between acid and base concentrations in the blood and body fluids.

buffers: compounds that help keep a solution's acidity or alkalinity constant.

acidosis (assi-DOE-sis): above-normal acidity in the blood and body fluids.

alkalosis (alka-LOE-sis): above-normal alkalinity (base) in the blood and body fluids.

Table 6–2

Examples of Hormones and Their Actions

Hormones	Actions
Growth hormone	Promotes growth.
Insulin and glucagon	Regulate blood glucose (see Chapter 4).
Thyroxin	Regulates the body's metabolic rate (see Chapter 7).
Calcitonin and parathormone	Regulate blood calcium (see Chapter 12).
Antidiuretic hormone	Regulates fluid and electrolyte balance (see Chapter 12).

Note: Hormones are chemical messengers that are secreted by endocrine glands in response to altered conditions in the body. Each travels to one or more specific target tissues or organs, where it elicits a specific response. For descriptions of many hormones important in nutrition, see Appendix A.

are contained inside the blood vessels (intravascular), within the cells (intracellular), and surrounding the cells (intercellular). Fluids can flow freely between these compartments, but the cells can't move fluids directly. They can manufacture proteins, though. Being large, proteins cannot pass freely across membranes; they are trapped on one side where they attract water. By making and keeping proteins, cells can retain fluids. Similarly, the cells can ship proteins out into the blood and intercellular spaces to maintain the fluid volume there. Should this system fail, too much fluid would collect outside the cells, causing edema.

Not only the quantity, but also the composition of body fluids depend on proteins. Special transport proteins maintain equilibrium in the surrounding fluids by moving molecules into and out of cells. Most of these proteins reside in cell membranes and act as "pumps," picking up compounds on one side of the membrane and depositing them on the other. In doing so, transport proteins enable cells to take up and release substances as needed. Each transport protein is specific for a certain compound or group of related compounds. Figure 6–10 illustrates how a membrane-bound transport protein maintains the sodium and potassium concentrations in the fluids inside and outside of the cells. The balance of these two electrolytes is critical to neural transmissions and muscle contractions; any disturbance triggers a major medical emergency. Such imbalances can cause irregular heartbeats, muscular weakness, kidney failure, and even death.

As Acid-Base Regulators Proteins also help to maintain the balance between acids and bases within the body fluids. Normal body processes continually produce acids and bases, which the blood carries to the kidneys and lungs for excretion. The challenge is to do this without upsetting the blood's acid-base balance.

In an acid solution, hydrogen ions abound; the more hydrogen ions, the more concentrated the acid. Proteins, which have negative charges on their surfaces, attract hydrogen ions, which have positive charges. By accepting and releasing hydrogen ions, proteins act as buffers, maintaining the acid-base balance of the blood and body fluids.

The blood's acid-base balance is tightly controlled. The extremes of acidosis and alkalosis lead to coma and death, largely because they denature working pro-

Figure 6–10

Transport Proteins

A transport protein within a cell membrane picks up substances on one side of the membrane and carries them to the other side without leaving the membrane. The substances being transported here are sodium and potassium. Maintaining a high concentration of potassium and a low concentration of sodium within the cells requires energy.

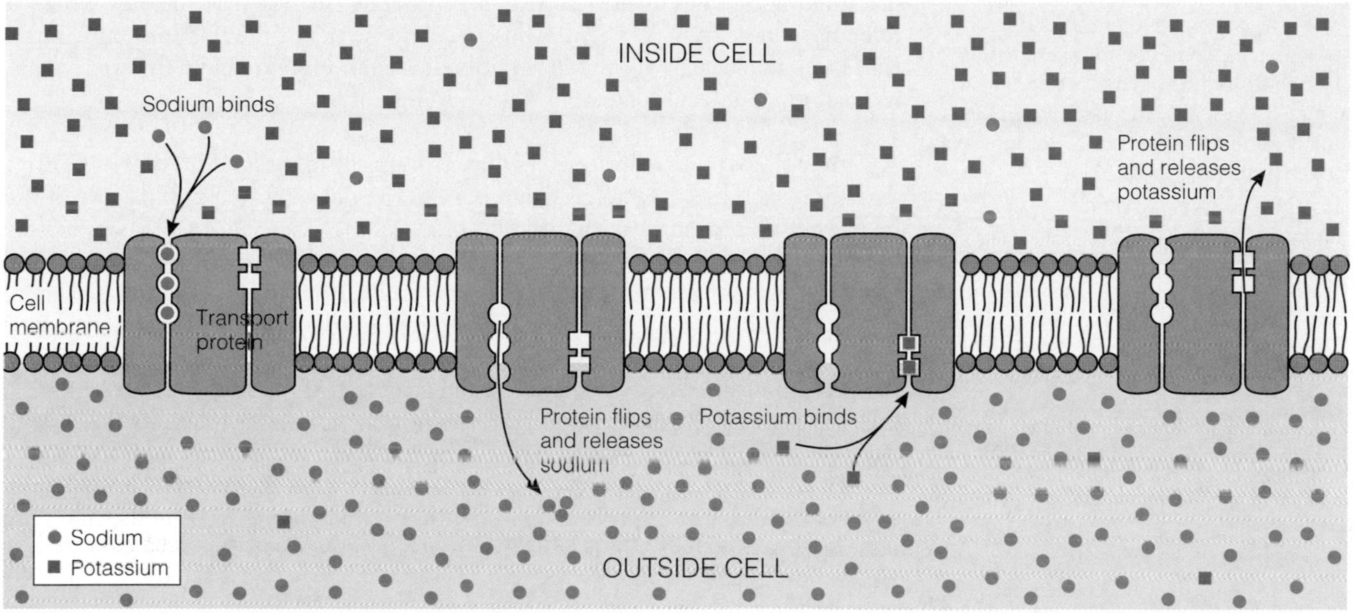

teins. Disturbing a protein's shape renders it useless. To give just one example, hemoglobin, when denatured, loses its capacity to carry oxygen.

As Transporters Some transport proteins are not attached to membranes, but move about in the body fluids, carrying nutrients and other molecules. The protein hemoglobin carries oxygen from the lungs to the cells. The lipoproteins transport lipids around the body. Special proteins carry vitamins and minerals.

The transport of the mineral iron provides an especially good illustration of these proteins' specificity and precision. When iron enters an intestinal cell, it is captured by a protein that will not let go unless the body needs iron. Before leaving the cell to enter the bloodstream, iron is attached to a carrier protein. The carrier, in turn, can pass iron on to a storage protein in the bone marrow or other tissues, which will hold it until it is needed. Then, when it is needed, iron is incorporated into proteins in the red blood cells and muscles that assist in oxygen transport and use.

The protein residing in the cells of the intestinal wall is **ferritin**; the carrier protein, **transferrin**; the storage protein, **ferritin** again; the red blood cell protein, **hemoglobin**; and the muscle cell protein, **myoglobin**.

As Antibodies Proteins also defend the body against disease. A virus—whether it is one that causes flu, smallpox, measles, or the common cold—enters the cells and multiplies there. One virus may produce 100 replicas of itself within an hour or so. Each replica can then burst out and invade 100 different cells, soon yielding 10,000 virus particles, which invade 10,000 cells. Left free to do their worst, they will soon overwhelm the body with disease.

antibodies: large proteins of the blood and body fluids, produced by the immune system in response to the invasion of the body by foreign molecules (usually proteins called *antigens*); antibodies combine with and inactivate the foreign invaders, thus protecting the body.

antigen: a substance that elicits the formation of antibodies or an inflammation reaction from the immune system. A bacterium, a virus, a toxin, and a protein in food that causes allergy are all examples of foreign antigens.

immunity: the body's ability to recognize and eliminate foreign invaders; see Highlight 18.

Fortunately, when the body detects invaders, it manufactures antibodies, giant protein molecules designed specifically to combat them. The antibodies work so swiftly and efficiently that in a normal, healthy individual, most diseases never have a chance to get started. Without sufficient protein, though, the body cannot maintain its resistance to disease.

Each antibody is designed to destroy just one invader. Once the body has manufactured antibodies against a particular antigen (such as the measles virus), it remembers how to make them. Consequently, the next time the body encounters that same invader, it will produce antibodies even more quickly. In other words, it develops a molecular memory, known as immunity.

Other Roles As mentioned earlier, proteins form integral parts of most body structures such as skin, muscles, and bones. They also participate in some of the body's most amazing activities such as blood clotting and vision. When a tissue is injured, a rapid chain of events leads to the production of fibrin, a stringy, insoluble mass of protein fibers that forms a clot from liquid blood. Later, more slowly, the protein collagen forms a scar to replace the clot and permanently heal the cut. The light-sensitive pigments in the cells of the retina are molecules of the protein opsin. Opsin responds to light by changing its shape, thus initiating the nerve impulses that convey the sense of sight to higher brain centers.

The protein functions discussed here are summarized in Table 6–3. They are only a few of the many roles proteins play, but they convey some sense of the immense variety of proteins and their importance in the body.

A PREVIEW OF PROTEIN METABOLISM

This section previews protein metabolism; Chapter 7 provides a full description. Cells have several metabolic options, depending on their amino acid needs.

Table 6–3

Summary of Proteins' Functions

- *Growth and maintenance*. Proteins form integral parts of most body structures such as skin, tendons, membranes, muscles, organs, and bones. As such, they support the growth and repair of body tissues.
- *Enzymes*. Proteins facilitate chemical reactions.
- *Hormones*. Proteins regulate body processes. (Some, but not all, hormones are made of protein.)
- *Antibodies*. Proteins inactivate foreign invaders, thus protecting the body against diseases.
- *Fluid and electrolyte balance*. Proteins help to maintain the fluid volume and the composition of body fluids.
- *Acid-base balance*. Proteins help maintain the acid-base balance of body fluids by acting as buffers.
- *Transportation*. Proteins transport substances, such as lipids, vitamins, minerals, and oxygen, around the body.
- *Energy*. Proteins provide some fuel for the body's energy needs.

Protein Turnover Within each cell, proteins are constantly being made and broken down. When proteins break down, they free amino acids to join the general circulation. Some of these amino acids may be promptly recycled into other proteins; others may be stripped of their nitrogen and used for energy. Together the constant synthesis and degradation of body proteins are known as protein turnover;[2] and the protein that participates in this flux is called endogenous protein.

protein turnover: the degradation and synthesis of endogenous protein.

endogenous protein: the protein in the body. In contrast, protein in foods is **exogenous protein.**
endo = within
gen = arising
exo = outside (the body)

Nitrogen Balance If the body maintains the same *amount* of protein in its tissues from day to day, it is in nitrogen balance. If the body adds protein, it is in positive nitrogen balance; if it loses protein, it is in negative nitrogen balance.

Normally, healthy adults receive enough protein to meet their needs, and they dispose of any excess. Their nitrogen intake equals their nitrogen output, and they are said to be in zero nitrogen balance, or nitrogen equilibrium. Growing infants and children, pregnant women, and people recovering from protein deficiency or illness are in positive nitrogen balance: their nitrogen intake exceeds their nitrogen output. They are building protein tissues—adding new blood, bone, skin, and muscle cells to their bodies. In contrast, people who are starving or suffering other severe stresses such as burns, injuries, infections, and fever are in negative nitrogen balance: nitrogen output exceeds nitrogen intake. During these times, the body loses protein as it breaks down body proteins for energy.

nitrogen balance: the amount of nitrogen consumed (N in) as compared with the amount of nitrogen excreted (N out) in a given period of time.*

Nitrogen equilibrium (zero nitrogen balance): N in = N out.
Positive nitrogen balance: N in > N out.
Negative nitrogen balance: N in < N out.

Using Amino Acids to Make Proteins or Nonessential Amino Acids Cells can assemble amino acids into the proteins they need to do their work. If a particular nonessential amino acid is not readily available, cells can dismantle another amino acid and combine the amino group with carbon fragments from glucose to make the needed one. If an essential amino acid is missing, the body may break down some of its own proteins to obtain it.

Using Amino Acids to Make Other Compounds Cells can also use amino acids to make other compounds. For example, the amino acid tyrosine is used to make the neurotransmitters norepinephrine and epinephrine, which relay nervous system messages throughout the body. Tyrosine can also be made into the pigment melanin, which is responsible for brown hair, eye, and skin color, or into the hormone thyroxin, which helps to regulate the metabolic rate. For another example, the amino acid tryptophan serves as a precursor for the neurotransmitter serotonin and the vitamin niacin.

neurotransmitters: chemicals that are released at the end of a nerve cell when a nerve impulse arrives there; they diffuse across the gap to the next cell and alter the membrane of that second cell to either inhibit or excite it.

Using Amino Acids for Energy Even though amino acids are needed to do the work that only they can perform—build vital proteins—they will be sacrificed to provide energy and glucose if need be. Without energy, cells die; without glucose, the brain and nervous system falter. When glucose or fatty acids are limited, cells are forced to use amino acids for energy and glucose. The body does not make a specialized storage form of protein as it does for carbohydrate and fat. Glucose is stored as glycogen and fat as triglycerides, but protein in the body is available only

*The genetic materials DNA and RNA contain nitrogen, but the quantity is insignificant compared with the amount in protein. The average amino acid weighs about 6.25 times as much as the nitrogen it contains, so scientists can estimate the amount of protein in a sample of food, body tissue, or other material by multiplying the weight of the nitrogen in it by 6.25.

Reminder: The making of glucose from noncarbohydrate sources such as amino acids is *gluconeogenesis*. The action of carbohydrate and fat in providing enough energy to allow amino acids to be used to build body proteins is known as the *protein-sparing action* of carbohydrate and fat.

deamination: removal of the amino (NH_2) group from a compound such as an amino acid.

Urea metabolism is described in Chapter 7.

as the working and structural components of the tissues. When the need arises, the body dismantles its tissue proteins and uses them for energy.[3] Thus, over time, energy deprivation (starvation) always incurs wasting of lean body tissue as well as fat loss. An adequate intake of carbohydrates and fats spares amino acids from being used for energy and allows them to perform their unique roles.

Deaminating Amino Acids When amino acids are broken down (as occurs when they are to be used in energy production), they are first deaminated—stripped of their nitrogen-containing amino groups. Deamination produces ammonia, which the cells release into the bloodstream. The liver picks up the ammonia, converts it into urea (a less toxic compound), and returns the urea to the blood. The kidneys filter urea out of the blood; thus the amino nitrogen ends up in the urine. Urea is produced from both exogenous and endogenous amino acids. The remaining carbon fragments may enter a number of metabolic pathways—for example, they may be used to make fat.

Using Amino Acids to Make Fat If a person eats more protein that the body needs, the amino acids are deaminated, the nitrogen is excreted, and the remaining carbon fragments are converted to fat and stored for later use.* In this way, valuable, expensive, protein-rich foods can contribute to obesity.

To summarize, proteins serve the body as building blocks in the growth and repair of tissues; as enzymes in metabolism; as hormones; as regulators of the body's fluid balances; as transporters; as antibodies; and in many other ways (see Table 6–4). In the process, the proteins themselves are constantly being synthesized and broken down as needed. The body's assimilation of amino acids into proteins and release of amino acids via protein degradation and excretion can be tracked by measuring nitrogen balance, which should be positive during growth and steady in adulthood. An energy deficit or an inadequate protein intake may force the body to use amino acids as fuel, causing negative nitrogen balance. Protein eaten in excess of need is degraded and stored as body fat.

Protein in Foods

In the United States, where nutritious foods are abundant, people eat protein in such large quantities that even if its amino acid balance is not perfect, they receive all the amino acids they need. Where people eat only marginal amounts of protein-rich foods, however, the quality of the protein becomes crucial to their health. Hence, the protein quality of the diet is of great concern when making nutrition recommendations in countries where malnutrition is widespread.

*Chemists sometimes classify amino acids according to the destinations of their carbon fragments after deamination. If the fragment leads to the production of glucose, the amino acid is called "glucogenic"; if it leads to the formation of ketone bodies, fat, and sterols, the amino acid is called "ketogenic." There is no sharp distinction between glucogenic and ketogenic amino acids, however. A few are both; most are considered glucogenic; only one (leucine) is clearly ketogenic. E. M. N. Hamilton and S. A. S. Gropper, *The Biochemistry of Human Nutrition—A Desk Reference* (St. Paul, Minn.: West, 1987), pp. 116–117.

PROTEIN QUALITY

Food proteins that provide an unbalanced assortment of amino acids, so that the body cannot make full use of them, are poor-quality proteins. In countries where food is scarce, or where the people receive marginal or inadequate amounts of protein, the quality of the dietary protein determines, in large part, how well the children grow and how well the adults maintain their health.

Limiting Amino Acids To make proteins, a cell must have all the needed amino acids available simultaneously. The liver can produce any nonessential amino acid that may be in short supply so that the cells can continue linking amino acids into protein strands. If an essential amino acid is missing, though, a cell must dismantle its own proteins to obtain it. Therefore, to prevent protein breakdown, dietary protein must supply at least the nine essential amino acids plus enough nitrogen-containing amino groups and energy for the synthesis of the others. If the diet supplies too little of any essential amino acid, protein synthesis will be limited. The body makes complete proteins only; if one amino acid is missing, the others cannot form a "partial" protein. The body has no storage site for extra amino acids and is forced to either waste them or use them for another purpose. An essential amino acid supplied in less than the amount needed to support protein synthesis is called a *limiting* amino acid.

limiting amino acid: the essential amino acid found in the shortest supply relative to the amounts needed for protein synthesis in the body. Four amino acids are most likely to be limiting:
- Lysine.
- Methionine (plus cysteine).
- Threonine.
- Tryptophan.

Complete Protein A complete dietary protein contains all the essential amino acids in relatively the same amounts as human beings require; it may or may not contain all the nonessential amino acids. Generally, proteins derived from animals (meat, fish, poultry, cheese, eggs, and milk) are complete, although gelatin is an exception (it lacks tryptophan and cannot support growth and health as a diet's sole protein). Proteins from plants (vegetables, grains, and legumes) have more diverse amino acid patterns, and some tend to be limiting in one or more essential amino acids. Some plant proteins (for example, corn protein) are notoriously incomplete. Others (for example, soy protein) are complete.[4]

complete protein: a dietary protein containing all the amino acids essential in human nutrition in amounts adequate for human use.

complementary proteins: two or more proteins whose amino acid assortments complement each other in such a way that the essential amino acids missing from one are supplied by the other.

mutual supplementation: the strategy of combining two protein foods in a meal so that each food provides the essential amino acid(s) lacking in the other. Mutual supplementation is the dietary strategy that brings complementary proteins together in a meal.

Complementary Proteins In general, plant proteins are of lower quality than animal proteins, and plants also offer less protein per unit (either weight or measure) of food. For this reason, many vegetarians combine plant-protein foods with different but complementary amino acid patterns to obtain the full array of essential amino acids in their diets. This strategy is called mutual supplementation, and it yields complementary proteins that contain all the essential amino

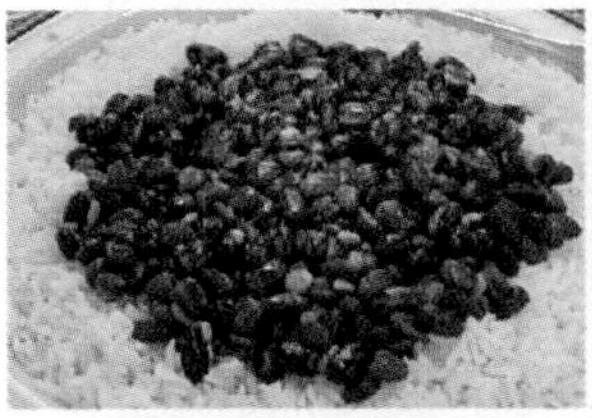

Black beans and rice is a favorite Hispanic combination that, together, provide a full array of amino acids.

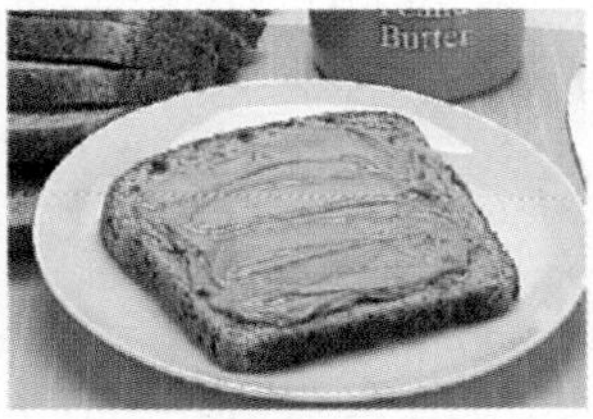

Another simple example of mutual supplementation: peanut butter on wheat bread, a North American tradition.

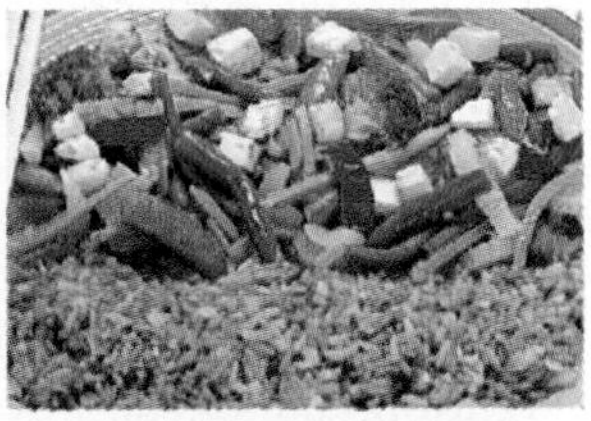

Tofu and stir-fried vegetables with rice offers the proteins of legumes, vegetables, and grains.

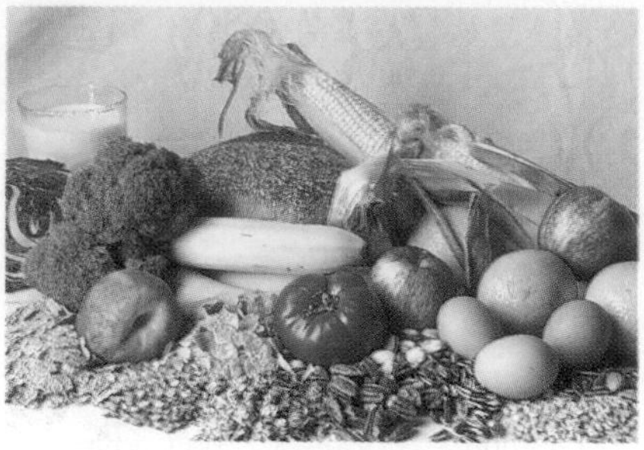

Vegetarians obtain their protein from legumes, nuts, whole grains, vegetables, and, in some cases, eggs and milk products.

acids in quantities sufficient to support health. The protein quality of the combination is greater than for either food alone.

Many people have long believed that mutual supplementation at every meal was critical to protein nutrition. For most healthy vegetarians, though, it is not necessary to balance amino acids at each meal when protein intake is varied and energy intake is sufficient.[5] Vegetarians can receive all the amino acids they need over the course of a day, if they eat a variety of grains, legumes, seeds, nuts, and vegetables. Protein deficiency will develop, however, when fruits and certain vegetables make up the core of the diet, severely limiting the *quantity* and *quality* of protein. Highlight 6 shows how to plan a nutritious vegetarian diet.

protein digestibility: a measure of the amount of amino acids absorbed from a given protein intake.

high-quality protein: an easily digestible, complete protein.

reference protein: standard against which to measure the quality of other proteins.

Digestibility Ideally, a protein is both complete and easily digestible, so that enough amino acids are available for protein synthesis. Such a protein is a high-quality protein. Digestibility depends on a protein's configuration, other foods eaten with it, and reactions that influence the release of amino acids.

Reference Protein One of the most complete and digestible proteins is egg protein. Until the early 1990s, egg protein was used as the standard for measuring protein quality; it was assigned a value of 100 and the quality of other food proteins was determined based on how they compared with egg. Such a standard is called a reference protein. Now, the Food and Agriculture Organization (FAO) of the United Nations and the World Health Organization (WHO) have established a new standard for the reference protein: the essential amino acid requirements of preschool-age children.

MEASURES OF PROTEIN QUALITY

Researchers have developed several methods for evaluating the quality of food proteins. The object of all of these methods is to identify high-quality proteins—that is, proteins that contain all of the essential amino acids in relatively the same proportion as human beings require. Proteins that are low in an essential amino acid cannot, by themselves, support protein synthesis. The following paragraphs briefly describe these measures; Appendix J provides more detail.

amino acid scoring: a method of evaluating protein quality by comparing a test protein's amino acid pattern with that of a reference protein; sometimes called chemical scoring.

Amino Acid Scoring The simplest way to evaluate a food protein's quality is to determine its amino acid composition and compare it with a reference protein. Scientists can easily identify the limiting amino acid—it is the one that falls shortest compared with the reference. If the test protein's limiting amino acid is 70 percent of the amount found in the reference protein, it receives a chemical score of 70. Such calculations fail to estimate digestibility, however.

biological value (BV): the amount of protein nitrogen that is retained for growth and maintenance, expressed as a percentage of the protein nitrogen that has been digested and absorbed; a measure of protein quality.

Biological Value The biological value (BV) of a protein measures its efficiency in supporting the body's needs. Scientists feed a given food protein to experimental animals as the sole protein in their diet and measure the animals' retention and loss of nitrogen. The more nitrogen retained, the higher the protein quality. (Recall that when an essential amino acid is missing, protein synthesis stops, and the remaining amino acids are deaminated and the nitrogen excreted.)

Biological value is expressed as a percentage of the absorbed nitrogen that is retained. For egg protein, the BV is 100 (all the absorbed protein is retained); the margin lists the BV of a few other proteins. Supplied in adequate quantity, a protein with a BV of 70 or greater can support human growth as long as energy intake is adequate.

BV of proteins:
- Egg 100
- Milk 93
- Beef 75
- Fish 75
- Corn 72

Net Protein Utilization Like BV, net protein utilization (NPU) measures nitrogen retention. Instead of measuring retention of absorbed nitrogen (as in BV), NPU measures retention of food nitrogen.

net protein utilization (NPU): the amount of protein nitrogen that is retained from a given amount of protein nitrogen eaten; a measure of protein quality.

Protein Efficiency Ratio The protein efficiency ratio (PER) measures the weight gain of a growing animal and compares it to the animal's protein intake. Until recently, PER was generally accepted as the official method used in the United States and Canada to assess protein quality.

protein efficiency ratio (PER): a measure of protein quality assessed by determining how well a given protein supports weight gain in growing rats; used to establish the protein quality for infant formulas and baby foods.

PDCAAS The protein-digestibility-corrected amino acid score or PDCAAS method compares the amino acid contents of a protein with human amino acid requirements and corrects for digestibility.[6] The protein's amino acid profile is determined as described earlier ("Amino Acid Scoring") and then it is compared against the amino acid requirements of preschool-aged children. This comparison reveals the most limiting amino acid. The rationale behind using the requirements of this age group is that if a protein will effectively support a young child's growth and development, then it will meet or exceed the requirements of older children and adults. Thus the PDCAAS method evaluates dietary protein quality for all age groups except infants. (The PER method described earlier is used to evaluate proteins for infants.)

To arrive at the PDCAAS, the amino acid score is multiplied by the food's protein digestibility percentage. Because the digestibility of many foods is similar in human beings and in rats, values for protein digestibility in rats are commonly used. Appendix J provides an example of how to calculate the PDCAAS and Table 6–4 lists the PDCAAS values of selected foods.

protein-digestibility-corrected amino acid score (PDCAAS): a measure of protein quality assessed by comparing the amino acid balance of a food protein with the amino acid requirements of preschool-aged children and then correcting for the true digestibility of the protein; recommended by the FAO/WHO and used to establish protein quality of foods for Daily Value percentages on food labels.

Table 6–4

PDCAAS Values of Selected Foods

Casein (milk protein)	1.00
Egg white	1.00
Soybean (isolate)	.99
Beef	.92
Pea flour	.69
Kidney beans (canned)	.68
Chick peas (canned)	.66
Pinto beans (canned)	.63
Rolled oats	.57
Lentils (canned)	.52
Peanut meal	.52
Whole wheat	.40

Note: 1.0 is the maximum PDCAAS a food protein can receive.

PROTEIN REGULATIONS FOR FOOD LABELS

The PDCAAS method has been integrated into the FDA's new labeling regulations.[7] The FDA determined that the PDCAAS method assesses protein quality more precisely for people over age one than the PER, which was used previously for labeling purposes. The PER method using casein as a standard has been retained to measure protein quality for infant formulas and baby foods.

All food labels must state the *quantity* of protein in gram amounts. The "% Daily Value" for protein is not mandatory on all labels, but is required whenever a food makes a protein claim or is intended for consumption by children under four years old.* Whenever the Daily Value percentage is declared, researchers must factor the quantity of the protein determined by using the PDCAAS method. Thus the "% Daily Value" for protein reflects both quantity and quality.

*For labeling purposes, the RDI (Reference Daily Intakes) for protein are as follows: for infants, 14 grams; for children under age 4, 16 grams; for older children and adults, 50 grams; for pregnant women, 60 grams; and for lactating women, 65 grams.

The quality of protein is of great importance in dealing with malnutrition worldwide. In the United States and Canada, protein deficiency is not common, but protein quality does play a crucial role in the growth of infants and the health of older adults. Protein quality becomes more important as consumers shift from a diet based on meat to a diet based on grains, vegetables, and fruits as recommended by the Daily Food Guide. All things considered, the best guarantee of amino acid adequacy is to eat mixtures of foods containing protein from a variety of sources in the presence of adequate amounts of vitamins, minerals, fiber, and energy. Protein quality scores of individual foods deserve little emphasis.

Health Effects and Recommended Intakes of Protein

No nutrient has been more intensely scrutinized than protein. As you know by now, it is indispensable to life. And it should come as no surprise that protein deficiency can have devastating effects on people's health. But like the other nutrients, protein in excess can also be harmful. This section examines the health effects and recommended intakes of protein.

PROTEIN-ENERGY MALNUTRITION

When people are deprived of protein, energy, or both, the result is protein-energy malnutrition (PEM). Although PEM touches many adult lives, it most often strikes early in childhood. It is the most widespread form of malnutrition in the world today, afflicting over 500 million children.[8] Most of the 40,000 children who die each day are malnourished.

Inadequate food intake leads to poor growth in children and to weight loss and wasting in adults. Children who are thin for their height may be suffering from acute PEM (recent severe food deprivation), whereas children who are short for their age have experienced chronic PEM (long-term food deprivation). Poor growth due to PEM is easy to overlook because a small child may look quite normal, but it is the most common sign of malnutrition.

PEM is most prevalent in Africa, Central America, South America, the Middle East, and East and Southeast Asia. In the United States, homeless people and those living in substandard housing in inner cities and rural areas have been diagnosed with PEM.[9] In addition to those living in poverty, elderly people who live alone and adults who are addicted to drugs and alcohol are frequently victims of PEM.[10] Adult PEM is also seen in people hospitalized with infections such as AIDS or tuberculosis; infections deplete body proteins, demand extra energy, induce nutrient losses, and alter metabolic pathways. PEM is also common in those suffering from the eating disorder anorexia nervosa. Prevention emphasizes frequent, nutrient-dense, energy-dense meals and, equally important, resolution of the underlying causes of PEM—poverty, infections, and illness.

protein-energy malnutrition (PEM), also called **protein-kcalorie malnutrition (PCM)**: a deficiency of both protein and energy; the world's most widespread malnutrition problem, including kwashiorkor, marasmus, and instances in which they overlap.

acute PEM: protein-energy malnutrition caused by recent severe food restriction; characterized in children by thinness for height (wasting).

chronic PEM: protein-energy malnutrition caused by long-term food deprivation; characterized in children by short height for age (stunting).

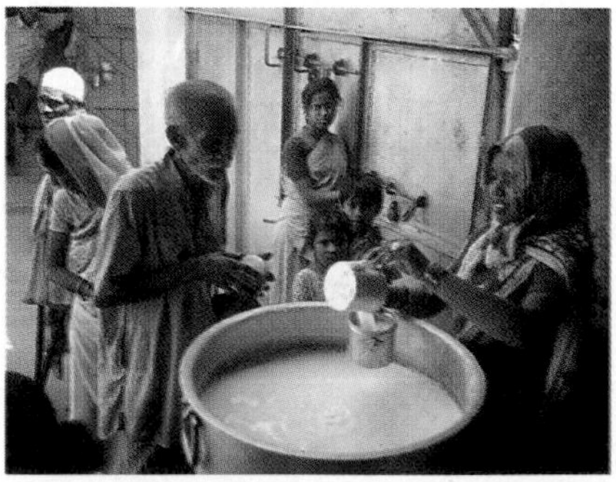

Donated food saves some people from starvation, but it is usually insufficient to meet nutrient needs or even to provide a full belly for every person who is hungry.

Classifying PEM Researchers have long believed that PEM occurs in two forms: marasmus and kwashiorkor, which differ in their clinical features (see Table 6–5). The child with marasmus looks emaciated, whereas the child with kwashiorkor looks swollen, particularly in the belly. Historically, marasmus was

Table 6–5

Features of Marasmus and Kwashiorkor in Children

Separating PEM into two classifications oversimplifies the condition, but at the extremes, marasmus and kwashiorkor exhibit marked differences. Marasmus-kwashiorkor mix presents symptoms common to both marasmus and kwashiorkor. In all cases, children are likely to develop diarrhea, infections, and multiple nutrient deficiencies.

Marasmus	Kwashiorkor
Infancy (less than 2 yr)	Older infants and young children (1 to 3 yr)
Severe deprivation, or impaired absorption, of protein, energy, vitamins, and minerals	Inadequate protein intake or, more commonly, infections
Develops slowly; chronic PEM	Rapid onset; acute PEM
Severe weight loss	Some weight loss
Severe muscle wasting, with fat	Some muscle wasting, with retention of some body fat
Growth: <60% weight-for-age	Growth: 60 to 80% weight-for-age
No detectable edema	Edema
No fatty liver	Enlarged fatty liver
Anxiety, apathy	Apathy, misery, irritability, sadness
Good appetite possible	Anorexia
Hair is sparse, thin, and dry; easily pulled out	Hair is dry and brittle; easily pulled out; changes color; becomes straight
Skin is dry, thin, and easily wrinkles	Skin develops lesions

thought to be caused by a lack of energy, with protein deficiency an indirect result. Kwashiorkor was thought to be caused by an inadequate amount or quality of protein in the presence of adequate energy. In reality, though, marasmus reflects a severe deprivation of food over a long time (chronic PEM) and therefore is caused by an inadequate energy *and* protein intake (and by inadequate vitamins and minerals as well). By comparison, kwashiorkor typically reflects a more sudden and recent deprivation of food (acute PEM). It too has probably been mischaracterized, because diets that are adequate in energy are rarely deficient in protein.[11] Some researchers maintain that marasmus and kwashiorkor are two stages of the same disease. Others suggest that kwashiorkor develops when malnourished children eat moldy grains.[12] Researchers continue to question the exact causes of kwashiorkor, but clearly, protein deficiency appears to be one of several factors involved. Most likely, dietary imbalances, multiple infections, parasitic diseases, and toxins together influence the development of kwashiorkor.[13] The following paragraphs describe three clinical syndromes—marasmus, kwashiorkor, and the combination of the two.

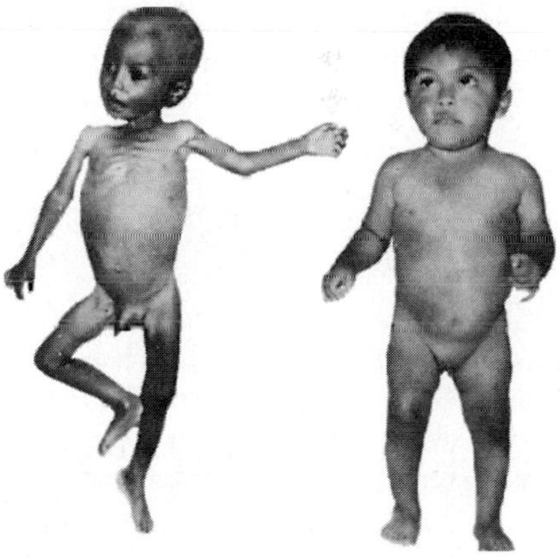

At left, a child suffering the severe wasting of marasmus. At right, the same child after nutritional therapy.

Marasmus Marasmus occurs most commonly in children from 6 to 18 months of age in all the overpopulated urban slums of the world. Children in impoverished nations simply do not have enough to eat and subsist on diluted cereal drinks that supply scant energy and protein of low quality; such food can barely sustain life, much less support growth. Consequently, marasmic children look like old people—just skin and bones.

marasmus (ma-RAZ-mus)**:** a form of PEM that results from a severe deprivation, or impaired absorption, of energy, protein, vitamins, and minerals.

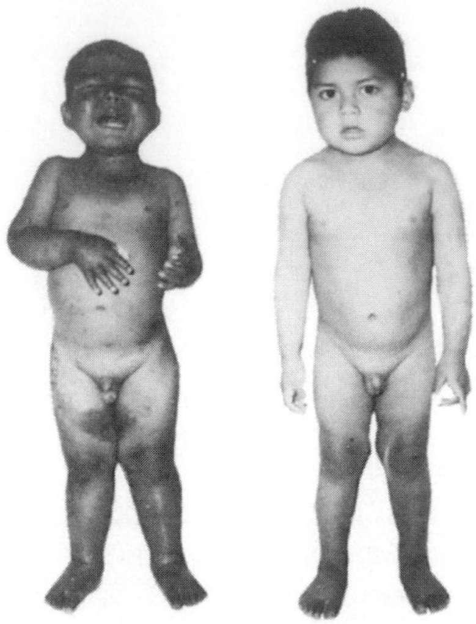

At left, a child swollen with the characteristic edema of kwashiorkor. At right, the same child after nutritional therapy.

Without adequate nutrition, muscles, including the heart, waste and weaken. Because the brain normally grows to almost its full adult size within the first two years of life, marasmus impairs brain development and learning ability. Reduced synthesis of key hormones slows metabolism and lowers body temperature. There is little or no fat under the skin to insulate against cold. Hospital workers find that children with marasmus need to be wrapped up and kept warm. They also need love because they have often been deprived of parental attention as well as food.

The starving child faces this threat to life by engaging in as little activity as possible—not even crying for food. The body musters all its forces to meet the crisis, so it cuts down on any expenditure of protein not needed for the heart, lungs, and brain to function. Growth ceases; the child is no larger at age four than at age two. Digestive enzymes are in short supply, the GI tract lining deteriorates, and absorption fails. The child can't assimilate what little food is eaten.

Kwashiorkor Kwashiorkor was originally a Ghanaian word meaning "the evil spirit that infects the first child when the second child is born." When a mother who has been nursing her first child bears a second child, she weans the first child and puts the second one on the breast. The first child, suddenly switched from nutrient-dense, protein-rich breast milk to a starchy, protein-poor cereal, soon begins to sicken and die. Kwashiorkor typically sets in between 18 months and two years.

kwashiorkor (kwash-ee-OR-core, kwash-ee-or-CORE)**:** a form of PEM that results from either inadequate protein intake or, more commonly, from infections.

Kwashiorkor usually develops rapidly as a result of protein deficiency or, more commonly, is precipitated by an illness such as measles or other infection.[14] As mentioned, some researchers believe that kwashiorkor and marasmus are two stages of the same disease. They point out that kwashiorkor and marasmus often exist side by side in the same community that consumes the same diet. They note that a child who has marasmus can later develop kwashiorkor. Some research indicates that marasmus represents the body's adaptation to starvation, and that kwashiorkor develops when adaptation fails.

Another possibility is that kwashiorkor may be a form of food poisoning superimposed on malnutrition. One supporting piece of evidence is that kwashiorkor seems to appear only in rainy, tropical communities. Many temperate regions have experienced widespread famine, yet have not had kwashiorkor. Another clue is that under hot, humid conditions, a common mold, *Aspergillus flavus*, produces aflatoxin, a toxin that inhibits protein synthesis. When malnourished children are forced to eat moldy grain for lack of other foods, their weakened bodies cannot defend against the toxin.

aflatoxin**:** potent cancer-causing toxin produced by the mold *Aspergillus flavus* that infects grains and peanuts. The USDA tests grains and peanuts grown in this country for aflatoxin contamination.

Reminder: *Edema* is the swelling of body tissue caused by excessive fluid in the interstitial spaces, seen in protein deficiency (among other conditions).

The loss of weight and body fat is usually not as severe in kwashiorkor as in marasmus, but there may be some muscle wasting. Proteins and hormones that previously maintained fluid balance diminish, and fluid leaks into the interstitial spaces. The child's limbs and face become swollen with edema, a distinguishing feature of kwashiorkor. The belly bulges with a fatty liver, caused by lack of the protein carriers that transport fat out of the liver. The fatty liver lacks enzymes to clear poisons from the body, so their toxic effects are prolonged. Without sufficient tyrosine to make melanin, the child's hair loses its color; inadequate protein synthesis leaves the skin patchy and scaly, often with sores that fail to heal.

Marasmus-Kwashiorkor Mix The combination of marasmus and kwashiorkor is characterized by the edema of kwashiorkor with the wasting of marasmus. Most often, the child is suffering the effects of both malnutrition and infections.

Infections In PEM, antibodies to fight off invading bacteria are degraded to provide amino acids for other uses, leaving the malnourished child vulnerable to infections. Blood proteins, including hemoglobin, are no longer synthesized, so the child becomes anemic and weak. Dysentery, an infection of the digestive tract, causes diarrhea, further depleting the body of nutrients. In the marasmic child, once infection sets in, kwashiorkor often follows.[15]

dysentery (DISS-en-terry): an infection of the digestive tract that causes diarrhea.

The combination of infections, fever, electrolyte imbalances, and anemia often leads to heart failure and occasionally sudden death. Infections combined with malnutrition are responsible for two-thirds of the deaths of young children in developing countries.[16] Measles, which might make a healthy child sick for a week or two, kills a child with PEM within two or three days.

Rehabilitation If caught in time, the life of a starving child may be saved by careful nutrition therapy. Diarrhea will have depleted the body's potassium and disturbed other electrolyte balances. Careful correction of fluid and electrolyte imbalances usually raises the blood pressure and strengthens the heartbeat. After the first 24 to 48 hours, protein and food energy may be given in small quantities, gradually increasing intakes as tolerated.

Reminder: The term *electrolyte balance* refers to the proper concentrations of salts within the body fluids (see Chapter 12 for details).

Experts assure us that we possess the knowledge, technology, and resources to end hunger. Programs that have involved the local people in the process of identifying problems and devising solutions have met with some success. But until those who have the food, technology, and resources make fighting hunger a priority, the war on hunger will not be won (see Chapter 20 for more on hunger).

HEALTH EFFECTS OF PROTEIN

While many of the world's people struggle to obtain enough food energy and protein, in developed countries both are so abundant that problems of excess are seen. Overconsumption of protein offers no benefits and may pose health risks.

The relationships between protein and chronic diseases are not clearly evident. Population studies have difficulty determining whether diseases correlate with animal proteins or with their accompanying saturated fats. Studies that rely on data from vegetarians must sort out the many lifestyle factors, other than a "no-meat diet," that might explain relationships between protein and health.

Heart Disease As mentioned, foods rich in animal protein tend to be rich in saturated fats. Consequently, it is not surprising to find a correlation between animal-protein intake and heart disease, although no independent effect has been demonstrated. On the other hand, substituting soy protein for animal protein lowers blood cholesterol, especially in those with high blood cholesterol.[17]

Recent research suggests that the amino acid homocysteine may be an independent risk factor for heart disease.[18] When compared with others, men with elevated homocysteine were three times as likely to have heart attacks.[19] Researchers do not yet know what role homocysteine plays in heart disease, nor do they understand what raises homocysteine in the blood. Elevated homocysteine is associated with suboptimal concentrations of B vitamins and can usually be corrected with vitamin B_{12}, vitamin B_6, and folate supplements.[20] Whether such treatments will reduce the risk of heart attacks remains unknown.

Cancer As in heart disease, the effects of protein and fats cannot be easily separated. Some studies have found a link between high-meat diets and colon cancer. Population studies suggest a correlation between high intakes of animal proteins and some types of cancer (notably, cancer of the colon, breast, pancreas, and prostate). One recent study has reported an increase in the risk of kidney cancer with a high consumption of red meat and high-protein foods.[21] A high protein intake increases the work of the kidneys and excretion of the end products of protein metabolism depends, in part, on an adequate fluid intake and healthy kidneys.

Other risk factors for adult bone loss (osteoporosis) are sex, age, and race, as Highlight 12 explains.

Adult Bone Loss (Osteoporosis) Do high protein intakes accelerate bone loss? Calcium excretion rises as protein intake increases; furthermore, calcium excretion appears to rise with intakes of animal-derived proteins, but not with plant-derived proteins.[22] Whether excess protein may deplete the bones of their chief minerals depends largely upon the ratio of protein to calcium intakes.[23] An ideal ratio has not been established, but a woman whose intake meets the RDA for both nutrients has a calcium-to-protein ratio of 16 to 1 (milligrams to grams). For most women in the United States, however, average calcium intakes are lower and protein intakes are higher, yielding a 9-to-1 ratio, which may produce calcium losses that compromise bone health.[24] In contrast, moderate increases in physical activity and calcium intake may protect against such losses.[25]

Table 6–6

Protein RDA as a Percentage of Energy RDA

When expressed as a percentage of energy intake, the protein requirement represents about 10 percent of the energy RDA.

Age (yr)	Protein RDA (g/kg)	Protein RDA (in kCalories) as a Percentage of Energy RDA (%)
0 to ½	2.2	8.0
½ to 1	1.6	6.5
1 to 3	1.2	4.9
4 to 6	1.1	5.3
7 to 10	1.0	5.6
Males		
11 to 14	1.0	7.2
15 to 18	0.9	7.9
19 to 24	0.8	8.0
25 to 50	0.8	8.7
51 +	0.8	11.0
Females		
11 to 14	1.0	8.4
15 to 18	0.8	8.0
19 to 24	0.8	8.4
25 to 50	0.8	9.1
51 +	0.8	10.5

Weight Control Protein-rich foods are often fat-rich foods that contribute to obesity with its accompanying health risks. Weight-loss gimmicks that encourage a high-protein diet are rarely useful; overweight people have better success with diets that provide adequate protein, minimal fat, and ample energy from carbohydrates. The higher a person's intake of protein-rich foods such as meat and milk, the more likely that fruits, vegetables, and grains will be crowded out, making the diet inadequate in other nutrients.

RECOMMENDED INTAKES OF PROTEIN

As mentioned earlier, the body continuously breaks down and loses its proteins and cannot store amino acids. To replace protein, the body needs dietary protein for two reasons: first, food protein is the only source of the *essential* amino acids; and second, it is the only practical source of *nitrogen* with which to build the nonessential amino acids and other nitrogen-containing compounds.

The *Diet and Health* report recommends that people's fat intakes should contribute 30 percent or less of total food energy, and carbohydrate, 55 percent or more—which leaves about 15 percent for protein. Current intakes in the United States and Canada, though higher than recommendations, do not seem to be high enough to cause harm. The *Diet and Health* report advises people to maintain moderate protein intakes—between the RDA and twice the RDA.

Protein RDA The protein RDA for healthy adults is 0.8 grams per kilogram of appropriate body weight per day. For infants and children, the RDA is higher. When compared to total energy intake, however, the protein RDA for infants and children is similar to that of adults as Table 6–6 shows. The RDA generously covers the needs for replacing worn-out tissue, so it increases for larger people; it also covers the needs for building new tissue during growth, so it increases for

How to Calculate Recommended Protein Intakes

To figure your protein RDA:

- Look up the appropriate weight for a person of your height (inside back cover). If your present weight falls within that range, use it for the following calculations. If your present weight falls outside the range, use the midpoint of the acceptable weight range as your reference weight.
- Convert pounds to kilograms, if necessary (pounds divided by 2.2 equals kilograms).
- Multiply kilograms by 0.8 to get your RDA in grams per day. (Males 18 years old and younger, multiply by 0.9.) Example:

$$\text{Weight} = 150 \text{ lb.}$$

$$150 \text{ lb} \div 2.2 \text{ lb/kg} = 68 \text{ kg (rounded off).}$$

$$68 \text{ kg} \times 0.8 \text{ g/kg} = 54 \text{ g protein (rounded off).}$$

115 ÷ 2.2
56 × 0.8

children and pregnant women. The accompanying box shows how to calculate your RDA for protein.

In setting the RDA, the committee assumes that people are healthy and do not have unusual metabolic needs for protein; that the protein eaten will be of mixed quality; and that the body will use the protein about as efficiently as it uses reference proteins. In addition, the committee assumes that the protein is consumed along with sufficient carbohydrate and fat to provide adequate energy and that other nutrients in the diet are adequate.

Protein recommendations for athletes are presented in Chapter 11.

Adequate Energy Note the qualification "adequate energy" in the preceding statement, and consider what happens if energy intake falls short of needs. An intake of 50 grams of protein, which is equal to 200 kcalories, provides about 10 percent of the total energy from protein, if the person receives 2000 kcalories a day. But if the person cuts energy intake drastically—to, say 800 kcalories a day—then an intake of 200 kcalories from protein is suddenly 25 percent of the total; yet it's still the same number of grams. The protein intake is reasonable, but the energy intake is not; the low energy intake will force the body to use the protein to meet energy needs rather than to replace lost body protein. Similarly, if the person's energy intake is high—say, 4000 kcalories—the 50-gram protein intake will represent only 5 percent of the total, yet it *still* is a reasonable protein intake. Again, the energy intake is unreasonable for most people, but in this case, it will permit the protein to be used to meet the body's needs.

*

Be careful when judging a protein intake as a percentage of energy. Always ascertain the number of grams as well, and compare it with the RDA or another standard stated in grams. A recommendation stated as a percentage of energy intake is useful only if the energy intake is within reason.

Protein in Abundance Many people tend to overvalue protein, perhaps because they have been so impressed with its many critical roles in the body. They think they need *lots* of protein, when, in fact, they are already receiving

Chapter 14 discusses athletes' nutrition needs further.

plenty. Even athletes typically don't need to increase their protein intakes. Most people in developed countries such as the United States and Canada receive much more protein than they need. This is not surprising considering the abundance of food eaten and the central role meats hold in the diet. A single ounce of meat delivers about 7 grams of protein, so one 8-ounce serving of meat alone supplies more than the RDA for an average-sized person. Besides meat, well-fed people eat many other nutritious foods, many of which also contain protein.

To illustrate how easy it is to overconsume protein, consider the *minimum* recommended servings for the Daily Food Guide. Six servings from the bread, cereal, rice, and pasta group provide about 18 grams of protein; 3 servings of vegetables deliver about 6 grams; 2 servings of milk offer 16 grams; and 2 servings of meat contain about 35 grams. This totals 75 grams of protein—higher than recommendations for most people. (The accompanying box describes how to estimate protein in foods.)

Just think how much more protein people receive when they eat additional servings. No wonder most people in the United States and Canada get more protein than they need. If they have an adequate *food* intake, they have a more-than-adequate protein intake. The key diet-planning principle to emphasize for protein is moderation. Even though most people receive plenty of protein, some feel compelled to take supplements as well, as the next section describes.

PROTEIN AND AMINO ACID SUPPLEMENTS

Health food stores and popular magazine articles advertise a wide variety of protein supplements, and people take these supplements for many different reasons, all of them unfounded. Athletes take them to build muscle. Dieters take them to spare their bodies' protein while losing weight. Women take them to strengthen their fingernails. People take individual amino acids, too—to cure herpes, to make themselves sleep better, to lose weight, and to relieve pain and depression.* Like many other magic solutions to health problems, protein and amino acid supplements don't work these miracles, and they can be harmful.

Muscle work builds muscle; protein supplements do not, and athletes do not need them. Instead, athletes need a well-balanced diet that provides sufficient dietary protein and adequate food energy. Food energy spares body protein; carbohydrate and fat serve this purpose equally well, and carbohydrate is safer. Fingernails are not affected by protein supplements, provided the diet is adequate. Normal, healthy people never need protein supplements.

Use of amino acids as dietary supplements is inappropriate, especially for:[29]

- All women of childbearing age.
- Pregnant or lactating women.
- Infants, children, and adolescents.
- Elderly people.
- People with inborn errors of metabolism that affect their bodies' handling of amino acids.
- Smokers.
- People on low-protein diets.
- People with chronic or acute mental or physical illnesses who take amino acids without medical supervision.

Furthermore, protein supplements are expensive, less completely digested than protein-rich foods, and, when used as replacements for such foods, often downright dangerous. The "liquid protein" diet, advocated some years ago for weight loss, caused deaths in many users; even some physician-supervised protein-sparing fasts based on liquid protein have caused abnormal heart rhythms. The Food and Drug Administration (FDA) warns that their use as a total diet without medical supervision "may cause serious illness or death."

Single amino acids do not occur naturally in foods and offer no benefit to the body; in fact, they can be harmful.[26] The body was not designed to handle the high concentrations and unusual combinations of amino acids found in supple-

*Canada allows single amino acid supplements to be sold only as drugs or as food additives.

How to Use the Exchange System to Estimate Protein

Exchange	Protein (g)
Milks	8
Meats	7
Starch	3
Vegetables	2
Fruits	—
Fats	—

The exchange system provides an easy way to estimate the protein a person consumes. The foods on the milk and meat lists supply protein in abundance: a cup of milk provides 8 grams of protein; an ounce of meat, 7 grams. A ½-cup portion of legumes provides 10 grams of protein in the exchange system (counted as one starch and one very lean meat exchange). The starch and vegetable lists contribute small amounts of protein, but they can add up to significant quantities; fruits and fats provide no protein.

To estimate the protein in this breakfast, you first need to recognize that this bowl of cereal contains 1 cup shredded wheat with 1 cup milk and ½ banana. Then you need to translate these portions into exchanges: 2 starches, 1 milk, and ½ fruit, respectively.

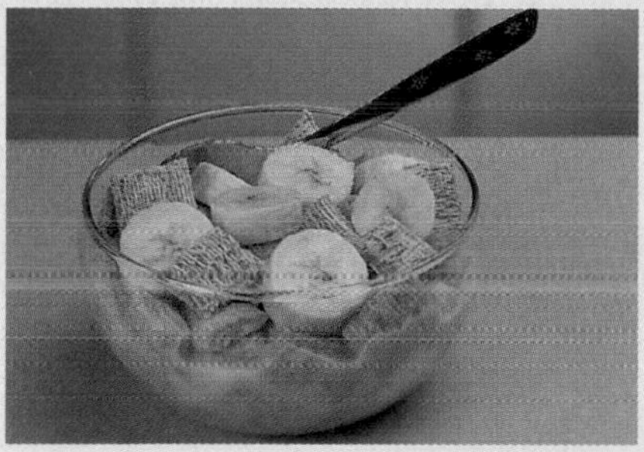

Breakfast		Exchange	Protein (g) Estimate	Protein (g) Actual
1 c shredded wheat	=	2 starch exchanges	6	5
1 c milk	=	1 milk exchange	8	8
½ banana	=	½ fruit exchange	—	1
			14	14

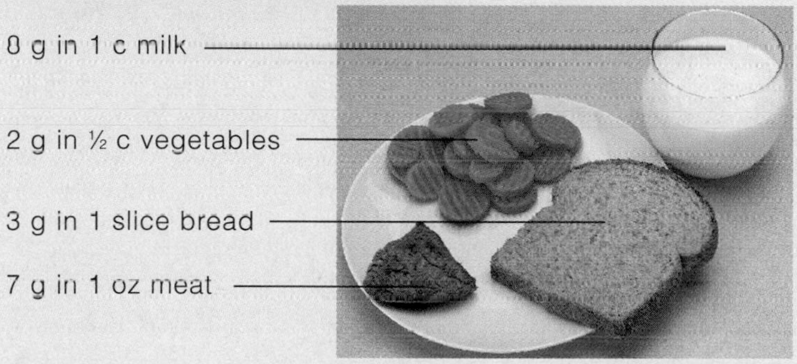

Milks and meats provide lots of protein; starch and vegetables contain a little; fruits and fats have none.

Using the exchange system to estimate, this breakfast provides about 14 grams of protein. A computer diet analysis program calculated the same. The exchange system sometimes over-or underestimates the protein contents of individual foods, but for most, its estimates of daily intakes are close. In any case, for nutrients eaten in such large quantities as protein, a difference of a few grams in a day's total is insignificant.

ments.[27] An excess of one amino acid can create such a demand for a carrier that it prevents the absorption of another amino acid, creating a deficiency. Those amino acids winning the competition enter in excess, creating the possibility of a toxicity. Toxicity of single amino acids in animal studies raises concerns about their use in human beings.[28] Anyone considering taking amino acid supplements should check with a physician first.

In two cases, recommendations for single amino acid supplements have led to widespread public use—lysine to prevent or relieve the infections that cause herpes cold sores on the mouth or genital organs, and tryptophan to relieve pain, depression, and insomnia. In both cases, enthusiastic popular reports and careful scientific experiments are at odds. Lysine does not relieve or cure herpes infections, and if long-term use helps prevent them, it does so only in some individuals and with unknown associated risks.

Tryptophan does have some interesting effects with respect to pain and sleep, but its use for these purposes is still experimental. More than 1500 people who elected to take tryptophan supplements developed a rare blood disorder known as eosinophilia myalgia syndrome (EMS). EMS is characterized by severe muscle pain, extremely high fever, and, in over three dozen cases, death. Treatment usually involves physical therapy and low doses of corticosteroids to relieve symptoms temporarily. Some evidence suggests that changes in procedures at a major Japanese tryptophan processing plant may have introduced contaminants that caused the disease.[30] Later research suggests multiple factors were involved, and the exact causes of EMS remain unknown. The FDA issued a recall of all products containing tryptophan.*

It is safest to obtain lysine, tryptophan, and all other amino acids in protein foods, eaten with carbohydrate to facilitate their use in the body. With all that we know about science, it is hard to improve on nature.

In summary, protein is indispensable to life and growth. Deficiencies arise from both energy-poor and protein-poor diets and lead to the devastating diseases of marasmus and kwashiorkor. Together these diseases are known as PEM (protein-energy malnutrition), the major form of malnutrition causing infections and death in children worldwide. Excesses of food energy and protein are also harmful. Optimally, the diet will be adequate in energy from carbohydrate and fat and will deliver 0.8 grams of protein per kilogram of normal body weight each day. U.S. and Canadian diets are typically more than adequate in this respect, and protein or amino acid supplements are superfluous.

---

*An EMS hotline (800-EMS-2829) has been established to disseminate information about the syndrome.

Study Questions

1. How does the chemical structure of proteins differ from the structures of carbohydrates and fats?
2. Describe the structure of amino acids, and explain how their sequence in proteins affects the proteins' shapes. What are essential amino acids?
3. Describe protein digestion and absorption.
4. Describe some of the roles proteins play in the human body.
5. What are enzymes? What roles do they play in chemical reactions? Describe the differences between enzymes and hormones.
6. How does the body use amino acids? What is deamination?
7. Describe protein synthesis.
8. What factors affect the quality of dietary protein? What is a complete protein?
9. How can vegetarians meet their protein needs without eating meat?
10. What are the health consequences of ingesting inadequate protein and energy? Describe marasmus and kwashiorkor. How can the two conditions be distinguished, and in what ways do they overlap?
11. How might protein excess, or the type of protein eaten, influence health?
12. What factors are considered in establishing recommended protein intakes? Define nitrogen balance. What conditions are associated with zero, positive, and negative balance?
13. Which food lists of the exchange system supply protein in abundance? In moderation? Not at all?
14. What are the benefits and risks of taking protein and amino acid supplements?

Problem Set appears on the next page

Notes

1. *Report of the Expert Advisory Committee on Amino Acids* (Ottawa: Health and Welfare Canada, 1990), p. 9.
2. J. C. Waterlow, Whole-body protein turnover in humans—Past, present, and future, *Annual Review of Nutrition* 15 (1995): 57–92.
3. V. R. Young and J. S. Marchini, Mechanisms and nutritional significance of metabolic responses to altered intakes of protein and amino acids, with reference to nutritional adaptation in humans, *American Journal of Clinical Nutrition* 51 (1990): 270–289.
4. V. R. Young, Soy protein in relation to human protein and amino acid nutrition, *Journal of the American Dietetic Association* 91 (1991): 828–835; J. W. Erdman and E. J. Fordyce, Soy products and the human diet, *American Journal of Clinical Nutrition* 49 (1989): 725–737.
5. V. R. Young and P. L. Pellett, Plant proteins in relation to human protein and amino acid nutrition, *American Journal of Clinical Nutrition* 59 (1994): 1203S–1212S; Position of The American Dietetic Association: Vegetarian diets, *Journal of the American Dietetic Association* 93 (1993): 1317–1319.
6. Protein quality evaluation, Report of the Joint FAO/WHO Expert Consultation, FAO Food and Nutrition Paper 51 (Rome: Food and Agriculture Organization of the United Nations, 1991); G. Sarwar and F. E. McDonough, Evaluation of protein digestibility–corrected amino acid score method for assessing protein quality of foods, *Journal of the Association of Official Analytical Chemists* 73 (1990): 347–356.
7. E. C. Henley, Food and Drug Administration's proposed labeling rules for protein, *Journal of the American Dietetic Association* 92 (1992): 293–296; V. R. Young and P. L. Pellett, Protein evaluation, amino acid scoring and the Food and Drug Administration's proposed food labeling regulation, *Journal of Nutrition* 121 (1991): 145–150.
8. M. C. Latham, Protein-energy malnutrition, in *Present Knowledge in Nutrition*, 6th ed., ed. M. L. Brown (Washington, D.C.: International Life Sciences Institute—Nutrition Foundation, 1990), pp. 39–46.
9. J. Wolgemuth and coauthors, Wasting malnutrition and inadequate nutrient intakes identified in a multiethnic homeless population, *Journal of the American Dietetic Association* 92 (1992): 834–839; E. Luder and coauthors, Health and nutrition survey in a group of urban homeless adults, *Journal of the American Dietetic Association* 90 (1990): 1387–1392.
10. B. Torún and F. Chew, Protein-energy malnutrition, in *Modern Nutrition in Health and Disease*, 8th ed., eds., M. E. Shils, J. A. Olson, and M. Shike (Philadelphia: Lea & Febiger, 1994), pp. 950–976.
11. C. Gopalan, The contribution of nutrition research to the control of undernutrition: The Indian experience, *Annual Review of Nutrition* 12 (1992): 1–17.
12. R. G. Hendrickse, Kwashiorkor: The hypothesis that incriminates aflatoxins, *Pediatrics* 88 (1991): 376–379.
13. D. B. Jelliffe and E. F. P. Jelliffe, Causation of kwashiorkor: Toward a multifactorial consensus, *Pediatrics* 90 (1992): 110–112.
14. J. C. Waterlow, Childhood malnutrition in developing nations: Looking back and looking forward, *Annual Review of Nutrition* 14 (1994): 1–19.
15. L. Lewinter-Suskind and coauthors, The malnourished child, in *Textbook of Pediatric Nutrition*, 2nd ed., eds., R. M. Suskind and L. Lewinter-Suskind (New York: Raven Press, 1993), pp. 127–140.
16. R. K. Chandra, 1990 McCollum Award Lecture: Nutrition and immunity: Lessons from the past and new insights into the future, *American Journal of Clinical Nutrition* 53 (1991): 1087–1101.
17. J. W. Anderson, B. M. Johnstone, and M. E. Cook-Newell, Meta-analysis of the effects of soy protein intake on serum lipids, *New England Journal of Medicine* 333 (1995): 276–282; K. K. Carroll, Review of clinical studies on cholesterol lowering response to soy protein, *Journal of the American Dietetic Association* 91 (1991): 820–827; K. Widhalm and coauthors, Effect of soy protein diet versus standard low fat, low cholesterol diet on lipid and lipoprotein levels in children with familial or polygenic hypercholesterolemia, *Journal of Pediatrics* 123 (1993): 30–34.
18. K. S. McCully, Micronutrients, homocysteine metabolism, and atherosclerosis, in *Micronutrients in Health and in Disease Prevention*, eds. A. Bendich and C. E. Butterworth, Jr. (New York: Marcel Dekker, 1991), pp. 69–93; J. Selhub and coauthors, Association between plasma homocysteine concentrations and extracranial carotid-artery stenosis, *New England Journal of Medicine* 332 (1995): 286–291; M. J. Stampfer and M. R. Malinow, Can lowering homocysteine levels reduce cardiovascular risk? *New England Journal of Medicine* 332 (1995): 328–329; J. B. Ubbink, Vitamin nutrition status and homocysteine: An atherogenic risk factor, *Nutrition Reviews* 52 (1994): 383–393.
19. M. J. Stampfer and coauthors, A prospective study of plasma homocyst(e)ine and risk of myocardial infarction in U.S. physicians, *Journal of the American Medical Association* 268 (1992): 877–881.
20. N. Pancharuniti and coauthors, Plasma homocyst(e)ine, folate, and vitamin B-12 concentrations and risk for early-onset coronary artery disease, *American Journal of Clinical Nutrition* 59 (1994): 940–948; J. B. Ubbink and coauthors, Vitamin B-12, vitamin B-6, and folate nutritional status in men with hyperhomocysteinemia, *American Journal of Clinical Nutrition* 57 (1993): 47–53; J. Selhub and coauthors, Vitamin status and intake as primary determinants of homocysteinemia in an elderly population, *Journal of the American Medical Association* 270 (1993): 2693–2698.

21. W. H. Chow and coauthors, Protein intake and risk of renal cell cancer, *Journal of the National Cancer Institute* 86 (1994): 1131–1139.
22. J. Hu and coauthors, Dietary intakes and urinary excretion of calcium and acids: A cross-sectional study of women in China, *American Journal of Clinical Nutrition* 58 (1993): 398–406.
23. Committee on Dietary Allowances, 1989, pp. 72–73; C. D. Arnaud and S. D. Sanchez, The role of calcium in osteoporosis, *Annual Review of Nutrition* 10 (1990): 397–414; R. P. Heaney, Protein intake and the calcium economy, *Journal of the American Dietetic Association* 93 (1993): 1259–1260.
24. J. A. Metz, J. J. B. Anderson, and P. N. Gallagher, Intakes of calcium, phosphorus, and protein, and physical activity level are related to radial bone mass in young adult women, *American Journal of Clinical Nutrition* 58 (1993): 537–542; Heaney, 1993.
25. R. R. Recker and coauthors, Bone gain in young adult women, *Journal of the American Medical Association* 268 (1992): 2403–2408.
26. V. Herbert, L-Tryptophan: A mediocolegal case against over-the-counter marketing of supplements of amino acids, *Nutrition Today*, March/April 1992, pp. 27–30.
27. H. N. Christensen, Amino acid nutrition: A two-step absorptive process, *Nutrition Reviews* 51 (1993): 95–100.
28. *Report of the Expert Advisory Committee on Amino Acids* (Ottawa: Health and Welfare Canada, 1990), p. 9.
29. S. A. Anderson and D. J. Raiten, eds., *Safety of Amino Acids Used as Supplements* (Bethesda, Md.: Federation of American Societies for Experimental Biology, 1992).
30. D. J. Clauw and P. Katz, Treatment of the eosinophilia-myalgia syndrome, *New England Journal of Medicine* 323 (1990): 417–418; E. A. Belongia, A. N. Myeno, and M. T. Osterholm, The eosinophilia-myalgia syndrome and tryptophan, *Annual Review of Nutrition* 12 (1992): 235–256.

Problem Set

1. Compare the nutritional values of various protein-rich foods.

   a. You might want to start this exercise by reviewing this list of foods and trying to guess which two foods are the most nutrient dense with respect to protein and which two are the least protein dense. Then look up these foods in Appendix H and record their energy and protein contents in the first two columns of this table. (Later you'll be asked to fill in column 3. The first line is done for you.)

Item No./Food	Energy (kcal)	Protein (g)	Protein per 100 kcal (g)
#602 Roast, oven cooked, prime rib, lean only, 4 oz	272	31	11
#611 Lamb chop, loin, broiled, lean and fat, 1	_____	_____	_____
#617 Bacon (pork), 3 medium slices	_____	_____	_____
#646 Roasted chicken breast, 1	_____	_____	_____
#647 Roasted chicken, drumstick, 1	_____	_____	_____
#653 Roasted turkey (white meat), 4 oz	_____	_____	_____
#1297 Beef bologna, 1 pce	_____	_____	_____
#720 Almonds (whole), dry roasted, 1 oz	_____	_____	_____
#740 Peanuts, oil roasted, 1 oz	_____	_____	_____
#854 Chickpeas (garbanzo beans), cooked, 1 c	_____	_____	_____
#860 Kidney beans, canned, 1 c	_____	_____	_____
#1288 Lentils (sprouted), stir-fried, 4 oz	_____	_____	_____
#94 2% low-fat milk, 1 c	_____	_____	_____
#144 Soy milk, 1 c	_____	_____	_____
#146 Plain, low-fat yogurt, 1 c	_____	_____	_____
#156 Egg, poached, 1	_____	_____	_____
#1681 Egg substitute, ½ c (equivalent to about 1½ regular, whole eggs)	_____	_____	_____
#925 Soybeans, ½ c	_____	_____	_____

Problem Set (continued)

b. Now it is time to fill in column 3 of the table. For people who have limited energy allowances, the fewer kcalories they have to spend meeting their protein needs, the better, because they will have more kcalories to spend on foods rich in other nutrients. So, for each food, how much protein can you "buy" for 100 kcal? As an example, the roast has 31 g protein in 272 kcal of energy. Let x = grams protein in 100 kcal:

$$\frac{31 \text{ g protein}}{272 \text{ kcal}} = \frac{x \text{ g protein}}{100 \text{ kcal}}$$

$$x = \frac{31 \text{ g protein} \times 100}{272 \text{ kcal}} = \frac{11.4 \text{ g protein}}{100 \text{ kcal}}$$

Round off column 3 to the nearest whole number: 11.4 g rounds off to 11 g protein per 100 kcal.

c. List here the three foods with the highest protein/100 kcal values, and the three with the lowest values.

Best protein buys: ______________ ______________ ______________

Worst protein buys: ______________ ______________ ______________

How do these answers compare with your initial guesses? ______________

d. Suppose you were a vegetarian who wanted to eat no meat or milk products. Select from the previous list, the lowest-fat nonmeat, nonmilk sources of protein. Which of the foods are the best sources of protein for the kcalories? ______________

2. Compute recommended protein intakes for people of different sizes. Refer to the box on p. 221 and compute the protein recommendation for the following people. The intake for a woman 5 ft 8 in tall is computed for you as an example.

A woman 5 ft 8 in tall is 68 in tall. From the table on the inside back cover, the midpoint in the blue area for this woman is 67 kg. (There are 8 blue rectangles, so the midpoint is between the 4th and 5th rectangles. If there were 7 rectangles, the midpoint would be the 4th rectangle.)

$0.8 \text{ g/kg} \times 67 \text{ kg} = 54 \text{ g protein per day.}$

a. A woman 5 ft 1 in tall: ______________

b. A man (18 years) 6 ft 4 in tall: ______________

3. Develop a perspective on the recommendation that protein should deliver 10% of daily kcalories. The chapter warns that this recommendation is not always appropriate. Consider a man 36 years old who is 5 ft 10 in tall, is moderately active, and eats 3500 kcal/day with 10% of the kcalories from protein.

a. What is this man's protein intake? Show your calculations: ______________

b. Is his protein intake appropriate? Too high? Too low? Justify your answer. ______________

4. Trade protein sources to increase fiber and reduce fat intake. The chapter says that an effective way to do this is to eat fewer animal sources of protein and more plant sources.

a. Start with a food choice based on meat, and then trade it for a serving of beans and rice, as follows (fill in the values):

(continued on the next page)

Problem Set (continued)

Item No./Food	Weight (g)	Energy (kcal)	Fat (g)	Fiber (g)
#598 Hamburger, 3 oz	______	______	______	______
#474 Hamburger bun, 1	______	______	______	______
#968 Catsup, 1 tbs	______	______	______	______
Totals:	______	______	______	______

b. Now replace the hamburger and bun with an approximately equal number of kcalories of beans and rice. Use salsa in place of catsup:

Item No./Food	Weight (g)	Energy (kcal)	Fat (g)	Fiber (g)
#796 Black beans, ½ c	______	______	______	______
#544 White rice, regular long grain, 1 c	______	______	______	______
#1347 Salsa, 1 tbs	______	______	______	______
Totals:	______	______	______	______

c. How much fat did you save by making this trade? ______ How many kcalories was that? ______ Show your calculations. ______________________________

d. How much fiber did you gain? ______________________________

e. What was the total weight of the hamburger meal? ______ The bean meal? ______________

This exercise is intended to help you see that when energy intake remains the same but you replace high-fat meat protein sources with high-fiber plant protein sources, you can eat considerably more food. This is one of the reasons why high-fiber items contribute satiety to a meal.

Vegetarian, Mediterranean, and Other Meat-Restricted Foodways

The waiter presents this evening's specials: a fresh spinach salad topped with mandarin oranges, raisins, and sunflower seeds, served with a bowl of pasta smothered in a mushroom and tomato sauce and topped with grated parmesan cheese. Then this one: a salad made of chopped parsley, scallions, celery, and tomatoes mixed with bulgar wheat and dressed with olive oil and lemon juice, served with a spinach and feta cheese pie. Do these meals sound good to you? Or is something missing . . . a pork chop or ribeye, perhaps?

Would vegetarian fare be acceptable to you some of the time? Most of the time? Ever? Perhaps it is helpful to recognize that dietary choices fall among a continuum—from one end, where people eat no meat or foods of animal origin, to the other end, where they eat generous quantities daily. Meat's place in the diet has been the subject of much research and controversy, as this highlight will reveal. One of the missions of this highlight, in fact, is to identify the *range* of meat intakes most compatible with health.

People who choose to exclude meat and other animal-derived foods from their diets today do so for many of the same reasons the Greek philosopher Pythagoras cited in the sixth century B.C.: physical health, ecological responsibility, and philosophical concerns. They might also cite world hunger issues, economic reasons, ethical concerns, or religious beliefs as motivating factors.

Vegetarians generally are categorized, not by their motivations, but by the foods they choose not to eat (see the glossary on p. 230). Some exclude red meat only; some also exclude chicken or fish; others also exclude eggs; and still others exclude milk and milk products as well. As you will see, though, the foods a person *excludes* are not nearly as important as the foods a person *includes* in the diet. Most vegetarian diets include a variety of grains, vegetables, legumes, and fruits, which offer abundant complex carbohydrates and fibers, an assortment of vitamins and minerals, and little fat—characteristics that reflect current dietary recommendations aimed at reducing obesity and the risks of several chronic diseases such as hypertension, heart disease, and cancer. Vegetarian diets that are well planned can offer sound nutrition and health benefits to adults.[1]

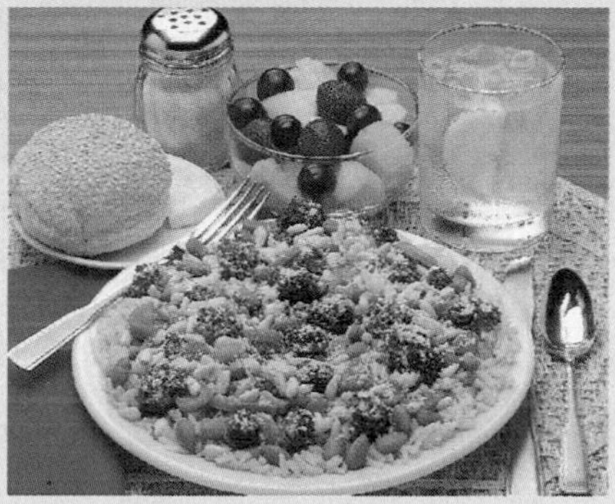

A balanced meal need not include meat to be nutritious.

This highlight first looks at the health benefits and potential problems of vegetarian diets and then shows how to plan a well-balanced vegetarian diet. It closes with a description of the Mediterranean diet—an ethnic pattern of eating that includes very little meat and exceeds current dietary recommendations for fat and alcohol, yet still seems to support good health.

HEALTH BENEFITS OF VEGETARIAN DIETS

Research on the health impacts of vegetarianism would be relatively easy if vegetarians differed from other people only in not eating meat. Many vegetarians, however, have adopted lifestyles that differ from those of meat eaters in many other ways. Compared with others, vegetarians are more likely to practice healthy habits: they typically maintain a healthy weight, use no tobacco or illicit drugs, use alcohol in moderation (if at all), and are physically active. Researchers must account for the effects of these lifestyle differences before they can pick out what aspects of health correlate just with diet. Even then, *correlations* are merely statements of what health factors *go with* the vegetarian diet; they do not show what health effects may be *caused by* the diet. Without more evidence, conclusions are only tentative. Still, with all these qualifications, research findings are intriguing. They seem to suggest that vegetarian diets offer some health benefits.

Weight Control

In general, vegetarians maintain a healthier body weight than nonvegetarians. Since obesity impairs health in a number of ways, this gives vegetarians a health advantage.

Glossary

lactovegetarians: people who include milk and milk products, but exclude meat, poultry, fish, seafood, and eggs from their diets.
lacto = milk

lacto-ovo-vegetarians: people who include milk, milk products, and eggs, but exclude meat, poultry, fish, and seafood from their diets.
ovo = egg

macrobiotic diets: extremely restrictive diets limited to a few cereals and fluids; based on metaphysical beliefs and not on nutrition.

meat replacement: products formulated to look and taste like meat, fish, or poultry; usually made of textured vegetable protein.

omnivores: people who have no formal restriction on the eating of any foods.
omni = all
vores = to eat

semivegetarians: people who include some, but not all, groups of animal-derived foods in their diets; they usually exclude red meat, but may occasionally include poultry, fish, and seafood; sometimes called **partial vegetarians.**

tempeh (TEM-pay)**:** a fermented soybean food, rich in protein and fiber.

textured vegetable protein: processed soybean protein used in vegetarian products such as soy burgers.

tofu (TOE-foo)**:** a curd made from soybeans, rich in protein and often fortified with calcium; used in many Asian and vegetarian dishes in place of meat.

vegans (VAY-guns or VEJ-ans)**:** people who exclude all animal-derived foods (including meat, poultry, fish, eggs, and dairy products) from their diets; also called **pure vegetarians**, **strict vegetarians**, or **total vegetarians**.

vegetarians: a general term used to describe people who exclude meat, poultry, fish, or other animal-derived foods from their diets.

Blood Pressure

Appropriate body weight helps to maintain a healthy blood pressure, as does a diet low in total fat and saturated fat and high in fiber, fruits, and vegetables.[2] In one group of volunteers, blood pressure declined during the period when they ate a vegetarian diet and rose again when they resumed eating meat.[3] Lifestyle factors also seem to influence blood pressure: smoking and alcohol intake raise blood pressure, and exercise lowers it.

Coronary Artery Disease

Fewer vegetarians suffer from diseases of the heart and arteries than meat eaters. The dietary factors most directly related to coronary artery disease is saturated fat, and in general, vegetarian diets are lower in total fat, saturated fat, and cholesterol than typical meat-based diets. Vegetarian diets are also higher in dietary fiber, another factor that helps control blood lipids.

When vegetarians are fed meat, which contains saturated fat, their blood lipid profiles change for the worse; when meat eaters are fed a low-fat vegetarian diet, their lipid profiles improve. In fact, one study reversed severe coronary artery disease without drugs by implementing a low-fat vegetarian diet, stress management, physical activity, and a no-smoking plan.[4] Another study compared two low-fat diets—one vegetarian and the other containing lean meats—and found that both diets lowered blood cholesterol, but the vegetarian diet's effects were greater.[5] People who eat meat can lower their blood cholesterol by keeping their intake to a minimum.[6] For example, one study found that semivegetarians who ate one to three servings of meat per week had blood lipids between the low blood lipids of vegetarians and the higher lipids of nonvegetarians.[7]

Cancer

Seventh-Day Adventists, a religious group whose foodways center on a lacto-ovo-vegetarian diet, have a significantly lower mortality rate from cancer than the rest of the population, even after all the cancers attributed to smoking and alcohol are discounted.[8] Their low cancer rates may be due to their vegetarian diets; evidence is overwhelming that high intakes of fruits and vegetables reduce the risks of cancer.[9]

Some scientific findings indicate that vegetarian diets are not only associated with lower cancer mortality in general, but with lower incidence of cancer at specific sites as well, most notably, colon cancer.[10] People with colon cancer seem to eat more meat, more saturated fat, and less fiber than others without cancer. High-protein, high-fat, low-fiber diets create an environment in the human colon that promotes the development of cancer in some people.[11]

In general, then, adults who eat vegetarian diets can reduce their risks of several chronic diseases, including obesity, high blood pressure, heart disease, and cancer. But there is nothing mysterious about the vegetarian diet; it simply includes ample fruits, vegetables, whole grains, and legumes—foods that are higher in fiber, richer in certain vitamins and minerals, and lower in fats than meat-based diets. Some people find it easier to meet today's dietary recommendations for health by following a vegetarian diet than by eating meals with meat. A meat eater can gain some of the same advantages by limiting meat intake to the recommended 5 to 7 ounces daily and selecting lean cuts, as well as including abundant grains, fruits, and vegetables.

Conversely, both vegetarian and meat-based diets can be detrimental to health when overloaded with fat. A vegetarian who dines on cheddar cheese, butter sauces, sour cream, and deep-fried vegetables invites the same health hazards as the person who overeats high-fat meats. And both diets, if not properly balanced, can lack nutrients. Poorly planned vegetarian diets typically lack iron, zinc, calcium, vitamin B_{12}, and vitamin D; without planning, the meat eater's diet may lack vitamin A, vitamin C, folate, and fiber, among others.

PROBLEMS ASSOCIATED WITH VEGETARIAN DIETS

The negative health aspects of any diet, including vegetarian diets, reflect poor diet planning. Careful attention to energy intake and specific problem nutrients can ensure adequacy. Diet planning during pregnancy, lactation, infancy, childhood, and illness, in particular, must provide for the increases in energy and nutrients needed during those times—when the consequences of poor nutrition can be great.

Adequacy of Most Vegetarian Diets

Vegetarians who include milk products and eggs have few nutrient-deficiency concerns. Such diets can adequately support the growth of children.

Inadequacy of Strict Vegetarian Diets

Achieving adequate energy and nutrient intakes may be difficult for the vegan who excludes all animal products, and particularly for growing children and pregnant and lactating women. Foods of plant origin generally offer much less energy per bite than foods of animal origin; while a diet that delivers a lot of food with relatively little energy may be advantageous for many adults, it can be detrimental for children who need energy-dense foods for growth. Vegan diets can fail to provide sufficient energy to support the growth of a child within a quantity of food small enough for the child to eat. A child's small stomach can hold only so much food, and a vegan child may feel full before eating enough to meet nutrient and energy needs. A vegan child's diet should emphasize cereals, legumes, and nuts to meet protein and energy needs in a small volume. Meat, which contains abundant protein, iron, and food energy in less bulk, supports the growth of children more efficiently. Compared with meat-eating children, vegan children tend to be smaller in height and lighter in weight; their low energy intakes can impair growth.[12]

When vegan children get their protein only from plant foods, they may need protein intakes higher than the RDA for normal growth and health. The standard protein recommendations may be inadequate to support the growth of vegan children, but specific recommendations have not been established.[13]

Approximately 2 out of every 15 households include one or more members who are vegetarians. These people number some 12 million nationwide, representing an eightfold increase over the past two decades.[14] Those who plan their diets carefully easily obtain all the nutrients they need to support good health.

VEGETARIAN DIET PLANNING

The vegetarian has the same meal-planning task as any other person—using a variety of foods that will deliver all the needed nutrients within an energy allowance that maintains a healthy body weight. An added challenge is to do so with fewer foods.

Well-planned vegetarian meals can provide adequate amounts of all the nutrients a person needs for good health. Vegetarians can follow the Daily Food Guide presented in Chapter 2 with a few modifications (see Table H6–1). Those who include milk products and eggs can follow the regular plan, using legumes and products made from them, such as peanut butter, tempeh, and tofu, in place of meat. Those who do not use milk can use soy milk fortified with calcium, vitamin D, and vitamin B_{12}. Vegetarian adults should include at least one cup of dark green vegetables daily to help meet iron needs and legumes to help meet zinc needs. In general, these tactics ensure adequate intakes of the main nutrients

Table H6–1

Daily Food Guide for Vegetarians

Food Group	Suggested Daily Servings	Serving Sizes
Breads, cereals and other grain products	6 or more	1 slice bread ½ bun, bagel, or English muffin ½ c cooked cereal, rice, or pasta 1 oz dry cereal
Vegetables	4 or more[a]	½ c cooked or 1 c raw
Fruits	3 or more	1 piece fresh fruit ¾ c fruit juice ½ c canned or cooked fruit
Legumes and other meat alternates	2 to 3	½ c cooked beans 4 oz tofu or tempeh 8 oz soy milk 2 tbs nuts or seeds (these tend to be high in fat, so use sparingly) 1 egg or 2 egg whites
Milk and milk products	2 to 3[b]	1 c low-fat or nonfat milk 1 c low-fat or nonfat yogurt 1½ oz low-fat cheese

[a]Include 1 cup of dark green vegetables daily to help meet iron requirements.

[b]People who do not use milk or milk products: use soy milk fortified with calcium, vitamin D, and vitamin B_{12}.

Source: Adapted with permission from Position of The American Dietetic Association: Vegetarian diets, *Journal of the American Dietetic Association* 93 (1993): 1318.

vegetarian diets might otherwise lack: iron, zinc, calcium, vitamin B_{12}, and vitamin D. In contrast, most vegetarians easily obtain large quantities of the nutrients that are abundant in plant foods: thiamin, riboflavin, folate, and vitamins B_6, C, A, and E.

Protein

Protein is not the problem it was once thought to be for vegetarian diets. People who use animal-derived foods such as milk and eggs receive high-quality proteins and are unlikely to develop protein deficiencies. Even those who eat only plant-derived foods are unlikely to develop protein deficiencies provided that energy intakes are adequate and the protein sources varied.[15] The proteins of whole grains, legumes, seeds, nuts, and vegetables can provide adequate amounts of all the amino acids. An advantage of many vegetarian protein foods is that they are generally lower in saturated fat than meats and are often higher in fiber and richer in some vitamins and minerals.

To ease meal preparation, vegetarians sometimes use meat replacements made of textured vegetable protein (soy protein). These foods are formulated to look and taste like meat, fish, or poultry. Many of these products are designed to match the known nutrient contents of animal-protein foods, but sometimes they fall short. A wise vegetarian does not rely on these products too heavily, but learns to use a variety of whole foods instead. Vegetarians may also use soybeans in the form of bean curds, or tofu, to bolster protein intake.

Iron

Getting enough iron can be a problem even for meat eaters, and those who eat no meat, must pay special attention to their iron intake. The iron in plant foods such as legumes, dark green leafy vegetables, iron-fortified cereals, and whole-grain breads and cereals is not readily absorbed. Iron absorption is enhanced by vitamin C, though, and vegetarians typically eat many vitamin C–rich fruits and vegetables, so that they suffer no more iron-deficiency anemia than other people do.[16]

Zinc

Zinc is similar to iron in that meat is its richest food source and zinc from plant sources is not well absorbed. In addition, soy, which is commonly used as a meat alternate, interferes with zinc absorption. Nevertheless, most vegetarian adults are not zinc deficient.[17] Perhaps the best advice to vegetarians regarding zinc is to eat a variety of nutrient-dense foods; include grains, nuts, and legumes such as black-eyed peas, pinto beans, and kidney beans; and maintain an adequate energy intake. For vegetarians who include seafood, oysters, crabmeat, and shrimp are rich in zinc.

Calcium

The calcium intakes of lactovegetarians are similar to those of the general population, but people who use no milk risk deficiency. Careful planners select calcium-rich foods, such as calcium-fortified juices or soy milk in ample quantities regularly. This is especially important for children. Soy formulas for infants are fortified with calcium and can be used in cooking, even for adults. Other good calcium sources include calcium-set tofu, some legumes, some green vegetables such as broccoli and turnip greens, some nuts such as almonds, and certain seeds such as sesame seeds.*[18] The choices should be varied because binders in some plant foods may limit absorption.

Vitamin B_{12}

The requirement for vitamin B_{12} is small, but this vitamin is found only in animal-derived foods. Fermented plant products such as tempeh, made from soybeans, may contain some vitamin B_{12} from the bacteria that did the fermenting, but unfortunately, much of the vitamin B_{12} found in these products may be an inactive form.[19] Vegans must rely on vitamin B_{12}–fortified sources (such as soy milk or breakfast cereals) or vitamin B_{12} supplements to ensure against deficiency.[20]

*Calcium salts are often added during processing to coagulate the tofu.

Vitamin D

For people who do not use vitamin D–fortified milk and who do not receive enough exposure to sunlight to synthesize adequate vitamin D, supplements may be warranted.[21] This is particularly important for children and older adults. In northern climates during winter months, young children on vegan diets can readily develop rickets, the vitamin D–deficiency disease.[22]

As you can see, vegetarianism is not a religion like Buddhism or Hinduism, but merely an eating plan that selects plant foods to deliver needed nutrients. The quality of the diet depends not on whether it includes meat, but on whether the food choices are nutritionally sound. Health experts would quickly add that one should also limit intakes of substances such as fat and alcohol that are harmful in excess—and vegetarians in this country typically do. Interestingly, the Mediterranean diet—a predominantly vegetarian diet with an ethnic flair—breaks these rules on moderation, yet still seems to have health advantages.

AN ALMOST-VEGETARIAN DIET: THE MEDITERRANEAN DIET

The Mediterranean diet is based on the traditional eating habits of people in a region of the world where the incidence of chronic disease is low and life expectancy is high.[23]*

*Much of the early research (late 1950s and early 1960s) focused on men living in farming communities on the Greek island of Crete.

The many countries that border the Mediterranean Sea each have their own culture, traditions, and dietary habits, but similarities are also evident.[24] The people dine on crusty breads, grains, potatoes, and pasta; a variety of vegetables; feta and mozzarella cheeses and yogurt; and ripe fruit.[25] They eat some fish and poultry, a few eggs, and very little meat.

Their principal source of fat is olive oil and they typically drink wine with meals. Consequently, traditional Mediterranean diets are:[26]

- Low in saturated fat.
- Rich in monounsaturated fat.
- Rich in carbohydrate and fiber.
- Rich in nutrients and nonnutrients that support good health.

Furthermore, because processed foods are used modestly in these countries, intakes of salt, refined sugars, and *trans*-fatty acids are low.[27] All in all, the Mediterranean diet has been gaining a reputation for its health benefits as well as its delicious flavors.

The Mediterranean Diet Pyramid

A few nutrition experts were so impressed with the Mediterranean diet and its health benefits that they created a renegade food pyramid.* Like the official USDA Food Guide Pyramid introduced in Chapter 2, their pyramid is based on breads,

*The Mediterranean diet pyramid was developed by the Harvard School of Public Health, the European office of the World Health Organization, and the Oldways Preservation & Trust in Boston.

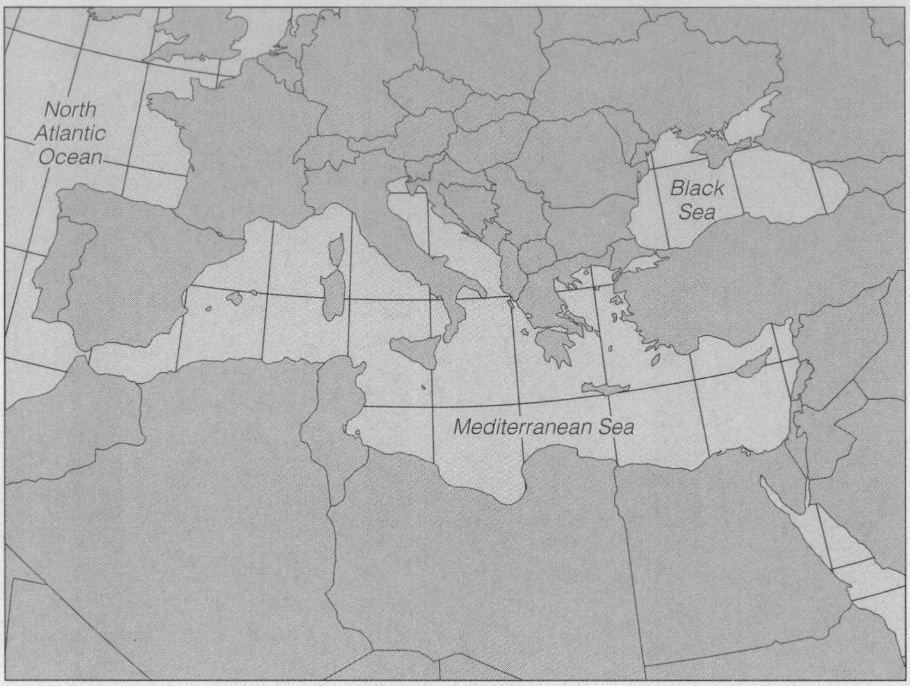

The people of the Mediterranean area eat plenty of fruits, vegetables, legumes, and grains; some dairy products, fish, and poultry; and very little red meat. Olive oil is their principal source of dietary fat.

cereals, rice, pasta, and other grains, and it places vegetables and fruits on the next level up. The Mediterranean pyramid introduces a small difference at this level in that it includes legumes with the vegetable group instead of with the meats, but greater differences become apparent farther up the pyramid. Olive oil sits just above the fruits, vegetables, and legumes, with cheese and yogurt above that; these foods are to be included daily. Fish, poultry, eggs, and sweets come next and are to be eaten a few times per week. Lean red meats sit at the tip of the pyramid, to be eaten only a few times per month. Figure H6–1 compares the two pyramids.

This Mediterranean pyramid contradicts many diet and health recommendations and is worth examining because it raises interesting issues. For example, although current dietary recommendations restrict fat to no more than 30 percent of daily kcalories, the traditional Mediterranean diet can deliver as much as 40 percent of a day's kcalories from fat. The Mediterranean plan does not restrict total fat, but it does limit *animal* fat—a distinction not made in the USDA plan. People following the USDA plan get most of their fat from red meat, poultry, eggs, milk, yogurt, and cheese; consequently much of their fat is saturated fat. Those following the Mediterranean plan use olive oil abundantly, and so receive most of their fat as monounsaturated vegetable oil. Their limited consumption of dairy products and meats provides less than 10 percent of their kcalories from saturated fats—a goal both plans agree on, but the USDA plan typically fails to meet.

The distinctions between types of fat have implications for chronic diseases, as Chapter 5 points out. The monounsaturated fats of olive oil and canola oil and the omega-3 polyunsaturated fats of fish may actually benefit heart health; in contrast, most, but not all, saturated fats are detrimental. Substituting unsaturated fats such as olive oil for saturated fats or *trans*-fatty acids improves blood lipids and reduces the risks of cardiovascular disease.[28] In addition to its beneficial fatty acid composition (high in monounsaturated and low in saturated fatty acids), olive oil contains vitamin E and other antioxidant compounds that protect against heart disease. These distinctions in types of fat are not evident in the USDA pyramid and dietary recommendations. People are simply advised to cut back on all fat so that they will cut back on saturated fat—the real culprit.

Many Mediterranean people drink wine with each meal, and the Mediterranean pyramid includes wine in moderation. Moderate alcohol consumption reduces the risk of cardiovascular disease and seems to be compatible with a healthy lifestyle.[29] The USDA pyramid does not address alcoholic beverages directly, but most diet and health recommendations advise people to drink alcoholic beverages in moderation, if at all.

Perhaps the hallmark of the Mediterranean diet is its abundance of vegetables, fruits, legumes, and whole grains—foods associated with lower risks of cardiovascular disease

Figure H6–1

Food Pyramids Compared

Mediterranean Diet Pyramid

This pyramid is based on the dietary traditions of Crete around 1960, structured in light of current nutrition research.

USDA Pyramid

This pyramid is based on the dietary guidelines established in 1992 by the U.S. Department of Agriculture.

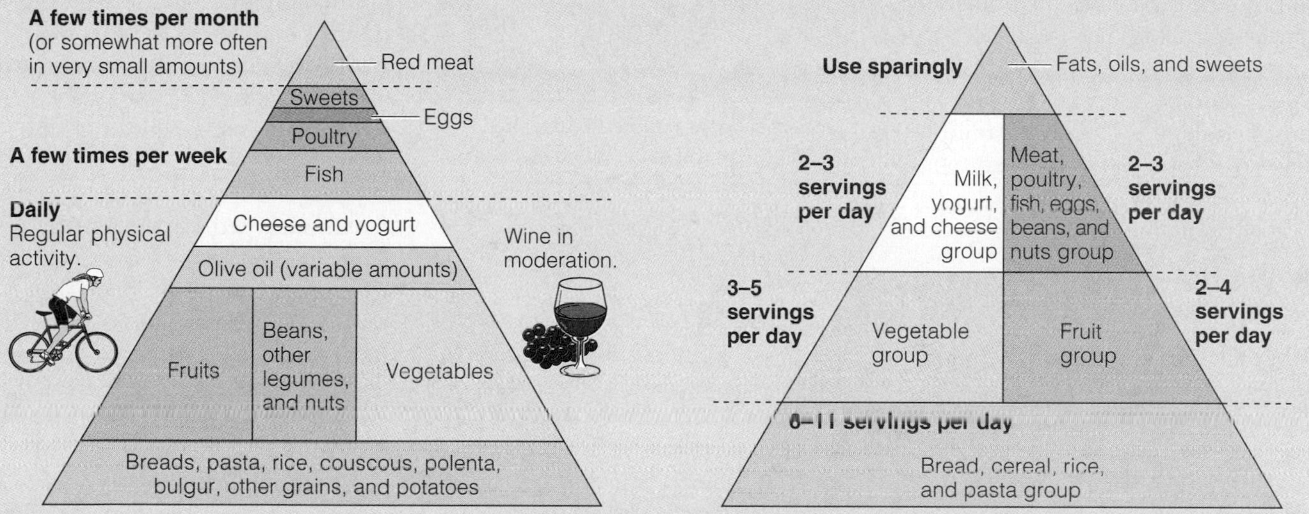

Sources: 1994 Oldways Preservation & Exchange Trust, U.S. Department of Agriculture.

and cancer.[30] The protective effects of these plant-derived foods are attributed not only to their lack of fat, but also to their abundance of nutrients and nonnutritents, many of which act as antioxidants (see Highlight 10).[31]

Some Concerns about the Mediterranean Plan

Critics of the Mediterranean Plan have expressed concerns that it may be inadequate in calcium and iron—two problem nutrients for many people, especially women. Because these nutrients are typically lacking in many people's diets, it seems unwise to restrict calcium selections to cheeses and yogurt and iron-rich meat consumption to a few times a month.

An Implication of the Mediterranean Plan: Limit Meat

Is it appropriate to suggest that people in the United States should adopt Mediterranean eating habits and begin indulging in olive oil and wine? Not really, for at least two reasons. First, diet is not the only, or even the most important, factor implicated in heart disease, as Chapter 18 points out. Many other differences between the lifestyles of the people living in the Mediterranean and those living here could account for the differences in life expectancy and disease risks. Furthermore, as Highlight 2 pointed out, all ethnic food patterns have pros and cons. Perhaps the most important suggestion to be taken from the Mediterranean Plan is to focus more on grains, vegetables, and fruits, and less on meats. The average daily consumption of meat in the United States is more than half a pound per person per *day*; in the Mediterranean region, it is about half a pound per person per *week*. The difference in meat intake, and therefore in saturated fat intake, is significant.

In general, at most, two 3-ounce servings of meat per day are needed.[32] This amount of meat alone provides most of a person's daily recommended protein intake—and other foods together can provide a similar amount. Some researchers argue that this much meat eaten daily is not compatible with good health; if any meat is eaten, they suggest it should be eaten infrequently and in small portions.[33] With the evidence pointing to the health advantages of a meat-restricted diet, perhaps between 0 and 6 ounces of meat daily would best serve the needs of most people; the USDA pyramid suggests 5 to 7 ounces of meat, poultry, or fish a day.

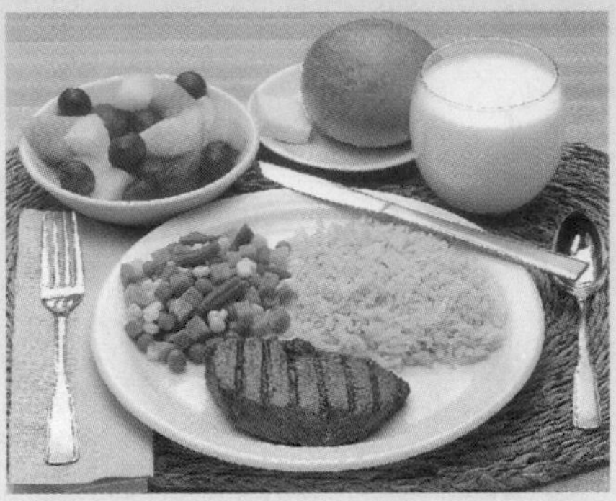

Two meat servings of the size depicted here represent the maximum daily meat intake suggested by the Daily Food Guide as health promoting.

PYRAMIDS—OFFICIAL AND OTHERWISE

What about this renegade pyramid? It seems almost sacrilegious to oppose the government's official word on nutrition, but it can be enlightening to take a peek at the politics involved in developing such recommendations.

For more than a century, government agencies have issued statements advising consumers about food choices. Dietary guidelines may originally have been developed purely for the public good, but now they underlie national policy in many areas. They are used to define curricula for nutrition education, establish regulations for food labels, develop new food products, regulate institutional foodservices, provide commodity foods, and create school menus. And because the guidelines encourage people to eat more of some foods and less of others, they exert a profound effect on food purchases. Inevitably, therefore, politics has become involved in the dietary guidelines.

Food producers did not complain when early dietary recommendations urged people to "Eat more" of their products to help prevent nutrient deficiencies. However, when recommendations began to urge people to "Eat less" of some products to help prevent chronic diseases, food producers became aroused. Now, lobbyists representing the food industry scurry about Capitol Hill trying to protect their interests and influence national policies that affect dietary intakes. Their efforts have been successful.

The influence of the meat industry on government policy makers provides a notable example.[34] In 1977, a dietary goal was to "Decrease consumption of meat." The "Eat less" guideline was changed in 1980 to "Choose lean meat." By 1990 the recommendation was stated even more favorably, "Have two or three servings, with a daily total of about 6 ounces." By 1992, when the pyramid was created, the daily total had been revised to "5 to 7 ounces." The design of the pyramid itself was delayed by a year and cost an additional million dollars, in large part because of protests from the meat industry.

The preceding paragraph was not written to pick on the meat industry. Lobbyists representing the dairy industry, the egg industry, the sugar industry, and every other food manufacturer try to influence dietary recommendations. The point is that people outside the world of nutrition science profoundly influence our nation's diet. Shifting our diet towards a healthier plan would require major changes in the agricultural and food manufacturing policies and practices of this nation.[35] One wonders what the government's nutrition advice would be if it were untainted by politics.

Having learned some of the relationships between diet and health, many people may discover that their strategies for planning meals need to change. In the past, they decided what cut of beef, ham, pork, lamb, poultry, or fish to prepare and then filled in the menu with an accompanying "starch" (potato, rice, or noodles), salad or other vegetable, and bread. Now, they fill their dinner plates with legumes, grains, vegetables, and fruits. Then they add small quantities of milk products, eggs, lean meat, fish, or poultry.

For the most part, it seems that nonmeat and low-meat diets can both support good health. Keep in mind, too, that diet is only one factor influencing health. Whatever a diet consists of, its context is also important: no smoking; alcohol consumption in moderation, if at all; regular physical activity; adequate rest; and medical attention when needed all contribute to a healthy life. Establishing these healthy habits early in life seems to be the most important step one can take to reduce the risks of later diseases.[36]

NOTES

1. Position of The American Dietetic Association: Vegetarian diets, *Journal of the American*

Dietetic Association 93 (1993): 1317–1319.
2. L. J. Beilin, Vegetarian and other complex diets, fats, fiber, and hypertension, *American Journal of Clinical Nutrition* 59 (1994): 1130S–1135S.
3. L. J. Beilin and coauthors, Vegetarian diet and blood pressure levels: Incidental or causal association? *American Journal of Clinical Nutrition* 48 (1988): 806–810.
4. D. Ornish and coauthors, Can lifestyle changes reverse coronary heart disease? *Lancet* 336 (1990): 129–133.
5. M. Kestin and coauthors, Cardiovascular disease risk factors in free-living men: Comparison of two prudent diets, one based on lacto-ovovegetarianism and the other allowing meat, *American Journal of Clinical Nutrition* 50 (1989): 280–287.
6. S. A. Morgan, A. J. Sinclair, and K. O'Dea, Effect on serum lipids of addition of safflower oil or olive oil to very-low-fat diets rich in lean beef, *Journal of the American Dietetic Association* 93 (1993): 644–648.
7. C. L. Melby, M. L. Toohey, and J. Cebrick, Blood pressure and blood lipids among vegetarian, semivegetarian, and nonvegetarian African Americans, *American Journal of Clinical Nutrition* 59 (1994): 103–109.
8. P. K. Mills and coauthors, Cancer incidence among California Seventh-Day Adventists, 1976–1982, *American Journal of Clinical Nutrition* 59 (1994): 1136S–1142S.
9. W. C. Willett, Micronutrients and cancer risk, *American Journal of Clinical Nutrition* 59 (1994): 1162S–1165S.
10. R. Frentzel-Beyme and J. Chang-Claude, Vegetarian diets and colon cancer: The German experience, *American Journal of Clinical Nutrition* 59 (1994): 1143S–1152S.
11. M. I. McBurney, P. J. Van Soest, and J. L. Jeraci, Colonic carcinogenesis: The microbial feast or famine mechanism, *Nutrition and Cancer* 10 (1987): 23–28.
12. T. A. B. Sanders and S. Reddy, Vegetarian diets and children, *American Journal of Clinical Nutrition* 59 (1994): 1176S–1181S.
13. P. B. Acosta, Availability of essential amino acids and nitrogen in vegan diets, *American Journal of Clinical Nutrition* 48 (1988): 868–874.
14. P. K. Johnson, Preface to the Second International Congress on Vegetarian Nutrition, *American Journal of Clinical Nutrition* (supplement) 59 (1994): vii.
15. V. R. Young and P. L. Pellett, Plant proteins in relation to human protein and amino acid nutrition, *American Journal of Clinical Nutrition* 59 (1994): 1203S–1212S; Position of The American Dietetic Association, 1993.
16. W. J. Craig, Iron status of vegetarians, *American Journal of Clinical Nutrition* 59 (1994): 1233S–1237S.
17. R. J. Gibson, Content and bioavailability of trace elements in vegetarian diets, *American Journal of Clinical Nutrition* 59 (1994): 1223S–1232S.
18. C. M. Weaver and K. L. Plawecki, Dietary calcium: Adequacy of a vegetarian diet, *American Journal of Clinical Nutrition* 59 (1994): 1238S–1241S.
19. V. Herbert, Vitamin B-12: Plant sources, requirements, and assay, *American Journal of Clinical Nutrition* 48 (1988): 852–858.
20. D. R. Miller and coauthors, Vitamin B-12 status in a macrobiotic community, *American Journal of Clinical Nutrition* 53 (1991): 524–529.
21. C. Lamberg-Allardt and coauthors, Low serum 25-hydroxyvitamin D concentrations and secondary hyperparathyroidism in middle-aged white strict vegetarians, *American Journal of Clinical Nutrition* 58 (1993): 684–689.
22. P. C. Dagnelie, High prevalence of rickets in infants on macrobiotic diets, *American Journal of Clinical Nutrition* 51 (1990): 202–208.
23. A. Keys, Mediterranean diet and public health: Personal reflections, *American Journal of Clinical Nutrition* 61 (1995): 1321S–1323S.
24. E. Helsing, Traditional diets and disease patterns of Mediterranean, circa 1960, *American Journal of Clinical Nutrition* 61 (1995): 1329S–1337S.
25. W. C. Willett and coauthors, Mediterranean diet pyramid: A cultural model of healthy eating, *American Journal of Clinical Nutrition* 61 (1995): 1402S–1406S.
26. A. P. Simopoulos, The Mediterranean Food Guide—Greek column rather than an Egyptian Pyramid, *Nutrition Today* 30 (1995): 54–61.
27. W. P. T. James, Nutrition science and policy research: Implications for Mediterranean diets, *American Journal of Clinical Nutrition* 61 (1995): 1324S–1328S.
28. M. B. Katan, P. L. Zock, and R. P. Mensink, Dietary oils, serum lipoproteins, and coronary heart disease, *Amerian Journal of Clinical Nutrition* 61 (1995): 1368S–1373S.
29. E. B. Rimm and R. C. Ellison, Alcohol in the Mediterranean diet, *American Journal of Clinical Nutrition* 61 (1995): 1378S–1382S.
30. A. Tavani and C. LaVecchia, Fruit and vegetable consumption and cancer risk in a Mediterranean population, *American Journal of Clinical Nutrition* (1995): 1374S–1377S; L. H. Kushi, E. B. Lenart, and W. C. Willett, Health implications of Mediterranean diets in light of contemporary knowledge. 1. Plant foods and dairy products, *American Journal of Clinical Nutrition* 61 (1995): 1407S–1415S.
31. W. P. T. James, G. G. Duthie, and K. W. J. Wahle, The Mediterranean diet: Protective or simply non-toxic? *European Journal of Clinical Nutrition* (supplement 2) 43 (1989): 31–41.
32. Members of the Committee on Diet and Health as quoted in *The Nation's Health*, a newsletter published by the American Public Health Association, April 1989, p. 15.
33. L. H. Kushi, E. B. Lenart, and W. C. Willett, Health implications of Mediterranean diets in light of contemporary knowledge. 2. Meat, wine, fats, and oils, *American Journal of Clinical Nutrition* 61 (1995): 1416S–1427S.
34. M. Nestle, Editorial: The politics of dietary guidance—A new opportunity, *American Journal of Public Health* 84 (1994): 713–715.
35. P. O'Brien, Dietary shifts and implications for US agriculture, *American Journal of Clinical Nutrition* 61 (1995): 1390S–1396S.
36. V. Følnnebø, The healthy Seventh-day Adventist lifestyle: What is the Norwegian experience? *American Journal of Clinical Nutrition* 59 (1994): 1124S–1129S.

Chapter 7

Metabolism: Transformations and Interactions

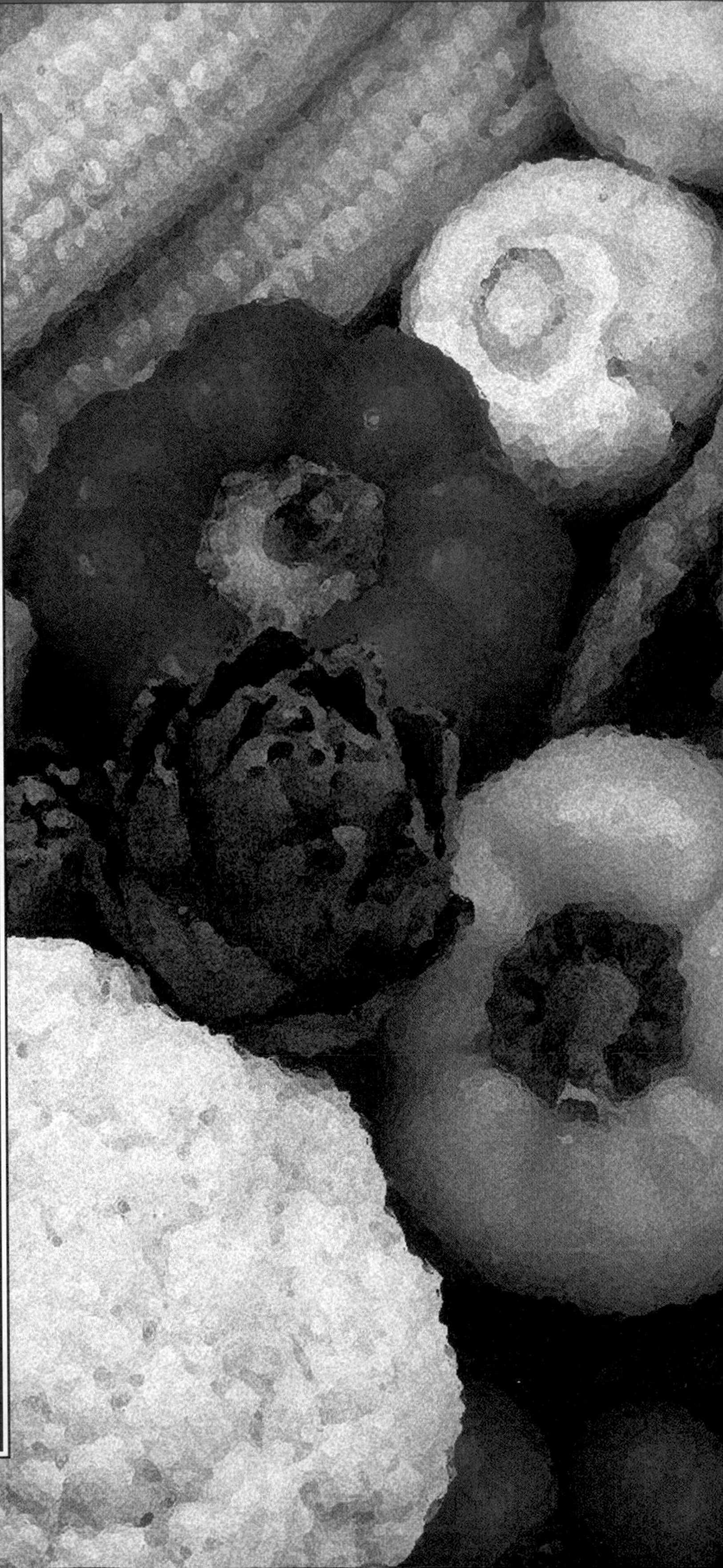

CONTENTS

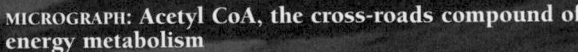

MICROGRAPH: Acetyl CoA, the cross-roads compound of energy metabolism

We are all solar creatures. Almost all living things depend on the sun's energy. Plants rely directly on the sun to provide the light energy that drives the reactions of photosynthesis—the process by which plants make carbohydrate from carbon dioxide and water using the energy from sunlight. That energy from the sun is captured in the energy that holds atoms together—the energy of chemical bonds. We humans, and all other animals, use the sun indirectly, for we cannot photosynthesize. We depend on plants, or on animals that eat plants, for the food that gives us our energy-yielding nutrients.

This chapter describes the processes in the human body that *release* energy from the chemical bonds in nutrients. In so doing, it lays the groundwork for understanding many of the daily realities examined in later chapters. Energy derived from the metabolism of nutrients enables people to ride bicycles, compose music, and do everything else they do. An excess of food energy makes people fat, though most people do not understand how it does this. Nor do most people understand exactly how physical activity speeds up energy use and fat loss. By studying metabolism, readers who are interested in losing weight will discover which foods contribute most to body fat and which to select when trying to lose weight safely. Physically active readers will discover which foods best support endurance activities and which to select when trying to build lean body mass.

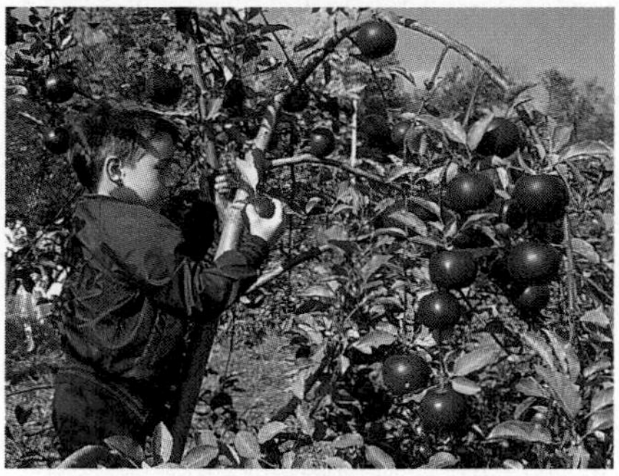

We receive energy from the sun by way of the foods we eat.

photosynthesis: the process by which green plants make carbohydrates from carbon dioxide and water using the green pigment chlorophyll to trap the sun's energy.
photo = light
synthesis = put together (making)

Chemical Reactions in the Body

Earlier chapters have already introduced some of the body's chemical reactions: examples are the making and breaking of the bonds in carbohydrates, lipids, and proteins. The sum of these and all the other chemical reactions that go on in living cells is known as metabolism; and *energy* metabolism includes all the ways the body obtains and spends energy from food.

Appendix B provides an overview of basic chemistry concepts.

metabolism: the sum total of all the chemical reactions that go on in living cells; **energy metabolism** includes all the reactions by which the body obtains and spends the energy from food.
meta = among
bole = change

Chapters 4, 5, and 6 laid the groundwork for the study of metabolism; a brief review may be helpful. During digestion, the body breaks down the three energy-yielding nutrients—carbohydrates, fats, and proteins—into four basic units that can be absorbed into the blood:

- From carbohydrates—glucose.
- From fats—glycerol and fatty acids.
- From proteins—amino acids.

Amino acids are not primarily energy nutrients, but they can flow into energy pathways if needed or if eaten in excess, so they are included.

Look for these four basic units to appear again and again in the metabolic reactions described in this chapter. Alcohol also enters many of the metabolic pathways; Highlight 7 focuses on how alcohol disrupts metabolism and how the body handles it.

Building Reactions—Anabolism The cells can use the basic units of energy-yielding nutrients to build body compounds. Glucose units may be joined together to make glycogen chains. Glycerol and fatty acids may be assembled into triglycerides. Amino acids may be linked together to make proteins. Each of these reactions starts with small, simple compounds and uses them as building

anabolism (an-ABB-o-lism): reactions in which small molecules are put together to build larger ones. Anabolic reactions require energy.
ana = up

Figure 7–1

Anabolic and Catabolic Reactions Compared

Note: You need not memorize a color code to understand the figures in this chapter but you may find it helpful to know that blue is used for carbohydrates, yellow for fats, and red for proteins.

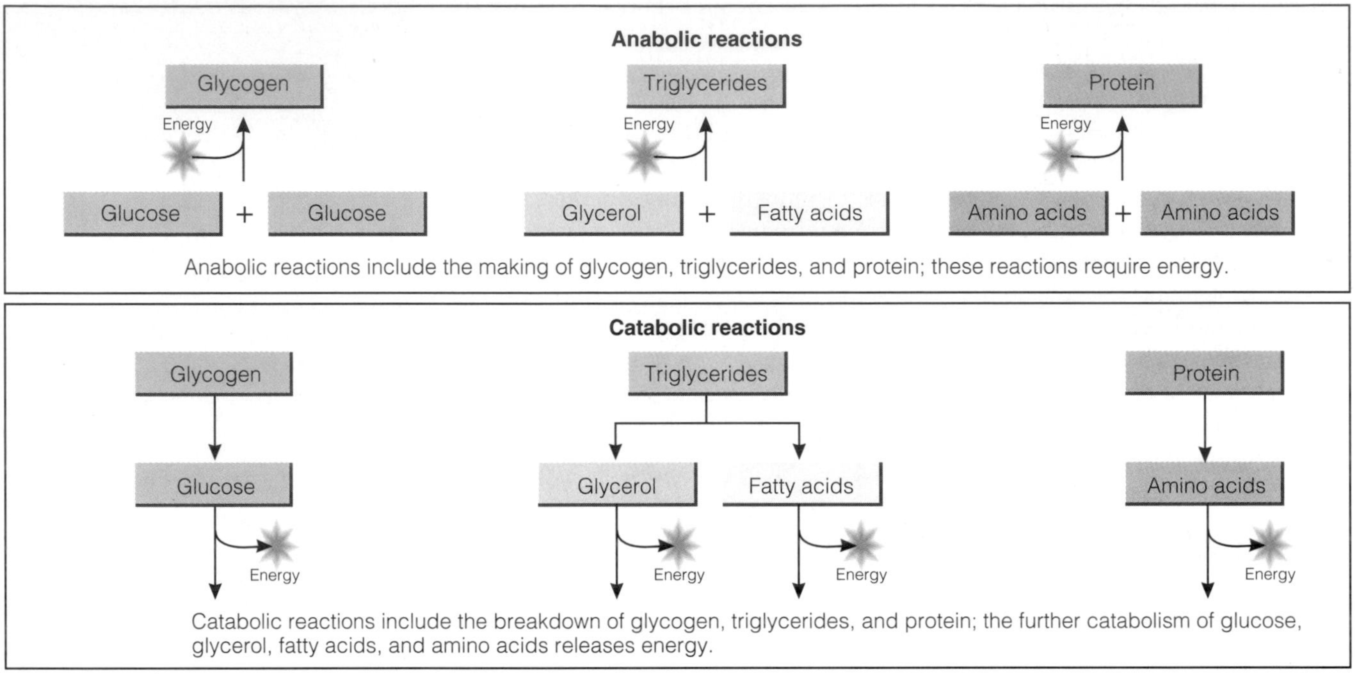
Anabolic reactions
Glycogen
Energy
Glucose + Glucose
Triglycerides
Energy
Glycerol + Fatty acids
Protein
Energy
Amino acids + Amino acids
Anabolic reactions include the making of glycogen, triglycerides, and protein; these reactions require energy.
Catabolic reactions
Glycogen
Glucose
Energy
Triglycerides
Glycerol
Fatty acids
Energy
Energy
Protein
Amino acids
Energy
Catabolic reactions include the breakdown of glycogen, triglycerides, and protein; the further catabolism of glucose, glycerol, fatty acids, and amino acids releases energy.

blocks to form larger, more complex structures. Such reactions involve doing work and so require energy. The building up of body compounds is known as anabolism; this book represents anabolic reactions, wherever possible, with "up" arrows in chemical diagrams (such as those shown in Figure 7–1).

catabolism (ca-TAB-o-lism): reactions in which large molecules are broken down to smaller ones. Catabolic reactions usually release energy.
kata = down

Breakdown Reactions—Catabolism The breaking down of body compounds is known as catabolism; catabolic reactions usually release energy and are represented, wherever possible, by "down" arrows in chemical diagrams (as in Figure 7–1). Catabolic reactions include the breakdown of glycogen to glucose, of triglycerides to fatty acids and glycerol, and of protein to amino acids. When the body needs energy, it breaks down any or all of these four basic units into even smaller units, as described later.

The Transfer of Energy in Reactions When a chemical bond breaks, energy can be released as heat, captured in another chemical bond, or both. Often, as one compound is broken apart, some of the energy is released as heat, and some is used to put together another compound. Such reactions, in which the breakdown of one compound provides energy for the building of another, are known as coupled reactions.

coupled reactions: pairs of chemical reactions in which energy released from the breakdown of one compound is used to create a bond in the formation of another compound.

The energy released during catabolism is often captured by go-between molecules that can easily transfer that energy to other compounds. These molecules are sometimes called the body's "common energy currency," or "high-energy compounds." One such compound is ATP (adenosine triphosphate). The breakdown of energy-nutrient molecules is coupled to the making of many ATP molecules, which capture much of the released energy in their bonds.

ATP, as its name indicates, contains three phosphate groups. The energy in the phosphate bonds is greater than the energy in most other chemical bonds. When energy is needed, hydrolysis readily breaks the high-energy bonds between ATP's phosphate groups, splitting off one or two of them and releasing their energy. These reactions, in turn, are coupled to other reactions that use that energy. Thus the body uses ATP to transfer the energy produced during catabolic reactions to power its anabolic reactions. Figure 7–2 explains how the body uses ATP to carry its energy currency, build body structures, do other work, or generate heat, as needed.

ATP (adenosine triphosphate): a common high-energy compound composed of a purine (adenine), a sugar (ribose), and three phosphate groups.

ATP = A–P~P~P.

(Each ~ denotes a "high-energy" bond.)

Reminder: *Hydrolysis* is the process by which a molecule is broken apart with the addition of water.

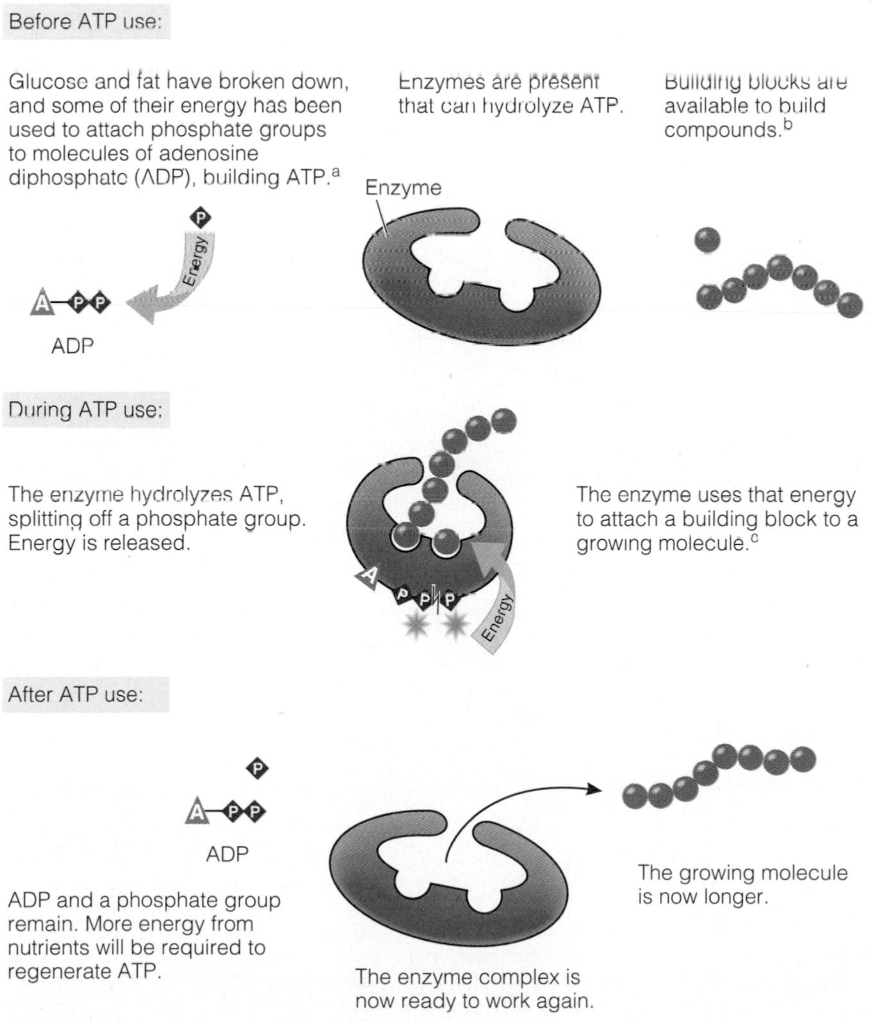
Before ATP use:
Glucose and fat have broken down, and some of their energy has been used to attach phosphate groups to molecules of adenosine diphosphate (ADP), building ATP.[a]
Enzymes are present that can hydrolyze ATP.
Building blocks are available to build compounds.[b]
Enzyme
Energy
ADP
During ATP use:
The enzyme hydrolyzes ATP, splitting off a phosphate group. Energy is released.
The enzyme uses that energy to attach a building block to a growing molecule.[c]
Energy
After ATP use:
ADP
ADP and a phosphate group remain. More energy from nutrients will be required to regenerate ATP.
The enzyme complex is now ready to work again.
The growing molecule is now longer.

Figure 7–2

ATP (Adenosine Triphosphate), One of the Body's Quick-Energy Molecules

[a]ADP (adenosine diphosphate) is lower in energy than ATP; AMP (adenosine monophosphate) is even lower.

[b]Compounds that ATP energy might be used to build include glycogen, fat, proteins, and hormones, among others.

[c]In all such reactions, half or more of the total original energy is lost as heat, accounting for the temperature-raising effect of metabolism. ATP can also break apart without doing work and release all of its energy as heat if needed.

Appendix A presents a brief summary of the structure and function of the cell.

The Site of Reactions—Cells The body's metabolic work is going on all the time within all the cells. Figure 7–3 illustrates a typical cell and shows where the major reactions of energy production take place. The type and extent of metabolic activity vary depending on the type of cell, but of all the body's cells, the liver cells are the most versatile and metabolically active. Table 7–1 offers insights into the liver's work.

Reminder: An *enzyme* is a special protein that serves as a catalyst for a chemical reaction and is not altered in the process.

coenzymes: small organic molecules that work with enzymes to facilitate the enzymes' activity. Many coenzymes have B vitamins as part of their structures (Figure 10–1 in Chapter 10 illustrates coenzyme action).

co = with

The Helpers in Reactions—Enzymes and Coenzymes Metabolic reactions almost always require enzymes to facilitate their action. In some cases, the enzymes need assistants to help them. Enzyme helpers are called coenzymes.

Coenzymes are small organic molecules that associate closely with most enzymes, but are not proteins themselves. The relationships between coenzymes and enzymes differ in detail, but one thing is true of all: without its coenzyme, an enzyme cannot function. Some of the B vitamins serve as coenzymes to the enzymes that release energy from glucose, glycerol, fatty acids, and amino acids. These B vitamin coenzymes stand alongside the metabolic pathways, so to speak, and help to keep the disassembly lines moving. Chapter 10 provides more details on the coenzyme actions of the B vitamins.

With these introductory remarks in mind, it is time to enter a cell and follow the various paths that glucose, glycerol, fatty acids, and amino acids take to yield

Figure 7–3

A Typical Cell (Simplified Diagram)

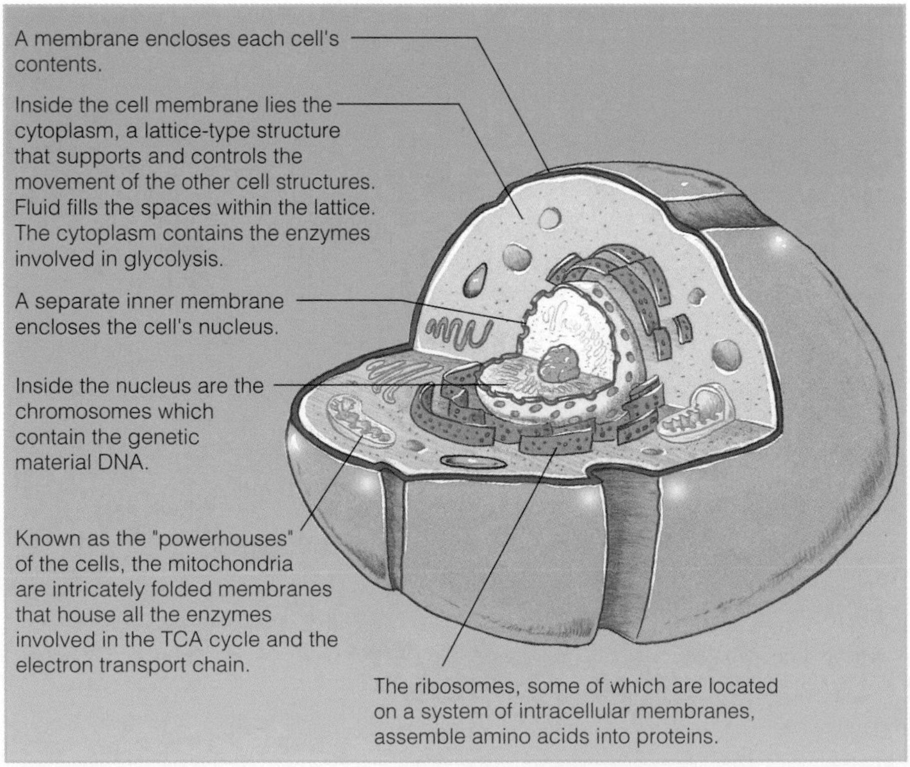
A membrane encloses each cell's contents.
Inside the cell membrane lies the cytoplasm, a lattice-type structure that supports and controls the movement of the other cell structures. Fluid fills the spaces within the lattice. The cytoplasm contains the enzymes involved in glycolysis.
A separate inner membrane encloses the cell's nucleus.
Inside the nucleus are the chromosomes which contain the genetic material DNA.
Known as the "powerhouses" of the cells, the mitochondria are intricately folded membranes that house all the enzymes involved in the TCA cycle and the electron transport chain.
The ribosomes, some of which are located on a system of intracellular membranes, assemble amino acids into proteins.

[a]Glycolysis is described on pp. 244–245.

[b]The TCA cycle and electron transport chain are described on p. 255.

energy. As you will see, each starts down a different path, but they all reach a common destination. At a certain point, they lose their individuality and most of their options—during catabolism all roads lead to energy.

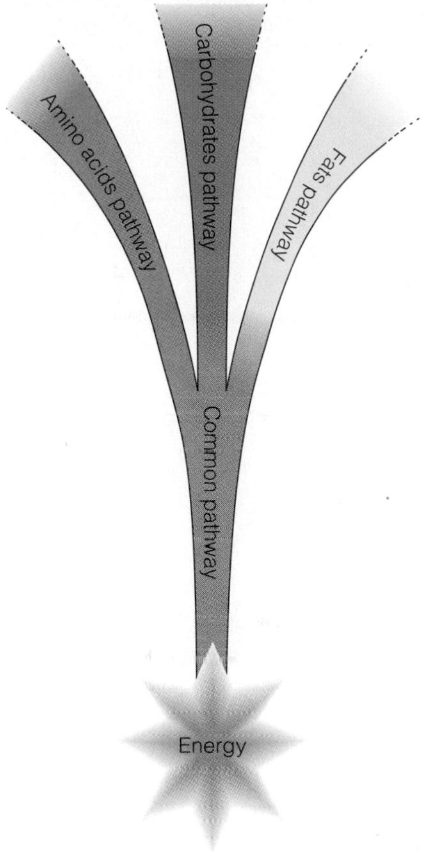

This simple overview introduces the metabolism that is presented in the upcoming text and detailed in Figure 7–18.

Table 7–1

Metabolic Work of the Liver

The liver is the most active processing center in the body. When nutrients enter the body, the liver receives them first; then it metabolizes, packages, stores, or ships them out for use by other organs. When alcohol, drugs, or poisons enter the body, they are also sent directly to the liver; here they are detoxified and their by-products shipped out for excretion. An enthusiastic anatomy and physiology professor once remarked that given the many vital activities of the liver, we should express our feelings for others by saying, "I love you with all my liver," instead of with all my heart. Granted, this declaration lacks romance, but it makes a valid point. Here are just *some* of the many jobs performed by the liver.

Carbohydrates:

- Converts fructose and galactose to glucose.
- Makes and stores glycogen.
- Breaks down glycogen and releases glucose.
- Breaks down glucose for energy when needed.
- Makes glucose from amino acids and glycerol when needed.

Lipids:

- Builds and breaks down triglycerides, phospholipids, and cholesterol as needed.
- Breaks down fatty acids for energy when needed.
- Packages extra lipids in lipoproteins for transport to other body organs.
- Manufactures bile to send to the gallbladder for use in fat digestion.
- Makes ketone bodies when necessary.

Proteins:

- Manufactures nonessential amino acids that are in short supply.
- Removes from circulation amino acids that are present in excess of need and deaminates them or converts them to other amino acids.
- Removes ammonia from the blood and converts it to urea to be sent to the kidneys for excretion.
- Makes other nitrogen-containing compounds the body needs (such as bases used in DNA and RNA).
- Makes plasma proteins such as clotting factors.

Other:

- Detoxifies alcohol, other drugs, and poisons; prepares waste products for excretion.
- Helps dismantle old red blood cells and captures the iron for recycling.
- Stores most vitamins and many minerals.
- Forms lymph.

To renew your appreciation for this remarkable organ, you might want to review Figure 3–8 on p. 98.

Breaking Down Nutrients for Energy

Glucose, glycerol, fatty acids, and amino acids are the basic units derived from food, but a molecule of each of these compounds is made of still smaller units, the atoms—carbons, nitrogens, oxygens, and hydrogens. During catabolism, the body separates these atoms from one another. To follow this action, recall how many carbons are in the "backbones" of these compounds.

- Glucose has 6 carbons:

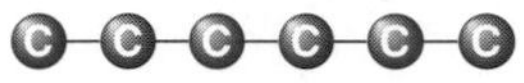

- Glycerol has 3 carbons:

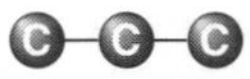

- A fatty acid usually has an even number of carbons, commonly 18 carbons or more:

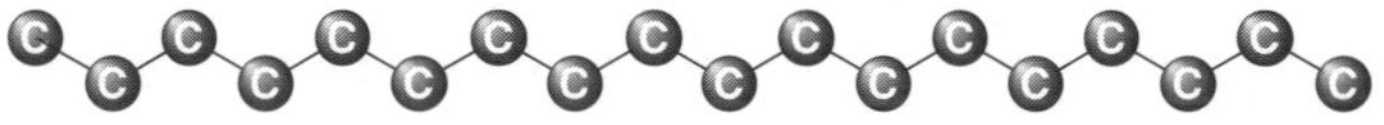

- An amino acid has 2, 3, or more carbons with a nitrogen attached:*

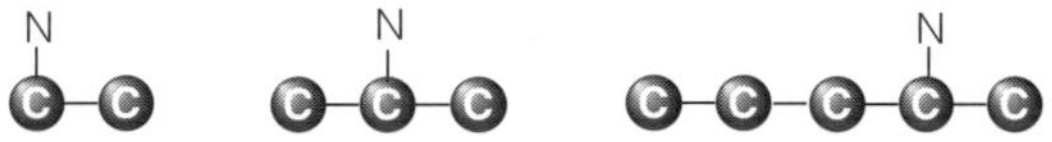

Full chemical structures and reactions appear both in the earlier chapters and in Appendix C; this chapter diagrams the reactions using just the compounds' carbon and nitrogen backbones.

What happens to these compounds inside cells can best be understood by starting with glucose. Two new names appear—pyruvate (a 3-carbon structure) and acetyl CoA (a 2-carbon structure with a coenzyme attached)—and the rest of the story falls into place around them. A major point to notice in the following discussion is that all compounds that can be converted to pyruvate can be used to make glucose. Compounds that are converted directly to acetyl CoA cannot make glucose, however.

pyruvate (PIE-roo-vate): pyruvic acid, a 3-carbon compound that, in metabolism, can be derived from glucose, certain amino acids, or glycerol. The term *pyruvate* means a salt of *pyruvic acid.* (Throughout this book, the ending *-ate* is used interchangeably with *-ic acid;* for our purposes they mean the same thing.)

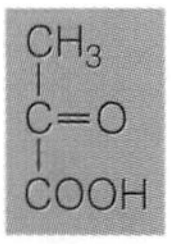

acetyl CoA (ASS-eh-teel, or ah-SEET-il, coh-AY): a 2-carbon compound (acetate, or acetic acid, shown in Figure 5–2 on p. 155) to which a molecule of CoA is attached.

CoA (coh-AY): coenzyme A; the coenzyme derived from the B vitamin pantothenic acid and central to the energy metabolism of nutrients.

GLUCOSE

The first pathway glucose takes on its way to yield energy is called glycolysis (glucose splitting).† Figure 7–4 shows a simplified drawing of glycolysis, which actually involves several steps and several enzymes (see Appendix C for details). Along the way, the 6-carbon glucose is split in half, forming two 3-carbon compounds. These 3-carbon compounds continue along the pathway until they are converted to pyruvate. Thus the net yield of one glucose molecule is two pyruvate

---

*The figures in this chapter usually show amino acids as compounds of 2, 3, or 5 carbons arranged in a straight line, but in reality amino acids may contain other numbers of carbons and assume other structural shapes (see Appendix C).

†Glycolysis takes place in the cytoplasm of the cell (see Figure 7–3).

The 6-carbon compound glucose is split into two interchangeable 3-carbon compounds that are converted to pyruvate in a series of reactions.

All of the other monosaccharides can enter the pathway at various points.

Glycolysis ends with the production of pyruvate (unless there is a shortage of oxygen, in which case pyruvate is converted to lactic acid, as a later section of the text describes).

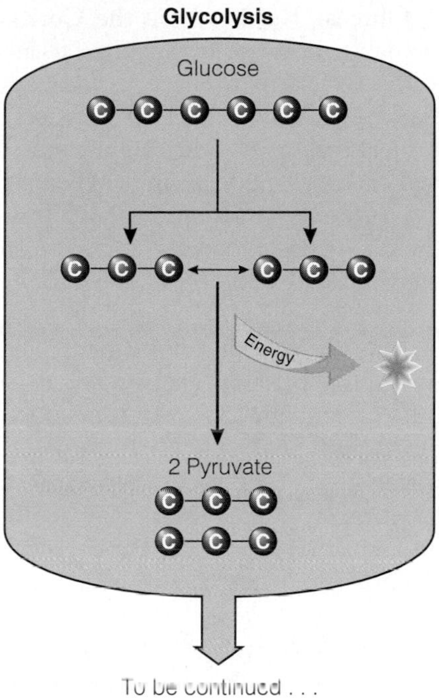

Figure 7–4

Glycolysis: Glucose-to-Pyruvate Pathway (Anaerobic)

Glucose splits to two 3-carbon compounds that become pyruvate. The pathway is called glycolysis (glucose splitting) and may occur in anaerobic conditions (does not require oxygen).

molecules. If they continue breaking down, both pyruvate molecules will release much of their energy to form ATP molecules and some of their energy as heat.

Glucose-to-Pyruvate, and Back Again After splitting glucose to pyruvate, a cell can make glucose again from pyruvate in a process similar to the reversal of glycolysis. Making glucose requires energy, however, and a few different enzymes. Still, glucose is retrievable from pyruvate, so the arrows between glucose and pyruvate are shown pointing up as well as down.

Glucose-to-Pyruvate, an Anaerobic Pathway To start the process of splitting glucose to pyruvate, the cell must use a little energy, but it then produces more energy than it had to invest initially.* No oxygen has been required thus far—that is, glycolysis is an anaerobic pathway. More energy can be released by taking pyruvate through additional metabolic reactions, but oxygen is needed for these reactions (they are aerobic).†

Pyruvate-to-Acetyl CoA If the cell needs energy and oxygen is available, it removes a carbon group (COOH) from pyruvate to produce acetyl CoA. The carbon group from pyruvate becomes carbon dioxide, which is released into the blood, circulated to the lungs, and breathed out. The remaining 2-carbon compound bonds with a molecule of CoA, becoming acetyl CoA. Figure 7–5 diagrams the pyruvate-to-acetyl CoA reaction.

glycolysis (gligh-COLL-ih-sis): the metabolic breakdown of glucose to pyruvate. Glycolysis does not require oxygen (anaerobic).
glyco = glucose
lysis = breakdown

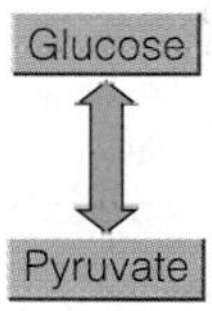

anaerobic (AN-air-ROE-bic): not requiring oxygen.
an = not

aerobic (air-ROE-bic): requiring oxygen.

*The cell uses 2 ATP to begin the breakdown of glucose to pyruvate, but then gains 4 ATP for a net gain of 2 ATP.

†With sufficient oxygen, pyruvate molecules enter the mitochondria of the cell (see Figure 7–3) where they will be converted to acetyl CoA.

Figure 7–5

Pyruvate-to-Acetyl CoA (Aerobic)
Each pyruvate loses a carbon as carbon dioxide and picks up a molecule of CoA, becoming acetyl CoA. The arrow goes only one way (down), because the step is not reversible. Result (from 1 glucose): 2 carbon dioxide and 2 acetyl CoA.

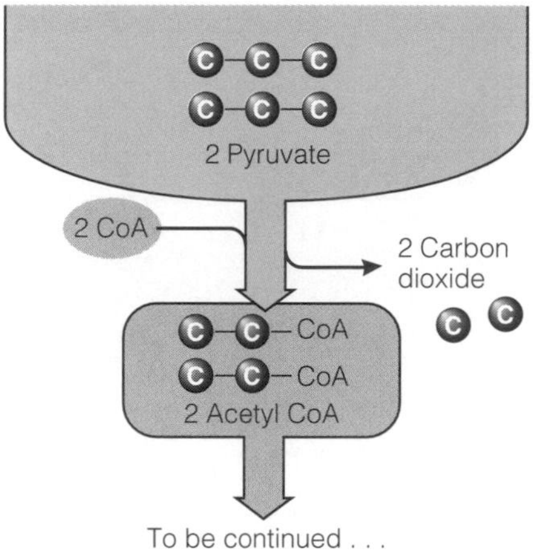

lactic acid: an acid produced from pyruvate during anaerobic metabolism.

Cori cycle: the path from muscle glycogen to glucose to pyruvate to lactic acid (which travels to the liver) to glucose (which can travel back to the muscle) to glycogen; named after the scientist who elucidated this pathway.

Glucose Retrieval via the Cori Cycle Alternatively, when less oxygen is available, pyruvate is converted to lactic acid. This anaerobic reaction occurs to a limited extent even at rest, but increases dramatically during high-intensity exercise—that is, whenever exertion exceeds the capacity of the heart and lungs to clear carbon dioxide from the muscles. With limited oxygen available and limited carbon dioxide clearance, lactic acid accumulates in muscles, causing burning pain and fatigue. (To relieve this pain, relax the muscles frequently so that the circulating blood can carry the lactic acid away to the liver.) The liver can convert lactic acid to glucose, a recycling process that is called the Cori cycle.

Muscles' Needs for Oxygen The role of oxygen in metabolism is worth noticing, for it helps make many things understandable. As you breathe oxygen into your lungs, the oxygen is attached to a carrier (hemoglobin) in your red blood cells that delivers it to the cells, making oxygen available for energy metabolism. You know you need to breathe harder when you are using energy faster (exercising), but you may not have realized why. Energy nutrients are being broken down to provide that energy, and oxygen is always ultimately involved in the process. As just mentioned, oxygen combines with the carbons of glucose to form carbon dioxide; later sections will describe how oxygen combines with the hydrogens to form water.

Chapter 14 will describe the body's use of the energy nutrients to fuel physical activity, but the facts just presented offer a sneak preview. The first pathway in glucose metabolism (glycolysis) yields some energy without oxygen (it is anaerobic), but the later pathways require oxygen (they are aerobic). Aerobic metabolism yields by far the *most energy* and so is crucial for endurance activities.

Pyruvate-to-Acetyl CoA, an Irreversible Step The step from pyruvate to acetyl CoA is metabolically irreversible: a cell cannot retrieve the shed carbons from carbon dioxide to remake pyruvate, and then glucose. It is a one-way step and is therefore shown with only a "down" arrow in Figure 7–6. Notice that acetyl CoA can be used as a building block for fatty acids, but it cannot be used to remake glucose.

Acetyl CoA-to-Carbon Dioxide: The TCA Cycle Once made, acetyl CoA has the option of taking different metabolic paths, depending on the cell's needs. If the cell needs energy, acetyl CoA may proceed through a series of reactions

Figure 7–6

The Paths of Pyruvate and Acetyl CoA
Pyruvate and acetyl CoA may follow several reversible paths, but the path from pyruvate to acetyl CoA is irreversible.

Amino acids that can be used to make glucose are called *glucogenic;* amino acids that are converted to acetyl CoA are called *ketogenic*.

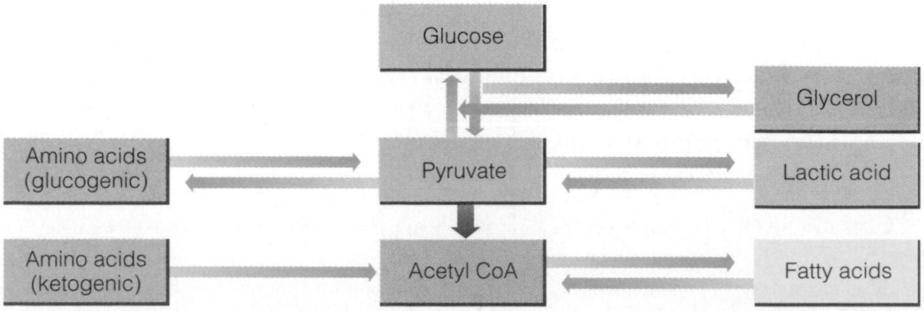

known as the TCA cycle. The TCA cycle converts the 2-carbon acetyl CoA to two carbon dioxide molecules and frees its coenzyme (CoA) to be reused (see Figure 7–7). In the process, much more energy is made available than during glycolysis (more details are given later).

Acetyl CoA-to-Fat If energy is not needed, acetyl CoA will not enter the TCA cycle, but will be used to make fatty acids instead. This explains how carbohydrate, eaten in excess of the body's needs, can lead to fat deposition. As you will see, fat or protein eaten in excess of immediate energy needs can take the same pathway to body fat.

Figure 7–8 (on p. 248) combines Figures 7–4, 7–5, and 7–7 and shows the whole sequence of steps in glucose breakdown. In summary, the main steps in the catabolism of glucose are:

Glucose
to
pyruvate
to
acetyl CoA
to
carbon dioxide.

Keep in mind that glucose can be retrieved only from pyruvate or compounds

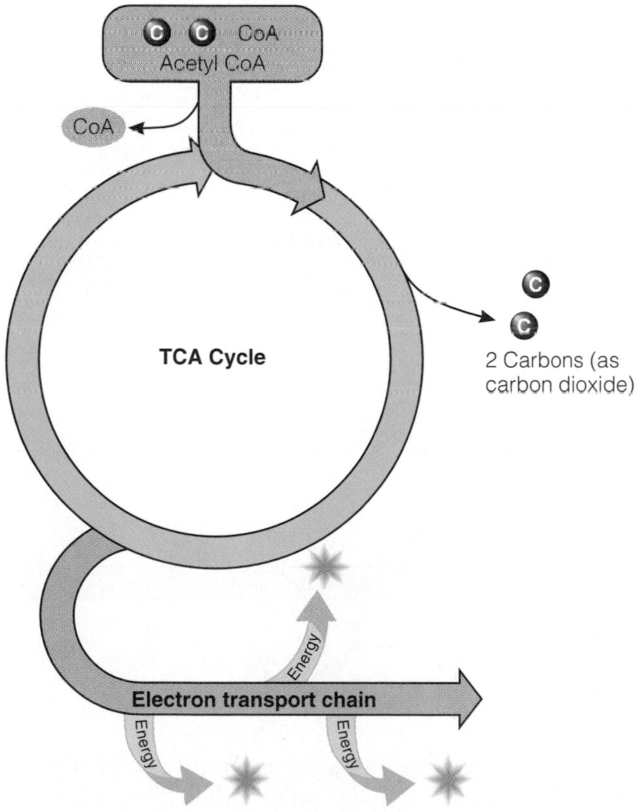

Figure 7–7

The Breakdown of Acetyl CoA

The complete oxidation of acetyl CoA is accomplished through the reactions of the **TCA** (tricarboxylic acid) **cycle,** or **Krebs cycle** (named for the biochemist who elucidated them), and the **electron transport chain.** In the TCA cycle, the acetyl CoA carbons are converted to carbon dioxide. Each CoA returns to pick up another acetate (coming from glucose, lipids, or protein).

The net result is that acetyl CoA splits, the carbons combine with oxygen, and the energy originally in the acetyl CoA is stored in ATP and similar compounds, thus becoming available for the body's use. Chapter 10 describes how the B vitamin coenzymes participate in these metabolic pathways. For more details, see the text and Appendix C.

Figure 7–8

Glucose-to-Energy Pathway
Through these processes, energy from glucose is made available to do the cells' work. Ultimately, glucose is completely disassembled to single-carbon fragments, and the fragments are combined with oxygen to form carbon dioxide. Much of the energy released is trapped and stored in ATP. Details of the TCA cycle and the electron transport chain are shown later and in Appendix C.

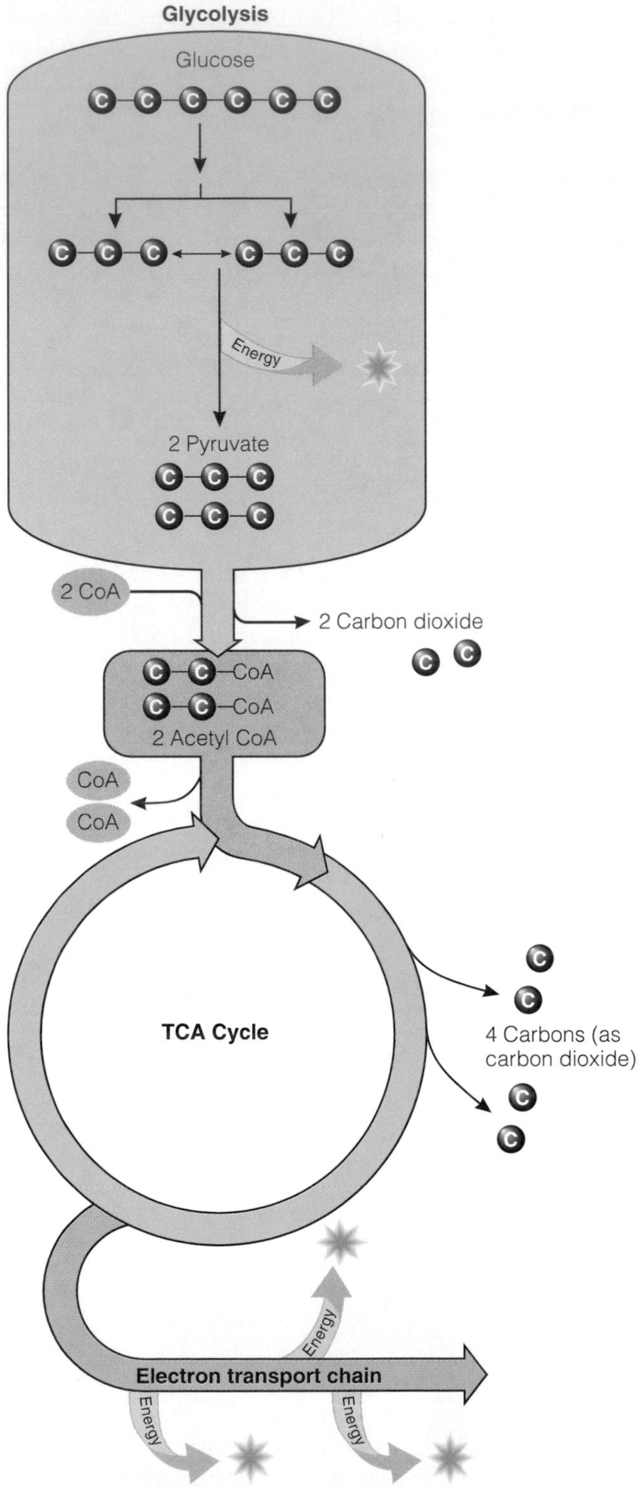

earlier in the pathway. Once the commitment to acetyl CoA is made, glucose is not retrievable; acetyl CoA can go on to carbon dioxide, fat, or other compounds but not back to glucose.

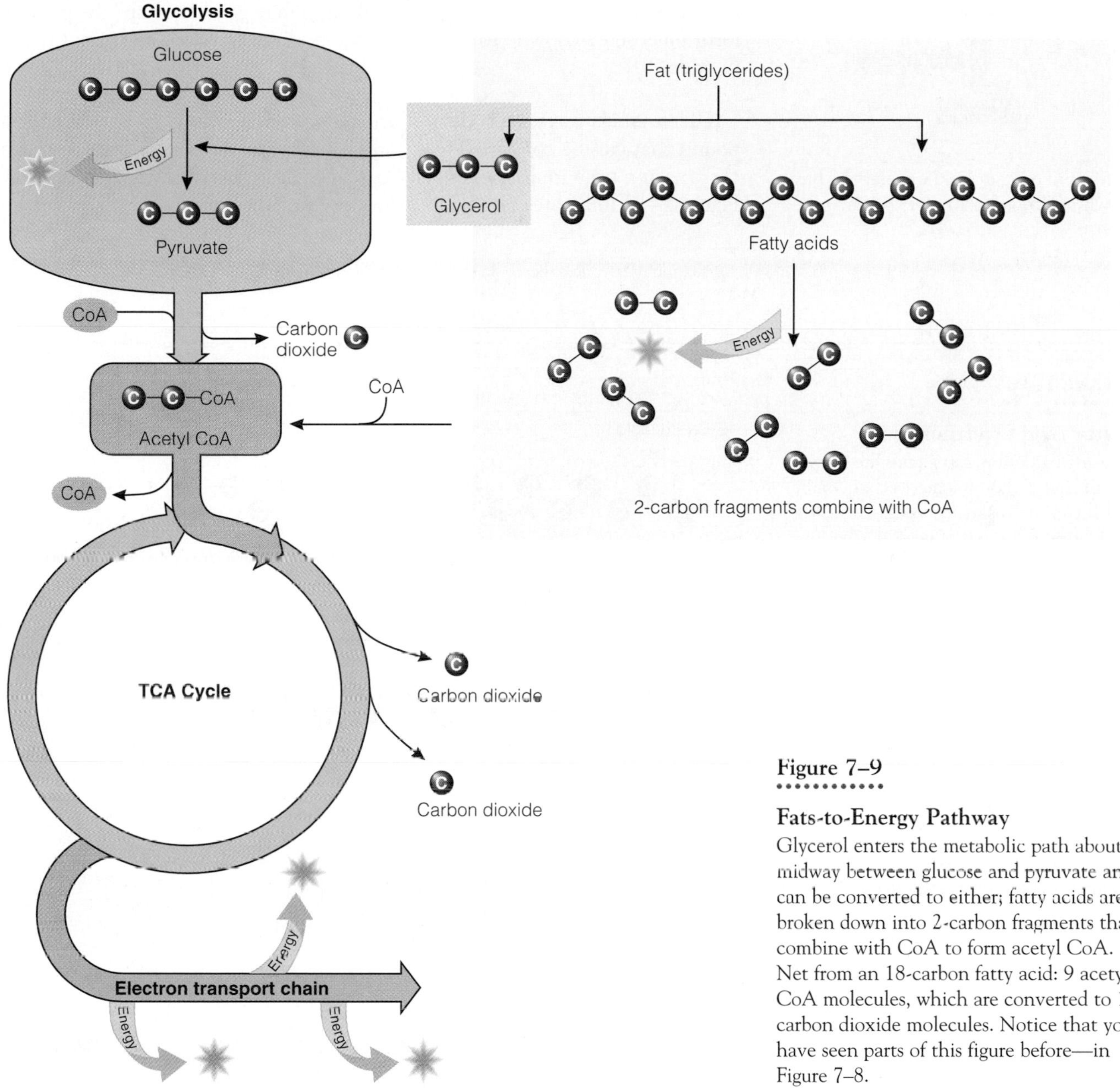

Figure 7–9

Fats-to-Energy Pathway
Glycerol enters the metabolic path about midway between glucose and pyruvate and can be converted to either; fatty acids are broken down into 2-carbon fragments that combine with CoA to form acetyl CoA. Net from an 18-carbon fatty acid: 9 acetyl CoA molecules, which are converted to 18 carbon dioxide molecules. Notice that you have seen parts of this figure before—in Figure 7–8.

GLYCEROL AND FATTY ACIDS

Once glucose breakdown is understood, fat and protein breakdown are easily learned, for all three share a common metabolic pathway. Recall that triglycerides can break down to glycerol and fatty acids. Figure 7–9 repeats the pathway that glucose follows and shows how glycerol and fatty acids enter into it.

Glycerol-to-Pyruvate Glycerol (a 3-carbon compound like pyruvate, but with a different arrangement of H and OH on the C) is easily converted to

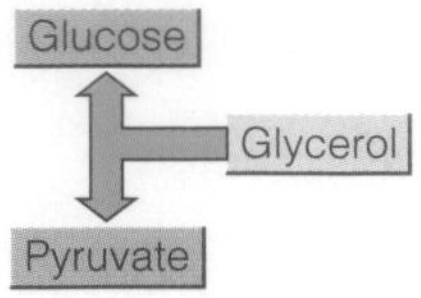

another 3-carbon compound. This compound may go either "up" the pathway to form glucose or "down" to form pyruvate and acetyl CoA and, finally, carbon dioxide.

fatty acid oxidation: the metabolic breakdown of fatty acids to acetyl CoA.

Fatty Acids-to-Acetyl CoA Unlike glycerol, which is a 3-carbon compound that can be converted to 3-carbon pyruvate, fatty acids are taken apart 2 carbons at a time in a series of aerobic reactions known as fatty acid oxidation.* Figure 7–10 illustrates fatty acid oxidation and shows that in the process, each

*Oxidation of fatty acids occurs in the mitochondria of the cells (see Figure 7–3).

Figure 7–10

Fatty Acid Oxidation
During oxidation, fatty acids are taken apart to 2-carbon fragments that combine with CoA to make acetyl CoA. Fatty acid oxidation is a series of aerobic reactions.

The fatty acid is first activated by coenzyme A.

A little energy is released each time a carbon-carbon bond is cleaved.

Another CoA joins the chain, and the bond at the second carbon (the beta-carbon) weakens. Acetyl CoA splits off, leaving a fatty acid that is two carbons shorter.

The shorter fatty acid enters the pathway and the cycle repeats. The molecules of acetyl CoA enter the TCA cycle, yielding abundant energy.

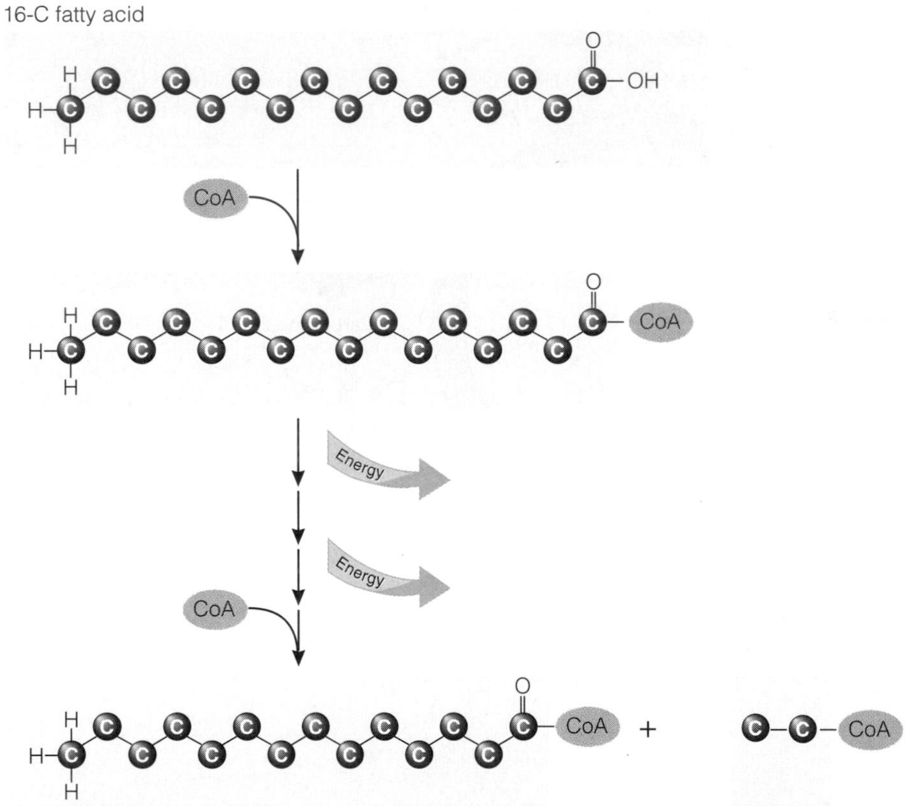

Net result from a 16-C fatty acid:	14-C fatty acid CoA	+	1 acetyl CoA
Cycle repeats, leaving:	12-C fatty acid CoA	+	2 acetyl CoA
Cycle repeats, leaving:	10-C fatty acid CoA	+	3 acetyl CoA
Cycle repeats, leaving:	8-C fatty acid CoA	+	4 acetyl CoA
Cycle repeats, leaving:	6-C fatty acid CoA	+	5 acetyl CoA
Cycle repeats, leaving:	4-C fatty acid CoA	+	6 acetyl CoA
Cycle repeats, leaving:	2-C fatty acid CoA*	+	7 acetyl CoA

*Notice that 2-C fatty acid CoA = acetyl CoA, so that the final yield from a 16-C fatty acid is 8 acetyl CoA.

2–carbon fragment splits off and combines with a molecule of CoA to make acetyl CoA. Each acetyl CoA then enters the TCA cycle in the same manner as acetyl CoA from glucose does (review Figure 7–9). A little energy is released each time a 2-carbon fragment breaks off from a fatty acid during oxidation, but when these 2-carbon units enter the TCA cycle as acetyl CoA, they yield nearly three times as much energy. If the cell does not need energy, the acetyl CoA molecules will combine with each other to make body fat, in the same way acetyl CoA produced from excess carbohydrate does.

Glucose Not Retrievable from Fatty Acids Cells can make glucose from pyruvate and other 3-carbon compounds, as mentioned earlier, but they cannot make glucose from the 2-carbon fragments of fatty acids. In chemical diagrams, the arrow between pyruvate and acetyl CoA always points only one way—down—and fatty acid fragments enter the metabolic path below this arrow (review Figure 7–6). Thus fatty acids cannot be used to make glucose.

The significance of this is that fat, for the most part, normally cannot provide energy for red blood cells or the brain and nervous system, which require glucose as fuel. Remember that almost all dietary fats are triglycerides, and that triglycerides contain only one small molecule of glycerol (3 carbons) with three fatty acids. The glycerol can yield glucose, but that represents only 3 of the 50 or so carbon atoms in the molecule—about 5 percent of its weight (see Figure 7–11). Thus fat is an insignificant source of glucose; about 95 percent of fat cannot be converted to glucose.

Reminder: The making of glucose from the glycerol of triglycerides (or from amino acids) is *gluconeogenesis*. About 5% of fat (the glycerol portion of a triglyceride) and most amino acids can be converted to glucose.

AMINO ACIDS

The preceding two sections have shown how the breakdown of carbohydrate and fat provides energy for the body's use. One energy-yielding nutrient remains: protein or, rather, the amino acids of protein.

Amino Acid Catabolism If amino acids are needed for energy, or if they are consumed in excess of the need to synthesize protein, they enter the metabolic pathway as shown in Figure 7–12 (on p. 252). First, amino acids are deaminated (that is, they lose their nitrogen as described in the next section), and then they are catabolized in a variety of ways. Some amino acids can be converted to pyruvate; others are converted to acetyl CoA; and still others enter the TCA cycle directly as compounds other than acetyl CoA.

Reminder: *Deamination* is the reaction that removes the nitrogen-containing amino group from an amino acid.

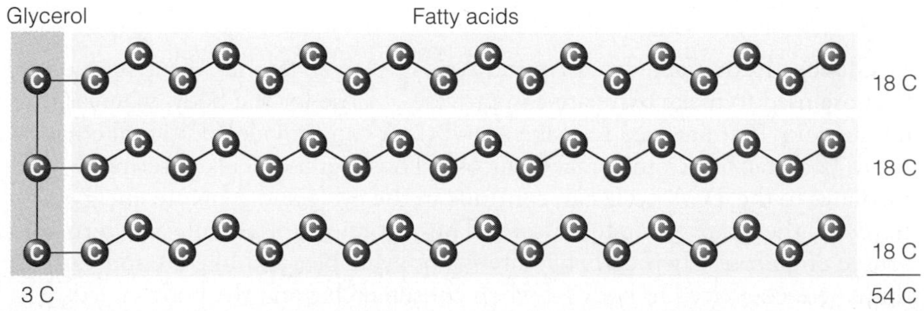

Figure 7–11

The Carbons of a Typical Triglyceride

A typical triglyceride contains only one small molecule of glycerol (3 C), but has three fatty acids (each about 18 C on the average, or about 54 C). Only the glycerol portion of a triglyceride can yield glucose.

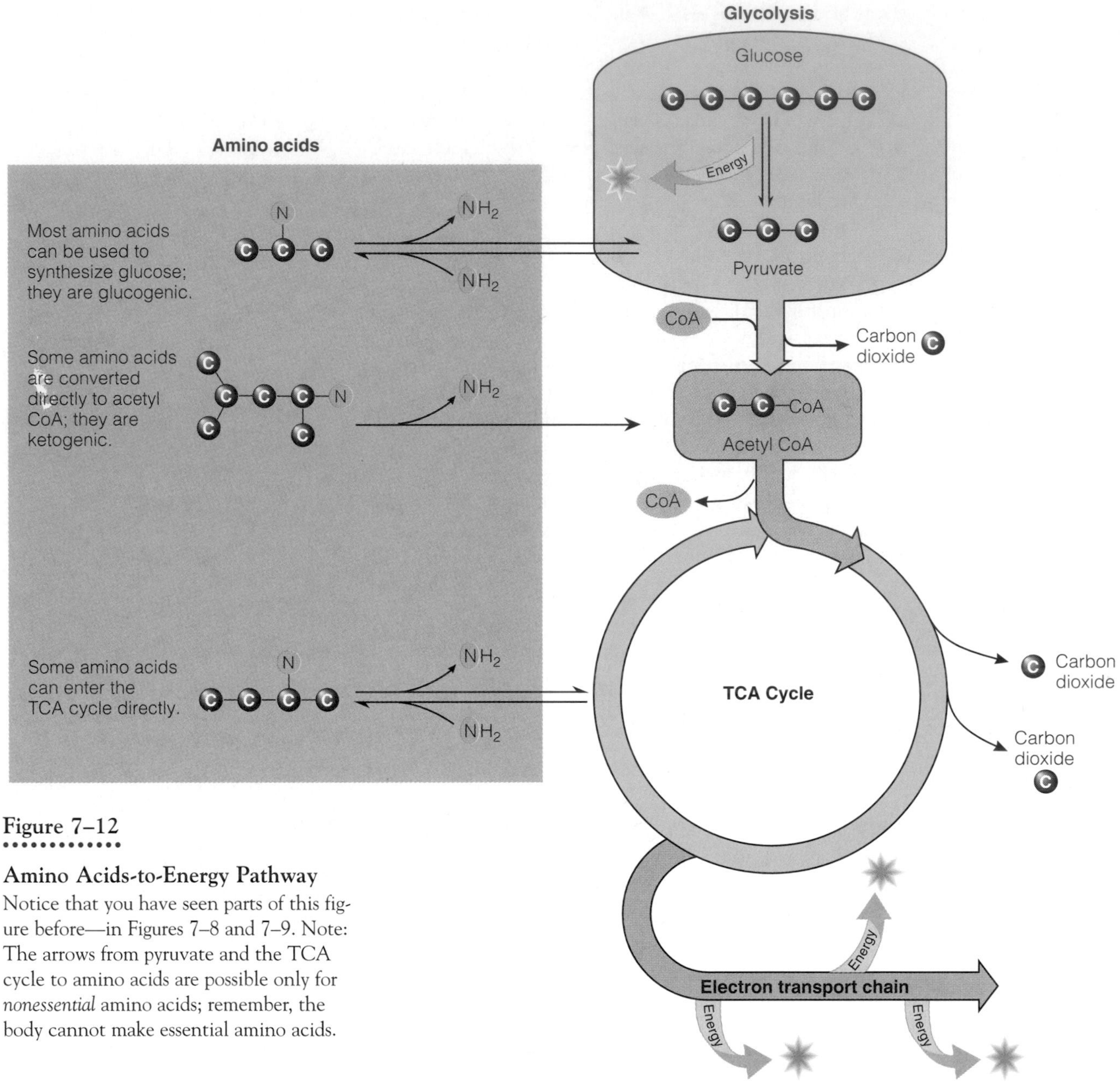

Figure 7–12

Amino Acids-to-Energy Pathway

Notice that you have seen parts of this figure before—in Figures 7–8 and 7–9. Note: The arrows from pyruvate and the TCA cycle to amino acids are possible only for *nonessential* amino acids; remember, the body cannot make essential amino acids.

Glucose Retrievable from Amino Acids As you might expect, amino acids that are used to make pyruvate can provide glucose for the body, whereas those amino acids that are used to make acetyl CoA can provide additional energy or make body fat but cannot make glucose. Those amino acids entering as intermediates to the TCA cycle can continue in the cycle and generate energy; alternatively, they can generate glucose. Thus protein, unlike fat, is a fairly good source of glucose when carbohydrate is not available; and like fat and carbohydrate, it is converted to body fat when consumed beyond the body's needs.

A key to understanding these metabolic pathways is learning which fuels can be converted to glucose and which cannot. The parts of protein and fat that can be converted to pyruvate *can* provide glucose for the body, whereas the parts that are converted to acetyl CoA *cannot* provide glucose, but can readily provide fat. You must have glucose to fuel your brain's activities, and if you don't obtain it from food, your body will devour its own lean tissue to provide it. Therefore, to keep this from happening, you need to supply fuels that can provide glucose—primarily carbohydrate. If you offer your body only fat, which delivers mostly acetyl CoA, you put your body in the position of having to break down protein tissue for glucose. If you offer your body only protein, you put your body in the position of having to convert protein to glucose. Clearly, the best diet supplies some protein, some fat, and abundant carbohydrate.

Reminder: Diet and health recommendations advise that daily energy intake provide:
- 55–60% carbohydrate.
- $\leq$ 30% fat.
- 10–15% protein.

Amino Acids-to-Fat Once amino acids have been converted to acetyl CoA, if energy is not needed, fatty acids are made and stored as triglycerides in adipose tissue. (Recall from Chapter 6 that the body cannot store surplus amino acids as such; it has to convert them to other compounds.) Thus protein can also add to fat stores if eaten in excess.

People who eat huge portions of meat and other protein-rich foods may wonder why they have weight problems. Not only does the fat in those foods lead to fat storage; the protein can, too, when energy intake exceeds energy needs. Many fad weight-loss diets encourage high-protein intakes based on the false assumption that protein builds only muscle, not fat.

Products of deamination:
- Keto acid.
- Ammonia.

Deamination When amino acids are metabolized for energy or used to make fat, they must be deaminated first. Two products result from deamination. One is, of course, the structure without its amino group—often a keto acid (see Figure 7–13). The other product is ammonia, a toxic compound chemically identical to the strong-smelling ammonia in bottled cleaning solutions. Ammonia is a base, and if the body produces larger quantities than it can handle, the blood's critical acid-base balance becomes upset.

keto acid: an organic acid that contains a carbonyl group (C=O).

ammonia: a compound with the chemical formula NH_3; produced during the deamination of amino acids.

Transamination As the discussion of protein in Chapter 6 pointed out, only some amino acids are essential; others can be made in the body, given a source of nitrogen. The body does this by transferring an amino group from one amino

transamination: the transfer of an amino group from one amino acid to a keto acid, producing a new nonessential amino acid and a new keto acid.

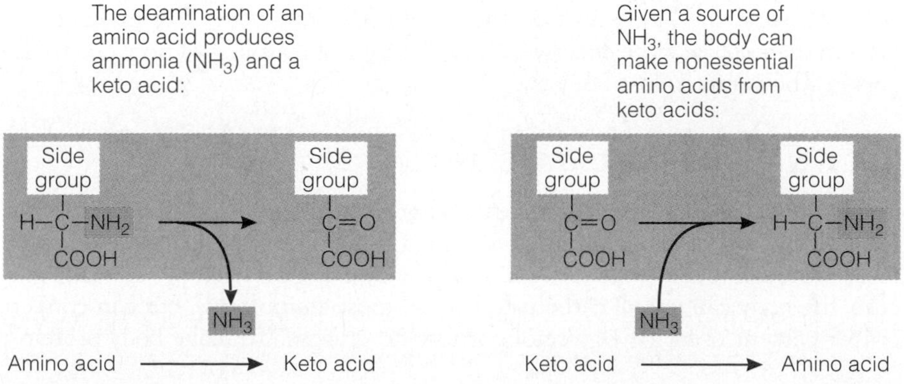

Figure 7–13

Keto Acids

Figure 7–14

Transamination to Make a Nonessential Amino Acid

The body can transfer amino groups from an amino acid to a keto acid, forming a new nonessential amino acid and a new keto acid.

Transamination reactions require the vitamin B_6 coenzyme.

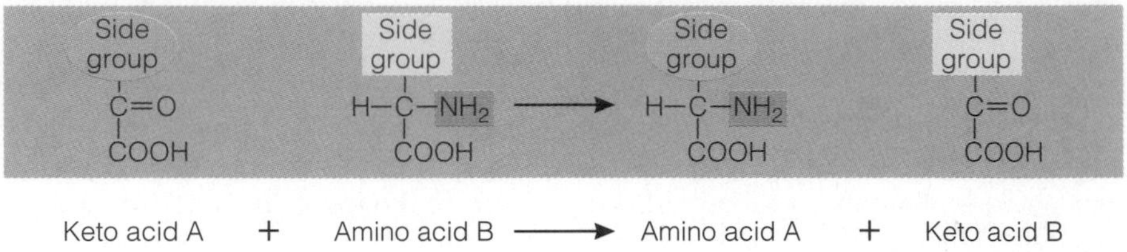

acid to its corresponding keto acid, producing a new amino acid and a new keto acid, as shown in Figure 7–14. Through many such reactions, involving many different keto acids, the liver cells can synthesize the nonessential amino acids.

urea (you-REE-uh): the principal nitrogen-excretion product of metabolism. Two ammonia fragments are combined with carbon dioxide to form urea.

Ammonia-to-Urea in the Liver The liver continuously produces small amounts of ammonia in deamination reactions. Some of this ammonia provides the nitrogen needed for the synthesis of nonessential amino acids. The liver quickly combines any unused ammonia with carbon dioxide to make urea, a much less toxic compound (see Figure 7–15). The diagram greatly oversimplifies the reactions; details are shown in Appendix C.

Urea Excreted via the Kidneys Liver cells release urea into the blood, where it circulates until it passes through the kidneys (see Figure 7–16 on the next page). The kidneys then remove urea from the blood for excretion in the urine. Normally, the liver efficiently scoops up all the ammonia, makes urea from it, and releases the urea into the blood; then the kidneys clear all the urea from the blood. This division of labor allows easy diagnosis of diseases of both organs. If the liver is sick, blood ammonia will be high; if the kidneys are sick, blood urea will be high.

Figure 7–15

Urea Synthesis

When amino nitrogen is stripped from amino acids, ammonia is produced. The liver detoxifies ammonia before releasing it into the bloodstream by combining it with another waste product, carbon dioxide, to produce urea. See Appendix C for details.

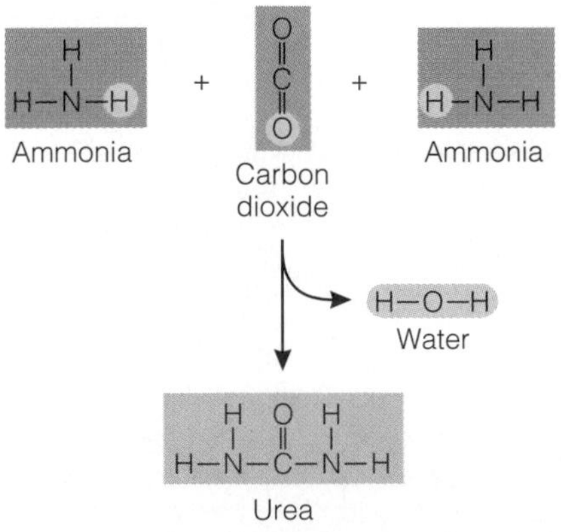

Water Needed to Excrete Urea Urea is the body's principal vehicle for excreting unused nitrogen, and the amount produced increases with protein intake. To keep urea in solution, the body needs water. For this reason, a person who regularly consumes a high-protein diet (say, 100 grams a day or more) must drink more water than usual; without extra water, the person risks an accumulation of urea in the blood. In fact, the weight loss from water loss makes high-protein diets *appear* to be effective, but water loss, of course, is of no value to the person who wants to lose body fat.

THE FINAL STEPS OF CATABOLISM

To review the ways the body can use the energy-yielding nutrients, see Table 7–2 (on p. 256). To obtain energy, the body uses glucose and fatty acids as its primary fuels, although it can use amino acids to provide energy if need be. To make glucose, the body can use all carbohydrates and most amino acids, but can convert only 5 percent of fat (the glycerol portion) to glucose. To make body proteins, the body needs amino acids. It can use glucose to make some amino acids when nitrogen is available; it cannot use fats to make body proteins. Finally, when energy is consumed beyond the body's needs, the body can convert all three energy-yielding nutrients to fat for storage.

The TCA Cycle To this point the discussion has followed each of the energy-yielding nutrients to the point where acetyl CoA enters the TCA cycle.* The TCA cycle serves as a busy traffic center through which these 2-carbon acetyl CoA molecules pass on their way to carbon dioxide, releasing their energy to other compounds as they go.

The TCA cycle is called a cycle, but that doesn't mean it regenerates acetyl CoA. Acetyl CoA goes one way only—to carbon dioxide and water, releasing energy as it goes. The TCA cycle is a circular path, though, in the sense that a 4-carbon carbohydrate-like compound does cycle around and around.† This compound picks up acetyl CoA (a 2-carbon compound), drops off one carbon (as carbon dioxide), then another carbon (as carbon dioxide), and returns to pick up another acetyl CoA. As for the acetyl CoA, its carbons go only one way—to carbon dioxide (see Appendix C for additional details).

As acetyl CoA molecules break down to carbon dioxide and water, hydrogen atoms with their electrons are removed from the compounds in the cycle. Coenzymes of the B vitamins niacin and riboflavin receive the hydrogens and their electrons and transfer them to the electron transport chain.

The Electron Transport Chain The electron transport chain (ETC) consists of a series of proteins that serve as electron "carriers." These carriers are mounted in sequence on a membrane inside the energy-generating organelles within the cell known as mitochondria (review Figure 7–3). As each carrier receives electrons, it releases a little energy and passes the electrons on to the next carrier. While some of the energy is released as heat, much of it is captured in the bonds of ATP molecules. These electron-transferring molecules continue passing electrons and giving up energy until, at the end of the chain, any usable energy has been captured in the body's ATP molecules. The last step is to donate the low-energy electrons with their hydrogen atoms (H) to oxygen (O), forming water (H_2O), from which the body cannot extract any more energy. Everyone knows that breathing oxygen is essential to life—now you understand why. Figure 7–17 provides a simple diagram of the process; see Appendix C for details.

Figure 7–16

Urea Excretion

The liver and kidneys both play a role in disposing of excess nitrogen. Can you see why the person with liver disease has high blood ammonia, while the person with kidney disease has high blood urea? (Figure 3–8 provides details of how the kidneys work.)

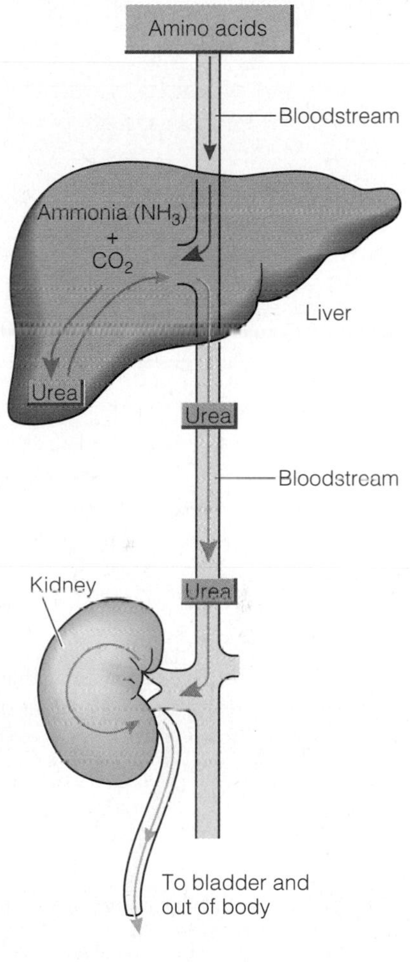

---

*The TCA cycle reactions take place in the mitochondria of the cell (see Figure 7–3).

†Actually, the 4-carbon compound does not cycle around as the same structure throughout; instead it travels through a series of reactions. On picking up acetyl CoA, it becomes a 6-carbon compound. On dropping off carbon dioxide, it becomes a 5- and then a 4-carbon compound. Each reaction changes the structure slightly until finally the original 4-carbon compound forms again and picks up another acetyl CoA, starting the series of reactions over again.

The carbons that enter the cycle in acetyl CoA may not be the ones that are given off as carbon dioxide. In one of the steps of the cycle, a 6-carbon compound of the cycle becomes symmetrical, both ends being identical. Thereafter it loses carbons to carbon dioxide at one end or the other. Thus only half of the carbons from acetyl CoA are given off as carbon dioxide in any one turn of the cycle; the other half become part of the compound that returns to pick up another acetyl CoA. It is true to say, though, that for each acetyl CoA that enters the TCA cycle, 2 carbons are given off as carbon dioxide. It is also true that with each turn of the cycle the energy equivalent of one acetyl CoA is released.

Table 7–2

Summary of Energy-Yielding Nutrient Metabolism

Nutrient	Yields Energy	Can Yield Glucose	Can Yield Amino Acids and Body Proteins	Can Yield Fat Stores
Carbohydrates (glucose)	Yes	Yes	Yes—when nitrogen is available, can yield *nonessential* amino acids	Yes
Lipids (triglycerides)	Yes	No—glycerol provides minimal amount	No	Yes
Proteins (amino acids)	Yes—if needed	Yes—when carbohydrate is unavailable	Yes	Yes

The TCA cycle and the ETC are both aerobic processes. They represent the body's most efficient means of capturing the energy from nutrients and transferring it into the bonds of ATP.

Summary All the details this chapter has presented so far are combined in Figure 7–18. After a balanced meal, the body handles the nutrients as shown. The digestion of *carbohydrate* yields glucose; some is stored as glycogen, and some

Figure 7–17

Electron Transport Chain

An important concept to remember is that an electron is not a fixed amount of energy. The electrons that bond the H to the B vitamin coenzyme have a relatively large amount of energy. In the series of reactions that follow, they lose this energy in small amounts, until at the end they are attached (with H) to oxygen (O) to make water (H_2O). In some of the steps, the energy they lose is captured into ATP in coupled reactions. Appendix C provides a more detailed explanation.

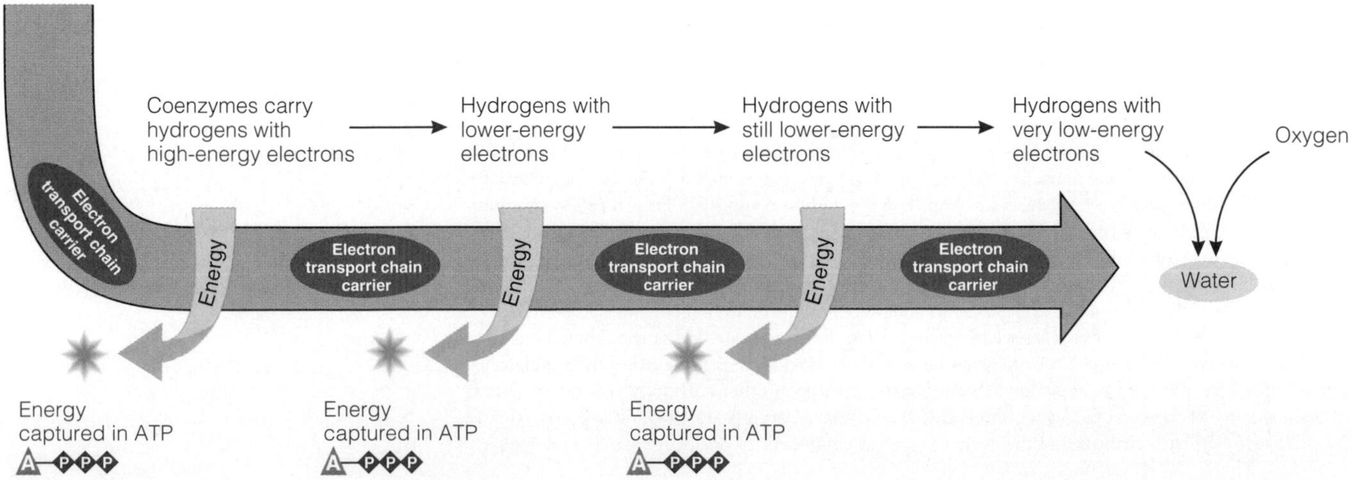

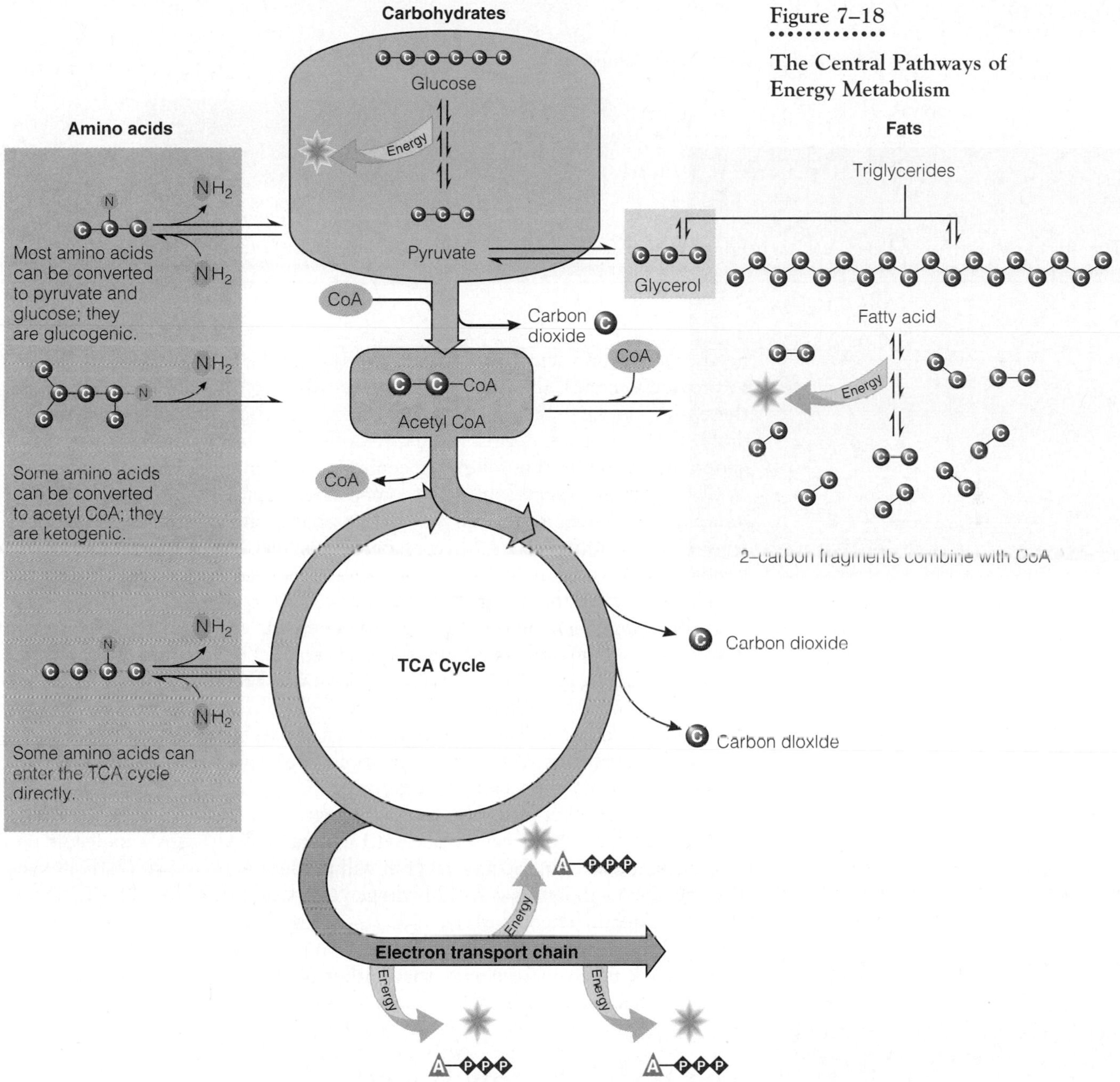

Figure 7–18

The Central Pathways of Energy Metabolism

is taken into the brain and other cells and broken down to pyruvate and acetyl CoA to provide energy. The acetyl CoA can then enter the TCA cycle and ETC to provide more energy. The digestion of *fat* yields glycerol and fatty acids; some are reassembled and stored as fat, and others are broken down to acetyl CoA, enter the TCA cycle and ETC, and provide energy. The digestion of *protein* yields amino acids, some of which are used to build body protein. If there is a surplus, however, or if not enough carbohydrate and fat are available to meet energy

Figure 7–19

Chemical Structures of a Fatty Acid and Glucose Compared

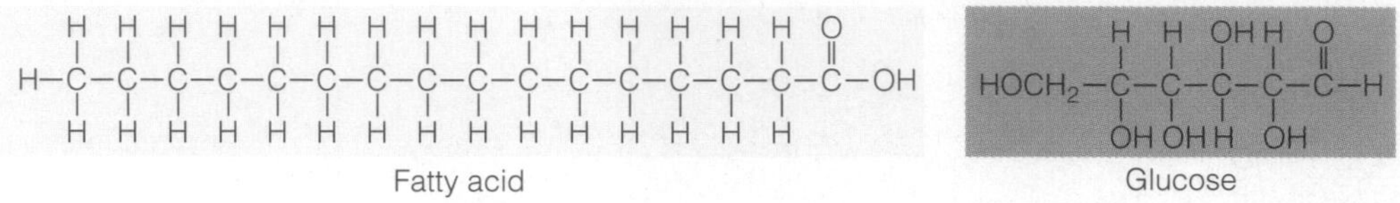

The structure shown here for glucose is not the ring structure shown in Chapter 4, but an alternative way of drawing its chemical structure.

needs, some amino acids are broken down through the same pathways as glucose to provide energy. Other amino acids enter directly into the TCA cycle, and these, too, can be broken down to yield energy. In summary, although carbohydrate, fat, and protein enter the TCA cycle by different routes, the energy-generating pathways that follow are common to all energy-yielding nutrients.

Of the various energy-containing compounds, fat provides the most energy for its weight. The reason this is so may be apparent from Figure 7–19, which compares a fatty acid molecule with a glucose molecule. Notice that nearly all the bonds in a fatty acid molecule are between carbons and hydrogens. Oxygen can be added to all of them (forming carbon dioxide with the carbons, and water with the hydrogens). As this happens, the energy in the fat is released. In glucose, on the other hand, an oxygen is already bonded to each carbon; thus there is less potential for oxidation, and less energy will become available when the remaining bonds are broken.

Because fat contains many hydrogen atoms and its bonds are readily oxidized, it generates abundant ATP during oxidation. This explains why fat yields more kcalories per gram than carbohydrate or protein. (Remember that each ATP holds energy and that kcalories measure energy; thus the more ATP generated, the more kcalories have been collected.) The more hydrogens a molecule of a fuel nutrient contains, the more ATP it will produce upon oxidation. For example, one glucose molecule with 12 hydrogen atoms will yield 38 ATP when completely oxidized. In comparison, one 16-carbon fatty acid molecule with 32 hydrogen atoms will yield 129 ATP when completely oxidized. Gram for gram, fat can pack much more energy than either of the other two energy-yielding nutrients, making it the body's preferred form of energy storage.

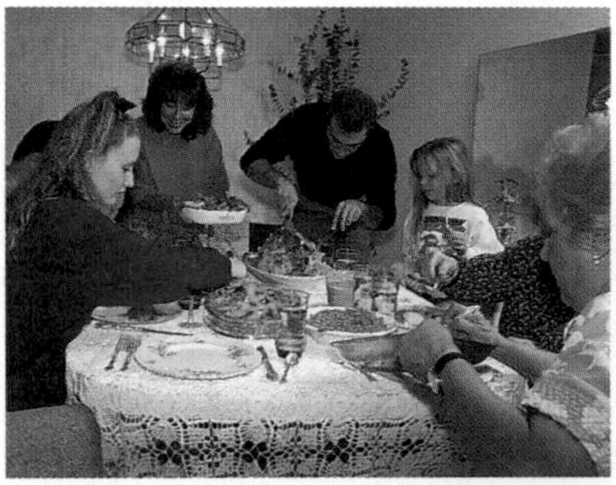

People can enjoy bountiful meals such as this without storing body fat, provided that they spend as much energy as they take in.

The Body's Energy Budget

The average person takes in close to a million kcalories a year and expends more than 99 percent of them, maintaining a stable weight for years on end. This remarkable achievement, which many people manage without even thinking about it, could be called the economy of maintenance. The body's energy budget is balanced. Some people, however, eat too much and get fat; others eat too little and get thin. The metabolic details have already been described; the next sections will review them from the perspective of the body fat gained or lost. The possible reasons why people eat too much or too little are explored in Chapter 8.

THE ECONOMICS OF FEASTING

Figure 7–20 shows how metabolism favors fat formation when a person eats too much of any energy-yielding nutrient. Carbohydrate, fat, and protein can all enlarge the body's fat stores.

Surplus Carbohydrate Surplus carbohydrate (glucose) is first stored as glycogen, but there is a limit to the capacity of the glycogen-storing cells. Once glycogen stores are filled, the overflow is routed to fat (part A of the figure). Fat cells enlarge as they fill with fat, and they seem to be able to multiply indefinitely. Thus excess carbohydrate can contribute to obesity.

Surplus Fat Surplus dietary fat moves efficiently into the body's fat stores. It may break down to fragments such as acetyl CoA, but if energy flow is already

---

Figure 7–20

How Carbohydrate, Fat, and Protein, Eaten in Excess, Contribute to Body Fat

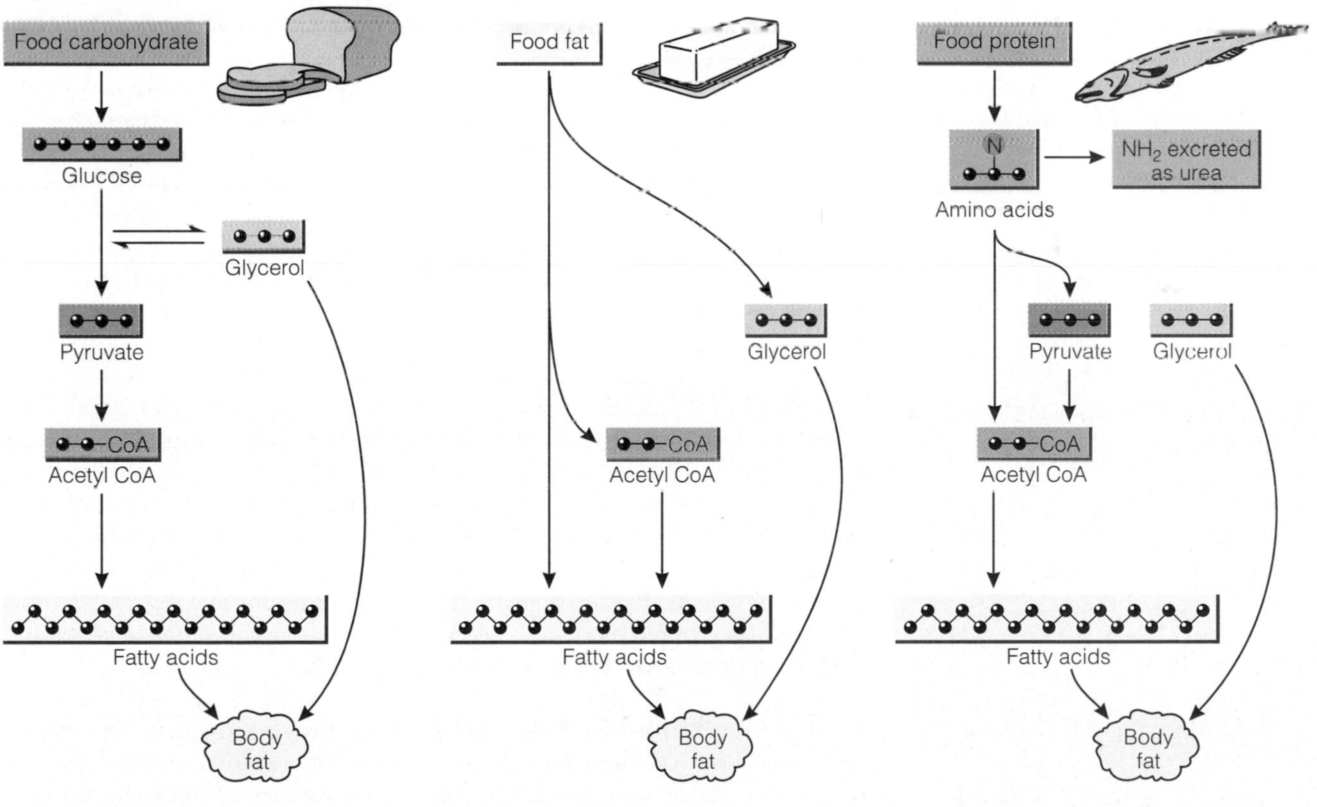

A. Carbohydrate, eaten in excess of need, is broken down to pyruvate and acetyl CoA; acetyl CoA molecules are then assembled into fatty acids, combined with glycerol, and stored as body fat.

B. Fat, eaten in excess of need, is either stored directly or broken down to glycerol and acetyl CoA, and then built up into different fat molecules.

C. Protein is broken down to amino acids. These, if not used to build body protein, are deaminated, and the nitrogen is excreted as urea; some carbon skeletons are converted to pyruvate and acetyl CoA and then to fat.

rapid enough to meet the demand, these fragments will not break down further. Instead, they will be routed to the assembly of triglycerides and stored in the fat cells (part B of Figure 7–20).

Surplus Protein Finally, surplus protein encounters the same fate (part C of Figure 7–20). If not needed to build body protein or to meet present energy needs, amino acids will be deaminated and their carbon skeletons converted through the intermediates, pyruvate and acetyl CoA, to triglycerides. Thus amino acids, too, expand the fat cells and add to body weight.

THE TRANSITION FROM FEASTING TO FASTING

After a meal, glucose, glycerol, and fatty acids from foods are either used or stored. Later, as the body shifts from a fed state to a fasting one, it begins drawing energy out of storage. Glycogen and fat are released from storage to provide more glucose, glycerol, and fatty acids to produce energy.

Energy is needed all the time. Even when a person is asleep and totally relaxed, the cells of many organs are hard at work. In fact, this work—the cells' work that maintains all life processes without any conscious effort—represents about two-thirds to three-fourths of the total energy a person spends in a day. The small remainder is the work that a person's muscles perform voluntarily during waking hours.

Reminder: The action of carbohydrate and fat in providing energy that allows protein to be used for other purposes is called *protein-sparing action*.

The body's top priority is to meet the cells' needs for energy, and it normally does this by periodic refueling—that is, by eating. When food is not available, the body turns to its own tissues for other fuel sources. If people choose not to eat, we say they are fasting; if they have no choice, we say they are starving. The body makes no such distinction. In either case, the body is forced to switch to a wasting metabolism, drawing on its reserves of carbohydrate and fat and, within a day or so, on its vital protein tissues as well. Figure 7–21 shows the metabolic pathways operating in the body as it shifts from feasting (part A) to fasting (parts B and C).

THE ECONOMICS OF FASTING

As Figure 7–21 shows, during fasting, all paths lead to energy—fuel must be delivered to every cell. As the fast begins, glucose from the liver's stored glycogen and fatty acids from the body's stored fat are both flowing into cells, then breaking down to yield acetyl CoA, and delivering energy to power the cells' work.* Several hours later, however, most of the glucose is used up—liver glycogen is exhausted and blood glucose begins to fall. The liver begins making glucose from lactic acid formed by red blood cells and muscles and from the amino acid alanine. Low blood glucose serves as a signal to promote further fat breakdown.

Glucose Needed for the Brain At this point, most of the cells are depending on fatty acids to continue providing their fuel. But red blood cells and the cells of the nervous system need glucose. Glucose is their major energy fuel, and even when other energy fuels are available, glucose must be present to permit the energy-metabolizing machinery of the nervous system to work. Normally, the brain and nerve cells consume about two-thirds of the total *glucose* used each

*The muscles' stored glycogen provides glucose only for the muscle in which the glycogen is stored.

Figure 7–21

Feasting and Fasting

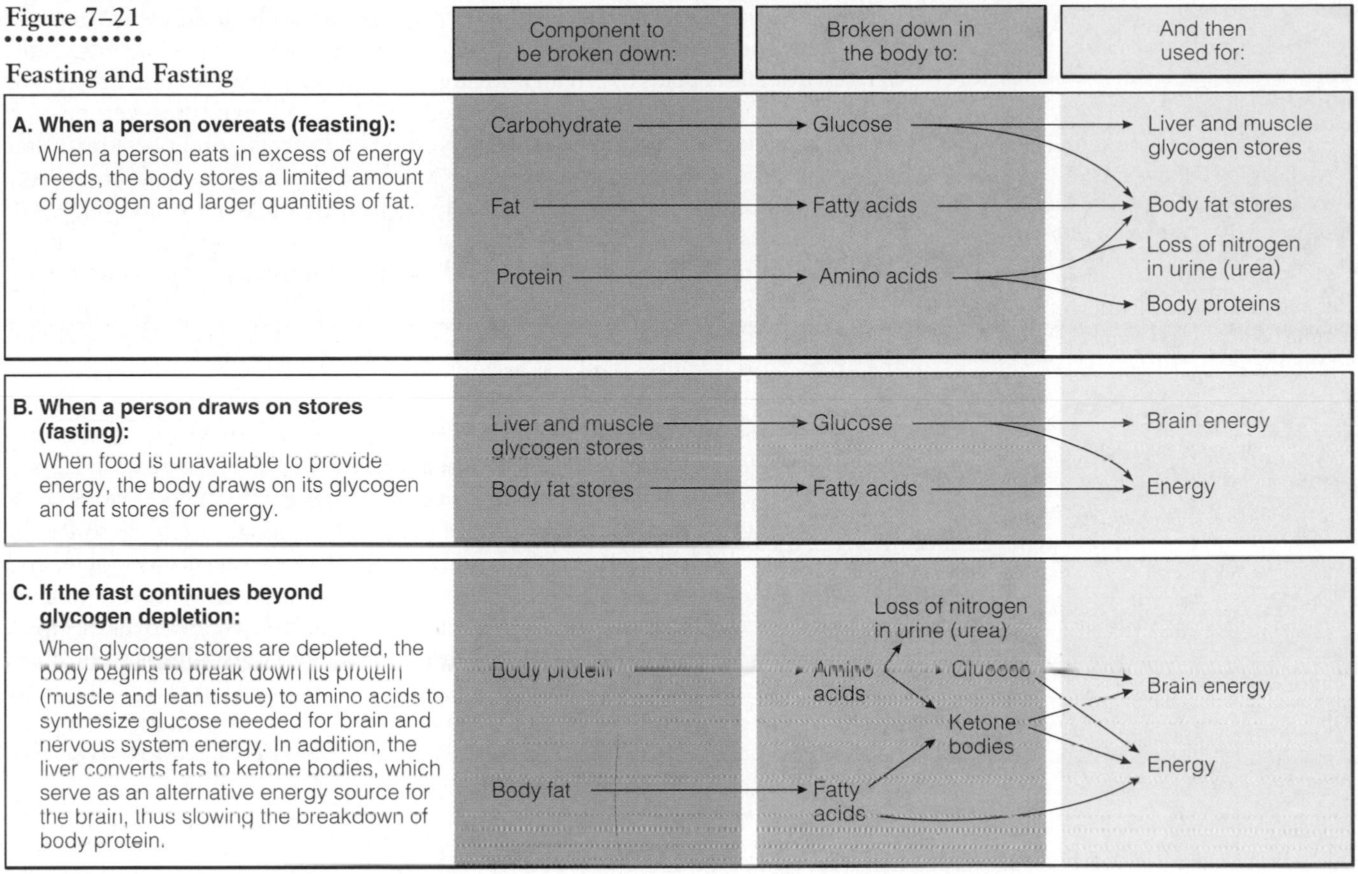
Component to be broken down:
Broken down in the body to:
And then used for:
A. When a person overeats (feasting):
When a person eats in excess of energy needs, the body stores a limited amount of glycogen and larger quantities of fat.
Carbohydrate
Glucose
Liver and muscle glycogen stores
Fat
Fatty acids
Body fat stores
Protein
Amino acids
Loss of nitrogen in urine (urea)
Body proteins
B. When a person draws on stores (fasting):
When food is unavailable to provide energy, the body draws on its glycogen and fat stores for energy.
Liver and muscle glycogen stores
Glucose
Brain energy
Body fat stores
Fatty acids
Energy
C. If the fast continues beyond glycogen depletion:
When glycogen stores are depleted, the body begins to break down its protein (muscle and lean tissue) to amino acids to synthesize glucose needed for brain and nervous system energy. In addition, the liver converts fats to ketone bodies, which serve as an alternative energy source for the brain, thus slowing the breakdown of body protein.
Loss of nitrogen in urine (urea)
Body protein
Amino acids
Glucose
Brain energy
Ketone bodies
Energy
Body fat
Fatty acids

day—about 400 to 600 kcalories. About one-fifth of the *energy* the body uses when it is at rest is used for the brain.

Protein Called on to Meet Glucose Needs The red blood cells' and brain's special requirements for glucose pose a problem for the fasting body. The body can use its stores of fat, which may be quite generous, to furnish most of its cells with energy, but the brain and nerves prefer energy in the form of glucose. For this reason, body protein tissues such as muscle and liver always break down to some extent during fasting. Amino acids that yield pyruvate can be used to make glucose; and to obtain them, body proteins must be broken down. The amino acids that can't be used to make glucose are used as an energy source for other body cells.

Fat's Small Glucose Contribution from Glycerol The breakdown of body protein is an expensive way to obtain glucose. In the first few days of a fast, body protein provides about 90 percent of the needed glucose; glycerol, about 10 percent. If body protein loss were to continue at this rate, death would ensue within three weeks, regardless of the quantity of fat a person had stored. Fortunately, fat breakdown also increases with fasting—in fact, fat breakdown almost doubles, providing energy for other body cells and glycerol for glucose production.[1]

Reminder: *Condensation* is the process by which two molecules are joined together with the removal of water.

Reminder: The group of ketones that are formed during the incomplete oxidation of fatty acids are *ketone bodies*. A *ketone* is a compound that contains a carbonyl group (C=O) between other carbons.

Reminder: The combination of elevated ketone bodies in the blood (ketonemia) and in the urine (ketonuria) is *ketosis*.

The Shift to Ketosis As the fast continues, the body finds a way to use its fat to fuel the brain. It adapts by condensing together acetyl CoA fragments derived from fatty acids to produce an alternate energy source, ketone bodies (see Figure 7–22). Normally produced and used only in small quantities, ketone bodies can provide fuel for some brain cells. Ketone body production rises until, after about 10 days of fasting, it is meeting much of the nervous system's energy needs.[2] Still, many areas of the brain rely exclusively on glucose, and body protein continues to be sacrificed to produce it.

When ketone bodies contain a COOH (acid) group, they are called keto acids. Small amounts of keto acids are a normal part of the blood chemistry; but when their concentration rises, the pH of the blood declines and ketone bodies spill into the urine. This is ketosis, and it is a sign that the body's chemistry is going awry.

Suppression of Appetite The starvation that produces ketosis also causes loss of appetite. Researchers have theorized that having no appetite is an advantage to a person without access to food, because the search for food would be a waste of energy. When the person finds food and eats again, the body shifts out of ketosis, the hunger center gets the message that food is again available, and the appetite returns. This chain of events has served as justification for weight-loss routines that induce ketosis, such as fasting and low-carbohydrate diets. However, any kind of food restriction, with or without ketosis, leads a person to adapt by losing appetite. A well-balanced low-kcalorie diet can induce the same effect. Therefore ketosis-producing diets offer no special advantage in terms of appetite suppression, and because ketosis can disrupt the body's acid-base balance, other weight-loss regimens are preferred to ketogenic diets.

Figure 7–22

Ketone Body Formation

1. The first step in the formation of ketone bodies is the condensation of two molecules of acetyl CoA and the removal of the CoA to form a compound that is converted to the first ketone body.
2. This ketone body may lose a molecule of carbon dioxide to become another ketone.
3. Or, the acetoacetate may add two hydrogens, becoming another ketone body (beta-hydroxybutyrate). See Appendix C for more details.

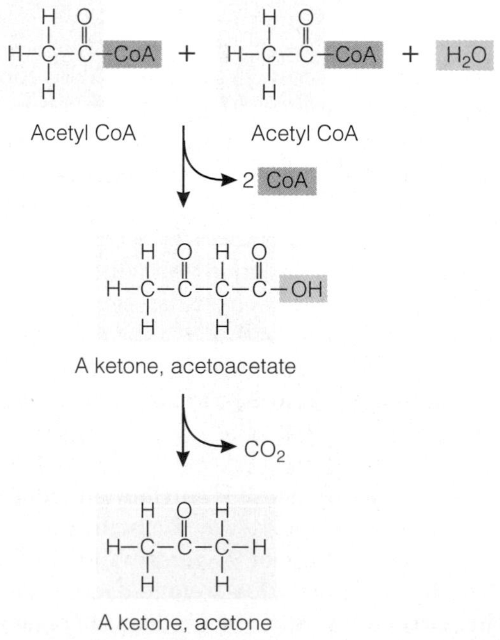

Slowing of Metabolism In any case, while the body is shifting to the use of ketone bodies, it simultaneously reduces its energy output and conserves both its fat and lean tissue. As the lean (protein-containing) organ tissues shrink in mass, they perform less metabolic work, reducing energy expenditures. As the muscles waste, they can do less work and so demand less energy, reducing expenditures further. The hormones of fasting slow metabolism even further in the effort to conserve lean body mass for as long as possible. Because of the slowed metabolism, the loss of fat falls to a bare minimum—less, in fact, than the fat that would be lost on a low-kcalorie diet. Thus, although *weight* loss during fasting may be quite dramatic, *fat* loss may be less than when at least some food is eaten.

Symptoms of Starvation The adaptations just described—slowing of energy output and reduction in fat loss—occur in the starving child, the hungry homeless adult, the fasting religious person, the person with anorexia nervosa, and the malnourished hospital client. Such adaptations help to prolong their lives and explain the physical symptoms of energy deprivation: wasting, slowed metabolism, lowered body temperature, and reduced resistance to disease.

The body's adaptations to fasting are sufficient to maintain life for a long time. Mental alertness need not be diminished, and even physical energy may remain unimpaired for a surprisingly long time. Still, fasting presents hazards. The same alterations in metabolism occur on a low-carbohydrate diet.

The Low-Carbohydrate Diet An economy similar to that of fasting prevails when a person consumes a low-carbohydrate diet. Once the body's available glycogen reserves are spent, the only significant remaining source of glucose is protein. The low-carbohydrate diet usually provides some protein from food, but some is still taken from body tissue. The onset of ketosis signals that this wasting process has begun.

Low-carbohydrate dieting – living on dietary protein and fat and on body protein and fat almost exclusively.

People are attracted to the low-carbohydrate diet because it brings a dramatic weight loss within the first few days. They would be disillusioned if they realized that much of this weight loss is a loss of glycogen and protein together with large quantities of water and important minerals. A dieter who boasts of losing 7 pounds in two days on a low-carbohydrate diet must be unaware that *at best*, a pound or two is fat, and 5 or 6 pounds are lean tissue, water, and minerals. Once the dieter begins to eat a balanced diet, the body will avidly devour and retain these needed materials, and the weight will zoom back, quite often to higher than the starting point.

These facts offer a warning: beware of quick-weight-loss schemes. Learn to distinguish between loss of *fat* and loss of *weight*.

The Protein-Sparing Fast A variant on fasting is the technique of ingesting only protein. The hope is that the protein will spare lean tissue and that the person will break down body fat at a maximal rate to meet other energy needs. The protein does spare the lean tissues to some extent, but then it is used to provide glucose, just as dietary carbohydrate would be.

Protein-sparing fasting = living on dietary protein and on body protein and fat.

Protein formulas (liquid and powdered) were popular weight-loss regimens during the late 1970s—until serious health risks, including deaths, emerged. Since then products have been reformulated to contain high-quality protein, carbohydrates, some fat, vitamins, and minerals. In addition, such formulas are sold only to doctors or hospitals for supervised use and must carry a "Protein Diet Warning" on their labels.[3] Even with more complete formulas, such weight-loss regimens present serious health risks and need to be carefully monitored. In addition to the health risks, protein fasts have a poor long-term success rate; most people regain the lost weight. Thus the protein-sparing fast has to be judged at best a moderate success and at worst a failure.

The term *protein sparing* has been used in another situation. Hospital clients enduring severe physical stresses such as cancer or major surgery also lose body protein. This is especially likely, and especially dangerous, if they are simultaneously fighting infection, which prevents the body from going into ketosis. Physicians make every effort to prevent the loss of vital lean tissue by supplying amino acids as well as glucose in some form—through a vein if the client can't eat. The effort to provide protein-sparing *therapy* for prevention of malnutrition should not be confused with the protein-sparing *fast* for weight loss.

This chapter has probed the intricate details of metabolism at the level of the cells, exploring the transformations of nutrients to energy and to storage compounds. Several chapters and highlights to come build on this information. The highlight that follows this chapter shows how alcohol disrupts normal metabolism. Chapter 8 describes how a person's intake and expenditure of energy is reflected in body composition. Chapter 9 examines the consequences of unbalanced energy budgets—overweight and underweight—and what to do about them. Chapter 10 shows the vital roles the B vitamins play as coenzymes assisting all the metabolic pathways described here. And Chapter 14 revisits metabolism to show how it supports the work of physically active people and how athletes can best apply that information in their choices of foods to eat.

We are all solar creatures, indeed. The sun's energy sparks every move that we make, and our beautifully designed bodies make use of it in astonishing ways.

Study Questions

1. Define metabolism, anabolism, and catabolism; give an example of each.
2. Name one of the body's quick-energy molecules, and describe how is it used.
3. What are coenzymes, and what service do they provide in metabolism?
4. Name the four basic units, derived from foods, used by the body in metabolic transformations. How many carbons are in the "backbones" of each?
5. Summarize the main steps in the metabolism of glucose, glycerol, fatty acids, and amino acids.
6. Define aerobic and anaerobic metabolism. How does insufficient oxygen influence metabolism?
7. How does the body dispose of excess nitrogen?
8. Describe how a surplus of the three energy nutrients contributes to body fat stores.
9. What adaptations does the body make during a fast? What are ketone bodies? Define ketosis.
10. Distinguish between a loss of *fat* and a loss of *weight*, and describe how both might happen.

Notes

1. M. G. Carlson, W. L. Snead, and P. J. Campbell, Fuel and energy metabolism in fasting humans, *American Journal of Clinical Nutrition* 60 (1994): 29–36.
2. M. C. Linder, Nutrition and metabolism of proteins, in *Nutrition Biochemistry and Metabolism*, ed. M. C. Linder (New York: Elsevier, 1991), pp. 87–109.
3. M. Segal, A sometime solution to a weighty problem, *FDA Consumer*, April 1990, pp. 11–15.

Alcohol and Nutrition

Social gatherings offer opportunities for people to share conversation, food, and drink. Among the beverages available are those that contain alcohol, and people must choose whether to drink them. Most people who drink manage their relationships with alcohol relatively safely.[1] Unfortunately, some 18 million people in the United States abuse alcohol to the point that their personal relationships, work, and health become impaired. With the understanding of metabolism gained from Chapter 7, you are in a position to understand how the body handles alcohol, how alcohol affects metabolism, and how alcohol can impair health.

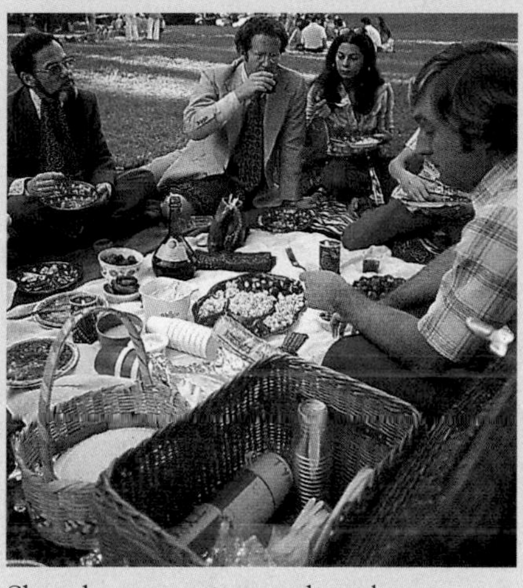

Shared conversations and meals sometimes include alcoholic beverages.

ALCOHOL IN BEVERAGES

To the chemist, *alcohol* refers to a class of organic compounds containing hydroxyl (OH) groups. The glycerol to which fatty acids are attached in triglycerides is an example of an alcohol to a chemist. But to most people, *alcohol* refers to the intoxicating ingredient in beer, wine, and hard liquor (distilled spirits). The chemist's name for this particular alcohol is *ethyl alcohol,* or *ethanol.* Glycerol has 3 carbons with 3 hydroxyl groups attached; ethanol has only 2 carbons and 1 hydroxyl group (see Figure H7–1). The remainder of this highlight talks about the particular alcohol, ethanol, but refers to it simply as *alcohol.*

Alcohols affect living things profoundly, partly because they act as lipid solvents. Their ability to dissolve lipids out of cell membranes allows them to penetrate rapidly into cells, destroying cell structures and thereby killing the cells. For this reason, most alcohols are toxic, or poisonous, in relatively small amounts; by the same token, because they kill microbial cells, they are useful as disinfectants.

Ethanol is less toxic than the other alcohols. Sufficiently diluted and taken in small enough doses, its action in the brain produces euphoria—a pleasing effect that people seek—not with zero risk, but with a low enough risk (if the doses are low enough) to be tolerable. Used to achieve this effect, alcohol is a drug—that is, a substance that modifies body functions. Like all drugs, alcohol offers both benefits and hazards. It must be used with caution, if used at all.

Alcohol arises naturally from carbohydrates when certain microorganisms metabolize them in the absence of oxygen—an anaerobic process called fermentation (the glossary on p. 266 defines fermentation and other alcohol-related terms). Since all plants contain carbohydrate, all can serve as the starting material for fermentation.

People have consumed wine, beer, and other fermented beverages for more than 5000 years. Different societies use different plants to produce alcoholic beverages; the most familiar are grapes and other berries (used to make wine), apples (fermented, or hard, cider), and grains (beer and various distilled liquors). Wines, ciders, and beers are ready for use after fermentation, whereas the liquors undergo further distilling to concentrate the alcohol. Thus grain mashes can be distilled further to yield the whiskeys—bourbon (at least half from corn), rye (from rye), scotch (from barley), vodka (from wheat, rye, corn, or potatoes), rum (from cane products such as molasses), and brandy (from wine). Distilled liquors are often served with mixers such as carbonated beverages or fruit juices (cocktails) or

Figure H7–1

Two Alcohols: Glycerol and Ethanol

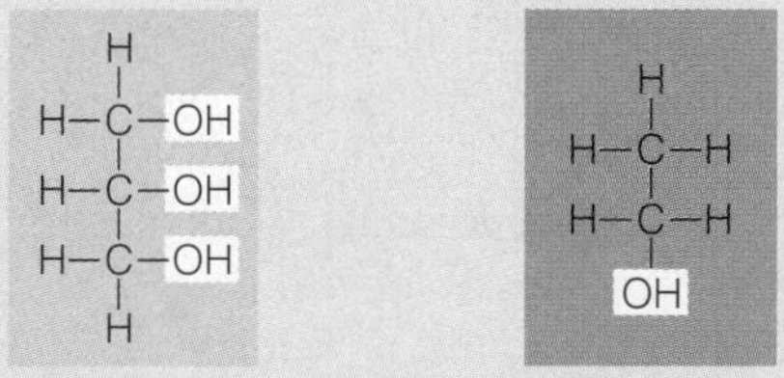

Glycerol is the alcohol used to make triglycerides.

Ethanol is the alcohol in beer wine, and distilled spirits.

Glossary

acetaldehyde (ass-et-AL-duh-hide): an intermediate in alcohol metabolism.

alcohol: a class of organic compounds containing hydroxyl (OH) groups.

alcohol dehydrogenase: an enzyme that converts ethanol to acetaldehyde. The MEOS also oxidizes alcohol (see *MEOS*).

antidiuretic hormone (ADH): a hormone produced by the pituitary gland in response to dehydration (or a high sodium concentration in the blood); it stimulates the kidneys to reabsorb more water and therefore to excrete less. This ADH should not be confused with the enzyme alcohol dehydrogenase, which is sometimes also abbreviated ADH.

beer: an alcoholic beverage brewed by fermenting malt and hops.

cirrhosis (seer-OH-sis): advanced liver disease in which liver cells turn orange, die, and harden, permanently losing their function; often associated with alcoholism.
cirrhos = an orange

distilled liquor: an alcoholic beverage made by fermenting and distilling grains; sometimes called *distilled spirits* or *hard liquor*.

drink: a dose of any alcoholic beverage that delivers ½ oz of pure ethanol:

- 4 to 5 oz of wine.
- 10 oz of wine cooler.
- 12 oz of beer.
- 1¼ oz of hard liquor (80 proof whiskey, scotch, rum, or vodka).

drug: a substance that can modify one or more of the body's functions.

ethanol: a particular type of alcohol found in beer, wine, and distilled spirits; also called *ethyl alcohol* (see Figure H7–1). Ethanol is the most widely used—and abused—drug in our society. It is also the only legal, nonprescription drug that produces euphoria.

euphoria (you-FORE-eh-uh): a feeling of great well-being, which people often seek through the use of drugs such as alcohol.
eu = good
phoria = bearing

fatty liver: an early stage of liver deterioration seen in several diseases, including kwashiorkor and alcoholic liver disease. Fatty liver is characterized by an accumulation of fat in the liver cells.

fermentation: the oxidation of carbohydrate in the absence of atmospheric oxygen, a process that yields alcohol as an end product.

fibrosis (fye-BROH-sis): an intermediate stage of liver deterioration seen in several diseases, including viral hepatitis and alcoholic liver disease. In fibrosis, the liver cells lose their function and assume the characteristics of connective tissue cells (fibers).

gout (GOWT): a painful condition in which uric acid crystals form in the joints.

MEOS (microsomal ethanol-oxidizing system): a system of enzymes in the liver that oxidize not only alcohol, but also several classes of drugs. (The *microsomes* are tiny particles of membranes with associated enzymes that can be collected from broken-up cells.)
micro = tiny
soma = body

moderation: in relation to alcohol consumption, not more than two drinks a day for the average-sized man and not more than one drink a day for the average-sized woman.

NAD (nicotinamide adenine dinucleotide): the main coenzyme form of the vitamin niacin; its reduced form is NADH.

narcotic (nor-KOT-ic): any drug that dulls the senses, induces sleep, and becomes addictive with prolonged use.

proof: a way of stating the percentage of alcohol in distilled liquor. Liquor that is 100 proof is 50% alcohol; 90 proof is 45%, and so forth.

wine: an alcoholic beverage made by fermenting grape juice.

---

flavored with herbs and spices to make liqueurs or after-dinner drinks.

Beer, wine, and liquor deliver different amounts of alcohol. The amount of alcohol in distilled liquor is stated as *proof:* distilled liquor of 100 proof is 50 percent alcohol, 80 proof liquor is 40 percent alcohol, and so forth. Regular wine (at 8 to 14 percent) and beer (at 4 to 6 percent) have less alcohol. (Some fortified wines and beers have more alcohol.)

Taken in moderation, alcohol can be compatible with good health. The term *moderation* is important in describing alcohol use. How many drinks constitute moderate use, and how much is "a drink"? First, a drink is any alcoholic beverage that delivers ½ ounce of *pure ethanol:*

- 4 to 5 ounces of wine.
- 10 ounces of wine cooler.
- 12 ounces of beer.
- 1¼ ounce of distilled liquor (80 proof whiskey, scotch, rum, or vodka).

Second, it is impossible to name an

exact amount of alcohol per day that is appropriate for everyone because people have different tolerances to alcohol. Authorities have attempted to set limits that are acceptable for most healthy people. An accepted definition of moderation is not more than two drinks a day for the average-sized man and not more than one drink a day for the average-sized woman. Notice that this advice is stated as a maximum, not as an average; seven drinks one night a week would not be considered moderate, even though one a day would be. Doubtless some people could consume slightly more; others could not handle nearly so much without risk. The amount a person can drink safely is highly individual, depending on genetics, health condition, sex, weight, age, and family history.

ALCOHOL IN THE BODY

From the moment an alcoholic beverage enters the body, it is treated as if it has special privileges. Unlike foods, which require time for digestion, alcohol needs no digestion and is quickly absorbed. About 20 percent is absorbed directly across the walls of an empty stomach and can reach the brain within a minute. Consequently, a person can immediately feel euphoric when drinking, especially on an empty stomach.

When the stomach is full of food, alcohol has less chance of touching the walls and diffusing through, so its influence on the brain is slightly delayed. This information leads to a practical tip: eat snacks when drinking alcoholic beverages. Carbohydrate snacks slow alcohol absorption and high-fat snacks slow peristalsis, keeping the alcohol in the stomach longer. Salty snacks make a person thirsty; to quench thirst, drink water instead of more alcohol.

The stomach begins to break down alcohol with its alcohol dehydrogenase enzyme. This action can reduce the amount of alcohol entering the blood by about 20 percent. Research shows that women produce less of this stomach enzyme than men, which partially explains why women become more intoxicated on less alcohol than men.[2] Women absorb about one-third more alcohol than men of the same size who drink the same amount of alcohol.

Alcohol is rapidly absorbed in the duodenum. From this point on, alcohol receives VIP (Very Important Person) treatment: it gets absorbed and metabolized before most nutrients.

ALCOHOL ARRIVES IN THE LIVER

The capillaries of the digestive tract merge into veins that carry the alcohol-laden blood to the liver. These veins branch and rebranch into capillaries that touch every liver cell. Liver cells are the only cells in the body that can make enough of the enzyme alcohol dehydrogenase to oxidize alcohol at an appreciable rate. The routing of blood through the liver cells gives them the chance to dispose of some alcohol before it moves on.

Alcohol affects every organ of the body, but the most dramatic evidence of its disruptive behavior appears in the liver. If liver cells could talk, they would describe the alcohol of intoxicating beverages as demanding, egocentric, and disruptive of the liver's efficient way of running its business. For example, liver cells normally prefer fatty acids as their fuel, and they like to package excess fatty acids into triglycerides and ship them out to other tissues. When alcohol is present, however, the liver cells are forced to metabolize alcohol and let the fatty acids accumulate, sometimes in huge stockpiles. Alcohol metabolism also permanently changes liver cell structure, which impairs the liver's ability to metabolize fats.[3] This explains why heavy drinkers develop fatty livers.

The liver can process about ½ ounce *ethanol* per hour (the amount in a typical drink), depending on the person's body size, previous drinking experience, food intake, and general health. This maximum rate of alcohol breakdown is set by the amount of alcohol dehydrogenase available. If more alcohol arrives at the liver than the enzymes can handle, the extra alcohol travels to all parts of the body, circulating again and again until liver enzymes are finally available to process it. Another practical tip derives from this information: drink slowly enough to allow the liver to keep up—no more than 1 drink per hour.

The amount of alcohol dehydrogenase enzyme present in the liver varies with individuals, depending on the genes they have inherited and on how recently they have eaten. Fasting for as little as a day forces the body to degrade its proteins, including the alcohol-processing enzyme, and this can slow the rate of alcohol metabolism by half. Drinking on an empty stomach thus causes the drinker to feel the effects more promptly for two reasons: rapid absorption and slowed breakdown. By maintaining higher blood alcohol concentrations for longer times, alcohol can anesthetize the brain more completely.

The alcohol dehydrogenase enzyme breaks down alcohol by removing hydrogens in two steps. (Figure H7–2 provides a simplified diagram of alcohol metabolism; Appendix C provides the chemical details.) In the first step, alcohol dehydrogenase oxidizes alcohol to acetaldehyde. High concentrations of acetaldehyde in the brain and other tissues are responsible for many of the punishing effects of alcohol abuse.

In the second step, a related enzyme, acetaldehyde dehydrogenase, oxidizes the acetaldehyde to acetyl CoA, the "crossroads" compound that can enter the TCA cycle to generate energy. These reactions produce hydrogen ions (acid). The B vitamin niacin (in its role as the coenzyme known as NAD) helpfully picks up these hydrogen ions (becoming NADH). Thus, whenever the body breaks down alcohol, NAD diminishes and NADH accumulates.

Figure H7–2

Alcohol Metabolism

The conversion of alcohol to acetyl CoA requires the B vitamin niacin in its role as NAD. When the enzymes oxidize alcohol, they remove H atoms and attach them to NAD. Thus NAD is used up, and NADH accumulates. (Note: More accurately, NAD^+ is converted to $NADH + H^+$. For simplicity's sake, the process has been described here as if one hydrogen were added to NAD, but, in reality, two are added.)

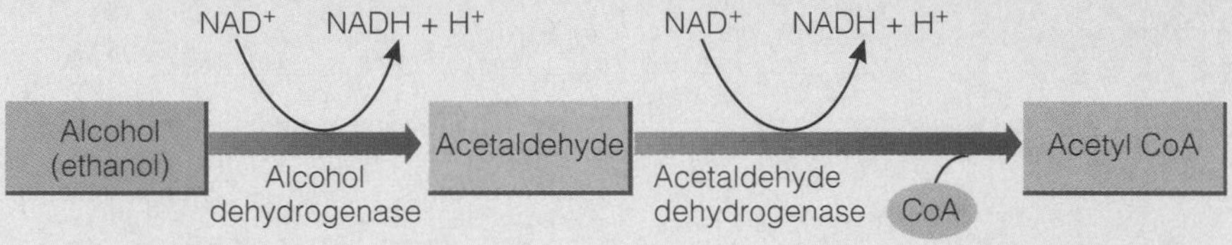

ALCOHOL DISRUPTS THE LIVER

During alcohol metabolism, NAD becomes unavailable for the multitude of other vital body processes for which it is required, including glycolysis, the TCA cycle, and the electron transport chain. Its presence is sorely missed in these energy pathways because it is the chief carrier of the hydrogens that travel with their electrons along the electron transport chain. Without NAD, the energy pathway is blocked. Traffic either backs up, or an alternate route is taken. Such changes in the normal flow from glucose to energy have striking physical consequences.

For one, the accumulation of hydrogen ions during alcohol metabolism shifts the body's acid-base balance toward acid. For another, the accumulation of NADH slows the TCA cycle, so pyruvate and acetyl CoA build up. Excess acetyl CoA then takes the route to fatty acid synthesis (as Figure H7–3 illustrates), and fat clogs the liver.

As you might expect, a liver clogged with fat cannot function properly. Liver cells become less effi-

Figure H7–3

Alternate Route for Acetyl CoA: To Fat

Acetyl CoA molecules are blocked from getting into the TCA cycle by the high level of NADH. Instead of being used for energy, the acetyl CoA molecules become building blocks for fatty acids.

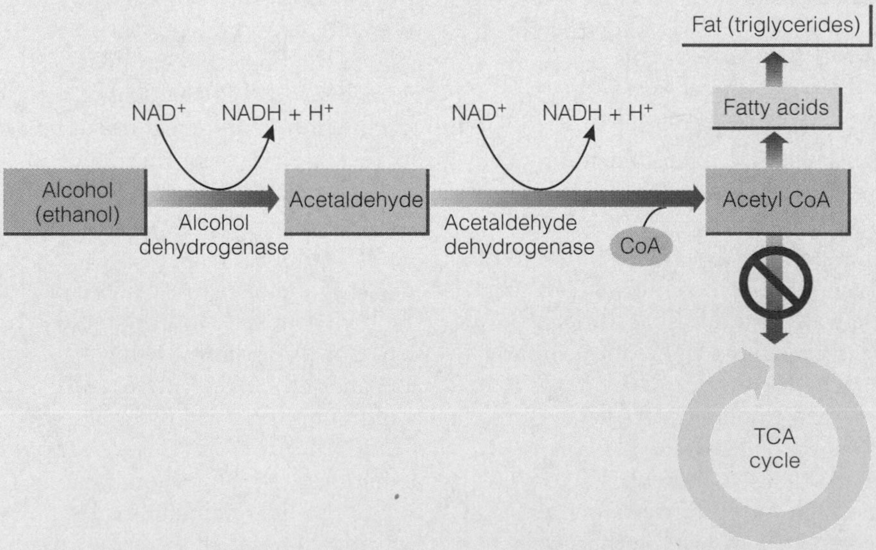

cient at performing a number of tasks. Much of this inefficiency impairs a person's nutritional health in ways that cannot be corrected by diet alone. For example, the liver has difficulty activating vitamin D, as well as producing and releasing bile. To overcome such problems, a person needs to stop drinking alcohol.

The synthesis of fatty acids accelerates with exposure to alcohol. Fat accumulation can be seen in the liver after a single night of heavy drinking. Fatty liver, the first stage of liver deterioration seen in heavy drinkers, interferes with the distribution of nutrients and oxygen to the liver cells. If the condition lasts long enough, the liver cells will die and form fibrous scar tissue—the second stage of liver deterioration, called fibrosis. Some liver cells can regenerate with good nutrition and abstinence from alcohol, but in the most advanced stage, cirrhosis, damage is the least reversible.

The fatty liver has difficulty generating glucose from protein. The lack of glucose together with the overabundance of acetyl CoA sets the stage for ketosis. The body uses the acetyl CoA to make ketone bodies, which push the acid-base balance further toward acid.

Excess NADH also promotes the making of lactic acid from pyruvate. The conversion of pyruvate to lactic acid uses the hydrogens from NADH and restores some NAD, but a lactic acid buildup has serious consequences of its own—it adds still further to the body's acid burden and interferes with the excretion of another acid, uric acid, causing goutlike symptoms.

Alcohol alters both amino acid and protein metabolism. Synthesis of proteins important in the immune system slows down, weakening the body's defenses against infection. Protein deficiency can develop, both from the depression of protein synthesis and from a poor diet. Normally, the cells would at least use the amino acids that a person happened to eat, but the drinker's liver deaminates the amino acids and uses the carbon fragments to make fat or ketones. Eating well does not protect the drinker from protein depletion; a person has to stop drinking alcohol.

The liver's VIP treatment of alcohol affects its handling of drugs as well as nutrients. In addition to the dehydrogenase enzyme already described, the liver possesses an enzyme system that metabolizes *both* alcohol and several types of other drugs. Called the MEOS (microsomal ethanol-oxidizing system), this system handles about one-fifth of the total alcohol a person consumes. At high blood alcohol concentrations, however, or if repeatedly exposed to alcohol, the MEOS grows larger.

As a person's blood alcohol rises, alcohol competes with—and wins out over—other drugs whose metabolism relies on the MEOS. If a person drinks and uses another drug at the same time, the drug will be metabolized more slowly and will therefore exert greater effects. The MEOS is busy disposing of alcohol, so the drug cannot be handled until later; the dose may build up so that its effects are greatly amplified—sometimes to the point of being fatal.

In contrast, once a heavy drinker stops drinking and alcohol is no longer competing with other drugs, the enlarged MEOS metabolizes drugs much faster than before. As a result, determining the correct dosages of medications can be confusing and tricky. The physician who prescribes sedatives every four hours, for example, unaware that the person has recently gone from being a heavy drinker to an abstainer, expects the MEOS to dispose of the drug at a certain predicted rate. The MEOS is adapted to metabolizing large quantities of alcohol, though, so it metabolizes the drug extra fast. The drug's effects wear off unexpectedly fast, leaving the client undersedated. Imagine the doctor's alarm should a patient wake up on the table during an operation! A skilled anesthesiologist always asks clients about their drinking patterns before putting them to sleep.

This discussion has emphasized the major way that the blood is cleared of alcohol—metabolism by the liver—but there is another way. About 10 percent of the alcohol leaves the body through the breath and in the urine. This is the basis for the breath and urine tests for drunkenness. The amounts of alcohol in the breath and in the urine are in proportion to the amount still in the bloodstream and brain. In nearly all states, legal drunkenness is set at 0.10 percent or less, reflecting the relationship between alcohol use and industrial and traffic accidents.

ALCOHOL ARRIVES IN THE BRAIN

Alcohol is a narcotic. People used it for centuries as an anesthetic because it can deaden pain. But alcohol was a poor anesthetic because one could never be sure how much a person would need and

Figure H7–4

Alcohol's Effects on the Brain

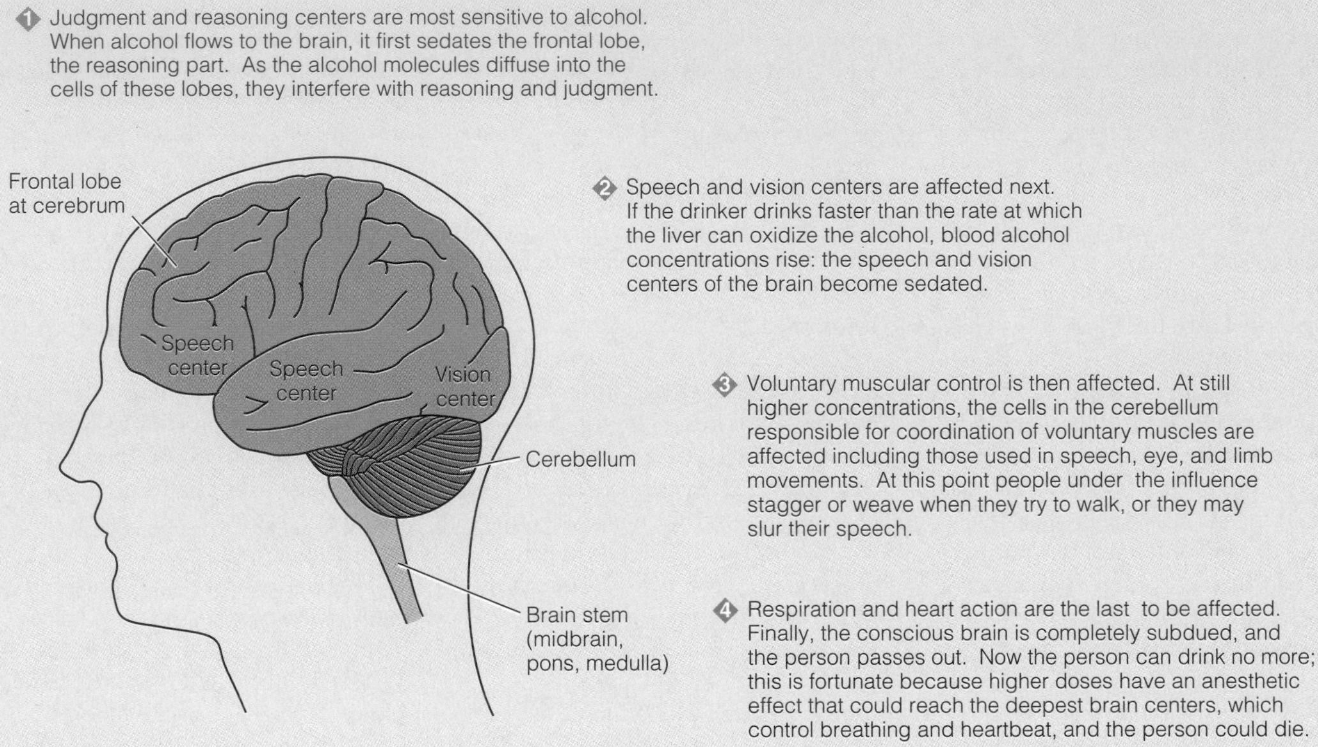
❶ Judgment and reasoning centers are most sensitive to alcohol. When alcohol flows to the brain, it first sedates the frontal lobe, the reasoning part. As the alcohol molecules diffuse into the cells of these lobes, they interfere with reasoning and judgment.
Frontal lobe at cerebrum
Speech center
Speech center
Vision center
Cerebellum
Brain stem (midbrain, pons, medulla)
❷ Speech and vision centers are affected next. If the drinker drinks faster than the rate at which the liver can oxidize the alcohol, blood alcohol concentrations rise: the speech and vision centers of the brain become sedated.
❸ Voluntary muscular control is then affected. At still higher concentrations, the cells in the cerebellum responsible for coordination of voluntary muscles are affected including those used in speech, eye, and limb movements. At this point people under the influence stagger or weave when they try to walk, or they may slur their speech.
❹ Respiration and heart action are the last to be affected. Finally, the conscious brain is completely subdued, and the person passes out. Now the person can drink no more; this is fortunate because higher doses have an anesthetic effect that could reach the deepest brain centers, which control breathing and heartbeat, and the person could die.

how much would be a fatal dose. Consequently, new, more predictable anesthetics have replaced alcohol. However, alcohol continues to be used today as a kind of social anesthetic to help people relax or to relieve anxiety. People think that alcohol is a stimulant because it seems to relieve inhibitions. Actually, though, it accomplishes this by sedating *inhibitory* nerves, which are more numerous than excitatory nerves. Ultimately, alcohol acts as a depressant and affects all the nerve cells. Figure H7–4 describes alcohol's effects on the brain.

It is lucky that the brain centers respond to a rising blood alcohol concentration in the order described in Figure H7–4 because a person usually passes out before managing to drink a lethal dose. It is possible, though, to drink so fast that the effects of alcohol continue to accelerate after the person has gone to sleep. Occasionally, a person dies from drinking enough to stop the heart before passing out. Table H7–1 shows the blood alcohol levels that correspond to progressively greater intoxication, and Table H7–2 shows the brain responses that occur at these blood levels.

Like liver cells, brain cells die with excessive exposure to alcohol. Liver cells may be replaced, but not all brain cells can regenerate. Thus some heavy drinkers suffer permanent brain damage.

People who drink alcoholic beverages may notice that they urinate more, but they may be unaware of the vicious cycle that results. Alcohol depresses production of antidiuretic hormone (ADH) by the pituitary gland in the brain. Loss of body water leads to thirst, and thirst leads to more drinking. The only fluid that will relieve dehydration is water, but the thirsty drinker may drink alcohol instead. This only worsens the problem. Such information provides another practical tip: drink water when thirsty and before each alcoholic drink.

Table H7–1

Alcohol Doses and Blood Levels

Number of Drinks[a]	Percentage of Blood Alcohol by Body Weight				
	100 lb	120 lb	150 lb	180 lb	200 lb
2	0.08	0.06	0.05	0.04	0.04
4	0.15	0.13	0.10	0.08	0.08
6	0.23	0.19	0.15	0.13	0.11
8	0.30	0.25	0.20	0.17	0.15
12	0.45	0.36	0.30	0.25	0.23
14	0.52	0.42	0.35	0.34	0.27

[a]Taken within an hour or so.
1 drink = 12 oz of 4.5% beer.
4 oz of 14% wine.
1 to 1½ oz of 50% liquor.

Note: In nearly all states, legal drunkenness is set at 0.10 percent or less.

The water loss caused by depressed ADH is accompanied by the loss of important minerals. As Chapters 12 and 13 will explain, these minerals are vital to the body's fluid balance and to many chemical reactions in the cells, including muscle action. For the person made sick by excessive alcohol intake and requiring detoxification, early repletion therapy attempts to restore mineral balance as quickly as possible.

ALCOHOL AND MALNUTRITION

For many moderate drinkers, alcohol does not suppress food intake, and in some cases, it may actually stimulate appetite. When alcohol is consumed as *added* energy, it can contribute body fat.[4] Metabolically, alcohol behaves like fat in promoting obesity; each ounce of alcohol represents about a half ounce of fat.[5] Chronic alcohol ingestion seems to have the opposite effect, however. Alcohol produces euphoria, which depresses appetite, so heavy drinkers tend to eat poorly and suffer malnutrition. Alcohol is rich in energy (7 kcalories per gram), but like pure sugar or fat, the kcalories are empty of nutrients. The more alcohol people drink, the less likely that they will eat enough food to obtain adequate nutrients. The more kcalories spent on alcohol, the fewer kcalories available to spend on nutritious foods. Table H7–3 (on p. 272) shows the kcalorie amounts of typical alcoholic beverages.

Chronic alcohol abuse not only displaces nutrients from the diet but also interferes with the body's metabolism of nutrients. Most dramatic is alcohol's effect on the B vitamin folate. When alcohol is present, the body behaves as if it were actively trying to expel folate. The liver, which normally contains enough folate to meet all needs, leaks folate into the blood. As blood folate rises, the kidneys are deceived into excreting it. Alcohol abuse causes a folate deficiency that

Table H7–2

Alcohol Blood Levels and Brain Responses

Blood Alcohol Concentration	Effect on Brain
0.05	Impaired judgment, relaxed inhibitions, altered mood, increased heart rate
0.10	Impaired coordination, delayed reaction time, exaggerated emotions, impaired peripheral vision, impaired ability to operate a vehicle
0.15	Slurred speech, blurred vision, staggered walk, seriously impaired coordination and judgment
0.20	Double vision, inability to walk
0.30	Uninhibited behavior, stupor, confusion, inability to comprehend
0.40 to 0.60	Unconsciousness, shock, coma, death (cardiac or respiratory failure)

Note: Blood alcohol concentration depends on a number of factors, including alcohol in the beverage, the rate of consumption, the person's gender, and body weight. For example, a 100-pound female can become legally drunk (0.10 concentration) by drinking three beers in an hour, whereas a 220-pound male consuming that amount at the same rate would have a 0.05 blood alcohol concentration.

Table H7–3

kCalories in Alcoholic Beverages and Mixers

Beverage	Amount (oz)	Energy (kcal)
Beer		
Regular	12	150
Light	12	100
Nonalcoholic	12	32–82
Distilled liquor (gin, rum, vodka, whiskey)		
80 proof	1½	100
86 proof	1½	105
90 proof	1½	110
Liqueurs		
Coffee liqueur	1½	175
Coffee and cream liqueur	1½	155
Crème de menthe	1½	185
Mixers		
Club soda	12	0
Cola	12	150
Cranberry juice cocktail	8	145
Diet drinks	12	2
Ginger ale	12	125
Grapefruit juice	8	95
Orange juice	8	110
Tomato or vegetable juice	8	45
Tonic	12	124
Wine		
Dessert	3½	160
Nonalcoholic	8	14
Red	3½	75
Rosé	3½	75
White	3½	70
Wine cooler	12	50

devastates digestive system function. The intestine normally releases and retrieves folate continuously, but it becomes damaged by folate deficiency and alcohol toxicity, so it fails to retrieve its own folate and misses any that may trickle in from food as well. Alcohol also interferes with the action of what little folate is left, and this inhibits the production of new cells, especially the rapidly dividing cells of the intestine and the blood. The combination of poor folate status and alcohol consumption has been implicated in promoting colorectal cancer.[6]

Acetaldehyde, an intermediate in alcohol metabolism, interferes with nutrient use, too. For example, acetaldehyde dislodges vitamin B_6 from its protective binding protein so that it is destroyed, causing a vitamin B_6 deficiency and, thereby, lowered production of red blood cells.

Malnutrition occurs not only because of lack of intake and altered metabolism, but because of direct toxic effects as well.[7] Alcohol causes stomach cells to oversecrete both gastric acid and histamine, an agent of the immune system that produces inflammation. Beer in particular stimulates gastric acid secretion, irritating the stomach and esophagus linings and making them vulnerable to ulcer formation.[8]

Nutrient deficiencies are virtually inevitable in alcohol abuse, not only because alcohol displaces food but also because alcohol directly interferes with the body's use of nutrients, making them ineffective even if they are present. Intestinal cells fail to absorb B vitamins, notably thiamin, folate, and vitamin B_{12}. Liver cells lose efficiency in activating vitamin D. Cells in the retina of the eye, which normally process the alcohol form of vitamin A (retinol) to its aldehyde form needed in vision, find themselves processing ethanol to acetaldehyde instead.

Over a lifetime, excessive drinking, regardless of dietary intake, creates deficits of all the nutrients mentioned in this discussion and more. No diet can compensate for the damage caused by heavy alcohol consumption.[9]

ALCOHOL'S SHORT-TERM EFFECTS

Heavy or binge drinking (defined as at least 4 to 5 drinks in a row) is widespread on college campuses and poses serious health and social consequences to both drinkers and nondrinkers alike.*[10] Alcohol is

*This definition of binge drinking, without specification of time elapsed, is consistent with standard practice in alcohol research among college students.

responsible for most accidental deaths, including automobile fatalities. Compared with nondrinkers or moderate drinkers, people who frequently binge drink (at least three times within two weeks) are more likely to engage in unprotected sex, damage property, and assault others.

Binge drinking is not limited to college campuses, of course, but that environment seems most accepting of such behavior despite its problems. Social acceptance may make it difficult for binge drinkers to recognize themselves as problem drinkers. For this reason, interventions must focus both on individuals and on the whole population. The damage alcohol causes only becomes worse if the pattern is not broken.

Table H7–4

Health Effects of Alcohol Consumption

Health Problem	Effects of Alcohol
Arthritis	Increases the risk of gouty arthritis.
Cancer	Increases the risk of cancer of the liver, pancreas, rectum, and breast; increases the risk of cancer of the mouth, pharynx, larynx, and esophagus, where alcohol interacts synergistically with tobacco.
Fetal alcohol syndrome	Causes physical and behavioral abnormalities in the fetus.
Heart disease	Raises blood pressure, blood lipids, and the risk of stroke and heart disease in heavy drinkers; when compared with those who abstain, heart disease risk is generally lower in light-to-moderate drinkers (see Chapter 18).
Hyperglycemia	Raises blood glucose.
Hypoglycemia	Lowers blood glucose, especially in people with diabetes.
Kidney disease	Enlarges the kidneys, alters hormone functions, and increases the risk of kidney failure.
Liver disease	Causes fatty liver, alcoholic hepatitis, and cirrhosis.
Malnutrition	Increases the risk of protein-energy malnutrition; low intakes of protein, calcium, iron, vitamin A, vitamin C, thiamin, vitamin B_6, and riboflavin; and impaired absorption of calcium, phosphorus, vitamin D, and zinc.
Nervous disorders	Causes neuropathy and dementia; impairs balance and memory.
Obesity	Increases energy intake, but is not a primary cause of obesity.
Psychological disturbances	Causes depression, anxiety, and insomnia.

Note: This list is by no means all-inclusive. Alcohol has direct toxic effects on all body systems.

ALCOHOL'S LONG-TERM EFFECTS

By far the longest-term effect of alcohol is the damage done to a child whose mother abused alcohol during pregnancy. The devastating effects of alcohol on the unborn, and the message that pregnant women should not drink alcohol, are presented in Highlight 15.

For nonpregnant adults, a drink or two sets in motion many destructive processes in the body, but the next day's abstinence reverses them. As long as the doses are moderate, time between them is ample, and nutrition is adequate, recovery is probably complete.

If the doses of alcohol are heavy and the time between them short, complete recovery cannot take place. Repeated onslaughts of alcohol gradually take a toll on all parts of the body (see Table H7–4). Compared with nondrinkers, heavy drinkers have significantly greater risks of dying from all causes.[11]

PERSONAL STRATEGIES

One obvious option available to people attending social gatherings is to enjoy the conversation, eat the food, and drink nonalcoholic beverages. Several nonalcoholic beverages are available that mimic the look and taste of their alcoholic counterparts. For those who enjoy champagne or beer, sparkling ciders and beers are available without alcohol. Instead of drinking a cocktail, a person can sip tomato juice with a slice of lime and a stalk of celery or just a plain cola beverage. Any of these drinks can ease conversation.

The person who chooses to drink alcohol should sip each drink slowly with food. The alcohol molecules should dribble slowly enough into the liver cells that the enzymes can handle the load. It is best to space drinks, too, allowing about an hour or so to metabolize each drink.

If you want to help sober up a friend who has had too much to drink, don't wear yourself out walking arm in arm around the block. Walking muscles have to work harder, but muscle cells can't metabolize alcohol; only liver cells can. Remember that each person has a limited amount of alcohol dehydrogenase that clears the blood at a steady rate. In short, time alone will do the job.

Nor will it help to give your friend a cup of coffee. Caffeine is a stimulant, but it won't speed up alcohol metabolism. The police say ruefully, "If you give a drunk a cup of coffee, you'll just have a wide-awake drunk on your hands." Table H7–5 presents other alcohol myths.

Table H7–5

Myths and Truths Concerning Alcohol

Myth:	Alcohol is legal; therefore, it is not a drug.
Truth:	Alcohol is legal, but it alters one or more of the body's functions and is medically defined as a depressant drug.
Myth:	A shot of alcohol warms you up.
Truth:	Alcohol diverts blood flow to the skin making you *feel* warmer, but it actually cools the body.
Myth:	Wine and beer are mild; they do not lead to addiction.
Truth:	Wine and beer drinkers worldwide have high rates of death from alcohol-related illnesses. It's not what you drink, but how much, that makes the difference.
Myth:	Mixing drinks is what gives you a hangover.
Truth:	Too much alcohol in any form produces a hangover.
Myth:	Alcohol is a stimulant.
Truth:	Alcohol depresses the activity of the brain.

Don't drive too soon after drinking. The lack of glucose for the brain's function and the length of time needed to clear the blood of alcohol make alcohol's adverse effects linger long after its blood concentration has fallen to zero. Driving coordination is still impaired the morning *after* a night of drinking, even if the drinking was moderate. Responsible aircraft pilots know that they must allow 24 hours for their bodies to clear alcohol completely, and they refuse to fly any sooner. The Federal Aviation Administration and major airlines enforce this rule.

Society also pays a high price when a drinker gets behind the wheel of an automobile. Traffic accidents are the number one cause of death among young people (ages 5 to 32), and almost half of all traffic fatalities involve alcohol. In 1991 close to 20,000 people were killed in alcohol-related traffic accidents.[12] This was the lowest incidence in a decade thanks to the educational efforts of MADD (Mothers Against Drunk Driving), the implementation of designated driver programs, a higher minimum drinking age in many states, and the severe legal consequences of driving while under the influence (DUI). In addition to traffic fatalities, alcohol use has been implicated in most of the other deaths in young people, including drownings, falls, suicides, and homicides.[13]

You may have heard the story of the woman who kept saying "Amen!" as the preacher ranted about one sin after another; but when he got to her favorite sin, she whispered to her husband that the preacher had "quit preachin' and gone to meddlin'. " We've tried to stick to scientific facts, so the only "meddlin'" we'll do is to urge you to look again at the drawing of the brain in Figure H7–4 and note that when someone drinks, judgment fails first. Judgment might tell a person to limit alcohol consumption to two drinks at a party, but if the first drink takes judgment away, many more drinks may follow. The failure to stop drinking as planned, on repeated occasions, is a danger sign warning that the person should not drink at all. Appendix F provides addresses for organizations that offer information about alcohol and alcohol abuse.

Ethanol interferes with a multitude of chemical and hormonal reactions in the body—many more than have been enumerated here. With heavy alcohol consumption, the potential for harm is great. The best way to escape the harmful effects of alcohol is, of course, to refuse alcohol altogether. If you do drink, do so with care, and in moderation.

NOTES

1. Secretary of Health and Human Services, Eighth Special Report to the U.S. Congress on Alcohol and Health (Rockville, Md.: U.S.

Department of Health and Human Services, 1993).

2. M. Frezza and coauthors, High blood alcohol levels in women: The role of decreased gastric alcohol dehydrogenase activity and first-pass metabolism, *New England Journal of Medicine* 322 (1990): 95–99.

3. C. S. Lieber, Herman Award Lecture, 1993: A personal perspective on alcohol, nutrition, and the liver, *American Journal of Clinical Nutrition* 58 (1993): 430–442.

4. B. J. Sonko and coauthors, Effect of alcohol on postmeal fat storage, *American Journal of Clinical Nutrition* 59 (1994): 619–625; P. M. Suter, Y. Schutz, and E. Jequier, The effect of ethanol on fat storage in healthy subjects, *New England Journal of Medicine* 326 (1992): 983–987.

5. J. P. Flatt, Body weight, fat storage, and alcohol metabolism, *Nutrition Reviews* 50 (1992): 267–270.

6. Folate, alcohol, methionine, and colon cancer risks: Is there a unifying theme? *Nutrition Reviews* 52 (1994): 18–20.

7. Lieber, 1993.

8. M. V. Singer, S. Teyssen, and V. E. Eysselein, Action of beer and its ingredients on gastric acid secretion and release of gastrin in humans, *Gastroenterology* 101 (1991): 935–942.

9. Lieber, 1993.

10. H. Wechsler and coauthors, Health and behavioral consequences of binge drinking in college: A national survey of students at 140 campuses, *Journal of the American Medical Association* 272 (1994): 1672–1677.

11. A. L. Klatsky, M. A. Armstrong, and G. D. Friedman, Alcohol and mortality, *Annals of Internal Medicine* 117 (1992): 646–654.

12. Alcohol-related traffic fatalities, *FDA Consumer,* March 1993, p. 26.

13. Committee on Substance Abuse, Alcohol use and abuse: A pediatric concern, *Pediatrics* 95 (1995): 439–442.

Chapter 8

Energy Balance and Body Composition

CONTENTS

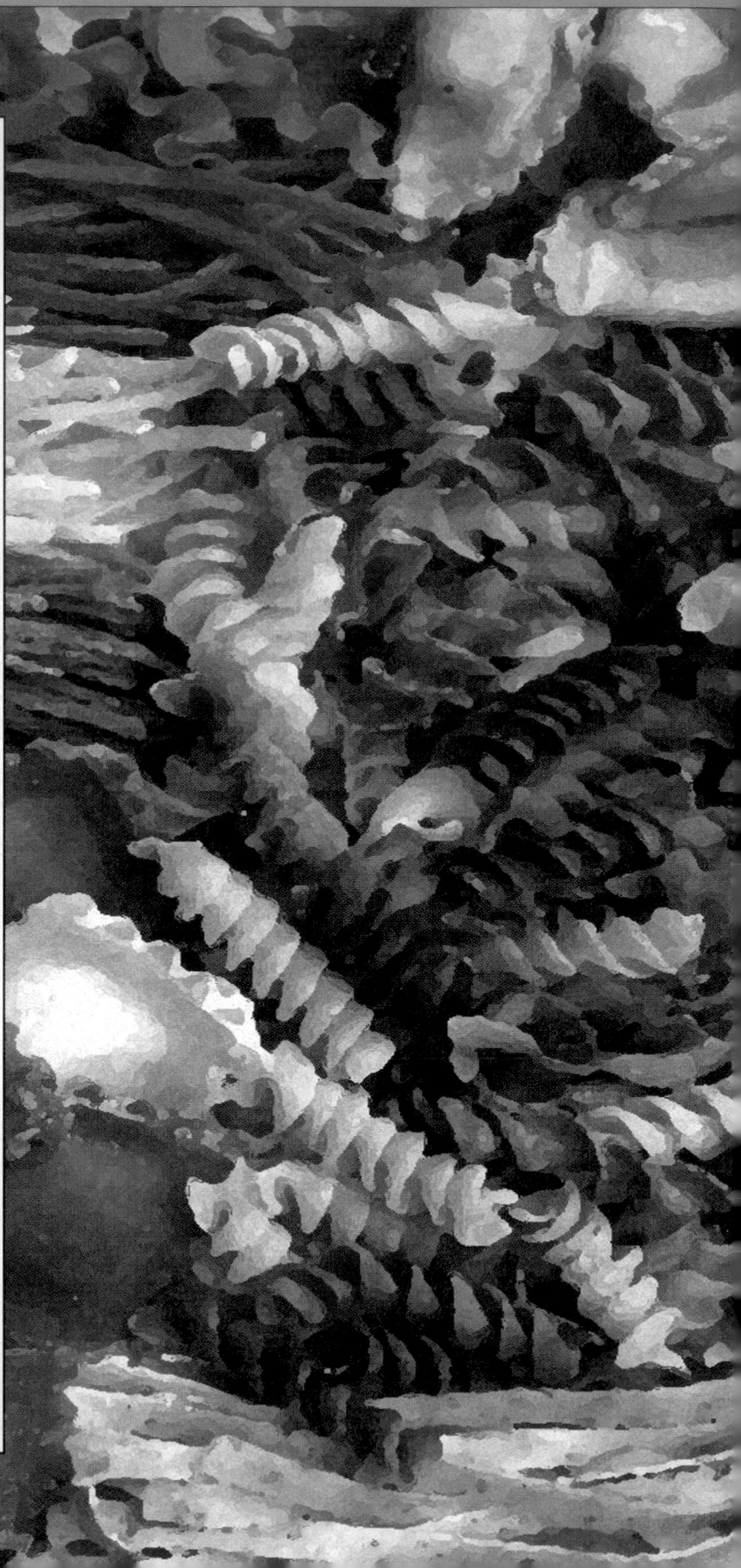

MICROGRAPH: Adenosine triphosphate, the body's common energy currency

The body's remarkable machinery can cope with many extremes of diet. As you have seen, it can convert both carbohydrate (glucose) and protein (amino acids) to fat. To some extent, it can convert amino acids to glucose. To a very limited extent, it can even convert fat (the glycerol portion) to glucose. But a grossly unbalanced diet imposes hardships on the body. If energy intake is too low or if too little carbohydrate or protein is supplied, the body must degrade its own lean tissue to meet its glucose and protein needs. If energy intake is too high or if fat is oversupplied, the body stores fat.

Overfatness and underweight both result from unbalanced energy budgets. The simple picture is as follows. Overfat people have consumed more food energy than they have spent and have banked the surplus in their body fat. To reduce fat reserves, overfat people need to spend more energy than they take in from food. In contrast, underweight people have consumed too little food energy to support their bodies' activities and so have depleted their bodies' fat stores and possibly their lean tissues as well. To gain weight, they need to take in more food energy than they expend. As you will see, though, the details of the body's weight regulation are quite complex. This chapter describes energy balance and body composition and examines the problems associated with having too much or too little body fat; the next chapter presents strategies toward resolving these problems.

The term *overfat* refers to an excess of body fat, which is not necessarily the same as *overweight*, as a later section of the chapter explains.

Energy Balance

People spend energy continuously and eat periodically to refuel. Ideally, their food intakes cover their energy needs without too much excess. Excess energy is stored as fat, and stored fat is used for energy between meals. The amount of body fat a person deposits in, or withdraws from, "savings" on any given day depends on the energy balance for that day—the amount consumed (energy in) versus the amount expended (energy out). When a person is maintaining weight, energy in equals energy out.

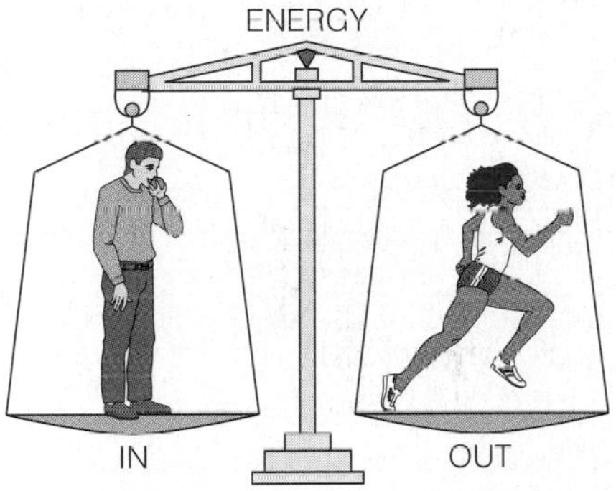

When energy in balances with energy out, a person's body weight is stable.

Most people maintain a steady energy balance over time. On any given day, they may eat a little more or a little less than usual, and their weight may go up or down a pound or two, but for the most part, they stay in balance. When the balance shifts, their weight changes.

A pound of body fat stores about 3500 kcalories. It stands to reason that a person who eats 3500 extra kcalories should gain a pound, and that a person who cuts 3500 kcalories should lose a pound, but this does not always happen. When a person overeats, much of the excess energy is stored, but some energy is spent to maintain the heavier body.[1] Furthermore, people seem to gain more body fat when they eat extra fat kcalories than when they eat extra carbohydrate kcalories, and they seem to lose body fat most efficiently when they limit kcalories specifically from fat.[2] Whether a person chooses extra potatoes or extra butter may make a great difference to body weight and body composition. Highlight 8 explores this research further.

1 lb body fat = 3500 kcal.
Body fat, or adipose tissue, is composed of a mixture of mostly fat, some protein, and water. A pound of body fat (454 g) is approximately 87% fat, or (454 × 0.87) 395 g, and 395 g × 9 kcal/g = 3555 kcal.

A reasonable rate of weight loss for overweight people is ½ to 1 pound a week. Even for obese people, a reasonable weight-loss rate is only 1 percent of body weight per week.[3] Such a gradual loss is more likely to stay off than rapid weight losses and can be achieved with a reasonable energy intake of about 10 kcalories per pound of body weight. If food energy is restricted too severely, dieters lose

Energy intake for weight loss:
10 kcal/lb body weight.

As Chapter 12 explains, water constitutes about 60% of an adult's body weight. Consequently, retention or losses of water influence body weight.

lean tissue and may not receive enough nutrients. In addition, restrictive eating may set in motion the unhealthy cycle of restrictive dieting and binge eating.

Besides, quick changes in weight are not just changes in fat. Weight gained or lost rapidly includes some fat, large amounts of fluid, and some lean tissues such as muscles and bone minerals. Even over the long term, the composition of weight gained or lost is normally about 75 percent fat and 25 percent lean. During starvation, losses of fat and lean are about equal. Invariably, though, *fat* gains and losses are gradual. The next two sections introduce the two sides of the energy-balance equation: energy in and energy out.

Energy In: The kCalories in Food

Foods and beverages are the "energy in" part of the energy-balance equation. How much energy a person receives depends on how much the person eats and drinks and on the composition of the foods and beverages.

FOOD COMPOSITION

bomb calorimeter (KAL-oh-RIM-eh-ter): an instrument that measures the *heat* energy released when foods are burned, thus providing an estimate of the potential energy of foods.
calor = heat
metron = measure

Reminder: A *kcalorie* is a unit of *heat* energy. One kcalorie is the amount of heat necessary to raise the temperature of 1 kg of water 1°C.

Food energy values can be determined by:
- **Direct calorimetry**, which measures the amount of heat released.
- **Indirect calorimetry**, which measures the amount of oxygen consumed.

The number of kcalories that the human body derives from a food, as contrasted with the number of kcalories determined by calorimetry, is the **physiological fuel value**.

Reminder:
- 1 g carbohydrate = 4 kcal.
- 1 g fat = 9 kcal.
- 1 g protein = 4 kcal.
- 1 g alcohol = 7 kcal.

To find out how many kcalories a food provides, a laboratory scientist can burn the food in a bomb calorimeter (see Figure 8–1). When the food burns, the chemical bonds between the carbon and hydrogen atoms break, releasing energy in the form of heat. The amount of heat given off provides a *direct* measure of the food's energy value (remember that kcalories are units of heat energy). In addition to releasing heat, these reactions generate carbon dioxide and water—just as the body's cells do when they metabolize the energy-yielding nutrients in a controlled version of this same process. When the food burns and the chemical bonds break, the carbons (C) and hydrogens (H) combine with oxygen (O) to form carbon dioxide (CO_2) and water (H_2O). The amount of oxygen consumed gives an *indirect* measure of the amount of energy released.

A bomb calorimeter measures the available energy in foods but overstates the amount of energy that the human body derives from foods. The body is less efficient than a calorimeter and cannot metabolize all of a food's energy-yielding nutrients all the way to carbon dioxide and water. Researchers who use calorimetry can correct for this discrepancy mathematically to make useful tables of the energy values of foods (such as Appendix H). These values are reasonable estimates, but do not reflect the *precise* amount of energy a person will derive from the foods consumed.

The energy values of foods can also be computed from the amounts of carbohydrate, fat, and protein (and alcohol, if present) in the foods.* For example, a food containing 8 grams protein, 12 grams carbohydrate, and 5 grams fat would provide 32 protein kcalories, 48 carbohydrate kcalories, and 45 fat kcalories, for a total of 125 kcalories.

FOOD INTAKE

To achieve energy balance, the body must meet its needs without storing too much or too little energy. Somehow the body must decide how often and how

*Some of the food energy values in the table of food composition in Appendix H were derived by bomb calorimetry, and many were calculated from their energy-yielding nutrient contents.

much to eat—when to start eating and when to stop. Eating is a complex behavior controlled by a variety of psychosocial, metabolic, and physiological factors.[4] The hypothalamus appears to be the control center, integrating messages about energy intake, expenditure, and storage from other parts of the brain and from the mouth, GI tract, and liver.

Short-Term Controls Some of these messages influence immediate food intake, controlling the size and frequency of meals. For example, the hunger message influences how much food will be eaten at one meal and how fast a person might eat. Palatability is also important: more is likely to be eaten when a meal is appetizing. Then satiety comes into play: receptors in the GI tract detect nutrients and signal satiety after each meal.[5] These receptors also influence when the next meal will be eaten.

Hunger People typically eat meals at roughly four-hour intervals; the stomach is ideally designed to handle periodic batches of food. Four hours after a meal, most, if not all, of the food has left the stomach and been absorbed by the intestine. When the stomach is empty, the hunger message is delivered to initiate eating. Most normal-weight people do not feel like eating until the stomach is either empty, or almost so. Even then, feelings of satiety may have disappeared quite a while before a person feels hungry. Hunger is also triggered by gastric contraction, the absence of nutrients in the small intestine, and GI hormones.

The body seems to be able to adapt its hunger response to accommodate changes in energy intake. People who restrict their energy intakes may feel pangs of hunger for the first few days, but these sensations diminish with time. After the body has adapted to a lower energy intake, eating a large, energy-rich meal makes the person feel uncomfortable. People can adapt to eating excessive amounts of food as well. Some research suggests that repeated binge eating enlarges the stomach's capacity.[6] Consequently the person may experience less satiety after a normal meal, setting the stage for another binge.

Receptors in the GI tract also adapt and change their responses depending on whether nutrient intake has been high or low. One study found that after two weeks on a high-fat diet, the digestion and absorption of a high-fat meal were accelerated.[7] The GI tract had adapted to handle this increase in fat intake efficiently, thus conserving energy. Such findings have interesting implications for the development of obesity.

Appetite Like hunger, appetite initiates eating, but it differs in that hunger is physiological (an inborn instinct), whereas appetite is psychological (a learned response to food). The two do not always coincide. A person may experience appetite without hunger, for example, when presented with a hot piece of homemade apple pie after having eaten a large Thanksgiving dinner. In contrast, a person may feel hungry but have no appetite for food when faced with a stressful situation or illness; in such circumstances eating becomes a chore. Figure 8–2 lists factors thought to be involved in hunger and appetite.

Satiety Most normal-weight people stop eating when they feel full or satisfied. Satiety occurs in response to gastric distention, nutrients in the small intestine, and GI hormones. Gastric distention can make a person feel too uncomfortable to eat, but it cannot by itself provide the comfortable sensation of satiety, which depends

Figure 8–1

Bomb Calorimeter

When food is burned, the chemical bonds between the carbons and hydrogens are broken, and energy is released in the form of heat. The amount of heat generated provides a direct measure of the amount of energy stored in the food's chemical bonds.

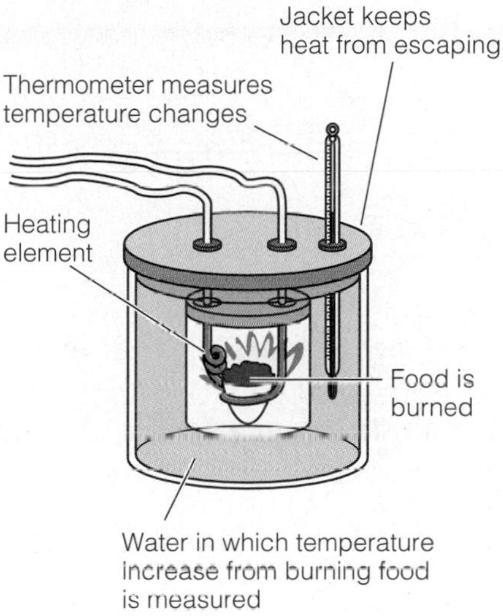

palatability: pleasing taste. When tasting foods, the tongue presses them against the *palate* (PAL-ut), or roof of the mouth.

hunger: the physiological need to eat, experienced as a drive to obtain food; an unpleasant sensation.

appetite: the psychological desire to eat or an interest in food; a positive sensation that accompanies the sight, smell, or thought of food.

satiety (sah-TIE-eh-tee)**:** the feeling of satisfaction and fullness that food brings.
sate = to fill

Figure 8–2

Hunger and Appetite

This is a partial list of the factors thought to affect hunger and appetite.

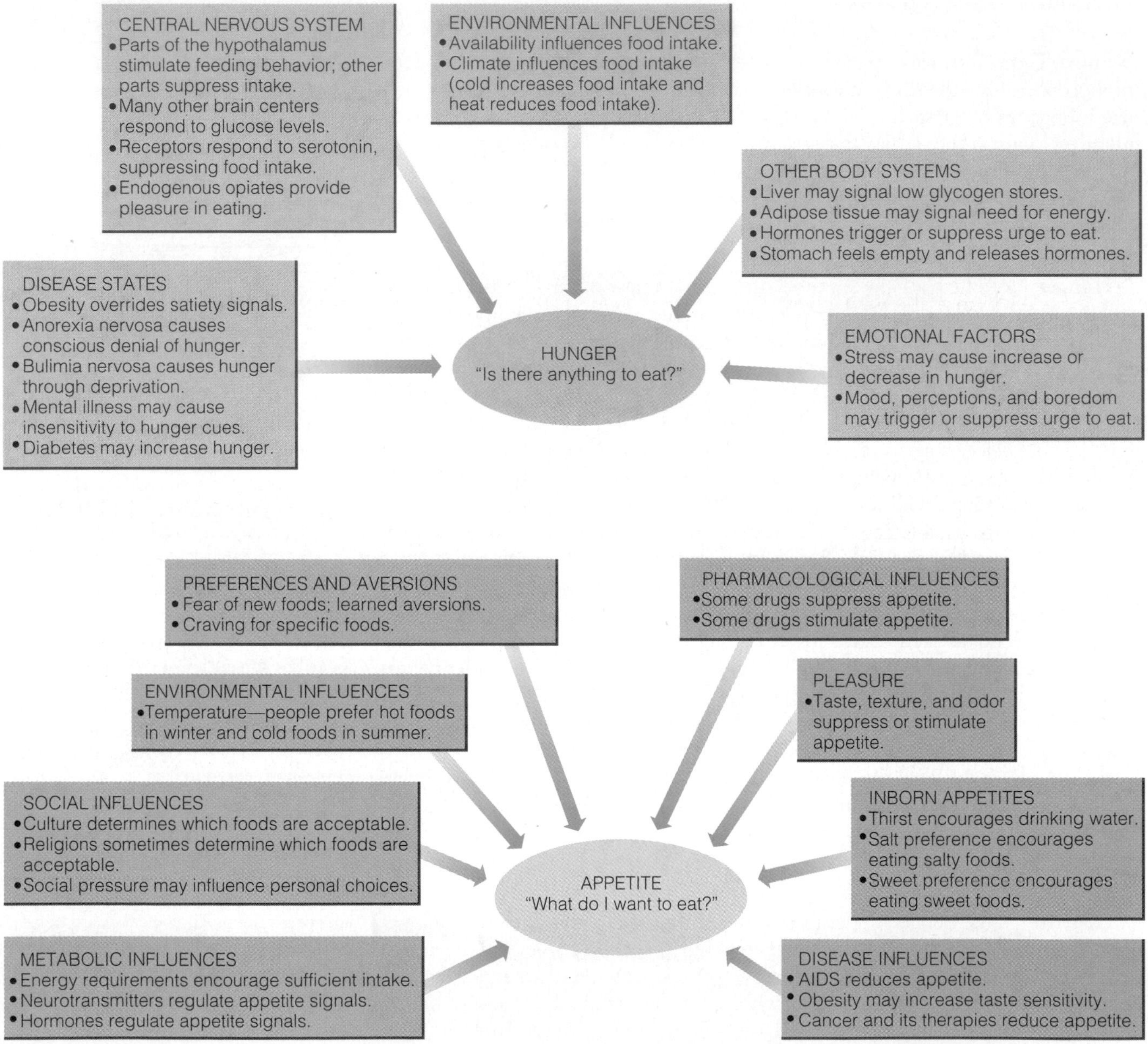

Source: Adapted from T. W. Castonguay and coauthors, Hunger and appetite: Old concept/new distinctions, *Nutrition Review* 41 (1983): 101–110.

on nutrients in the small intestine. Foods rich in carbohydrates and fibers delay the absorption of nutrients and extend the duration of satiety.[8] Nutrients in the small intestine also trigger the release of GI hormones (such as cholecystokinin) and the stimulation of nerves, sending messages about food intake to the hypothalamus. Eating in response to social schedules instead of hunger may override satiety, however, and contribute to overeating.[9]

Overriding Hunger and Satiety Signals Eating is intimately connected to emotional needs such as the primitive fear of starvation and the infant's association of food with mother love. Not surprisingly, eating can be triggered by signals other than hunger, even when food is not needed. Some people experience food cravings when they are bored or anxious.[10] In fact, they may eat in response to any kind of stress, negative or positive. (What do I do when I'm grieving? Eat. What do I do when I'm celebrating? Eat!) Some people respond to external stimuli such as the time of day ("It's time to eat") or the availability, sight, and taste of food ("I'd love a piece of chocolate even though I am stuffed!"). Being presented with a variety of foods stimulates eating; people eating one food until satisfied may begin eating enthusiastically again when given a fresh selection of different foods. Such behavior can easily lead to weight gain.

Eating in response to arousal is called **stress eating**.

The theory that some people eat in response to such external factors as the presence of food or the time of day rather than to such internal factors as hunger is known as the **external cue theory**.

Eating can also be suppressed by signals other than satiety, even when a person is hungry. People with the eating disorder anorexia nervosa, for example, use tremendous discipline to ignore the pangs of hunger. Some people simply cannot eat during times of stress, negative or positive. (I'm too sad to eat. I'm too excited to eat!) Why some people overeat in response to stress and others cannot eat at all remains a bit of a mystery. Factors that appear to be involved include how the person perceives the stress and whether normal eating behaviors are restrained.

Long-Term Controls Other types of messages influence longer-term food intakes. Such is the case with metabolic signals from nutrients and hormones, which reflect the overall balance between energy intake and energy needs over spans of several days. Some metabolic signals, such as those arising in a pregnant woman or an athlete, may influence food intake for several months.

In summary, a mixture of signals governs people's eating behavior. Hunger, appetite, and satiety each result from stimuli generated by the nervous and hormonal systems. Superimposed on these are complex factors involving emotions, habit, and other aspects of human functioning that are poorly understood.

Energy Out: The kCalories the Body Spends

The body converts the energy of food to the energy currency of ATP molecules with about 50 percent efficiency, radiating the rest as heat. Then, when ATP energy is used to do work, again about 50 percent is lost as heat. Thus the overall efficiency of the human body in converting food energy to work is 25 percent; the other 75 percent is released as heat. The work itself, as it is done, generates heat as well, so that a body's total heat production reflects the amount of energy it is spending.

The body's generation of heat is known as thermogenesis, and it can be measured to determine the amount of energy expended. This measurement of heat output is known as *direct calorimetry*. Alternatively, a person's energy expenditure can be calculated by measuring the amount of oxygen consumed and carbon dioxide expelled, *indirect calorimetry*.

thermogenesis: the generation of heat; used in physiology and nutrition studies as an index of how much energy the body is spending. The total energy a body spends reflects three main categories of thermogenesis:

- Basal thermogenesis (metabolism).
- Exercise-induced thermogenesis (physical activity).
- Diet-induced thermogenesis (thermic effect of food).

A fourth category is sometimes involved:

- Adaptive thermogenesis (energy of adaptation).

direct calorimetry (cal-o-RIM-uh-tree)**:** the measurement of energy output as heat energy.

indirect calorimetry: the estimation of energy output from measures of the amount of oxygen used and carbon dioxide eliminated.

COMPONENTS OF ENERGY EXPENDITURE

People spend energy when they are physically active, of course, but they also spend energy when they are resting quietly. In fact, quiet metabolic activities account for the lion's share of most people's energy expenditures, as Figure 8–3 shows.

basal metabolism: the energy needed to maintain life when a body is at complete rest after a 12-hour fast (to exclude the thermic effect of the previous meal).

basal metabolic rate (BMR): the rate of energy use for metabolism under basal conditions, usually expressed as kcalories per kilogram body weight per hour. (Table 8–3 on p. 285 provides equations for estimating BMR.)

A similar measure of energy output is the **resting energy expenditure (REE)**. The REE measure is usually less precise than the BMR because the criteria for rest and fasting are less strict, but the difference is usually less than 10% and can be discounted for most purposes.

Basal Metabolism At least two-thirds of the energy the average person spends in a day supports the body's metabolic activities. Metabolic activities maintain the body temperature and keep the lungs inhaling and exhaling air, the bone marrow making new red blood cells, the heart beating 100,000 times a day, the kidneys filtering wastes—in short, they support all the basic processes of life.

The basal metabolic rate (BMR) is the rate at which the body spends energy for these maintenance activities. The rate may vary dramatically from person to person and may vary for the same individual with a change in circumstances or physical condition.[11] The rate is slowest when a person is sleeping undisturbed, but it is usually measured in a room with a comfortable temperature when the person is lying still after a restful sleep and is not digesting any food.

In general, the more a person weighs, the more *total* energy is required, but the amount of energy *per pound* of body weight may be lower. For example, an adult's BMR might be 1500 kcalories and an infant's only 500, but compared with their body weights, the infant's BMR is more than twice as fast. Similarly, a normal-weight adult may have a metabolic rate one and a half times that of an obese adult when compared to body weight.

Table 8–1 summarizes the factors that raise and lower the BMR. For the most part, the BMR is highest in people with considerable lean body mass (growing children, physically active people, pregnant women, and males). One way to increase the BMR then is to participate in endurance and strength-building activities regularly to maximize lean body tissue.[12] The BMR is also high in people who are tall and so have a large surface area for their weight, in people with fever or under stress, and in people with highly active thyroid glands.

The BMR declines during adulthood as lean body mass diminishes. This change in body composition occurs, in part, because some hormones that influence metabolism become more, or less, active as a person ages. Voluntary activity tends to be reduced as well, bringing the average decline in energy expenditure to

Figure 8–3

Components of Energy Expenditure
The amount of energy spent in a day differs for each individual, but in general, basal metabolism is the largest component of energy expenditure (60 to 65%), and the thermic effect of food is the smallest (only 10%). The amount spent in voluntary physical activities has the greatest variability, depending on a person's activity patterns.

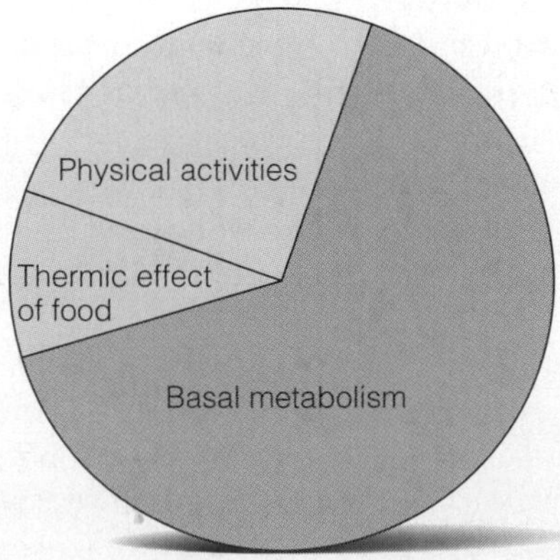

Table 8–1

Factors That Affect the BMR

Factor	Effect on BMR
Age	Lean body mass diminishes with age, slowing the BMR.[a]
Height	In tall, thin people, the BMR is higher.[b]
Growth	In children and pregnant women, the BMR is higher.
Body composition	The more lean tissue, the higher the BMR (which is why males usually have a higher BMR than females). The more fat tissue, the lower the BMR.
Fever	Fever raises the BMR.[c]
Stresses	Stresses (including many diseases and certain drugs) raise the BMR.
Environmental temperature	Both heat and cold raise the BMR.
Fasting/starvation	Fasting/starvation lowers the BMR.[d]
Malnutrition	Malnutrition lowers the BMR.
Hormones	The thyroid hormone thyroxin, for example, can speed up or slow down the BMR.[e]
Smoking	Nicotine increases energy expenditure.
Caffeine	Caffeine increases energy expenditure.
Sleep	BMR is lowest when sleeping.

[a]The BMR begins to decrease in early adulthood (after growth and development cease) at a rate of about 2 percent/decade. A reduction in voluntary activity as well brings the total decline in energy expenditure to 5 percent/decade.

[b]If two people weigh the same, the taller, thinner person will have the faster metabolic rate, reflecting the greater skin surface, through which heat is lost by radiation, in proportion to the body's volume (see margin drawing).

[c]Fever raises the BMR by 7 percent for each degree Fahrenheit.

[d]Prolonged starvation reduces the total amount of metabolically active lean tissue in the body, although the decline occurs sooner and to a greater extent than body losses alone can explain. More likely, the neural and hormonal changes that accompany fasting are responsible for changes in the BMR.

[e]The thyroid gland releases hormones that travel to the cells and influence cellular metabolism. Thyroid hormone activity can speed up or slow down the rate of metabolism by as much as 50%.

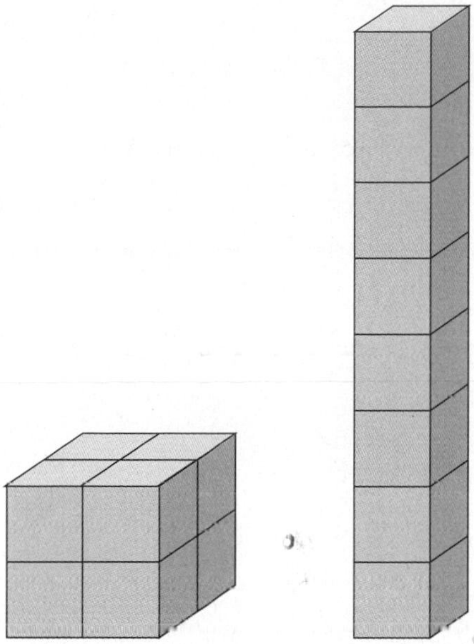

Notice that each of these structures is made of 8 blocks. They weigh the same, but they are arranged differently. If you were to count the sides of these structures, you would see that the short, wide one has 24 sides and the tall, thin one has 34. Because the tall, thin structure has a greater surface area it will lose more heat (expend more energy) than the short, wide one. Similarly, two people of different heights might weigh the same, but the taller, thin one will have a higher BMR (expending more energy) because of the greater skin surface.

about 5 percent per decade.[13] This decline in the BMR that occurs when a person reduces voluntary activity reflects the loss of lean body mass and may be prevented with ongoing physical activity. The BMR also slows down during fasting and malnutrition.[14]

Physical Activity The second component of a person's energy output is physical activity: voluntary movement of the skeletal muscles and support systems. Physical activity is the most variable component of energy expenditure. Consequently, its influence on both weight gain and weight loss can be significant.[15]

During physical activity, the muscles need extra energy to move, and the heart and lungs need extra energy to deliver nutrients and oxygen and dispose of wastes. The amount of energy needed for any activity, whether playing tennis or studying for an exam, depends on three factors: muscle mass, body weight, and

voluntary activities: the component of a person's daily energy expenditure that involves conscious and deliberate muscular work—walking, lifting, climbing, or other physical activity. In contrast, **involuntary activities** occur independently, without conscious will or knowledge—heart beating, lungs breathing, glands secreting, GI tract muscles contracting, and other activities critical to maintaining life.

activity. The larger the muscle mass required and the heavier the weight of the body part being moved, the more energy is spent. Table 8–2 gives average energy expenditures for people of different body weights engaged in various activities

Table 8–2

Energy Spent on Various Activities

Activity	kCal/lb/min[a]	kCalories per Minute at Different Body Weights				
		110 lb	125 lb	150 lb	175 lb	200 lb
Aerobic dance (vigorous)	.062	6.8	7.8	9.3	10.9	12.4
Basketball (vigorous, full court)	.097	10.7	12.1	14.6	17.0	19.4
Bicycling						
13 mph	.045	5.0	5.6	6.8	7.9	9.0
15 mph	.049	5.4	6.1	7.4	8.6	9.8
17 mph	.057	6.3	7.1	8.6	10.0	11.4
19 mph	.076	8.4	9.5	11.4	13.3	15.2
21 mph	.090	9.9	11.3	13.5	15.8	18.0
23 mph	.109	12.0	13.6	16.4	19.0	21.8
25 mph	.139	15.3	17.4	20.9	24.3	27.8
Cross-country skiing						
8 mph	.104	11.4	13.0	15.6	18.2	20.8
Golf (carrying clubs)	.045	5.0	5.6	6.8	7.9	9.0
Handball	.078	8.6	9.8	11.7	13.7	15.6
Horseback riding (trot)	.052	5.7	6.5	7.8	9.1	10.4
Rowing (vigorous)	.097	10.7	12.1	14.6	17.0	19.4
Running						
5 mph	.061	6.7	7.6	9.2	10.7	12.2
6 mph	.074	8.1	9.2	11.1	13.0	14.8
7.5 mph	.094	10.3	11.8	14.1	16.4	18.8
9 mph	.103	11.3	12.9	15.5	18.0	20.6
10 mph	.114	12.5	14.3	17.1	20.0	22.9
11 mph	.131	14.4	16.4	19.7	22.9	26.2
Soccer (vigorous)	.097	10.7	12.1	14.6	17.0	19.4
Studying	.011	1.2	1.4	1.7	1.9	2.2
Swimming						
20 yd/min	.032	3.5	4.0	4.8	5.6	6.4
45 yd/min	.058	6.4	7.3	8.7	10.2	11.6
50 yd/min	.070	7.7	8.8	10.5	12.3	14.0
Table tennis (skilled)	.045	5.0	5.6	6.8	7.9	9.0
Tennis (beginner)	.032	3.5	4.0	4.8	5.6	6.4
Walking (brisk pace)						
3.5 mph	.035	3.9	4.4	5.2	6.1	7.0
4.5 mph	.048	5.3	6.0	7.2	8.4	9.6

[a]To calculate kcalories spent per minute of activity for your own body weight, multiply kcal/lb/min by your exact weight and then multiply that number by the number of minutes spent in the activity. For example, if you weigh 142 pounds, and you want to know how many kcalories you spent doing 30 minutes of vigorous aerobic dance: 0.062 × 142 = 8.8 kcalories per minute; 8.8 × 30 (minutes) = 264 total kcalories spent.

Source: Values for swimming, bicycling, and running have been adapted with permission of Ross Laboratories, Columbus, Ohio 43216, from G. P. Town and K. B. Wheeler, Nutrition concerns for the endurance athlete, *Dietetic Currents* 13 (1986): 7–12. Copyright 1986 Ross Laboratories. Values for all other activities have been adapted with permission from Consumer Reports Books, 1983. *Physical Fitness for Practically Everybody: The Consumer's Union Report on Exercise*. Copyright 1983 by Consumers Union of U.S. Inc., Yonkers, NY 10703–1057.

and shows that a heavy person usually uses more energy per minute to perform a task than a light person does. The activity's duration, frequency, and intensity also influence energy cost: the longer, the more frequent, and the more intense the activity, the more kcalories spent per minute.

Chapter 14 describes how the activity's duration, frequency, and intensity also influence the body's fuel mix of carbohydrate and fat.

Thermic Effect of Food The body uses some energy to process food. When a person eats, the GI tract muscles speed up their rhythmic contractions, and the cells that manufacture and secrete digestive juices begin their tasks. This acceleration of activity produces heat and is known as the thermic effect of food (TEF).

The thermic effect of food is proportional to the food energy taken in and is usually estimated at 10 percent of energy intake. Thus a person who ingests 2000 kcalories in a day probably spends about 200 kcalories on the thermic effect of food. Because the thermic effect of food reflects the body's digestion and absorption activities, it is influenced by factors such as meal size, frequency, and composition; in general, the thermic effect of food is greater for high-carbohydrate foods than for high-fat foods and for a meal eaten all at once rather than spread out over a couple of hours.[16] For most purposes, however, the thermic effect of food can be ignored because its contribution to total energy output is smaller than the probable errors involved in estimating overall energy intake and output.

thermic effect of food (TEF): an estimation of the energy required to process food (digest, absorb, transport, metabolize, and store ingested nutrients); also called *diet-induced thermogenesis (DIT)*, the *specific dynamic effect (SDE)* of food, or the *specific dynamic activity (SDA)* of food.

Adaptive Thermogenesis Some additional energy is spent when a person must adapt to dramatically changed circumstances (adaptive thermogenesis). When the body has to adapt to physical conditioning, cold, overfeeding, starvation, trauma, or other types of stress, it has extra work to do, building the tissues and producing the enzymes and hormones necessary to cope with the demand. In some circumstances this energy makes a considerable difference in the total energy spent. Because this component of energy expenditure is so variable and specific to individuals, the Committee on Dietary Allowances does not include it when calculating energy requirements.

adaptive thermogenesis: adjustments in energy expenditure related to changes in environment such as cold and to physiological events such as overfeeding, trauma, and changes in hormone status.

ESTIMATING ENERGY REQUIREMENTS

In calculating the energy RDA, the Committee on Dietary Allowances considered the following components of energy expenditure:

- Energy spent on basal metabolism.
- Energy spent on physical activities.
- Energy spent on digesting and metabolizing food.

These three components vary, depending on a person's age, sex, body size, heredity, state of health, and other factors. The committee first estimated energy spent on basal metabolism for each age-sex group. Then the committee added increments for physical activity, assuming the average person would be lightly to moderately active. Finally, it added increments for the influence of food, assuming that each person would meet energy needs by eating a mixed diet of ordinary foods.

To estimate energy spent on basal metabolism, the committee used an equation that considers age, sex, and weight as shown in Table 8–3. (The box on p. 287 shows a sample calculation.)

Table 8–3

Equations for Estimating BMR from Body Weight

Sex and Age (yr)	Equation to Derive BMR in kCal/day
Males	
0–3	(60.9 × wt[a]) − 54
3–10	(22.7 × wt) + 495
10–18	(17.5 × wt) + 651
18–30	(15.3 × wt) + 679
30–60	(11.6 × wt) + 879
>60	(13.5 × wt) + 487
Females	
0–3	(61.0 × wt) − 51
3–10	(22.5 × wt) + 499
10–18	(12.2 × wt) + 746
18–30	(14.7 × wt) + 496
30–60	(8.7 × wt) + 829
>60	(10.5 × wt) + 596

[a]Weight expressed in kilograms.

Source: Reprinted with permission from *Recommended Dietary Allowances*, 10th edition. Copyright 1989 by National Academy of Sciences. Published by the National Academy Press, Washington, D.C.

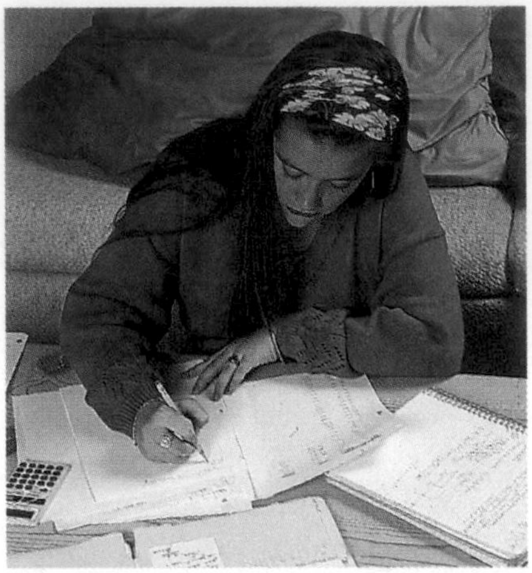

It feels like work and it may make you tired, but studying requires only a kcalorie or two per minute.

To estimate the energy spent on physical activity, the committee did not use individual values such as those presented in Table 8–2. This process is too time-consuming and impractical to be useful for estimating the energy needs of a population. Instead the committee clustered various activities according to intensity of effort (under the headings of light, moderate, and heavy activity). Then they determined an "activity factor" for each level of intensity for each sex (see Table 8–4). Again, the box on p. 287 shows a sample calculation.

To summarize, a person takes in energy from food and, on average, spends most of it on basal metabolic activities, some of it on physical activities, and a little on the thermic effect of food. When the energy consumed equals the energy expended, the person is in energy balance and body weight is stable. If more energy is taken in than is expended, the person gains weight. If more energy is spent than is taken in, the person loses weight. Changes in body weight reflect changes in body composition.

Body Weight, Body Composition, and Health

body composition: the proportions of muscle, bone, fat, and other tissue that makes up a person's total body weight.

A person 5 feet 10 inches tall who weighs 150 pounds may carry only about 30 of those pounds as fat. The rest is mostly water and lean tissues—muscles, organs such as the heart and liver, and the bones of the skeleton. Direct measures of body composition are impossible in living human beings; instead, researchers assess body composition indirectly based on the following assumption:

Body weight = fat + lean tissue (including water).

Table 8–4

Estimating Daily Energy RDA at Various Levels of Physical Activity

Level of Intensity	Type of Activity	Activity Factor (× BMR)	Energy Expenditure (kcal/kg/day)
Very light	Seated and standing activities, painting trades, driving, laboratory work, typing, sewing, ironing, cooking, playing cards, playing a musical instrument	1.3 (men) 1.3 (women)	31 30
Light	Walking on a level surface at 2.5 to 3 mph, garage work, electrical trades, carpentry, restaurant trades, housecleaning, child care, golf, sailing, table tennis	1.6 (men) 1.5 (women)	38 35
Moderate	Walking 3.5 to 4 mph, weeding and hoeing, carrying a load, cycling, skiing, tennis, dancing	1.7 (men) 1.6 (women)	41 37
Heavy	Walking with a load uphill, tree felling, heavy manual digging, basketball, climbing, football, soccer	2.1 (men) 1.9 (women)	50 44
Exceptional	Athletes training in professional or world-class events	2.4 (men) 2.2 (women)	58 51

Source: Adapted with permission from *Recommended Dietary Allowances*, 10th edition. Copyright 1989 by the National Academy of Sciences. Published by the National Academy Press, Washington, D.C.

How to Estimate Energy Output

Basal Metabolism

One way to estimate your energy output for basal metabolism is to use Table 8–3.* For example, a 20-year-old male who weighed 160 pounds would select the equation appropriate for his sex and age range:

$$(15.3 \times \text{wt}) + 679.$$

First, he would convert his weight from pounds to kilograms:

$$160 \text{ lb} \div 2.2 \text{ lb/kg} = 72.7 \text{ kg}.$$

Then, he would insert his weight into the equation:

$$(15.3 \times 72.7 \text{ kg}) + 679 = 1791 \text{ kcal/day}.$$

The estimated energy expenditure to cover basal metabolism for a 20-year-old male who weighs 160 pounds is 1791 kcalories/day.

A shortcut method uses an easy-to-remember formula for estimating basal energy needs. Round off 72.7 kg to 73 and use the factor 1 kcal/kg/hr for men (or 0.9 for women). For example:

$$1 \text{ kcal} \times 73 \text{ kg} \times 24 \text{ hr} = 1752 \text{ kcal/day}.$$

The difference between 1791 and 1752 is insignificant and acceptable in estimations such as these.

Basal Metabolism and Voluntary Physical Activity

To account for the energy used in physical activities as well, review the activities listed in Table 8–4 and determine which level of intensity typifies your average daily activity. Then multiply the selected activity factor by your value for basal metabolism. For example, if the man introduced above engages in mostly light activity, his activity factor would be 1.6. Multiply this factor by his basal metabolism kcalories:

$$1.6 \times 1791 = 2866 \text{ kcal/day}.$$

The result, 2866 kcalories/day, expresses his *total* daily energy needs.

Alternatively, total energy expenditure can be estimated in one step based on body weight as shown in the last column of Table 8–4. As an example, for a 160-pound man engaged in mostly light activity:

$$38 \text{ kcal} \times 73 \text{ kg} = 2774 \text{ kcal/day}.$$

Keep in mind that these estimates of energy output are just that—*estimates*. The difference between 2866 and 2774 is insignificant and acceptable. Either way, the man's total energy needs are about 2800 kcalories/day.

---

* In the United States, many researchers use another set of equations known as the Harris-Benedict method to determine BMR. The values calculated from the two sets of equations do not differ significantly. Harris-Benedict equations:

For men: $\text{BMR} = 66 + (13.7 \times \text{wt in kg}) + (5 \times \text{ht in cm}) - (6.8 \times \text{age in yr})$.

For women: $\text{BMR} = 655 + (9.6 \times \text{wt in kg}) + (1.8 \times \text{ht in cm}) - (4.7 \times \text{age in yr})$.

See Appendix D for equations to convert kg and cm.

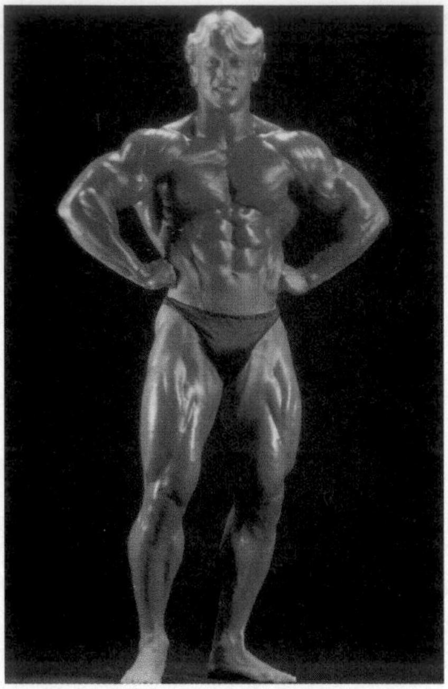

At 5 feet 7½ inches and 200 pounds, Andreas Cahling would be considered over*weight* by most height-weight standards, but he is clearly not over*fat*. In fact, his body fat is only 10 percent.

Weight gains and losses tell us nothing about how the body's composition may have changed, yet that is the measure most people use to judge their "fatness." For many people, overweight means overfat. This is not always the case, though. Athletes with dense bones and well-developed muscles may be overweight by an arbitrary standard such as weight-for-height tables, but have little body fat. Conversely, inactive people may seem to have acceptable weights, when, in fact, they may have too much body fat.

DEFINING HEALTHY BODY WEIGHT

How much should a person weigh? How can a person know if her weight is appropriate for her height and age? How can a person know if his weight is jeopardizing his health? Such questions seem so simple, yet even the experts can't agree on the answers. Most often, they try to identify the weights associated with lowest mortality.[17] With this in mind, healthy body weight is defined by three criteria:[18]

- A weight within the suggested range for height, as shown in Table 8–5.
- A fat distribution pattern that is associated with a low risk of illness or death.
- Freedom from all medical conditions that would suggest a need for weight loss.

People who meet all of these criteria may not gain any health advantage by changing their weights. Those who mistakenly think of themselves as overweight even though they meet these criteria for healthy weight may need to revise their self-image. Such people may still want to improve their eating and exercise habits, but they should do so to reap the rewards of being physically fit, not for the sake of weight loss. Anyone who does not meet all of the above criteria may want to consult with a health care professional, who should carefully consider each criterion in relation to the others.[19] The rest of the chapter examines these three criteria in more detail.

BODY WEIGHT AND ITS STANDARDS

Health care professionals often compare people's weights with standard weight-for-height tables, such as the table issued by the Metropolitan Life Insurance Company in 1983, which specifies weights for height, sex, and frame size. Normally, the assessor uses the midpont of the weight range for a person of a given height and assumes a medium build. If the person's actual weight is 10 to 20 percent above that, then the person is considered overweight; if 20 percent or more above the standard, the person is obese; and if 10 percent below the standard, the person is underweight.

frame size: the size of a person's bones and musculature. Appendix E describes how to take measures to estimate body frame size and provides tables of standards used in assessment.

overweight: body weight above some standard of acceptable weight that is usually defined in relation to height (such as the weight-for-height tables).

underweight: body weight below some standard of acceptable weight that is usually defined in relation to height (such as the weight-for-height tables).

The 1983 Metropolitan Height and Weight table appears in Appendix E.

Changing Weight Standards Standards for desirable weights have steadily increased over the past 35 years. In 1990, the dietary guidelines included a set of suggested weights (shown in Table 8–5) that were more permissive than the Metropolitan Life standards of 1983—and those in turn were more generous than the company's previous standards issued in 1959.

Disagreements over Standards Authorities argued over which weight standards were most appropriate. Some criticized, and some praised, the 1990 standards because they allowed people ages 35 and older to be heavier and to gain

Table 8–5

Suggested Weights for Adults

1990 Guidelines					1995 Guidelines (proposed)		
Height[a]	Weight (lb)[a]				Height[a]	Weight (lb)[a]	
	19 TO 34 YEARS		35 YEARS AND OVER			ADULTS OF ALL AGES	
	MIDPOINT	RANGE	MIDPOINT	RANGE		MIDPOINT	RANGE
					4′10″	105	91–119
					4′11″	109	94–124
5′0″	112	97–128	123	108–138	5′0″	112	97–128
5′1″	116	101–132	127	111–143	5′1″	116	101–132
5′2″	120	104–137	131	115–148	5′2″	120	104–137
5′3″	124	107–141	135	119–152	5′3″	124	107–141
5′4″	128	111–146	140	122–157	5′4″	128	111–146
5′5″	132	114–150	144	126–162	5′5″	132	114–150
5′6″	136	118–155	148	130–167	5′6″	136	118–155
5′7″	140	121–160	153	134–172	5′7″	140	121–160
5′8″	144	125–164	158	138–178	5′8″	144	125–164
5′9″	149	129–169	162	142–183	5′9″	149	129–169
5′10″	153	132–174	167	146–188	5′10″	153	132–174
5′11″	157	136–179	172	151–194	5′11″	157	136–179
6′0″	162	140–184	177	155–199	6′0″	162	140–184
6′1″	166	144–189	182	159–205	6′1″	166	144–189
6′2″	171	148–195	187	164–210	6′2″	171	148–195
6′3″	176	152–200	192	168–216	6′3″	176	152–200
6′4″	180	156–205	197	173–222	6′4″	180	156–205
6′5″	185	160–211	202	177–228	6′5″	185	160–211
6′6″	190	164–216	208	182–234	6′6″	190	164–216

Note: The higher weights in the ranges generally apply to men, who tend to have more muscle and bone; the lower weights more often apply to women, who have less muscle and bone.

[a]Without shoes or clothes.

Source: Nutrition and Your Health: Dietary Guidelines for Americans, 3rd ed. (Washington, D.C.: U.S. Government Printing Office, 1990); *Report of the Dietary Guidelines Advisory Committee on the Dietary Guidelines for Americans*, 1995.

weight as they aged.[20] Some approved, and some disapproved, of the 1990 weight tables for not specifying recommendations by sex; the tables simply stated that higher weights in the ranges generally apply to men and lower weights more often apply to women. Fueling the debate were findings that higher weights within the normal range may increase cardiovascular disease risks in women.[21]

Changing Weight Standards—Again By 1995, the proposed dietary guidelines had discarded the 1990 position that allowed weight gain with age; the 1995 suggested weight standards for all adults are the same as those issued in 1990 for young adults (see Table 8–5). As the 1995 guidelines explain, "health risks due to excess weight appear to be the same for older as for younger adults."

As long as there have been tables of recommended weights, debates have raged over their validity and usefulness. The Metropolitan tables were not unanimously accepted either. They were criticized for grouping all adults together without considering that appropriate weights may vary with age. Furthermore, recommended weights were based on insurance data, which underrepresent the lower socioeconomic class, minorities, and the elderly. Insurance-based weight-for-height tables are specifically inadequate for identifying the weights most closely associated with minimal health risks.

body mass index (BMI): an index of a person's weight in relation to height, determined by dividing the weight (in kilograms) by the square of the height (in meters).

Body Mass Index Many health professionals prefer to use a standard derived by manipulating the height and weight measures mathematically—the body mass index (BMI):

$$\text{BMI} = \frac{\text{weight (kg)}}{\text{height (m)}^2}$$

A person who takes measurements in pounds and inches can convert them to metric units or can use this modified equation:*[22]

$$\text{BMI} = \frac{\text{weight (lb)} \times 705}{\text{height (in)}^2}.$$

Appendix E presents a nomogram that permits people to scan for their BMI rather than calculating it. The inside back cover shows weight ranges for various heights using the BMI to define underweight, acceptable weight, overweight, and obesity.

Overweight may then be defined by a BMI between 25 and 30 and obesity as a BMI above 30.[23] The average BMI of adults in the United States is 26.3.[24] Figure 8–4 presents visual images associated with various BMI values.

- BMI <20 = underweight.
- BMI 20 to 25 = normal.
- BMI 25 to 30 = overweight.
- BMI >30 = obese.

A person whose BMI reflects an unacceptable health risk can choose a desired BMI and then calculate an appropriate body weight for it by using Table 8–6. For

*The conversion factor 705 was selected because it is a whole number that is relatively easy to remember; it does overestimate BMI by 0.06 percent, however, and some experts have suggested that 703 might be a better value.

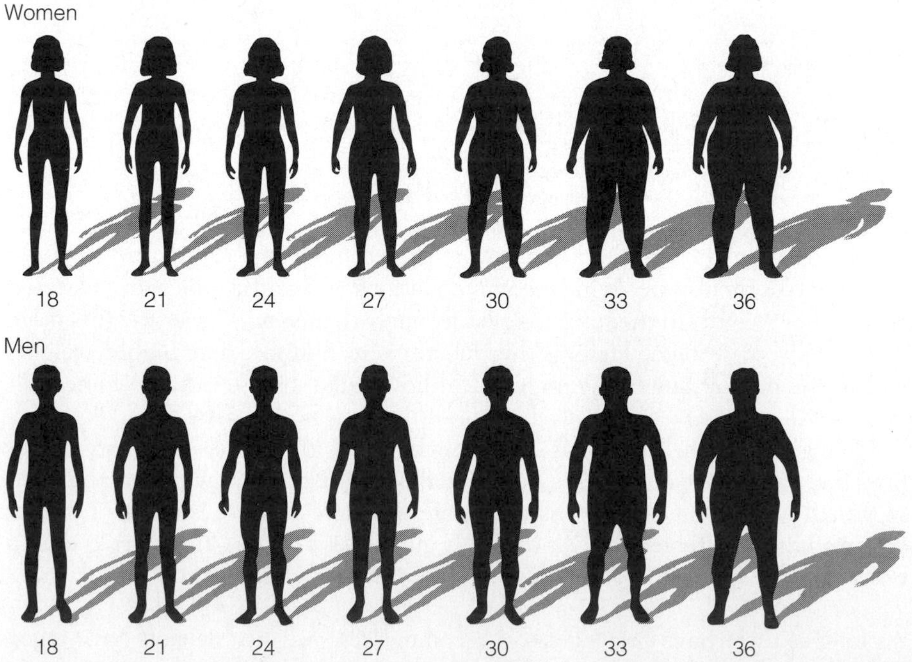

Figure 8–4

Silhouettes and BMI

Source: Reprinted from material of the Canadian Dietetic Association.

example, a person who is 5 feet 5 inches tall and weighs 165 pounds has a BMI of 27.5. To reach a BMI of 24, the person would need to weigh about 145 pounds (24 ÷ 0.166). Such a calculation can help a person to determine realistic weight goals using health risks as a guide.

Weight measures are inexpensive, easy to take, and highly accurate. Unfortunately, they fail to reveal two valuable pieces of information in assessing disease risk: how much of the weight is fat and where the fat is located.

BODY FAT AND ITS DISTRIBUTION

The ideal amount of body fat depends partly on the person. A normal-weight man may have from 10 to 25 percent body fat; a woman, because of her greater quantity of indispensable fat, 18 to 32 percent.

Some People Need Less For many athletes, a lower percentage of body fat may be ideal—just enough fat to provide fuel, insulate and protect the body, assist in nerve impulse transmissions, and support normal hormone activity, but not so much as to burden the muscles with excess weight to carry. For athletes, then, ideal body fat might be 5 to 10 percent for men and 15 to 20 percent for women.[25] (You may want to review the photo of Andreas Cahling on p. 288 to appreciate what 10 percent body fat looks like.)

Some People Need More For an Alaskan fisherman, a higher percentage of body fat is probably beneficial because fat provides an insulating blanket to prevent excessive loss of body heat in cold climates. A woman starting a pregnancy needs sufficient body fat to support conception and fetal growth. Below a certain

Table 8–6

Weight Needed for a Certain BMI

To obtain the weight needed for a certain BMI, divide the desired BMI by the height factor appropriate for your height.

Height	Height Factor	Height	Height Factor	Height	Height Factor
4′7″	0.232	5′3″	0.177	5′11″	0.139
4′8″	0.224	5′4″	0.172	6′0″	0.136
4′9″	0.216	5′5″	0.166	6′1″	0.132
4′10″	0.209	5′6″	0.161	6′2″	0.128
4′11″	0.202	5′7″	0.157	6′3″	0.125
5′0″	0.195	5′8″	0.152	6′4″	0.122
5′1″	0.189	5′9″	0.148	6′5″	0.119
5′2″	0.183	5′10″	0.143	6′6″	0.116

Source: R. P. Abernathy, Body mass index: Determination and use. Copyright the American Dietetic Association. Reprinted by permission from *Journal of the American Dietetic Association* 91 (1991): 843.

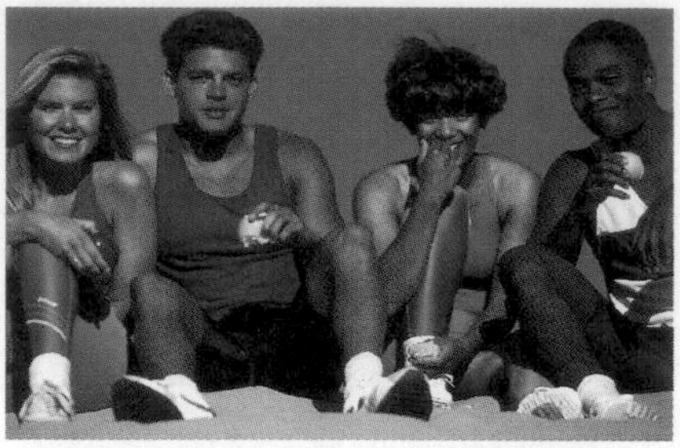

A healthy body contains enough lean tissue to support health and the right amount of fat to meet body needs.

threshold for body fat, hormone synthesis falters, and individuals may become infertile, develop depression, experience abnormal hunger regulation, or become unable to keep warm. These thresholds differ for each function and for each individual; much remains to be learned about them.

The Criterion of Health In asking what is ideal, people often mistakenly turn to fashion for the answer. Keep in mind that fashion is fickle; body shapes that society values change with time and have little in common with health. Fashion models whose careers depend on body shape often develop eating disorders.

Clearly, the most important criterion for determining how much a person should weigh and how much body fat a person needs is health. Ideally, a person has enough fat to meet basic needs but not so much as to incur health risks. Researchers find health problems develop when body fat exceeds 22 percent in young men, 25 percent in older men, 32 percent in younger women, and 35 percent in older women; these are the values used to define obesity, and age 40 is the dividing line.[26]

intra-abdominal fat: fat stored within the abdominal cavity in association with the internal abdominal organs, as opposed to the fat stored directly under the skin (subcutaneous fat).

central obesity: excess fat around the trunk of the body; also called **abdominal fat** or **upper-body fat**.

Fat Distribution The distribution of fat on the body may be more critical than fatness alone. Intra-abdominal fat that is stored around the organs of the abdomen presents a greater risk to health than fat elsewhere on the body and increases the risk of premature death.[27] This distribution of fat is referred to as central obesity or upper-body fat, and independently of total body fat, is associated with increased risks of heart disease, stroke, diabetes, hypertension, and some types of cancer.[28]

Abdominal fat is common in women past menopause and even more common in men. Even when total body fat is similar, men have more abdominal fat than either premenopausal or postmenopausal women.[29] Interestingly, people with central obesity smoke more and drink alcohol more than the average. A smoker may weigh less than the average nonsmoker, but the smoker's central obesity may be greater, leading researchers to think that smoking may directly affect fat distribution.[30] Exercise, in contrast, correlates negatively with central obesity.

Popular articles sometimes call bodies with upper-body fat "apples" and those with lower-body fat, "pears." Researchers sometimes refer to upper-body fat as "android" (manlike) obesity and to lower-body fat as "gynoid" (womanlike) obesity.

Fat around the hips and thighs, sometimes referred to as lower-body fat, is most common in women in their reproductive years and seems relatively harmless. In fact, people who are overweight, but who do not have excessive fat around the abdomen "seem robust" and less susceptible to health problems than overweight people with central obesity; theirs is a benign obesity.[31]

Exactly how abdominal fat influences disease development remains unknown. Researchers are studying the links between abdominal fat stores, blood lipids, blood pressure, and glucose metabolism. Abdominal fat seems to be more active than lower body fat. When mobilized, abdominal fat goes directly to the liver rather than emptying into the general circulation, as other fat does. The liver then packages this fat into VLDL, and these become LDL, the lipoprotein most implicated in heart disease. As blood lipids rise, the nervous system responds by releasing hormones and neurotransmitters that accelerate the heart rate and raise the blood pressure, aggravating heart problems and hypertension. Fat metabolism interferes with the liver's ability to clear insulin from the bloodstream.[32] As a consequence, blood glucose and insulin levels remain elevated, setting the stage for diabetes.

Fatfold Measures Health care professionals use several techniques to estimate body fat and its distribution. Fatfold measures provide a good estimate of total body fat and a fair assessment of the fat's location.[33] About half of the fat in the body lies directly beneath the skin, so the thickness of this subcutaneous fat reflects total body fat. On some parts of the body, such as the back and the back of the arm over the triceps muscle, this fat is loosely attached; a skilled assessor can measure its thickness and then compare the measurement with standards (see Appendix E).

If a person gains body fat, the fatfold increases proportionately; if the person loses fat, it decreases. Measures taken from central-body sites (around the abdomen) better reflect changes in fatness than those taken from upper sites (arm and back).

A major limitation of the fatfold test is that fat may be thicker under the skin in one area than in another. This limitation can be overcome by taking fatfold measurements at three or more different places on the body (including both central- and lower-body sites) and comparing each measurement with standards for that site. Most often, however, the triceps fatfold measurement alone is used because it is easily accessible.

Fatfold measurements correlate directly with the risk of heart disease.[34] They assess central obesity and its associated risks better than do weight measures such as the BMI.

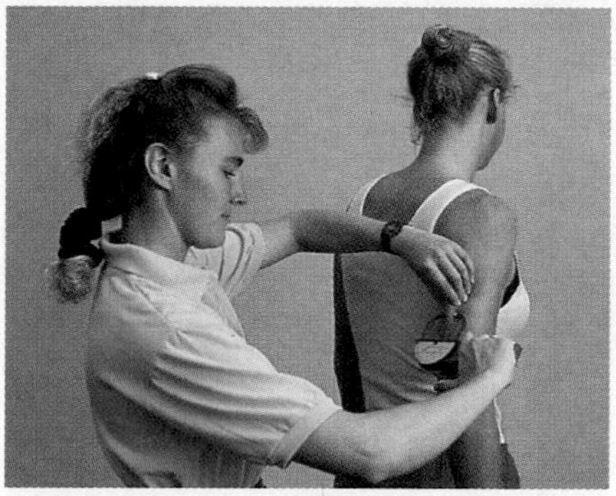

Obtaining an accurate fatfold measure requires training in the use of a caliper that has been calibrated.

fatfold measure: a clinical estimate of total body fatness in which the thickness of a fold of skin on the back of the arm (over the triceps muscle), below the shoulder blade (subscapular), or in other places is measured with a caliper. (The older, less preferred, term is **skinfold test**.)

Waist-to-Hip Ratio Another valuable indicator of fat distribution is the waist-to-hip ratio: the waist circumference divided by the hip circumference. Many clinicians use the waist-to-hip method to assess abdominal obesity, but this ratio may not be appropriate for women, older people, and some racial or ethnic groups.[35] Furthermore, it may not be useful in assessing *changes* in body fat. When people lose weight, they readily lose fat from the abdominal region, most likely because it is metabolically more active than lower-body fat. But while the fat distribution changes with weight loss, the waist-to-hip ratio seems to remain fairly stable.[36]

To calculate the waist-to-hip ratio, divide the waistline measurement by the hip measurement. For example, a woman with a 28-inch waist and 38-inch hips would have a ratio of:

$$28 \div 38 = 0.74.$$

In general, women with a ratio of 0.80 or greater and men with a ratio of 0.95 or greater are at high risk of obesity-related health problems.

Other Measures of Body Composition Other techniques for estimating body fat include hydrodensitometry and bioelectrical impedance analysis. To estimate body density using hydrodensitometry, the person is weighed twice—first on land and then again when submerged under water. The difference between the person's actual weight and underwater weight provides a measure of the body's volume. A mathematical equation using two measurements (volume and actual weight) allows the assessor to calculate body density, from which the percentage of body fat can be estimated. Underwater weighing usually generates a good estimate of body fat and is useful in research, although the technique has drawbacks: it requires bulky, expensive, and nonportable equipment. Furthermore, submerging some people (especially those who are very young, very old, ill, or fearful) underwater is not always practical.

hydrodensitometry (HI-dro-DEN-see-TOM-eh-tree): a method of measuring body density in which the person is first weighed and then submerged in water.

To measure body fat using the bioelectrical impedance technique, a very-low-intensity electrical current is briefly sent through the body by way of electrodes placed on the wrist and ankle. Since electrolyte-containing fluids, which readily conduct an electrical current, are found primarily in lean body tissues, the leaner

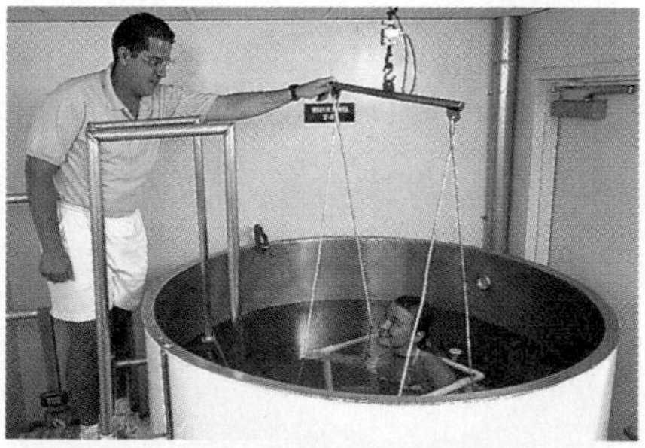

Researchers may use hydrodensitometry to estimate the percentage of body fat.

bioelectrical impedance: a method for estimating body fat using low-intensity electrical current.

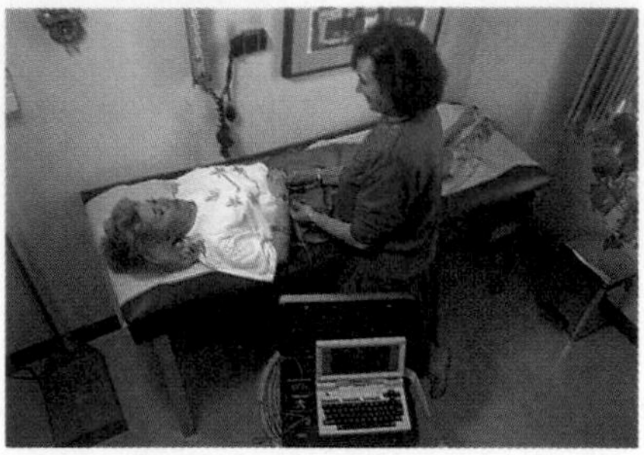

Bioelectrical impedance provides a simple and painless way to estimate body fat.

the person, the less resistance to the current. The measurement of electrical resistance is then used in a mathematical equation to estimate the percentage of body fat.

In addition to anthropometric measures, energy expended in leisure-time physical activities can be used to predict body density and body fat.[37] An increase in activity correlates with an increase in body density and a decrease in body fat. Appendix E provides more details and includes many of the tables and charts routinely used in assessment procedures.*

HEALTH RISKS ASSOCIATED WITH BODY WEIGHT AND BODY FAT

BMI values correlate with disease risks.[38] Most people with a BMI between 20 and 25 have few health risks; risks increase as BMI falls below 20 or rises above 25, indicating that both too little and too much body fat impair health.[39] Factors such as blood pressure or smoking habits raise risks independently of BMI.

Similarly, epidemiological data show a J-shaped relationship between body weights and mortality (see Figure 8–5).[40] People who are underweight or extremely overweight carry high risks of early deaths; people whose weights fall within the acceptable to slightly overweight range live longest.

Health Risks of Underweight It has long been known that thin people die first during a seizure or a famine. Overly thin people are also at a disadvantage in the hospital, where they sometimes receive little, if any, food so that they can undergo tests or surgery. Underweight also increases the risk for any person fighting a wasting disease such as cancer, especially when accompanied by undernutrition. A person without adequate nutrient and energy reserves will have a particularly tough battle against such medical stresses. In fact, many people with cancer die, not from the cancer itself, but from malnutrition. Underweight women become infertile, and those who do conceive may give birth to unhealthy infants. An underweight woman can improve her chances of having a healthy infant by gaining weight prior to conception, during pregnancy, or both. For all these reasons, underweight people are urged to gain some body fat as an energy reserve and to acquire protective amounts of all the nutrients that can be stored.

Figure 8–5

Body Mass Index and Mortality
Both underweight and overweight present risks of a premature death. This J-shaped curve describes the relationship between body mass index (BMI) and mortality and shows that optimal BMI is between 21 and 25 (some researchers extend this range from 19 to 27).

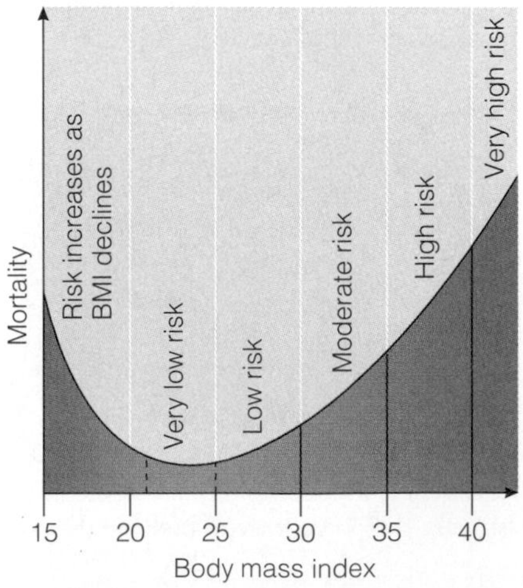

Health Risks of Overweight As for excessive body fat, the health risks are so many that it has been declared a disease: obesity.[41] Among the health risks of obesity are diabetes, hypertension, cardiovascular disease, sleep apnea (abnormal ceasing of breathing during sleep), osteoarthritis, abdominal hernias, some cancers, varicose veins, gout, gallbladder disease, arthritis, respiratory problems (including Pickwickian syndrome, a breathing blockage linked with sudden death), liver malfunction, complications in pregnancy and surgery, flat feet, and even a high accident rate. The costs of these obesity-related illnesses were estimated at more than $39 billion in 1986.[42] The costs in terms of lives is also great. Mortality increases as excess weight increases; people with a BMI greater than 35 are twice as likely to die prematurely as others.[43]

*Researchers sometimes estimate body composition using these methods: total body water, radioactive potassium count, dual-energy X-ray absorptiometry, near-infrared spectrophotometry, ultrasound, computed tomography, and magnetic resonance imaging. Each has advantages and disadvantages with respect to cost, technical difficulty, and precision of estimating body fat (see Appendix E for a comparison).

Cardiovascular Disease The relationship between obesity and cardiovascular disease risk is strong, with links to both blood cholesterol and blood pressure. Central obesity may raise the risk of heart disease as much as the leading three risk factors (high blood cholesterol, hypertension, and smoking) do.[44] Weight loss is effective in preventing and treating hypertension in overweight people.[45] Of course, lean and normal-weight people may also have high blood pressure, and hypertension is just as dangerous in lean people as it is in obese people.

Cardiovascular disease risk factors associated with obesity:
- High LDL cholesterol.
- Low HDL cholesterol.
- High blood pressure (hypertension).
- Diabetes.

Chapter 18 provides many more details.

Diabetes Diabetes (NIDDM) is three times more likely to develop in an obese person than in a nonobese person. Furthermore, the diabetic person often has central obesity. Central-body fat cells appear to be larger and more insulin-resistant than lower-body fat cells, and insulin resistance is a major risk factor for the development of NIDDM.[46] For those who are overweight, weight loss is effective in improving glucose tolerance and insulin resistance.

Reminder: *NIDDM* refers to noninsulin-dependent diabetes, the most common form of diabetes in which the body's cells fail to respond to insulin (insulin resistance).

Cancer The risk of cancer increases with body weight, but researchers do not fully understand the relationship. One possible explanation may be that obese people have elevated levels of hormones that could influence cancer development. For example, adipose tissue is the major site of estrogen synthesis in women, obese women have elevated levels of estrogen, and estrogen has been implicated in the development of cancers of the female reproductive system. These cancers account for half of all cancers in women.[47]

In summary, controversy surrounds the setting of standards for body weight. The standard currently considered most valid as an index of health is based on the body mass index (BMI) and rises with advancing age. The weight appropriate for an individual depends largely on factors specific to that individual, including body fat distribution, family health history, occupation, and current health status. At the extremes, overweight and underweight carry clear risks to health, and the attempt to correct them is worthwhile.

Excess body fat is implicated in many of today's chronic diseases. Most health authorities urge people to achieve and maintain a healthy weight, yet they are baffled by the question why people become fat. For some reason, people who are overweight consume more food energy than they use each day and store that energy as fat—their energy budget is unbalanced. The highlight that follows shows how food fat gets preferentially stored as body fat.

Study Questions

1. What are the consequences of an unbalanced energy budget?
2. Define hunger, appetite, and satiety and describe how each influences food intake.
3. Describe each component of energy expenditure. What factors influence each? How can energy expenditure be estimated?
4. Distinguish between body weight and body composition. What assessment techniques are used to measure each?
5. What problems are involved in defining "ideal" body weight?
6. What risks are associated with excess body weight and excess body fat?
7. What is central obesity, and what is its relationship to disease?

Problem Set appears on pp. 298–299

Notes

1. A. Tremblay and coauthors, Overfeeding and energy expenditures in humans, *American Journal of Clinical Nutrition* 56 (1992): 857–862.
2. M. Shah and R. W. Jeffery, Is obesity due to overeating and underactivity, or to a defective metabolic rate? A review, *Annals of Behavioral Medicine* 13 (1991): 73–81.
3. A. J. Stunkard, Address presented at the North American Association for the Study of Obesity and Emory University School of Medicine conference on Obesity Update: Pathophysiology, Clinical Consequences, and Therapeutic Options, Atlanta, Georgia, August 31–September 2, 1992.
4. N. Read, S. French, and K. Cunningham, The role of the gut in regulating food intake in man, *Nutrition Reviews* 52 (1994): 1–10; P. Norton, G. Falciglia, and D. Gist, Physiologic control of food intake by neural and chemical mechanisms, *Journal of the American Dietetic Association* 93 (1993): 450–454.
5. D. J. Shide and coauthors, Accurate energy compensation for intragastric and oral nutrients in lean males, *American Journal of Clinical Nutrition* 61 (1995): 754–764.
6. A. Geliebter and coauthors, Gastric capacity, gastric emptying, and test-meal intake in normal and bulimic women, *American Journal of Clinical Nutrition* 56 (1992): 656–661.
7. K. M. Cunningham and coauthors, Gastrointestinal adaptation to diets of differing fat composition in human volunteers, *Gut* 32 (1991): 483–486.
8. A. Raben and coauthors, Decreased postprandial thermogenesis and fat oxidation but increased fullness after a high-fiber meal compared with a low-fiber meal, *American Journal of Clinical Nutrition* 59 (1994): 1386–1394; J. E. Blundell, S. Green, and V. Burley, Carbohydrates and human appetite, *American Journal of Clinical Nutrition* 59 (1994): 728S–734S; W. H. Turnbull, J. Walton, and A. R. Leeds, Acute effects of mycoprotein on subsequent energy intake and appetite variables, *American Journal of Clinical Nutrition* 58 (1993): 507–512; S. J. French and N. W. Read, Effect of guar gum on hunger and satiety after meals of differing fat content: Relationship with gastric emptying, *American Journal of Clinical Nutrition* 59 (1994): 87–91.
9. J. Rodin, Determinants of food intake regulation in obesity, in *Obesity*, eds. P. Björntorp and B. N. Brodoff (Philadelphia: J. B. Lippincott, 1992), pp. 220–230.
10. A. J. Hill, C. F. Weaver, and J. E. Blundell, Food craving, dietary restraint and mood, *Appetite* 17 (1991): 187–197.
11. L. O. Schulz and D. A. Schoeller, A compilation of total daily energy expenditures and body weights in healthy adults, *American Journal of Clinical Nutrition* 60 (1994): 676–681.
12. T. J. Horton and C. A. Geissler, Effect of habitual exercise on daily energy expenditure and metabolic rate during standardized activity, *American Journal of Clinical Nutrition* 59 (1994): 13–19.
13. W. J. Carter, Macronutrient requirements for elderly persons, in *Geriatric Nutrition: The Health Professional's Handbook*, ed. R. Chernoff (Gaithersburg, Md.: Aspen Publishers, 1991), pp. 11–24.
14. S. Krug-Wispé, Nutritional assessment, in *Handbook of Pediatric Nutrition*, eds. P. M. Queen and C. E. Lang (Gaithersburg, Md.: Aspen Publishers, 1991), pp. 26–76; J. C. Waterlow, Childhood malnutrition in developing nations: Looking back and looking forward, *Annual Review of Nutrition* 14 (1994): 1–19.
15. A. C. King and D. L. Tribble, The role of exercise in weight regulation in nonathletes, *Sports Medicine* 11 (1991): 331–349.
16. R. S. Schwartz and coauthors, The thermic effect of carbohydrate versus fat feeding in man, *Metabolism* 34 (1985): 285–293; M. M. Tai, P. Castillo, and F. X. Pi-Sunyer, Meal size and frequency: Effect on the thermic effect of food, *American Journal of Clinical Nutrition* 54 (1991): 783–787.
17. R. F. Kushner, Body weight and mortality, *Nutrition Reviews* 51 (1993): 127–136.
18. U.S. Department of Agriculture and U.S. Department of Health and Human Services, Home and Garden Bulletin No. 232, *Nutrition and Your Health: Dietary Guidelines for Americans*, 3rd ed. (Washington, D.C.: U.S. Government Printing Office, 1990).
19. C. W. Callaway, New weight guidelines for Americans, *American Journal of Clinical Nutrition* 54 (1991): 171–172.
20. W. C. Willett and coauthors, New weight guidelines for Americans: Justified or injudicious? *American Journal of Clinical Nutrition* 53 (1991): 1102–1103; Callaway, 1991; G. A. Bray and R. L. Atkinson, New weight guidelines for Americans, *American Journal of Clinical Nutrition* 55 (1992): 481–483; R. B. Abernathy, New weight guidelines for Americans, *American Journal of Clinical Nutrition* 56 (1992): 1066–1067.
21. W. C. Willett and coauthors, Weight, weight change, and coronary heart disease in women, *Journal of the American Medical Association*, 273 (1995): 461–465.
22. S. H. Stensland and S. Margolis, Simplifying the calculation of body mass index for quick reference, *Journal of the American Dietetic Association* 90 (1990): 856.
23. Committee on Diet and Health, Food and Nutrition Board,

Diet and Health: Implications for Reducing Chronic Disease Risk (Washington, D.C.: National Academy Press, 1989), pp. 99–135.
24. R. J. Kuczmarski and coauthors, Increasing prevalence of overweight among US adults, *Journal of the American Medical Association* 272 (1994): 205–211.
25. T. G. Lohman, Body composition assessment in sports medicine, *Sports Medicine Digest,* September 1990, pp. 1–2.
26. G. A. Bray, An approach to the classification and evaluation of obesity, in *Obesity,* eds. P. Björntorp and B. N. Brodoff (Philadelphia: J. B. Lippincott, 1992), pp. 294–308; G. A. Bray, Definition and characterization of obesity, an address presented at the North American Association for the Study of Obesity and Emory University School of Medicine conference on Obesity Update: Pathophysiology, Clinical Consequences, and Therapeutic Options, Atlanta, Georgia, August 31–September 2, 1992.
27. P. Björntorp, Regional adiposity, in *Obesity,* eds. P. Björntorp and B. N. Brodoff (Philadelphia: J. B. Lippincott, 1992), pp. 579–586.
28. M. Zamboni and coauthors, Obesity and regional body fat distribution in men: Separate and joint relationships to glucose tolerance and plasma lipoproteins, *Amerian Journal of Clinical Nutrition,* 60 (1994): 682–687; E. M. Emery and coauthors, A review of the association between abdominal fat distribution, health outcome measures, and modifiable risk factors, *American Journal of Health Promotion* 7 (1993): 342–353; F. X. Pi-Sunyer, Health implications of obesity, *American Journal of Clinical Nutrition* 53 (1991): 1595S–1603S.
29. S. Lemieux and coauthors, Sex differences in the relation of visceral adipose tissue accumulation to total body fatness, *American Journal of Clinical Nutrition* 58 (1993): 463–467; C. J. Ley, B. Lees, and J. C. Stevenson, Sex- and menopause-associated changes in body-fat distribution, *American Journal of Clinical Nutrition* 55 (1992): 950–954.
30. R. J. Troisi, Cigarette smoking, dietary intake, and physical activity: Effects on body fat distribution—The Normative Aging study, *American Journal of Clinical Nutrition* 53 (1991): 1104–1111.
31. Björntorp, 1992.
32. Björntorp, 1992.
33. C. Orphanidou and coauthors, Accuracy of subcutaneous fat measurement: Comparison of skinfold calipers, ultrasound, and computed tomography, *Journal of the American Dietetic Association* 94 (1994): 855–858.
34. R. P. Donahue and coauthors, Central obesity and coronary heart disease in men, *Lancet,* April 11, 1987, pp. 821–824.
35. J. B. Croft, Waist-to-hip ratio in a biracial population: Measurement, implications, and cautions for using guidelines to define high risk for cardiovascular disease, *Journal of the American Dietetic Association* 95 (1995): 60–64.
36. K. van der Kooy and coauthors, Waist-hip ratio is a poor predictor of changes in visceral fat, *American Journal of Clinical Nutrition* 57 (1993): 327–333; M. Zamboni and coauthors, Effect of weight loss on regional body fat distribution in premenopausal women, *American Journal of Clinical Nutrition* 58 (1993): 29–34.
37. A. W. Gardner and E. T. Poehlman, Physical activity is a significant predictor of body density in women, *American Journal of Clinical Nutrition* 57 (1993): 8–14.
38. G. A. Bray, Pathophysiology of obesity, *American Journal of Clinical Nutrition* 55 (1992): 488S–494S.
39. Committee on Diet and Health, 1989, pp. 563–592.
40. T. B. VanItallie, Body weight, morbidity, and longevity, in *Obesity,* eds. P. Björntorp and B. N. Brodoff (Philadelphia: J. B. Lippincott, 1992), pp. 361–369.
41. Pi-Sunyer, 1991.
42. G. A. Colditz, Economic costs of obesity, *American Journal of Clinical Nutrition* 55 (1992): 503S–507S.
43. L. V. Sjöström, Mortality of severely obese subjects, *American Journal of Clinical Nutrition* 55 (1992): 516S–523S.
44. C. Bouchard, G. A. Bray, and V. S. Hubbard, Basic and clinical aspects of regional fat distribution, *American Journal of Clinical Nutrition* 52 (1990): 946–950.
45. J. Wylie-Rosett and coauthors, Trial of Antihypertensive Intervention and Management: Greater efficacy with weight reduction than with a sodium-potassium intervention, *Journal of the American Dietetic Association* 93 (1993): 408–415; S. A. Corrigan and coauthors, Weight reduction in the prevention and treatment of hypertension: A review of representative clinical trials, *American Journal of Health Promotion* 5 (1991): 208–214.
46. S. Lillioja and coauthors, Insulin resistance and insulin secretory dysfunction as precursors of non-insulin-dependent diabetes mellitus: Prospective Studies of Pima Indians, *New England Journal of Medicine* 329 (1993): 1988–1992.
47. A. P. Simopoulos, Characteristics of obesity, in *Obesity,* eds. P. Björntorp and B. N. Brodoff (Philadelphia: J. B. Lippincott, 1992), pp. 308–319.

Problem Set

1. Estimate various people's basal metabolic energy needs per day. Refer to Table 8–3 and calculate the BMR in kcalories per day for the following people. For example, calculate the energy needs of a 10-year-old boy who weighs 75 lb (34 kg).

   Using the range for ages 10–18: $(17.5 \times 34) + 651 = 1246$ kcal/day.

   Using the range for ages 3–10: $(22.7 \times 34) + 495 = 1267$ kcal/day.

   These two answers are similar. The boy needs about 1250 kcal/day for basal metabolism.

   a. A 10-year-old girl of the same weight. (Use either range. If you try them both, you'll find about a 100-kcalorie difference, but 10-year-old girls' energy needs vary by even more than this.) ______________ or ________________

   b. An 18-year-old man who weighs 150 lb (68 kg). Again, use either range, and again, if you use both, you'll find about a 100-kcalorie difference: __________________________ or ______________________

   c. A 35-year-old man who weighs 200 lb (91 kg): ____

   d. A 50-year-old woman who weighs 115 lb (52 kg): ______________ Add other examples of your own.

2. Compare the energy a person might spend on various physical activities. Refer to Table 8–2, and compute how much energy a person who weighs 142 lb would spend doing each of the following. Show your calculations. The first example is done for you. You may want to compare various activities based on your weight.

   30 min vigorous aerobic dance: 0.062 kcal/lb/min $\times$ 142 lb $= 8.8$ kcal/min.

   8.8 kcal/min $\times$ 30 min $= 264$ kcal.

   a. 2 hr golf, carrying clubs: ____

   b. 20 min running at 9 mph: ____

   c. 45 min swimming at 20 yd/min: ____

   d. 1 hr walking at 3.5 mph: ____

3. Consider the effect of age on BMR. An infant who weighs 20 lb has a BMR of 500 kcal/day; an adult who weighs 170 lb has a BMR of about 1500. Based on body weight, who has the faster BMR (show your calculations)? ____

4. Compute daily energy needs for a woman, age 20, who is 5 ft 6 in tall, weighs 130 lb, and is lightly active.

   a. From Table 8–3, what is her energy need for basal metabolism (show your calculations)? ______________

   b. From Table 8–4, estimate her daily energy expenditure, using her activity factor: ______________ and using her weight: ____________________

5. Discover what weight is needed to achieve a desired BMI. Refer to Table 8–6 and consider a person who is 5 ft 4 in tall. Suppose this person wants to have a BMI of 21. What should this person weigh? Show your calculations. ____

Problem Set (continued)

6. Calculate safe weight-loss rates for people of different sizes. The recommended rate is only 1% of body weight per week.

   a. Calculate what this rate would be for a person who weighs 120 lb. Show your calculations: ___________

   b. What would the safe rate be for a person who weighs 250 lb? Show your calculations: ___________

7. Calculate the energy intakes appropriate for weight loss. The suggested minimum energy intake for anyone is 10 kcal per pound of body weight.

   a. How many kcalories per day is this minimum for a person who weights 130 lb? ___________

   b. How many kcalories for a person who weighs 250 lb? ___________

8. Convert body fat into kcalorie values. Suppose a man is 5 ft 3 in tall and weighs 150 lb, and 30% of that weight is fat.

   a. How many pounds of fat does he have? ___________

   b. Assuming that the energy value of body fat is 3500 kcal per pound, how many kcalories does this person have stored in his body fat? ___________

   c. Suppose he loses 15 lb. For purposes of this question, assume that he exercised enough to retain virtually all of his lean tissue. Now he weighs 135 lb. How many pounds of this is fat? ______ What percentage of his body weight is now fat (show your calculations)? ___________

   d. How many kcalories does a 15-pound loss of fat represent? ___________

   e. If a diet and exercise plan provides a deficit of 500 kcal/day (that is, 500 kcal less each day is eaten than is spent), how many days (or weeks or months) will it take to lose that much fat? ___________

The Fattening Power of Fat

The people of the United States have grown fatter over the past century. By comparison, people of other nations such as China consume more food energy per body weight than we do, yet they remain lean. The favored explanation has been that our sedentary lifestyle is responsible. Alternatively, perhaps our excessive diet is responsible: we have been taking in more energy than we need. Most likely, it is a combination of the two as Chapter 9 describes. Of particular interest is recent research suggesting that when the excess energy derives from fat, it is more fattening than when it comes from carbohydrates.

This highlight explores the possible roles that fat, carbohydrate, and the balance between them may play in the development of obesity. (Protein's contribution to both dietary intake and energy expenditure is relatively minor and fairly constant; the making of body fat depends primarily on the intake and oxidation of carbohydrate and fat.) This discussion explores the following questions: (1) Do people eating foods high in fat simply consume too many kcalories? (2) Or do they make more fat from fat than from carbohydrate? To rephrase that second question: (3) If energy intake exceeds energy need by 100 kcalories, and those kcalories are from fat, do they contribute more body fat than 100 extra kcalories from carbohydrate? Researchers have followed several leads in attempting to discover whether dietary fat influences body fatness more than its energy contribution alone can explain.

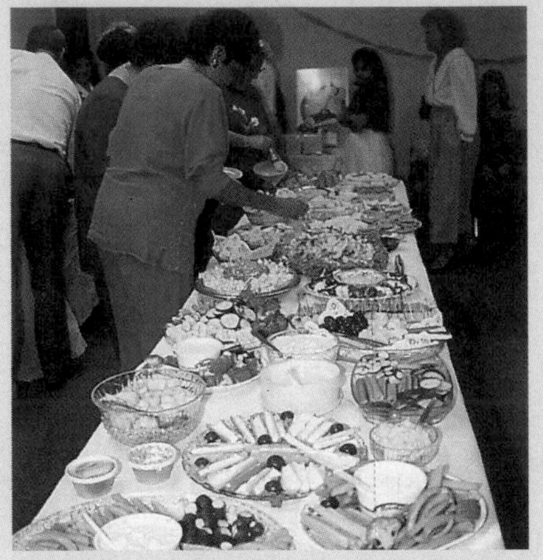

Many people are selecting low-fat snacks to help them control weight.

HIGH-FAT DIETS PROMOTE OVEREATING AND WEIGHT GAIN

A study using rats found that a fat-rich diet did *not* necessarily lead them to overeat.[1] Rats fed a high-fat diet (42 percent of the kcalories from fat) voluntarily ate less food than rats given a lower-fat control diet, so that they received the same number of kcalories as the controls. The rats behaved as though they had internal kcalorie counters that determined how much food they needed to eat to meet their energy needs.

Even with similar energy intakes, however, the rats eating the fat-rich diet became severely obese. Their body composition changed to more than 50 percent body fat, whereas the control rats remained at 30 percent body fat. In rats, then, the fat content of the diet seems to play a role, independently of kcalories, in obesity development.

When researchers asked if *people* on high-fat diets would adjust their food intakes to maintain constant energy intakes, the answer was slightly different. One study allowed average-weight women to eat freely from three different plans: a low-fat diet (15 to 20 percent of kcalories from fat), a medium-fat diet (30 to 35 percent), and a high-fat diet (45 to 50 percent).[2] The women followed each plan for two weeks. The foods in each plan were similar in taste and appearance; they differed only in the percentages of kcalories from fat (and, of course, the foods that were higher in fat were lower in carbohydrate).

Like the rats, the women ate less food when their diet supplied more fat. Unlike the rats, though, the women did not adjust their food intakes enough to compensate fully for the high-fat diet's excess kcalories. To fully compensate for the extra kcalories of fat in milk, for example, a person drinking whole milk instead of nonfat milk would need to drink 40 percent less milk, and the women failed to make such adjustments.

Body weight changes at the end of each two-week session were consistent with fat and energy intakes. The average weight change was a loss of almost 1 pound on the low-fat diet, and a gain of almost ¾ pound on the high-fat diet. A ¾-pound weight gain seems small, but repeated every two weeks, it would amount to some 20 pounds a year. Such a course is the path to obesity.

The answer to question 1, then, is yes: people eating diets high in fat typically eat more kcalories. Why don't people accurately compensate their intakes?

Some people do seem to compensate quite accurately, although it seems to be the exception rather than the rule. One study fed yogurt with different amounts of fat and carbohydrate to men and women 30 minutes before allowing them to eat as much as they liked for lunch. Only the normal-weight men who were unconcerned about their eating habits and body weight accurately adjusted their intakes at lunch to compensate for the energy of the yogurt.[3] Most of the others ate about the same amount for lunch, regardless of the type of yogurt eaten earlier.

HIGH-CARBOHYDRATE DIETS PROVIDE SATIETY

Findings that high-fat diets lead people to overeat and gain weight suggest that fat may be less satisfying than carbohydrate.[4] In one study, lean people were given a breakfast supplemented with either carbohydrate or fat.[5] Both breakfasts provided the same food energy, but the carbohydrate-supplemented one suppressed the eaters' appetites both at breakfast and later, when a midmorning snack was offered. Another study confirmed that a high-carbohydrate snack offers more satiety and limits food intake at the next meal more than a high-fat snack does.[6]

In another study, eight men of normal weight ate freely from either a high-fat or a mixed diet.[7] When the men consumed the high-fat diet, they overate, taking in over 1000 kcalories per day more than when they were eating the mixed diet. Not only were their fat intakes high, but their *carbohydrate* intakes were also high; they seemed to continue to eat until they attained a desired amount of carbohydrate, as if they were deriving their satiety from carbohydrate. Perhaps the satiety mechanism ensures that the body will receive a threshold amount of carbohydrate. After all, all the body's cells require some carbohydrate in their fuel mix, and the body cannot make carbohydrate from fat.

If people do, indeed, eat to obtain a certain amount of carbohydrate, then the higher the diet is in fat relative to carbohydrate, the more fat and total energy (kcalories) they will have to eat before they are satisfied. Thus people restricting their carbohydrate intakes may unwittingly head toward obesity by eating excess fat in order to get enough carbohydrate.

HIGH-FAT DIETS DEPOSIT BODY FAT

Now for question 2. How does the diet's fat content affect body composition? Using seven-day diet records, researchers found that 155 obese men were consuming the "typical American diet"—about 16 percent of total kcalories from protein, 38 percent from carbohydrate, 41 percent from fat, and 6 percent from alcohol.[8] Their total food energy intakes (2570 kcalories per day) fell short of current energy recommendations (2900 kcalories per day).[9] This might indicate that the men's intakes were appropriate to their needs and would not lead to weight gain.

When the researchers compared the dietary data to body weight and body composition measures, they noticed two particularly interesting findings. They found no correlation between total food energy intakes and the men's body fat measurements. They did, however, find a positive correlation between the men's *dietary fat* intakes and their *body fat* measurements: the more fat a man ate, the greater his body fat. The researchers also found a negative correlation between body fat and carbohydrate, plant-protein, and fiber intake: the less legumes, grains, fruits, and vegetables a man ate, the greater his body fat. These findings suggest that when people eat diets high in fat, they tend to store body fat efficiently, even with moderate food energy intakes.

Other studies comparing body compositions and the diets of adults have confirmed that people who eat high-fat foods have higher body fat and greater weight gains than total energy intake alone would predict.[10] Again and again, the data suggest that dietary fat influences body fatness independently of total energy intakes, and that fat people tend to eat more fat.[11]

In still another study, researchers provided either high-fat or mixed diets to men who were attempting to gain weight and found that those eating the high-fat diets gained the same amount of weight, but in *less time* and with *fewer kcalories* than did those eating the mixed diets.[12] In addition, the men eating the mixed diets needed to continue consuming high-kcalorie diets to maintain their weight gains, whereas those who gained weight on the high-fat diets were able to maintain their weight gains at the same energy intakes as they had consumed before the study.

In general, it seems that high-fat diets promote weight gain; this is especially evident in people with a genetic predisposition for obesity.[13] Apparently, even with moderate food energy intakes, people can convert large percentages of their dietary fat to body fat.[14] Immediately after a meal, when blood lipids are high, fat-storage cells eagerly take their fill. Once deposited in storage, fat becomes a less readily available energy source than it was before. To move fat out of storage requires spending energy and that means physical activity. It seems that the body is quite efficient in its storage of fat.

FAT IS EFFICIENTLY METABOLIZED

As Chapter 8 mentioned, when the body processes a meal, some energy immediately escapes as heat—the *thermic effect of food (TEF)*. Only the energy that remains after the TEF is spent is available to the body.

On average, a person spends about 10 percent of energy intake on the TEF, but this percentage varies considerably, depending on the composition of the meal. The more dietary carbohydrate consumed, the more heat the body gives off. A high-carbohydrate meal even enhances the heat given off after the next meal eaten. In contrast, as the percentage of fat in the diet increases, TEF heat production declines. So a high-fat diet both loses less energy to the TEF and provides more energy for the body's use and storage.

Figure H8–1 shows how much more efficient fat metabolism is than carbohydrate metabolism. To convert a dietary triglyceride to a triglyceride in adipose tissue, the body simply removes two of the fatty acids from the glycerol backbone, absorbs the parts, and puts them (and others) together again. To convert a molecule of sucrose, however, the body has to split glucose from fructose, absorb them, dismantle them to pyruvate and acetyl CoA, assemble many acetyl CoA molecules into fatty acid chains, and finally attach fatty acids to a glycerol backbone to make a triglyceride for storage in adipose tissue. Quite simply, the body uses less energy to convert dietary fat to body fat than it does to convert dietary carbohydrate to body fat. Estimates in the literature differ slightly, but in general, storing dietary fat in body fat uses only 3 percent of the ingested energy intake, but storing dietary carbohydrate in body fat requires an expenditure of 23 percent of ingested energy intake.[15] The body chooses the thrifty option. After a meal, glucose is preferentially oxidized and fat is preferentially stored.[16]

As Chapter 8 mentioned, maintaining energy balance and body weight requires keeping energy intake and output equal, but the composition of the diet may be just as important in determining fat storage as total energy intake or output.[17] If energy intake *exceeds* the body's energy needs—regardless of whether the excess is from fat or carbohydrate—the result will be weight gain. The difference is that excess dietary fat leads to a greater accumulation of body fat.[18] Thus the answer to question 3 appears to be yes: the efficiency with which the body uses or stores energy may vary considerably, depending on the diet's composition.

CARBOHYDRATE DISPLACES DIETARY FAT WITHOUT ADDING FAT

In general, as dietary fat intake falls, carbohydrate intake rises and vice versa. Perhaps it is possible to control body fat accumulation simply by eating enough carbohydrate to displace most of the diet's fat. But if carbohydrate intake soared, would body fat still remain relatively constant? Or would excess carbohydrate also contribute to body fat? Let us look more closely at the metabolism of carbohydrate.

The body handles abundant quantities of carbohydrate by storing it as glycogen. Just as dietary fat efficiently becomes body fat, dietary carbohydrate efficiently becomes glycogen. Excess glucose can be converted to fat, but this is a minor pathway.[19] Converting glucose to fat is energetically expensive and does not appear to occur until after glycogen stores have filled—and glycogen stores do not fill to capacity under normal eating conditions.[20] Even then, new fat is not made from carbohydrate.[21] Weight gain that accompanies an excess of dietary carbohydrate reflects a shift in energy expenditure: fat oxidation decreases as carbohydrate oxidation increases. Furthermore, the elevated insulin that accompanies a high-carbohydrate intake stimulates the deposition of *dietary fat* into storage.

Returning to the question asked earlier, what would happen if a person simply replaced fat kcalories with carbohydrate kcalories and kept total intake the same? A study did this and found that it made no difference in either energy expenditure or body composition.[22] Complaints from participants in this study, however, were noteworthy: they had to eat much more food when on the low-fat, high-carbohydrate diet than they were accustomed to eating. Weight loss that typically accompanies a low-fat diet seems to occur, then, not because of a magical carbohydrate to fat ratio, but because a high-carbohydrate diet

Figure H8–1

Two Pathways to Body Fat Compared

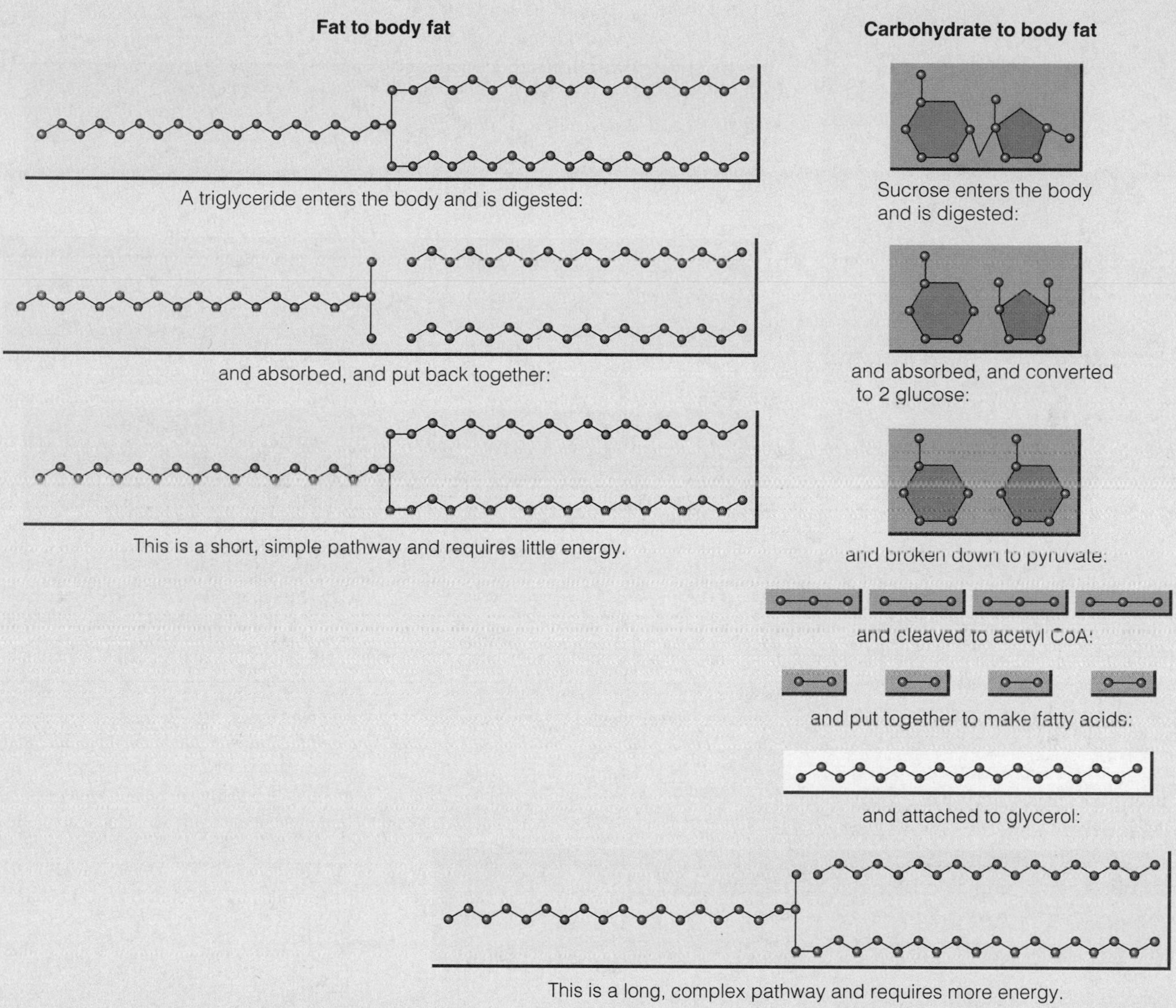
Fat to body fat
Carbohydrate to body fat
A triglyceride enters the body and is digested:
Sucrose enters the body and is digested:
and absorbed, and put back together:
and absorbed, and converted to 2 glucose:
This is a short, simple pathway and requires little energy.
and broken down to pyruvate:
and cleaved to acetyl CoA:
and put together to make fatty acids:
and attached to glycerol:
This is a long, complex pathway and requires more energy.

is more likely to provide satiety and a lower energy intake.

TENTATIVE ANSWERS

Given the size of the body's glycogen stores (800 kcalories) and its fat stores (140,000 kcalories), dietary carbohydrate has a much greater influence on daily balances than does dietary fat.[23] Because glycogen stores are limited and dwindle quickly, glucose is used frugally when the diet supplies only small amounts and freely when stores are abundant.[24] In other words, the body maintains its glycogen stores by adjusting oxidation to dietary intake.[25]

In contrast, dietary fat intake does not promote oxidation.[26] Instead, fat storage or oxidation occurs in response to daily changes in energy balance. When the body

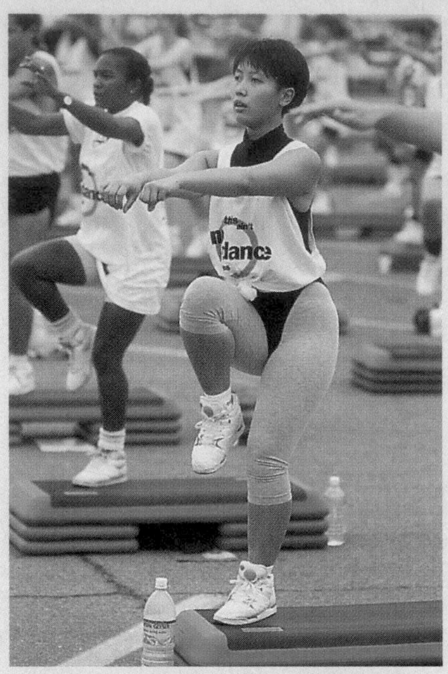

Physical activity is the key to losing body fat.

receives more dietary fat than is being oxidized, it expands its fat stores. If the body expends more energy than it takes in, it oxidizes more fat and draws on its fat stores.[27] The rule is simply "don't eat more fat than you burn."[28] To limit fat deposits, eat a low-fat diet. To use up body fat stores, exercise, especially by engaging in prolonged aerobic activity of low-to-moderate intensity.

Clearly, from all of the experiments reported here, a diet's total kcalories are important, but they are not the only variable that predicts whether fat will be stored. The total fat, the total carbohydrate, and the fat-to-carbohydrate ratio of the diet also matter.

This highlight has focused narrowly on the body's efficiency in handling various fuels from the diet. Other factors such as genetics, age, smoking, and alcohol intake also influence the body's metabolic efficiency. From what we now know about food fat, though, it is clearly wise for people concerned with weight control to habitually select low-fat, high-carbohydrate foods and to exercise regularly. This is the recommendation of every leading nutrition authority. It is one of the best ways to lower risks from diseases and to meet the body's needs for nutrients. Now we can add that it is probably the best way to control body fatness, too.

NOTES

1. L. B. Oscai, M. M. Brown, and W. C. Miller, Effect of dietary fat on food intake, growth and body composition in rats, *Growth* 48 (1984): 415–424.
2. L. Lissner and coauthors, Dietary fat and the regulation of energy intake in human subjects, *American Journal of Clinical Nutrition* 46 (1987): 886–892.
3. B. J. Rolls and coauthors, Satiety after preloads with different amounts of fat and carbohydrate: Implications for obesity, *American Journal of Clinical Nutrition* 60 (1994): 476–487.
4. R. J. Stubbs and coauthors, Covert manipulation of dietary fat and energy density: Effect on substrate flux and food intake in men eating ad libitum, *American Journal of Clinical Nutrition* 62 (1995): 316–329.
5. J. E. Blundell and coauthors, Dietary fat and the control of fat on meal size and post-meal satiety, *American Journal of Clinical Nutrition* 57 (1993): 772S–778S.
6. Rolls and coauthors, 1994.
7. A. Tremblay and coauthors, Impact of dietary fat content and fat oxidation on energy intake in humans, *American Journal of Clinical Nutrition* 49 (1989): 799–805.
8. D. M. Dreon and coauthors, Dietary fat: Carbohydrate ratio and obesity in middle-aged men, *American Journal of Clinical Nutrition* 47 (1988): 995–1000.
9. Committee on Dietary Allowances, *Recommended Dietary Allowances*, 10th ed. (Washington, D.C.: National Academy Press, 1989), p. 33.
10. W. C. Miller and coauthors, Diet composition, energy intake, and exercise in relation to body fat in men and women, *American Journal of Clinical Nutrition* 52 (1990): 426–430; I. Romieu and coauthors, Energy intake and other determinants of relative weight, *American Journal of Clinical Nutrition* 47 (1988): 406–412; G. Haus and coauthors, Key modifiable factors in weight maintenance: Fat intake, exercise, and weight cycling, *Journal of the American Dietetic Association* 94 (1994): 409–413; R. C. Klesges and coauthors, A longitudinal analysis of the impact of dietary intake and physical activity on weight changes in adults, *American Journal of Clinical Nutrition* 55 (1992): 818–822; Tremblay and coauthors, 1989; R. L. Atkinson, Role of diet in obesity treatment, an address presented at the North American Association for the Study of Obesity and Emory University School of Medicine conference on Obesity Update: Pathophysiology, Clinical Consequences, and Therapeutic Options, Atlanta, Georgia, August 31–September 2, 1992.
11. W. C. Miller and coauthors, Dietary fat, sugar, and fiber predict body fat content, *Journal of the American Dietetic Association* 94 (1994): 612–615; C. D. Thomas and coauthors, Nutrient balance and energy expenditure during ad libitum feeding of high-fat and high-carbohydrate diets in humans, *American Journal of Clinical Nutrition* 55 (1992): 934–942; K. R. Westerterp, Food quotient, respiratory quotient, and energy balance, *American Journal of Clinical Nutrition* 57 (1993): 759S–765S.
12. E. Danforth, Diet and obesity, *American Journal of Clinical Nutrition* 41 (1985): 1132–1145.
13. B. L. Heitmann and coauthors, Dietary fat intake and weight gain in women genetically predisposed for obesity, *American Journal of Clinical Nutrition* 61 (1995): 1213–1217.
14. K. Donato and D. M. Hegsted, Efficiency of utilization of various sources of energy for growth, *Proceedings of the National Academy of Sciences* 82 (1985): 4866–4870.
15. Danforth, 1985; G. A. Leveille and P. F. Cloutier, Isocaloric diets: Effects of dietary changes, *American Journal of Clinical Nutrition* 45 (1987): 158–163.
16. O. E. Owen and coauthors, Oxidative and nonoxidative macronutrient disposal in lean and obese men after mixed meals, *American Journal of Clinical Nutrition* 55 (1992): 630–636.
17. Miller and coauthors, 1990.
18. T. J. Horton and coauthors, Fat and carbohydrate overfeeding in humans: Different effects on energy storage, *American Journal of Clinical Nutrition* 62 (1995): 19–29.
19. M. K. Hellerstein and coauthors, Measurement of de novo hepatic lipogenesis in humans using stable isotopes, *Journal of Clinical Investigation* 87 (1991): 1841–1852.

20. K. J. Acheson and coauthors, Glycogen storage capacity and de novo lipogenesis during massive carbohydrate overfeeding in man, *American Journal of Clinical Nutrition* 48 (1988): 240–247.
21. B. Swinburn and E. Ravussin, Energy balance or fat balance? *American Journal of Clinical Nutrition* 57 (1993): 766S–771S.
22. L. R. Roust, K. D. Hammel, and M. D. Jensen, Effects of isoenergetic, low-fat diets on energy metabolism in lean and obese women, *American Journal of Clinical Nutrition* 60 (1994): 470–475.
23. G. A. Bray, The nutrient balance approach to obesity, *Nutrition Today*, May/June 1993, pp. 13–18.
24. J. P. Flatt, Effect of carbohydrate and fat intake on postprandial substrate oxidation and storage, *Topics in Clinical Nutrition* 2 (1987): 15–27.
25. Horton, 1995; P. S. Shetty and coauthors, Alterations in fuel selection and voluntary food intake in response to isoenergetic manipulation of glycogen stores in humans, *American Journal of Clinical Nutrition* 60 (1994): 534–543. W. G. H. Abbott and coauthors, Short-term energy balance: Relationship with protein, carbohydrate, and fat balances, *American Journal of Physiology* 255 (1988): 332–337.
26. Horton, 1995; J. P. Flatt, Use and storage of carbohydrate and fat, *American Journal of Clinical Nutrition* 61 (1995): 952S–959S.
27. C. Bennett and coauthors, Short-term effects of dietary-fat ingestion on energy expenditure and nutrient balance, *American Journal of Clinical Nutrition* 55 (1992): 1071–1077.
28. J. P. Flatt, The biochemistry of energy expenditure, in *Obesity*, eds. P. Björntorp and B. N. Brodoff (Philadelphia: J. B. Lippincott, 1992), pp. 100–116.

Chapter 9

Weight Control: Overweight and Underweight

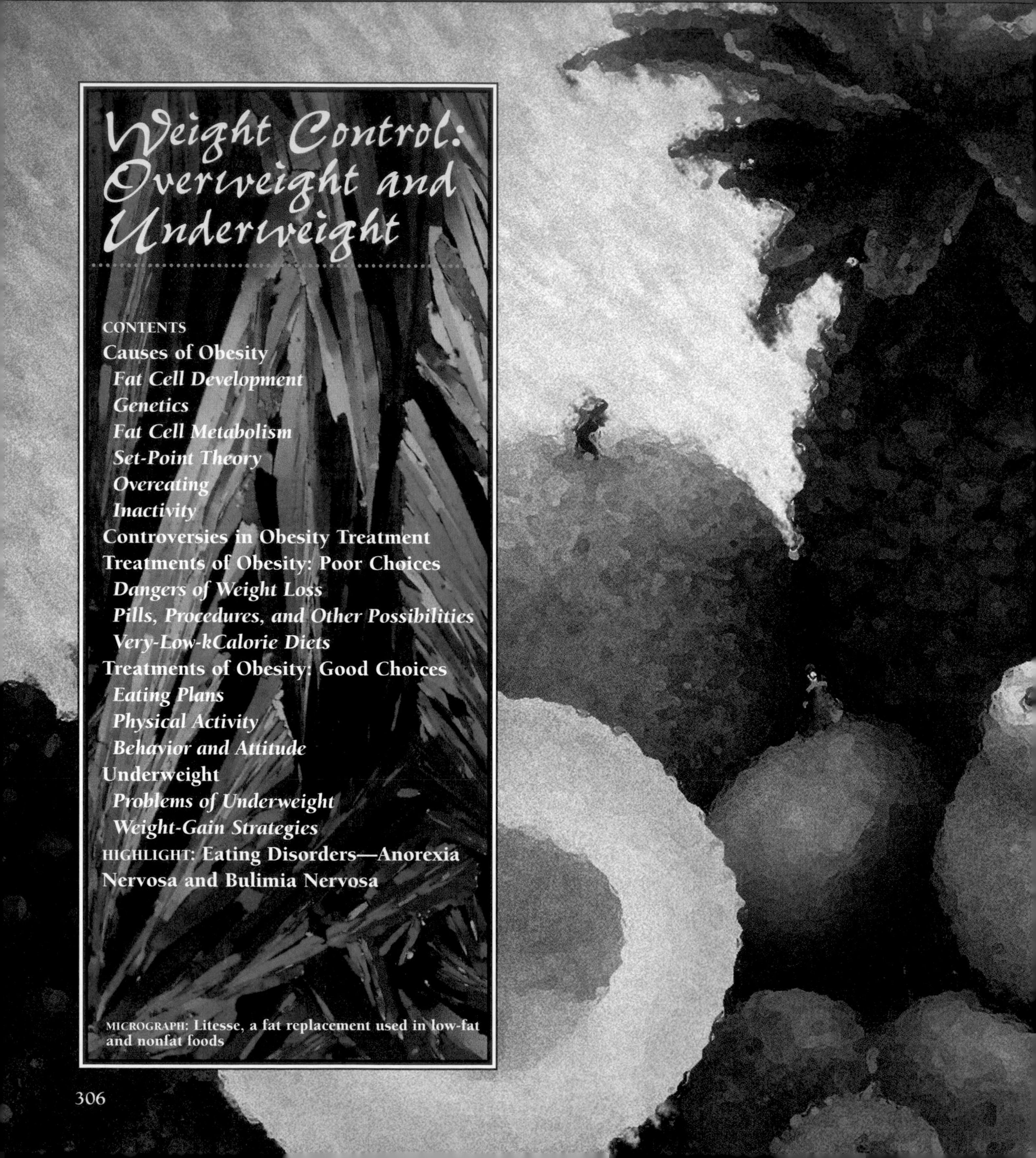

CONTENTS

MICROGRAPH: Litesse, a fat replacement used in low-fat and nonfat foods

Are you pleased with your body weight? If you answered yes, you are a rare individual. Nearly all people in our society think they should weigh more or less (mostly less) than they do. Usually, their primary reason is appearance, but they often perceive, correctly, that physical health is also somehow related to weight. At the extremes, both overweight and underweight present health risks.

This chapter emphasizes the problems of overweight, partly because they have been more intensively studied and partly because they are a widespread health problem in the developed countries. Information on underweight is presented wherever appropriate. The highlight that follows this chapter delves into the eating disorders anorexia nervosa and bulimia nervosa.

Despite our nation's preoccupation with body image and weight loss, the incidence of obesity continues to rise dramatically (see Figure 9–1). Approximately one out of three adults and one out of five teenagers in the United States are now overweight.*[1] The prevalance of overweight has been increasing and is especially high among women, the poor, and some ethnic groups.[2]

HEALTHY PEOPLE 2000: Reduce overweight to a prevalence of no more than 20% among people aged 20 years and older and maintain prevalence at no more than 15% among adolescents aged 12 and 19 years.

Figure 9–1

Prevalence of Obesity among Adults in the United States

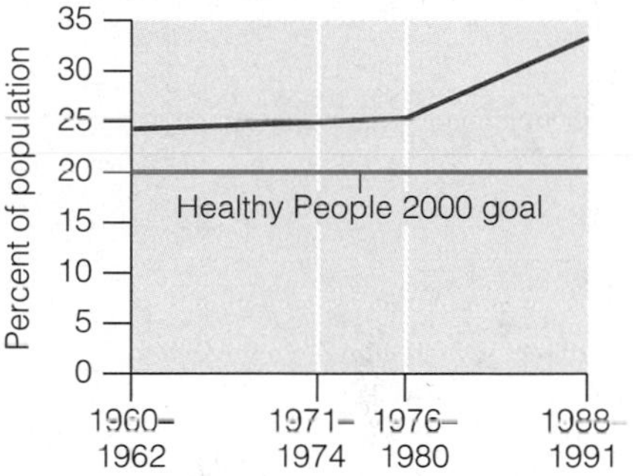

Causes of Obesity

Excess body fat accumulates when people consistently take in more food energy than they spend. Why do they do this? Is it genetic? Environmental? Cultural? Behavioral? Socioeconomic? Psychological? Metabolic? All of these? Most likely, obesity has many interrelated causes; some experts in the field speak of many different *obesities*. Why an imbalance between energy intake and energy expenditure occurs is unclear; the next sections summarize possible explanations.

FAT CELL DEVELOPMENT

When more energy is consumed than is spent for whatever reason, much of the excess energy is stored in fat cells. The amount of fat on a person's body reflects both the *number* and the *size* of the fat cells. The number of fat cells increases most rapidly during the growing years of late childhood and early puberty.[3] Fat cell number increases more rapidly in obese children than in lean children, and obese children entering their teen years may already have as many fat cells as do adults of normal weight.

The fat cells can expand in size. When the cells reach their maximum size, they may also divide. Thus obesity develops when a person's fat cells increase in number, in size, or quite often both. Figure 9–2 illustrates fat cell development.

Obesity due to an increase in the *number* of fat cells is **hyperplastic obesity**. Obesity due to an increase in the *size* of fat cells is **hypertrophic obesity**.

With fat loss, the fat cells shrink in size, but not in number. For this reason, people with extra fat cells may tend to regain lost weight rapidly; they may be able to shrink their cells, but not reduce the number. When they gain weight, their many fat cells readily expand. In contrast, people with a normal number of

*Overweight is defined as BMI ≥ 27.8 for men and ≥ 27.3 for women.

Figure 9–2

Fat Cell Development

Fat cells are capable of increasing their size by 20-fold and their number by several thousandfold.

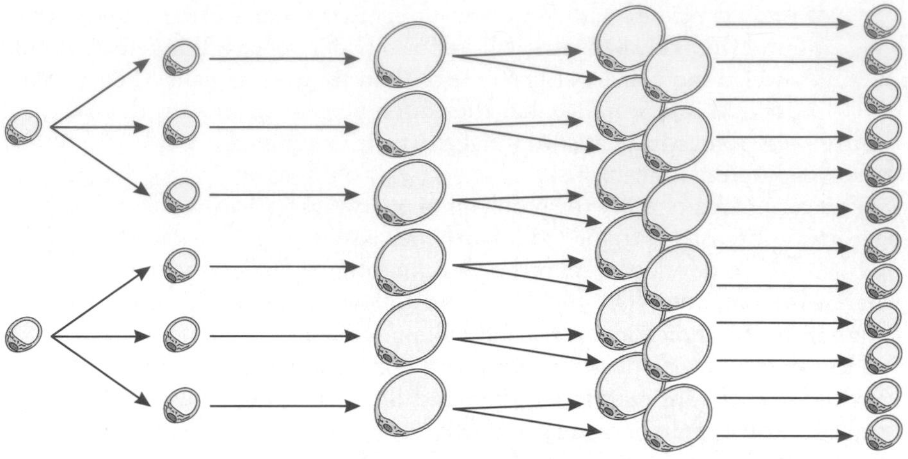

enlarged fat cells may be more successful in maintaining weight losses; when their cells shrink, both cell size and number are normal. Prevention of obesity is most critical, then, during the growing years when cell number is increasing.

During growth, fat cells increase in number.
When energy intake exceeds expenditure, fat cells increase in size.
When fat cells have reached their maximum size and energy intake continues to exceed energy expenditure, fat cells increase in number again.
With fat loss, the size of the fat cells shrinks, but not the number.

Studies of body weight regulation have noted differences between the body's white adipose tissue and its brown adipose tissue: regular white fat primarily stores fat, whereas brown fat produces heat. When white fat is oxidized, some of the energy is released in heat and some is captured in ATP, but brown fat oxidation is uncoupled from ATP formation; it produces heat only. Radiating energy away as heat enables the body to spend, rather than store, energy. The heat is particularly important in newborns and in animals who hibernate or live in cold climates; they have plenty of brown adipose tissue. In contrast, human adults have small amounts of brown fat in strategic locations, and its role is poorly understood. Some researchers have speculated that the lack of brown fat in adults may contribute to obesity, but its role in weight regulation remains unknown.[4]

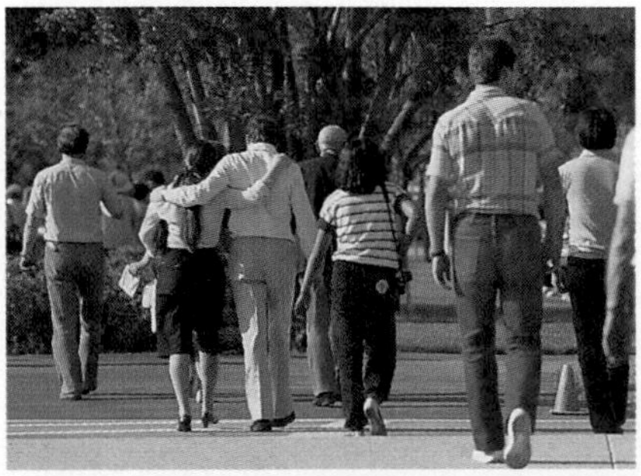

Heredity is the most significant determinant of each person's weight.

GENETICS

Genetics plays an important role in determining a person's body weight and body composition. When both parents are obese, the chances that their children will be obese are quite high (80 percent), whereas when neither parent is obese, the chances are relatively small (less than 10 percent). Adoption studies show that biological parents and their natural children tend to be similar in weight, but that adoptive parents and their adopted children do not. Studies of more than 600 pairs of twins yield similar findings: identical twins are twice as likely to weigh the same as fraternal twins—even when reared apart.[5]

Similarly, some people have the genetic tendency to *gain* more weight than others on comparable energy intakes.[6] When several sets of identical twins ate an extra 1000 kcalories a day for 100 days, some of the pairs gained 9 pounds while others gained up to 29 pounds. Within each pair, the amount of weight gained, percentage of body fat, and distribution of fat were similar.

Genetics may also influence the way energy is *spent*. Differences in BMR among individuals are greater than can be explained by age, sex, and body composition alone. Similarities within families suggest a genetic influence on BMR, and a low metabolic rate is a major risk factor for weight gain.[7]

Recently, researchers have discovered a gene in humans that they have named the *obese* gene.[8] Mice with a defective version of the gene weigh up to three times as much as normal mice. Scientists believe that when the gene is functioning, it is active in fat-storage cells and may signal the body to stop eating. Like all genes, the obese gene instructs cells to make a particular protein, perhaps a hormone that slows down eating as the body accumulates fat. Scientists are currently working on determining the protein's exact role, and they are hopeful it will lead them to an understanding of how the body controls its weight.

FAT CELL METABOLISM

Some of the research investigating the genetic influence on obesity focuses on the enzyme lipoprotein lipase (LPL), which promotes fat storage in both fat and muscle cells. People with high LPL activity are especially efficient at storing fat. As you might expect, obese people have much more LPL activity in their fat cells than lean people (muscle cell LPL activity is similar).[9] Consequently, even modest excesses in energy intake have a more dramatic impact on obese people than on lean people.

Reminder: The enzyme *lipoprotein lipase (LPL)* promotes fat storage.

The activity of LPL is partially regulated by sex-specific hormones—estrogen in women and testosterone in men. In women, fat cells in the breasts, hips, and thighs produce abundant LPL, putting fat away in those body sites; in men, fat cells in the abdomen produce abundant LPL. This explains why men tend to develop central obesity whereas women more readily develop lower-body fat.

The activity of LPL may explain why lost weight is so easily regained.[10] One group of researchers measured the LPL in nine obese people before they followed a very-low-kcalorie diet and again after they had lost an average of 90 pounds. The researchers found that LPL activity *rose* after weight loss, and that it rose highest in the people who had been fattest prior to weight loss. Researchers speculate that weight loss serves as a signal to the gene that produces the LPL enzyme, saying "Make more enzyme to store fat." This response to weight loss helps explain why obese people easily regain weight after having lost it, and why their repeated efforts at weight loss are so difficult—they are battling against enzymes that want to store fat. The activity of LPL also supports the theory that some inner mechanism sets a person's weight or body composition and that if anything is done to change it, the body will adjust to restore the set point.

SET-POINT THEORY

Many internal physiological variables, such as blood glucose, blood pH, and body temperature, remain fairly stable under a variety of conditions. The hypothala-

set point: the point at which controls are set (for example, on a thermostat). The set-point theory proposes that the body tends to maintain a certain weight by means of its own internal controls.

mus and other regulatory centers constantly monitor and delicately adjust conditions so as to maintain homeostasis. The stability of such complex systems may depend on set-point regulators that maintain variables within specified limits.

Research on the regulation of body weight has been influenced by this set-point concept. Unlike body temperature, however, people's weight ranges vary widely. For example, a reasonable weight for an adult woman, 5 feet 4 inches tall, is about 135 pounds. Yet it is easy to find women of that height who weigh less than 100 pounds and others who weigh more than 200 pounds. These large variations within a population may seem inconsistent with a tightly regulated set-point system, but they aren't; it is the variation within an *individual* that is fairly narrow over long time spans.

Researchers speculate that the body sends out signals to *defend* the established body weight when it is challenged. Recent research confirms that the body adjusts its metabolism whenever it gains or loses weight—in the direction that returns to the initial body weight: energy expenditure increases with weight gain and decreases with weight loss.[11] These changes in energy expenditure are greater than those predicted based on body composition and help to explain why it is so difficult for an obese person to maintain weight losses.

The set-point theory remains controversial and unproven, but many researchers seem to agree that the body somehow (probably by way of genetics) stabilizes its weight. Research is focusing on whether and how a person can lower an elevated set point by manipulating environmental factors such as diet and exercise.

OVEREATING

One obvious, although not necessarily accurate, explanation for obesity is that overweight people overeat. Yet diet histories from obese people reveal energy intakes that are similar to, or even less than, those of others.[12] Diet histories may not, however, be accurate records of actual intakes. Misreporting of diet and exercise patterns occurs among nonobese as well as obese people.[13]

Some obese people report that even when they follow an energy-restricted diet, they cannot lose weight. But studies have found that these people may actually be eating more and exercising less than they think they are.[14] Furthermore, they tend to believe that their obesity is caused by genetic and metabolic factors, and not by their overeating. Some clinicians dub this "denial" and say that it prevents people from recognizing and taking responsibility for their behaviors.[15]

The long-held belief that obese people do not overeat but simply have low energy needs has been challenged. Compared with others, obese people who report being unable to lose weight despite energy-restrictive dieting do not have lower measures of basal metabolic rate, thermic effect of food, or metabolic response to exercise.[16] Such findings have led some experts to conclude that obese people simply eat more and exercise less than nonobese people.[17]

INACTIVITY

People may be obese, not because they eat too much, but because they spend too little energy.[18] Some obese people are so extraordinarily inactive that even when they eat less than lean people, they still have an energy surplus. Reducing their food intake further would jeopardize health and incur nutrient deficiencies.

Physical activity, then, is a necessary component of nutritional health. People must be physically active if they are to eat enough food to deliver all the nutrients needed without unhealthy weight gain.

One hundred years ago, 30 percent of the energy used in farm and factory work came from muscle power; today only 1 percent does.[19] Modern technology has replaced physical activity at home, at work, and in transportation. Underactivity is probably the single most important contributor to obesity. In turn, television watching may contribute most to physical inactivity.[20]

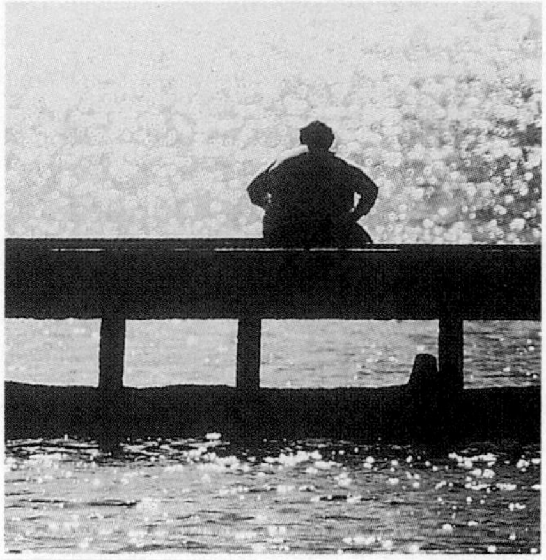
Lack of physical activity fosters obesity.

Watching television contributes to obesity in several ways. First, television viewing requires little energy beyond the resting metabolic rate; in fact, one study reports that television viewing actually *lowers* energy expenditure.[21] Second, it replaces time spent in more vigorous activities. Third, watching television correlates with between-meal snacking, eating the high-kcalorie, high-fat foods most heavily advertised on programs, and influencing family food purchases. Nonnutritious foods and beverages appear not only in commercials, but also within the television programs themselves. People, especially children, may miss the message that eating and drinking these foods will bring about weight gain when they see television stars indulging in such behavior and remaining thin.

Children who watch the most television have the greatest prevalence of obesity: obesity increases by 2 percent for each additional hour of television viewed per day.[22] The relationship between television and obesity remains strong when control variables such as prior obesity and socioeconomic class are considered.

Like all the other "causes" of obesity, inactivity alone fails to explain it fully. Fat cell development, genetics, metabolism, set point, and overeating all offer possible, but still incomplete, explanations. Most likely, obesity has not one cause, but different causes and combinations of causes in different people. After all, no two people are alike either physically or psychologically. Some causes may be within a person's control and some may be beyond it. In recent years, the view has been gaining ground that obesity is no one's "fault"—it is not a matter of undisciplined gluttony. Philosophies of weight control and treatment have been evolving to square with this view.

Controversies in Obesity Treatment

An estimated 30 to 40 percent of all U.S. women (and 20 to 25 percent of U.S. men) are trying to lose weight at any given time, spending up to $30 to $40 billion each year to do so.[23] Many of these people do not even need to lose weight. Others need to lose weight, but are not successful. People have attached so many dreams of happiness to weight loss that they are willing to risk huge sums of money for the slightest chance of success. As a result, weight-loss schemes are one of the leading forms of fraud in the United States.

Many people assume that every overweight person can achieve slenderness and should pursue that goal. First consider that most overweight people cannot—for whatever reason—become slender: only 5 percent of all people who try to lose weight are able to maintain their losses.[24] Then consider the prejudice involved in that assumption. People come with varying weight tendencies just as they come with varying potentials for height and degrees of intelligence, yet we do not

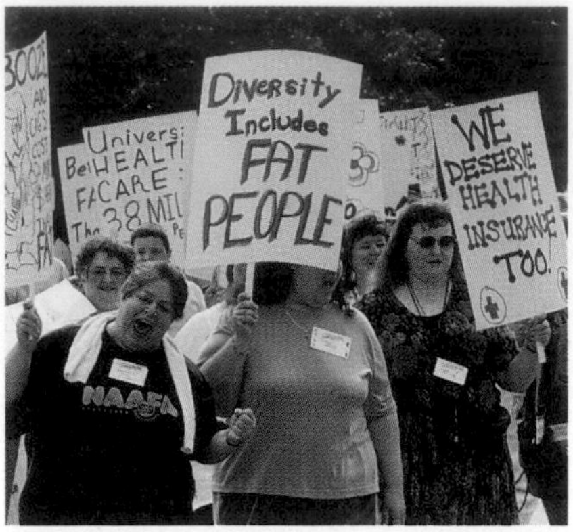

Members of the National Association to Advance Fat Acceptance protest rampant discrimination.

expect tall people to shrink or smart people to stop thinking in an effort to become "normal."

Our society places such enormous value on thinness that many overweight people face prejudice and discrimination: they are judged on their appearance more than on their character. Socially, overweight people are stereotyped as lazy, stupid, and lacking in self-control. They are less likely to be married than those who are not overweight.[25] Overweight people pay more for insurance and for clothing; they are also less likely to be admitted to college or hired for employment, even when they are qualified. This is especially true for women—a 250-pound man can equally easily be a lumberjack or a corporate executive, but a woman that size faces numerous obstacles. Psychologically, fat people may suffer embarrassment when others treat them with hostility and contempt, and some have even learned to view their own bodies as grotesque and loathsome.[26] Parents and friends may chide them about their weight and lack of discipline to resolve the problem. All of this hurts self-esteem. Many overweight people today are tired of our nation's obsession with weight control and simply want to be accepted as they are. Health care professionals, including dietitians, are among the chief offenders, and some of them are calling for action to stop stigmatizing obesity and to extend the Americans with Disabilities Act to include the obese.[27] To free our nation of its obsession with body weight and prejudice against obesity we must first learn to judge others for who they are and not for what they weigh.[28]

Still, traditional medical advice urges all obese people to reduce their weight to reduce associated health risks. Obese people die younger from a host of causes, including heart attacks, strokes, certain types of cancer, and complications of diabetes (the non-insulin-dependent type).*[29] Even after the effects of diagnosed diseases are discounted, the risk of death remains twice as high for obese people, especially for those with lifelong obesity, than would otherwise be expected.

Encouraging weight loss may be justified when health benefits are clear. For example, a 30-year-old man with a BMI of 40 may be able to avoid the diabetes that runs in his family by losing 75 pounds. The effort required to do so may be great, but it is far less than the effort and consequences of living with diabetes. Sometimes health benefits appear with less weight loss. A 60-year-old man the same size may be able to improve the arthritis in his knees by losing 25 pounds, for example. In this case, the effort to lose more weight may not pay off.[30] Often a person's motivations for weight loss have nothing to do with health: for example, when a 20-year-old woman with a BMI of 25 wants to lose a few pounds for spring break. Sometimes a person may be healthier *not* losing weight. Such is the case in people with anorexia nervosa who want to lose weight in spite of the devastating medical consequences (see Highlight 9).

In summary, the question whether a person should lose weight depends on many factors: the extent of overweight, age, health, and genetic makeup among them. Not all obesity will cause disease or shorten life expectancy, and just as there are normal-weight people who are unhealthy, there are obese people who are

*The greater the degree of overweight, the higher the death rate, especially in the young.

healthy. The concept of "healthy obese" people is relatively new, yet it has become generally accepted; the debate focuses on how to characterize this group's health status and risks.[31] Weight-loss advice, then, does not apply equally to all overweight people. Some people may risk more in the process of losing weight than in remaining obese.

Treatments of Obesity: Poor Choices

Most obesity treatments are ineffective and possibly risky. The negative effects must be carefully considered before embarking on any weight-loss program.

DANGERS OF WEIGHT LOSS

Many states have developed a consumer bill of rights to help protect potential weight-loss clients. Such a document explains the risks associated with weight-loss programs and provides honest predictions of success (see Table 9–1). Physical problems may arise from fad diets and "yo-yo" dieting, and psychological problems may emerge from repeated "failures."[32]

Fad Diets Fad diets espouse exaggerated or false theories of weight loss and advise consumers to follow inadequate diets. Some fad diets are more hazardous to health than obesity itself. Adverse reactions can be as minor as headaches, nausea, and dizziness or as serious as death. Of 29,000 claims, treatments, and

Chapter 7 describes the metabolic consequences of a low-carbohydrate diet and the protein-sparing fast.

Table 9–1

Weight-Loss Consumer Bill of Rights (An Example)

1. *WARNING:* Rapid weight loss may cause serious health problems. Rapid weight loss is weight loss of more than 1½ pounds to 2 pounds per week or weight loss of more than 1 percent of body weight per week after the second week of participation in a weight-loss program.
2. Consult your personal physician before starting any weight-loss program.
3. Only permanent lifestyle changes, such as making healthful food choices and increasing physical activity, promote long-term weight loss and successful maintenance.
4. Qualifications of this provider are available upon request.
5. *YOU HAVE A RIGHT TO:*
   - Ask questions about the potential health risks of this program and its nutritional content, psychological support, and educational components.
   - Receive an itemized statement of the actual or estimated price of the weight-loss program, including extra products, services, supplements, examinations, and laboratory tests.
   - Know the actual or estimated duration of the program.
   - Know the name, address, and qualifications of the dietitian or nutritionist who has reviewed and approved the weight-loss program.

Figure 9–3

The Weight-Cycling Effect of Repeated Dieting

Each round of dieting is followed by a rebound of weight to a higher level than before.

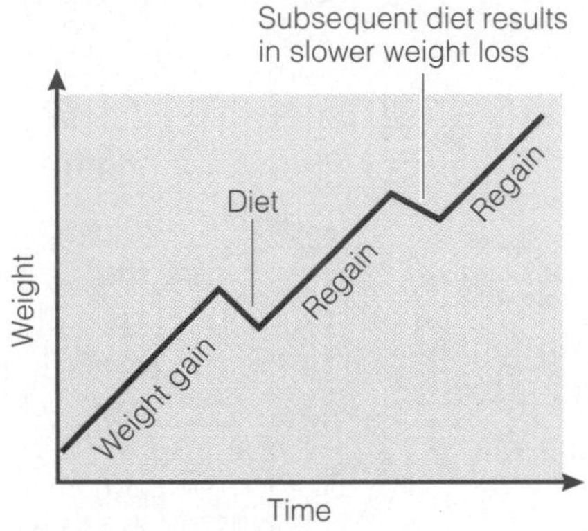

weight cycling: repeated cycles of weight loss and gain. The weight-cycling pattern is popularly called the **ratchet effect** or **yo-yo effect** of dieting.

Losing 10 pounds and keeping them off may be beneficial, but losing 100 pounds and regaining them may be quite harmful.

Figure 9–4

The Psychology of Weight Cycling

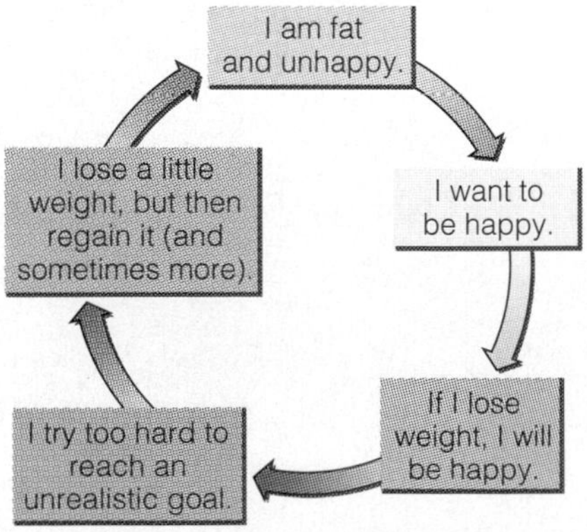

Source: Adapted with permission from J. P. Foreyt and G. K. Goodrick, *Living without Dieting* (Houston: Harrison Publishing, 1992).

theories for losing weight, fewer than 6 percent of them are effective—and 13 percent are downright dangerous. The accompanying box offers guidelines for identifying weight-loss scams. Some of the nation's largest diet programs have misled consumers with unsubstantiated claims and deceptive testimonials.[33] Furthermore, they fail to provide an assessment of the short- and long-term results of their treatment plans, even though such evaluations are possible and would permit consumers to make informed decisions.[34]

Weight Cycling Many people who try to lose weight become trapped in weight cycling, the endless repeating rounds of weight loss and regain from "yo-yo" dieting (see Figure 9–3). When people repeatedly lose weight only to regain it, their bodies become very efficient at making and storing fat. This increased efficiency shows itself in a way familiar to dieters who have lost and gained—and lost and gained again. With each attempt, it becomes harder and takes longer to lose weight and easier and quicker to gain it back. In fact, previous weight-cycling history can predict a person's success (or lack thereof) in maintaining weight loss.[35]

Such fluctuations in body weight do not appear to produce permanent changes in body composition, but they do increase the risks of diabetes, hypertension, high blood lipids, and even death, independent of the obesity itself.[36] Some research indicates that maintaining a stable weight, even if it is overweight, may be less harmful to health than repeated bouts of weight gains and losses. Such concerns should not deter obese people who want to lose weight from trying, but rather should encourage them to commit to lifelong changes that will maintain weight losses.[37]

Psychological Problems Some weight-loss programs are better than others in terms of cost, approach, and customer satisfaction, but none are particularly successful in helping people keep lost weight off. Most programs assume that the problem can be solved simply by applying willpower and hard work. If determination were the only factor involved, though, the success rate would be far greater than 5 percent. Overweight people may readily assume the blame for their failures to lose weight and maintain the losses when, in fact, the programs have failed to deliver on their promises.[38] Ineffective treatment and its associated sense of failure add to a person's psychological burden.[39] Figure 9–4 illustrates how the devastating psychological effects of obesity and dieting perpetuate themselves.

PILLS, PROCEDURES, AND OTHER POSSIBILITIES

A number of alternative strategies for losing weight have been set forth. Some are of limited usefulness, some are not useful at all, and some are actually harmful.

Diuretics Temporary water retention may add several pounds on the scale, but obesity does not cause water retention.* In fact, obese people have a *smaller*

*Many women experience temporary water retention around the time of the menstrual period. Oral contraceptives may also cause water retention and may even promote fat gain in some women. A woman who has this problem should consult her physician about switching brands.

How to Identify Unsound Weight Loss Schemes and Diets

1. They promise dramatic, rapid weight loss (i.e., substantially more than 1 percent of total body weight per week).
2. They promote diets that are nutritionally unbalanced or extremely low in kcalories. Diets should provide:
   - A reasonable number of kcalories (not fewer than 1200 kcalories per day).
   - Enough, but not too much, protein (between the RDA and twice the RDA).
   - Enough, but not too much fat (between 20 and 30 percent of daily energy intake from fat).
   - Enough carbohydrate to spare protein and prevent ketosis (about 100 grams).
   - A balanced assortment of vitamins and minerals from a variety of foods from each of the food groups.
3. They use liquid formulas rather than foods and provide too little energy.
4. They attempt to make clients dependent upon special foods or devices rather than teaching them how to make good choices from the conventional food supply.
5. They fail to encourage permanent, realistic lifestyle changes, including regular exercise and behavior modification.
6. They misrepresent salespeople as "counselors" supposedly qualified to give guidance in nutrition and/or general health. Even if adequately trained, such "counselors" would still be objectionable because of the obvious conflict of interest that exists when providers profit directly from products they recommend and sell.
7. They collect large sums of money at the start or require that clients sign contracts for expensive, long-term programs. Programs should be reasonably priced and on a pay-as-you-go basis.
8. They fail to inform clients of the risks associated with weight loss in general or the specific program being promoted. They provide no information about drop-out rates or long-term success of their clients.
9. They promote unproven or spurious weight-loss aids such as human chorionic gonadotrophin hormone (HCG), starch blockers, diuretics, sauna belts, body wraps, passive exercise, ear stapling, acupuncture, electric muscle-stimulating (EMS) devices, spirulina, amino acid supplements (e.g., arginine, ornithine), glucomannan, methylcellulose (a "bulking agent"), "unique" ingredients, and so forth.
10. They fail to provide for weight maintenance after the program ends.

Source: Adapted from *National Council Against Health Fraud Newsletter,* March/April 1987, National Council Against Health Fraud, Inc.

diuretic (dye-you-RET-ic): a drug that promotes water excretion; popularly, a "water pill."
dia = through
ure = urine

percentage of body water than people of normal weight. When people take diuretics, they lose water, not fat. The weight loss lasts only half a day or so, and the price is dehydration and mineral imbalances.

Amphetamines Years ago physicians routinely prescribed amphetamines (pep pills) to reduce the appetite. Not only are amphetamines of little value in weight loss, but they are also highly addictive. Many dieters who used them remained overweight and were left with the additional problem of getting off the drugs. Common side effects of amphetamines include dizziness, irritability, blurred vision, nausea, vomiting, and diarrhea. Amphetamines are no longer approved by the FDA for weight loss.

Other Prescription Drugs Most prescription drugs either suppress appetite and so curb food intake or speed up energy metabolism and the use of fat for fuel.*[40] Most drugs that suppress appetite can be addictive and lose their effectiveness after a few weeks of use.[41] Drugs that accelerate energy expenditure also have serious side effects and lose their effectiveness with time.† One compound currently under investigation because of its action in reducing fat synthesis and enhancing fat utilization is DHEA—a product made in the body during the synthesis of steroid hormones.‡[42] A hormone called leptin that regulates body fat is being studied in obese mice and has proven successful in causing them to lose a third of their weight in two weeks.

Another new drug currently under testing acts on the small intestine's fat-digesting enzymes to prevent digestion and absorption of about a third of the fat consumed. The drug, tetrahydrolipostatin, faces years of rigorous study before it can be approved by the FDA.

One nonaddicting drug, dexfenfluramine, shows promise in reducing hunger and improving dietary compliance.[43] The drug works by stimulating the brain to release the neurotransmitter serotonin, which depresses appetite. Several other appetite-suppressing drugs are also under study and may one day prove their worth. Side effects vary with each obesity drug, but the overall incidence is relatively modest.

While some drugs have proved effective in promoting initial weight loss, the long-term effects of their use are unknown.[44] Government regulations restrict the use of prescription drugs for obesity to a three-month limit due to fears of potential abuse and previous indiscriminate prescription; some research indicates that long-term treatment may be beneficial.[45] In either case, drugs should be used only as one component of a comprehensive weight-loss program.

Over-the-Counter Products The FDA has given approval to two over-the-counter medications to help with weight loss. One contains phenylpropanolamine, which suppresses appetite and enhances weight loss when used with a low-kcalorie diet.[46] The other contains benzocaine (in a candy form), which anesthetizes the tongue, reducing taste sensations.

---

*Examples of drugs that suppress food intake include naltrexone, chlorocitric acid, cholecystokinin-octapeptide, and serotonergic agents.

†Examples of drugs that stimulate fat utilization include idazoxon, atpamezole, phenoxybenzamine, and thermogenic agents.

‡DHEA stands for dehydroepiandrosterone.

Manufacturers of many other diet products have been making weight-loss claims without having to prove their effectiveness or safety.* One company marketed guar gum, the soluble fiber commonly used as a thickener in many food products, as a weight-loss product. Guar gum forms a gel when taken with water, and in several cases (including one that led to death), people developed esophageal blockages and GI obstructions after swallowing guar tablets. Upon learning of these problems, the FDA banned the sale of guar tablets. Consumers can best protect themselves from hazards like these by remembering that weight loss does not come in tablet form.

Other Gimmicks Other gimmicks don't help with weight loss either. Hot baths do not speed up the basal metabolic rate so that pounds can be lost in hours. Steam and sauna baths do not melt the fat off the body, although they may dehydrate people so that their weights change dramatically. Machines that jiggle parts of the body while people lean passively on them provide pleasant stimulation, but no exertion and so no expenditure of energy. Brushes, sponges, and massages intended to move, burn, or break up "cellulite" do nothing of the kind, because there is no such thing as cellulite.

Surgery Surgery, as an approach to weight loss, is justified in some specific cases of clinically severe obesity. Guidelines for client evaluation, selection, care, and follow-up have been published.[17] The person contemplating surgery for weight loss should consider all the health implications before submitting to it.

Two gastric partitioning procedures have gained wide acceptance and are illustrated in Figure 9–5.[48] Both procedures effectively limit food intake by reducing the size of the stomach's pouch. They reduce the size of the outlet as well, so they delay the passage of food from the stomach into the intestine for digestion and absorption. The long-term safety and effectiveness of gastric

*To obtain a list of ineffective diet aids, write to FDA, HFE-20, 5600 Fishers Lane, Rockville, MD 20857.

cellulite (SELL-you-light or SELL-you-leet): supposedly, a lumpy form of fat; actually, a fraud. The lumpy appearance in fatty areas of the body is caused by strands of connective tissue that attach the skin to underlying muscles. These points of attachment may pull tight where the fat is thick, making lumps appear between them. The fat itself is not different from fat anywhere else in the body. So, if the fat in these areas is lost, the lumpy appearance disappears.

clinically severe obesity: a BMI of 40 or greater or 100 pounds or more overweight for an average adult. A less preferred term used to describe the same condition is *morbid obesity*.

gastric partitioning: a surgical procedure used to treat clinically severe obesity. The operation limits food intake by reducing the size of the stomach and delays gastric emptying by restricting the outlet.

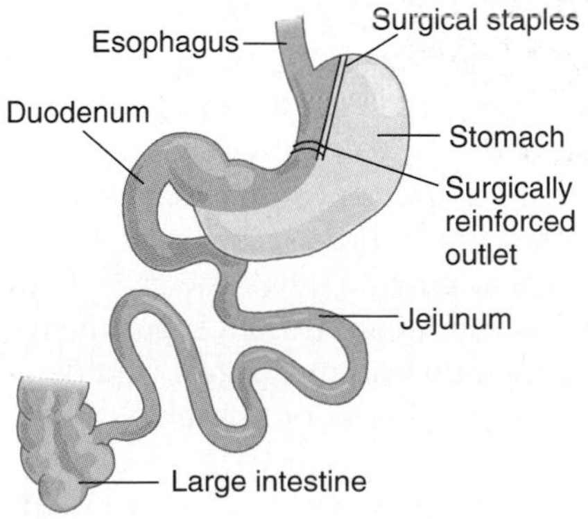

In vertical banded gastroplasty, the surgeon constructs a small gastric pouch and restricts the outlet from the stomach to the intestine.

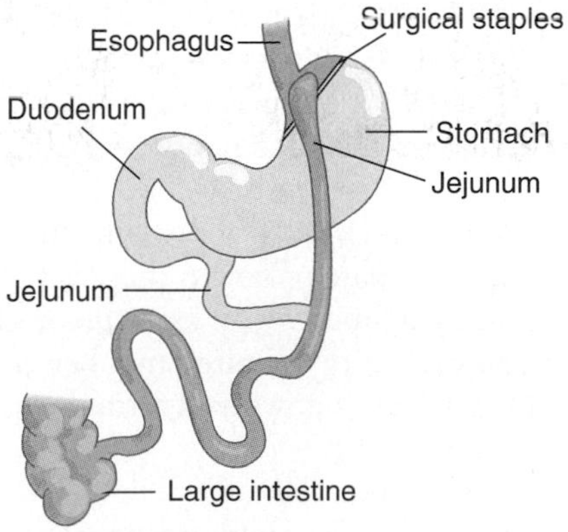

In gastric bypass, the surgeon constructs a small gastric pouch and creates an outlet directly to the jejunum.

Figure 9–5

Surgical Procedures Used in the Treatment of Severe Obesity

The dark pink areas highlight the flow of food through the GI tract. Notice that the first procedure maintains a relatively normal flow whereas the second one bypasses most of the stomach, all of the duodenum, and some of the jejunum. The pale pink areas indicate the sections that have been bypassed.

surgery depend, in large part, on compliance with dietary instructions. Common immediate postsurgical complications include infections, nausea, vomiting, and dehydration; in the long term, vitamin and mineral deficiencies and psychiatric disorders are common.[49] Lifelong medical supervision is necessary for those who choose the surgical route, but in suitable candidates the benefits of weight loss prove worth the risks.[50]

Another surgical procedure is used, not to treat obesity, but to remove the evidence. Plastic surgeons can extract some fat deposits by suction lipectomy, or "liposuction." This cosmetic procedure has little effect on body weight, but can alter body shape slightly in specific areas.

Gastric Balloons A physician can position and inflate a balloon inside the stomach so that a person who eats too much food will feel uncomfortable. Risks of gastric ulcer, internal bruising, and intestinal blockage commonly occur during the fourth month of use, so the FDA requires removal of these balloons after three months.

Jaw Wiring Desperation leads some people to request that their jaws be wired shut so that they will be forced to consume a liquid diet. This does bring about weight loss, but when the wires are removed, most people promptly regain the lost weight because they have not learned the new eating habits that will support weight maintenance.

VERY-LOW-KCALORIE DIETS

For many obese people, compliance with a well-balanced, nutritionally adequate, energy-restricted diet offers slow results compared with the number of pounds they have to lose. Quite often, they become frustrated and lose hope before significant changes become apparent. For these people, very-low-kcalorie diets (VLCD) offered by medical centers provide rapid weight loss (sort of a "jump start" on the journey). For the duration of the VLCD, they need make no decisions about what foods to buy, how to prepare them, or how much to eat. They need only drink a formula as prescribed.

Recommended criteria for people on VLCD:[51]

- Motivated.
- Moderately to severely obese (BMI>30).
- No heart, kidney, gallbladder, or liver disease; cancer; or alcoholism.
- No psychiatric disorders (including eating disorders).

This break from food may help a person establish a new relationship with food. Unlike a recovering alcoholic, who can abstain from alcohol altogether, or a smoker, who can throw away all cigarettes, a person cannot give up food "cold turkey." A VLCD provides a break from poor eating habits and an opportunity to begin good eating habits when the VLCD ends.

VLCD plans provide 800 kcalories, at least 1 gram per kilogram of body weight of high-quality protein, little or no fat, and a little carbohydrate (not enough to spare protein); there is no advantage to providing less energy.[52] They are accompanied by an assortment of vitamins and minerals from supplements. Meals consist of a limited number of foods (primarily lean meats, fish, and poultry) each day, a powdered formula available by prescription, or a combination of the two.

VLCD formulas are designed to be nutritionally adequate, but the body responds to this severe energy restriction as if the person were starving—conserving energy and preparing to regain weight at the first opportunity. As Chapter 7 described, several changes occur in hormone concentrations, metabolic activities, fluid and electrolyte balances, and organ functions in the effort to meet the challenge of living on a much-less-than-adequate energy intake. For these reasons, a VLCD is appropriate only for short-term use (four months) and under close medical supervision.[53] Table 9–2 lists common side effects of VLCD.

Without doubt, weight losses on VLCD are dramatic. Unfortunately, weight regains are almost certain.[54] With the weight loss comes a slower BMR and slower fat oxidation—conditions that favor weight gain.[55] Such rapid losses and steady gains are detrimental to both physical and mental health. People undertaking VLCD should be forewarned that the hard part begins at the end of the diet,

Table 9–2

Possible Physical Consequences of Very-Low-kCalorie Diets

Blood	Immunity
• Blood carotene concentrations increase. • Blood cholesterol concentrations increase. • Blood urea concentrations increase.	• Immune response diminishes. • White blood cells decrease in number.
Cardiovascular/respiratory	**Metabolic**
• Blood pressure declines. • Carbon dioxide production declines. • Cardiac output declines. • Heart muscle atrophies. • Heartbeat becomes irregular. • Low blood pressure develops. • Oxygen consumption declines. • Pulse rate declines. • Respiratory rate declines.	• Basal metabolism declines. • Bone mineral content shifts. • Cold intolerance occurs. • Dehydration may occur. • Gout may occur. • Ketosis develops. • Lean body tissues are lost. • Mineral and electrolyte imbalances occur. • Nitrogen balance becomes negative.
Digestive	**Other**
• Gallstones and kidney stones form. • GI tract motility declines. • Liver inflammation and fibrosis develop. • Nausea, vomiting, diarrhea, abdominal discomfort, and constipation occur. **Hormonal** • Menstrual irregularity develops. • Sex drive is lost.	• Body and breath odor (from ketone excretion) may become apparent. • Cold intolerance develops. • Hair falls out. • Headaches occur. • Lethargy, fatigue, and loss of stamina set in. • Skin dries out. • Sleeplessness may occur. • Sudden death becomes possible.

Sources: Evidence on metabolic rate, lean body tissue, liver, gallstone, heartbeat, bones, and nitrogen balance, from various authors in *American Journal of Clinical Nutrition* 56 (1992): supplement; immune failure reported in C. J. Field, R. Gougeon, and E. B. Marliss, Changes in circulating leukocytes and mitogen responses during very-low-energy all-protein reducing diets, *American Journal of Clinical Nutrition* 54 (1991): 123–129; reduced oxygen consumption reported in K. N. Pavlou and coauthors, Exercise as an adjunct to weight loss and maintenance in moderately obese subjects, *American Journal of Clinical Nutrition* 49 (1989): 1115–1123; low blood pressure, headache, atrophy of heart muscle, and hormonal effects from R. L. Atkinson, Low calorie diets and obesity, in Biotechnology and Nutrition, eds. D. D. Bills and S. D. Kung (Boston: Butterworth-Heinemann, 1992), pp. 29–45.

when they have to learn to maintain their weight loss. A weight-maintenance phase is an essential part of every VLCD program.[56]

In summary, weight-loss efforts often are misguided, and when pursued via unwise weight-loss techniques, they can be downright dangerous. This is not to say, though, that no one should attempt to lose weight. Weight loss is highly desirable for those whose health will benefit from it, who can do it, and who pursue it using safe and effective techniques.

Treatments of Obesity: Good Choices

Dietary recommendations state that for good health, a person should "achieve and maintain appropriate body weight." The goal is not weight loss, but health gains. Weight loss can improve control of diabetes and reduce the risks of heart disease by lowering blood pressure and blood cholesterol, especially for those with upper-body fat.[57] For these reasons, parameters such as blood pressure, blood cholesterol, or even self-esteem are more useful than body weight in marking success. Of course, the same eating and exercise habits that improve health often lead to an appropriate body weight and composition as well. Whether the goal is health or weight loss, expectations need to be reasonable. Unreachable targets ensure failure. It is better to aim for realistic and achievable goals. Then, if success is greater than expected, there will be rewards instead of disappointments.

- Weight-loss pointer: Adopt reasonable expectations about health and weight goals and about how long it will take to achieve them.

In pursuing good health, keep in mind that it is a lifelong journey. Most adults are keenly aware of their body weights and shapes and realize that what they eat and what they do can make a difference to some extent. Those who are most successful at preventing weight gain or maintaining weight loss seem to have fully incorporated healthful eating and physical activity into their lives. Their approach is not "on-again-off-again," but a routine part of their daily lives. And it is a multifaceted approach, involving diet, physical activity, behavior, and attitude.

HEALTHY PEOPLE 2000: Increase to at least 50% the proportion of overweight people aged 12 years and older who have adopted sound dietary practices combined with regular physical activity to attain an appropriate body weight.

EATING PLANS

- Weight-loss pointer: Be involved in planning.

No one food plan is magical, and no specific food must be included or avoided. In designing a plan, people need only consider foods that they like or can learn to like, that are available, and that are within their means.

Realistic Energy Intake The main characteristic of a weight-loss diet is that it provides less energy than the person needs to maintain present body weight. Restricting energy intake too severely, however, may have only short-term effects and can be counterproductive.[58] Rapid weight loss means excessive loss of lean tissue. Initially, overweight people should only try to stop binge eating and start eating normally—say, three meals a day—and then examine energy intake.

Energy intake should provide nutritional adequacy without excess—that is, somewhere between kcalorie-restricted dieting and complete freedom to eat everything in sight. A rule of thumb is that a person needs at least 10 kcalories per pound of current weight each day to lose fat efficiently while retaining lean tissue. For example, a 140-pound woman would start by setting her energy intake at 1400 kcalories a day. Then as she lost weight, she would adjust her energy intake downward.

- Weight-loss pointer: Adopt a realistic plan.

Nutritional Adequacy Nutritional adequacy is difficult to achieve on fewer than 1200 kcalories a day, and most healthy adults should not consume any less than that. Consider that 1200 kcalories a day allows a person who weighs 120 pounds to lose weight, yet hardly anyone who weighs 120 pounds is overweight. People weighing more can lose weight on higher energy intakes. A plan that provides an adequate intake supports a healthier and more successful weight loss than a restrictive plan that creates feelings of starvation and deprivation, which can lead to an irresistible urge to binge.

- Weight-loss pointer: Make nutritional adequacy a high priority.

Take a look at Table 9–3 and notice that the 1200-kcalorie food plan represents the minimum servings suggested in the Daily Food Guide (introduced in Chapter 2) and allows a teaspoon of fat at each of three meals. Such an intake would allow most people to lose weight gradually and still meet their nutrient needs with careful, nutrient-dense food selections. (Women might need an iron supplement.) The other patterns provide for higher energy intakes.

- Weight-loss pointer: Emphasize nutrient-dense foods.

Small Portions Overweight people usually need to learn to eat less food at each meal—one piece of chicken for dinner instead of two, a teaspoon of butter on the vegetables instead of a tablespoon, and a cookie for dessert instead of six. The goal is to eat enough food for energy, nutrients, and pleasure, but not so much as to have an excess. This amount should leave a person feeling satisfied—not necessarily full. Keep in mind that even low-fat foods can deliver a lot of kcalories when a person eats large quantities. A low-fat cookie or two can be a sweet treat even on a weight-loss diet, but a whole box would clearly be excessive.

- Weight-loss pointer: Eat small portions of foods at each meal.

Carbohydrates, Not Fats Center meals and snacks on complex carbohydrate foods. Fresh fruits, vegetables, legumes, and whole grains offer abundant

- Weight-loss pointer: Make legumes, grains, vegetables, and fruits central to your diet plan.

Table 9–3

Diet Patterns for Different Energy Intakes

Exchange	Energy Level (kcal)						
	1200	1500	1800	2000	2200	2600	3000
Starch	6	7	8	9	11	13	15
Meat (lean)	4	5	6	6	6	7	8
Vegetable	3	4	5	5	5	6	6
Fruit	2	3	4	4	4	5	6
Milk (nonfat)	2	2	2	3	3	3	3
Fat	3	5	6	7	8	10	12

Note: These patterns follow the Daily Food Guide plan and supply less than 30 percent of kcalories as fat.

vitamins, minerals, and fiber but little fat. They also require effort to eat—an added bonus. People who eat these foods in abundance spontaneously eat for longer times and take in fewer kcalories than when eating foods of high energy density. The satiety signal indicating fullness is sent after a 20-minute lag, so a person who slows down and savors each bite eats less before the signal reaches the brain.

- Weight-loss pointer: Eat slowly.

Satiety plays a key role in weight-loss diets. Researchers compared a diet in which fat was restricted, but complex carbohydrates were eaten freely, with a more conventional energy-restricted diet.[59] Moderately obese women in both diet groups lost weight, but those who ate the low-fat, complex carbohydrate-rich diet rated it higher in terms of satiety and taste. They also gave higher ratings to "quality of life," perhaps because they felt less deprived when allowed to eat unrestricted quantities of low-fat, complex carbohydrate foods.

- Weight-loss pointer: Eat complex carbohydrates in abundance.

Findings from several other studies agree: restricting fat is effective in, and may even be more effective than, restricting energy for weight loss.[60] Furthermore, body composition may improve on a low-fat diet. Rats who had been on a high-fat diet were switched to a diet that provided fewer kcalories, with each group receiving either a low-, medium-, or high-fat diet.[61] Compared with rats on the low-fat diet, the rats on the high-fat diet lost less weight and kept much more of their body fat. Even worse, their LPL activity increased compared with rats that remained on the initial high-fat diet. This study suggests that body *fat* will not be lost by following a low-kcalorie diet alone, even when weight is lost—dietary fat must also be reduced.

- Weight-loss pointer: Select low-fat foods regularly.

Similarly, women who followed a low-fat diet (20 percent kcalories from fat) lost both weight and body fat.[62] In fact, the only way the women could *maintain* weight was to raise their total energy intakes. Clearly then, to lose weight and improve body composition, measure fat with extra caution. A slip of the butter knife adds more kcalories than a slip of the sugar spoon. Less fat in the diet means less fat in the body (review Highlight 8 for more evidence). Be careful not to take this advice to the extreme, however; too little fat in the diet or in the body carries health risks as well.

Speaking of empty kcalories, a person trying to achieve or maintain a healthy weight needs to pay attention not only to fat, but to sugar and alcohol, too. Using them for pleasure on occasion is compatible with health as long as most daily choices are of nutrient-dense foods.

- Weight-loss pointer: Limit concentrated sweets and alcoholic beverages.

Adequate Water Learn to satisfy thirst with water. Water fills the stomach between meals and dilutes the metabolic wastes generated from the breakdown of fat. It meets the water need that was formerly met by eating extra food (remember that foods provide water).

- Weight-loss pointer: Drink plenty of water (8 glasses or more a day).

Adopt a lifelong "eating plan for good health" rather than a "diet for weight loss." That way, you will be able to keep the lost weight off.

- Weight-loss pointer: Learn, practice, and follow a healthful eating plan for the rest of your life.

PHYSICAL ACTIVITY

People who combine diet and exercise are more likely to lose more fat and less likely to regain weight than those who only diet.[63] People who include physical activity in their weight control program seem to follow their diet plan more

- Fitness pointer: Participate in some form of physical activity regularly.

closely than those who do not exercise.[64] Consequently they benefit from both a little less energy input and the added energy output of physical activity. Table 8–2 (on p. 284) shows how much energy each of several activities uses. The table also shows that the number of kcalories spent in an activity depends more upon body weight than on how fast the exercise is done. For example, a person who weighs 150 pounds and runs a mile in 6 minutes spends about 103 kcalories. That same person walking a mile in 15 minutes uses almost the same amount—about 92 kcalories. Similarly, a 220-pound person spends about 150 kcalories on the 6-minute mile, and only a little less—about 135 kcalories—on the 15-minute walk. Whether a person chooses to run or walk the distance, the same energy will be spent; walking will just take longer. To lose fat, expend as much energy as your time allows.[65]

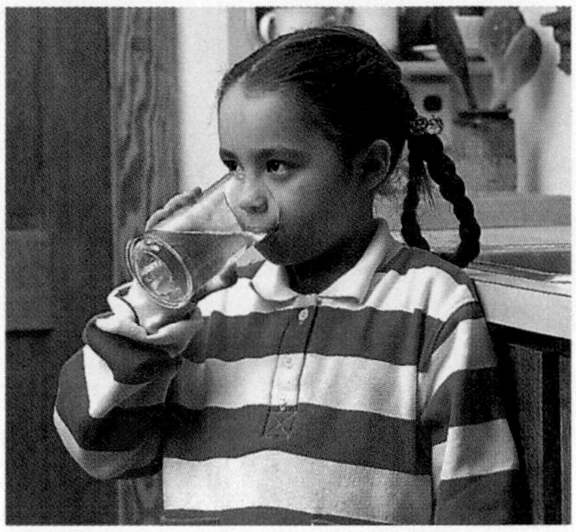

Drinking water is a healthy habit.

Activity and the BMR Activity also contributes to energy output in an indirect way—by speeding up basal metabolism. It does this both immediately and over the long term. On any given day, basal metabolism remains elevated for several hours after intense and prolonged exercise. Over the long term, daily vigorous activity for many weeks gradually changes body composition toward more lean tissue. Metabolic rate rises accordingly, and this makes a contribution toward continued weight loss or maintenance.

The raised metabolic rate continues for as long as the person keeps exercising regularly. The more energy expended in metabolic activities, the greater the energy requirement. This means that a person can eat more without gaining weight, which in turn brings both pleasure and nutrients.

Activity and Appetite Control Physical activity also helps to control appetite. People think that exercising will make them hungry, but this is not entirely true. Yes, active people do have healthy appetites, but immediately after a good workout, most people do not feel like eating. They may be thirsty and want to shower, but they are not hungry. The reason is that the body has released fuels from storage to support the exercise, so glucose and fatty acids are abundant in the blood. At the same time, the body has suppressed its digestive functions. Hard physical work and eating are not compatible. A person must calm down, put energy fuels back in storage, and relax before eating. Thus exercise helps curb appetite, especially the inappropriate appetite that accompanies boredom, anxiety, or depression and might prompt a person to eat when not hungry. Weight-control programs encourage people to use this strategy to overcome their urge to eat when not hungry: go out and exercise instead. The activity passes time, relieves anxiety, and prevents inappropriate eating.

Benefits of physical activity in a weight-control program:

- Short-term increase in energy expenditure (from exercise and from a slight rise in BMR).
- Long-term increase (slight) in BMR.
- Appetite control.
- Stress reduction and control of stress eating.
- Physical, and therefore psychological, well-being.
- High self-esteem.

Activity and Psychological Benefits Activity also helps reduce stress. Since stress itself is a cue to inappropriate eating for many people, activity can help here, too. Activity offers still more psychological advantages. The fit person looks and feels healthy and, as a result, gains self-esteem. High self-esteem motivates a person to persist in seeking weight control and fitness, which continues the beneficial cycle.

Choosing Activities Clearly, physical activity is a plus in a weight-control program. What kind of physical activity is best? People seeking to lose weight

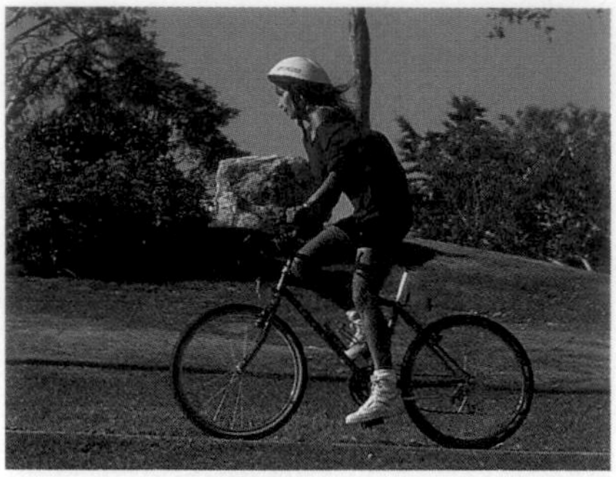

Regular physical activity, such as bicycling or walking briskly, will help to burn fat.

should choose activities that they enjoy and that they are willing to do regularly. Sustained physical activities of moderate intensity (aerobic exercises) are more effective in weight control than short bursts of vigorous exercise.[66] In addition to exercise, there are hundreds of ways to incorporate energy-spending activities into daily routines: take the stairs instead of the elevator, walk to the neighbor's apartment instead of making a phone call, and rake the grass clippings instead of using a bagger. Remember that sitting uses more kcalories than lying down, standing uses more kcalories than sitting, and moving uses more kcalories than standing. A 175-pound person who replaces a 30-minute television program with a 2-mile walk a day can spend enough energy to lose (or not gain) 18 pounds in a year. Walk a mile. Run a race. Swim a lap. Dance a jig. Ride a bike. Climb a mountain. Do whatever you enjoy doing—and do it often.

Spot Reducing People sometimes ask about "spot reducing." Unfortunately, muscles do not "own" the fat that surrounds them. Fat cells all over the body release fat in response to demand, and the fat is then used by whatever muscles are active. No exercise can remove the fat from any one particular area—and, incidentally, neither can massage machines that claim to break up fat on trouble spots. Being moved passively by machines or pounded by massages neither increases energy output nor takes off fat.

Exercise can help with trouble spots in another way, though. Strengthening muscles in a trouble area can help to improve their tone; stretching to gain flexibility can help with associated posture problems. Thus aerobic, strength, and flexibility workouts can improve fitness and physical appearance.

BEHAVIOR AND ATTITUDE

Behavior and attitude are important supporting factors to achieving and maintaining appropriate body weight and composition. Behavior modification changes the hundreds of small behaviors of overeating and underexercising that lead to, and perpetuate, obesity. Making these changes requires time and effort, so you must be prepared to invest in yourself. Furthermore, it is important to adopt the right attitude. Healthy eating and activity choices are not intolerable tasks that demand herculean willpower to achieve. They are an essential part of healthy living and should simply be incorporated into the day. "They are just things one has to do"[67]—much like brushing one's teeth or wearing a seat belt.

- Behavior change pointer: A record of diet and exercise habits reveals problem areas, the first step toward improving behaviors.

Becoming Aware of Behaviors A person who is aware of all the behaviors that created a problem has a head start toward solving it. Thus the first step in changing behaviors is to record present eating and exercise behaviors (see Figure 9–6). Keeping a diary will help the individual identify behaviors that may need changing and establish a baseline against which to measure future progress.

behavior modification: the changing of behavior by the manipulation of *antecedents* (cues or environmental factors that trigger behavior), the *behavior* itself, and *consequences* (the penalties or rewards attached to behavior).

Making Small Changes Behavior-modification strategies encourage making many small changes in daily behaviors. Behavior-modification experts see each behavior as the second part of a three-part sequence. Its antecedents precede it, and its consequences follow it:

A (antecedents) → B (behavior) ↔ C (consequences)

Time	Place	Activity or food eaten	People present	Mood
10:30–	School	6 peanut	by myself	Starved
10:40	vending	butter crackers		
	machine	and 12 oz. cola		
12:15–	Restaurant	Sub sandwich	friends	relaxed
12:30		and 12 oz. cola		& friendly
3:00–	Gym	Weight	work out	tired
3:45		training	partner	
4:00–	Snack bar	Small	by myself	OK
4:10		frozen		
		yogurt		

Figure 9–6

Food Diary

The entries in a food diary should include the times and places of meals and snacks, the types and amounts of foods eaten, the persons present when food is eaten, and a description of the individual's feelings when eating. The diary should also record physical activities: the kind, the intensity level, the duration, and the person's feelings about them.

A behavior occurs in response to antecedents (cues or stimuli); the more intense the antecedents are, the more likely the behavior will occur. The behavior in turn leads to consequences. The more intense these consequences are, positively or negatively, the more or less likely the behavior is to occur again.

Applying Behavior-Modification Strategies The box on pp. 326–327 shows how a person might apply behavior-modification strategies to a weight-control program. The strategies are designed to encourage the repeated occurrence of desired eating and exercise behaviors and to eliminate the occurrence of unwanted behaviors. A particularly attractive feature of these strategies is that they do not involve blaming oneself or putting oneself down—an important element in fostering self-esteem.

With so many possible behavior changes available, a person can choose where to begin. Start simply and don't try to master them all at once. Attempting too many changes at one time is never successful; a person must set priorities. Pick one trouble area that is manageable and start there. Practice a desired behavior until it is habitual and automatic. Then select another trouble area to work on, and so on. Another bit of advice along the same lines: don't try to tackle weight loss during a particularly stressful time of life.

Maintaining Weight Finally, be aware that it can be hard to maintain weight loss. Maintenance is only possible if the eating and activity behaviors that led to weight loss continue. If, on arriving at goal weight after months of self-discipline, the victorious weight loser "celebrates" by resuming old eating habits, then maintenance will not be successful.

Obesity is not "cured" by simply attaining a reasonable body weight; eating wisely and staying active must continue to be part of life's daily routines. Ongoing membership in a weight-control organization and regular, continued physical activity can provide indispensable support for the formerly overweight person who wants to remain trim.

- Behavior change pointer: Adopt permanent lifestyle changes to achieve and maintain a healthy weight.

How to Apply Behavior-Modification Strategies to Weight Loss

1. To eliminate inappropriate eating cues:
   - Buy foods that are low in fat.
   - Shop when you are not hungry.
   - Serve low-fat meals.
   - Let other family members buy, store, and serve their own sweets (monitor children's intakes).
   - Change channels or look away when food commercials appear on television.
   - Shop only from a list and stay away from convenience stores.
   - Carry appropriate snacks from home and avoid vending machines.
2. To suppress the cues you cannot eliminate:
   - Eat only in one place (at a table), and in one room; use plates, bowls, and eating utensils.
   - Clear plates directly into the garbage.
   - Create obstacles to the eating of problem foods (for example, make it necessary to unwrap, cook, and serve each one separately).
   - Minimize contact with excessive food (serve individual plates, don't put serving dishes on the table, and leave or clean the table when you have finished eating).
   - Make small portions of food look large by spreading food out and serving on small plates.
   - Control deprivation (eat regular meals, don't skip meals, avoid getting tired, avoid boredom by keeping cues to fun activities in sight).
3. To strengthen the cues to appropriate eating and exercise:
   - Encourage others to eat appropriate foods with you.
   - Keep your favorite appropriate foods in the front of the refrigerator.

Personal Attitude Being overweight becomes a part of a person's identity. For many people, overeating and being overweight have become integral aspects of their lives, involving social, marital, and family relationships; community activities; work; health; self-concept; and emotional states. Changing diet and exercise behaviors without attention to a person's self-concept invites failure. People who fully understand their personal relationships with food are best prepared to make healthful changes in eating and exercise behaviors.

Sometimes habitual behaviors that are hazardous to health, such as smoking or drinking alcohol, contribute positively by helping people adapt to stressful situations. Similarly, many people overeat to cope with the stresses of life. To break out of that pattern, they must first identify the particular stressors that trigger the urge to overeat. Then, when faced with these situations, they must learn and practice problem-solving skills. These skills will help them to respond appropriately to difficult situations.

All this is not to imply that psychological therapy holds the magic answer to a weight problem. Still, efforts to improve one's general well-being may result in

- Learn appropriate portion sizes and prepare one portion at a time.
- Establish specific times for meals and snacks.
- Prepare foods attractively.
- Keep your walking shoes (ski poles, tennis racket) by the door.

4. To engage in desired eating or exercise behaviors:
   - Eat only at planned times; plan not to eat after a specified time (say, 7:00 or 8:00 P.M.).
   - Slow down (pause several times during a meal, put down utensils between mouthfuls, chew thoroughly before swallowing, swallow before reloading the fork, always use utensils).
   - Leave some food on the plate.
   - Engage in no other activities while eating (such as reading or watching television).
   - Move more (shake a leg, pace, fidget, flex your muscles).
   - Join in and exercise with a group of active people.
5. To arrange or emphasize negative consequences of inappropriate eating:
   - Eat your meals with other people.
   - Ask that others respond neutrally when you deviate from your plan (make no comment). This is a negative consequence because it withholds attention.
   - If you slip, don't punish yourself.
6. To arrange or emphasize positive consequences of appropriate behaviors:
   - Update records of food intake, exercise, and weight change regularly.
   - Arrange for rewards for each unit of behavior change or weight loss.
   - Ask family and friends for reinforcement (praise and encouragement).

weight control even when weight loss is not the primary goal. When the problems that trigger the urge to overeat are dealt with in alternative ways, people may find they eat less and that their eating behavior begins to respond appropriately to internal cues of hunger rather than inappropriately to external signals of stress. Sound emotional health supports a person's ability to take care of health in all ways—including nutrition, weight control, and fitness.

- Behavior change pointer: Learn alternative ways to deal with emotions and stresses.

Self-esteem underlies emotional health and facilitates personal growth. Overweight people who have low self-esteem can learn to feel better about themselves even before they lose the first pound. A person can enhance self-esteem by fostering a positive view of the inner self and by developing a healthy relationship with the outer self, the body. To view the inner self positively, practice positive thinking, make affirmative statements about oneself, and visualize success. People who believe they can lose weight are more successful at losing weight than those who expect to fail; people who view themselves as "physically fit" are more successful at maintaining weight loss than those who view themselves as "fat" or even as "formerly fat."

- Behavior change pointer: Use positive self-talk—"You can do it!"
- Behavior change pointer: Believe that you can succeed in spite of past failures.

- Behavior change pointer: Attend support groups regularly or develop supportive relationships with others.

Support Groups Group support is important when making life changes. Some people find it helpful to join a group that provides support in efforts to lose weight, such as Take Off Pounds Sensibly (TOPS), Weight Watchers (WW), Overeaters Anonymous (OA), or others. A modest expenditure for health is well worthwhile, but people need to avoid rip-offs, of course; review the box on p. 315 for help in identifying unsound weight-loss schemes. Many dieters find it helpful to form their own self-help groups.

HEALTHY PEOPLE 2000: Increase to at least 50% the proportion of worksites with 50 or more employees that offer nutrition education and/or weight management programs for employees.

A surefire remedy for obesity has yet to be found, although many people find a combination of the approaches just described to be most effective. Diet and exercise shift energy balance so that more energy is being spent than is taken in. The physical activity maintains or even builds the lean body so that fat is preferentially lost and metabolic energy needs remain high. The behavior modification retrains habits so that once the weight is lost, it will not return; and the improvement in inner self helps a person to manage life without a dependency on food. This treatment package requires time, individualization, and sometimes the assistance of skilled health care professionals.

Underweight

Reminder: *Underweight* is a body weight so low as to have adverse health effects; it is generally defined as 10% or more below the standard or BMI <20.

Underweight is a far less prevalent problem than overweight, affecting no more than 10 percent of U.S. adults. Whether the underweight person needs to gain weight is a question of health and, like weight loss, a highly individual matter. People who are healthy at their present weights, may stay there; those who are at risk for malnutrition and illness should try to gain. Medical advice can help make the distinction.

Some people are unalterably thin by reason of heredity or early physical influences. They may find gaining weight difficult. People who wish to gain weight for appearance's sake or to improve their athletic performance need to be aware that healthful weight gains can be achieved only by physical conditioning combined with high energy intakes. On a high-kcalorie diet alone, a person will gain weight, but it will be mostly fat. Even if the gain improves appearance, it can be as detrimental to health as being slightly underweight. For an athlete, such a weight gain might impair performance. Therefore, in weight gain, as in weight loss, physical activity and energy intake are essential components of a sound plan.

PROBLEMS OF UNDERWEIGHT

The causes of underweight may be as diverse as those of overweight—hunger, appetite, and satiety irregularities; psychological traits; metabolic factors; and hereditary tendencies. Habits learned early in childhood, especially food aversions, may perpetuate themselves.

The demand for energy to support physical activity and growth often contributes to underweight. An active, growing boy may need more than 4000 kcalories a day to maintain his weight and may be too busy to take time to eat. Underweight people find it hard to gain weight—due, in part, to their expenditure of energy in adaptive thermogenesis. So much energy may be spent adapting to a higher food intake that at first as many as 750 to 800 extra kcalories a day may be needed to gain a pound a week. Like those who want to lose weight, people who want to gain must learn new habits and learn to like new foods. They are also similarly vulnerable to potentially harmful schemes and would be wise to review the consumer bill of rights on p. 313, using the term "weight gain" instead of "weight loss" where appropriate.

WEIGHT-GAIN STRATEGIES

Weight-gain strategies center on eating foods that provide many kcalories in a small volume and exercising to build muscle. Conventional advice to the bodybuilder is to eat enough foods to provide about 700 to 1000 kcalories a day above normal energy needs and to exercise to build lean tissue.

- Weight-gain pointer: Expect weight gain to take time (1 pound per month would be reasonable).

Energy-Dense Foods Energy-dense foods (the very ones eliminated from a successful weight-loss diet) hold the key to weight gain. Pick the highest-kcalorie items from each food group—that is, milk shakes instead of nonfat milk, salmon instead of snapper, avocados instead of cucumbers, a cup of grape juice instead of a small apple, and whole-wheat muffins instead of whole-wheat bread. Because fat contains more than twice as many kcalories per teaspoon as sugar does, fat adds kcalories without adding much bulk.

- Weight-gain pointer: Eat energy-dense foods regularly.

Be aware that a low-fat diet plan is recommended because the general U.S. population is overweight and at risk for heart disease. Consumption of high-fat foods is not healthy for most people, but may be essential for an underweight individual who needs to gain weight. An underweight person who is physically active and eating a nutritionally adequate diet can afford a few extra kcalories from fat. For health's sake, it would be wise to select monounsaturated and polyunsaturated fats instead of those with saturated fats: for example, sautéing vegetables in olive oil instead of butter.

Regular Meals Daily People who are underweight need to make meals a priority and take the time to plan, prepare, and eat each meal. They should eat at least three healthy meals every day and learn to eat more food within the first 20 minutes of a meal. Another suggestion is to eat meaty appetizers or the main course first and leave the soup or salad until later.

- Weight-gain pointer: Eat at least three meals a day.

Large Portions It is also important to learn to eat more food at each meal. Put extra slices of ham and cheese on the sandwich for lunch, drink milk from a larger glass, and eat cereal from a larger bowl.

- Weight-gain pointer: Eat large portions of foods and expect to feel full.

The person should expect to feel full. Most underweight individuals are accustomed to small quantities of food. When they begin eating significantly more, they feel uncomfortable. This is normal and passes over time.

- Weight-gain pointer: Eat snacks between meals.

Extra Snacks Since a substantially higher energy intake is needed each day, in addition to eating more food at each meal, it is necessary to eat more frequently. Between-meal snacking offers a solution. For example, a student might make three sandwiches in the morning and eat them between classes in addition to the day's three regular meals.

- Weight-gain pointer: Drink plenty of juice and milk.

Juice and Milk Beverages provide an easy way to increase energy intake. Consider that 6 cups of cranberry juice add almost 1000 kcalories to the day's intake. kCalories can be added to milk by mixing in powdered milk or packets of instant breakfast.

For people who are underweight due to illness, concentrated liquid formulas are often recommended because a weak person can swallow them easily. A physician or registered dietitian can recommend high-protein, high-kcalorie formulas to help the underweight person maintain or gain. Used in addition to regular meals, these can help considerably.

- Weight-gain pointer: Exercise and eat to build muscles.

Exercising to Build Muscles To gain weight, use strength training primarily and increase energy intake to support that exercise. Eating extra food will then support a gain of both muscle and fat.

In theory, it takes an excess of about 2000 to 2500 kcalories to support the gain of a pound of pure lean tissue.[68] The rate at which the body can build muscle tissue also depends on the person. Men and women have mixtures of both male and female hormones; people with more male hormones build muscle more easily than others, but it is not known what the limits are. (Highlight 14 provides cautions on the use of steroid hormones.) About 700 to 1000 kcalories a day above normal energy needs is enough to support both the exercise and the building of muscle.

The problem of underweight is less prevalent than overweight. To gain weight a person must train physically and increase energy intake by selecting energy-dense foods, eating regular meals, taking larger portions, and consuming extra snacks and beverages.

An extreme underweight condition known as anorexia nervosa is sometimes seen in people who employ heroic self-denial in order to control their weight. They go to such extremes that they become severely undernourished, achieving final body weights of 70 pounds or even less. The distinguishing feature of a person with anorexia nervosa, as opposed to other underweight people, is that the starvation is intentional. Anorexia nervosa is a major eating disorder seen in our society today. Another is bulimia nervosa—compulsive overeating and purging. Eating disorders are the subject of the highlight that follows this chapter.

Study Questions

1. What factors contribute to obesity?
2. List several ill-advised ways to lose weight and explain why such methods are not recommended.
3. Discuss dietary strategies suitable for achieving and maintaining a healthy body weight.
4. What are the benefits of increased physical activity in a weight-loss program?
5. Describe the behavior-modification techniques recommended for changing an individual's dietary habits. What role does personal attitude play?
6. Describe strategies for successful weight gain.

Problem Set

1. Critique a commercial weight-loss plan. Consumers spend billions of dollars a year on weight-loss programs such as Slim-Fast, Sweet Success, Weight Watchers, Nutri/System, Jenny Craig, Optifast, Medifast, and Formula One. One such plan calls for a milk shake in the morning, noon, and afternoon snack, and "a sensible, balanced, low-fat dinner" in the evening. One shake mixed in 8 oz of vitamin A– and D–fortified nonfat milk offers 190 kcal; 32 g of carbohydrate, 13 g of protein, and 1 g of fat; at least one-third of the Daily Value for all RDA vitamins and minerals; plus 2 g of fiber.

a. Calculate the kcalories and grams of carbohydrate, protein, and fat that three shakes provide: ________

b. How do these values compare with the criteria listed in the second item in the box on p. 315? ________

c. Plan "a sensible, balanced, low-fat dinner" that will help make this weight loss plan adequate and balanced. Now, how do the day's totals compare with the criteria in item #2 on p. 315? ________

d. Critique this plan using the other criteria described on p. 315 as a guide. ________

2. Evaluate a weight-gain attempt. People attempting to gain weight sometimes have a hard time because they choose low-kcalorie, high-bulk foods that make it hard to consume enough energy. Consider the following lunch: a chef's salad consisting of 2 c iceberg lettuce, 1 whole tomato, 1 oz swiss cheese, 1 oz roasted ham (lean and fat), 1 hard-boiled egg, ½ cucumber, and ¼ c mayonnaise-type salad dressing. If you analyzed the gram weights of these foods, you'd find that they totaled 551 g. This is a pretty filling meal.

a. How much does this meal weigh in pounds? ________

b. The meal provides 541 kcal. What is the energy density of this meal, expressed in kcalories per gram? Show your calculations. ________

c. To gain weight, this person is advised to eat an additional 500 kcal at this meal. Using foods with this same energy density, how much more chef's salad will this person have to eat? ________

d. Suppose a person simply can't do this. Try to reduce the bulk of this meal by replacing some of the lettuce with more energy-dense foods. Delete 1 c lettuce from the salad and add 1 oz roast beef and 1 oz cheddar cheese. Show how these changes influence the weight and kcalories of this meal:

Item No./Food	Weight (g)	Energy (kcal)
Original totals:	551	541
Minus:		
# 867 Lettuce, 1 c	– ________	– ________
Plus:		
# 603 Roast beef, 1 oz	+ ________	+ ________
#37 Cheddar cheese, 1 oz	+ ________	+ ________
Totals:	________	________

e. How many kcalories did the changes add? ____

f. How much more *weight* of food did these changes add? ________

This exercise should reveal why people attempting to gain weight are advised to add high-fat items, within reason, to their daily meals.

Notes

1. R. J. Kuczmarski and coauthors, Increasing prevalence of overweight among US adults: The National Health and Nutrition Examination Surveys, 1960 to 1991, *Journal of the American Medical Association* 272 (1994): 205–211; Data from the 1988–1991 National Health and Nutrition Examination Survey (NHANES III) as reported in National Heart, Lung, and Blood Institute Obesity Education Summary Report, September 1994; Prevalence of overweight among adolescents—United States, 1988–1991, *Morbidity and Mortality Weekly Report* 43 (1994): 818–821.

2. NIH Technology Assessment Conference Panel, Methods for voluntary weight loss and control, *Annals of Internal Medicine* 116 (1992): 942–949.
3. G. A. Bray, An approach to the classification and evaluation of obesity, in *Obesity*, eds. P. Björntorp and B. N. Brodoff (Philadelphia: J. B. Lippincott, 1992), pp. 294–308.
4. G. Ailhaud, P. Grimaldi, and R. Négrel, Cellular and molecular aspects of adipose tissue development, *Annual Review of Nutrition* 12 (1992): 207–233.
5. A. J. Stunkard and coauthors, The body-mass index of twins who have been reared apart, *New England Journal of Medicine* 322 (1990): 1483–1487.
6. C. Bouchard, The response to long-term overfeeding in identical twins, *New England Journal of Medicine* 322 (1990): 1477–1482.
7. E. Ravussin and C. Bogardus, A brief overview of human energy metabolism and its relationship to essential obesity, *American Journal of Clinical Nutrition* 55 (1992): 242S–245S.
8. Y. Zhang and coauthors, Positional cloning of the mouse *obese* gene and its human homologue, *Nature* 372 (1994): 425–431.
9. R. H. Eckel, Lipoprotein lipase regulation in obesity and after weight loss, an address presented at the North American Association for the Study of Obesity and Emory University School of Medicine conference on Obesity Update: Pathophysiology, Clinical Consequences, and Therapeutic Options, Atlanta, Georgia, August 31–September 2, 1992.
10. P. A. Kern and coauthors, The effects of weight loss on the activity and expression of adipose-tissue lipoprotein lipase in very obese humans, *New England Journal of Medicine* 322 (1990): 1053–1059.
11. R. L. Leibel, M. Rosenbaum, and J. Hirsch, Changes in energy expenditure resulting from altered body weight, *New England Journal of Medicine* 332 (1995): 621–628; P. Pasquet and M. Apfelbaum, Recovery of initial body weight and composition after long-term massive overfeeding in men, *American Journal of Clinical Nutrition* 60 (1994): 861–863.
12. Committee on Diet and Health, *Diet and Health: Implications for Reducing Chronic Disease Risk* (Washington, D.C.: National Academy Press, 1989), p. 144.
13. E. Danforth and E. A. H. Sims, Obesity and efforts to lose weight, *New England Journal of Medicine* 327 (1992): 1947–1948.
14. S. W. Lichtman and coauthors, Discrepancy between self-reported and actual caloric intake and exercise in obese subjects, *New England Journal of Medicine* 327 (1992): 1893–1898.
15. A. Laws, Actual versus self-reported intake and exercise in obesity (letter), *New England Journal of Medicine* 328 (1993): 1494–1495.
16. Lichtman and coauthors, 1992.
17. G. B. Forbes, Diet and exercise in obese subjects: Self-report versus controlled measurements, *Nutrition Reviews* 51 (1993): 296–300.
18. R. Rising and coauthors, Determinants of total daily energy expenditure: Variability in physical activity, *American Journal of Clinical Nutrition* 59 (1994): 800–804.
19. A. P. Simopoulos, Characteristics of obesity, in *Obesity*, eds. P. Björntorp and B. N. Brodoff (Philadelphia: J. B. Lippincott, 1992), pp. 309–319.
20. S. L. Gortmaker, W. H. Dietz, Jr., and L. W. Y. Cheung, Inactivity, diet, and the fattening of America, *Journal of the American Dietetic Association* 90 (1990): 1247–1255; E. Obarzanek and coauthors, Energy intake and physical activity in relation to indexes of body fat: The National Heart, Lung, and Blood Institute Growth and Health study, *American Journal of Clinical Nutrition* 60 (1994): 15–22.
21. R. C. Klesges, M. L. Shelton, and L. M. Klesges, Effects of television on metabolic rate: Potential implications for childhood obesity, *Pediatrics* 91 (1993): 281–286.
22. W. H. Dietz, Jr., and S. L. Gortmaker, Do we fatten our children at the television set? Obesity and television viewing in children and adolescents, *Pediatrics* 75 (1985): 807–812.
23. NIH Technology Assessment Conference Panel, 1992.
24. R. L. Atkinson and V. S. Hubbard, Report on the NIH Workshop on Pharmacologic Treatment of Obesity, *American Journal of Clinical Nutrition* 60 (1994): 153–156; F. M. Kramer and coauthors, Long-term follow-up of behavioral treatment for obesity: Patterns of weight regain among men and women, *International Journal of Obesity* 13 (1989): 123–136; T. A. Wadden and coauthors, Treatment of obesity by very low calorie diet, behavior therapy, and their combination: A five year prospective, *International Journal of Obesity* (supplement) 13 (1989): 39–46.
25. S. L. Gortmaker and coauthors, Social and economic consequences of overweight in adolescence and young adulthood, *New England Journal of Medicine* 329 (1993): 1008–1012.
26. A. J. Stunkard and T. A. Wadden, Psychological aspects of human obesity, in *Obesity*, eds. P. Björntorp and B. N. Brodoff (Philadelphia: J. B. Lippincott, 1992), pp. 352–360.
27. H. Oberrieder and coauthors, Attitude of dietetics students and registered dietitians toward obesity, *Journal of the American Dietetic Association* 95 (1995): 914–915; A. J. Stunkard and T. I. A. Sørensen, Obesity and socioeconomic status—A complex relation, *New England Journal of Medicine* 329 (1993): 1036–1037.
28. J. A. Cassell, Social anthropology and nutrition: A different look at obesity in America, *Journal of the American Dietetic Association* 95 (1995): 424–427.
29. L. V. Sjöström, Mortality of severely obese subjects, *American Journal of Clinical Nutrition* 55 (1992): 516S–523S.
30. J. S. Garrow, Treatment of obesity, *The Lancet* 340 (1992): 409–413.
31. R. J. Garrison, Healthy adiposity in women: The Framingham Offspring Study, *Journal of the American College of Nutrition* 12 (1993): 357–362.
32. K. A. Petersmarck, The Michigan approach: Building consensus for safe weight loss, *Journal of the American Dietetic Associ-*

ation 92 (1992): 679–680.
33. FTC accuses five diet programs of deceptive advertising, *FDA Consumer*, December 1993, p. 3.
34. Committee to Develop Criteria for Evaluating the Outcomes of Approaches to Prevent and Treat Obesity, Food and Nutrition Board, Institute of Medicine, National Academy of Sciences, *Journal of the American Dietetic Association* 95 (1995): 96–105; T. A. Wadden and coauthors, A multicenter evaluation of a proprietary weight reduction program for the treatment of marked obesity, *Archives of Internal Medicine* 152 (1992): 961–966.
35. G. Haus and coauthors, Key modifiable factors in weight maintenance: Fat intake, exercise, and weight cycling, *Journal of the American Dietetic Association* 94 (1994): 409–413.
36. K. van der Kooy and coauthors, Effect of a weight cycle on visceral fat accumulation, *American Journal of Clinical Nutrition* 58 (1993): 853–857; A. M. Prentice and coauthors, Effects of weight cycling on body composition, *American Journal of Clinical Nutrition* 56 (1992): 209S–216S; L. Lissner and coauthors, Variability of body weight and health outcomes in the Framingham population, *New England Journal of Medicine* 324 (1991): 1839–1844; L. Lissner and K. D. Brownell, Weight cycling, mortality, and cardiovascular disease: A review of epidemiologic findings, in *Obesity*, eds. P. Björntorp and B. N. Brodoff (Philadelphia: J. B. Lippincott, 1992), pp. 653–661.
37. National Task Force on the Prevention and Treatment of Obesity, Weight cycling, *Journal of the American Medical Association* 272 (1994): 1196–1202; Garrow, 1992.
38. E. S. Parham, Applying a philosophy of nutrition education to weight control, *Journal of Nutrition Education* 22 (1990): 194–197.
39. S. C. Wooley and D. M. Garner, Obesity treatment: The high cost of false hope, *Journal of the American Dietetic Association* 91 (1991): 1248–1251.
40. G. A. Bray, Drug treatment of obesity, *American Journal of Clinical Nutrition* 55 (1992): 538S–544S; A. Astrup and coauthors, The effect of ephedrine/caffeine mixture on energy expenditure and body composition in obese women, *Metabolism: Clinical and Experimental* 41 (1992): 686–688.
41. C. D. Berdanier, Dehydroepiandrosterone (DHEA): Useful or useless as an antiobesity agent? *Nutrition Today*, November/December 1993, pp. 34–38.
42. Berdanier, 1993.
43. S. Heshka, Dexfenfluramine for the long-term management of obesity, in *Obesity: New Directions in Assessment and Management*, eds. T. B. VanItallie and A. P. Simopoulos (Philadelphia: The Charles Press, 1995), pp. 227–233; M. M. Kogon and coauthors, Psychological and metabolic effects of dietary carbohydrates and dexfenfluramine during a low-energy diet in obese women, *American Journal of Clinical Nutrition* 60 (1994): 488–493; Dexfenfluramine influences dietary compliance and eating behaviors of obese subjects, *Nutrition Reviews* 52 (1994): 65–68; L. M. H. Mathus-Vliegen and A. M. A. Res, Dexfenfluramine influences dietary compliance and eating behavior, but dietary instruction may overrule its effect on food selection in obese subjects, *Journal of the American Dietetic Association* 93 (1993): 1163–1165; N. Finer, F. Finer, and P. Naoumova, Drug therapy after very-low-calorie diets, *American Journal of Clinical Nutrition* 56 (1992): 195S–198S.
44. R. L. Atkinson, Treatment of obesity (editorial), *Nutrition Reviews* 50 (1992): 338–345.
45. D. J. Goldstein and J. H. Potvin, Long-term weight loss: The effect of pharmacologic agents, *American Journal of Clinical Nutrition* 60 (1994): 647–657.
46. D. E. Schteingart, Phenylpropanolamine in the management of moderate obesity, in *Obesity: New Directions in Assessment and Management*, eds. T. B. VanItallie and A. P. Simopoulos (Philadelphia: The Charles Press, 1995), pp. 220–226.
47. Gastrointestinal surgery for severe obesity: National Institutes of Health Consensus Development Conference Statement, *American Journal of Clinical Nutrition* 55 (1992): 615S–619S.
48. Gastrointestinal surgery for severe obesity, 1992.
49. Gastrointestinal surgery for severe obesity, 1992; W. J. Pories, Surgical approaches to the treatment of the morbidly obese, an address presented at the North American Association for the Study of Obesity and Emory University School of Medicine conference on Obesity Update: Pathophysiology, Clinical Consequences, and Therapeutic Options, Atlanta, Georgia, August 31–September 2, 1992.
50. A. M. C. Macgregor and C. S. W. Rand, Gastric surgery in morbid obesity: Outcome in patients aged 55 years and older, *Archives of Surgery* 128 (1993): 1153–1157.
51. National Task Force on the Prevention and Treatment of Obesity, *Journal of the American Medical Association* 270 (1993): 967–974.
52. G. D. Foster and coauthors, A controlled comparison of three very-low-calorie diets: Effects on weight, body composition, and symptoms, *American Journal of Clinical Nutrition* 55 (1992): 811–817.
53. T. A. Wadden, T. B. Van Itallie, and G. L. Blackburn, Responsible and irresponsible use of very-low-calorie diets in the treatment of obesity, *Journal of the American Medical Association* 263 (1990): 83–85.
54. National Task Force on Prevention and Treatment of Obesity, 1993; A. C. Shovic and coauthors, Effectiveness and dropout rate of a very-low-calorie diet program, *Journal of the American Dietetic Association* 93 (1993): 583–584.
55. F. Froidevaux and coauthors, Energy expenditure in obese women before and during weight loss, after refeeding, and in the weight-relapse period, *American Journal of Clinical Nutrition* 57 (1993): 35–42.
56. F. X. Pi-Sunyer, The role of very-low-calorie diets in obesity, *American Journal of Clinical Nutrition* 56 (1992): 240S–243S.
57. J. A. Kanaley and coauthors, Differential health benefits of weight loss in upper-body and lower-body obese women,

American Journal of Clinical Nutrition 57 (1993): 20–26.
58. J. P. Foreyt and G. K. Goodrick, Weight management without dieting, *Nutrition Today*, March/April 1993, pp. 4–9.
59. M. Shah and coauthors, Comparison of a low-fat ad libitum complex-carbohydrate diet with a low-energy diet in moderately obese women, *American Journal of Clinical Nutrition* 59 (1994): 980–984.
60. L. Lissner, Dietary fat and the regulation of energy intake in human subjects, *American Journal of Clinical Nutrition* 46 (1987): 886–892; A Kendall and coauthors, Weight loss on a low-fat diet: Consequences of the imprecision of the control of food intake in humans, *American Journal of Clinical Nutrition* 53 (1991): 1124–1129; L. Sheppard, A. R. Kristal, and L. H. Kushi, Weight loss in women participating in a randomized trial of low-fat diets, *American Journal of Clinical Nutrition* 54 (1991): 821–828.
61. C. N. Boozer, A. Brasseur, and R. L. Atkinson, Dietary fat affects weight loss and adiposity during energy restriction in rats, *American Journal of Clinical Nutrition* 58 (1993): 846–852.
62. Sheppard, Kristal, and Kushi, 1991; T. E. Prewitt and coauthors, Changes in body weight, body composition, and energy intake in women fed high- and low-fat diets, *American Journal of Clinical Nutrition* 54 (1991): 304–310.
63. R. Ross, H. Pedwell, and J. Rissanen, Effects of energy restriction and exercise on skeletal muscle and adipose tissue in women as measured by magnetic resonance imaging, *American Journal of Clinical Nutrition* 61 (1995): 1179–1185; S. B. Racette and coauthors, Effects of aerobic exercise and dietary carbohydrate on energy expenditure and body composition during weight reduction in obese women, *American Journal of Clinical Nutrition* 61 (1995): 486–494; D. D. Hensrud and coauthors, A prospective study of weight maintenance in obese subjects reduced to normal body weight without weight-loss training, *American Journal of Clinical Nutrition* 60 (1994): 688–694; Haus and coauthors, 1994; S. Kayman, W. Bruvold, and J. S. Stern, Maintenance and relapse after weight loss in women: Behavioral aspects, *American Journal of Clinical Nutrition* 52 (1990): 800–807.
64. S. B. Racette and coauthors, Exercise enhances dietary compliance during moderate energy restriction in obese women, *American Journal of Clinical Nutrition* 62 (1995): 345–349.
65. M. Grediagin and coauthors, Exercise intensity does not effect body composition change in untrained, moderately overfat women, *Journal of the American Dietetic Association* 95 (1995): 661–665.
66. J. P. Flatt, Biochemistry of energy expenditure, in *Obesity*, eds. P. Björntorp and B. N. Brodoff (Philadelphia: J. B. Lippincott, 1992), pp. 100–116.
67. Garrow, 1992.
68. W. D. McArdle, F. I. Katch, and V. L. Katch, *Exercise Physiology: Energy, Nutrition, and Human Performance*, 2nd ed. (Philadelphia: Lea & Febiger, 1991), pp. 634–655.

Eating Disorders—Anorexia Nervosa and Bulimia Nervosa

For some people, dieting to lose weight progresses to a dangerous and obsessive point. An estimated 2 million people in the United States, primarily girls and young women, suffer from the eating disorders anorexia nervosa and bulimia nervosa (the glossary on p. 336 defines these and related terms). Many more do not meet the specific criteria that define these disorders but have "dieted" to the point of endangering health. Psychologists refer to these cases as "eating disorders not otherwise specified."[1]

Why do so many people in our society suffer from these disorders? Some researchers speculate that our society's excessive pressure to be thin is to blame. By making thinness the ideal, society pushes people to view normal healthy body weight as fat. Then healthy people who perceive themselves as fat adopt unhealthy eating behaviors to battle this imaginary problem. Some researchers have uncovered neurological links with depression and impulsive behaviors, and still others believe the cause to be an inability to cope. They agree that the disorders are most likely multifactorial and that treatment requires a multidisciplinary approach that addresses two sets of issues and behaviors: those relating to food and weight and those involving relationships with oneself and others.[2] The nutrition component of treatment requires both dietary intervention and education.

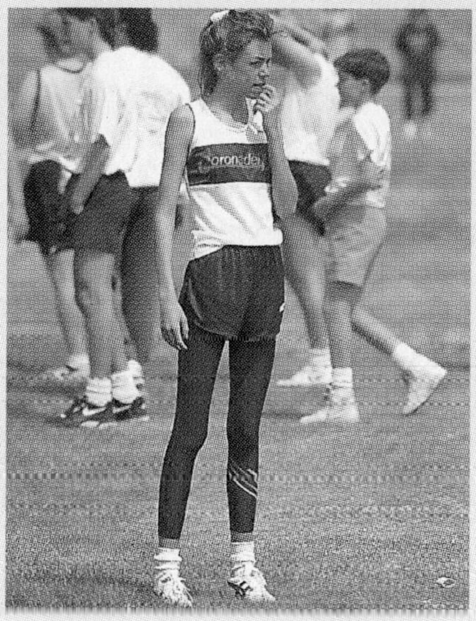

People with anorexia nervosa see themselves as fat, even when they are dangerously underweight.

ANOREXIA NERVOSA

Julie is 18 years old. She is a superachiever in school and a fine dancer. She watches her diet with great care, and she exercises and practices ballet daily, maintaining a heroic schedule of self-discipline. She is thin, but she is not satisfied with her weight and is determined to lose more. She is 5 feet 6 inches tall and weighs 85 pounds. She has anorexia nervosa.

Julie is unaware that she is undernourished, and she sees no need to obtain treatment. She stopped menstruating (developed amenorrhea) several months ago and has become moody and easily depressed. She insists that she is too fat, although her eyes are sunk in deep hollows in her face. She has recently been told by her dance master that her performance is not up to her potential; she blames this on a stress fracture that is slow to heal.[3] Julie denies that she is ever tired, although she is close to physical exhaustion, and she no longer sleeps easily. Her family is concerned, and though reluctant to push her, they have finally insisted that she see a psychiatrist. Julie's psychiatrist has diagnosed anorexia nervosa and prescribed group therapy as a start, but warns that if she does not begin to gain weight soon she will need to be hospitalized.

Characteristics of Anorexia Nervosa

Most people with anorexia nervosa are women and girls from educated, middle- or upper-class families. Men account for only about 5 to 10 percent of cases, although many more report that their most powerful fear is of gaining weight or becoming fat.[4] Among male athletes and dancers, eating disorders are much more common, possibly equaling the incidence among their female peers.[5] Athletes, in general, seem to be vulnerable to eating disorders.[6] To succeed in competition, athletes must often meet stringent weight requirements. Competitors often report being terrified of becoming fat, being obsessed with food, and using laxatives in an attempt to control weight.[7] Ballet dancers, jockeys, wrestlers, distance runners, gymnasts, and others whose body weight and appearance are frequently judged in comparison with an "ideal" are especially prone to develop problems. Chapter 14 revisits the topic of eating disorders in athletes.

Coaches, trainers, and especially parents contribute to eating disorders.[8] Such authority figures are likely to be critical and to overvalue outward appearances while under-

Glossary

anorexia nervosa: an eating disorder characterized by a refusal to maintain a minimally normal body weight and a distortion in perception of body shape and weight, most commonly seen in teenage girls and young women.
an = without
orex = mouth
nervos = of nervous origin

bulimia nervosa: an eating disorder characterized by repeated episodes of binge eating usually followed by self-induced vomiting, misuse of laxatives or diuretics, fasting, or excessive exercise.
buli = ox

cathartic: a strong laxative.

eating disorder: a disturbance in eating behavior that jeopardizes a person's physical or psychological health.

emetic (em-ETT-ic): an agent that causes vomiting.

valuing inner self-esteem. Family patterns often include parents who oppose one another's authority and vacillate between defending the anorexic child's behavior and condemning it, confusing the child and disrupting normal parental control.[9] In the extreme, parents may even be abusive. Julie is a perfectionist, and her parents expect perfection. She works hard to please her parents and identifies so strongly with their ideals and goals that she sometimes feels she has no identity of her own. She feels controlled by others, yet she earnestly desires to control her own destiny. When she does not eat, she gains control.

How can a person as thin as Julie continue to starve herself? Julie uses tremendous discipline to strictly limit her portions of low-kcalorie foods. She will deny her hunger, telling you how full she is after having eaten only a half-dozen carrot sticks. She can recite the kcalorie cost of dozens of foods and of as many exercises. If she feels that she has gained an ounce of weight, she runs or jumps rope until she is sure she has exercised it off. If she fears she has eaten too much, she takes laxatives to hasten the passage of food from her system. Her other ways of staying thin are so effective that she is unaware that laxatives have no effect on body fat. She is desperately hungry. In fact, she is starving, but she doesn't eat because her need for self-control dominates. Her obsession with dieting accelerates; the more weight she loses, the more she wants to lose.

Many people, on learning of this disorder, say they wish they had "a touch" of it to get thin. They mistakenly think that people with anorexia nervosa feel no hunger. They also fail to comprehend the psychological and physical pain associated with the condition.

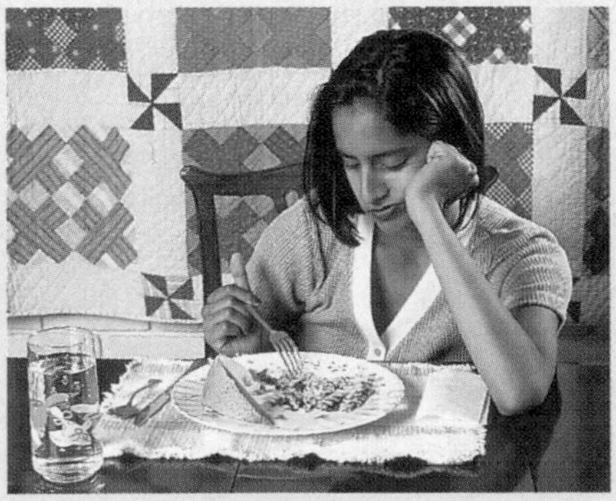

People with anorexia nervosa may reluctantly eat small amounts of low-kcalorie foods.

Central to the diagnosis of anorexia nervosa is a distorted body image that overestimates the person's own body fatness. When Julie looks at herself in the mirror, she sees her 85-pound body as fat. The more Julie overestimates her body size, the more resistant she is to treatment, and the more unwilling to examine her faulty values and misconceptions. Malnutrition itself is known to affect brain functioning and judgment in this way. Table H9–1 shows the criteria that professionals use to diagnose anorexia nervosa.

Anorexia nervosa cannot be self-diagnosed. Nearly everyone in our society is engaged in the pursuit of thinness, and denial runs high among people with anorexia nervosa. Some women have all the attitudes and behaviors associated with the condition, but without the weight loss.

Anorexia nervosa damages the body much as starvation does. In fact, after a few months, most people with anorexia nervosa have protein-energy malnutrition (PEM) that is similar to marasmus.[10] Victims are dying to be thin—quite literally. In young people, growth ceases and normal development falters. They lose so much lean tissue that basal metabolic rate slows, an effect that may remain even after treatment and regain of weight.[11] In athletes, the loss of lean tissue affects physical performance unfavorably. Hormonal changes and nutrient deprivation compromise bone density and lead to stress fractures.[12] Losses of bone density are especially pronounced in female athletes who cease menstruating because of overtraining. In fact, eating disorders, premature bone loss, and irregular menstruation are a common triple threat to

Table H9–1

Criteria for Diagnosis of Anorexia Nervosa

A person with anorexia nervosa demonstrates the following:

A. Refusal to maintain body weight at or above a minimal normal weight for age and height (e.g., weight loss leading to maintenance of body weight less than 85% of that expected; or failure to make expected weight gain during period of growth, leading to body weight less than 85% of that expected).

B. Intense fear of gaining weight or becoming fat, even though underweight.

C. Disturbance in the way in which one's body weight or shape is experienced, undue influence of body weight or shape on self-evaluation, or denial of the seriousness of the current low body weight.

D. In females past puberty, amenorrhea, i.e., the absence of at least three consecutive menstrual cycles. (A woman is considered to have amenorrhea if her periods occur only following hormone, e.g., estrogen, administration.)

Two types:

Restricting type: During the episode of anorexia nervosa, the person does not regularly engage in binge eating or purging behavior (i.e., self-induced vomiting or the misuse of laxatives, diuretics, or enemas).

Binge eating/purging type: During the episode of anorexia nervosa, the person regularly engages in binge eating or purging behavior (i.e., self-induced vomiting or the misuse of laxatives, diuretics, or enemas).

Source: Reprinted with permission from the *Diagnostic and Statistical Manual of Mental Disorders*, 4th ed. (Washington, D.C.: American Psychiatric Association, 1994).

overtrained female athletes.[13] Additionally, the heart pumps inefficiently and irregularly, the heart muscle becomes weak and thin, the chambers diminish in size, and the blood pressure falls. Electrolytes that help to regulate heartbeat become unbalanced. Many deaths occur due to multiple organ system failure.

Starvation brings other physical consequences: impaired immune response, anemia, and a loss of digestive functions that worsens malnutrition. Peristalsis becomes sluggish, the stomach empties slowly, and the lining of the intestinal tract atrophies. The deteriorated GI tract fails to provide sufficient absorptive surfaces and digestive enzymes for handling any food the victim may eat. The pancreas slows its production of digestive enzymes. The person who resumes eating ample food may have diarrhea, further worsening malnutrition.

Other effects of starvation include altered blood lipids, high blood vitamin A and vitamin E, low blood proteins, dry thin skin, abnormal nerve functioning, reduced bone density, low body temperature, low blood pressure, and the development of fine body hair (the body's attempt to keep warm). The electrical activity of the brain becomes abnormal, and insomnia is common. Both women and men lose their sex drives.

Women with anorexia nervosa develop amenorrhea (it is one of the diagnostic criteria). In one-third to one-half of all cases, that symptom precedes the weight loss.[14] Anorexia nervosa delays the onset of menstruation in young girls. Menstrual periods typically resume with recovery, although some women never restart even after they have gained weight. Should an underweight woman with anorexia nervosa become pregnant, she is likely to give birth to an underweight baby—and low-birthweight babies face many health problems (as Chapter 15 explains).[15]

Treatment in Anorexia Nervosa

Treatment artfully combines medical, psychosocial, and dietary facets to initiate and sustain weight gain with psychological techniques to resolve personal and family problems. Teams of physicians, nurses, psychiatrists, family therapists, and dietitians work together to treat people with anorexia nervosa.

The diet needs to be tailored individually to each client's needs; appropriate diet is crucial to recovery. Clients are seldom willing to feed themselves, but if they are, they may recover without other interventions. Table H9–2 (on p. 338) lists principles of nutrition intervention in anorexia nervosa.

Because anorexia nervosa is like starvation physically, health care professionals classify clients based on indicators of protein-energy malnutrition.* Low-risk clients need nutrition counseling. Intermediate-risk clients may need supplements such as high-kcalorie, high-protein formulas in addition to regular meals, but they may not have to be

*Indicators of protein-energy malnutrition: a low percentage of body fat, low serum albumin, low serum transferrin, and impaired immune reactions.

Table H9–2

Principles of Nutrition Intervention in Anorexia Nervosa

- Increase food energy intake slowly (adding 200 kcal/week).
- Prescribe well-balanced diets, with *some* individual variations according to client preferences (e.g., vegetarian).
- Give multiple vitamin-mineral supplements at RDA levels.
- Enhance elimination with dietary fiber from grain sources.
- Reduce sensations of bloating with small, frequent feedings.
- In behavioral programs, link rewards to food energy intake, not to weight gain.
- Use liquid supplements when the client cannot achieve desired intake with solid food.
- Reduce satiety sensations by offering cold or room-temperature foods and finger foods (e.g., snacks).
- Provide interactive nutrition counseling as an ongoing process.
- Reduce excessive caffeine intake.
- Provide parenteral nutritional support only in severe states of ill health, malnutrition, and wasting.

Source: Adapted from C. L. Rock and J. Yager, Nutrition and eating disorders: A primer for clinicians, *International Journal of Eating Disorders* 6 (1987): 276, as cited in *Nutrition and the M.D.*, July 1988, with permission. Reprinted with permission of John Wiley & Sons, Inc., copyright 1987.

hospitalized. High-risk clients may requires hospitalization, and tube feeding may be necessary to forestall death. This step causes psychological trauma.[16] Drugs are commonly prescribed, but to date, they play a limited role in treatment.

The goals of treatment are simultaneously to facilitate weight gain and to resolve underlying personal and family problems. The first dietary objective is to stop weight loss while establishing regular eating patterns. The diet should include foods from each of the food groups, with portion sizes gradually increasing as energy intake increases. Because body weight is low and fear of weight gain is high, initial food intake may be small. At first, energy intake may be as low as whatever the person has become accustomed to, but ideally it will at least meet basal metabolic needs. As eating becomes more comfortable, energy intake should increase gradually. Vitamin and mineral supplements may be necessary to restore nutrient losses. Physicians and clients need to realize that weight gain may be difficult, especially during the first week of treatment, perhaps because the resting metabolic rate of people with anorexia nervosa is so high.[17]

Denial is so common among those with anorexia nervosa that few seek treatment on their own. Of those who are treated, about half recover fully.[18] They can maintain a healthy body weight, and many of the women begin menstruating again, although weight gain alone is not always sufficient in restoring menstruation.[19] The other half have poor or fair treatment outcomes, relapsing back into abnormal eating behaviors to some extent.[20] Over 10 percent of those treated for anorexia nervosa die—most commonly from starvation, electrolyte imbalance, or suicide.

Before drawing conclusions about someone who is extremely thin or who eats very little, remember that diagnosis and treatment require professional attention. People who are seeking help with anorexia nervosa, either for themselves or for others, can call the National Association of Anorexia Nervosa and Associated Disorders for information.*

BULIMIA NERVOSA

Kelly is a charming, intelligent, 20-year-old flight attendant of normal weight who thinks constantly about food. She alternates between starving herself and secretly binge eating; then, when she has eaten too much, she makes herself vomit. Few people would fail to recognize these symptoms as those of bulimia nervosa.

Bulimia nervosa is distinct from anorexia nervosa and is more prevalent, although the true incidence is difficult to establish because denial is equally common in this disease.[21] More men suffer from bulimia nervosa than from anorexia nervosa, but it is still more common in women.[22] The secretive nature of bulimic behaviors makes recognition of the problem difficult; once recognized, diagnosis is based on the criteria listed in Table H9–3.

Families of bulimic people often have unusually close emotional ties between members. They may be overcontrolling and intermeshed in ways that stifle individual growth and development.[23] If the member with bulimia nervosa begins taking

*Phone numbers and addresses are in Appendix F.

Table H9–3

Criteria for Diagnosis of Bulimia Nervosa

A person with bulimia nervosa demonstrates the following:

A. Recurrent episodes of binge eating. An episode of binge eating is characterized by both of the following:
   1. Eating, in a discrete period of time (e.g., within any two-hour period), an amount of food that is definitely larger than most people would eat during a similar period of time and under similar circumstances.
   2. A sense of lack of control over eating during the episode (e.g., a feeling that one cannot stop eating or control what or how much one is eating).

B. Recurrent inappropriate compensatory behavior in order to prevent weight gain, such as self-induced vomiting; misuse of laxatives, diuretics, enemas, or other medications; fasting; or excessive exercise.

C. Binge eating and inappropriate compensatory behaviors both occur, on average, at least twice a week for three months.

D. Self-evaluation unduly influenced by body shape and weight.

E. The disturbance does not occur exclusively during episodes of anorexia nervosa.

Two types:

Purging type: The person regularly engages in self-induced vomiting or the misuse of laxatives, diuretics, or enemas.

Nonpurging type: The person uses other inappropriate compensatory behaviors, such as fasting or excessive exercise, but does not regularly engage in self-induced vomiting or the misuse of laxatives, diuretics, or enemas.

Source: Reprinted with permission from *Diagnostic and Statistical Manual of Mental Disorders*, 4th ed. (Washington, D.C.: American Psychiatric Association, 1994).

steps toward recovery, others in the family may feel threatened. Changes in the family structure often meet with resistance, even if such changes would greatly benefit the person with bulimia nervosa. Additionally, the family may have secrets that are hidden from outsiders. Many people with bulimia nervosa report having been abused sexually or physically by family members or family friends.

Characteristics of Bulimia Nervosa

Like the typical person with bulimia nervosa, Kelly is single, female, and white. She is well educated and close to her ideal body weight, although her weight fluctuates 10 pounds or so—up and down—over a few weeks. As a flight attendant, she is required to "make weight"—that is, to weigh no more than a certain cutoff weight slightly below the weight that her body maintains naturally.

Kelly seldom lets her eating disorder interfere with work or other activities, although many bingers do. From early childhood she has been a high achiever and emotionally dependent on her parents. As a young teen, Kelly cycled on and off crash diets but could never maintain an appropriate weight. Kelly feels anxious at social events and cannot easily establish personal relationships. She is sometimes depressed and is often impulsive. Some people with bulimia nervosa abuse drugs, steal compulsively (kleptomania), or are sexually promiscuous.

Like the person with anorexia nervosa, the person with bulimia nervosa spends much time thinking about her body weight and food. Her preoccupation with food manifests itself in secretive binge-eating episodes, which usually progress through several emotional stages: anticipation and planning, anxiety, urgency to begin, rapid and uncontrollable consumption of food, relief and relaxation, disappointment, and finally shame or disgust.

A bulimic binge is not like normal eating. It is not primarily a response to hunger; it is a compulsion to eat. Food is not consumed for its nutritional value. A typical binge occurs periodically, in secret, usually at night, and lasts an hour or more. A binge frequently follows a period of rigid dieting, so that eating is accelerated by hunger. During a binge, Kelly consumes thousands of kcalories of food. She typically chooses cookies, cakes, and ice cream—and she eats the entire bag of cookies, the whole cake, and every last spoonful of ice cream. These foods are easy-to-eat, low-fiber, smooth-textured, high-fat, and especially, high-carbohydrate foods. After the binge, Kelly pays the price with swollen hands and feet, bloating, fatigue, headache, nausea, and pain.

Binges are typically followed by self-induce vomiting, fasting, or the misuse of laxatives, diuretics, or enemas. These purging behaviors are often accompanied by feelings of shame or guilt. Hence a vicious cycle develops: negative self-perceptions followed by dieting, binging, and purging, which in turn lead to negative self-perceptions (see Figure H9–1).[24] Bulimic behaviors often begin in late adolescence or early adulthood after a long series of various unsuccessful weight-reduction diets. People with bulimia nervosa commonly follow a pattern of restrictive dieting interspersed with binge eating and purging behaviors and experience weight fluctuations of more than 10 pounds up and down over short periods of time.

On first glance, purging seems to offer a quick and easy solution to the problems of unwanted kcalories and body weight. Many people perceive such behavior as neutral or even positive, when, in fact, binge eating and purging have serious physical consequences.[25] Signs of subclinical malnutrition are evident in a compromised immune system.[26] Fluid and electrolyte imbalance caused by vomiting or diarrhea can lead to abnormal heart rhythms and injury to the kidneys, which have to cope with the altered balance. Urinary tract infections can lead to kidney failure. Vomiting causes irritation and infection of the pharynx, esophagus, and salivary glands; erosion of the teeth; and dental caries. The esophagus may rupture or tear, as may the stomach. Sometimes the eyes become red from pressure during vomiting. The hands may be bruised or cut by the teeth while inducing vomiting. Some people induce vomiting by using emetics—drugs that are intended as first aid for poisoning. Overuse of emetics can lead to heart failure. Others use cathartics—strong laxatives that can injure the lower intestinal tract.

Unlike Julie, Kelly is aware that her behavior is abnormal, and she is deeply ashamed of it. Feeling inadequate ("I can't even control by eating"), she tends to be passive and to look to others, primarily men, for confirmation of her sense of worth. When she is rejected either in reality or in her imagination, her bulimia nervosa becomes worse. Then Kelly's depression may deepen, and she may seek solace in drug or alcohol abuse.

Figure H9–01

The Vicious Cycle of Restrictive Dieting and Binge Eating

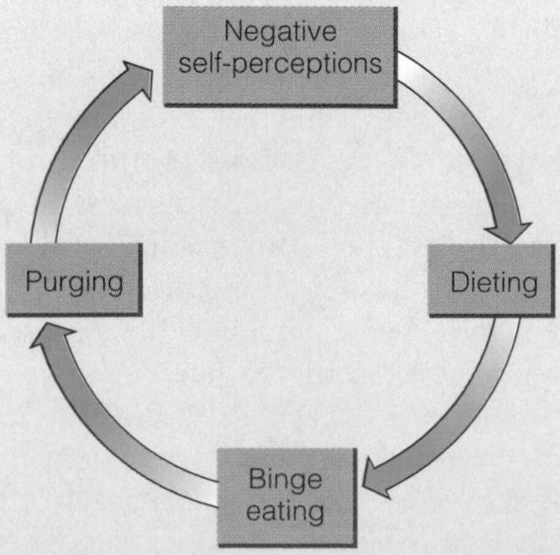

Treatment in Bulimia Nervosa

The dietary goals of treatment are to help clients gain control over food, establish regular eating patterns, and restore nutritional health.

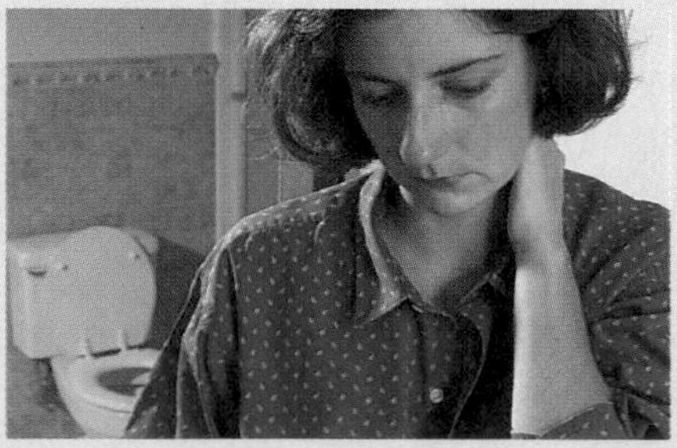

Bulimic binges are often followed by self-induced vomiting and feelings of shame or disgust.

Energy intake should not be severely restricted because restrictive weight-loss dieting is a strong trigger to binge. Rather than cyclic weight gains and losses, maintenance is a must for recovery. The person needs to learn to eat a quantity of nutritious food sufficient to nourish the body. Table H9–4 offers diet recommendations for the treatment of bulimia nervosa.

A mental health professional should be on the treatment team. Clinical depression is common in people with bulimia nervosa, and the rates of alcohol, marijuana, and cigarette abuse are high.[27] Some physicians prescribe the antidepressant drug fluoxetine in the treatment of bulimia nervosa.* Another drug that may be useful in the management of bulimia nervosa is naloxone, an opiate antagonist that suppresses the consumption of sweet and high-fat foods in binge-eaters.[28]

Anorexia nervosa and bulimia nervosa are distinct eating disorders, yet they sometimes overlap in important ways.[29] Victims of both disorders share an overconcern with body weight and the tendency to drastically undereat; many perceive foods as "forbidden" and "give in" to an eating binge. The two disorders can also appear in the same person, or one can lead to the other.

BINGE-EATING DISORDER

Cheryl is a 40-year-old schoolteacher who has been overweight all her life. Her friends and family are forever encouraging her to lose weight, and she has come to believe

*Fluoxetine is marketed under the trade name Prozac.

Table H9–4

Diet Recommendations for Bulimia Nervosa

- Avoid finger foods; eat foods that require the use of utensils.
- Enhance satiety by eating warm foods.
- Include vegetables, salad, and/or fruit at meals to prolong eating time.
- Choose whole-grain and high-fiber breads and cereals to maximize bulk.
- Eat a well-balanced diet and meals, consisting of a variety of foods.
- Use foods that are naturally divided into portions, such as potatoes (rather than rice or pasta); 4- and 8-ounce containers of yogurt or cottage cheese; precut steak or chicken parts; and frozen entreés.
- Include foods containing ample complex carbohydrates (for satiety) and some fat (to slow gastric emptying).
- Eat meals and snacks sitting down.
- Plan meals and snacks, and record plans in a food diary prior to eating.

Source: Adapted from C. L. Rock and J. Yager, Nutrition and eating disorders: A primer for clinicians, *International Journal of Eating Disorders* 6 (1987): 276, as cited in *Nutrition and the M.D.*, July 1988, with permission. Reprinted with permission of John Wiley & Sons, Inc., copyright 1987.

that if she only had more willpower, dieting would work. She periodically gives dieting her best shot—restricting energy intake for a day or two only to succumb to uncontrollable cravings, especially for high-fat foods. Like Cheryl, up to half of the obese people who try to lose weight periodically binge; unlike people with bulimia nervosa, however, they typically do not purge. Such an eating disorder does not meet the criteria for either anorexia nervosa or bulimia nervosa—yet such compulsive overeating is a problem. The 1994 American Psychiatric Association's manual includes binge eating under the category "eating disorders not otherwise specified." Table H9–5 (on p. 342) lists criteria for unspecified eating disorders, including binge eating. Obesity alone is not an eating disorder.

Clinicians note differences between people with bulimia nervosa and those with binge-eating disorder. People with binge eating disorder consume less during a binge, rarely purge, and exert less restraint during times of dieting. Similarities also exist, including feeling out of control, disgusted, depressed, embarrassed, guilty, or distressed because of their self-perceived gluttony.[30]

There are also differences between obese binge eaters and obese people who do not binge. Those with the binge eating disorder report higher rates of self-loathing, disgust about body size, depression, and anxiety.[31] Their eating habits differ as well. Obese binge eaters tend to consume more kcalories and more dessert and snack-type foods during regular meals and binges than obese people who do not binge.[32]

Binge eating is a behavioral disorder that can be resolved with treatment. Resolving such behavior may not bring weight loss, but it may make participation in weight-control programs easier. It also improves physical health, mental health, and the chances of success in breaking the cycle of rapid weight losses and gains.

EATING DISORDERS IN SOCIETY

Eating disorders have complex causes. A person's psychological problems develop within the context of society. Proof that society plays a role in eating disorders is found in their demographic distribution—they are known only in developed nations, and they become more prevalent as wealth increases and food becomes plentiful.

Some people point to the vomitoriums of ancient times and claim that bulimia nervosa is not new, but the two are actually distinct. Ancient people were eating for pleasure, without guilt, and in the company of others; they vomited so that they could rejoin the feast. Bulimia nervosa is a disorder of isolation and is often accompanied by low self-esteem.

A food-centered society that favors thinness puts people in a bind. Families may encourage hearty eating and socializing around the dinner table. Party hosts take pride in the delicacies they serve, and guests are obliged to indulge. A child raised in such a setting and also encouraged to aspire to a thin ideal may see little alternative but to celebrate by indulging in food and then to vomit, crash diet, or starve to "undo" possible weight gain. Then, starving and guilty, but still reluctant to appear to be a glutton, the child may begin eating uncontrollably to relieve a desperate hunger.

There is no doubt that our society sets unrealistic ideals for body

Table H9–5

Unspecified Eating Disorders, including Binge Eating Disorder

Criteria for Diagnosis of Unspecified Eating Disorders, in General

Many people have eating disorders but do not meet all the criteria to be classified as having anorexia nervosa or bulimia nervosa. Some examples include those who:

A. Meet all of the criteria for anorexia nervosa, except irregular menses.
B. Meet all of the criteria for anorexia nervosa, except that their current weights fall within the normal ranges.
C. Meet all of the criteria for bulimia nervosa, except that binges occur less frequently than stated in the criteria.
D. Are of normal body weight and who compensate inappropriately for eating small amounts of food (example: self-induced vomiting after eating two cookies).
E. Repeatedly chew food, but spit it out without swallowing.
F. Have recurrent episodes of binge eating but who do not compensate as do those with bulimia nervosa.

Criteria for Diagnosis of Binge-Eating Disorder, Specifically

A person with a binge-eating disorder demonstrates the following:

A. Recurrent episodes of binge eating. An episode of binge eating is characterized by both of the following:
   1. Eating, in a discrete period of time (e.g., within any two-hour period) an amount of food that is definitely larger than most people would eat in a similar period of time under similar circumstances.
   2. A sense of lack of control over eating during the episode (e.g., a feeling that one cannot stop eating or control what or how much one is eating).
B. Binge-eating episodes are associated with at least three of the following:
   1. Eating much more rapidly than normal.
   2. Eating until feeling uncomfortably full.
   3. Eating large amounts of food when not feeling physically hungry.
   4. Eating alone because of being embarrassed by how much one is eating.
   5. Feeling disgusted with oneself, depressed, or very guilty after overeating.
C. The binge eating causes marked distress.
D. The binge eating occurs, on average, at least twice a week for six months.
E. The binge eating is not associated with the regular use of inappropriate compensatory behaviors (e.g., purging, fasting, excessive exercise) and does not occur exclusively during the course of anorexia nervosa or bulimia nervosa.

Source: Reprinted with permission from American Psychiatric Association, *Diagnostic and Statistical Manual of Mental Disorders*, 4th ed. (Washington, D.C.: American Psychiatric Association, 1994).

weight, especially in women, and devalues those who do not conform to them. Even professionals, including physicians and dietitians, are prone to praise people for losing weight and to suggest weight loss to people who do not need it for their health. As a result, even beautiful, normal-weight preteen girls are already worried that they are too fat. Two-thirds of adolescent girls and one-third of adolescent boys are dissatisfied with their body weight and shape.[33] Characteristics of disordered eating such as restrained eating, fasting, binge eating, purging, fear of fatness, and distortion of body image are extraordinarily common among young, white, middle- and upper-class girls.[34] Most are "on diets," and many are poorly nourished. Some eat too little food to support normal growth; thus they miss out on their adolescent growth spurts and may never catch up. Many eat so little that hunger propels them into binge-purge cycles. Magazines, newspapers, and television all convey the message that to be thin is to be beautiful and happy. Anorexia nervosa and bulimia nervosa are not a form of rebellion against these unreasonable expectations, but rather an exaggerated acceptance of them.

Perhaps a person's best defense against these disorders is to learn to appreciate his or her own uniqueness. When people discover and honor the body's real needs, they become unwilling to sacrifice health for conformity. The author Eda LeShan described her recovery from overeating this way: "Deep inside there had always been a small child begging for my attention. All I gave her was food. Now I give her love."[35] To respect and value oneself may be lifesaving.

NOTES

1. American Psychiatric Association: *DSM-IV* (Washington, D.C.: American Psychiatric Association, 1994).

2. Position of The American Dietetic Association: Nutrition intervention in the treatment of anorexia nervosa, bulimia nervosa, and binge

eating, *Journal of the American Dietetic Association* 94 (1994): 902–907.
3. N. T. Frusztajer and coauthors, Nutrition and the incidence of stress fractures in ballet dancers, *American Journal of Clinical Nutrition* 51 (1990): 779–783.
4. American Psychiatric Association, 1994; A. R. Lucas and D. M. Huse, Behavioral disorders affecting food intake: Anorexia nervosa and bulimia nervosa, in *Modern Nutrition in Health and Disease*, eds. M. E. Shils, J. A. Olson, and M. Shike (Philadelphia: Lea & Febiger, 1994), pp. 977–983; M. J. Devlin and B. T. Walsh, Anorexia nervosa and bulimia, in *Obesity*, eds. P. Björntorp and B. N. Brodoff (Philadelphia: J. B. Lippincott, 1992), pp. 436–444; S. N. Collier and coauthors, Assessment of attitudes about weight and dieting among college-aged individuals, *Journal of the American Dietetic Association* 90 (1990): 276–278.
5. "Anorexia athletica," Special report on nutrition and the athlete, *Sports Medicine Digest*, 1989, p. 10; S. N. Steen and K. D. Brownell, Patterns of weight loss and regain in wrestlers: Has the tradition changed? *Medicine and Science in Sports and Exercise* 22 (1990): 762–768.
6. K. K. Yeager and coauthors, The female athlete triad: Disordered eating, amenorrhea, osteoporosis, *Medicine and Science in Sports and Exercise* 25 (1993): 775–777.
7. J. L. Walbery and C. S. Johnston, Menstrual function and eating behavior in female recreational weight lifters and competitive body builders, *Medicine and Science in Sports and Exercise* 23 (1991): 30–36.
8. M. T. Depalma and coauthors, Weight control practices of lightweight football players, *Medicine and Science in Sports and Exercise* 25 (1993): 694–701; B. J. Larson, Relationship of family communication patterns to Eating Disorder Inventory scores in adolescent girls, *Journal of the American Dietetic Association* 91 (1991): 1065–1067.
9. G. Szmukler and C. Dare, Family therapy of early-onset, short-history anorexia nervosa, in *Family Approaches in Treatment of Eating Disorders*, eds. D. B. Woodside and L. Shekter-Wolfson (Washington, D.C.: American Psychiatric Press, 1991), pp. 25–47.
10. P. Barbe and coauthors, Sex-hormone-binding globulin and protein-energy malnutrition indexes as indicators of nutritional status in women with anorexia nervosa, *American Journal of Clinical Nutrition* 57 (1993): 319–322.
11. R. C. Casper and coauthors, Total daily energy expenditure and activity level in anorexia nervosa, *American Journal of Clinical Nutrition* 53 (1991): 1143–1150; L. Scalfi and coauthors, Bioimpedance analysis and resting energy expenditure in undernourished and refed anorectic patients, *European Journal of Clinical Nutrition* 47 (1993): 61–67.
12. R. B. Mazess, H. S. Barden, and E. S. Ohlrich, Skeletal and body-composition effect of anorexia nervosa, *American Journal of Clinical Nutrition* 52 (1990): 438–441; L. K. Bachrach and coauthors, Decreased bone density in adolescent girls with anorexia nervosa, *Pediatrics* 86 (1990): 440–447.
13. R. C. Henderson, Bone health in adolescence: Anorexia and athletic amenorrhea, *Nutrition Today*, March/April 1991, pp. 25–29; F. Munning, Tackling women's health issues, *Physician and Sportsmedicine*, September 1992, p. 33.
14. M. A. Balaa and D. A. Drossman, Anorexia nervosa and bulimia: The eating disorders, *Disease a Month* (Chicago: Year Book Medical Publishers, June 1985), pp. 1–52.
15. Committee on Nutritional Status during Pregnancy and Lactation, *Nutrition during Pregnancy* (Washington, D.C.: National Academy Press, 1990).
16. B. R. Carruth, Adolescence, in *Present Knowledge in Nutrition*, ed. M. L. Brown (Washington, D.C.: International Life Sciences Institute, 1990), pp. 325–332.
17. M. V. Solanto and coauthors, Rate of weight gain of inpatients with anorexia nervosa under two behavioral contracts, *Pediatrics* 93 (1994): 989–991; E. Obarzanek, M. D. Lesem, and D. C. Jimerson, Resting metabolic rate of anorexia nervosa patients during weight gain, *American Journal of Clinical Nutrition* 60 (1994): 666–675.
18. Devlin and Walsh, 1992.
19. E. A. Weltman and coauthors, Weight and menstrual function in patients with eating disorders and cystic fibrosis, *Pediatrics* 85 (1990): 282–287.
20. American Psychiatric Association Workgroup on Eating Disorders, Practice guidelines for eating disorders, I. Disease definition, epidemiology, and natural history, *American Journal of Psychiatry* 150 (1993): 212–228.
21. D. M. Stein, The prevalence of bulimia: A review of empirical research, *Journal of Nutrition Education* 23 (1991): 205–213.
22. American Psychiatric Association, 1994; Devlin and Walsh, 1992.
23. L. G. Roberto, Impasses in the family treatment of bulimia, in Woodside and Shekter-Wolfson, 1991, pp. 69–85.
24. Adapted from D. Newmark-Sztainer, R. Butler, and H. Palti, Dieting and binge eating: Which dieters are at risk? *Journal of the American Dietetic Association* 95 (1995): 586–589.
25. P. W. Meilman, F. A. von Hippel, and M. S. Gaylor, Self-induced vomiting in college women: Its relation to eating, alcohol use, and Greek life, *College Health* 40 (1991): 39–41.
26. A. Marcos, Evaluation of immunocompetence and nutritional status in patients with bulimia nervosa, *American Journal of Clinical Nutrition* 57 (1993): 65–69.
27. J. A. Bushnell and coauthors, Bulimia comorbidity in the general population and in the clinic, *Psychological Medicine* 24 (1994): 605–611; C. M. Bulik, Alcohol use and depression in women with bulimia, *American Journal of Drug and Alcohol Abuse* 13 (1987): 343–355; D. B. Herzog, Are anorexic and bulimic patients depressed? *American Journal of Psychiatry* 141 (1984): 1594–1597.
28. A. Drewnowski and coauthors, Naloxone, an opiate blocker, reduces the consumption of sweet high-fat foods in obese and lean female binge-eaters, *American Journal of Clinical Nutrition* 61 (1995): 1206–1212.
29. C. G. Fairburn and G. T. Wilson, Binge eating: Nature, assessment, and treatment (New York: Guilford Press, 1993).
30. J. P. Foreyt and G. K. Goodrick, Weight management without dieting, *Nutrition Today*, March/April 1993, pp. 4–9; R. L. Spitzer and coauthors, Binge eating disorder: A multisite field trial of the diagnostic criteria, *International Journal of Eating Disorders* 11 (1992): 191–203.
31. American Psychiatric Association, 1994.
32. S. Z. Yanovski and coauthors, Food selection and intake of obese women with binge-eating disorder, *American Journal of Clinical Nutrition* 56 (1992): 975–980.
33. D. C. Moore, Body image and eating behavior in adolescents, *Journal of the American College of Nutrition* 12 (1993): 505–510.
34. Moore, 1993; L. M. Mellin, C. E. Irwin, and S. Scully, Prevalence of disordered eating in girls: A survey of middle-class children, *Journal of the American Dietetic Association* 92 (1992): 851–853.
35. E. LeShan, *Winning the Losing Game: Why I Will Never Be Fat Again* (New York: Crowell, 1979).

Chapter 10

The Water-Soluble Vitamins: B Vitamins and Vitamin C

CONTENTS

MICROGRAPH: Vitamin C, the water-soluble vitamin known for its antioxidant actions

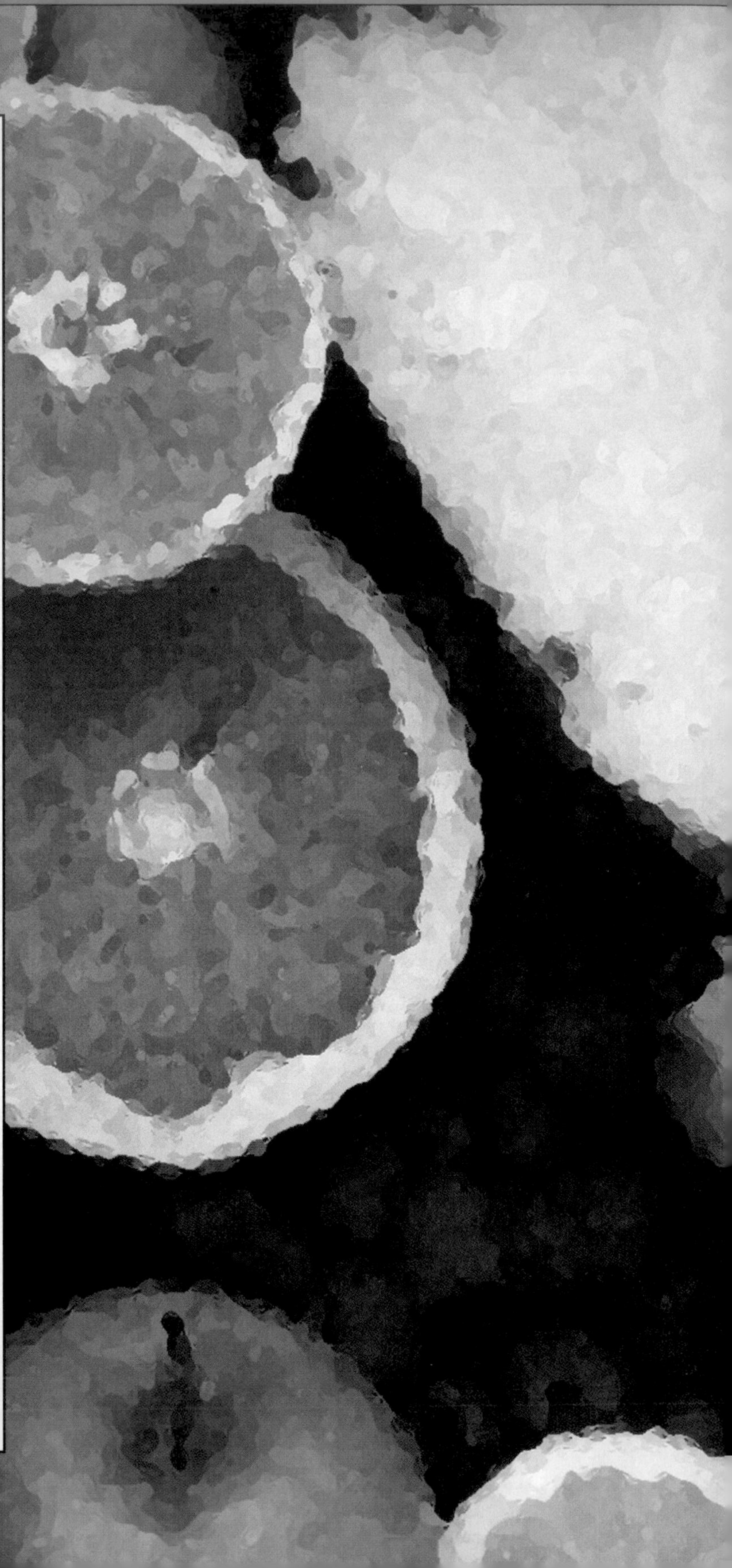

Earlier chapters focused on the energy-yielding nutrients, which play leading roles in the body. The vitamins and minerals are their supporting cast. This chapter begins with an overview of the vitamins and then examines each of the water-soluble vitamins; the next chapter features the fat-soluble vitamins.

The Vitamins—An Overview

The vitamins are powerful substances, as their absence attests. Vitamin A deficiency can cause blindness; a lack of niacin can cause symptoms of mental illness; and a lack of vitamin D can retard bone growth. The consequences of deficiencies are so dire, and the effects of restoring the needed vitamins so dramatic, that people spend billions of dollars every year on vitamin pills to cure a host of ailments (see Highlight 10). Vitamins certainly contribute to sound nutritional health, but they do not cure all ills. Furthermore, vitamin supplements do not offer the many benefits that come from vitamin-rich foods.

Reminder: The *vitamins* are organic, essential nutrients required in minute amounts to perform specific functions that promote growth, reproduction, or the maintenance of health and life.
vita = life
amine = containing nitrogen (the first vitamins discovered contained nitrogen)

The *presence* of the vitamins also attests to their power. Vitamin C not only prevents the deficiency disease scurvy, but also seems to protect against certain types of cancer. Similarly, vitamin E seems to help protect against some facets of cardiovascular disease. The B vitamin folate helps to prevent birth defects. As you will see, the vitamins' roles in supporting optimal health extend far beyond preventing deficiency diseases. In fact, some of the credit given to low-fat diets in preventing disease actually belongs to the vitamins that such diets deliver (see Highlight 11 for more on vitamins in disease prevention). A diet that includes plenty of vegetables, fruits, and grain products is like a coin—the two sides are different but it spends the same. On the one side, such a diet is low in fat; on the other, it provides vitamins in abundance. Both attributes help to maintain health and slow the progression of disease.

The vitamins differ from the carbohydrates, fats, and proteins in the following ways:

- *Structure*. Vitamins are individual units; they are not linked in long chains.
- *Function*. Vitamins do not yield usable energy when broken down; they assist the enzymes that release energy from carbohydrates, fats, and proteins.
- *Food contents*. The amounts of vitamins people ingest daily and the amounts they require are measured in *micrograms* or *milligrams*, rather than grams.

The vitamins are similar to the energy-yielding nutrients, though, in that they are all vital to life, organic, and available in foods.

Precursors Some of the vitamins are available from foods in an inactive form known as precursors, or provitamins. Once inside the body, precursors are changed chemically to an active form of the vitamin. Thus, in measuring a person's vitamin intake, it is important to count both the amount of the active vitamin and the potential amount available from its precursors. The summary tables throughout this chapter and the next identify which vitamins have precursors.

precursors: substances that precede others; with regard to vitamins, compounds that can be converted into active vitamins; also known as **provitamins**.

Organic Nature Because vitamins are organic, they can be destroyed. They can break down and become unable to perform their duties; therefore, they must be handled with care during storage and in cooking. The water-soluble vitamins thiamin, riboflavin, and vitamin C are especially vulnerable. Prolonged heating may destroy as much as 40 percent of the thiamin in food. Riboflavin can be destroyed by the ultraviolet rays of the sun or by fluorescent light; foods stored in transparent glass containers are most likely to lose riboflavin. Oxygen destroys vitamin C, so losses are closely related to the extent to which foods are cut or broken and thereby exposed to air.

The body treats vitamins with respect. It makes special provisions to absorb them, it provides most of them with special protein carriers, and it provides special enzymes to alter their forms so that they can perform different roles.

Solubility As you may recall, carbohydrates and proteins are hydrophilic and lipids are hydrophobic. The vitamins divide along the same lines—the hydrophilic, water-soluble ones are the B vitamins and vitamin C; the hydrophobic, fat-soluble ones are vitamins A, D, E, and K.

Solubility is apparent in the food sources and it affects the body's absorption, transport, storage, and excretion of the vitamins. The water-soluble vitamins are found in the watery compartments of foods; the fat-soluble vitamins usually occur together in the fats and oils of foods. On being absorbed, the water-soluble vitamins move directly into the blood; like fats, the fat-soluble vitamins must first enter the lymph, then the blood. Once in the blood, many of the water-soluble vitamins travel freely; many of the fat-soluble vitamins require protein carriers for transport. Upon reaching the cells, water-soluble vitamins freely circulate in the water-filled compartments of the body; fat-soluble vitamins tend to become trapped in the cells associated with fat. The kidneys, monitoring the blood that flows through them, detect and remove excess water-soluble vitamins, but do not "see" the fat-soluble vitamins. These tend to remain in fat-storage sites in the body rather than being excreted, and so are more likely to reach toxic levels when consumed in excess.

Because the body stores fat-soluble vitamins, they can be eaten in large amounts once in a while and still meet the body's needs over time. Water-soluble vitamins are retained for varying periods in the body; a single day's omission from the diet does not bring on a deficiency, but still, the water-soluble vitamins must be eaten more regularly than the fat-soluble vitamins.

In summary, the vitamins are essential nutrients that are needed in tiny amounts in the diet to both prevent deficiency diseases and support optimal health. The water-soluble vitamins are the B vitamins and vitamin C; the fat-soluble vitamins are vitamins A, D, E, and K. Table 10–1 summarizes the differences between the water-soluble and fat-soluble vitamins.

As each vitamin was discovered, it was given a name and sometimes a letter and number as well. Many of the water-soluble vitamins have multiple names, which has led to some confusion. Table 10–2 lists the standard names; summary tables throughout this chapter provide the common alternative names.[1]

The discussion of B vitamins that follows begins with a brief description of each of them, then offers a look at the ways they work together. Thus a preview of the "trees" is followed by a survey of the "forest."

Table 10–1

Water-Soluble and Fat-Soluble Vitamins Compared

Exceptions occur, but these differences between the water-soluble and fat-soluble vitamins are valid generalizations.

	Water-Soluble Vitamins: B Vitamins and Vitamin C	Fat-Soluble Vitamins: Vitamins A, D, E, and K
Absorption	Directly into the blood.	First into the lymph, then the blood.
Transport	Travel freely.	Many require protein carriers.
Storage	Freely circulate in water-filled parts of the body.	Trapped in the cells associated with fat.
Excretion	Kidneys detect and remove excess in urine.	Less readily excreted; tend to remain in fat-storage sites.
Toxicity	Unlikely to reach toxic levels when consumed in excess.	Likely to reach toxic levels when consumed in excess.
Requirements	Needed in frequent, small doses.	Needed in periodic doses.

Table 10–2

The Water-Soluble Vitamins

- B vitamins
  - Thiamin
  - Riboflavin
  - Niacin
  - Biotin
  - Pantothenic acid
  - Vitamin B_6
  - Folate
  - Vitamin B_{12}
- Vitamin C

The B Vitamins—As Individuals

Despite advertisements that claim otherwise, the vitamins are not fuels that give you energy. The energy-yielding nutrients—carbohydrate, fat, and protein—are used for fuel; the B vitamins help the body to use that fuel.

It is true, though, that without B vitamins the body would lack energy. Many of the B vitamins serve as coenzymes to the enzymes that release energy from carbohydrate, fat, and protein. Figure 10–1 illustrates coenzyme action.

Other B vitamins play other indispensable roles in metabolism. One assists enzymes that metabolize amino acids; two others help cells to multiply. Among

- The B vitamins that serve in coenzymes in energy pathways: thiamin, riboflavin, niacin, pantothenic acid, and biotin.
- The B vitamin that serves in coenzymes in amino acid metabolism: vitamin B_6.

Figure 10–1

Coenzyme Action

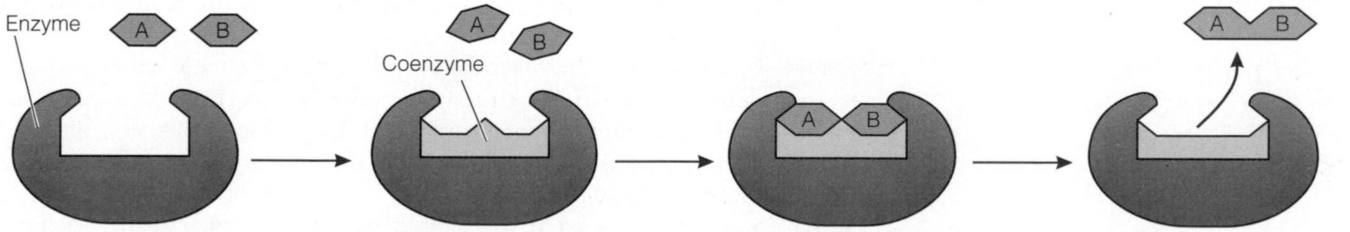

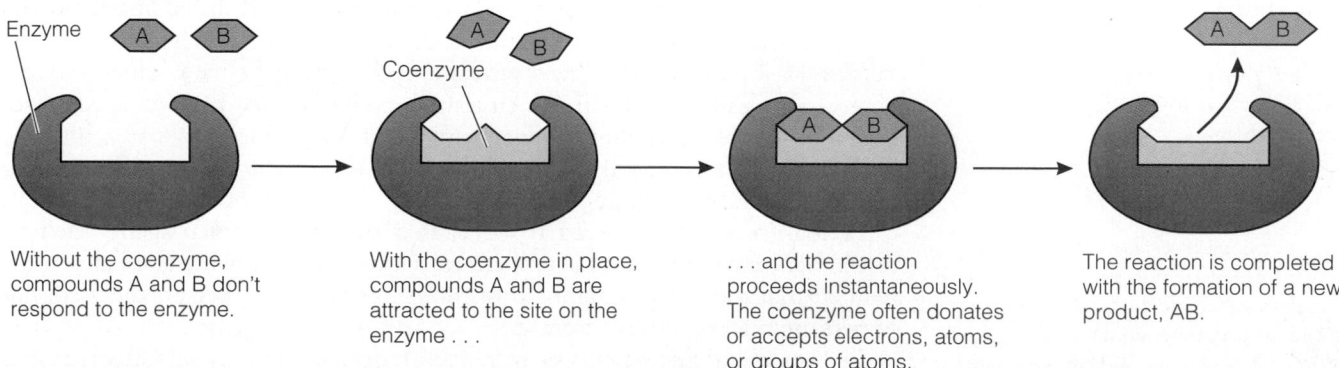

Without the coenzyme, compounds A and B don't respond to the enzyme.

With the coenzyme in place, compounds A and B are attracted to the site on the enzyme . . .

. . . and the reaction proceeds instantaneously. The coenzyme often donates or accepts electrons, atoms, or groups of atoms.

The reaction is completed with the formation of a new product, AB.

- The B vitamins that help cells to divide: folate and vitamin B_{12}.

Reminder: A *coenzyme* is a small organic molecule that associates closely with many enzymes; many B vitamins form an integral part of coenzymes.

these cells are the red blood cells and the cells lining the GI tract—cells that deliver energy to all the others.

The vitamin portion of a coenzyme allows a chemical reaction to take place; the remaining portion of the coenzyme binds to the enzyme. Without its coenzyme, an enzyme cannot function. Thus symptoms of B vitamin deficiencies directly reflect the disturbances of metabolism incurred by a lack of coenzymes.

The following sections describe individual B vitamins and note many coenzymes and metabolic pathways. Keep in mind that a later section will assemble these pieces of information into a whole picture.

THIAMIN

thiamin (THIGH-ah-min): a B vitamin; the coenzyme form is TPP (thiamin pyrophosphate).

Researchers first isolated the coenzyme form of thiamin in 1926. Since then, the world of vitamins and enzyme action has opened up, revealing its intricacies and permitting medicine and science to put vitamins and enzymes to use in a multitude of ways.

Thiamin is the vitamin part of the coenzyme TPP, which assists in energy metabolism. The TPP coenzyme promotes the conversion of pyruvate to acetyl CoA. The reaction removes one carbon from the 3-carbon pyruvate to make the 2-carbon acetyl CoA and carbon dioxide. Later TPP promotes a similar step in the TCA cycle where it helps convert a 5-carbon compound to a 4-carbon compound. Besides playing these pivotal roles in the energy metabolism of all cells, thiamin occupies a special site on the membranes of nerve cells. Processes in nerves and in their responding tissues, the muscles, depend heavily on thiamin.

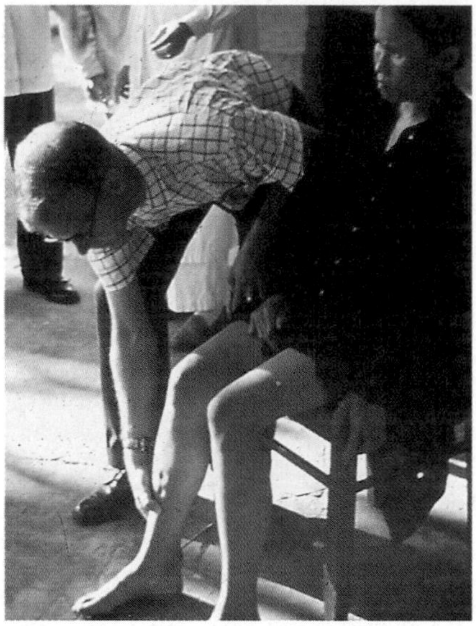

Beriberi may be characterized as "wet" (referring to edema) or "dry" (with muscle wasting, but no edema). Physical examination confirms that this woman has wet beriberi. Notice how the impression of the doctor's thumb remains on her leg.

Thiamin Recommendations Because thiamin is essential in energy metabolism, the RDA is stated in milligrams per 1000 kcalories of food energy. Generally, if a person eats enough food to meet energy needs and obtains that energy from thiamin-containing foods, thiamin needs will be met. This is true even for an athlete with high energy needs because almost any nutrient-dense food supplies thiamin, and people with greater energy needs eat more food. A person who is fasting or is on a very-low-kcalorie diet still needs at least 1 milligram thiamin a day to support the body's ongoing metabolic activities.

Thiamin Deficiency People who fail to meet energy needs risk thiamin deficiency, a condition that seems to be reappearing among the nation's malnourished and homeless people. Similarly, people who derive most of their energy from empty-kcalorie items, like alcohol, risk thiamin deficiency. Alcohol contributes energy, but provides no nutrients and often displaces food. In addition, alcohol enhances thiamin excretion in the urine, doubling the risk of deficiency.

beriberi: the thiamin-deficiency disease; it pointed the way to discovery of the first vitamin, thiamin.
beri = weakness
beriberi = "I can't, I can't"

Prolonged thiamin deficiency can result in the disease beriberi, which was first observed in East Asia when the custom of polishing rice became widespread. Rice provided 80 percent of the energy intake of the people of that area, and rice hulls were their principal source of thiamin. When the hulls were removed, beriberi spread like wildfire.

The **Wernicke-Korsakoff** (VER-nee-key KORE-sah-koff) syndrome commonly seen in malnourished alcohol abusers is characterized by symptoms similar to those seen in thiamin deficiency and can be treated with thiamin supplements.

Beriberi was first believed to be caused by an infectious agent. Medical researchers wasted much time and energy seeking a microbial cause before they realized that the cause of beriberi was not something that was in the food, but something that was absent from it.

Because thiamin participates in nerve processes, paralysis sets in when it is lacking. The symptoms of beriberi include damage to the nervous system as well

Table 10–3

Thiamin—A Summary

Other Names	Deficiency Disease Name
Vitamin B_1	Beriberi
Adult RDA	**Deficiency Symptoms**
0.5 mg/1000 kcal/day (1mg/day minimum) Men (19–50 yr): 1.5 mg/day Women (19–50 yr): 1.1 mg/day	BLOOD/CIRCULATORY SYSTEM Edema, enlarged heart, abnormal heart rhythms, heart failure NERVOUS/MUSCULAR SYSTEMS Degeneration, wasting, weakness, painful calf muscles, low morale, difficulty walking, loss of ankle and knee-jerk reflexes, mental confusion, paralysis
Chief Functions in the Body	
Part of the coenzyme TPP (thiamin pyrophosphate) used in energy metabolism; supports normal appetite and nerve function	
Significant Sources	
Occurs in all nutritious foods in moderate amounts; pork, ham, bacon, liver, whole-grain or enriched breads and cereals, legumes, nuts	

as to the heart and other muscles. Table 10–3 summarizes thiamin's deficiency symptoms, main functions, and food sources.

Thiamin Food Sources Before examining Figure 10–2, you may want to read the box on p. 350 that describes the many features found in this and similar figures in this chapter and the next three chapters. When you look at Figure 10–2, notice that thiamin occurs in small quantities in many nutritious foods. The long red bars near the bottom of the graph represent meats that are exceptionally rich in thiamin—those in the pork and ham family.

As mentioned earlier, prolonged cooking can destroy thiamin. Also, like other water-soluble vitamins, thiamin leaches into water when foods are boiled or blanched. Cooking methods that require little or no water such as steaming and microwave heating conserve thiamin and other water-soluble vitamins.

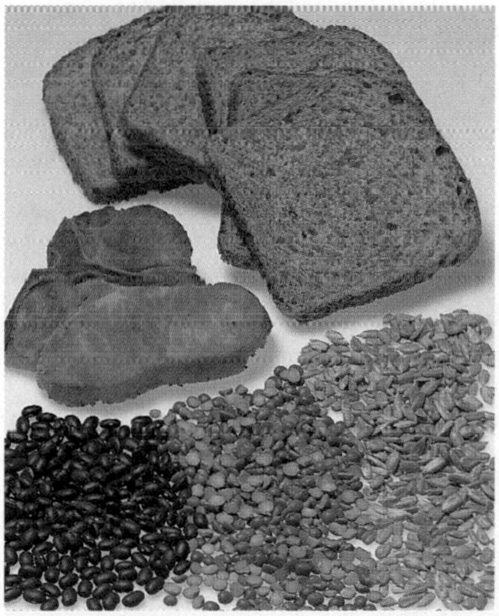

Meats (especially pork and ham), legumes such as black beans and split peas, sunflower seeds, and whole-wheat bread are thiamin-rich foods.

RIBOFLAVIN

Like thiamin, riboflavin helps enzymes to facilitate the release of energy from nutrients in all body cells. The coenzyme forms of riboflavin are FMN and FAD; both can accept and then donate two hydrogens (see Figure 10–3 on p. 352). During energy metabolism, FAD picks up two hydrogens (with their electrons) from the TCA cycle and delivers them to the electron transport chain (see Chapter 7).

riboflavin (RYE-boh-flay-vin): a B vitamin; the coenzyme forms are FMN (flavin mononucleotide) and FAD (flavin adenine dinucleotide).

Riboflavin Recommendations Like thiamin's RDA, riboflavin's RDA is stated in milligrams per 1000 kcalories of food energy, so recommendations vary accordingly for different age and sex groups. Growing infants and children have

How to Look to Foods for Single Nutrients

Figure 10–2 is the first of a series of figures in this and the next three chapters that present the vitamins and minerals in foods. Each figure presents the same 45 foods, which were selected to ensure a variety of choices representative of each of the food groups as suggested by the Daily Food Guide Pyramid. From the base of the pyramid, for example, a bread, a cereal, a rice, and a pasta were chosen. Other Pyramid suggestions were also considered: to include dark-green leafy vegetables (spinach, broccoli); deep-yellow vegetables (carrots, sweet potatoes); starchy vegetables (potatoes, corn, green peas); legumes (navy, pinto, kidney, and garbanzo beans); and other vegetables (green beans). The selection of fruits followed the Pyramid suggestions to use whole fruits (apples, bananas); citrus fruits (oranges, grapefruit juice); melons (watermelon); and berries (strawberries). Items were selected from the milk and meat groups in a similar way. In addition to the 45 foods that appear in all of the figures, five different foods were selected for each of the nutrients. These five foods were chosen to add variety and often reflect excellent, and sometimes unusual, sources of the specific nutrient.

Notice that the figures list the food, the serving size, and the food energy (kcalories) on the left and graph the amount of the nutrient per serving on the right along with the RDA for adults, so you can see how many servings would be needed to meet recommendations. Serving sizes reflect those used by the Daily Food Guide plan. The colored bars show at a glance which food groups best provide a nutrient: gold for breads and cereals; green for vegetables; purple for fruits; white for milk and milk products; brown for legumes; and red for meat, fish, and poultry. (Because the Pyramid mentions legumes with both the meat group and the vegetable group and because legumes are especially rich in many vitamins and minerals, they have been given their own color to highlight their nutrient contributions.) Notice how the bar graphs shift in the various figures. Careful study of all of the figures taken together will confirm that variety is the key to nutrient adequacy.

Another way to evaluate foods for their nutrient contributions is to consider their nutrient density (their calcium *per 100 kcalories*, for example). Quite often, vegetables rank higher on a nutrient-per-100 kcalories list than they do on a nutrient-per-serving list. Both listings offer valuable information, though, especially when combined with a realistic appraisal. For example, turnip greens provide more calcium per kcalorie than milk, but milk offers more calcium per serving. What matters most is which are you more likely to consume—1½ cups of turnip greens or 1 cup of milk? Both provide about 300 milligrams of calcium, but the greens save you about 50 kcalories. The left column in the figure highlights in yellow the foods that offer the best deal for your energy "dollar" (the kcalorie). Notice how many of them are vegetables.

Realistically, people cannot eat for single nutrients. All the figures taken together permit a conclusion to be drawn in Highlight 13 about how to combine foods into nourishing meals.

Figure 10–2 Thiamin in Selected Foods

Food	Serving size (kcalories)
Bread, whole wheat	1 slice (64 kcal)
Corn flakes, fortified	1 oz (108 kcal)
White rice	1/2 c cooked (134 kcal)
Spaghetti pasta	1/2 c cooked (99 kcal)
Oatmeal	1/2 c cooked (73 kcal)
Tortilla, flour	1 8"-round (115 kcal)
Spinach	1 c raw (12 kcal)
Broccoli	1/2 c cooked (22 kcal)
Carrots	1/2 c shredded raw (24 kcal)
Green peas	1/2 c cooked (62 kcal)
Corn	1/2 c cooked (66 kcal)
Green beans	1/2 c cooked (22 kcal)
Sweet potatoes	1/2 c cooked (117 kcal)
Potato	1 baked w/skin (220 kcal)
Tomato juice	3/4 c (31 kcal)
Apple	1 medium raw (81 kcal)
Banana	1 medium raw (104 kcal)
Orange	1 medium raw (62 kcal)
Strawberries	1/2 c fresh (23 kcal)
Raisins	1/4 c (109 kcal)
Watermelon	1 slice (154 kcal)
Grapefruit juice	3/4 c fresh (72 kcal)
Avocado	1/4 (85 kcal)
Milk	1 c low-fat 2% (121 kcal)
Yogurt, plain	1 c low-fat (143 kcal)
Cheddar cheese	1½ oz (171 kcal)
Cottage cheese	1/2 c low-fat 2% (101 kcal)
Swiss cheese	1 1/2 oz (159 kcal)
Ice cream	1/2 c, 10% fat (134 kcal)
Navy beans	1/2 c cooked (129 kcal)
Pinto beans	1/2 c cooked (117 kcal)
Kidney beans	1/2 c cooked (109 kcal)
Garbanzo beans	1/2 c cooked (134 kcal)
Peanut butter	2 tbs (190 kcal)
Sunflower seeds	1 oz dry (159 kcal)
Tofu (soybean curd)	1/2 c (94 kcal)
Shrimp	3 oz boiled (85 kcal)
Ground beef, lean	3 oz broiled (239 kcal)
Chicken breast	3 oz roasted (141 kcal)
Cod	3 oz poached (88 kcal)
Ham, lean	3 oz roasted (123 kcal)
Sirloin steak, lean	3 oz broiled (171 kcal)
Tuna, canned in water	3 oz (99 kcal)
Bologna, beef	2 slices (144 kcal)
Egg	1 hard cooked (77 kcal)
Additional 5 foods:	
Pork chop, lean	3 oz broiled (166 kcal)
Chorizo sausage	3 oz (387 kcal)
Soy milk	1/2 c (79 kcal)
Pistachios, shelled	1 oz dried (164 kcal)
Squash, acorn	1/2 c baked (68 kcal)

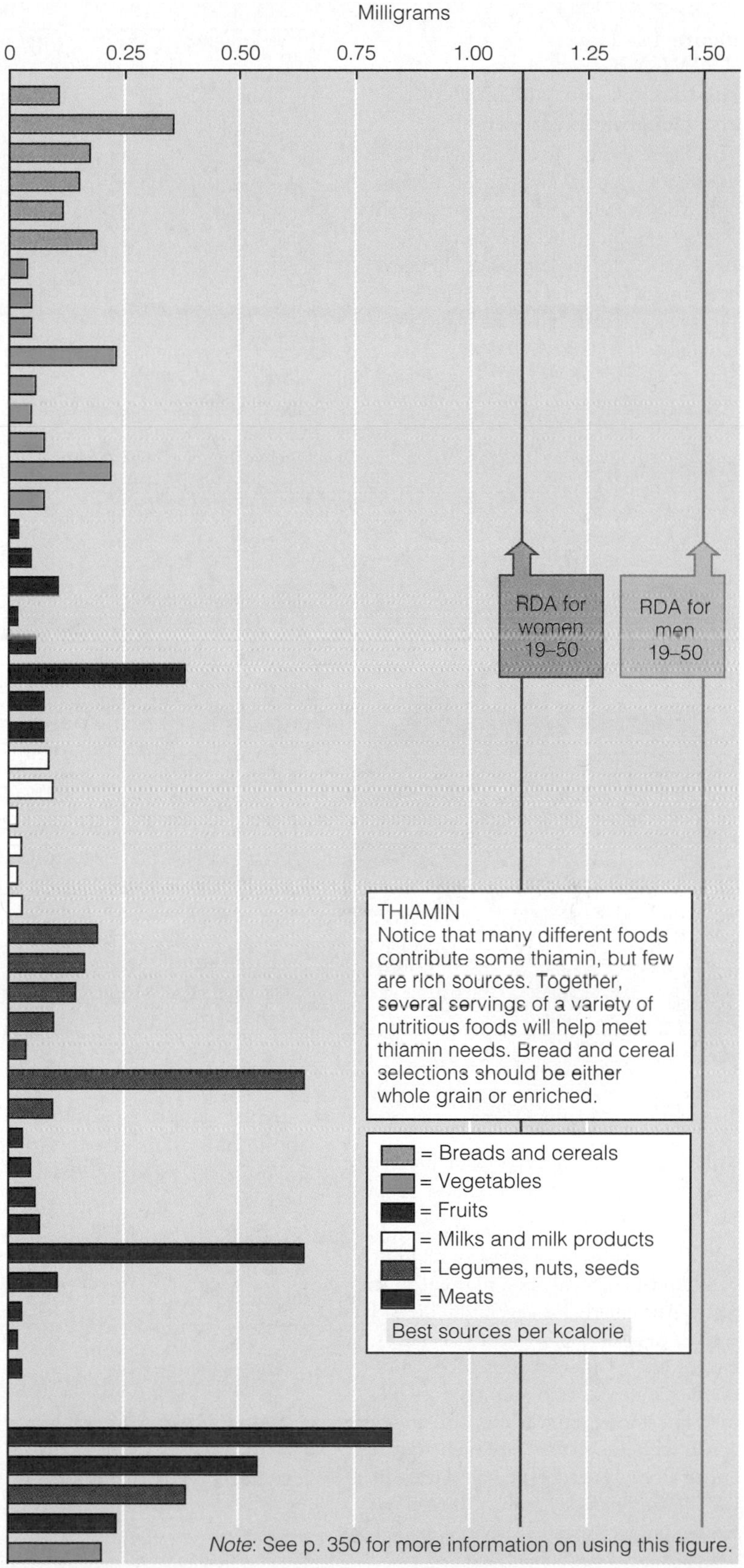
Milligrams
0
0.25
0.50
0.75
1.00
1.25
1.50
RDA for women 19–50
RDA for men 19–50
THIAMIN
Notice that many different foods contribute some thiamin, but few are rich sources. Together, several servings of a variety of nutritious foods will help meet thiamin needs. Bread and cereal selections should be either whole grain or enriched.
= Breads and cereals
= Vegetables
= Fruits
= Milks and milk products
= Legumes, nuts, seeds
= Meats
Best sources per kcalorie
Note: See p. 350 for more information on using this figure.

Figure 10–3

Riboflavin Coenzyme, Accepting and Donating Hydrogens
This figure shows the chemical structure of the riboflavin portion of the coenzyme only; the remainder of the coenzyme structure is represented by dotted lines (see Appendix C for the complete chemical structure of FAD and FMN). The reactive sites that accept and donate hydrogens are highlighted in white.

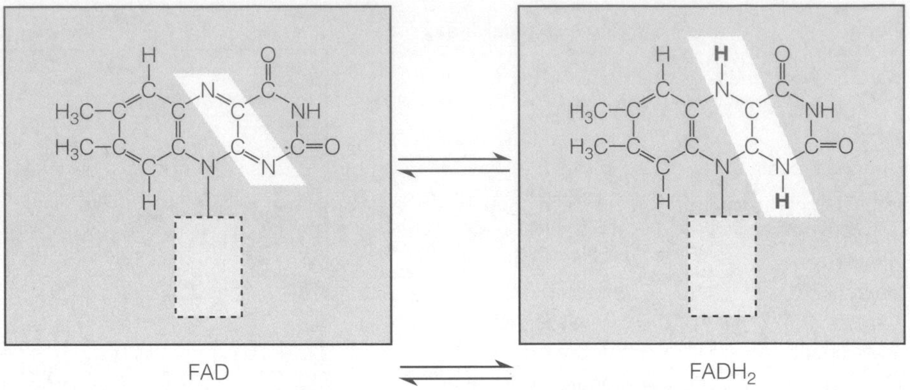

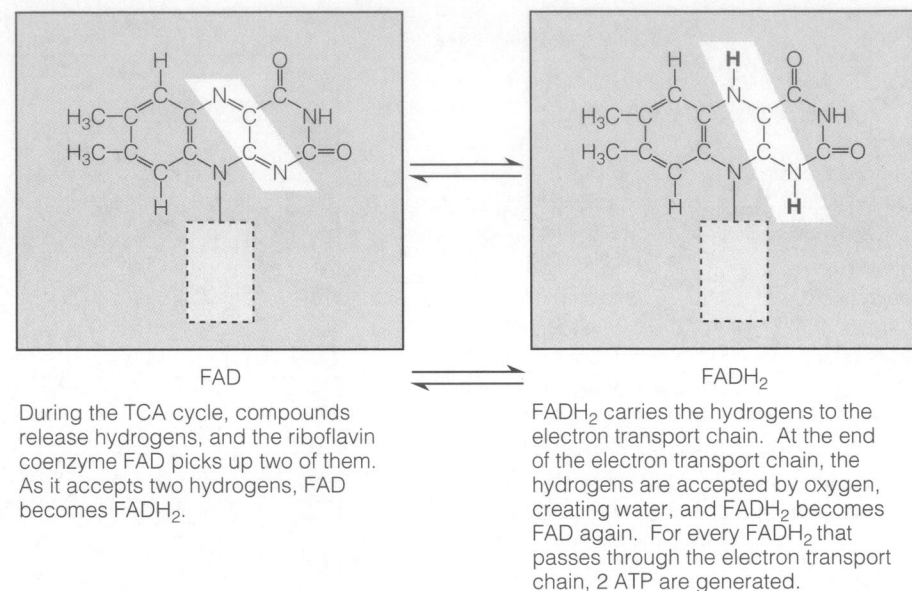

During the TCA cycle, compounds release hydrogens, and the riboflavin coenzyme FAD picks up two of them. As it accepts two hydrogens, FAD becomes $FADH_2$.

$FADH_2$ carries the hydrogens to the electron transport chain. At the end of the electron transport chain, the hydrogens are accepted by oxygen, creating water, and $FADH_2$ becomes FAD again. For every $FADH_2$ that passes through the electron transport chain, 2 ATP are generated.

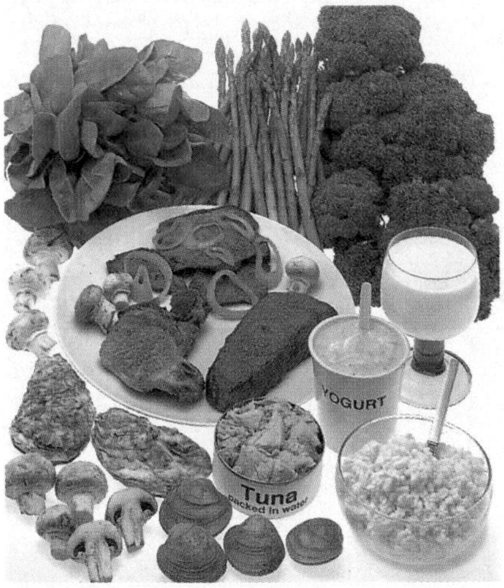

Milk and milk products provide much of the riboflavin in the diets of most people.

nutritional yeast: a preparation of yeast cells grown especially as a nutrient supplement, particularly for vegetarian diets. The type of yeast used is brewer's yeast, not baker's yeast. Different species of yeasts produce different compounds; yeast cells used in brewing produce alcohol, proteins, and B vitamins as they grow. The nutrients are removed from beer and wine in the filtering process. Yeast cells used in baking produce mostly carbon dioxide, which causes bread dough to rise.

high riboflavin needs; so do pregnant women. The riboflavin RDA is generous enough to cover the needs of most physically active people and so does not differ from the RDA for sedentary people of the same age and sex.[2]

Riboflavin Deficiency No one disease is associated with riboflavin deficiency. Lack of the vitamin affects the facial skin, eyes, and GI tract. Table 10–4 lists riboflavin's deficiency symptoms, chief roles, and food sources.

Riboflavin Food Sources Clearly, milk, milk products such as cheese, and liver dominate the riboflavin list (see Figure 10–4 on p. 354). The need for riboflavin is a major reason for including milk and milk products in every day's meals; no other commonly eaten food can make such a substantial contribution in a single serving.

Most people easily meet their riboflavin RDA. On the average, they derive about half their riboflavin from milk and milk products, about a fourth from meats, and most of the rest from green vegetables (such as broccoli, turnip greens, asparagus, and spinach) and whole-grain or enriched bread and cereal products. A list of riboflavin sources ranked per 100 kcalories includes many dark green, leafy vegetables high on the list (notice those foods highlighted in yellow in the left column of the figure). Vegetarians who don't use milk must rely on ample servings of dark greens for riboflavin. Nutritional yeast is another rich source.

Light and irradiation destroy riboflavin. For these reasons, precautions are taken when vitamin D is added to milk by irradiation.* Also, milk is seldom sold in transparent glass or plastic containers; cardboard or opaque plastic containers are preferred. In contrast, riboflavin is stable to heat, so cooking does not destroy it.

*Vitamin D can be added to milk by feeding cows irradiated yeast or by irradiating the milk itself.

Table 10–4

Riboflavin—A Summary

Other Names	Deficiency Disease Name
Vitamin B_2	Ariboflavinosis (ay-RYE-boh-FLAY-vin-oh-sis)
Adult RDA	**Deficiency Symptoms**
	MOUTH, GUMS, TONGUE
0.6 mg/1000 kcal/day (1.2 mg/day minimum) Men (19–50 yr): 1.7 mg/day Women (19–50 yr): 1.3 mg/day	Cracks and redness at corners of mouth;[a] painful, smooth, purplish-red tongue[b]
Chief Functions in the Body	NERVOUS SYSTEM AND EYES
Part of coenzymes FMN (flavin mononucleotide) and FAD (flavin adenine dinucleotide) used in energy metabolism; supports normal vision and skin health	Inflamed eyelids and sensitivity to light,[c] reddening of cornea
	OTHER
Significant Sources	Skin rash
Milk, yogurt, cottage cheese, meat, leafy green vegetables, whole-grain or enriched breads and cereals	

[a]Cracks at the corners of the mouth are termed *cheilosis* (kee-LOH-sis).
[b]Smoothness of the tongue is caused by loss of its surface structures and is termed *glossitis* (gloss-EYE-tis).
[c]Hypersensitivity to light is *photophobia*.

NIACIN

The name niacin describes two chemical structures: nicotinic acid and nicotinamide (also known as niacinamide). The body can easily convert nicotinic acid to nicotinamide, which is the major form of niacin in the blood. The two coenzyme forms of niacin, NAD and NADP, participate in numerous metabolic activities. They are central in energy-transfer reactions, especially the metabolism of glucose, fat, and alcohol. NAD is similar to riboflavin coenzymes in that it carries hydrogens (and their electrons) during metabolic reactions, including the pathway from the TCA cycle to the electron transport chain.

niacin (NIGH-a-sin): a B vitamin. Niacin can be eaten preformed or made in the body from its precursor, tryptophan, one of the amino acids. The active coenzyme forms are NAD (nicotinamide adenine dinucleotide) and NADP (the phosphate form of NAD).

Niacin Recommendations Niacin is unique among the B vitamins in that the body can make it from the amino acid tryptophan. To make 1 milligram of niacin requires approximately 60 milligrams of dietary tryptophan. For this reason, recommended niacin intakes are stated in "equivalents." A food containing 1 milligram of niacin and 60 milligrams of tryptophan provides the equivalent of 2 milligrams of niacin, or 2 niacin equivalents (NE). Like the RDA for thiamin and riboflavin, the RDA for niacin is based on energy intake.

1 NE = 1 mg niacin.
1 NE = 60 mg tryptophan.

The box on p. 356 describes how to calculate niacin equivalents in the diet.

niacin equivalents: the amount of niacin present in food, including the niacin that can theoretically be made from its precursor, tryptophan, present in the food.

Niacin Deficiency The niacin-deficiency disease, pellagra, produces the symptoms of diarrhea, dermatitis, dementia, and eventually death. In the early 1900s, pellagra caused widespread misery and some 87,000 deaths in the U.S. South, where many people subsisted on a low-protein diet centered on corn. This

pellagra (pell-AY-gra): the niacin-deficiency disease.
pellis = skin
agra = rough

Figure 10–4 Riboflavin in Selected Foods

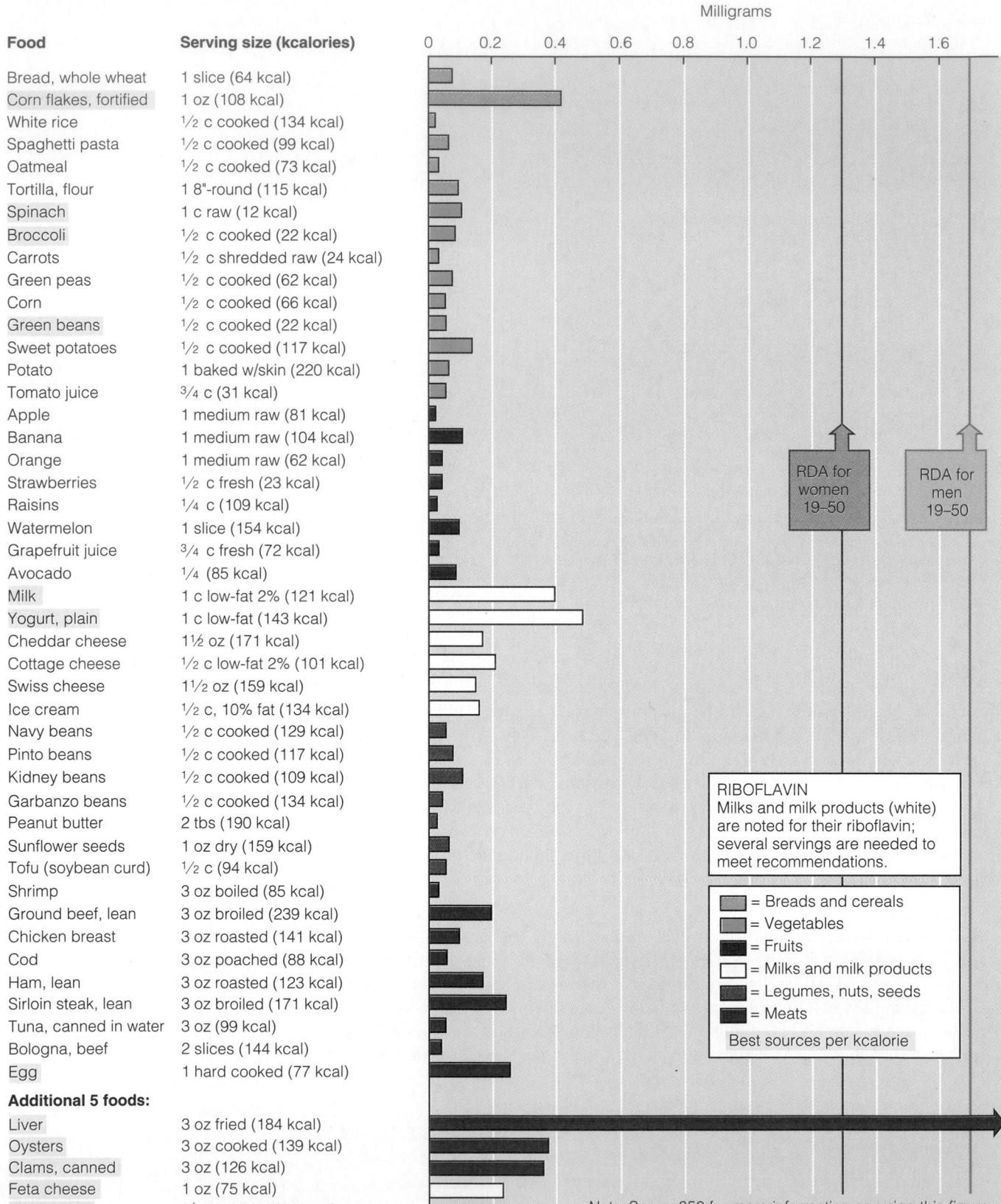

Food	Serving size (kcalories)
Bread, whole wheat	1 slice (64 kcal)
Corn flakes, fortified	1 oz (108 kcal)
White rice	½ c cooked (134 kcal)
Spaghetti pasta	½ c cooked (99 kcal)
Oatmeal	½ c cooked (73 kcal)
Tortilla, flour	1 8"-round (115 kcal)
Spinach	1 c raw (12 kcal)
Broccoli	½ c cooked (22 kcal)
Carrots	½ c shredded raw (24 kcal)
Green peas	½ c cooked (62 kcal)
Corn	½ c cooked (66 kcal)
Green beans	½ c cooked (22 kcal)
Sweet potatoes	½ c cooked (117 kcal)
Potato	1 baked w/skin (220 kcal)
Tomato juice	¾ c (31 kcal)
Apple	1 medium raw (81 kcal)
Banana	1 medium raw (104 kcal)
Orange	1 medium raw (62 kcal)
Strawberries	½ c fresh (23 kcal)
Raisins	¼ c (109 kcal)
Watermelon	1 slice (154 kcal)
Grapefruit juice	¾ c fresh (72 kcal)
Avocado	¼ (85 kcal)
Milk	1 c low-fat 2% (121 kcal)
Yogurt, plain	1 c low-fat (143 kcal)
Cheddar cheese	1½ oz (171 kcal)
Cottage cheese	½ c low-fat 2% (101 kcal)
Swiss cheese	1½ oz (159 kcal)
Ice cream	½ c, 10% fat (134 kcal)
Navy beans	½ c cooked (129 kcal)
Pinto beans	½ c cooked (117 kcal)
Kidney beans	½ c cooked (109 kcal)
Garbanzo beans	½ c cooked (134 kcal)
Peanut butter	2 tbs (190 kcal)
Sunflower seeds	1 oz dry (159 kcal)
Tofu (soybean curd)	½ c (94 kcal)
Shrimp	3 oz boiled (85 kcal)
Ground beef, lean	3 oz broiled (239 kcal)
Chicken breast	3 oz roasted (141 kcal)
Cod	3 oz poached (88 kcal)
Ham, lean	3 oz roasted (123 kcal)
Sirloin steak, lean	3 oz broiled (171 kcal)
Tuna, canned in water	3 oz (99 kcal)
Bologna, beef	2 slices (144 kcal)
Egg	1 hard cooked (77 kcal)
Additional 5 foods:	
Liver	3 oz fried (184 kcal)
Oysters	3 oz cooked (139 kcal)
Clams, canned	3 oz (126 kcal)
Feta cheese	1 oz (75 kcal)
Mushrooms	½ c cooked (21 kcal)

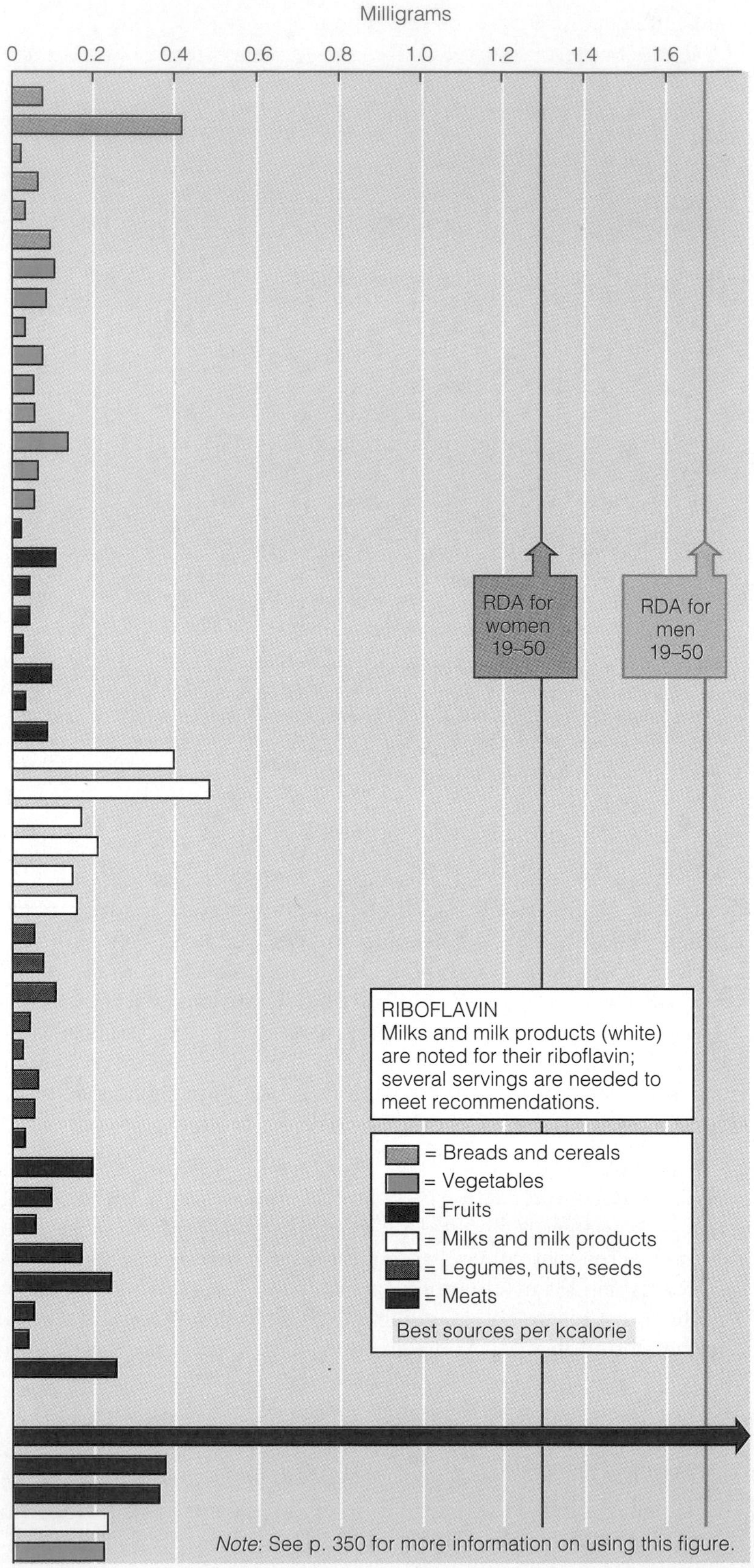

Note: See p. 350 for more information on using this figure.

diet supplied neither enough niacin nor enough tryptophan. At least 70 percent of the niacin in corn is unavailable. Furthermore, corn is high in the amino acid leucine, which may contribute to the development of pellagra.[3] (See Table 10–5 for niacin's deficiency and toxicity symptoms as well as its various names, functions, and food sources.)

See p. 356 for a photo of the dermatitis of pellagra.

Niacin Toxicity Large doses of niacin exert a druglike effect on the nervous system and on blood lipids and blood glucose. When niacin in the form of nicotinic acid is taken in doses ten times the RDA or more, it dilates the capillaries and causes a tingling sensation that can be painful, an effect known as the "niacin flush." The nicotinamide form does not produce this effect.

Physicians can effectively lower blood cholesterol with large doses of niacin, but such therapy must be closely monitored because of its adverse side effects (liver damage and peptic ulcers, among others).[4] Pharmacological doses of nicotinamide are currently being tested in a large international study to prevent diabetes (IDDM).[5]

When a normal dose of a nutrient (levels commonly found in foods and not exceeding 150% of the RDA) provides a normal blood concentration, the nutrient is having a **physiological effect**. When a large dose (two to ten times greater than the RDA) overwhelms some body system and acts like a drug, the nutrient is having a **pharmacological effect**.

physio = natural

pharma = drug

Table 10–5

Niacin—A Summary

Other Names	Deficiency Disease Name	
Nicotinic acid, nicotinamide, niacinamide, vitamin B_3; precursor is dietary tryptophan	Pellagra	
Adult RDA	**Deficiency Symptoms**	**Toxicity Symptoms**
6.6 mg NE/1000 kcal/day (13 NE minimum) Men (19–50 yr): 19 mg NE/day Women (19–50 yr): 15 mg NE/day	DIGESTIVE SYSTEM	
	Diarrhea	Diarrhea, heartburn, nausea, ulcer irritation, vomiting
Chief Functions in the Body	MOUTH, GUMS, TONGUE	
Part of coenzymes NAD (nicotinamide adenine dinucleotide) and NADP (its phosphate form) used in energy metabolism; supports health of skin, nervous system, and digestive system	Inflamed, swollen, smooth tongue[a]	
	NERVOUS SYSTEM	
Significant Sources	Irritability, loss of appetite, weakness, dizziness, mental confusion progressing to psychosis or delirium	Fainting, dizziness
Milk, eggs, meat, poultry, fish, whole-grain and enriched breads and cereals, nuts, and all protein-containing foods	SKIN	
	Bilateral symmetrical determatitis, especially on areas exposed to sun	Painful flush and rash ("niacin-, flush")excessive sweating
	OTHER	
		Liver damage, low blood pressure

[a]Smoothness of the tongue is caused by loss of its surface structures and is termed *glossitis* (gloss-EYE-tis).

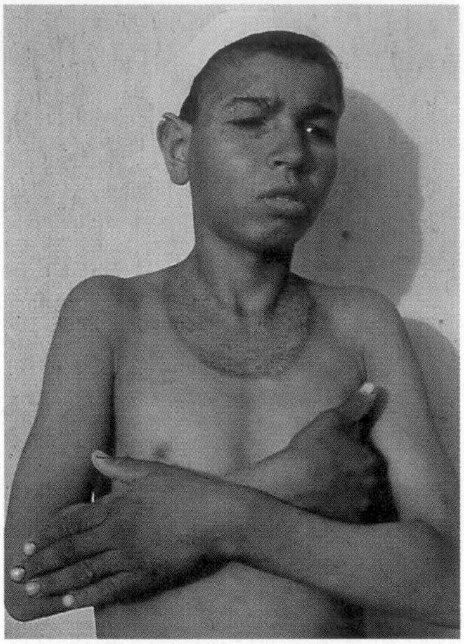

In the dermatitis of pellagra, the skin darkens and flakes away as if it were sunburned. Kwashiorkor also produces a "flaky paint" dermatitis, but the two are easily distinguished. The dermatitis of pellagra is bilateral and symmetrical and occurs only on those parts of the body exposed to the sun.

How to Determine Niacin Intake

To obtain a rough approximation of niacin intake:

1. Calculate total protein consumed (grams).
2. Assuming that the RDA amount of protein will be used first to make body protein, subtract the RDA to obtain "leftover" protein available to make niacin (grams). (Actually, the RDA provides a generous protein allowance, so "leftover" protein may be even greater than this.)
3. About 1 gram of every 100 grams of protein is tryptophan, so divide by 100 to obtain the tryptophan in this leftover protein (grams).
4. Multiply by 1000 to express this amount of tryptophan in milligrams.
5. Divide by 60 to get niacin equivalents (milligrams).
6. Finally, add the amount of preformed niacin obtained in the diet (milligrams).

Niacin Food Sources Tables of food composition typically list preformed niacin only, but people also obtain the vitamin from protein, which almost invariably contains the niacin precursor, tryptophan. Hence diets that are high in protein are never deficient in niacin. The accompanying box shows how to calculate the total amount of niacin available from the diet. The average diet supplies enough preformed niacin to meet daily needs, and dietary tryptophan usually meets about half the need.

The predominance of red bars in Figure 10–5 explains why meat, poultry, and fish contribute about half the niacin equivalents most people receive. About a fourth of most people's niacin comes from enriched breads and cereals. Mushrooms, asparagus, and leafy green vegetables are among the richest vegetable sources (per kcalorie) and can provide abundant niacin to the person who eats generous amounts of them.

Niacin is less vulnerable to losses during food preparation and storage than other water-soluble vitamins. Being fairly heat-resistant, niacin can withstand reasonable cooking times, but like other water-soluble vitamins, it will leach into cooking water.

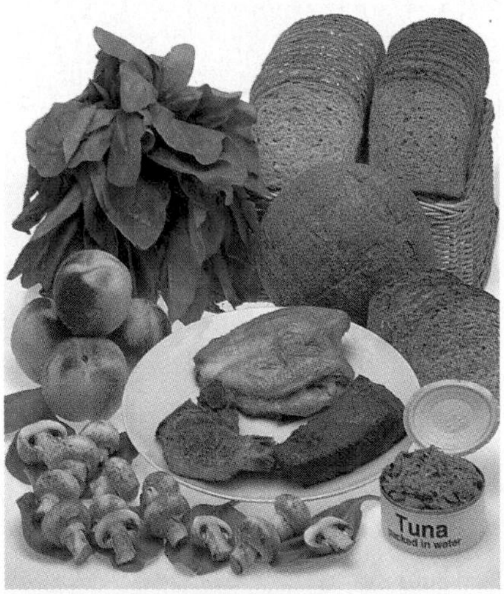

Protein-rich foods such as tuna fish and chicken contribute much of the niacin in people's diets. Enriched breads and cereals, leafy green vegetables, and a few fruits are also rich in niacin.

BIOTIN

Biotin plays an important role in metabolism as a coenzyme that carries carbon dioxide. This role is critical to the TCA cycle: biotin delivers a carbon to 3-carbon pyruvate, thus replenishing the 4-carbon compound needed to combine with acetyl CoA to keep the TCA cycle turning. The biotin coenzyme also serves crucial roles in gluconeogenesis, fatty acid synthesis, and the breakdown of certain fatty acids and amino acids.

biotin (BY-oh-tin): a B vitamin that functions as a coenzyme in the metabolism of carbohydrates and fats.

Biotin Recommendations Biotin is needed in very small amounts. Recommendations for daily intakes have not been established; instead, "estimated safe and adequate daily dietary intakes" have been set.

Figure 10–5 Niacin in Selected Foods

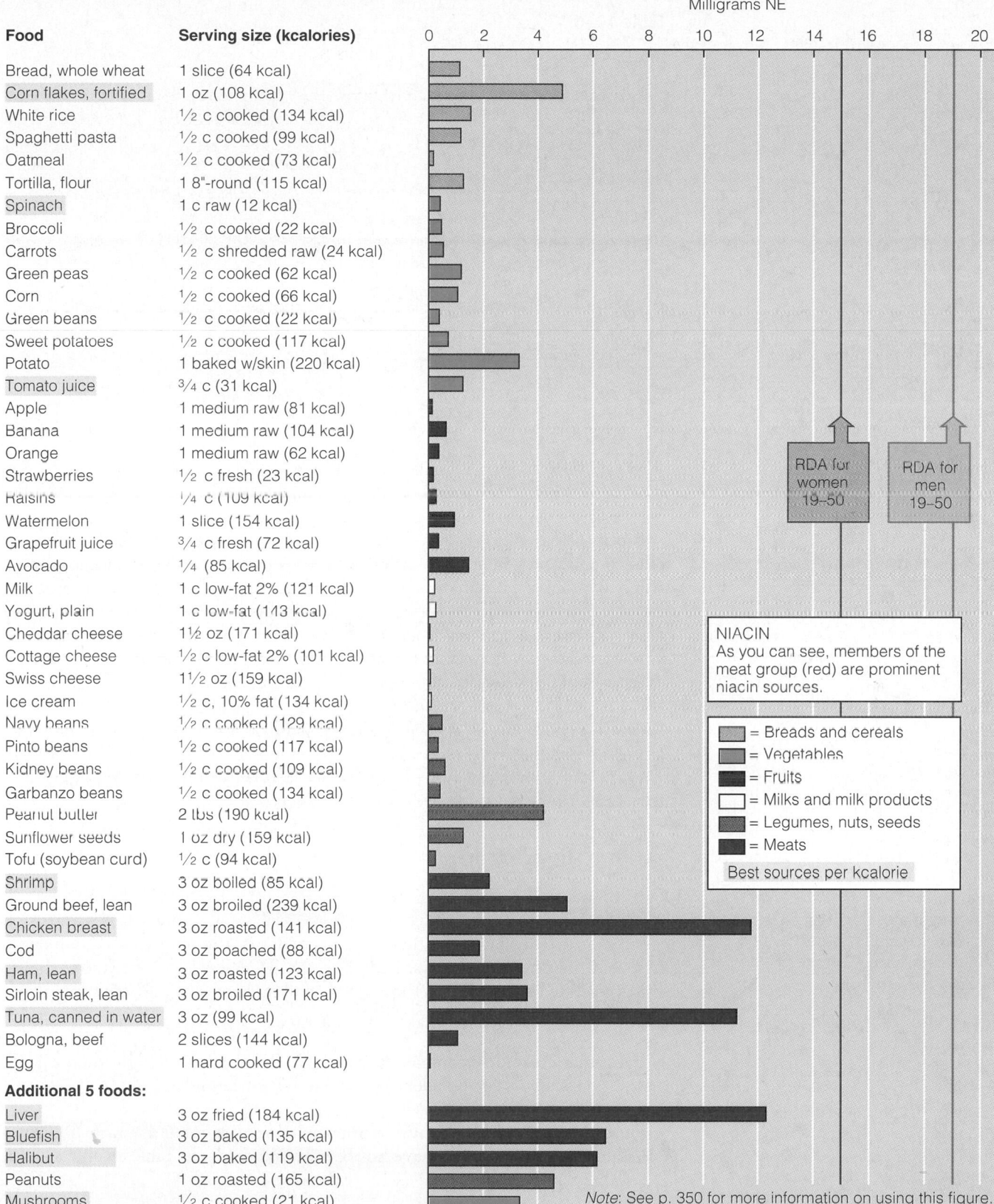

Food	Serving size (kcalories)
Bread, whole wheat	1 slice (64 kcal)
Corn flakes, fortified	1 oz (108 kcal)
White rice	1/2 c cooked (134 kcal)
Spaghetti pasta	1/2 c cooked (99 kcal)
Oatmeal	1/2 c cooked (73 kcal)
Tortilla, flour	1 8"-round (115 kcal)
Spinach	1 c raw (12 kcal)
Broccoli	1/2 c cooked (22 kcal)
Carrots	1/2 c shredded raw (24 kcal)
Green peas	1/2 c cooked (62 kcal)
Corn	1/2 c cooked (66 kcal)
Green beans	1/2 c cooked (22 kcal)
Sweet potatoes	1/2 c cooked (117 kcal)
Potato	1 baked w/skin (220 kcal)
Tomato juice	3/4 c (31 kcal)
Apple	1 medium raw (81 kcal)
Banana	1 medium raw (104 kcal)
Orange	1 medium raw (62 kcal)
Strawberries	1/2 c fresh (23 kcal)
Raisins	1/4 c (109 kcal)
Watermelon	1 slice (154 kcal)
Grapefruit juice	3/4 c fresh (72 kcal)
Avocado	1/4 (85 kcal)
Milk	1 c low-fat 2% (121 kcal)
Yogurt, plain	1 c low-fat (143 kcal)
Cheddar cheese	1½ oz (171 kcal)
Cottage cheese	1/2 c low-fat 2% (101 kcal)
Swiss cheese	1 1/2 oz (159 kcal)
Ice cream	1/2 c, 10% fat (134 kcal)
Navy beans	1/2 c cooked (129 kcal)
Pinto beans	1/2 c cooked (117 kcal)
Kidney beans	1/2 c cooked (109 kcal)
Garbanzo beans	1/2 c cooked (134 kcal)
Peanut butter	2 tbs (190 kcal)
Sunflower seeds	1 oz dry (159 kcal)
Tofu (soybean curd)	1/2 c (94 kcal)
Shrimp	3 oz boiled (85 kcal)
Ground beef, lean	3 oz broiled (239 kcal)
Chicken breast	3 oz roasted (141 kcal)
Cod	3 oz poached (88 kcal)
Ham, lean	3 oz roasted (123 kcal)
Sirloin steak, lean	3 oz broiled (171 kcal)
Tuna, canned in water	3 oz (99 kcal)
Bologna, beef	2 slices (144 kcal)
Egg	1 hard cooked (77 kcal)
Additional 5 foods:	
Liver	3 oz fried (184 kcal)
Bluefish	3 oz baked (135 kcal)
Halibut	3 oz baked (119 kcal)
Peanuts	1 oz roasted (165 kcal)
Mushrooms	1/2 c cooked (21 kcal)

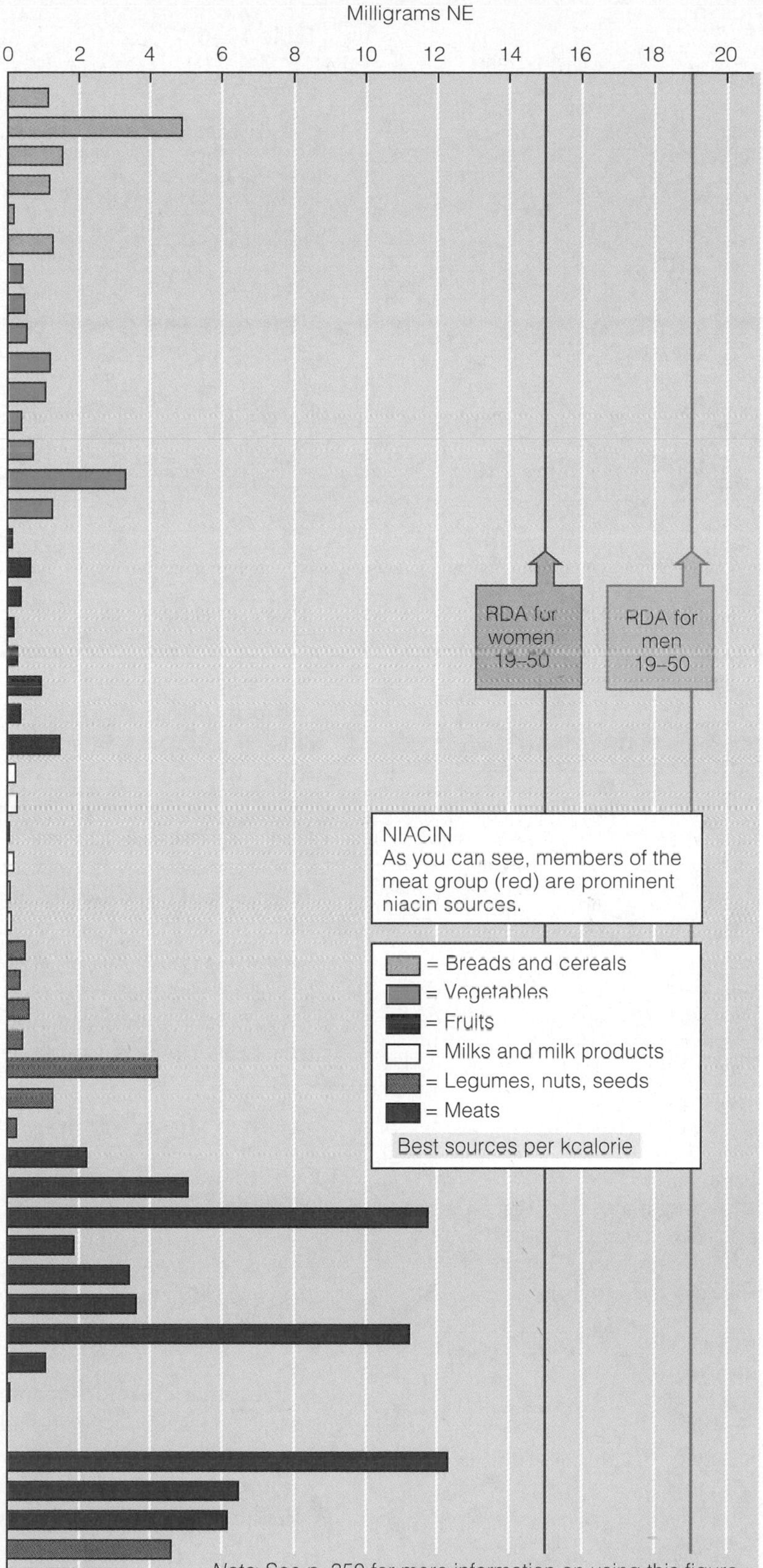

Note: See p. 350 for more information on using this figure.

Table 10–6

Biotin—A Summary

Estimated Safe and Adequate Intake	Deficiency Symptoms
Adults: 30 to 100 μg/day	BLOOD/CIRCULATORY SYSTEM Abnormal heart action
Chief Functions in the Body	DIGESTIVE SYSTEM Loss of appetite, nausea
Part of a coenzyme used in energy metabolism, fat synthesis, amino acid metabolism, and glycogen synthesis	NERVOUS/MUSCULAR SYSTEMS
Significant Sources	Depression, hallucinations, muscle pain, weakness, fatigue
Widespread in foods	SKIN Drying, scaly dermatitis, hair loss

The protein **avidin** in egg whites binds biotin.
avid = greedy

Biotin Deficiency Biotin deficiencies rarely occur. Researchers can induce a biotin deficiency in animals or human beings by feeding them raw egg whites, which contain a protein that binds biotin and thus prevents its absorption. Biotin-deficiency symptoms include scaly dermatitis, hair loss, loss of appetite, nausea, hallucinations, and depression. More than two dozen egg whites must be consumed daily to produce these effects, however, and the eggs have to be raw; cooking denatures the binding protein.

Biotin Food Sources Biotin is widespread in foods (including egg yolks), so eating a variety of foods protects against deficiencies. Biotin is also synthesized by GI tract bacteria, but how much of it is absorbed is unknown. A brief summary of biotin facts is provided in Table 10–6.

PANTOTHENIC ACID

pantothenic (PAN-toe-THEN-ick) **acid:** a B vitamin; the principal active form is part of coenzyme A, called "CoA" throughout Chapter 7.
pantos = everywhere

Pantothenic acid is involved in more than 100 different steps in the synthesis of lipids, neurotransmitters, steroid hormones, and hemoglobin.[6] It serves as part of coenzyme A—the same CoA that forms acetyl CoA, the "crossroads" compound in several metabolic pathways, including the TCA cycle. Coenzyme A helps shuttle acetate (as acetyl CoA) and other small molecules along pathways in glucose, fatty acid, and energy metabolism.

Pantothenic Acid Recommendations No RDA exists for pantothenic acid. Instead, estimated safe and adequate intakes have been set.

Pantothenic Acid Deficiency Pantothenic acid deficiency is rare. Its symptoms involve a general failure of all the body's systems (see Table 10–7).

Table 10–7

Pantothenic Acid—A Summary

Estimated Safe and Adequate Intake	Deficiency Symptoms	Toxicity Symptoms
Adults: 4 to 7 mg/day	DIGESTIVE SYSTEM	
Chief Functions in the Body	Vomiting, intestinal distress	Occasional diarrhea
Part of coenzyme A, used in energy metabolism	NERVOUS SYSTEM	
Significant Sources	Insomnia, fatigue	
Widespread in foods	OTHER	
		Water retention (rare)

Pantothenic Acid Food Sources Pantothenic acid is widespread in foods, and typical diets seem to provide adequate intakes. Meat, fish, poultry, whole-grain cereals, and legumes are particularly good sources. Pantothenic acid loss during food preparation can be substantial because it is readily destroyed by heat.

VITAMIN B_6

Vitamin B_6 occurs in three forms—pyridoxal, pyridoxine, and pyridoxamine. All three can be converted to the coenzyme PLP.

vitamin B_6: a family of compounds—pyridoxal, pyridoxine, and pyridoxamine; the primary active coenzyme form is PLP (pyridoxal phosphate).

The PLP coenzyme is active in amino acid metabolism because it can transfer amino groups. This feature permits the body to synthesize nonessential amino acids when amino groups are available (review Figure 7–14 on p. 254). The ability to add and remove amino groups makes PLP valuable in protein and urea metabolism as well. The conversion of the amino acid tryptophan to niacin or to the neurotransmitter serotonin also depends on PLP as does the synthesis of heme, nucleic acids, and lecithin.

serotonin (SER-oh-tone-in)**:** a neurotransmitter important in sleep and sensory perception; it is synthesized from the amino acid tryptophan with the help of vitamin B_6.

A surge of vitamin B_6 research in the last decade has revealed that vitamin B_6 influences cognitive development, immune function, and steroid hormone activity.[7] Unlike other water-soluble vitamins, vitamin B_6 is stored extensively in muscle tissue.

Among the many drugs that interact with vitamin B_6, alcohol stands out. As Highlight 7 described, when the body breaks down alcohol, it first produces acetaldehyde. If allowed to accumulate, acetaldehyde has toxic effects, and so it must quickly be broken down further. Acetaldehyde dislodges PLP from its enzymes; once loose, PLP breaks down and is excreted. Thus alcohol actively promotes the destruction and loss of vitamin B_6 from the body.

Another drug that acts as a vitamin B_6 antagonist is INH, a drug that inhibits the growth of the tuberculosis bacterium.* INH has saved countless lives, but as a vitamin B_6 antagonist, it binds and inactivates the vitamin, inducing a defi-

antagonist: a competing factor that counteracts the action of another factor. When a drug displaces a vitamin from its site of action, the drug renders the vitamin ineffective and thus acts as a vitamin antagonist.

*INH stands for *isonicotinic acid hydrazide*.

ciency. Whenever INH is used to treat tuberculosis, vitamin B_6 supplements must be given to protect the person from deficiency.

Vitamin B_6 Recommendations Because the vitamin B_6 coenzymes play many roles in amino acid metabolism, dietary needs are roughly proportional to protein intakes. The RDA for vitamin B_6 is high enough to handle at least 100 grams of protein per day for men and 60 grams of protein per day for women. Research does not support claims that large doses of vitamin B_6 enhance physical endurance. Pills cannot compete with a nutritious diet.

Vitamin B_6 Deficiency People given a vitamin B_6–deficient diet first experience weakness, irritability, and insomnia. Advanced symptoms include growth failure, impaired motor function, and convulsions. Immune function is also impaired in vitamin B_6 deficiency.[8]

Common PMS symptoms:
- Headaches.
- Breast swelling and tenderness.
- Water retention.
- Weight gain.
- Irritability.
- Anxiety.
- Fatigue.
- Depression.
- Appetite changes and food cravings.
- Backaches.
- Acne.
- Constipation.

carpal tunnel syndrome: a pinched nerve at the wrist, causing pain or numbness in the hand.

Vitamin B_6 Toxicity The first major report of vitamin B_6 toxicity appeared in 1983. Until that time, everyone (including researchers and dietitians) believed that, like the other water-soluble vitamins, vitamin B_6 could not reach toxic concentrations in the body. The report told of seven women who had been taking more than 2 grams of vitamin B_6 daily (the RDA for women is less than 2 *milli*grams) for two months or more.

Most of these women were attempting to treat the symptoms of premenstrual syndrome (PMS). PMS is a cluster of physical, emotional, and psychological symptoms that some women experience prior to menstruation. In about 5 percent of women with PMS, at least one physical or psychological symptom can reach such severity as to be temporarily disabling.[9]

Specific PMS symptoms vary from woman to woman, but their timing is predictable: they begin seven to ten days prior to menstruation and wane after menstruation begins. The cause of PMS remains undefined, although researchers generally agree that the hormonal changes of the menstrual cycle must be responsible. Without a full understanding of PMS causes, medical treatments flounder, and quack treatments abound. Among nutritional approaches, the taking of vitamin B_6 has received much attention, but seems to have done more harm than good.

Some people have taken vitamin B_6 supplements in an attempt to cure carpal tunnel syndrome and sleep disorders; at least one study reports that vitamin B_6 may be effective in treating carpal tunnel syndrome.[10] Self-prescribing is ill-advised, however, because large doses of vitamin B_6 taken for months or years can cause irreversible nerve damage. (Table 10–8 lists common symptoms of both deficiency and toxicity as well as chief functions and food sources of vitamin B_6.)

That vitamin B_6 is both essential and harmful may seem surprising, but the same is true of most vitamins and minerals. The effects of every substance depend on its dose, and this is one reason consumers should not self-prescribe vitamins for their own ailments. See the box, "Dose Levels and Effects," (on p. 362) for a perspective on doses.

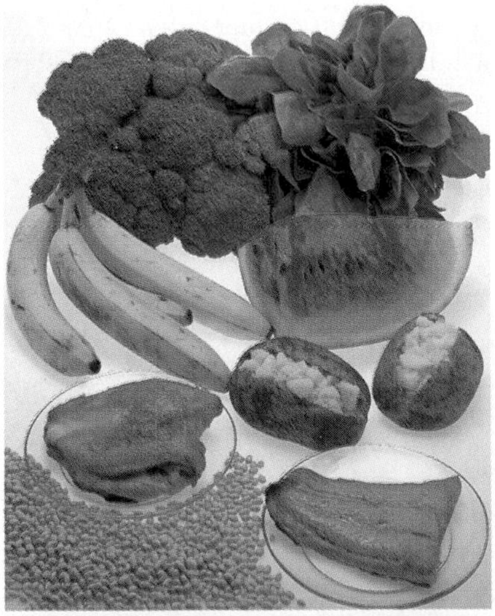

Most protein-rich foods provide ample vitamin B_6; some vegetables and fruits are good sources, too.

Vitamin B_6 Food Sources As you can see from Figure 10–7 (on p. 363), meats, fish, and poultry (red), potatoes and a few other vegetables (green), and fruits (purple) offer vitamin B_6. As is true of most of the other vitamins, vegetables would rank considerably higher if foods were ranked by nutrient density

Table 10–8

Vitamin B_6—A Summary

Other Names	Deficiency Symptoms	Toxicity Symptoms
Pyridoxine, pyridoxal, pyridoxamine	BLOOD/CIRCULATORY SYSTEM	
	Anemia (small-cell type)[a]	Bloating
Adult RDA	MOUTH, GUMS, TONGUE	
0.016 mg/g protein/day Men: 2.0 mg/day Women: 1.6 mg/day	Smooth tongue,[b] cracked corners of the mouth[c]	
Chief Functions in the Body	NERVOUS/MUSCULAR SYSTEMS	
Part of coenzymes PLP (pyridoxal phosphate) and PMP (pyridoxamine phosphate) used in amino acid and fatty acid metabolism; helps to convert tryptophan to niacin; helps to make red blood cells	Abnormal brain wave pattern, irritability, muscle twitching, convulsions	Depression, fatigue, irritability, headaches, nerve damage leading to numbness and muscle weakness
	SKIN	
	Irritation of sweat glands, dermatitis	
Significant Sources	OTHER	
Green and leafy vegetables, meats, fish, poultry, shellfish, legumes, fruits, whole grains	Kidney stones	Bone pain

[a]Small-cell–type anemia is *microcytic anemia*.
[b]Smoothness of the tongue is caused by loss of its surface structures and is termed *glossitis* (gloss-EYE-tis).
[c]Cracks at the corners of the mouth are termed *cheilosis* (kee-LOH-sis).

(vitamin B_6 per 100 kcalories). Several servings of vitamin B_6–rich foods are needed to meet recommended intakes.

Foods lose vitamin B_6 when heated. Information is limited, but research shows that vitamin B_6 bioavailability from plant-derived foods is lower than from animal-derived foods; fiber does not appear to hamper absorption.

bioavailability: the rate and extent to which a nutrient is absorbed.

FOLATE

Folate, also known as folic acid or folacin, has a chemical name that would fit a flying dinosaur: pteroylglutamic acid (PGA for short). Its primary coenzyme form is THF. THF serves as part of an enzyme complex that handles one-carbon compounds that arise during metabolism. This action helps convert vitamin B_{12} to one of its coenzyme forms and helps synthesize the DNA required for all rapidly growing cells.

folate (FOLE-ate)**:** a B vitamin; also known as folic acid, folacin, or pteroylglutamic (tare-o-EEL-glue-TAM-ick) acid (PGA). The coenzyme forms are DHF (dihydrofolate) and THF (tetrahydrofolate).

Foods deliver folate mostly in the "bound" form—that is, combined with a string of amino acids (glutamate), known as polyglutamate (see Appendix C for the chemical structure). The intestine prefers to absorb the "free" folate form—folate with only one glutamate attached (the monoglutamate form). Enzymes on the intestinal cell surfaces hydrolyze the polyglutamate to monoglutamate and then attach a methyl group. Special transport systems deliver the monoglutamate form to the liver and other body cells.

How to Understand Dose Levels and Effects

A substance may have a beneficial or harmful effect, but a critical thinker would not conclude that the substance itself was beneficial or harmful without first asking what dose was used. Two corollaries to this statement might be the following:

- A substance that is poisonous at a high concentration may be an essential nutrient at a lower concentration.
- A nutrient needed at a low concentration may be toxic at a high concentration.

Figure 10–6 shows three possible relationships between dose levels and effects. The third diagram represents the situation with nutrients—more is better up to a point, but beyond that point, still more is harmful.

Figure 10–6

Dose Levels and Effects

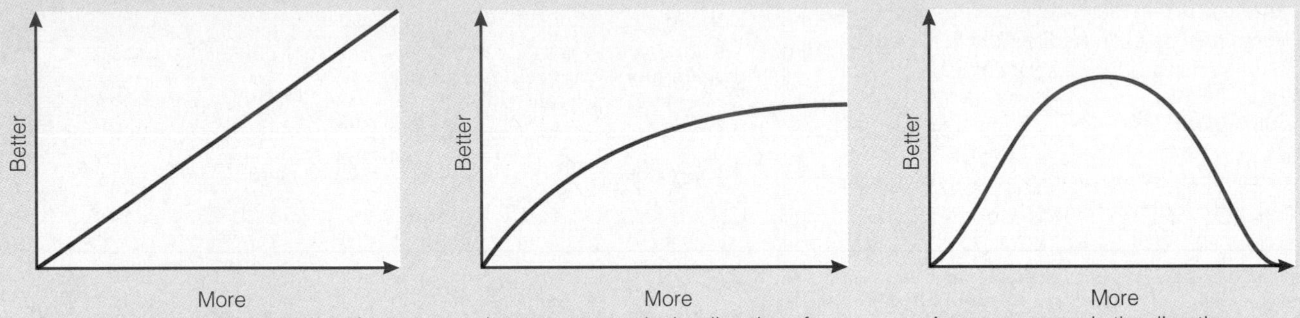

As you progress in the direction of more, the effect gets better and better, with no end in sight (real life is seldom, if ever, like this).

As you progress in the direction of more, the effect reaches a maximum and then a plateau, becoming no better with higher doses.

As you progress in the direction of more, the effect reaches an optimum at some intermediate dose and then declines, showing that more is better up to a point and then harmful. That too much is as harmful as too little represents the situation with nutrients.

To store folate, cells add glutamate, converting it back to the polyglutamate form. To release it, they hydrolyze it back to monoglutamate again. To dispose of excess folate, the liver secretes most of it into bile and ships it to the gallbladder, whence it returns to the intestine—an enterohepatic circulation route like that of bile itself (review Figure 5–15 on p. 170).

In order for the folate coenzyme to function, the methyl group needs to be removed from methyl-THF. The enzyme that removes the methyl group requires the help of vitamin B_{12}. Without that help, folate becomes trapped inside cells in its methyl form, unavailable to support DNA synthesis and cell growth (see Figure 10–8 on p. 364).

This complicated system for handling folate is vulnerable to GI tract injuries. Since folate is actively secreted back into the intestinal tract with bile, it has to be reabsorbed repeatedly. If the GI tract cells are harmed, then folate is rapidly lost from the body. Such is the case in alcohol abuse; folate deficiency rapidly develops and, ironically, damages the GI tract further. The folate coenzymes, remem-

Figure 10–7 Vitamin B_6 in Selected Foods

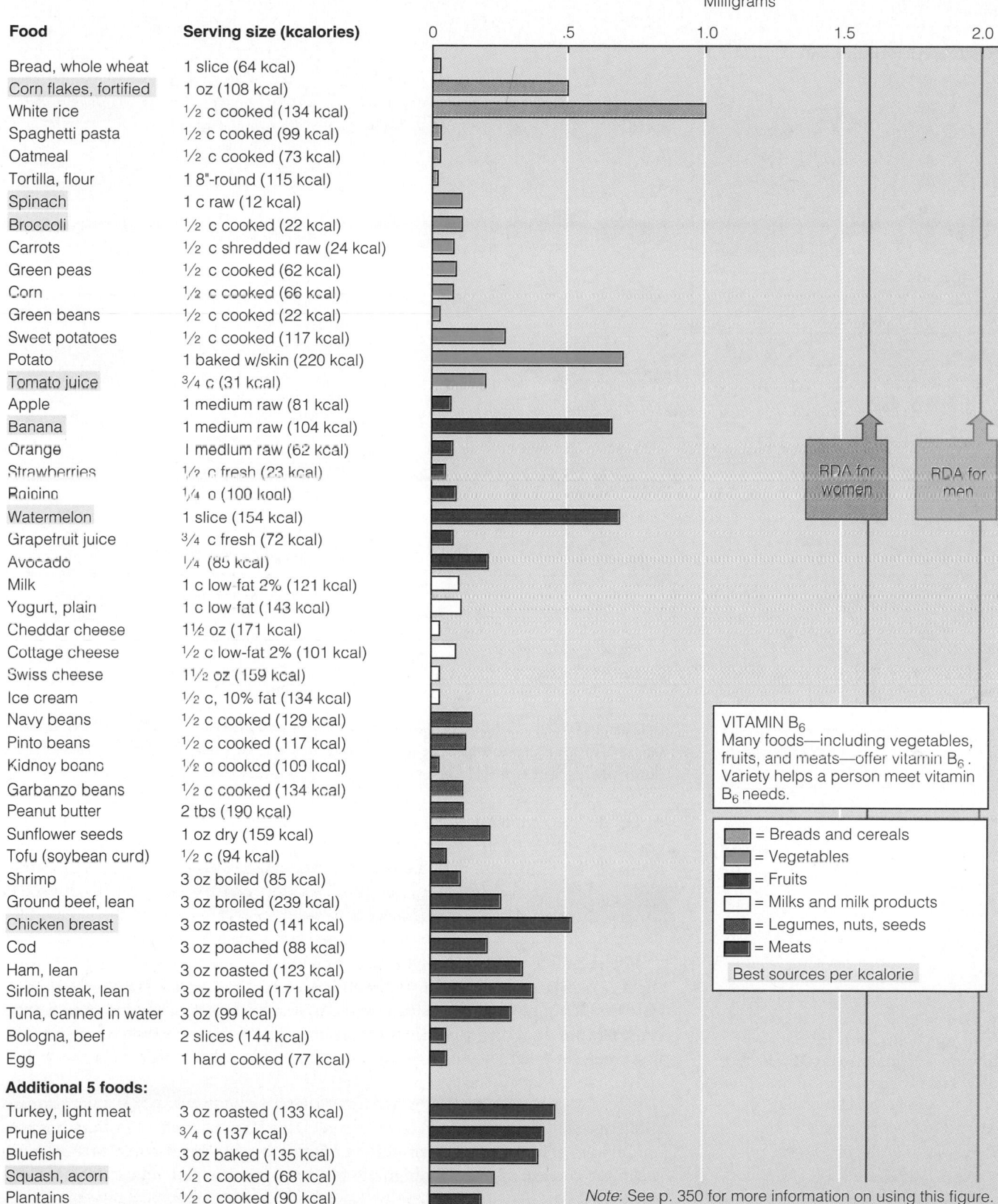

Food	Serving size (kcalories)
Bread, whole wheat	1 slice (64 kcal)
Corn flakes, fortified	1 oz (108 kcal)
White rice	1/2 c cooked (134 kcal)
Spaghetti pasta	1/2 c cooked (99 kcal)
Oatmeal	1/2 c cooked (73 kcal)
Tortilla, flour	1 8"-round (115 kcal)
Spinach	1 c raw (12 kcal)
Broccoli	1/2 c cooked (22 kcal)
Carrots	1/2 c shredded raw (24 kcal)
Green peas	1/2 c cooked (62 kcal)
Corn	1/2 c cooked (66 kcal)
Green beans	1/2 c cooked (22 kcal)
Sweet potatoes	1/2 c cooked (117 kcal)
Potato	1 baked w/skin (220 kcal)
Tomato juice	3/4 c (31 kcal)
Apple	1 medium raw (81 kcal)
Banana	1 medium raw (104 kcal)
Orange	1 medium raw (62 kcal)
Strawberries	1/2 c fresh (23 kcal)
Raisins	1/4 c (100 kcal)
Watermelon	1 slice (154 kcal)
Grapefruit juice	3/4 c fresh (72 kcal)
Avocado	1/4 (85 kcal)
Milk	1 c low-fat 2% (121 kcal)
Yogurt, plain	1 c low fat (143 kcal)
Cheddar cheese	1½ oz (171 kcal)
Cottage cheese	1/2 c low-fat 2% (101 kcal)
Swiss cheese	1 1/2 oz (159 kcal)
Ice cream	1/2 c, 10% fat (134 kcal)
Navy beans	1/2 c cooked (129 kcal)
Pinto beans	1/2 c cooked (117 kcal)
Kidney beans	1/2 c cooked (109 kcal)
Garbanzo beans	1/2 c cooked (134 kcal)
Peanut butter	2 tbs (190 kcal)
Sunflower seeds	1 oz dry (159 kcal)
Tofu (soybean curd)	1/2 c (94 kcal)
Shrimp	3 oz boiled (85 kcal)
Ground beef, lean	3 oz broiled (239 kcal)
Chicken breast	3 oz roasted (141 kcal)
Cod	3 oz poached (88 kcal)
Ham, lean	3 oz roasted (123 kcal)
Sirloin steak, lean	3 oz broiled (171 kcal)
Tuna, canned in water	3 oz (99 kcal)
Bologna, beef	2 slices (144 kcal)
Egg	1 hard cooked (77 kcal)
Additional 5 foods:	
Turkey, light meat	3 oz roasted (133 kcal)
Prune juice	3/4 c (137 kcal)
Bluefish	3 oz baked (135 kcal)
Squash, acorn	1/2 c cooked (68 kcal)
Plantains	1/2 c cooked (90 kcal)

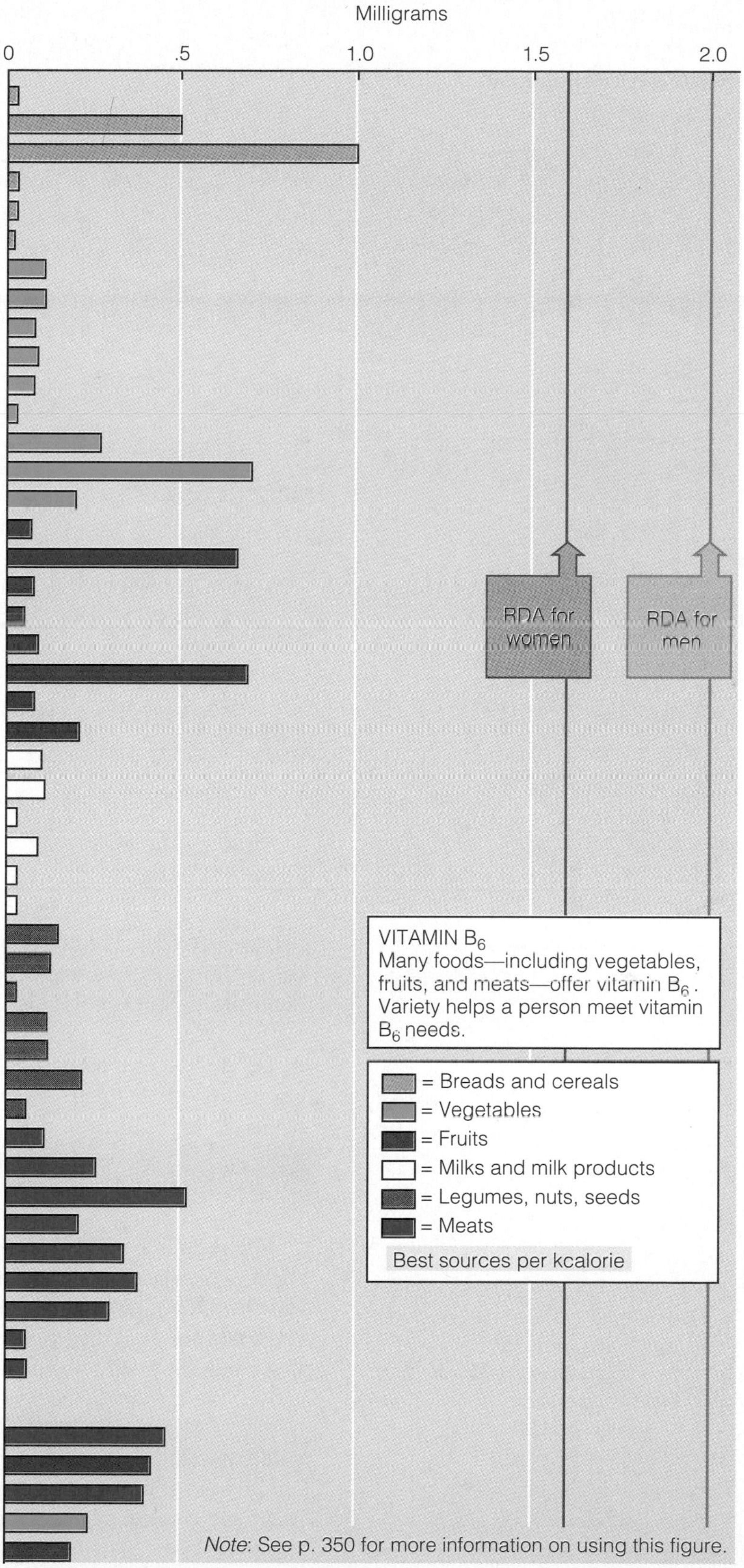

Figure 10–8

Folate's Absorption and Activation

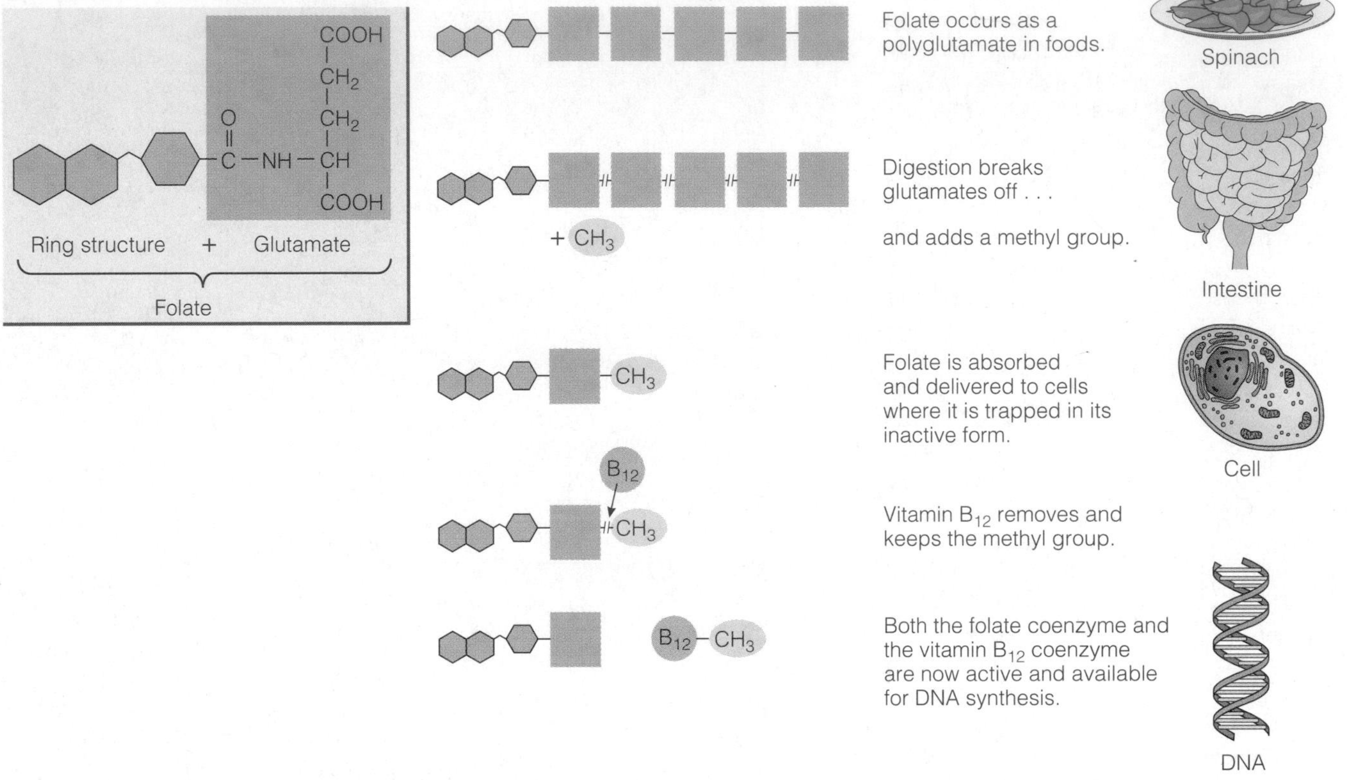
COOH
CH2
CH2
O
C—NH—CH
COOH
Ring structure + Glutamate
Folate
Folate occurs as a polyglutamate in foods.
Spinach
Digestion breaks glutamates off . . .
+ CH3
and adds a methyl group.
Intestine
CH3
Folate is absorbed and delivered to cells where it is trapped in its inactive form.
Cell
B12
CH3
Vitamin B12 removes and keeps the methyl group.
B12 CH3
Both the folate coenzyme and the vitamin B12 coenzyme are now active and available for DNA synthesis.
DNA

ber, are active in cell multiplication—and the cells lining the GI tract are among the most rapidly renewed cells in the body. Unable to make new cells, the GI tract deteriorates and not only loses folate, but also fails to absorb other nutrients.

Folate Recommendations Recommendations for daily intake are set high enough to cover folate's poor bioavailability. Only about half of dietary folate is available for use in the body. The need for folate rises considerably during pregnancy and whenever cells are multiplying, so the recommendations for pregnant women are considerably higher than for other adults.

Folate and Neural Tube Defects Several research studies have focused on the role of folate in preventing neural tube defects. The neural tube is the embryonic tissue from which the central nervous system develops. Neural tube defects cause serious disabilities and infant mortality. The defects commonly arise in the first weeks of pregnancy before a woman may realize she is pregnant.

Recent evidence suggests that folate supplements taken one month before conception and continued throughout the first trimester of pregnancy can prevent neural tube defects.[11] For this reason, the Public Health Services has recommended that all women of childbearing age who are capable of becoming pregnant should take 0.4 milligrams (400 micrograms) of folate daily.[12] This

The brain and spinal cord develop from the neural tube, and defects in its orderly formation during early gestation may result in various central nervous system disorders. The two main types of neural tube defects are *spina bifida* (literally, "split spine,") and *anencephaly* ("no brain").

For perspective, the folate RDA for women 15 years and older is 180 μg/day.

amount of folate can be met through diet rather easily—all one needs to do is eat the suggested minimum five servings of fruits and vegetables daily. But many women typically eat too few fruits and vegetables and receive only 0.2 milligrams of folate from foods daily.

For this reason, and because most pregnancies are unplanned, the Food and Drug Administration has proposed that some staple food, perhaps flour, be fortified to deliver folate to the U.S. population. Fortification is expected to prevent half of the 4000 neural tube defects each year, but it raises safety concerns as well.[13] Because high intakes of folate complicate the diagnosis of a vitamin B_{12} deficiency, folate consumption should not exceed 1 milligram daily.[14] Whether it is wise to fortify our food supply with folate is the subject of much debate.[15]

Folate's role in preventing neural tube defects is unclear. Most women whose babies develop neural tube defects are not deficient in folate and women with severe folate deficiencies typically do *not* give birth to infants with neural tube defects—so other factors must also be involved. Researchers speculate that "folate deficiency must act on an underlying nutrient-sensitive genetic defect to yield a defective newborn."[16]

Folate Deficiency Folate deficiency impairs cell division and protein synthesis—processes critical to growing tissues. In a folate deficiency, the replacement of red blood cells and GI tract cells falters. Not surprisingly then, two of the first symptoms of a folate deficiency are anemia and GI tract deterioration.

The anemia of folate deficiency is characterized by large, immature blood cells. Without folate, DNA synthesis slows and the cells lose their ability to divide. The nucleus of the cell is not released as normally occurs during development. As a result, the immature blood cells are enlarged and oval-shaped. They cannot carry oxygen or travel through the capillaries as efficiently as normal red blood cells. (Table 10–9 provides a summary of information about folate.)

anemia: literally, "too little blood." Anemia is any condition in which too few red blood cells are present, or the red blood cells are immature (and therefore large) or too small or contain too little hemoglobin to carry the normal amount of oxygen to the tissues. It is not a disease itself but can be a symptom of many different disease conditions, including many nutrient deficiencies, bleeding, excessive red blood cell destruction, and defective red blood cell formation.

an = without
emia = blood

The large-cell anemia of a folate deficiency is known as **macrocytic** or **megaloblastic** anemia.

macro = large
cyte = cell
mega = large

Folate deficiencies may develop from inadequate intake and have been reported in babies fed goat's milk, which is notoriously low in folate. Folate deficiency may also result from impaired absorption or an unusual metabolic need for the vitamin. Metabolic needs increase wherever cell multiplication must speed up: in pregnancies involving twins and triplets; in cancer; in skin-destroying diseases such as chicken pox and measles; and in burns, blood loss, GI tract damage, and the like.

Of all the vitamins, folate appears to be most vulnerable to interactions with drugs. Some drugs have a chemical structure similar to folate and can displace the vitamin from enzymes and interfere with normal metabolism. Many anticancer drugs are of this type. Cancer cells, like all cells, need the real vitamin to multiply; without it, they die. Unfortunately, other cells in the body also need folate, and vitamin deficiency develops.

Aspirin and antacids also interfere with the body's handling of folate. Healthy adults who use these drugs to relieve an occasional headache or upset stomach need not be concerned, but people who rely heavily on aspirin or antacids should be aware of the nutrition consequences. Oral contraceptives also impair folate status, as does smoking.[17] Abnormalities in the cervical cells of oral contraceptive users and in the lung cells of smokers seem to indicate a "localized" folate deficiency. Folate deficiency aggravates the risk of cervical cancer,[18] although it is not certain that folate supplements can normalize cervical cells.

Table 10–9

Folate—A Summary

Other Names	Folic acid, folacin, pteroylglutamic acid (PGA)
Adult RDA	3 μg/kg body weight/day Men: 200 μg/day Women: 180 μg/day
Chief Functions in the Body	Part of coenzymes THF (tetrahydrofolate) and DHF (dihydrofolate) used in DNA synthesis and therefore important in new cell formation
Significant Sources	Leafy green vegetables, legumes, seeds, liver

	Deficiency Symptoms	Toxicity Symptoms
BLOOD/CIRCULATORY SYSTEM	Anemia (large-cell type)[a]	
DIGESTIVE SYSTEM	Heartburn, diarrhea (loss of villi and their enzymes), constipation	
IMMUNE SYSTEM	Suppression, frequent infections	
MOUTH, GUMS, TONGUE	Smooth, red tongue[b]	
NERVOUS SYSTEM	Depression, mental confusion, fainting, fatigue	
OTHER		Masks vitamin B_{12}–deficiency symptoms

[a]Large-cell–type anemia is known as either *macrocytic* or *megaloblastic anemia.*

[b]Smoothness of the tongue is caused by loss of its surface structures and is termed *glossitis* (gloss-EYE-tis).

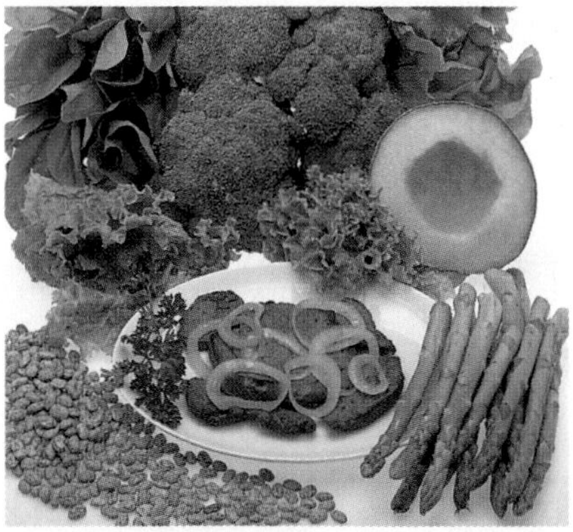

Leafy green vegetables, legumes, liver, and some fruits are rich in folate.

vitamin B_{12}: a B vitamin characterized by the presence of cobalt (see Figure 13–7 on p. 500); the active forms of coenzyme B_{12} are methylcobalamin and deoxyadenosylcobalamin.

Folate Food Sources Figure 10–9 shows that folate is especially abundant in legumes and vegetables. The vitamin's name suggests the word *foliage*, and indeed, leafy green vegetables are outstanding sources. The lack of red and white bars illustrates that meats, milk, and milk products are poor folate sources. Heat and oxidation during cooking and storage can destroy as much as half of the folate in foods.[19]

VITAMIN B_{12}

Vitamin B_{12} and folate are closely related: each depends on the other for activation. Recall that vitamin B_{12} removes a methyl group to activate the folate coenzyme; similarly, folate donates a methyl group to activate the vitamin B_{12} coenzyme (review Figure 10–8). The regeneration of the amino acid methionine and the synthesis of DNA and RNA depend on the folate coenzyme and therefore on both folate and vitamin B_{12}.* In addition, without any help from folate, vitamin

*In the body, the essential amino acid methionine serves as a methyl (CH_3) donor. In doing so, methionine can be converted to other amino acids. While some of these amino acids can regenerate methionine, a continuous supply of methionine is still needed in the diet.

Figure 10–9 Folate in Selected Foods

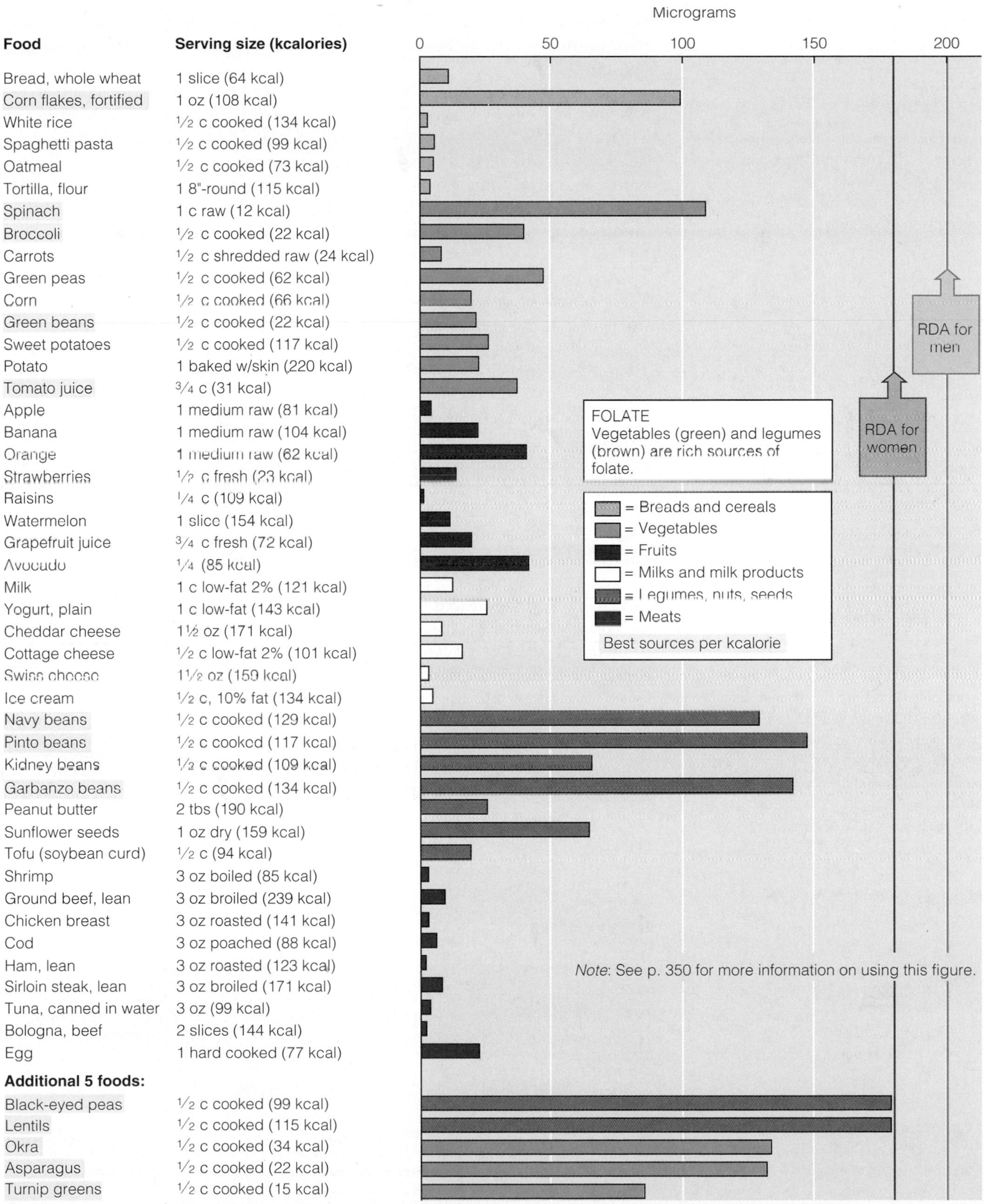
Micrograms
0
50
100
150
200
Food
Serving size (kcalories)
Bread, whole wheat 1 slice (64 kcal)
Corn flakes, fortified 1 oz (108 kcal)
White rice 1/2 c cooked (134 kcal)
Spaghetti pasta 1/2 c cooked (99 kcal)
Oatmeal 1/2 c cooked (73 kcal)
Tortilla, flour 1 8"-round (115 kcal)
Spinach 1 c raw (12 kcal)
Broccoli 1/2 c cooked (22 kcal)
Carrots 1/2 c shredded raw (24 kcal)
Green peas 1/2 c cooked (62 kcal)
Corn 1/2 c cooked (66 kcal)
Green beans 1/2 c cooked (22 kcal)
Sweet potatoes 1/2 c cooked (117 kcal)
Potato 1 baked w/skin (220 kcal)
Tomato juice 3/4 c (31 kcal)
Apple 1 medium raw (81 kcal)
Banana 1 medium raw (104 kcal)
Orange 1 medium raw (62 kcal)
Strawberries 1/2 c fresh (23 kcal)
Raisins 1/4 c (109 kcal)
Watermelon 1 slice (154 kcal)
Grapefruit juice 3/4 c fresh (72 kcal)
Avocado 1/4 (85 kcal)
Milk 1 c low-fat 2% (121 kcal)
Yogurt, plain 1 c low-fat (143 kcal)
Cheddar cheese 1½ oz (171 kcal)
Cottage cheese 1/2 c low-fat 2% (101 kcal)
Swiss cheese 1½ oz (159 kcal)
Ice cream 1/2 c, 10% fat (134 kcal)
Navy beans 1/2 c cooked (129 kcal)
Pinto beans 1/2 c cooked (117 kcal)
Kidney beans 1/2 c cooked (109 kcal)
Garbanzo beans 1/2 c cooked (134 kcal)
Peanut butter 2 tbs (190 kcal)
Sunflower seeds 1 oz dry (159 kcal)
Tofu (soybean curd) 1/2 c (94 kcal)
Shrimp 3 oz boiled (85 kcal)
Ground beef, lean 3 oz broiled (239 kcal)
Chicken breast 3 oz roasted (141 kcal)
Cod 3 oz poached (88 kcal)
Ham, lean 3 oz roasted (123 kcal)
Sirloin steak, lean 3 oz broiled (171 kcal)
Tuna, canned in water 3 oz (99 kcal)
Bologna, beef 2 slices (144 kcal)
Egg 1 hard cooked (77 kcal)
Additional 5 foods:
Black-eyed peas 1/2 c cooked (99 kcal)
Lentils 1/2 c cooked (115 kcal)
Okra 1/2 c cooked (34 kcal)
Asparagus 1/2 c cooked (22 kcal)
Turnip greens 1/2 c cooked (15 kcal)
RDA for men
RDA for women
FOLATE
Vegetables (green) and legumes (brown) are rich sources of folate.
= Breads and cereals
= Vegetables
= Fruits
= Milks and milk products
= Legumes, nuts, seeds
= Meats
Best sources per kcalorie

Note: See p. 350 for more information on using this figure.

B_{12} maintains the sheath that surrounds and protects nerve fibers and promotes their normal growth. Bone cell activity and metabolism also seem to depend on vitamin B_{12}.

After ingestion, vitamin B_{12} is released from the proteins to which it was attached in foods by hydrochloric acid and the enzyme pepsin in the stomach. Then the vitamin binds with an "intrinsic factor" for absorption from the intestinal tract into the bloodstream. The genes carry the code for this factor, which is synthesized in the stomach. After the intrinsic factor attaches to vitamin B_{12}, the complex passes to the small intestine, where the vitamin is gradually absorbed. Transport of vitamin B_{12} in the blood depends on specific binding proteins.

intrinsic: inside the system. The intrinsic factor is a glycoprotein (a protein with short polysaccharide chains attached) made in the stomach that aids in the absorption of vitamin B_{12}.

Vitamin B_{12} Recommendations According to the RDA, adults need about 2 micrograms of vitamin B_{12} a day—only two-millionths of a gram. The ink in the period at the end of this sentence may weigh about 2 micrograms. But tiny though this amount appears to the human eye, it contains billions of molecules of vitamin B_{12}, enough to provide coenzymes for all the enzymes that need its help.

Vitamin B_{12} Deficiency Most vitamin B_{12} deficiencies reflect inadequate absorption, not poor intake. Inadequate absorption typically occurs for one of two reasons: a lack of hydrochloric acid or a lack of intrinsic factor. Many people, especially those over 60, develop atrophic gastritis, a condition characterized by inadequate hydrochloric acid. Consequently, even with adequate intake, their vitamin B_{12} status diminishes: the vitamin is not released from the dietary proteins and so is not available for binding with the intrinsic factor.

atrophic gastritis: chronic inflammation of the stomach accompanied by a diminished size and functioning of the mucosa and glands.
atrophy = wasting
gastro = stomach
itis = inflammation

Some people inherit a defective gene for the intrinsic factor. Without the intrinsic factor, they develop deficiency symptoms, even though they are receiving enough vitamin B_{12} from foods. In some cases, or when the stomach has been injured and cannot produce enough of the intrinsic factor, vitamin B_{12} must be injected to bypass the need for intestinal absorption. The vitamin B_{12} deficiency caused by lack of intrinsic factor is known as pernicious anemia.

pernicious (per-NISH-us) anemia: a blood disorder that reflects a vitamin B_{12} deficiency caused by lack of intrinsic factor and characterized by a deficit of red blood cells, muscle weakness, and neurological disturbances.
pernicious = destructive

Because vitamin B_{12} is required to convert folate to its active form, one of the most obvious vitamin B_{12}–deficiency symptoms is the anemia of folate deficiency. This anemia is characterized by large, immature red blood cells, which are indicative of slow DNA synthesis and an inability to divide (see Figure 10–10). When folate is trapped in its inactive (methyl folate) form due to vitamin B_{12} deficiency, or is unavailable due to folate deficiency itself, DNA synthesis slows.

First to be affected in vitamin B_{12} or folate deficiency are the rapidly growing blood cells. Either vitamin B_{12} or folate will clear up the anemia, but if folate is given when vitamin B_{12} is needed, the result is disastrous: devastating neurological symptoms. Remember that vitamin B_{12}, but not folate, maintains the sheath that surrounds and protects nerve fibers and promotes their normal growth. Folate "cures" the *blood* symptoms of a vitamin B_{12} deficiency, but allows the *nerve* symptoms to progress. By doing so, folate "masks" a vitamin B_{12} deficiency. A deficiency of vitamin B_{12} causes a creeping paralysis of the nerves and muscles, which begins at the extremities and works inward and up the spine. Early detection and correction are necessary to prevent permanent nerve damage and paralysis. With sufficient folate in the diet, the neurological symptoms of vitamin B_{12} deficiency can develop without evidence of anemia. Such interactions between folate and vitamin B_{12} highlight some of the safety issues surrounding

Figure 10–10

Normal and Anemic Blood Cells

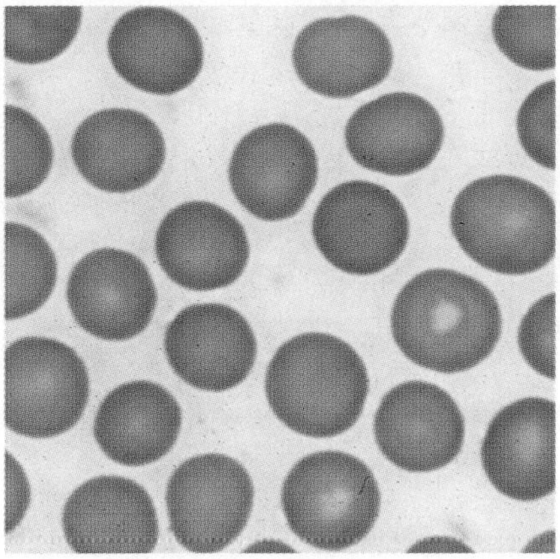

Normal blood cells. The size, shape, and color of the red blood cells show that they are normal. Mature red blood cells have lost their nuclei.

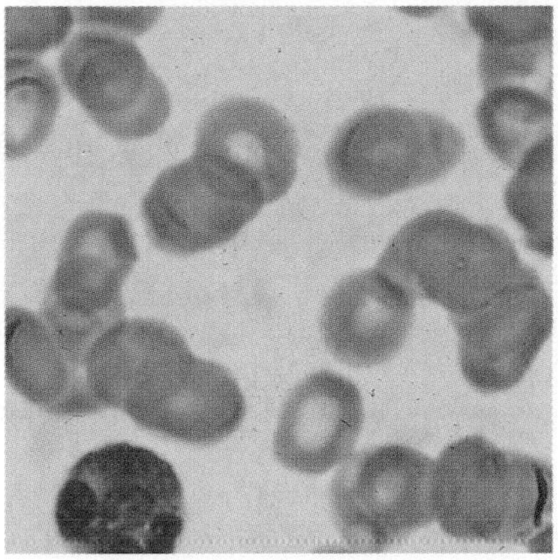

Blood cells in pernicious anemia (megaloblastic). Megaloblastic blood cells are arrested at an immature stage of development, so they still have their nuclei. For this reason, they are slightly larger than normal red blood cells, and their shapes are irregular.

the use of supplements and fortification of the food supply. Table 10–10 provides a summary of information about vitamin B_{12}.

Vitamin B_{12} Food Sources Vitamin B_{12} is unique among the nutrients in being found almost exclusively in foods derived from animals. Anyone who eats reasonable amounts of meat is guaranteed an adequate intake, and vegetarians who use milk, cheese, and eggs are also protected from deficiency. Fermented soy products such as miso (a soybean paste) or sea algae such as spirulina do *not* provide vitamin B_{12} in its active form. Extensive research shows that the amounts listed on the labels of these plant products are inaccurate and misleading, because the vitamin B_{12} is in an inactive, unavailable form. Vegans need a reliable source, such as vitamin B_{12}–fortified soy "milk," meat replacements, or vitamin B_{12} supplements. Yeast that is grown on a vitamin B_{12}–enriched medium and mixed with that medium provides some vitamin B_{12}, but yeast itself does not contain active vitamin B_{12}.

Reminder: *Meat replacements* are textured vegetable-protein products formulated to look and taste like meat, fish, or poultry and often fortified with nutrients commonly found in meats.

People who stop eating foods containing vitamin B_{12} may take up to 20 years to develop deficiencies because the body recycles much of its vitamin B_{12}, reabsorbing it over and over again. Even when the body fails to absorb vitamin B_{12}, deficiency may take up to three years to develop because the body conserves its supply.

VITAMIN IMPOSTORS

The compounds inositol, choline, and lipoic acid are sometimes called B vitamins. Researchers are exploring the possibility that these substances may be essential and one day might be considered for an RDA. Some research indicates

inositol (in-OSS-ih-tall)**:** a nonessential nutrient that can be made in the body from glucose. Inositol is used in cell membranes.

Table 10–10

Vitamin B_{12}—A Summary

Other Names	Deficiency Disease Name
Cobalamin (and related forms)	Pernicious anemia[a]
Adult RDA	**Deficiency Symptoms**
2 µg/day (0.002 mg, or two-millionths of a gram)	BLOOD/CIRCULATORY SYSTEM Anemia (large-cell type)[b]
Chief Functions in the Body	MOUTH, GUMS, TONGUE Smooth tongue[c]
Part of coenzymes methylcobalamin and deoxyadenocobalamin used in new cell synthesis; helps to maintain nerve cells; re-forms folate coenzyme; helps to break down some fatty acids and amino acids	NERVOUS SYSTEM Fatigue, degeneration of peripheral nerves progressing to paralysis
Significant Sources	SKIN
Animal products (meat, fish, poultry, shellfish, milk, cheese, eggs)	Hypersensitivity

[a]The name *pernicious anemia* refers to the vitamin B_{12} deficiency caused by lack of intrinsic factor, but not to that caused by inadequate dietary intake.
[b]Large-cell–type anemia is known as either *macrocytic* or *megaloblastic anemia*.
[c]Smoothness of the tongue is caused by loss of its surface structures and is termed *glossitis* (gloss-EYE-tis).

choline (KOH-leen)**:** a nonessential nutrient that can be made in the body from an amino acid. Choline is used to make the phospholipid lecithin and the neurotransmitter acetylcholine.

lipoic (lip-OH-ick) **acid:** a nonessential nutrient.

that they are conditionally essential under certain circumstances.[20] Even if they are essential, though, supplements are unnecessary because these compounds are abundant in foods.

Some vitamin companies include these compounds in their formulations to make their vitamin pills look more "complete" than others, but these compounds confer no advantage. For a rational way to compare different vitamin-mineral supplements, read Highlight 10.

Medical practitioners have reported overdoses of choline and its relative lecithin (which contains choline as part of its structure as Figure 5–9 on p. 164 shows). Taken in excess, these components cause short-term discomforts such as GI distress, sweating, salivation, and anorexia, as well as long-term health hazards such as injury to the nervous and cardiovascular systems.

Other substances have been mistaken for essential nutrients for human beings because they are needed for growth by bacteria or other forms of life. Among them are PABA (para-aminobenzoic acid), the bioflavonoids (vitamin P or hesperidin), and ubiquinone (coenzyme Q_{10}). Other names associated wrongly with vitamins are "vitamin B_5" (another name for pantothenic acid), "vitamin B_{15}" (also called "pangamic acid," a hoax), "vitamin B_{17}" (Laetrile, an alleged "cancer cure" and not a vitamin by any stretch of the imagination), and "vitamin B_T" (carnitine, an important piece of cell machinery, but not a vitamin because it can be made by the body as needed).

In summary, the B vitamins serve as coenzymes that facilitate the work of every cell. They are active in carbohydrate, fat, and protein metabolism and in the making of DNA and thus new cells. Historically famous B vitamin deficiency diseases are beriberi (thiamin), pellagra (niacin), and pernicious anemia (vitamin B_{12}). Pellagra can be prevented by adquate protein because the amino acid tryptophan can be converted to niacin in the body. A high intake of folate can mask the blood symptom of a vitamin B_{12} deficiency but it will not prevent the associated nerve damage. Vitamin B_6 participates in amino acid metabolism and can be toxic in excess. Biotin and pantothenic acid serve important roles in energy metabolism and are abundant in food. Many substances that people claim as B vitamins are not (including inositol, lipoic acid, and choline).

The B Vitamins—In Concert

Figure 10–11 (on p. 372) is intended to convey an *impression* of the ways B vitamins busily work in metabolic pathways all over the body. They are involved in every crucial step. Metabolism is the body's work, and the B vitamin coenzymes are indispensable to it. In scanning the pathways of metabolism depicted in the figure, note the abbreviations for the coenzymes that keep the processes going.

Roles of the B Vitamin Coenzymes Look at the first step in the now-familiar pathway of glucose breakdown. To break down glucose to pyruvate, the cells must have certain enzymes. For the enzymes to work, they must have the niacin coenzyme NAD. To make NAD, the cells must be supplied with niacin (or enough of the amino acid tryptophan to make niacin). They can make the rest of the coenzyme without outside help.

The next step in glucose catabolism is the breakdown of pyruvate to acetyl CoA. The enzymes involved in this step require NAD plus the thiamin coenzyme, TPP. The cells can manufacture the TPP they need from thiamin, if thiamin is in the diet.

Another coenzyme needed for this step is CoA. Predictably, the cells can make CoA except for an essential part that must be obtained in the diet—pantothenic acid. Another coenzyme requiring biotin serves the enzyme complex involved in converting pyruvate to a compound that can combine with acetyl CoA in the TCA cycle.

These and other coenzymes are involved throughout all the metabolic pathways. When the diet provides riboflavin, the body synthesizes FAD—a needed coenzyme in the TCA cycle. Vitamin B_6 is an indispensable part of PLP—a coenzyme required for many amino acid conversions, for a crucial step in the making of the iron-containing portion of hemoglobin for red blood cells, and for many other reactions. Folate becomes THF—the coenzyme required for the synthesis of new genetic material and therefore new cells. The vitamin B_{12} coenzyme, in turn, regenerates THF to its active form; thus vitamin B_{12} is also necessary for the formation of new cells.

Thus each of the B vitamin coenzymes is involved, directly or indirectly, in energy metabolism. Some are facilitators of the energy-releasing reactions themselves; others help build new cells to deliver the oxygen and nutrients that permit the energy pathways to run.

Figure 10–11

Metabolic Pathways Involving B Vitamins

These metabolic pathways were introduced in Chapter 7 and are presented here to highlight the many coenzymes that facilitate the reactions. These coenzymes depend on the following vitamins:

- NAD and NADP: niacin.
- TPP: thiamin.
- CoA: pantothenic acid.
- B_{12}: vitamin B_{12}.
- FMN and FAD: riboflavin.
- THF: folate
- PLP: vitamin B_6.
- Biotin.

For further details, see Appendix C.

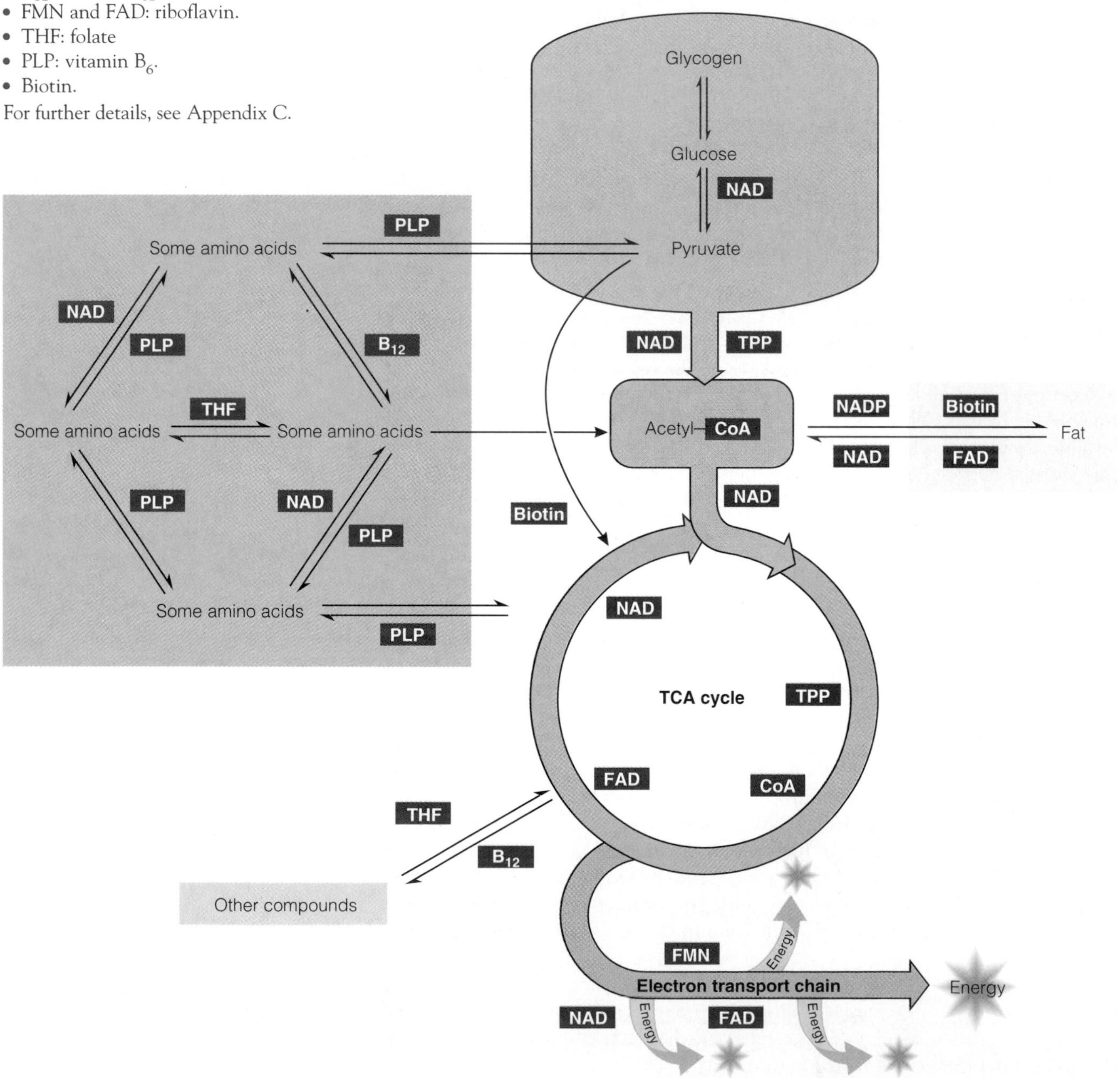

Effects of a Deficiency Now suppose the body's cells lack one of these B vitamins—niacin, for example. Without niacin, the cells cannot make NAD. Without NAD, the enzymes involved in every step of the glucose-to-energy pathway cannot function. Then, since all the body's activities require energy, literally everything begins to grind to a halt. This is no exaggeration. The deadly disease pellagra, caused by niacin deficiency, produces the "devastating *D*s": dermatitis, which reflects a failure of the skin; dementia, a failure of the nervous system; diarrhea, a failure of digestion and absorption; and eventually, as would be the case for any severe nutrient deficiency, death. These symptoms are the obvious ones, but a niacin deficiency affects all other organs, too, because all are dependent on the energy pathways. In short, niacin is like the horseshoe nail for want of which a war was lost. All the vitamins are like horseshoe nails.

For want of a nail, a horseshoe was lost.
For want of a horseshoe, a horse was lost.
For want of a horse, a soldier was lost.
For want of a soldier, a battle was lost.
For want of a battle, the war was lost,
And all for the want of a horseshoe nail!

—Mother Goose

B VITAMIN INTERACTIONS

This chapter has described some of the impressive ways that vitamins work individually, as if their many actions in the body could easily be disentangled. In fact, oftentimes it is difficult to tell which vitamin is truly responsible for a given effect because the nutrients are interdependent; the presence or absence of one affects another's absorption, metabolism, and excretion. You have already seen this interdependence with folate and vitamin B_{12}.

Riboflavin and vitamin B_6 are another example of a B vitamin relationship. One of the riboflavin coenzymes, FMN, assists the enzyme that converts vitamin B_6 to its coenzyme form PLP.[21] Consequently, a severe riboflavin deficiency can impair vitamin B_6 activity. Thus a deficiency of one nutrient may alter the action of another. Furthermore, a deficiency of one nutrient may create a deficiency of another. For example, a vitamin B_6 deficiency hinders calcium absorption and enhances magnesium excretion.[22] These interdependent relationships are evident in many of the B vitamin deficiencies.

B VITAMIN DEFICIENCIES

With any B vitamin deficiency, many body systems become deranged, and similar symptoms may appear. Removing "horseshoe nails" can have disastrous and far-reaching effects.

Deficiencies of single B vitamins seldom show up in isolation. After all, people do not eat nutrients singly; they eat foods, which contain mixtures of nutrients. Only in two cases described earlier—beriberi and pellagra—have dietary deficiencies associated with single B vitamins been observed on a large scale in human populations. Even in these cases, the deficiencies were not pure. Both diseases were attributed to deficiencies of single vitamins, but both were likely to have been deficiencies of several vitamins in which one vitamin stood out above the rest. When foods containing the vitamin known to be needed were provided, the vitamins that may have been in short supply came as part of the package.

Significantly, these deficiency diseases were eliminated by supplying foods—not pills. Vitamin pill advertisements make much of the fact that vitamins are indispensable to life, but human beings obtained their nourishment from foods for centuries before vitamin pills existed. If the diet lacks a vitamin, the solution is to adjust food intake to obtain that vitamin.

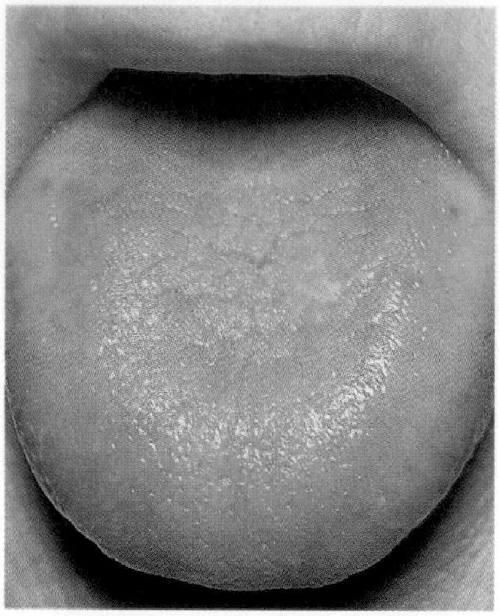

Tongue symptoms of B vitamin deficiency. The tongue is smooth due to atrophy of the tissue (glossitis).

Manufacturers of so-called *natural* vitamins boast that their pills are purified from real foods rather than synthesized in a laboratory. Think back on the course of human evolution; it is not *natural* to take any kind of pill. In reality, the finest, most complete vitamin "supplements" available are meat, fish, poultry, eggs, legumes, nuts, milk and milk products, vegetables, fruits, and grain products.

The skin and the tongue appear to be especially sensitive to B vitamin deficiencies, but note that listing them in the summary tables gives them undue emphasis. Remember that these two body parts are readily visible in a physical examination. If the skin is degenerating, other tissues beneath it may be, too. Similarly, the mouth and tongue are the visible part of the digestive system; if they are abnormal, there may well be an abnormality throughout the GI tract. The impact of a vitamin deficiency is felt inside the cells of the body; what the physician sees and reports are the deficiency's outward manifestations. The accompanying box offers other insights into symptoms and their causes.

Major deficiency diseases of epidemic proportions such as pellagra and beriberi are no longer seen in the United States and Canada, but lesser deficiencies of nutrients, including the B vitamins, sometimes are observed. When they occur, it is usually in people whose food choices are poor because of poverty, ignorance, illness, or poor health habits like alcohol abuse (review Highlight 7 to fully appre-

How to Distinguish Symptoms and Causes

It is more and more apparent that no one can observe a symptom and automatically jump to a conclusion regarding its cause. The summary tables in this chapter show that deficiencies of riboflavin, niacin, and vitamin B_6 can all cause skin rashes. But so can deficiencies of protein, linoleic acid, or vitamin A. Because skin is on the outside and easy to see, it is a useful indicator of things-going-wrong-in-cells. But by itself, a skin symptom says nothing about its possible cause.

The same is true of anemia. Anemia is often caused by iron deficiency, but it can also be caused by a folate or vitamin B_{12} deficiency; by digestive tract failure to absorb any of these nutrients; or by such nonnutritional causes as infections, parasites, cancer, or loss of blood. Again, no specific nutrient will always cure a given symptom.

A person who feels chronically tired may be tempted to self-diagnose iron-deficiency anemia and self-prescribe an iron supplement. But this will relieve tiredness only if the cause is indeed iron-deficiency anemia. If the cause is a folate deficiency, taking iron will only prolong the tiredness. A person who is better informed may decide to take a vitamin supplement with iron, covering the possibility of a vitamin deficiency. But the symptom may have a nonnutritional cause. If the cause of the tiredness is actually hidden blood loss due to cancer, the postponement of a diagnosis may be equivalent to suicide. When tiredness is caused by a lack of sleep, of course, no nutrient or combination of nutrients can replace a good night's rest. A person who is chronically tired should see a physician rather than self-prescribe.

ciate how alcohol induces vitamin deficiencies and interferes with energy metabolism). Remember from Chapter 1 that deficiencies can arise not only from deficient intakes (primary causes), but also for other (secondary) reasons.

B VITAMIN TOXICITIES

Toxicities of the B vitamins are uncommon but do occur when people overuse supplements. When the cells become oversaturated with a vitamin, they must work to eliminate the excess. The cells remove water-soluble vitamins by excreting excesses in the urine, but sometimes fail to regain homeostasis. On the other hand, B vitamin toxicities from foods alone are unknown.

B VITAMIN FOOD SOURCES

The food figures presented in this chapter, taken together, sing the praises of the balanced diet. The meat group serves thiamin, niacin, vitamin B_6, and vitamin B_{12} well. The milk and milk products group stands out for riboflavin and vitamin B_{12}. The fruit and vegetable groups excel in folate. The cereal and bread group delivers thiamin, riboflavin, and niacin. A diet that offers a variety of foods from each group, prepared with reasonable care, serves up ample B vitamins.

The B vitamin coenzymes work together in energy metabolism. Some are facilitators of the energy-releasing reactions themselves; others help build cells to deliver the oxygen and nutrients that permit the energy pathways to run. These vitamins depend on each other to function optimally; a deficiency of any of them creates multiple problems. Fortunately a variety of foods from each of the five food groups will provide an adequate supply of all of the B vitamins.

Vitamin C

Two hundred and fifty years ago, any man who joined the crew of a seagoing ship knew he had only half a chance of returning alive—not because he might be slain by pirates or die in a storm, but because he might contract the dread disease scurvy. As many as two-thirds of a ship's crew might die of scurvy on a long voyage. Only men on short voyages, especially around the Mediterranean Sea, were free of scurvy. No one knew the reason: that on long ocean voyages, the ship's cook used up the fresh fruits and vegetables early and then served cereals and meats until the return to port.

scurvy: the vitamin C–deficiency disease.

The first nutrition experiment ever performed on human beings was devised in 1747 to find a cure for scurvy. James Lind, a British physician, divided 12 sailors with scurvy into six pairs. Each pair received a different supplemental ration: cider, vinegar, sulfuric acid, seawater, oranges and lemons, or a purgative mixed with spices. Those receiving the citrus fruits quickly recovered, but sadly, it was 50 years before the British navy required all vessels to provide every sailor with lime juice daily. This tradition gave British sailors the nickname "limeys."

purgative: a strong laxative.

The antiscurvy "something" in limes and other foods was dubbed the antiscorbutic factor. Nearly 200 years later, the factor was isolated from lemon juice and found to be a 6-carbon compound similar to glucose; it was named ascorbic

antiscorbutic factor: the original name for vitamin C.
anti = against
scorbutic = causing scurvy

ascorbic acid: one of the two active forms of vitamin C (see Figure 10–12). Many people refer to vitamin C by this name.
a = without
scorbic = having scurvy

acid. Shortly thereafter, it was synthesized, and today hundreds of millions of vitamin C pills are produced in pharmaceutical laboratories each year and sold for a few dollars a bottle.

VITAMIN C ROLES

Vitamin C parts company with the B vitamins in its mode of action. In some settings, vitamin C helps a specific enzyme perform its job, but in others, it acts in a more general way as an antioxidant.

antioxidant: a compound that protects others from oxidation by being oxidized itself. An antioxidant donates electrons to another substance; that substance becomes reduced as the antioxidant simultaneously becomes oxidized. Chemists describe the antioxidant action of vitamin C as maintaining the "oxidation-reduction equilibrium," or "redox state."

Highlight 11 discusses the role of antioxidant nutrients in disease prevention in more detail. Chapter 13 provides more details on the relationship between vitamin C and iron.

Reminder: *Collagen* is the protein material from which connective tissues such as scars, tendons, ligaments, and the foundations of bones and teeth are made.

As an Antioxidant An antioxidant is any substance that prevents or inhibits the oxidation of another substance. In doing so, the antioxidant becomes oxidized itself, but this is useful because it protects the other substance from being altered or even destroyed by oxidation. Vitamin C is like a bodyguard for water-soluble substances; it stands ready to sacrifice its own life to save theirs. Figure 10–12 illustrates how vitamin C's structure can change, so that it can serve as an antioxidant.

Because of vitamin C's antioxidant property, manufacturers sometimes add it to foods as a preservative. In the cells and body fluids, vitamin C helps to prevent damage to tissues, which may be important in preventing disease. In the intestines, vitamin C protects iron from oxidation and so promotes iron absorption.

In Collagen Formation Vitamin C helps to form the fibrous structural protein known as collagen, the single most important protein of connective tissues. Collagen serves as the matrix on which bones and teeth are formed. When a person is wounded, collagen glues the separated tissues together, forming scars. Cells are held together largely by collagen; this is especially important in the artery walls, which must expand and contract with each beat of the heart, and in the thin capillary walls, which must withstand a pulse of blood every second or so without giving way.

The body makes all proteins by stringing together chains of amino acids. In collagen, the amino acids proline and lysine appear in abundance. During the synthesis of collagen, each time a proline or lysine is added to the growing protein chain, an enzyme hydroxylates it (adds an OH group to it), making the

Figure 10–12

Active Forms of Vitamin C

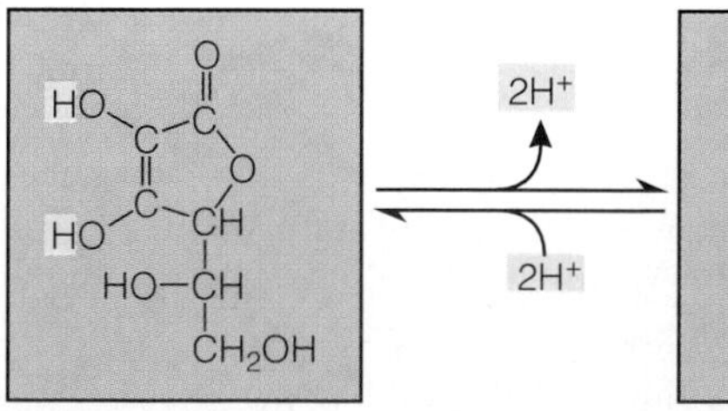

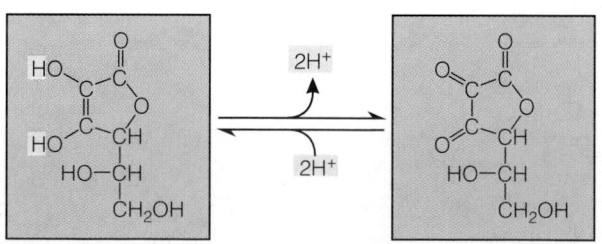

Ascorbic acid is the reduced form of vitamin C. Ascorbic acid can easily give up two hydrogens with their electrons, thereby becoming dehydroascorbic acid. Molecules with unpaired electrons (free radicals) combine with antioxidants such as vitamin C instead of causing oxidative damage to the cells.

Dehydroascorbic acid is the oxidized form of vitamin C. The reversibility of this reaction is key to vitamin C's role as an antioxidant.

amino acids hydroxyproline or hydroxylysine, respectively. Figure 10–13 illustrates the conversion of proline to hydroxyproline. This hydroxylase enzyme requires both vitamin C and iron. Iron works as a cofactor in the reaction, and vitamin C maintains iron in the form that allows it to do so. Without them, the hydroxylation step does not occur. Hydroxyproline and hydroxylysine facilitate the binding together of collagen fibers to make strong, ropelike structures.

cofactor: a mineral element that, like a coenzyme, works with an enzyme to facilitate a chemical reaction. The cofactor maintains the structural integrity of the enzyme and may also facilitate the enzyme's catalytic activity.

In Stress Vitamin C assists in the metabolism of several amino acids, some of which are used to make hormones—notably, the hormones norepinephrine and thyroxin. The adrenal glands are richer in vitamin C than any other organ in the body, and during stress, these glands release the vitamin, together with hormones, into the blood.

The vitamin's exact role in the stress reaction is unclear. Psychological stress alone does not appear to raise needs above the RDA, but some physical stresses such as infections, wound healing, and exposure to cold raise vitamin C needs. When immune system cells are called into action, they use a lot of oxygen and produce oxidants that can damage the cells themselves.[23] Thus vitamin C is used as an antioxidant whenever the immune system becomes active. The hormone thyroxin (made with vitamin C's help) regulates the metabolic rate, which speeds up under extreme stress and also when the body needs to produce extra heat—for example, in fever or cold weather.

Figure 10–13

Vitamin C's Role in Hydroxyproline Synthesis

Collagen is unique among body proteins because it contains large amounts of the amino acid hydroxyproline. The hydroxylase enzyme, which forms hydroxyproline by adding a hydroxyl group to the amino acid proline, requires vitamin C and iron.

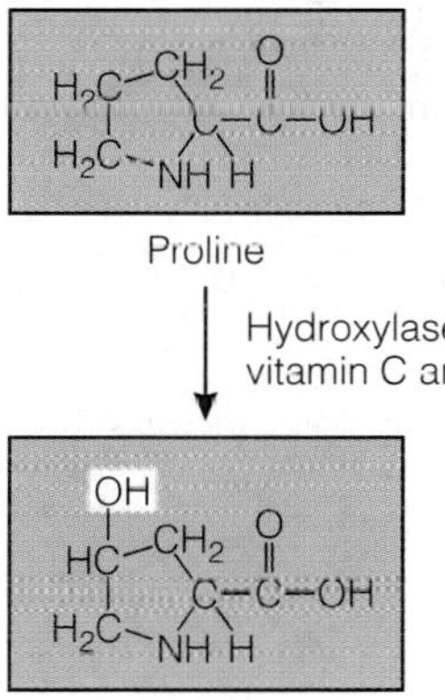

As a Cure for the Common Cold and Respiratory Infections Newspaper headlines touting vitamin C as a cure for colds have appeared frequently over the years, but researchers have found little, if any, support for such claims. A major review of the research on vitamin C in the treatment and prevention of the common cold revealed a significant difference of one-tenth of a cold per year and an average difference in duration of one-tenth of a day per cold in favor of those taking vitamin C. The term *significant* means that *statistical* analysis suggests that the findings probably didn't arise from a chance event, but from the experimental treatment being tested. The *human* significance of the findings, however, is apparent only when considered in a real-life context: the typical cold lasts about a week, and one-tenth of a day is only 2½ hours. Is that enough savings to warrant routine supplementation? Scientists think not; supplement users seem to think so.

Interestingly, findings from one study revealed that those who received the placebo *but thought they were receiving vitamin* C had fewer colds than the group who received vitamin C *but thought they were receiving the placebo*. (Never underestimate the healing power of faith!)

Recent discoveries of the ways vitamin C works in the body provide possible links between the vitamin and the common cold. Some research suggests that vitamin C (2 grams taken daily for two weeks) reduces blood histamine.[24] Anyone who has ever had a cold knows the discomfort of a runny or stuffed-up nose. Nasal congestion develops in response to elevated blood histamine, and people commonly take antihistamines for relief. Like an antihistamine, vitamin C comes to the rescue and deactivates histamine.[25]

Vitamin C also appears to protect the lungs.[26] Researchers exploring the relationship between vitamin C and upper respiratory infections found that vitamin C supplements significantly improved symptoms of respiratory infections.[27] In a study of runners, vitamin C supplements reduced the incidence of respiratory symptoms after participation in a marathon.[28] Earlier studies had shown that

Figure 10–14

Vitamin C Intake (mg)

Recommendations differ, but all are generously above the minimum requirement and below the toxicity level. In contrast, megadoses of 2 grams a day are clearly way up in the clouds.

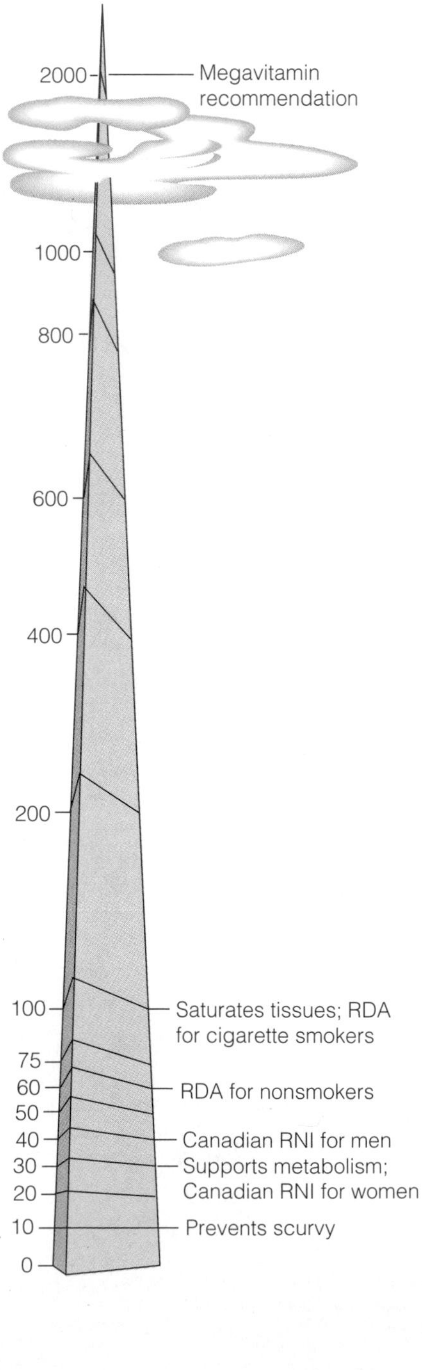

marathon and ultramarathon competitors have a high incidence of upper respiratory symptoms immediately following a race.

In Disease Prevention The role of vitamin C in the prevention of, or therapy for, cancer and other diseases is still being studied, and findings are presented in Highlight 11. An epidemiological study of over 11,000 U.S. adults reported an inverse relationship between all causes of death and vitamin C intake up to a few hundred milligrams.[29] The relationship was stronger for men that for women and remained apparent after controlling for confounding variables such as age, sex, cigarette smoking, disease history, race, and education.

VITAMIN C RECOMMENDATIONS

How much vitamin C is enough? Allowances set by different nations are based on similar research findings, but vary from 30 milligrams per day in Great Britain and Canada to 60 in the United States and 100 in Japan.[30] As Figure 10–14 illustrates, all the different recommendations fall within a broad range of possible safe intakes.

The requirement—the amount needed to prevent the overt symptoms of scurvy—is well known to be only 10 milligrams daily. However, 10 milligrams a day does not saturate all the body tissues; larger intakes increase the body's total vitamin C. At about 60 milligrams per day, the tissues in the average person stop responding to further increases in intake, and at 100 milligrams per day, 95 percent of the population probably reaches tissue saturation. After the tissues are saturated, excess vitamin C is readily excreted.

The RDA for vitamin C, like all the RDA, is intended to maintain health in healthy people, not to restore health in sick people. A variety of physical stresses deplete the body's vitamin C supply and may make higher intakes desirable. Among the stresses known to increase vitamin C needs are infections; burns; extremely high or low temperatures; intakes of toxic heavy metals such as lead, mercury, and cadmium; the chronic use of certain medications, including aspirin, barbiturates, and oral contraceptives; and cigarette smoking. Cigarette smoke contains oxidants, which greedily consume this potent antioxidant. Exposure to cigarette smoke, especially when accompanied by low intakes of vitamin C, depletes the body's pool in both active and passive smokers.[31] Whereas the RDA for nonsmokers is 60 milligrams a day, the RDA for people who smoke cigarettes regularly is 100 milligrams; the Canadian RNI provides a similar increase for those who smoke.

After oral surgery, dentists may prescribe supplemental vitamin C to hasten healing. After major operations or extensive burns, when a tremendous amount of scar tissue must form during healing, the amount needed to be as high as 1000 milligrams (1 gram) a day or even more. In individual cases, a physician may prescribe vitamin C supplements for certain conditions; self-medication is not recommended under any circumstances.

VITAMIN C DEFICIENCY

Two of the most notable signs of a vitamin C deficiency reflect its role in maintaining the integrity of blood vessels. The gums bleed easily around the teeth, and capillaries under the skin break spontaneously, producing pinpoint hemorrhages. Atherosclerotic plaques grow rapidly in the arteries. Table 10–11 reviews vitamin C information.

When the vitamin C pool falls to about a fifth of its optimal size (this may take several weeks on a diet lacking vitamin C), scurvy symptoms begin to appear. Failure to promote normal collagen synthesis causes further hemorrhaging. Muscles, including the heart muscle, degenerate. The skin becomes rough,

Table 10–11

Vitamin C—A Summary

Other Names	Ascorbic acid
Deficiency Disease Name	Scurvy
Adult RDA	60 mg/day Smokers: 100 mg/day
Chief Functions in the Body	Collagen synthesis (strengthens blood vessel walls, forms scar tissue, provides matrix for bone growth), antioxidant, thyroxin synthesis, amino acid metabolism, strengthens resistance to infection, helps in absorption of iron
Significant Sources	Citrus fruits, cabbage-type vegetables, dark green vegetables, cantaloupe, strawberries, peppers, lettuce, tomatoes, potatoes, papayas, mangoes

	Deficiency Symptoms	Toxicity Symptoms
BLOOD/CIRCULATORY SYSTEM	Anemia (small-cell type),[a] atherosclerotic plaques, pinpoint hemorrhages	
DIGESTIVE SYSTEM		Nausea, abdominal cramps, diarrhea
IMMUNE SYSTEM	Suppression, frequent infections	
MOUTH, GUMS, TONGUE	Bleeding gums, loosened teeth	
NERVOUS/MUSCULAR SYSTEMS	Muscle degeneration and pain, hysteria, depression	Headache, fatigue, insomnia
SKELETAL SYSTEMS	Bone fragility, joint pain	
SKIN	Rough skin, blotchy bruises	Hot flashes, rashes
OTHER	Failure of wounds to heal	Interference with medical tests, aggravation of gout symptoms, urinary tract problems, kidney stones[b]

[a]Small-cell-type anemia is *microcytic anemia*.
[b]People who have a tendency toward gout and those who have a genetic abnormality that alters the breakdown of vitamin C are prone to forming kidney stones. Vitamin C is inactivated and degraded by several routes, sometimes producing oxalate, which can form stones in the kidneys.

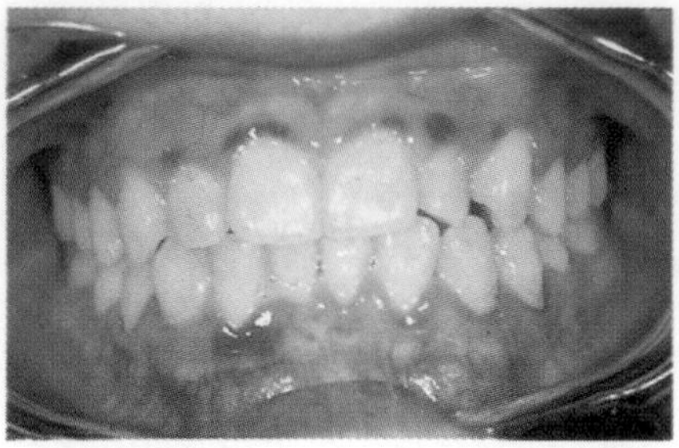

Scorbutic gums. Unlike other lesions of the mouth, scurvy presents a symmetrical appearance without infection.

brown, scaly, and dry. Wounds fail to heal because scar tissue will not form. Bone rebuilding falters; the ends of the long bones become softened, malformed, and painful, and fractures appear. The teeth become loose as the cartilage around them weakens. Anemia and infections are common. There are also characteristic psychological signs, including hysteria and depression. Sudden death is likely, occasioned by severe atherosclerosis or by massive bleeding into the joints and body cavities.

Once diagnosed, scurvy is readily reversed by vitamin C. Moderate doses in the neighborhood of 100 milligrams per day are sufficient, curing the scurvy within about five days. Such an intake is easily achieved by including vitamin C–rich foods in the diet.

VITAMIN C TOXICITY

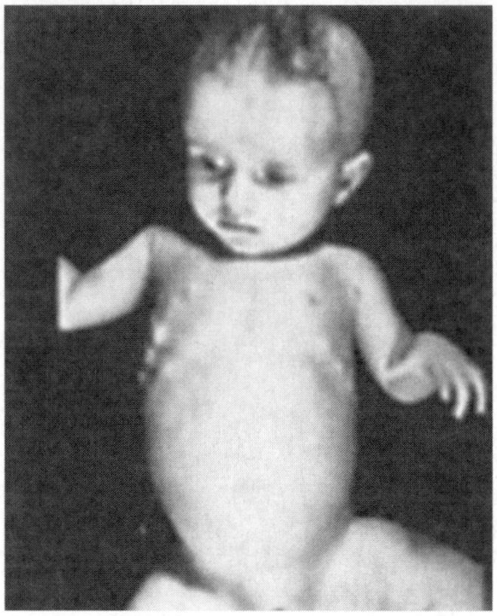

Infant scurvy. This is the characteristic "scorbutic pose," with legs bent and thighs rotated open. The infant's joints are painful, and she will cry if made to move.

The easy availability of vitamin C supplements and the publication of books recommending vitamin C to prevent colds and cancer have led thousands of people to take large doses of vitamin C. Not surprisingly, instances of vitamin C's causing harm have surfaced.

Toxic effects such as nausea, abdominal cramps, and diarrhea are often reported. Several instances of interference with medical regimens are also known. Large amounts of vitamin C excreted in the urine obscure the results of tests used to detect diabetes, giving a false positive result in some instances and a false negative in others. People taking anticlotting medications may unwittingly abolish the effect if they also take massive doses of vitamin C.* Those who have a tendency toward gout and those who have a genetic abnormality that alters vitamin C's breakdown to its excretion products are prone to forming kidney stones if they take large doses of vitamin C.† Vitamin C supplements are dangerous for people with iron overload; vitamin C enhances iron absorption and releases iron from body stores.[32]

A person who has taken large doses of vitamin C for a long time (say, ten times the RDA daily for several weeks) may adapt by limiting absorption and destroying and excreting more of the vitamin than usual. If the person then suddenly reduces intake to normal, the accelerated disposal system may not be able to put on its brakes fast enough to avoid destroying too much of the vitamin. It has been suggested that adults who stop taking large doses may develop scurvy on intakes that would protect most adults, but evidence is scanty on this point. If scurvy does develop, the situation is similar to withdrawal reaction seen in drug and alcohol abusers when they discontinue drug use. When people cease taking vitamin C in excessive doses, they might be wise to do so gradually.

Few instances warrant consuming more than 100 to 300 milligrams of vitamin C a day. For adults who dose themselves with 1 to 2 grams a day, the risks may not be great; those taking more than 2 grams, and especially those taking amounts above 8 grams per day, should be aware of the distinct possibility of harm.

false positive: a test result indicating that a condition is present (positive) when in fact it is not (therefore false).

false negative: a test result indicating that a condition is *not* present (negative) when in fact it is present (therefore false).

Reminder: *Gout* is a metabolic disease in which uric acid crystals precipitate in the joints.

*Vitamin C interferes with such anticoagulants as warfarin, dicumarol, heparin, and coumadin. It is unclear whether vitamin C inhibits the absorption or the action of these drugs.

†Vitamin C is inactivated and degraded by several routes, and sometimes oxalate, which can form kidney stones, is produced along the way. People may also develop oxalate crystals in their kidneys regardless of vitamin C status.

In conclusion, the range of safe vitamin C intakes seems to be broad, as is typical for water-soluble vitamins. Between the absolute minimum of 10 milligrams a day and a reasonable maximum of perhaps 300 milligrams, nearly everyone can find a suitable intake. People who venture outside these limits may be taking health risks.

withdrawal reaction: a reaction to removal of a substance (usually of a drug) that reveals that the user has become dependent. One infant is reported to have been born of a mother who took massive doses of vitamin C. The infant developed **rebound scurvy** on an intake that would have been adequate for the average infant.

VITAMIN C FOOD SOURCES

Fruits and vegetables can easily provide a generous intake of vitamin C. A cup of orange juice at breakfast, a salad for lunch, and a stalk of broccoli and a potato for dinner alone provide more than 300 milligrams. Clearly, a person making such food choices needs no vitamin C pills.

Figure 10–15 (on p. 382) shows the amounts of vitamin C in various common foods. The overwhelming abundance of purple and green bars reveals that not only are the citrus fruits highly famous for being rich in vitamin C, but other fruits and vegetables are in the same league. A single serving of broccoli, green pepper, cauliflower, cantaloupe, and strawberries provides more than 50 milligrams of the vitamin (and an array of other nutrients) for less than 60 kcalories. Because vitamin C is vulnerable to heat, raw fruits and vegetables usually have a higher nutrient density than their cooked counterparts.

The potato is an important source of vitamin C, not because one potato by itself meets the daily need, but because potatoes are such a common staple that they make significant contributions.[33] In fact, scurvy was unknown in Ireland until the potato blight of the mid-1840s when some two million people died of malnutrition and infection.[34] Potatoes provide about 20 percent of all the vitamin C in the U.S. diet.

The lack of gold, white, brown, and red bars in Figure 10–15 confirms that grains, milk (except breast milk), legumes, and meats are notoriously poor sources of vitamin C. Organ meats (liver, kidneys, and others) and raw meats contain some vitamin C, but most people don't eat large quantities of these. Raw meats and fish contribute enough vitamin C to be significant in parts of Alaska, Canada, and Japan, but elsewhere, fruits and vegetables are necessary to supply sufficient vitamin C.

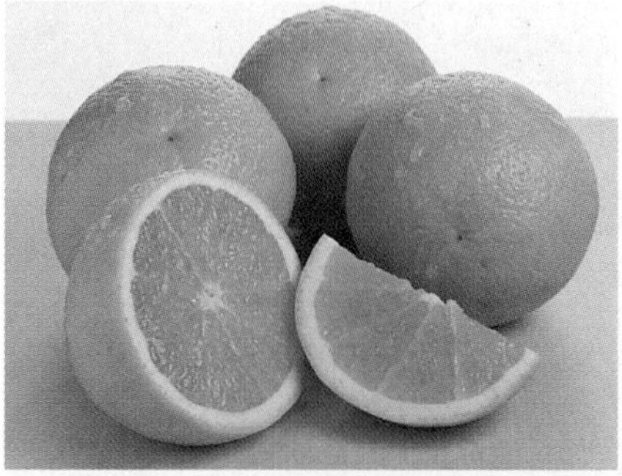

When nutritionists say "vitamin C," people think "oranges."

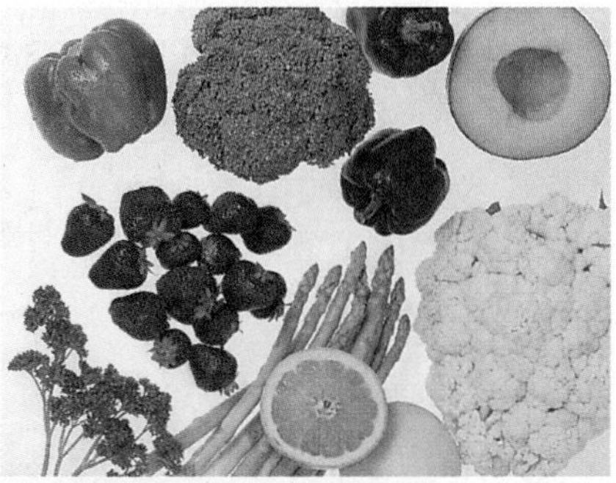

But these foods are also rich in vitamin C.

To protect the vitamin C in foods:

- Store cut produce in airtight wrappers and juices in closed containers (it's easily oxidized).
- Refrigerate produce, and avoid high temperatures and long cooking times (it's vulnerable to heat).
- Use a microwave oven or steam vegetables in a small amount of water (it's lost in the liquid).

Figure 10–15 Vitamin C in Selected Foods

Food	Serving size (kcalories)
Bread, whole wheat	1 slice (64 kcal)
Corn flakes, fortified	1 oz (108 kcal)
White rice	1/2 c cooked (134 kcal)
Spaghetti pasta	1/2 c cooked (99 kcal)
Oatmeal	1/2 c cooked (73 kcal)
Tortilla, flour	1 8"-round (115 kcal)
Spinach	1 c raw (12 kcal)
Broccoli	1/2 c cooked (22 kcal)
Carrots	1/2 c shredded raw (24 kcal)
Green peas	1/2 c cooked (62 kcal)
Corn	1/2 c cooked (66 kcal)
Green beans	1/2 c cooked (22 kcal)
Sweet potatoes	1/2 c cooked (117 kcal)
Potato	1 baked w/skin (220 kcal)
Tomato juice	3/4 c (31 kcal)
Apple	1 medium raw (81 kcal)
Banana	1 medium raw (104 kcal)
Orange	1 medium raw (62 kcal)
Strawberries	1/2 c fresh (23 kcal)
Raisins	1/4 c (109 kcal)
Watermelon	1 slice (154 kcal)
Grapefruit juice	3/4 c fresh (72 kcal)
Avocado	1/4 (85 kcal)
Milk	1 c low-fat 2% (121 kcal)
Yogurt, plain	1 c low-fat (143 kcal)
Cheddar cheese	1½ oz (171 kcal)
Cottage cheese	1/2 c low-fat 2% (101 kcal)
Swiss cheese	1 1/2 oz (159 kcal)
Ice cream	1/2 c, 10% fat (134 kcal)
Navy beans	1/2 c cooked (129 kcal)
Pinto beans	1/2 c cooked (117 kcal)
Kidney beans	1/2 c cooked (109 kcal)
Garbanzo beans	1/2 c cooked (134 kcal)
Peanut butter	2 tbs (190 kcal)
Sunflower seeds	1 oz dry (159 kcal)
Tofu (soybean curd)	1/2 c (94 kcal)
Shrimp	3 oz boiled (85 kcal)
Ground beef, lean	3 oz broiled (239 kcal)
Chicken breast	3 oz roasted (141 kcal)
Cod	3 oz poached (88 kcal)
Ham, lean[a]	3 oz roasted (123 kcal)
Sirloin steak, lean	3 oz broiled (171 kcal)
Tuna, canned in water	3 oz (99 kcal)
Bologna, beef[a]	2 slices (144 kcal)
Egg	1 hard cooked (77 kcal)
Additional 5 foods:	
Red bell pepper	1 c raw chopped (27 kcal)
Kiwi	1 (46 kcal)
Mango	1 (134 kcal)
Brussels sprouts	1/2 c cooked (30 kcal)
Snow peas	1/2 c stir fry (35 kcal)

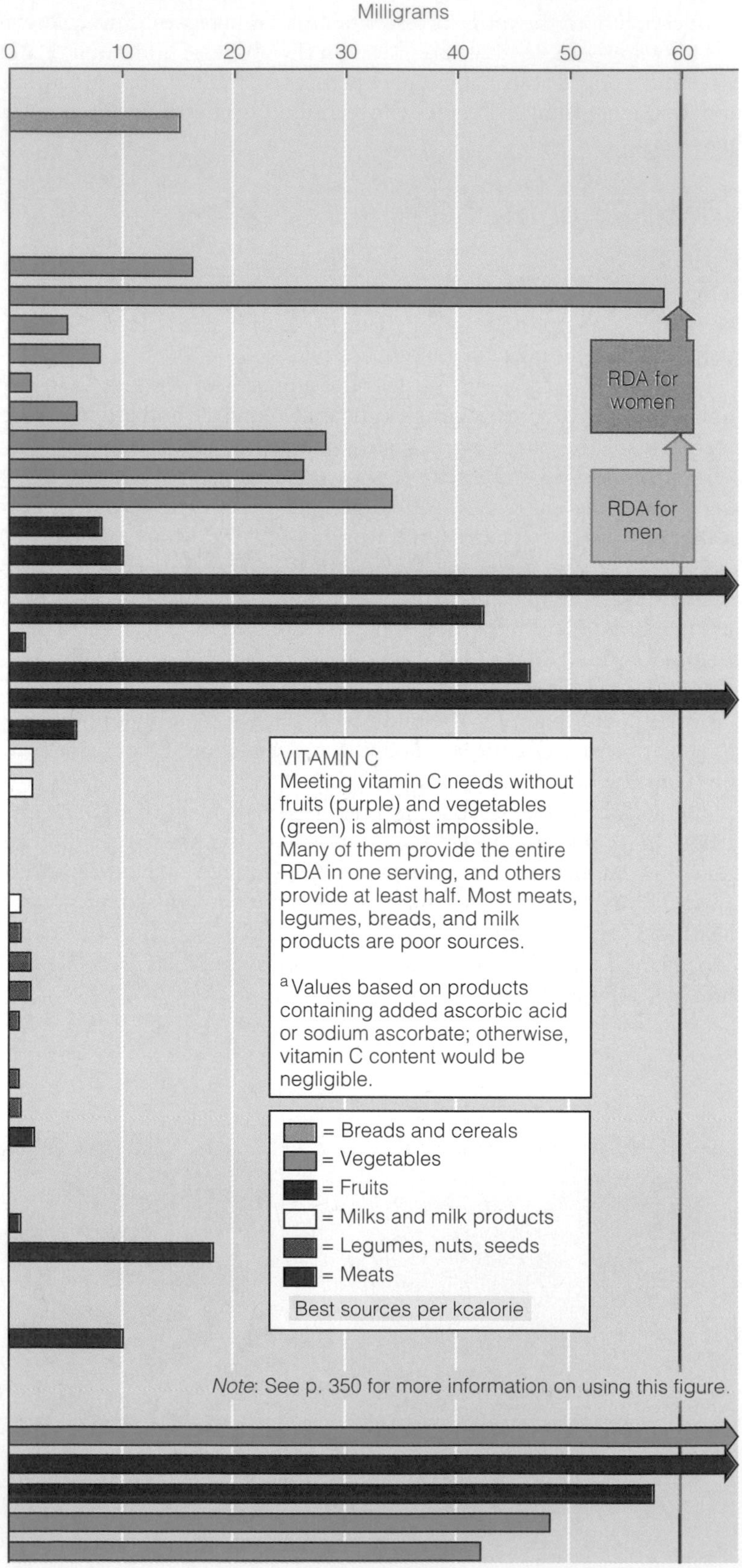

Milligrams
0
10
20
30
40
50
60
RDA for women
RDA for men
VITAMIN C
Meeting vitamin C needs without fruits (purple) and vegetables (green) is almost impossible. Many of them provide the entire RDA in one serving, and others provide at least half. Most meats, legumes, breads, and milk products are poor sources.
[a] Values based on products containing added ascorbic acid or sodium ascorbate; otherwise, vitamin C content would be negligible.
= Breads and cereals
= Vegetables
= Fruits
= Milks and milk products
= Legumes, nuts, seeds
= Meats
Best sources per kcalorie

Note: See p. 350 for more information on using this figure.

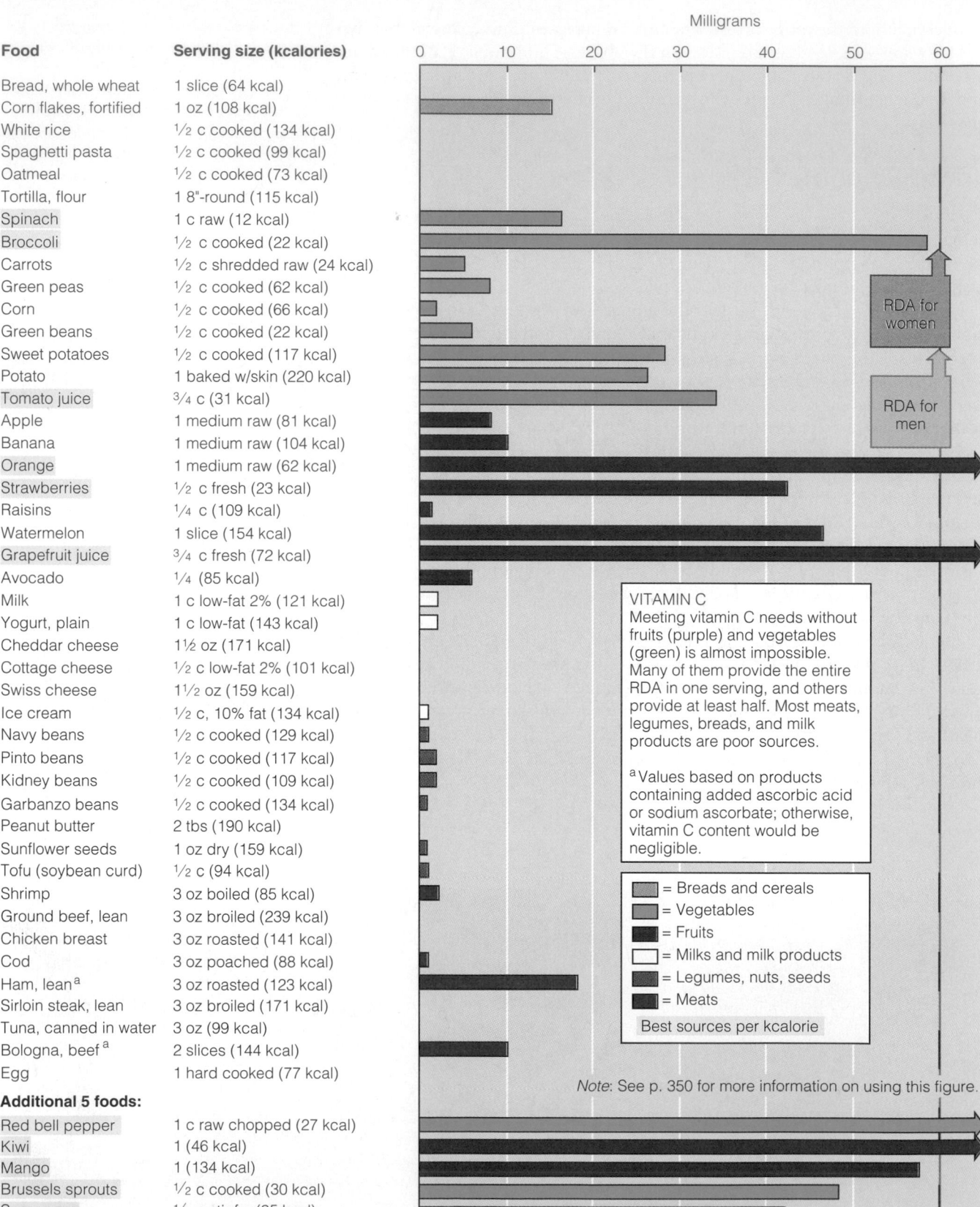

Vita means life. After this discourse on the vitamins, who could dispute that they deserve their name? Their regulation of metabolic processes makes them vital to normal growth, development, and maintenance of the body. The remarkable roles of the vitamins continue in the next chapter.

Study Questions

1. How do the vitamins differ from the energy nutrients?
2. Describe some general differences between fat-soluble and water-soluble vitamins.
3. Which B vitamins are involved in energy metabolism? Protein metabolism? Cell division?
4. For thiamin, riboflavin, niacin, biotin, pantothenic acid, vitamin B_6, folate, vitamin B_{12}, and vitamin C, state:
   - Its chief function in the body.
   - Its characteristic deficiency symptoms.
   - Its significant food sources.
5. What is the relationship of tryptophan to niacin?
6. Describe the relationship between folate and vitamin B_{12}.
7. What risks are associated with high doses of niacin? Vitamin B_6? Vitamin C?

Problem Set appears on the next page

Notes

1. The vitamin names used here are those established by the International Union of Nutritional Sciences Committee on Nomenclature, in Nomenclature policy: Generic descriptors and trivial names for vitamins and related compounds, *Journal of Nutrition* 117 (1987): 7–15.
2. Committee on Dietary Allowances, *Recommended Dietary Allowances*, 10th ed. (Washington, D.C.: National Academy Press, 1989), pp. 132–137.
3. D. A. Bender, *Nutritional Biochemistry of the Vitamins* (Cambridge: Cambridge University Press, 1992), pp. 184–222.
4. R. B. Colletti and coauthors, Niacin treatment of hypercholesterolemia in children, *Pediatrics* 92 (1993): 78–82; Y. Henkin, K. C. Johnson, and J. P. Segrest, Rechallenge with crystalline niacin after drug-induced hepatitis from sustained-release niacin, *Journal of the American Medical Association* 264 (1990): 241–243.
5. M. T. Behme, Nicotinamide and diabetes prevention, *Nutrition Reviews* 53 (1995): 137–139.
6. W. O. Song, Pantothenic acid: How much do we know about this B-complex vitamin? *Nutrition Today*, March/April 1990, pp. 19–25.
7. T. R. Guilarte, Vitamin B_6 and cognitive development: Recent research findings from human and animal studies, *Nutrition Reviews* 51 (1993): 193–198; S. N. Meydani and coauthors, Vitamin B_6 deficiency impairs interlukin 2 production and lymphocyte proliferation in elderly adults, *American Journal of Clinical Nutrition* 53 (1991): 1275–1280.
8. L. C. Rall and S. N. Meydani, Vitamin B_6 and immune competence, *Nutrition Reviews* 51 (1993): 217–225.
9. R. L. Reid, Premenstrual syndrome, *New England Journal of Medicine* 324 (1991): 1208–1210.
10. A. L. Bernstein and J. S. Dineson, Effect of pharmacologic doses of vitamin B_6 on carpal tunnel syndrome, electroencephalographic results, and pain, *Journal of the American College of Nutrition* 12 (1993): 73–76.
11. Committee on Genetics, Folic acid for the prevention of neural tube defects, *Pediatrics* 92 (1993): 493–494; M. M. Werler, S. Shapiro, and A. A. Mitchell, Periconceptional folic acid exposure and risk of occurrent neural tube defects, *Journal of the American Medical Association* 269 (1993): 1257–1261; A. E. Czeizel and I. Dudás, Prevention of the first occurrence of neural-tube defects by periconceptual vitamin supplementation, *New England Journal of Medicine* 327 (1992): 1832–1835.
12. From the Centers for Disease Control and Prevention, Recommendations for use of folic acid to reduce number of spina bifida cases and other neural tube defects, *Journal of the American Medical Association* 269 (1993): 1233–1238.
13. R. D. Williams, FDA proposes folic acid fortification, *FDA Consumer*, May 1994, pp. 11–14.
14. Folate and neural tube defects: US policy evolves, *Nutrition Reviews* 51 (1993): 358–361.
15. M. Nestle, Folate fortification and neural tube defects: Policy implications, *Journal of Nutrition Education* 26 (1994): 287–293; A. Bendich, Folic acid and prevention of neural tube birth defects: Critical assessment of FDA proposals to increase folic acid intakes, *Journal of Nutrition Education* 26 (1994): 294–299.

16. V. Herbert, Folate and neural tube defects, *Nutrition Today*, November/December 1992, pp. 30–33.
17. C. L. Krumdieck, Folic acid, in *Present Knowledge in Nutrition* 6th ed., ed. M. L. Brown (Washington, D.C.: Nutrition Foundation, 1990), pp. 179–188.
18. C. E. Butterworth and coauthors, Folate deficiency and cervical dysplasia, *Journal of the American Medical Association* 267 (1992): 528–533.
19. Committee on Dietary Allowances, 1989, pp. 150–158.
20. Choline: A conditionally essential nutrient for humans, *Nutrition Reviews* 50 (1992): 112–114; C. D. Berdanier, Is inositol an essential nutrient? *Nutrition Today*, March/April 1992, pp. 22–26.
21. D. B. McCormick, Riboflavin, in *Present Knowledge in Nutrition*, 1990, pp. 146–154.
22. J. R. Turnlund and coauthors, Vitamin B-6 depletion followed by repletion with animal- or plant-source diets and calcium and magnesium metabolism in young women, *American Journal of Clinical Nutrition* 56 (1992): 905–910.
23. G. Wolf, Uptake of ascorbic acid by human neutrophils, *Nutrition Reviews* 11 (1993): 337–338.
24. C. S. Johnston, L. J. Martin, and X. Cai, Antihistamine effect of supplemental ascorbic acid and neutrophil chemotaxis, *Journal of the American College of Nutrition* 11 (1992): 172–176.
25. A. R. Sherman and N. A. Hallquist, Immunity, in *Present Knowledge in Nutrition*, 1990, pp. 463–476.
26. J. Schwartz and S. T. Weiss, Relationship between dietary vitamin C intake and respiratory function in the First National Health and Nutrition Examination Survey (NHANES I), *American Journal of Clinical Nutrition* 59 (1994): 110–114.
27. C. Bucca, G. Rolla, and J. C. Farina, Effect of vitamin C on transient increase of bronchial responsiveness in conditions affecting the airways, *Annals of the New York Academy of Sciences* 669 (1992): 175–186.
28. E. M. Peters and coauthors, Vitamin C supplementation reduces the incidence of postrace symptoms of upper-respiratory-tract infection in ultramarathon runners, *American Journal of Clinical Nutrition* 57 (1993): 170–174.
29. J. E. Enstrom, L. E. Kanim, and M. A. Klein, Vitamin C intake and mortality among a sample of the United States population, *Epidemiology* 3 (1992): 194–202.
30. S. N. Gershoff, Vitamin C (ascorbic acid): New roles, new requirements, *Nutrition Reviews* 11 (1993): 313–326.
31. D. L. Tribble, L. J. Giuliano, and S. P. Fortmann, Reduced plasma ascorbic acid concentrations in nonsmokers regularly exposed to environmental tobacco smoke, *American Journal of Clinical Nutrition* 58 (1993): 886–890.
32. V. Herbert, Vitamin C supplements are dangerous for iron-overloaded persons, *Journal of the American Dietetic Association* 93 (1993): 526–527.
33. G. B. Forbes, Potatoes: A reliable source of vitamin C (Scorbutus nauticus cured without citrus), *Nutrition Today*, January/February 1993, pp. 33–35.
34. A. Nikiforuk, The Irish famine: A blighted fable, in *The Fourth Horseman: A Short History of Epidemics, Plagues, Famine and Other Scourges* (New York: M. Evans & Company, 1993), pp. 110–125.

Problem Set

1. Review the units in which vitamins are measured (a spot check).

a. For each of these vitamins, note the unit of measure:

Thiamin: ____________________

Riboflavin: ____________________

Niacin: ____________________

Vitamin B_6: ____________________

Folate: ____________________

Vitamin B_{12}: ____________________

Vitamin C: ____________________

b. Recall from the chapter's description of people's self-dosing with vitamin B_6 that people who suffer toxicity symptoms may be taking doses as high as 2 grams a day, whereas the RDA is about 2 *milli*grams. How much higher than 2 mg is 2 g? ______

c. Vitamin B_{12} is measured in micrograms. How many micrograms are in a gram? _____ How many grams are in a teaspoon of a granular powder?_____ How many micrograms does that represent?_____ What is your RDA for vitamin B_{12}?_____ This exercise should convince you that the amount of vitamin B_{12} a person needs is indeed quite small—yet still essential.

Problem Set (continued)

2. This exercise presents a day's meals that you will look at again from other points of view in each of the next three chapters. This time the focus is on the water-soluble vitamins. The day's meals have been simplified, and the foods have been sorted into groups to ease your task in analyzing their vitamin contents. The foods selected fit the pattern suggested in the Daily Food Guide, presented in Chapter 2, which suggests 6 to 11 servings a day of grains, 3 to 5 servings of vegetables including dark green vegetables and legumes, 2 to 4 servings of fruits, 2 to 3 servings of meat and meat alternates, and 2 servings of milk and milk products.

a. Record the energy and vitamin amounts in these foods. (Note the number of servings—for example, 6 slices of bread.)

Item No./Food	Ener (kcal)	Thia (mg)	Ribo (mg)	Niacin (mg NE)	Vit B_6 (mg)	Folate (μg)	Vit C (mg)
• Grains (6)							
# 357 Wheat bread, 6 slices	____	____	____	____	____	____	____
Total in grains:	____	____	____	____	____	____	____
• Vegetables (3)							
# 920 Spinach, cooked from fresh, ¼ c	____	____	____	____	____	____	____
# 891 Green peas, cooked from frozen, ½ c	____	____	____	____	____	____	____
# 834 Carrots, cooked from fresh, ½ c	____	____	____	____	____	____	____
Total in vegetables:	____	____	____	____	____	____	____
• Fruits (2)							
# 269 Orange juice, fresh, 1 c	____	____	____	____	____	____	____
# 264 Cantaloupe melon, ½	____	____	____	____	____	____	____
Total in fruits:	____	____	____	____	____	____	____
• Meats (2 to 3)							
# 1045 Bass fish, baked, 4 oz	____	____	____	____	____	____	____
# 598 Hamburger, lean, 4 oz	____	____	____	____	____	____	____
Total in meats:	____	____	____	____	____	____	____
• Milks (2)							
# 98 Milk, nonfat, 2 c	____	____	____	____	____	____	____
Total in milks:	____	____	____	____	____	____	____

b. Which *class* of foods offered the most thiamin? ______Riboflavin? ______Niacin? ______Vitamin B_6?______Folate?______Vitamin C?______

c. Which vitamin(s) tended to cluster in one or two food groups? ____________________Which was (were) most evenly distributed among the food groups?________________________________

3. Be aware of how niacin intakes are affected by dietary protein availability.

a. Refer to the box on p. 356, and calculate how much niacin a woman receives from a diet that delivers 90 g protein and 9 mg niacin. (Assume her RDA for protein is 46 g/day.) Show your calculations: ____________

b. Is this woman getting her RDA of niacin (15 mg NE)? ______

(continued on the next page)

Problem Set (continued)

4. Appreciate the need to eat a variety of many nutritious foods every day for thiamin. Following is a list of foods selected for their thiamin contents per serving.

   a. How many servings (and kcalories) of any one of these foods would you have to eat to get 100% of the Daily Value of 1.5 mg thiamin? Calculate your answer in the last two columns of the table (round your answers up); the first one is done for you.

Item No./Food		Energy (kcal)	Thiamin (mg)	Servings	kCalories
# 98	Nonfat milk, 1 c	85	.09	1.5 ÷ .09 = 16.7 c	17 c = 1445 kcal
# 206	Apple, fresh, 3¼″	______	______	______	______
# 37	Cheddar cheese, 1 oz	______	______	______	______
# 820	Broccoli, cooked from fresh, chopped, 1 c	______	______	______	______
# 357	Whole-wheat bread, 1 slice	______	______	______	______
# 606	Sirloin steak, lean, 4 oz	______	______	______	______
# 871	Mushrooms, raw, sliced, ½ c	______	______	______	______
# 623	Pork chop, lean broiled, 1 ea	______	______	______	______
# 750	Sunflower seeds, dry, ¼ c	______	______	______	______
# 891	Green peas, cooked from frozen, ½ c	______	______	______	______

   b. Would it be practical to get *all* of your thiamin from some one of these foods every day? ______

   c. Now review problem 2 and determine how much thiamin the eater obtained by eating the recommended number of servings of nutritious foods from each food group:

   From the grains: ______
   From the vegetables: ______
   From the fruits: ______
   From the meats: ______
   From the milks: ______
   Total thiamin: ______

   d. Does the total meet the 1.5 mg Daily Value for thiamin? ______

This exercise should demonstrate to your satisfaction that the way to meet your thiamin needs each day is to select many different nutritious foods from each of the food groups in reasonable serving sizes each.

Vitamin and Mineral Supplements

Approximately 40 percent of the U.S. population takes vitamin and mineral supplements regularly, spending billions of dollars on them each year.[1] Some people take supplements as dietary insurance, "in case" they are not meeting their nutrient needs from foods alone—as kind of an all-purpose extra food. Some people take supplements as health insurance to protect against certain diseases—as kind of an all-purpose extra drug.

One out of every five people take multinutrient pills daily.[2] Others take large doses of single nutrients, most commonly, vitamin C, iron, and calcium. In many cases, taking supplements is a costly but harmless practice; sometimes, it is both costly and harmful to health.

For the most part, people self-prescribe supplements, taking them on the advice of friends, television, or books that may or may not be reliable. Sometimes, they take supplements on the recommendation of a physician. When such advice follows a valid nutrition assessment, supplementation may be warranted, but even then the preferred course of action is to improve food choices and eating habits. Without an assessment, the advice to take supplements may be inappropriate.

When people think of supplements, they often think only of vitamins, but minerals are important, too, of course. People whose diets lack vitamins, for whatever reason, probably lack several minerals as well. Vitamin-mineral supplements may be appropriate in some circumstances.

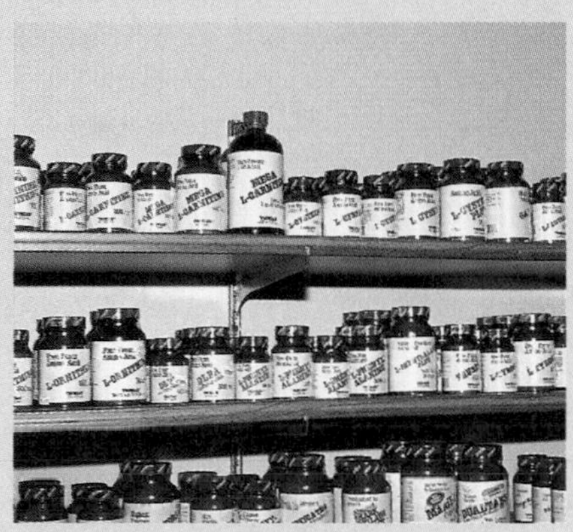

Supplements are available in a number of shapes and flavors, but none offer the full array of nutrients that a variety of foods can provide.

This highlight examines several questions related to supplement taking. What are the arguments for taking supplements? What are the arguments against taking them? Finally, if people do take supplements, how can they choose the appropriate ones?

ARGUMENTS FOR SUPPLEMENTS

Supplements do have appropriate uses. In some cases, they can correct deficiencies; in others, they can reduce the risk of diseases.

Correct Overt Deficiencies

Vitamin deficiency diseases such as scurvy, pellagra, and beriberi are rare, but they do still occur. Correcting an overt deficiency disease may require therapeutic doses two to ten times the RDA of a nutrient. When doses exceed the amounts of nutrients commonly found in foods, the supplements are being used more as drugs than as foods.

Improve Nutrition Status

In contrast to the classical deficiencies, which present a multitude of symptoms and are easy to recognize, subclinical deficiencies are subtle and easy to overlook—and they are also more likely to occur. People whose energy intakes are too low to deliver the needed amounts of nutrients, such as habitual dieters, strict vegetarians, and the elderly, risk developing subclinical deficiencies. If there is no way for these people to eat enough nutritious foods to meet their needs, then vitamin-mineral supplements may be appropriate to help prevent nutrient deficiencies.

While most nutrients can be obtained from a well-balanced diet, sometimes even a well-planned diet falls short of meeting the RDA for key nutrients. A person must not only follow guidelines such as the Food Guide Pyramid, but must also carefully select foods within that framework. While few people receive all of the RDA for all nutrients every day, most people receive at least their average needs for all nutrients. Supplements can help people to receive the intakes recommended by government and health authorities on a regular basis.

Consider the case of a woman who loses a lot of blood and therefore a lot of iron and other blood-building nutrients during menstruation each month. Such a woman may be able to eat well enough to make up for all nutrient deficits except that of iron: she may need an iron supplement. Chapter 13 shows ways for women to try to obtain enough iron in their diets, but also observes that it is hard to do. It also cautions that nutrition assessment is a necessary prerequisite to making the decision whether supplementation is appropriate.

Reduce Disease Risks

Many people, especially those who are intolerant to lactose or allergic to milk, may not receive enough calcium to forestall the bone degeneration of old age, osteoporosis. For them, nonmilk calcium-rich foods are especially valuable, but calcium supplements may also be appropriate (Highlight 12 provides more details).

Support Increased Nutrient Needs

Nutrient needs increase during certain stages of the life cycle, making it difficult to meet those needs without supplementation. For example, women of childbearing age may need folate supplements to reduce the risks of neural tube defects. Pregnant women and women who are breastfeeding their infants have exceptionally high nutrient needs and so usually need special supplements of iron, calcium, and folate. Newborns routinely receive a single dose of vitamin K at birth. Infants may need other supplements as well, depending on whether they are breastfed or receiving formula, and on whether their water contains fluoride.

Improve Body's Defenses

Health care professionals may provide special supplementation to people being treated for addictions to alcohol or other drugs and to people with prolonged illnesses, extensive injuries, or other severe stresses such as surgery. Nutrient intakes are reduced in people with illnesses that interfere with appetite, eating, or nutrient absorption. Nutrient needs are increased by diseases or drugs that speed or alter nutrient metabolism. In all these cases, supplements are appropriate.

ARGUMENTS AGAINST SUPPLEMENTS

Supplement taking is risky, and the higher the dose, the greater the risk of harm. People's tolerances for high doses of nutrients vary, just as their risks of deficiencies do. Amounts that some can tolerate may be harmful for others, and no one knows who falls where along the spectrum. It is impossible to say just how much of a nutrient is enough—or too much. Assuming, however, that it is best to err on the conservative side, Table H10–1 presents suggested limits for vitamins and minerals from supplements.

Toxicity

The extent and severity of supplement toxicity remain unclear. Only a few alert health care professionals can recognize toxicity, even when it is acute. When it is chronic, with the effects developing subtly and progressing slowly, it often goes unrecognized. In one case, a woman took just 1000 RE (5000 IU) of vitamin A a day, an amount typically found in vitamin-mineral supplements, daily for ten years. She was diagnosed with liver disease. Only when she discontinued the supplement did the condition clear up.[3] In view of the potential hazards, some authorities believe supplements should bear warning labels, advising consumers that large doses may be toxic.

Toxic overdoses of vitamins and minerals in children are more readily recognized and, unfortunately, fairly common. Poison control centers receive more than 30,000 reports a year of children under the age of six swallowing excessively large doses of supplements. Fruit-flavored, chewable vitamins shaped like cartoon characters entice young children to eat them like candy in amounts that can cause poisoning. Iron-containing supplements are especially toxic and are the leading cause of accidental ingestion fatalities among children.[4] Even mild overdoses cause GI distress, nausea, and black diarrhea that reflects gastric bleeding. Severe overdoses result in bloody diarrhea, shock, liver damage, coma, and death.

Life-Threatening Misinformation

Another problem arises when people who are ill come to believe that high doses of vitamins or minerals can be therapeutic. These claims are exceedingly common, as this report by a watchdog consumer group illustrates:

> In 1989, volunteers of the Consumer Health Education Council (CHEC) telephoned 41 Houston-area health food stores and asked to speak with the person who provided nutritional advice. The callers explained that they had a brother sick with AIDS. . . . All 41 retailers offered products they said could strengthen the brother's immune system. . . . Thirty said they sold products that would cure AIDS."[5]

Other such inquiries led to wrongheaded advice from salespeople urging that customers use supplements to treat headaches, dizziness, fatigue,

Table H10–1

Vitamin and Mineral Doses from Supplements

Nutrient	Safe Range of Intakes
Vitamins	
Vitamin A	75 to 750 RE[a]
Vitamin D	10 μg[a] (up to age 18); 5 μg[a] (adults)
Vitamin E	6 to 30 mg[a]
Thiamin	1 to 2 mg
Riboflavin	1 to 2 mg
Niacin (as niacinamide)	10 to 20 mg
Vitamin B_6	1.5 to 2.5 mg
Folate	0.1 to 0.4 mg (in multivitamin form)
Vitamin B_{12}	3 to 10 μg
Pantothenic acid	5 to 20 mg (in multivitamin form)
Biotin	Not recommended in supplement form
Vitamin C	50 to 100 mg
Minerals	
Calcium	400 to 800 mg
Phosphorus	No need to supplement
Magnesium	No need to supplement
Iron	10 to 39 mg (women)
Zinc	10 to 25 mg (adults)
Iodine	Not recommended in supplement form

[a]Some supplements are measured in International Units (IU). To convert to RDA-compatible units, see Appendix D.

Source: Parts adapted from the American Medical Association's Council on Scientific Affairs, Vitamin preparations as dietary supplements and as therapeutic agents, *Journal of the American Medical Association* 257 (1987): 1929–1936; Committee on Dietary Allowances, *Recommended Dietary Allowances*, 10th ed. (Washington, D.C.: National Academy Press, 1989); PHS recommends folic acid for women of childbearing age, *FDA Consumer*, December 1992, p. 3.

kidney stones, abnormal thirst (a diabetes warning sign), glaucoma (a progressive eye-destroying disease), and sudden weight loss (a serious medical symptom), as well as to prevent contracting the virus that causes AIDS. None of the salespeople recommended that the callers obtain medical advice.

Unknown Needs

Another argument against the use of supplements is that no one knows exactly how to formulate the "ideal" supplement. What nutrients should be included? How much of each? On whose needs should the choices be based? How should an individual choose a supplement, since no individual's needs are exactly like anyone else's? Surveys have repeatedly shown little relationship between the supplements people take and the nutrients they actually need. Often people take supplements containing the nutrients they need least and still miss out on the nutrients their diets are failing to deliver.

False Sense of Security

Another argument against supplements is that they may lull people into a false sense of security. A person might eat irresponsibly, thinking, "My supplement will cover my needs." Or, experiencing a warning symptom of a disease, a person might postpone seeking a diagnosis, thinking, "I probably need a nutrient supplement to make this go away." Such self-diagnosis is always dangerous.

Other Invalid Reasons

Other invalid reasons why people might take supplements include:

- The belief that the food supply contains inadequate nutrients.
- The belief that supplements can provide energy.
- The belief that supplements can enhance athletic performance or build lean body tissues without physical work or faster than work alone.
- The belief that supplements will help them cope with stress.
- The belief that supplements can prevent, treat, or cure symptoms of diseases ranging from the common cold to cancer.

Ironically, people with health problems are more likely to take supplements than others, yet today's health problems are more likely to be due to overnutrition and poor lifestyle choices than to nutrient deficiencies. The truth—that most people need to change their eating and exercise habits—is harder to swallow than a supplement.

Bioavailability and Antagonistic Actions

In general, the body absorbs nutrients best from foods in which the nutrients are diluted and dispersed among other ingredients that may facilitate their absorption. Taken in pure, concentrated form, nutrients are likely to interfere with one another's absorption or with the absorption of nutrients in foods eaten at the same time. Documentation of these effects is particularly extensive for minerals: zinc hinders copper and calcium absorption, iron hinders zinc absorption, calcium hinders magnesium and iron absorption, and magnesium hinders the absorption of calcium and iron. The same interference takes place when people use foods that are fortified with added minerals; thus the consumer who wants the benefits of optimal absorption of nutrients should use ordinary foods, selected for nutrient density and variety.

Although minerals provide the most familiar and best-documented examples, other types of interference among nutrients are now being seen. The vitamin A precursor beta-carotene, long thought to be completely nontoxic, has recently been shown to interfere with vitamin E metabolism when taken over the long term as a dietary supplement.[6] Vitamin E, on the other hand, antagonizes vitamin K activity, and so should not be used by people being treated for blood-clotting disorders.

In view of all the negatives associated with supplement taking, several professional nutrition societies have indicated that people ordinarily should *not* use supplements. Whenever a person's diet is inadequate the person should first attempt to improve it so as to obtain the needed nutrients from foods. If that is truly impossible, then the person needs a multivitamin-mineral supplement that supplies between 50 and 150 percent of the RDA amount for each of the nutrients. These amounts reflect the ranges commonly found in foods and therefore are compatible with the body's normal handling of nutrients (its physiologic tolerance). Some pointers can assist in the selection of an appropriate supplement.

SELECTION OF SUPPLEMENTS

Whenever a physician prescribes a supplement, consider it medicine and follow directions carefully. When selecting a supplement yourself, look for a single, balanced vitamin-mineral supplement.

If you decide to take a vitamin-mineral supplement, you may find yourself bewildered in front of a drugstore counter, reading the clever, and usually deceptive, ads on labels—"Energize your body!" "Specifically formulated for infants!" "For active lives!" "Reduce your stress!" Of course, each ad insists only *that* particular supplement can deliver the promised benefit. To evade the clutches of Madison Avenue advertising agencies, take an imaginary bottle of white paint and blot out the pictures of young people running on the beach and the meaningless generalities like "new and improved." With the art and claims gone, all you have left is the form they are in, the list of ingredients, and the price. Here's where the truth lies, and from it you can make a rational decision based on facts.

Form

You have two basic questions to answer. The first question: What form do you want—chewable, liquid, or pills? If you'd rather drink your supplements then chew them, fine. (If you choose a chewable form, though, be aware that chewable vitamin C can dissolve tooth enamel.)

If you choose pills, look for statements about the disintegration time. The U.S. Pharmacopoeia (USP) suggests that supplements should completely disintegrate within 30 to 45 minutes.* Obviously, supplements that don't dissolve have little chance of entering the bloodstream, so look for a brand that claims to meet USP disintegration standards.

Contents

The second question: What vitamins and minerals do *you* need? The RDA (on the inside front cover, left) and the RNI for Canadians (Appendix I) are standards appropriate for virtually all healthy people. Generally, an appropriate supplement provides vitamins and minerals in amounts smaller than, equal to, or very close to these recommendations. Avoid supplements that, in a daily dose, provide more than the RDA of vitamin A, vitamin D, or any mineral or more than ten times the RDA for *any* nutrient. Avoid preparations with more than 10 milligrams iron per dose, except for menstruating women. Iron is hard to get rid of once it's in the body, so an excess of iron can cause problems, just as a deficiency can (Chapter 13).

As a rule, steer clear of high doses. Think of your ancestors who depended only on foods for life and health. If the foods available to them *could* have supplied the

---

*The USP establishes standards for quality, strength, and purity of supplements.
V. Srinivasan and coauthors, Standards setting for nutritional supplements—A new approach, *Nutrition Today*, November/December 1993, pp. 26–33.

amount of a nutrient you see in a supplement, then perhaps it is safe to ingest that amount. By this standard, the doses some people take are clearly excessive. For example, to obtain 840 milligrams of vitamin E from its best food source, wheat germ, you would have to eat 15 *pounds* of wheat germ—yet some people take supplements containing more than 840 milligrams of vitamin E every day. To obtain 5 grams of vitamin C, you would have to eat 19 pounds of oranges, yet some people consume more than that much daily from supplements.

Our ancestors survived for centuries without nutrient supplements and arrived successfully at the point of producing us. On this basis alone, it can be argued that we must need no more vitamins or minerals than *we* can obtain from food. That much, but not more, would be reasonable to look for in a supplement.

Misleading Claims

Ignore "organic" or "natural" claims. Such supplements are no better than standard types and often cost more. The word *synthetic* may sound like "fake," but to synthesize just means to put together. Whether vitamins are synthesized in a laboratory or synthesized by plants and animals, your body uses them similarly. Only your wallet can tell the difference.

Avoid products that make "high potency" claims. More is not better. The RDA is more than enough. Remember that foods are also providing these nutrients. Nutrients can build up and cause unexpected problems. For example, a man who takes vitamins and begins to lose his hair may think his hair loss means he needs *more* vitamins, when in fact it may be the early sign of a vitamin A overdose.

Be wise to preparations that contain items not needed in human nutrition, such as choline and inositol. Such ingredients reveal a marketing strategy aimed at your pocket, not at your health. The manufacturer wants you to believe that its pills contain the latest "new" nutrient that other brands omit, but in reality, the nutrients we need are known and are in the RDA and RNI tables.

Realize that the claim that supplements "relieve stress" is another marketing ploy. If you give even passing thought to what people mean by "stress," you'll realize manufacturers could never design a supplement to meet everyone's needs. Is it stressful to take an exam? Well, yes. Is it stressful to survive a major car wreck with third-degree burns and multiple bone fractures? Definitely yes. The body's responses to these stresses are different. The body does use vitamins and minerals in mounting a stress response, but a body fed a well-balanced diet can meet the needs of most minor stresses. As for the major ones, medical intervention is needed. In any case, taking a vitamin supplement won't make life any less stressful.

Other marketing tricks to sidestep are "green" pills that contain dehydrated, crushed parsley, alfalfa, and other vegetable matter. The nutrients can be obtained from a serving of vegetables more easily and for less money. Such pills may also provide enzymes, but these are inactivated in the stomach during digestion.

Be aware that most geriatric "tonics" are poor in vitamins and minerals, yet so high in alcohol as to threaten inebriation. The liquids designed for infants are more complete.

Recognize the latest nutrition buzzwords. Manufacturers were marketing "antioxidant" supplements before the print had time to dry on the first scientific reports of antioxidant vitamins' action in preventing cancer and cardiovascular disease. Remember, too, that high doses can alter a nutrient's action in the body. An antioxidant in physiological quantities may be beneficial, but in pharmacological quantities, it may produce harmful by-products.[7]

Cost

When shopping for supplements, remember that local or store brands are just as good as nationally advertised brands. If they are less expensive, it is not because they are inferior, but because the price does not have to cover the cost of national advertising. (One full-page color ad in a national magazine costs upwards of $95,000—not to mention the high cost of 30 seconds of national television time.) The less expensive pills are in fact often from the same batch as the higher priced ones—only the packages differ.

REGULATION OF SUPPLEMENTS

The Dietary Supplement Health and Education Act of 1994 enables customers to make more informed choices about nutrient supplements. The new regulations subject supplements to the same general labeling requirements that apply to foods.[8] Specifically:

- Nutrition labeling for dietary supplements is now required.
- Labels may describe nutrient contents (as "high" or "low") accord-

ing to specific criteria.

- The FDA will authorize health claims that are supported by significant scientific agreement and are not brand specific. To date, two health claims have been approved: that folate may reduce the risk of neural tube defects and that calcium may reduce the risk of osteoporosis.
- Health claims have *not* been authorized for the following nutrient-disease relationships: dietary fiber and cancer, dietary fiber and cardiovascular disease, antioxidant vitamins and cancer, omega-3 fatty acids and coronary heart disease, and zinc and immune deficiency in the elderly.
- Products may not claim to diagnose, treat, cure, or relieve a specific disease.
- Labels may describe the role a nutrient plays in the body, explain how the nutrient performs its function, and indicate that consuming the nutrient is associated with general well-being.

The $4-billion-a-year supplement industry has launched a massive public campaign to "keep the FDA from taking away our vitamins." The industry is expected to continue fighting against regulations by trying to get overruling legislation.

Part of the battle over FDA regulation involves a proposal to create a new regulatory category for "nutraceuticals"—a term not recognized by the FDA that refers to compounds that supposedly provide medical and health benefits (see the accompanying glossary).[9] Proponents are urging the FDA to loosen its criteria for health claims and to allow manufacturers to make exclusive claims based on their own research—without being required to make the research public. Such exclusivity of health claims on products based on private research would be contrary to the open sharing of information that is fundamental to nutrition science. It would also be confusing and misleading for consumers. If a "nutraceutical" company could claim that its Brand X beta-carotene prevents lung cancer, then consumers would need to be aware that other brands have a similar effect and that many foods provide beta-carotene as well. Furthermore, consumers would need to know that such a claim is backed by sound scientific research—and that's what FDA approval provides.

If all the nutrients we need can come from food, why not just eat food? Foods have so much more to recommend them than supplements do. Nutrients in foods come in an infinite variety of combinations with a multitude of different carriers and absorption facilitators. They come with water, fiber, and a host of beneficial and interesting nonnutrients. Foods stimulate the GI tract to keep it healthy. They provide energy, and since you need energy each day, why not ask nutritious foods to deliver it? They offer pleasure, satiety, and opportunities for socializing while eating. In no way can nutrient supplements hold a candle to foods as a means of meeting human health needs. For further proof, read Highlight 11.

Glossary

nutraceuticals: substances that supposedly provide medical and health benefits; a term not recognized by the FDA.

supplements: pills, liquids, or powders that contain purified nutrients, or foods with purified nutrients added in amounts per serving greater than 50% above a standard considered sufficient for all healthy people.

NOTES

1. M. M. Bender and coauthors, Trends in prevalence and magnitude of vitamin and mineral supplement usage and correlation with health status, *Journal of the American Dietetic Association* 92 (1992): 1096–1101.
2. M. J. Slesinski, A. F. Subar, and L. L. Kahle, Trends in use of vitamin and mineral supplements in the United States: The 1987 and 1992 National Health Interview Surveys, *Journal of the American Dietetic Association* 95 (1995): 921–923.
3. R. Oren and Y. Ilan, Reversible hepatic injury induced by long-term vitamin A ingestion, *American Journal of Medicine* 93 (1992): 703–704.
4. T. Litovitz and A. Manoguerra, Comparison of pediatric poisoning hazards: An analysis of 3.8 million exposure incidents (A report from the American Association of Poison Control Centers), *Pediatrics* 89 (1992): 999–1006.
5. Advice from health food stores, *Priorities*, Spring 1992, p. 31.
6. M. J. Xu and coauthors, Reduction in plasma or skin alpha-tocopherol concentration with long-term oral administration of beta-carotene in humans and mice, *Journal of the National Cancer Institute* 84 (1992): 1559–1565.
7. V. Herbert, The antioxidant supplement myth, *American Journal of Clinical Nutrition* 60 (1994): 157–158.
8. Dietary supplements: Recent chronology and legislation, *Nutrition Reviews* 53 (1995): 31–36.
9. J. R. Hunt, Nutritional products for specific health benefits—Foods, pharmaceuticals, or something in between? *Journal of the American Dietetic Association* 94 (1994): 151–153.

Chapter 11

The Fat-Soluble Vitamins: A, D, E, and K

CONTENTS

MICROGRAPH: Beta-carotene, the vitamin A precursor found in fruits and vegetables

The fat-soluble vitamins A, D, E, and K differ from the water-soluble vitamins in several significant ways (review Table 10–1 on p. 347). The fat-soluble vitamins are found in the fats and oils of foods. They are insoluble in water, so they require bile for digestion and chylomicrons for absorption. Upon absorption, fat-soluble vitamins enter the lymphatic system before entering the bloodstream, where many of them require protein carriers for transport. The fat-soluble vitamins are stored in the liver and adipose tissue until they are needed; they are not readily excreted, as most of the water-soluble vitamins are. Having stored these vitamins, people can eat less than their daily need for days, weeks, or even months or years without ill effects. Blood concentrations are maintained because the body retrieves the vitamins from storage as needed; thus a person need only ensure that over time *average* daily intakes approximate the RDA. By the same token, because fat-soluble vitamins are stored, the risk of toxicity is greater than it is for the water-soluble vitamins.

Vitamin A and Beta-Carotene

Reminder: A *precursor* is a compound that can be converted into an active vitamin.

beta-carotene (BAY-tah KARE-oh-teen): an orange pigment and vitamin A precursor found in plants.

retinol (RET-ih-nol): the alcohol form of vitamin A.

retinal (RET-ih-nal): the aldehyde form of vitamin A, active in the eye.

retinoic (RET-ih-no-ick) **acid:** the acid form of vitamin A.

retinoids: chemically related compounds with biologic activity similar to retinol; metabolites of retinol.

preformed vitamin A: dietary vitamin A in its active form.

carotenoids: pigments commonly found in plants and animals, some of which have provitamin A activity. Carotenoids are among the best-known **phytochemicals**—plant chemicals that are not nutrients but have biological activity in the body (see Highlight 11 for more details).

retinol-binding protein (RBP): the specific protein responsible for transporting retinol.

Vitamin A was the first fat-soluble vitamin to be recognized. More than 75 years later, vitamin A and its precursor, beta-carotene, continue to intrigue researchers with their diverse roles and profound effects on health.

Three different forms of vitamin A are active in the body: retinol, retinal, and retinoic acid. Collectively, these compounds are known as retinoids. Foods derived from animals provide preformed vitamin A as compounds (retinyl esters) that are easily hydrolyzed to retinol in the intestine. Foods derived from plants provide carotenoids, some of which have vitamin A activity. The most important of the carotenoids is beta-carotene, which can be split to form retinol in the intestine and liver. Beta-carotene's absorption and conversion are less efficient than those of preformed vitamin A. Figure 11–1 illustrates the structural similarities and differences of these vitamin A compounds.

The cells can convert retinol and retinal to the other active forms as needed. The oxidation of retinol to retinal is reversible, but the further oxidation of retinal to retinoic acid is irreversible. This irreversibility is significant because each form of vitamin A performs a function that the others cannot (see Figure 11–2).

A special transport protein, retinol-binding protein (RBP), picks up vitamin A from the liver, where it is stored, and carries it in the blood. Cells that will use vitamin A have special protein receptors for it, as if the vitamin were fragile and had to be passed carefully from hand to hand without being dropped. Each form of vitamin A has its own receptor protein (retinol has several) within the cell.

ROLES IN THE BODY

Vitamin A is a versatile vitamin. Its major roles include:

- Promoting vision.
- Promoting cell differentiation (and thereby maintaining the health of epithelial tissues and skin).
- Supporting the immune system.
- Promoting growth and bone remodeling.

Figure 11–1

Forms of Vitamin A

In this diagram, corners represent carbon atoms, as in all previous diagrams in this book. A further simplification here is that methyl groups (CH_3) are understood to be at the ends of the lines extending from corners. (See Appendix C for complete structures.)

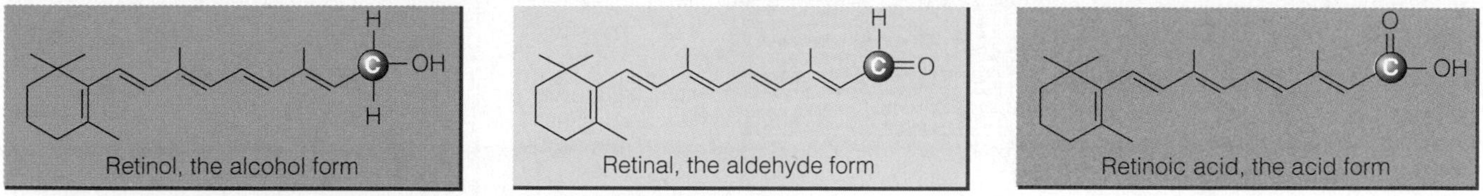

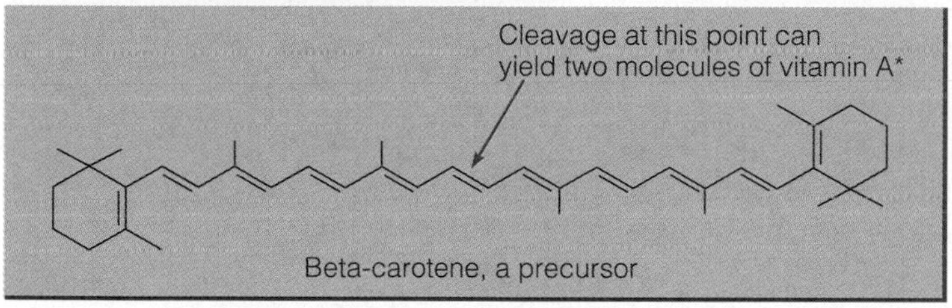

*Sometimes cleavage occurs at other points as well, so that one molecule of beta-carotene may yield only one molecule of vitamin A. Furthermore, not all beta-carotene is converted to vitamin A, and absorption of beta-carotene is not as efficient as vitamin A. For these reasons, 6 μg of beta-carotene are equivalent to 1 μg of vitamin A. Conversion of other carotenoids to vitamin A is even less efficient.

Each form of vitamin A performs specific tasks. Retinol supports reproduction and is the major transport and storage form of the vitamin. Retinal is active in vision and is also an intermediate in the conversion of retinol to retinoic acid. Retinoic acid acts like a hormone, regulating cell differentiation, growth, and embryonic development.[1] Animals raised on retinoic acid as their sole source of vitamin A can grow normally, but they become blind, because retinoic acid cannot be converted to retinal.[2]

Vitamin A in Vision Vitamin A plays two indispensable roles in the eye: it helps maintain a crystal-clear outer window, the cornea, and it participates in the transportation of light energy into nerve impulses at the retina (see Figure 11–3). When light falls on the eye, it passes through the clear cornea and strikes the cells of the retina. Pigment molecules inside the cells of the retina absorb light. (The glossary on p. 397 describes these molecules—rhodopsin, iodopsin, and others.) Each pigment molecule is composed of a protein called opsin bonded to a molecule of retinal. When light energy enters the eye, the retinal portion of the pigment

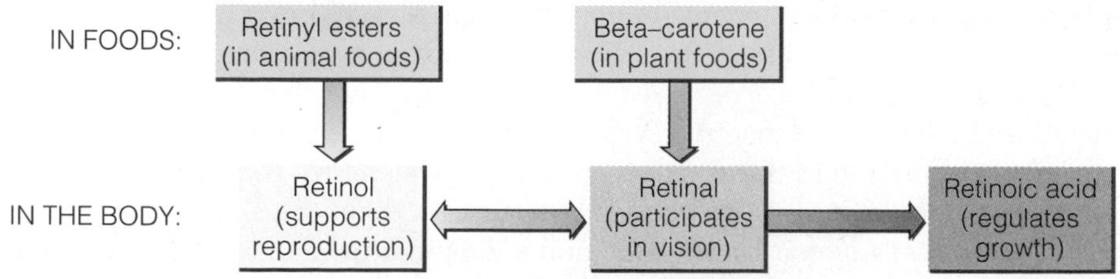

Figure 11–2

Conversion of Vitamin A Compounds

Notice that the conversion from retinol to retinal is reversible, whereas the pathway from retinal to retinoic acid is not.

Figure 11–3

Vitamin A's Role in Vision

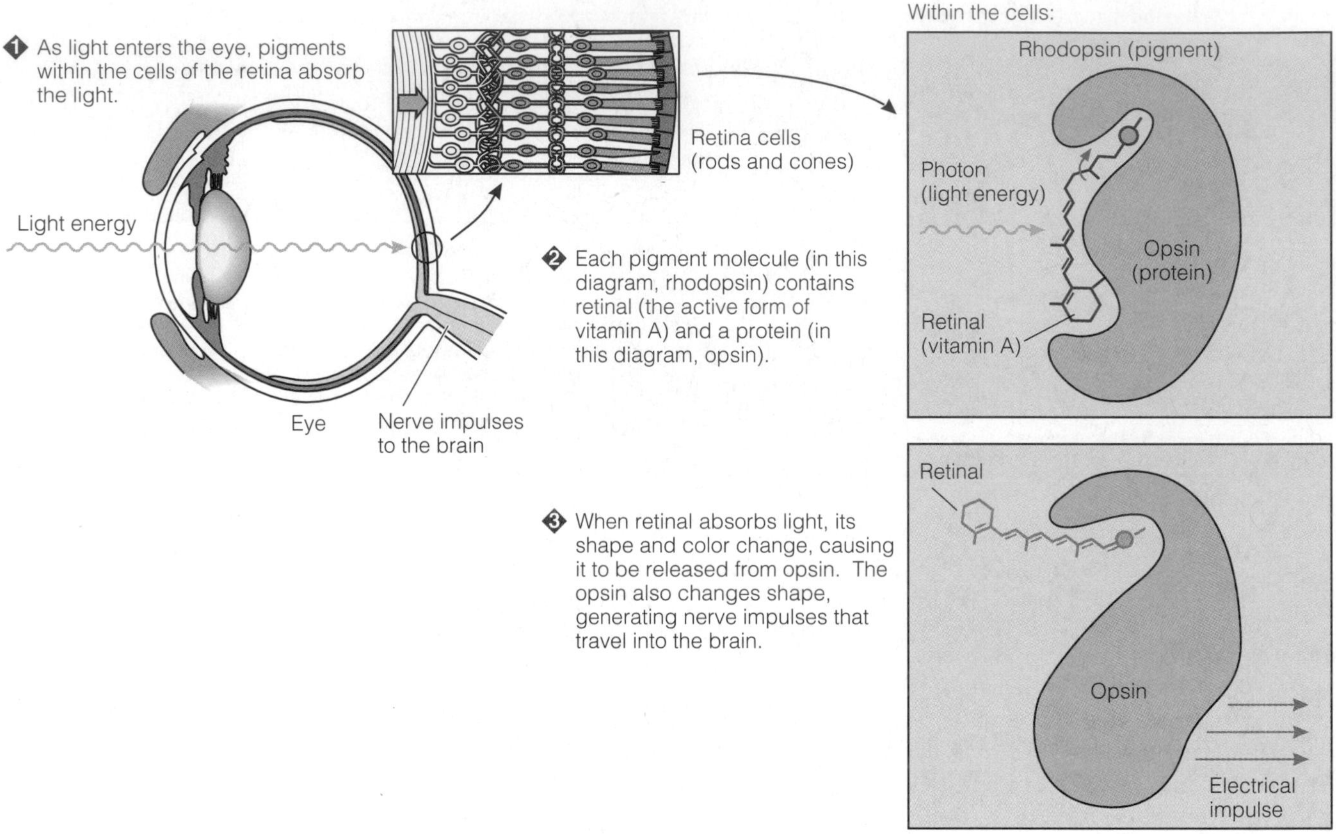
Within the cells:
Rhodopsin (pigment)
1 As light enters the eye, pigments within the cells of the retina absorb the light.
Retina cells (rods and cones)
Photon (light energy)
Light energy
2 Each pigment molecule (in this diagram, rhodopsin) contains retinal (the active form of vitamin A) and a protein (in this diagram, opsin).
Opsin (protein)
Retinal (vitamin A)
Eye
Nerve impulses to the brain
Retinal
3 When retinal absorbs light, its shape and color change, causing it to be released from opsin. The opsin also changes shape, generating nerve impulses that travel into the brain.
Opsin
Electrical impulse

molecule absorbs the photon and responds by changing shape: it shifts from a *cis* to a *trans* configuration as fatty acids do during hydrogenation (see p. 160). In the process, the retinal also changes color, becoming bleached. In its altered form, retinal cannot remain bonded to opsin and is released. This alters the shape of the opsin molecule.

The change in opsin's shape has further effects: it disturbs the membrane of the cell, generating an electrical impulse that travels along the cell's length. At the other end of the cell, the impulse is transmitted to a nerve cell, which conveys it deeper into the brain. Thus the message is sent. After sending the message, much of the retinal is converted back to its original form and rejoined to opsin to regenerate the pigment rhodopsin. Some retinal, however, may be oxidized to retinoic acid, a biochemical dead end for the visual process.

A genius could not have designed a better system. Light itself cannot be conducted through the solid material of the brain, but nerve impulses can be. To preserve the information in the different colors, or wavelengths, that light comes in, the eye uses the color-sensitive cone cells to receive them. Blue light is absorbed by one set of cells, green by another, and yellow-red by a third. By day, cones receive these colors and convey the full range of color vision to the optic center

Glossary of Vision Terms

cones: the cells of the retina that respond to bright light and are responsible for color vision.

cornea (KOR-nee-uh)**:** the transparent membrane covering the outside of the eye.

iodopsin (eye-o-DOP-sin)**:** the light-sensitive pigment of the cones in the retina. Both rhodopsin and iodopsin contain retinal; the protein portions of the pigments differ.

opsin (OP-sin)**:** the protein portion of the visual pigment molecule.

photon (FOE-ton)**:** a unit of light energy. Depending on its wavelength, a photon conveys different colors of light.

pigment: a molecule capable of absorbing certain wavelengths of light, so that it reflects only those that we perceive as a certain color.

retina (RET-in-uh)**:** the layer of light-sensitive nerve cells lining the back of the inside of the eye; consists of rods and cones.

rhodopsin (ro-DOP-sin)**:** the light-sensitive pigment of the rods in the retina; it contains the retinal form of vitamin A.
rhod = rod-shaped cells
opsin = visual protein

rods: the cells of the retina that respond to dim light and convey black-and-white vision.

---

in the brain. By night, the light entering the eye is of low intensity and can be received only by the rod cells; so by night a person can normally discern only the presence of light, not its color.

About 6 to 7 million cone cells and 100 million rod cells reside in the retina, and each contains about 30 million molecules of retinal-containing visual pigment. Visual activity leads to repeated small losses of retinal and necessitates its constant replenishment from retinol in the blood, which brings a new supply from the body stores. Ultimately, vitamin A and its relatives in foods are the source of all the retinal in the pigments of the eye.

A lot of retinal can be destroyed at night. If the body's vitamin A stores are marginal, the use of the eyes at night can lead to a vitamin A deficiency and the early, tell-tale symptom of night blindness. The eye is especially vulnerable to retinal destruction at night for three reasons. First, the pupil opens wide at night, so as to allow as much light as possible to enter the eye. Second, a shadowing pigment that protects the rods by day withdraws at night, leaving them exposed. Third, there are many more rods than cones. Hence, if a bright light suddenly shines at night through the wide-open pupil onto the unprotected rods, much of the pigment in them is bleached and momentarily inactivated. More retinal than usual is released, and more is lost. A moment passes before the pigments regenerate and sight returns. You no doubt have been temporarily "blinded" on occasion by a light shining directly into your eyes. Normally, of course, you quickly recover your ability to see.

night blindness: slow recovery of vision after flashes of bright light at night or an inability to see in dim light; an early symptom of vitamin A deficiency.

differentiation: development of specific functions different from those of the original.

epithelial (ep-i-THEE-lee-ul) **cells:** cells on the surface of the skin and mucous membranes.

epithelial tissues: the layers of the body that serve as selective barriers between the body's interior and the environment (examples are the cornea, the skin, the respiratory lining, and the lining of the digestive tract).

Vitamin A in Cell Differentiation Despite its important role in vision, only one-thousandth of the body's vitamin A is in the retina. Much more is in the cells lining the body's surfaces, where the vitamin participates in cell differentiation.[3]

All body surfaces, both inside and out, are covered by layers of cells known as epithelial cells. The epithelial tissue on the outside of the body is, of course, the mucous membranes: the membranes, composed of mucus-secreting cells, that line the surfaces of body tissues.

urethra (you-REE-thruh): the tube through which urine from the bladder passes out of the body.

Reminder: *Goblet cells* in the epithelium of the GI tract and lungs secrete mucus.

Reminder: *Mucus* is a slippery substance secreted by the goblet cells of mucous membranes.

skin. The epithelial tissues that line the inside of the body are the mucous membranes: the linings of the mouth, stomach, and intestines; the linings of the lungs and the passages leading to them; the linings of the urinary bladder and urethra; the linings of the uterus and vagina; and the linings of the eyelids and sinus passageways. Within the body, the mucous membranes of the GI tract alone line an area larger than a quarter of a football field, and vitamin A helps to maintain their integrity (see Figure 11–4).

Vitamin A promotes differentiation of both epithelial cells and goblet cells, one-celled glands that synthesize and secrete mucus. Mucus coats and protects the epithelial cells from invasive microorganisms and other harmful substances, such as gastric juices.

Vitamin A in Immunity Vitamin A's maintenance of healthy epithelial tissues helps to fight infection by preventing the invasion of bacteria and viruses. In addition, vitamin A appears to play a direct role in immunity itself.[4] Children with even mild vitamin A deficiency develop respiratory infections and diarrhea at two and three times the rate of children with normal vitamin A status.

Vitamin A in Growth As mentioned, vitamin A supports growth. Growth failure is common in children with vitamin A deficiency. When they are given vitamin A supplements, they gain weight and grow taller.

The growth of bones illustrates that growth is a complex phenomenon of remodeling. To convert a small bone into a large bone, the bone-remodeling cells must "undo" some parts of the bone as they go, and vitamin A participates in the undoing. The cells that break down bone contain sacs of degradative enzymes. With the help of vitamin A, these enzymes eat away at selected sites in the bone, removing the parts that are not needed. A similar process occurs when a human embryo loses its tail and becomes human-shaped; the tail "grows" shorter and shorter until it disappears. The process depends on vitamin A.

remodeling: the dismantling and re-formation of a structure, in this case, bone.

The cells that destroy bone during growth are osteoclasts; those that build bone are osteoblasts.
osteo = bone
clast = break
blast = build

The sacs of degradative enzymes are lysosomes (LYE-so-zomes).

Beta-Carotene as an Antioxidant Beta-carotene functions in the body as a vitamin A precursor, but it also has roles of its own. Not all dietary beta-carotene is converted to active vitamin A. Some beta-carotene acts as an antioxidant capable of protecting the body against disease. Highlight 11 discusses some recent findings related to this protection.

Figure 11–4

Mucous Membrane Integrity

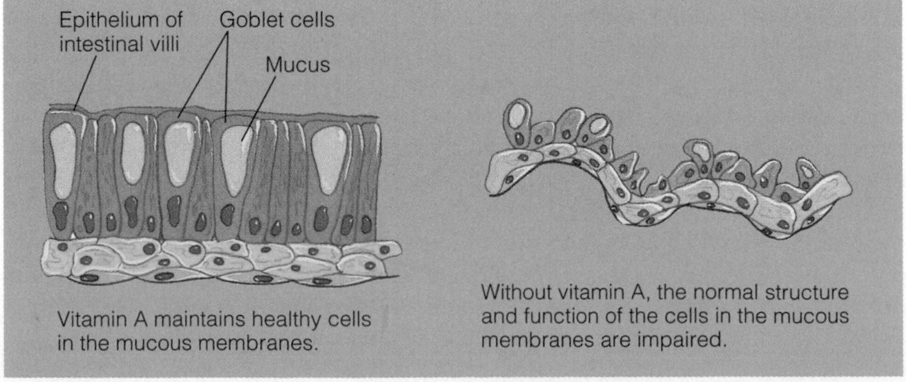

Epithelium of intestinal villi
Goblet cells
Mucus
Vitamin A maintains healthy cells in the mucous membranes.
Without vitamin A, the normal structure and function of the cells in the mucous membranes are impaired.

VITAMIN A RECOMMENDATIONS

Because the body can derive vitamin A either preformed or from beta-carotene, its contents in foods and its recommendations are expressed as retinol equivalents or RE. Some products still report their vitamin A contents using international units (IU), an older system of measurement that is based on some assumptions now known to be inaccurate. To evaluate vitamin A intake expressed in IU requires some computing: 1 RE is roughly equivalent to 3.33 IU of vitamin A from animal tissues or 10 IU from plant tissues.[5] Newer tables of food composition, including Appendix H in this book, report the vitamin A activity of foods in RE.

Vitamin A intakes can range widely before deficiency or toxicity symptoms appear (see Figure 11–5 on p. 401). Recommended intakes in both the United States and Canada are set at about double the minimum necessary to prevent deficiency. Doubtless, many people need not consume amounts this high; other countries and international agencies recommend lower values.[6] The exact upper limit of safety cannot be determined because people's tolerances to overdoses vary. Several authorities agree that the RDA are the best guidelines for safety and that higher intakes offer no benefits.[7]

RE (retinol equivalent): a measure of vitamin A activity; the amount of retinol that the body will derive from a food containing preformed retinol or its precursor beta-carotene.

1 RE = 1 μg retinol.
= 6 μg beta-carotene.
= 12 μg of other vitamin A precursor carotenes.

international units (IU): a measure of vitamin activity, determined by such biological methods as feeding a compound to vitamin-deprived animals and measuring growth. This system was used to measure vitamin A before direct chemical analysis was possible.

1 RE = 3.33 IU (retinol from animal foods).
= 10.00 IU (beta-carotene from plant foods).
≈ 5.00 IU (on average).

VITAMIN A DEFICIENCY

Vitamin A status depends mostly on the adequacy of vitamin A stores, 90 percent of which are in the liver. Vitamin A status also depends on a person's having adequate protein, because protein provides the vitamin's carriers for inside-the-body transport. If a healthy adult were to stop eating vitamin A–rich foods, deficiency symptoms would not begin to appear until after stores were depleted, which would take one to two years; it would take less time in a growing child. Then, however, the consequences would be profound and severe. Table 11–1 (on pp. 400–401) itemizes deficiency symptoms as well as toxicity symptoms, functions in the body, and food sources.

Vitamin A deficiency is one of the developing world's major nutrition problems. More than 100 million children worldwide have some degree of vitamin A deficiency, and so are vulnerable to infectious diseases.[8]

Infectious Diseases Since the early 1980s, several large studies conducted in Indonesia, India, Nepal, and Sudan have found that supplementing children with vitamin A can reduce death rates significantly.[9] This evidence prompted the World Health Organization (WHO) and UNICEF (the United Nations International Children's Emergency Fund) to make the control of vitamin A deficiency a major goal in their quest to improve child survival throughout the developing world.

In developing countries throughout the world, measles is a devastating infectious disease, killing as many as 2 million children each year.[10] The severity of the illness often correlates with the degree of vitamin A deficiency; deaths are usually due to related infections such as pneumonia and severe diarrhea.[11] Children with measles who receive vitamin A supplements recover faster from pneumonia and other infections than children who do not receive supplements.[12] Providing large doses of vitamin A to children hospitalized with severe measles can reduce their risk of dying by at least 50 percent.[13]

Of historical interest is a similar trial carried out in London in 1932 that showed remarkably consistent results: children hospitalized with measles who

Table 11–1

Vitamin A—A Summary

Other Names	Deficiency Disease Name	Toxicity Disease Name
Retinol, retinal, retinoic acid; precursor is provitamin A carotenoids such as beta-carotene	Hypovitaminosis A	Hypervitaminosis A[a]
Adult RDA	**Deficiency Symptoms**	**Toxicity Symptoms**
Men: 1000 μg RE/day Women: 800 μg RE/day	BONES/TEETH	
Chief Functions in the Body	Cessation of bone growth, painful joints, impaired enamel formation, cracks in teeth, tendency to decay, atrophy of dentin-forming cells	Increased activity of osteoclasts[b] causing decalcification, joint pain, fragility, stunted growth, and thickening of long bones; increase of pressure inside skull, mimicking brain tumor; headaches
Vision; maintenance of cornea, epithelial cells, mucous membranes, skin; bone and tooth growth; reproduction; immunity	BLOOD	
Significant Sources	Anemia, often masked by dehydration	Loss of hemoglobin and potassium by red blood cells, cessation of menstruation, slowed clotting time, easily induced bleeding
Retinol: fortified milk, cheese, cream, butter, fortified margarine, eggs, liver Beta-carotene: spinach and other dark leafy greens; broccoli, deep orange fruits (apricots, cantaloupe) and vegetables (squash, carrots, sweet potatoes, pumpkin)	EYES[c]	
	Night blindness, changes in epithelial tissue (hyperkeratinization), drying (xerosis), triangular gray spots on eye (Bitot's spots), irreversible drying (keratomalacia), and corneal degeneration (blindness)	
	SKIN	
	Plugging of hair follicles with keratin, forming white lumps (hyperkeratosis)	Dryness; itching; peeling; rashes; dry, scaling lips; cracking and bleeding of lips; nosebleeds; loss of hair; brittle nails

[a] A related condition, *hypercarotenemia*, is caused by the accumulation of too much of the vitamin A precursor beta-carotene in the blood, which turns the skin noticeably yellow. Hypercarotenemia is not, strictly speaking, a toxicity symptom.
[b] *Osteoclasts* are the cells that destroy bone during its growth. Those that build bone are *osteoblasts*.
[c] The eyes' symptoms of vitamin A deficiency are collectively known as *xerophthalmia*.

were given daily doses of cod liver oil (a rich source of vitamin A) died at a rate only half that of similar children not given the oil.[14] WHO now recommends routine vitamin A supplementation for all children with measles in areas where vitamin A deficiency is a problem or where the measles death rate is high.[15] In the United States, the American Academy of Pediatrics recommends vitamin A supplementation for certain groups of measles-infected infants and children.[16]

Night Blindness Night blindness is one of the first detectable signs of vitamin A deficiency and permits early diagnosis of the condition. In night blindness, the blood bathing the cells of the retina does not supply sufficient retinal to rapidly regenerate visual pigments bleached by light. The person loses the

Table 11–1

Vitamin A—A Summary (continued)

Deficiency Symptoms	Toxicity Symptoms
DIGESTIVE SYSTEM	
Changes in lining, diarrhea	Nausea, vomiting, abdominal pain, diarrhea, weight loss
IMMUNE SYSTEM	
Suppression of immune reactions; frequent respiratory, digestive, bladder, vaginal, and kidney infections	Overstimulation of immune reactions
NERVOUS/MUSCULAR SYSTEMS	
Brain and spinal cord growth too fast for stunted skull and spine	Loss of appetite, irritability, fatigue, insomnia, restlessness, headaches, blurred vision, nausea, vomiting, muscle weakness, interference with thyroxin
OTHER	
Kidney stones	Amenorrhea,[d] jaundice,[e] enlargement of liver[f] and spleen, massive accumulation of fat and vitamin A in liver

[d]Elevated serum carotene concentrations are associated with amenorrhea.

[e]*Jaundice* (JAWN-dice) is a symptom of liver disease, in which bile and related pigments spill into the bloodstream and the skin yellows.

[f]If liver impairment is severe, the "classic" signs seen in skin and hair may be masked.

ability to recover promptly from the temporary blinding that occurs following a flash of bright light at night or simply to see after the lights go out. In many parts of the world, after the sun goes down, vitamin A–deficient children become night-blind: they cannot find their shoes or toys and often cling to others or sit still, afraid that they may trip and fall or lose their way if they try to go home alone. In many developing countries, night blindness due to vitamin A deficiency is so common that the people have special words to describe it. In Indonesia, the term is *buta ayam,* which means "chicken eyes" or "chicken blindness." (Chickens do not have rods in their eyes and therefore cannot see at night.) Vitamin A–deficient children, like chickens, stumble after dark. Figure 11–6 shows the eyes' slow recovery in response to a flash of bright light in night blindness.

Blindness (Xerophthalmia) Beyond night blindness lies total blindness—failure to see at all. Night blindness is caused by a lack of vitamin A at the back of the eye, the retina; total blindness is caused by a lack in the front of the eye, the cornea. Vitamin A deficiency is the major cause of childhood blindness in the world, causing more than half a million preschool children to lose their sight each year. Blindness due to vitamin A deficiency, known as xerophthalmia, progresses. First, the cornea becomes dry and hard, a condition known as xerosis.

Figure 11–5

Vitamin A Deficiency and Toxicity

As the dose increases from zero, normalcy is reached. A wide range of intakes is safe, and then toxicity is reached.

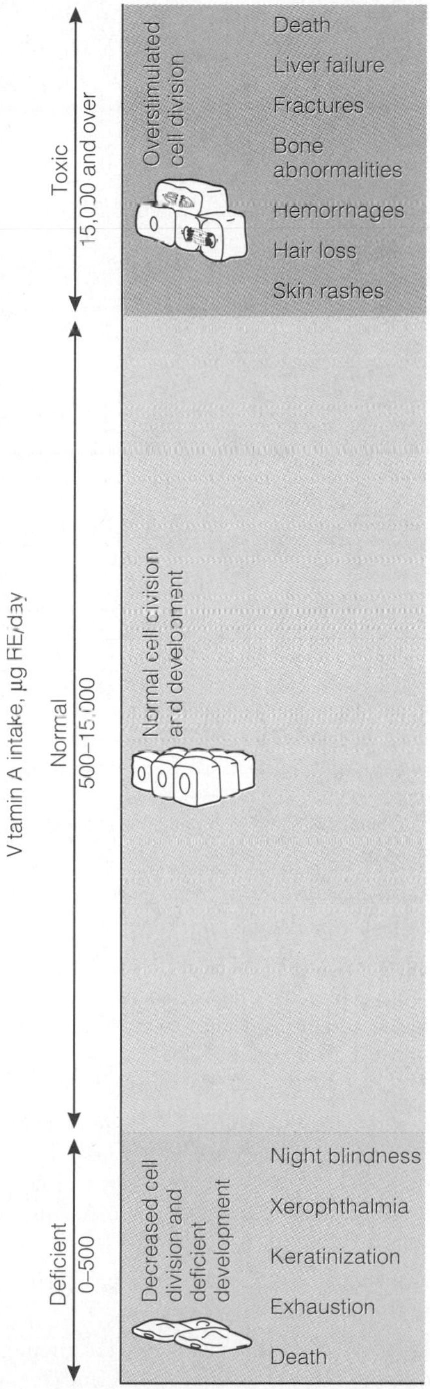

Figure 11–6

Night Blindness

These photographs illustrate the eyes' slow recovery in response to a flash of bright light at night. In animal research studies, the response rate is measured with electrodes.

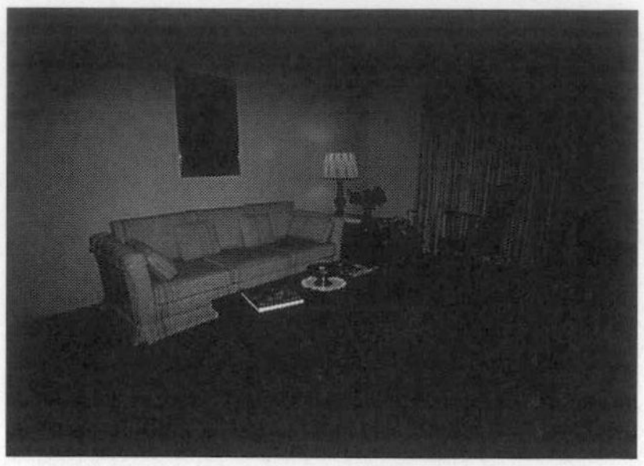

A. In dim light, you can make out the details in this room. You are using your rods for vision.

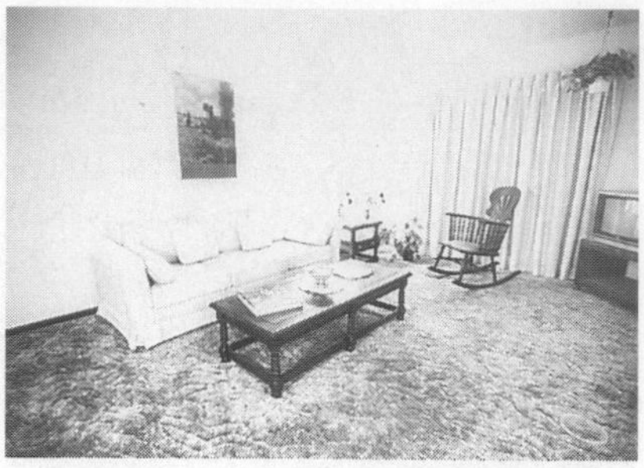

B. A flash of bright light momentarily blinds you as the pigment in the rods is bleached.

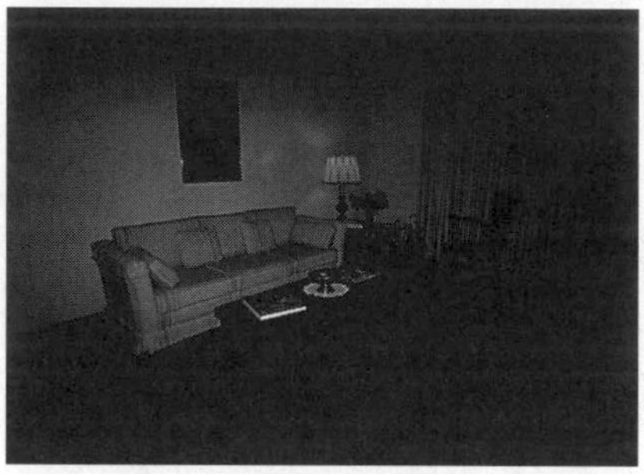

C. You quickly recover and can see the details again in a few seconds.

D. With inadequate vitamin A, you do not recover but remain blinded for many seconds.

---

xerophthalmia (zer-off-THAL-mee-uh)**:** progressive blindness caused by vitamin A deficiency.
xero = dry
ophthalm = eye

xerosis (zee-ROW-sis)**:** drying of the cornea; a sign of vitamin A deficiency.

keratomalacia (KARE-ah-toe-ma-LAY-shia)**:** softening of the cornea seen in severe vitamin A deficiency that leads to irreversible blindness.

keratin (KERR-uh-tin)**:** a water-insoluble protein; the normal protein of hair and nails. Keratin-producing cells may replace mucus-producing cells in vitamin A deficiency.

hair follicle (FOLL-i-cul)**:** a group of cells in the skin from which a hair grows.

keratinization: accumulation of keratin in a tissue; a sign of vitamin A deficiency.

Corneal xerosis can quickly progress to keratomalacia, the softening of the cornea that leads to irreversible blindness. Dietary vitamin A reduces the risk of xerophthalmia significantly.[17]

Keratinization Elsewhere in the body, vitamin A deficiency affects other surfaces. Without vitamin A, the goblet cells in the stomach and intestines diminish in number and activity, limiting the secretion of mucus. With less mucus, the normal digestion and absorption of nutrients are hindered, and this, in turn, worsens the deficiency by impairing the absorption of whatever vitamin A the diet may deliver. Similar changes in the cells of other epithelial tissues weaken defenses, making infections of the respiratory tract, the GI tract, the urinary tract, the vagina, and possibly the inner ear likely. On the body's outer surface, the epithelial cells change shape and begin to secrete the protein keratin—the hard, inflexible protein of hair and nails. The skin becomes dry, rough, and scaly as lumps of keratin accumulate around each hair follicle (keratinization).

VITAMIN A TOXICITY

Just as a deficiency of vitamin A affects all body systems, so does a toxicity. Symptoms begin to develop when all the binding proteins are swamped, and free vitamin A damages the cells. Such effects are unlikely when a person depends on a balanced diet for nutrients, but if the person takes large amounts of the preformed vitamin from animal foods or supplements, toxicity is a real possibility.

Beta-carotene, which is found in a wide variety of plant foods, is not converted efficiently enough in the body to cause vitamin A toxicity; instead, it is stored in fat depots under the skin. Overconsumption of beta-carotene may turn the skin yellow, but this is not harmful.

Children are most vulnerable to toxicity because they need less and are more sensitive to overdoses. Serious toxicity is seen in infants and young children when they are given more than ten times the recommended amount every day for weeks at a time. A child who regards vitamin pills as candy may easily self-overdose.

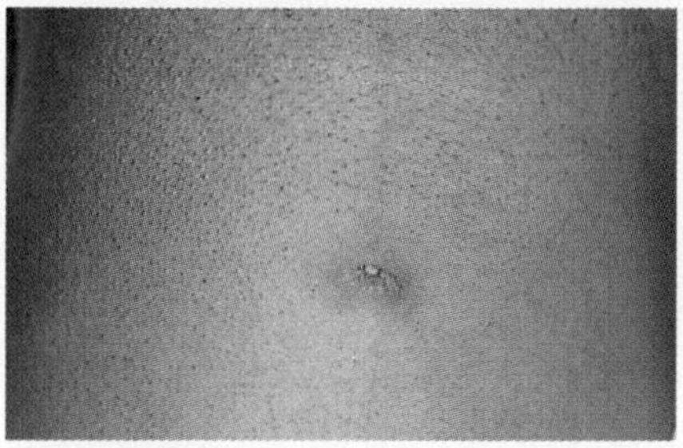

In vitamin A deficiency, the epithelial cells secrete the protein keratin in a process known as *keratinization*. (Keratinization doesn't occur in the GI tract, but mucus-producing cells dwindle, and mucus production declines.) The progression of this condition to the extreme is *hyperkeratinization* or *hyperkeratosis*. When keratin accumulates around each hair follicle, the condition is known as *follicular hyperkeratosis*.

Birth Defects In animals, large doses of vitamin A during pregnancy produce malformations in all organ systems. Although a clear-cut cause-and-effect relationship between excessive vitamin A intakes during pregnancy and birth defects is not confirmed in human beings, several reports implicate excess vitamin A as a factor. Most convincing was the case of a woman who ingested a single massive dose of vitamin A (about 100 times greater than the RDA) during the second month of her pregnancy.[18] Her infant was born with numerous birth defects, including eye malformations. The lowest intake of vitamin A that causes birth defects is uncertain, but several agencies suggest limiting supplements to less than 3 times the RDA for pregnant women.[19]

Not for Acne Adolescents need to know that massive doses of vitamin A have no corrective effect on acne, but may cause toxicity. The prescription medicine Accutane is made from vitamin A but is chemically altered. Taken orally, Accutane is effective against the deep lesions of cystic acne. It is highly toxic, however, especially during growth, and has caused birth defects in infants when women have taken it during their pregnancies. For this reason, women taking Accutane must begin using an effective form of contraception at least a month before starting to take the drug and continue using contraception a month after discontinuing its use.

acne: a chronic inflammation of the skin's follicles and oil-producing glands, which leads to an accumulation of oils inside the ducts that surround hairs; usually associated with the maturation of young adults.

Another vitamin A relative, Retin-A, fights acne, the wrinkles of aging, and other skin disorders. Applied topically, this ointment smooths and softens skin; it also lightens skin that has become darkly pigmented after inflammation.[20] During treatment, the skin becomes red and tender and peels. Although the Food and Drug Administration (FDA) has approved Retin-A, several questions remain unanswered: Does it have long-term toxic effects? How does it work? What is the minimum effective dose? How long do the benefits last?

Not for Cancer Beta-carotene and the retinoids may help prevent cancer, but the retinoids are so toxic as to preclude their use in supplement form.[21] Still, gullible people take massive doses of vitamin A in the hope of preventing cancer. As a result, more cases of vitamin A toxicity may be reported in the years to come. Highlight 11 discusses the role of beta-carotene in cancer prevention.

VITAMIN A IN FOODS

The richest source of preformed vitamin A are foods of animal origin—liver, fish liver oils, milk and milk products, butter, and eggs. Plants contain no preformed vitamin A, but many vegetables and some fruits contain provitamin A carotenoids, the red and yellow pigments of plants. Only a few carotenoids have vitamin A activity. The carotenoid with the greatest vitamin A activity is beta-carotene.

The Colors of Vitamin A Foods Recommendations to eat dark green and deep orange vegetables and fruits help people to meet their vitamin A needs (see Figure 11–7). A 1-cup serving of carrots, sweet potatoes, or dark greens such as spinach provides such liberal amounts of carotenoids that even allowing for inefficient absorption and conversion, the intake of the vitamin is sufficient for many days. Alternatively, a diet including more or larger servings of medium sources also ensures an ample intake.

Most foods with vitamin A activity are brightly colored—green, yellow, orange, and red. Any plant food with significant vitamin A activity must have some color, since carotene is a rich, deep yellow, almost orange compound. The dark green, leafy vegetables contain abundant amounts of the green pigment chlorophyll, which masks the carotene in them. An attractive meal includes foods of different colors; such a meal most likely supplies vitamin A as well.

On the other hand, colorful vegetables do not invariably provide vitamin A activity. Beets and corn, for example, derive their colors from the red and yellow xanthophylls, which have no vitamin A activity. On the third hand (this chapter has three hands), white plant foods such as potatoes, cauliflower, pasta, and rice also possess little or no vitamin A activity.

vitamin A activity: a term useful for referring to both the preformed vitamin A and carotene contents of foods without distinguishing between them.

carotene: a vitamin A precursor found in plants; an orange pigment.

chlorophyll: the green pigment of plants, which absorbs photons and transfers their energy to other molecules, thereby initiating photosynthesis.

xanthophylls (ZAN-tho-fills)**:** pigments found in plants; responsible for the color changes seen in autumn leaves.

Typical Intakes In the typical United States diet, about half of the vitamin A activity comes from vegetables and fruits, and half of this comes from the dark leafy greens (like spinach—not celery or cabbage) and the rich yellow or deep orange vegetables (such as winter squash, cantaloupe, carrots, and sweet potatoes—not corn or bananas). The other half of the vitamin A activity in foods is from preformed vitamin A in milk, cheese, butter, and other dairy products; eggs; and liver. Since vitamin A is fat soluble, it is lost when milk is skimmed. To compensate, nonfat milk is often fortified so as to supply about 40 percent of the RDA per quart.* Margarine is usually fortified so as to provide the same amount of vitamin A as butter.

Vitamin A–Poor Fast Foods Fast foods often lack vitamin A. Anyone who dines frequently on hamburgers, french fries, and colas is advised to emphasize vegetables at other meals.

Vitamin A–Rich Liver Liver is a rich source of preformed vitamin A, because in animals just as in humans, vitamin A is stored there.† People sometimes wonder if eating liver too frequently can cause vitamin A toxicity. Arctic explorers who have eaten large quantities of polar bear liver have become ill with symptoms suggesting vitamin A toxicity. Closer to home, vitamin A toxicity symptoms were reported in young children who regularly ate a chicken liver

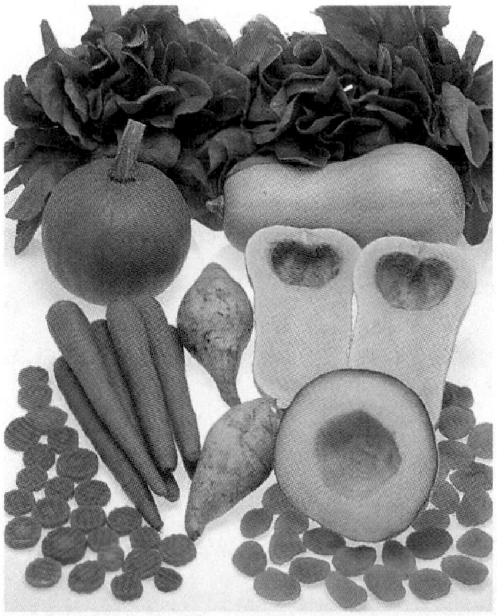

The carotenoids bring colors to meals; the retinoids allow us to see them.

*Vitamin A fortification of milk in Canada follows a similar standard.

†The liver is not the only organ that stores vitamin A. The kidneys, adrenals, and other organs do, too, but the liver stores the most and is the one most commonly eaten.

Figure 11–7 Vitamin A in Selected Foods

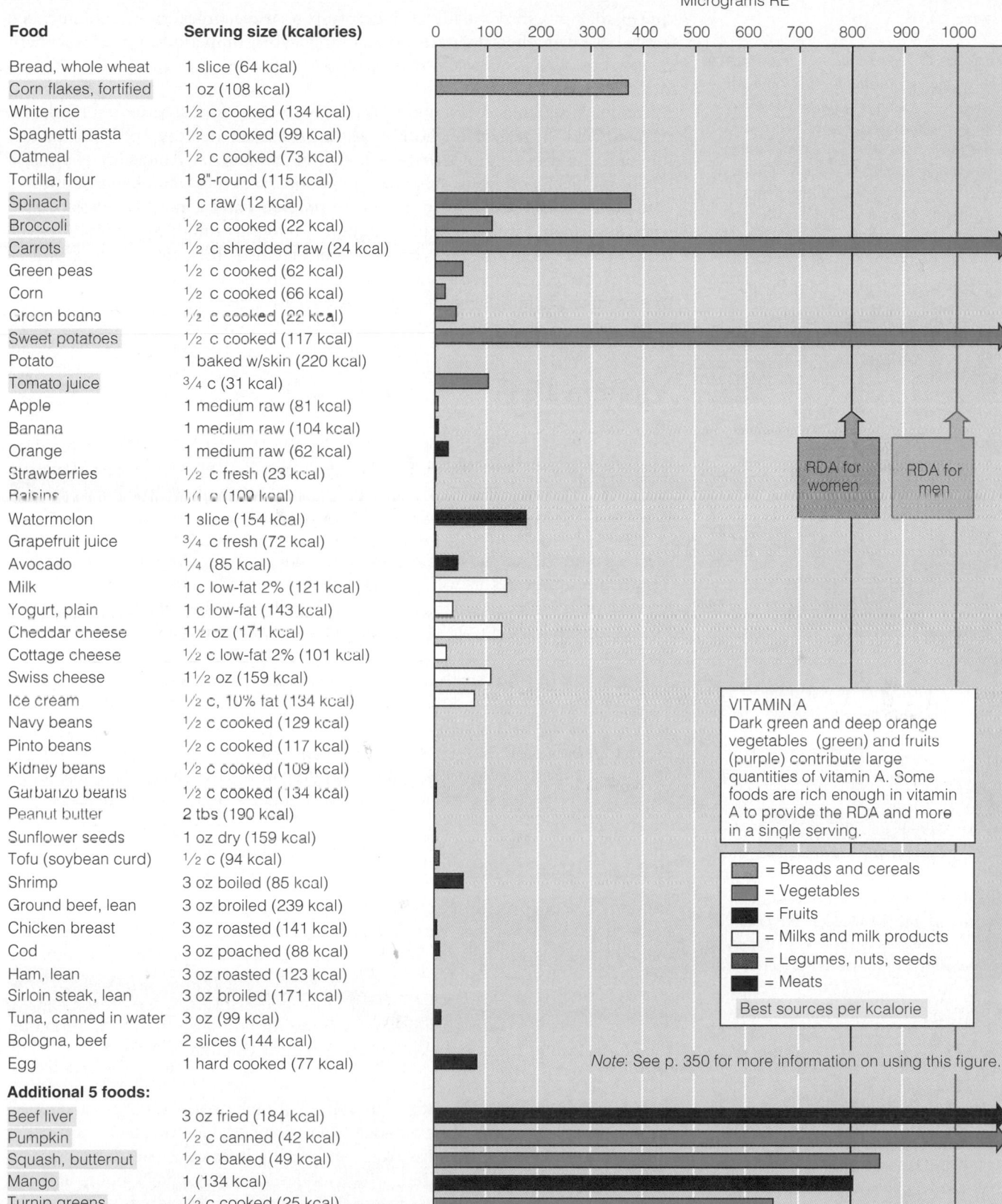

Food	Serving size (kcalories)
Bread, whole wheat	1 slice (64 kcal)
Corn flakes, fortified	1 oz (108 kcal)
White rice	1/2 c cooked (134 kcal)
Spaghetti pasta	1/2 c cooked (99 kcal)
Oatmeal	1/2 c cooked (73 kcal)
Tortilla, flour	1 8"-round (115 kcal)
Spinach	1 c raw (12 kcal)
Broccoli	1/2 c cooked (22 kcal)
Carrots	1/2 c shredded raw (24 kcal)
Green peas	1/2 c cooked (62 kcal)
Corn	1/2 c cooked (66 kcal)
Green beans	1/2 c cooked (22 kcal)
Sweet potatoes	1/2 c cooked (117 kcal)
Potato	1 baked w/skin (220 kcal)
Tomato juice	3/4 c (31 kcal)
Apple	1 medium raw (81 kcal)
Banana	1 medium raw (104 kcal)
Orange	1 medium raw (62 kcal)
Strawberries	1/2 c fresh (23 kcal)
Raisins	1/4 c (109 kcal)
Watermelon	1 slice (154 kcal)
Grapefruit juice	3/4 c fresh (72 kcal)
Avocado	1/4 (85 kcal)
Milk	1 c low-fat 2% (121 kcal)
Yogurt, plain	1 c low-fat (143 kcal)
Cheddar cheese	1 1/2 oz (171 kcal)
Cottage cheese	1/2 c low-fat 2% (101 kcal)
Swiss cheese	1 1/2 oz (159 kcal)
Ice cream	1/2 c, 10% fat (134 kcal)
Navy beans	1/2 c cooked (129 kcal)
Pinto beans	1/2 c cooked (117 kcal)
Kidney beans	1/2 c cooked (109 kcal)
Garbanzo beans	1/2 c cooked (134 kcal)
Peanut butter	2 tbs (190 kcal)
Sunflower seeds	1 oz dry (159 kcal)
Tofu (soybean curd)	1/2 c (94 kcal)
Shrimp	3 oz boiled (85 kcal)
Ground beef, lean	3 oz broiled (239 kcal)
Chicken breast	3 oz roasted (141 kcal)
Cod	3 oz poached (88 kcal)
Ham, lean	3 oz roasted (123 kcal)
Sirloin steak, lean	3 oz broiled (171 kcal)
Tuna, canned in water	3 oz (99 kcal)
Bologna, beef	2 slices (144 kcal)
Egg	1 hard cooked (77 kcal)
Additional 5 foods:	
Beef liver	3 oz fried (184 kcal)
Pumpkin	1/2 c canned (42 kcal)
Squash, butternut	1/2 c baked (49 kcal)
Mango	1 (134 kcal)
Turnip greens	1/2 c cooked (25 kcal)

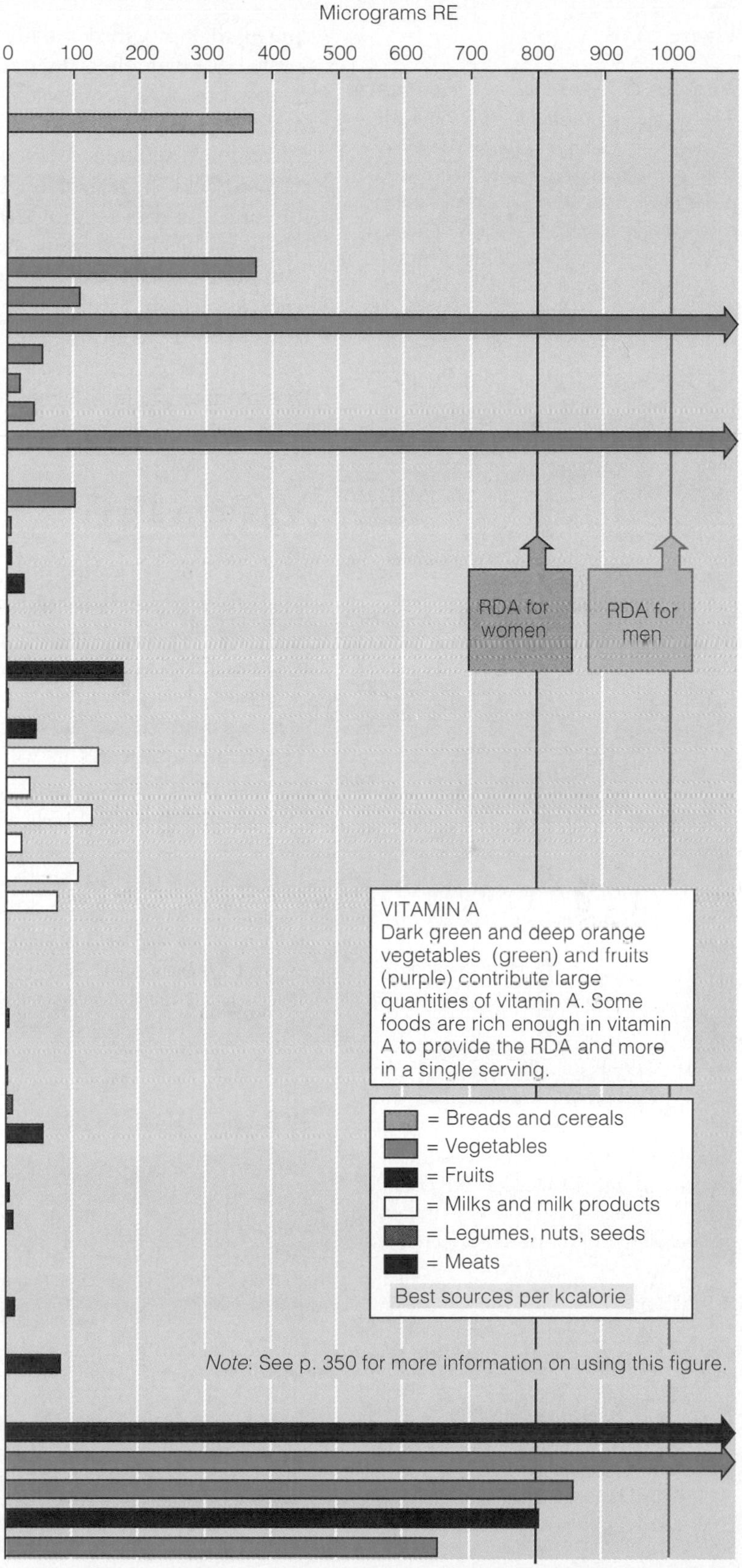

Note: See p. 350 for more information on using this figure.

Figure 11–8

Vitamin D Synthesis and Activation
The precursor of vitamin D is 7-dehydrocholesterol, which is made in the liver from cholesterol (see Figure 5–10 on p. 165 and Appendix C). This is one of the body's many "good" uses for cholesterol. The final product, active vitamin D, is 1,25-dihydroxycholecalciferol (or calcitriol). The hydroxylation of vitamin D to its active form is a closely regulated process.

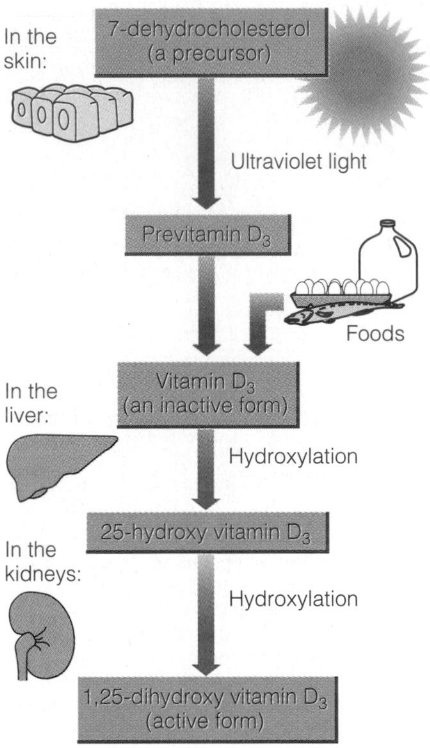

Vitamin D is also known as **vitamin D_3** or **cholecalciferol** (KO-lee-kal-SIF-er-ol). The plant version is known as **vitamin D_2** or **ergocalciferol** (er-go-kal-SIF-er-ol).

spread that provided a daily average of up to three times their recommended intake.[22] Liver offers many nutrients, and eating it periodically may benefit health, but once every week or so is often enough.

In summary, vitamin A is found in the body in three forms: retinol, retinal, and retinoic acid. Together, they are essential to vision, healthy epithelial tissues, immunity, and bone growth and remodeling. Vitamin A deficiency is a major health problem worldwide, leading to infections, blindness, and keratinization of epithelial tissues. Toxicity can also cause problems and is most often associated with supplement abuse. Preformed vitamin A is found primarily in animal-derived foods such as liver and milk, whereas the precursor beta-carotene is found in brightly colored plant foods such as spinach, carrots, and pumpkins. In addition to providing vitamin A, beta-carotene acts as an antioxidant in the body.

Vitamin D

Vitamin D is different from all the other nutrients in that the body can synthesize it, with the help of sunlight, from a precursor that the body makes from cholesterol. Therefore, vitamin D is not an essential nutrient: given enough time in the sun, people need no vitamin D from foods.

Figure 11–8 diagrams the pathway by which active vitamin D is made. Ultraviolet rays from the sun hit the precursor in the skin and convert it to previtamin D_3. This compound works its way back into the interior of the body and slowly, over the next 36 hours, is converted to vitamin D_3 with the help of the body's heat. The biological activity of the active vitamin is 500- to 1000-fold higher than that of its precursor.

Regardless of whether the body manufactures vitamin D_3 or obtains it from food, two hydroxylation steps must occur before the vitamin becomes fully active. First, the liver adds an OH group, and then the kidneys add another OH group to produce the active vitamin. A review of Figure 11–8 shows how diseases affecting either the liver or the kidneys can impair the transformation of inactive vitamin D to its active form and therefore produce symptoms of deficiency.

ROLES IN THE BODY

Vitamin D acts like a hormone—a compound manufactured by one organ of the body that affects another part. Vitamin D can enter a cell, cross the nuclear membrane, attach to specific receptors on the DNA or its protein wrapping, and promote cell differentiation.[23] The best-known vitamin D target organs are the intestines, the kidneys, and the bones. All respond to vitamin D by making calcium available for bone growth. For example, in animals, vitamin D promotes the elongation of intestinal villi, which enhances calcium absorption.

Vitamin D in Bone Growth Vitamin D is a member of a large and cooperative bone-making and maintenance team composed of nutrients and other compounds, including vitamins A, C, and K; the hormones parathormone and calcitonin; the protein collagen, which underlies and supports bone; and the minerals calcium, phosphorus, magnesium, and fluoride, which compose the inorganic part of bone. The special function of vitamin D is to promote normal bone mineralization. It helps to make calcium and phosphorus available in the blood that bathes the bones, to be deposited as the bones harden, or mineralize.

mineralization: the process in which calcium, phosphorus, and other minerals crystallize on the collagen matrix of a growing bone, hardening the bone.

Vitamin D raises blood concentrations of these minerals in three ways. It stimulates their absorption from the GI tract, it stimulates their retention by the kidneys, and it helps to withdraw them from bones into the blood. The star of the show is calcium itself; vitamin D is a director. The vitamin may work alone, as it does in the GI tract, or in combination with parathormone, as it does in the bones and kidneys. Details of how calcium moves from food into the blood and into and out of bone appear in Chapter 12.

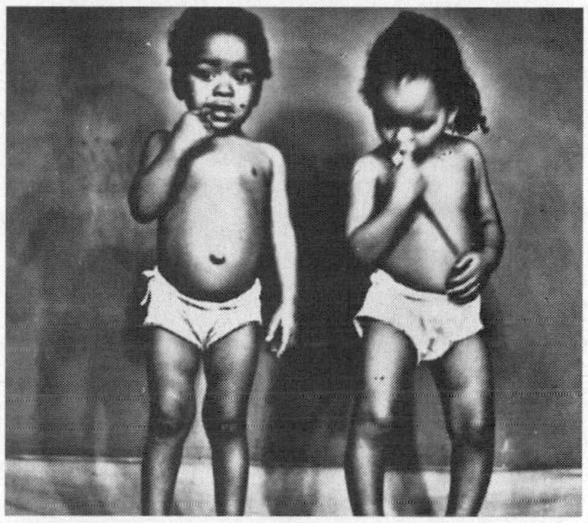

As Table 11–2 points out, rickets affects many areas of the body. The child on the left has the characteristic protruding belly resulting from lax abdominal muscles. The child on the right has the bowed legs commonly seen in rickets.

Vitamin D in Other Roles Scientists have recently discovered many other vitamin D target tissues, including the brain and nervous system, pancreas, skin, muscles and cartilage, reproductive organs, immune cells, and some cancer cells.[24] These discoveries suggest that vitamin D has numerous functions and may be valuable in treating a number of disorders, including cancer.[25]

VITAMIN D DEFICIENCY

In vitamin D deficiency, production of the calcium-binding protein in the intestinal cells slows. Thus even when calcium in the diet is adequate, it passes through the GI tract unabsorbed, leaving the bone undersupplied. The symptoms of a vitamin D deficiency are those of calcium deficiency, shown in Table 11–2 (on p. 408).

Rickets Worldwide, the vitamin D–deficiency disease rickets still affects large numbers of children. The bones fail to calcify normally, causing growth retardation and skeletal abnormalities. The bones become so weak that they bend when they have to support the body's weight. A child with rickets who is old enough to walk characteristically develops bowed legs, often the most obvious sign of the disease. Another obvious sign is the protruding belly that results from lax abdominal muscles.

rickets: the vitamin D–deficiency disease in children characterized by inadequate mineralization of bone (manifested in bowed legs or knock-knees, outward-bowed chest, and knobs on ribs). A rare type of rickets, *not* caused by vitamin D deficiency, is known as **vitamin D–refractory rickets**.

Osteomalacia Adult rickets, or osteomalacia, occurs most often in women who have low calcium intakes and little exposure to sun and who go through repeated pregnancies and periods of lactation. The bones of the legs may soften to such extent that a young woman who is tall and straight at 20 may be condemned by repeated pregnancies to become bent, bowlegged, and stooped before she is 30.

osteomalacia (os-tee-o-mal-AY-shuh)**:** a bone disease characterized by softening of the bones; symptoms include bending of the spine and bowing of the legs. The disease occurs most often in adult women.
osteo = bone
malacia = softening

Any failure to synthesize adequate vitamin D sets the stage for the mobilization of calcium from the bones and retardation of bone remodeling. This combination leads to a loss of bone mass, which can result in fractures. Highlight 12 describes the many factors that lead to osteoporosis, a condition of reduced bone density.

VITAMIN D TOXICITY

Whereas vitamin D deficiency depresses calcium absorption, blood calcium, and bone mineralization, an excess of the vitamin does the opposite, as shown in Table 11–2. It enhances calcium absorption, produces high blood calcium, and

High blood calcium is known as **hypercalcemia** and may develop from a variety of disorders, including vitamin D toxicity. It does *not* develop from a high calcium intake.

Table 11–2

Vitamin D—A Summary

Other Names	Deficiency Disease Names		Toxicity Disease Name
Calciferol, cholecalciferol, dihydroxy vitamin D; precursor is the body's own cholesterol	Rickets, osteomalacia		Hypervitaminosis D
Adult RDA	**Deficiency Symptoms**		**Toxicity Symptoms**
10 μg/day (19–24 yr) 5 μg/day (25 and over)	BONES/TEETH		BONES/TEETH
Chief Functions in the Body	**Rickets in Children** Faulty calcification, resulting in misshapen bones (bowing of legs) and retarded growth; enlargement of ends of long bones (knees, wrists); deformities of ribs (bowed, with beads or knobs);[a] delayed closing of fontanel, resulting in rapid enlargement of head (see figure); slow eruption of teeth; malformed, decay-prone teeth	**Osteomalacia in Adults** Softening effect: deformities of limbs, spine, thorax, and pelvis; demineralization; pain in pelvis, lower back, and legs; bone fractures	Increased calcium withdrawal
Promotes mineralization of bones (raises blood calcium and phosphorus by increasing absorption from digestive tract, withdrawing calcium from bones, stimulating retention by kidneys)			
Significant Sources	BLOOD		BLOOD
Self-synthesis with sunlight; fortified milk, fortified margarine, egg yolk, liver, fatty fish		Decreased calcium and/or phosphorus, increased alkaline phosphatase[b]	Increased calcium and phosphorus concentration
	NERVOUS/MUSCULAR SYSTEMS		NERVOUS/MUSCULAR SYSTEMS
	Lax muscles resulting in protrusion of abdomen; muscle spasms	Involuntary twitching, muscle spasms	Loss of appetite, headache, weakness, fatigue, excessive thirst, irritability, apathy
	EXCRETORY SYSTEM		EXCRETORY SYSTEM
	Increased calcium in stools, decreased calcium in urine		Increased excretion of calcium in urine, kidney stones, irreversible renal damage
	OTHER		OTHER
	Abnormally high secretion of parathormone		Calcification of soft tissues (blood vessels, kidneys, heart, lungs, tissues around joints), death

Fontanel
A fontanel is an open space in the top of a baby's skull before the bones have grown together. In rickets, closing of the fontanel is delayed.

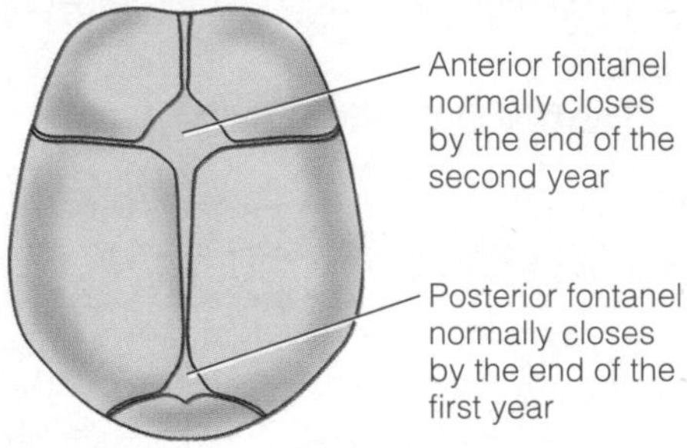

Anterior fontanel normally closes by the end of the second year
Posterior fontanel normally closes by the end of the first year

[a]Bowing of the ribs causes the symptoms known as *pigeon breast*. The beads that form on the ribs resemble rosary beads; thus this symptom is known as *rachitic* (ra-KIT-ik) *rosary* ("the rosary of rickets").

[b]Alkaline phosphatase is an enzyme in the blood that rises during bone resorption.

promotes the return of bone calcium into the blood. Excess blood calcium tends to precipitate in the soft tissue, forming stones, especially in the kidneys where calcium is concentrated in the effort to excrete it. Calcification may also harden the blood vessels and is especially dangerous in the major arteries of the heart and lungs, where it can cause death.

The range of safe intakes of vitamin D is narrower than that of vitamin A. Half the recommended intake is too little, but more than a few times the recommended intake may be too much. In fact, vitamin D is the most likely of the vitamins to have toxic effects when consumed in even small amounts above the RDA on a continuous basis. The amounts of vitamin D in foods available in the United States and Canada are well within safe limits, but pills containing the vitamin in concentrated form should be kept out of the reach of children and used cautiously by adults. During the warm months of the year, when sunlight exposure may be frequent, vitamin D supplements can harm healthy children and adults who drink at least 2 glasses of vitamin D–fortified milk per day.[26] Vitamin D toxicity has also been reported in people who drank milk that was fortified with too much vitamin D by mistake.[27]

VITAMIN D RECOMMENDATIONS AND SOURCES

The recommendation for vitamin D for rapidly growing children is twice as high as that for mature adults. Neither cow's milk nor human breast milk supplies enough vitamin D to meet human needs reliably; hence cow's milk is fortified, and infants are given either fortified formula or supplements.

Vitamin D activity was previously expressed in international units (IU), but is now expressed in micrograms of cholecalciferol. To convert, use the following factor: 1 IU = 0.025 μg cholecalciferol. For example:

- 100 IU = 2.5 μg.
- 400 IU = 10 μg.

Vitamin D in Foods Only a few foods supply significant amounts of vitamin D, notably those derived from animals: egg yolks, liver, fatty fish, butter, and fortified milk. The fortification of milk with vitamin D is the best guarantee that people will meet their needs and underscores the importance of milk in a well-balanced diet.* For those who use margarine in place of butter, fortified margarine is a significant source. A plant version of vitamin D may yield an active compound on irradiation, but its contribution is minor. Without adequate sunshine, fortification, or supplementation, a strict vegetarian diet cannot meet vitamin D needs.[28]

Most adults, especially in sunny regions, need not make special efforts to obtain vitamin D from food. People who are not outdoors much or who live in northern or predominantly cloudy or smoggy areas are advised to drink at least 2 cups of vitamin D–fortified milk a day.

Vitamin D from the Sun Most of the world's population relies on natural exposure to sunlight to maintain adequate vitamin D nutrition. The sun imposes no risk of vitamin D toxicity; prolonged exposure to sunlight degrades the vitamin D precursor in the skin, preventing its conversion to the active vitamin. Even lifeguards on southern beaches are safe from vitamin D toxicity from the sun.

Prolonged exposure to sunlight does, however, prematurely wrinkle the skin and present the risk of skin cancer. Sunscreens help reduce these risks, but unfor-

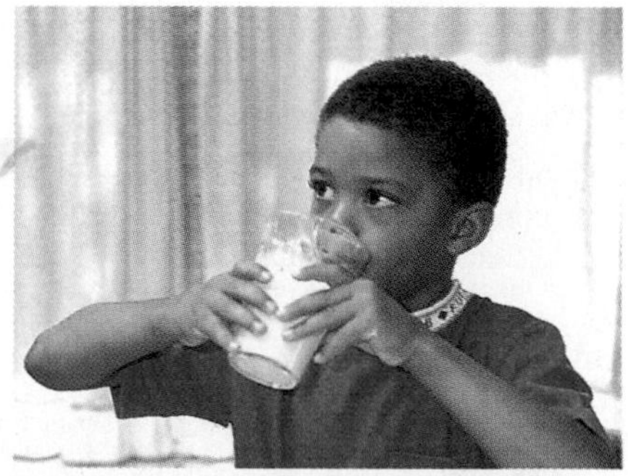

A cool glass of milk refreshes as it replenishes the bone-building nutrients.

*Vitamin D fortification of milk in the United States is 10 micrograms cholecalciferol (400 IU) per quart; in Canada, 360 IU per liter.

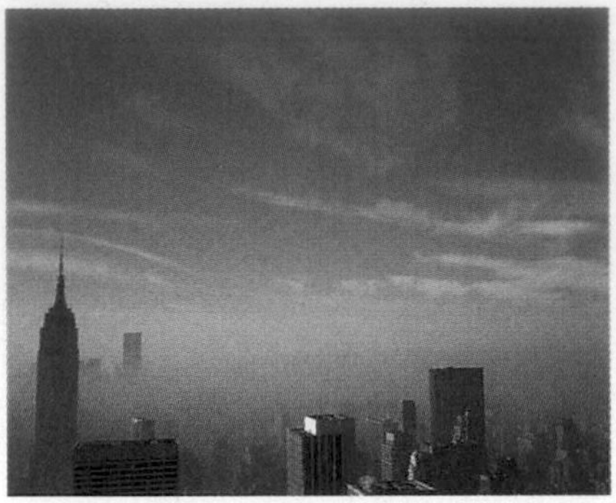

Smog filters out ultraviolet rays of the sun.

tunately, sunscreens with sun protection factors (SPF) of 8 and above also prevent vitamin D synthesis. A strategy to avoid this dilemma is to apply sunscreen after enough time has elapsed to provide sufficient vitamin D synthesis. For most people, exposing hands, face, and arms on a clear summer day for 10 to 15 minutes a few times a week should be sufficient to maintain vitamin D nutrition.

Dark-skinned people require longer sunlight exposure than light-skinned people, but by three hours, vitamin D synthesis in heavily pigmented skin arrives at the same plateau as in fair skin in 30 minutes. The ultraviolet rays of the sun that promote vitamin D synthesis are blocked by heavy clouds, smoke, or smog. Differences in skin pigmentation and smog may account for the finding that dark-skinned people in northern, smoggy cities are more prone to rickets. For these people, and for those who are unable to go outdoors frequently, dietary vitamin D is most important. Deficiency is especially likely in older adults because they typically drink little or no milk, their exposure to sunlight is limited, and the skin and kidneys lose their ability to make and activate vitamin D with advancing age.

The ultraviolet rays from tanning lamps and tanning booths may also stimulate vitamin D synthesis, but the hazards outweigh any possible benefits. The FDA warns that if the lamps are not properly filtered, people using tanning booths risk burns, damage to the eyes and blood vessels, and skin cancer.[29]

To summarize, vitamin D can be synthesized in the body with the help of sunlight or obtained from animal foods. It sends signals to three primary target sites: the GI tract to absorb more calcium, the bones to release more, and the kidneys to retain more. These actions support bone formation and maintenance. A deficiency causes rickets in childhood and osteomalacia in later life. Fortified milk is an important food source.

Vitamin E

In 1922, researchers discovered a component of vegetable oils necessary for reproduction in rats. This antisterility factor was named tocopherol, which means "to bring forth offspring."[30] A few years later, the compound was named vitamin E. When chemists isolated four different tocopherol compounds, they designated them by the first four letters of the Greek alphabet: alpha, beta, gamma, and delta. The tocopherols consist of a complex ring structure and a long saturated side chain (see Appendix C).* The numbers and positions of methyl groups on the ring distinguish one tocopherol from another. The most abundant and biologically active tocopherol in nature is alpha-tocopherol.

tocopherol (tuh-KOFF-er-all)**:** a general term for several chemically related compounds, most of which have vitamin E activity (see Appendix C for chemical structures).

alpha-tocopherol: the most biologically active vitamin E compound.

Reminder: An *antioxidant* is a compound that protects other compounds from oxidation by being oxidized itself.

VITAMIN E AS AN ANTIOXIDANT

Vitamin E is a fat-soluble antioxidant and one of the body's primary defenders against oxidation, protecting the lipids and other vulnerable components of the cells and their membranes from destruction. Within the mitochondria of cells,

*Another group of chemically related compounds, the tocotrienols (TOE-koe-try-EEN-ols), have unsaturated side chains. The tocotrienols are less abundant, less active, and less important in nutrition than the tocopherols are.

Table 11–3

Vitamin E—A Summary

Other Names	Deficiency Symptoms	Toxicity Symptoms
Alpha-tocopherol, tocopherol, tocotrienol	BLOOD/CIRCULATORY SYSTEM	
Adult RDA	Red blood cell breakage,[a] anemia	Augments effects of anticlotting medication
Men: 10 mg α-TE/day Women: 8 mg α-TE/day	DIGESTIVE SYSTEM	
Chief Functions in the Body		General discomfort
Antioxidant, stabilization of cell membranes, regulation of oxidation reactions, protection of PUFA and vitamin A	NERVOUS/MUSCULAR SYSTEMS	
Significant Sources	Degeneration, weakness, difficulty walking, severe pain in calf muscles	
Polyunsaturated plant oils (margarine, salad dressings, shortenings), green and leafy vegetables, wheat germ, whole-grain products, liver, egg yolks, nuts, seeds		

[a]The breaking of red blood cells is called *erythrocyte hemolysis*.

vitamin E protects a part of the metabolic equipment that transforms energy fuels into ATP. Vitamin E is especially effective in preventing the oxidation of the polyunsaturated fatty acids (PUFA), but it protects all other lipids and related compounds (for example, vitamin A) as well. Table 11–3 presents a summary of vitamin E's functions, deficiency symptoms, toxicity symptoms, and food sources.

Vitamin E exerts an especially important antioxidant effect in the lungs, where the exposure of cells to oxygen is maximal. Several kinds of cells benefit from the vitamin's protection: the red and white blood cells that pass through the lungs and the cells of the lung tissue itself. Vitamin E also protects the lungs from air pollutants such as nitrogen dioxide or ozone that can initiate damaging reactions.

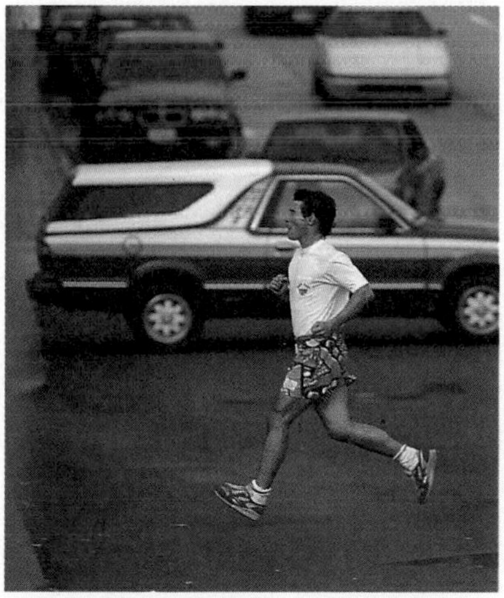

Vitamin E helps to protect the lungs against air pollutants, especially when a person is breathing hard during exercise.

Vitamin E protects white as well as red blood cells and thus participates in the body's immune defenses. Recent studies have found that vitamin E supplementation significantly above the RDA improves the immune response of healthy, older adults.[31] The researchers speculate that vitamin E's support of immunity may be due to its protection of cell lipids. Highlight 11 provides more on vitamin E's role in protecting against chronic disease.

While research continues to reveal possible roles for vitamin E, it also has clearly discredited claims that vitamin E improves physical performance, enhances sexual performance, or cures sexual dysfunction in males. Vitamin E does not slow or prevent the processes of aging such as hair turning gray or skin wrinkling. Nor does it slow the progression of Parkinson's disease.[32]

VITAMIN E DEFICIENCY

In human beings, dietary vitamin E deficiency is rare; deficiency is usually associated with diseases of fat malabsorption such as cystic fibrosis. When the blood concentration of vitamin E falls below a certain critical level, the red blood cells tend to break open and spill their contents, probably due to oxidation of the PUFA in their membranes. This classic sign of vitamin E deficiency, known as erythrocyte hemolysis, is seen in premature infants, born before the transfer of vitamin E from the mother to the infant that takes place in the last weeks of pregnancy. Vitamin E treatment corrects erythrocyte hemolysis.

Prolonged vitamin E deficiency also causes neuromuscular dysfunction involving the spinal cord and retina. Common symptoms include loss of muscle coordination and reflexes and impaired vision and speech. Vitamin E treatment corrects these neurological symptoms of vitamin E deficiency.

The neuromuscular weakness and atrophy that accompany a vitamin E deficiency can be cured by reintroducing the vitamin into the diet, but vitamin E does *not* prevent or cure the herditary muscular dystrophy that afflicts children. Children with hereditary muscular dystrophy do not benefit from vitamin E treatment and usually die at an early age when their respiratory muscles deteriorate.

Two other conditions seem to respond to vitamin E therapy, although results are inconsistent. One is a nonmalignant breast disease (fibrocystic breast disease), and the other is an abnormality of blood flow that causes cramping in the legs (intermittent claudication).

erythrocyte hemolysis: the breaking open of red blood cells; a symptom of vitamin E–deficiency disease in human beings.

erythrocyte (eh-REETH-ro-cite)**:** red blood cell.
erythro = red
cyte = cell

hemolysis (he-MOLL-uh-sis)**:** bursting of red blood cells.
hemo = blood
lysis = breaking

muscular dystrophy (DIS-tro-fee)**:** a hereditary disease in which the muscles gradually weaken; its most debilitating effects arise in the lungs.

fibrocystic breast disease: a harmless condition in which the breasts develop lumps, sometimes associated with caffeine consumption. In some, it responds to treatment by abstinence from caffeine; in others, it can be treated with vitamin E.
fibro = fibrous tissue
cyst = closed sac

intermittent claudication: severe calf pain caused by inadequate blood supply; it occurs when walking and subsides during rest.
intermittent = at intervals
claudicare = to limp

VITAMIN E TOXICITY

Even though many claims have been discredited, many people continue to take vitamin E supplements for all kinds of reasons. In fact, vitamin E supplement use has risen recently as its antioxidant action against disease has been recognized. Still, toxicity is not as common, and its effects are not as detrimental, as with vitamins A and D. Extremely high doses of vitamin E may interfere with the blood-clotting action of vitamin K and enhance effects of drugs used to oppose blood clotting, causing hemorrhage.

VITAMIN E RECOMMENDATIONS

Tocopherols occur in two forms, D and L, of which the D form is more active. The most active vitamin E compound is D-alpha-tocopherol. Different tocopherols vary in their vitamin E activity; to reconcile them, recommended intakes are expressed in tocopherol equivalents (TE). One TE equals the amount of vitamin E activity in 1 milligram of D-alpha-tocopherol.*

A person who consumes a large amount of PUFA needs more vitamin E. Fortunately, vitamin E and PUFA tend to occur together in the same foods.

D, L: *D* stands for *dextro*, or "right-handed," and *L*, for *levo*, or "left-handed," referring to the shapes of the molecules, which are mirror images of each other.

tocopherol equivalents (TE): the units in which vitamin E activity is measured. One TE equals the amount of vitamin E activity in 1 milligram of D-alpha-tocopherol.

*The activities of beta- and gamma-tocopherol and alpha-tocotrienol are one-half, one-tenth, and one-third the activity of D-alpha-tocopherol, respectively.

Figure 11–9 Vitamin E in Selected Foods

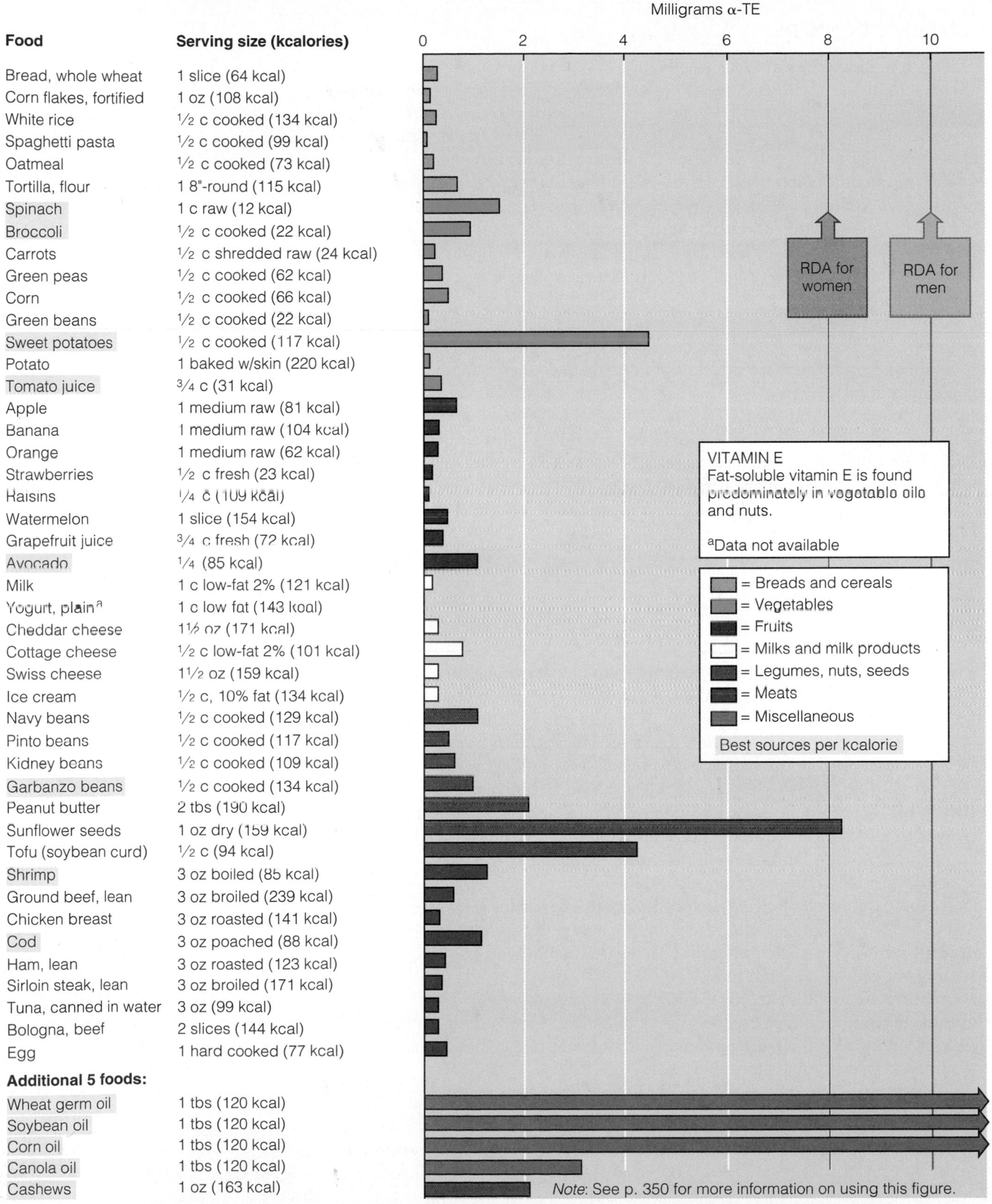
Milligrams α-TE
0
2
4
6
8
10
Food
Serving size (kcalories)
Bread, whole wheat 1 slice (64 kcal)
Corn flakes, fortified 1 oz (108 kcal)
White rice ½ c cooked (134 kcal)
Spaghetti pasta ½ c cooked (99 kcal)
Oatmeal ½ c cooked (73 kcal)
Tortilla, flour 1 8"-round (115 kcal)
Spinach 1 c raw (12 kcal)
Broccoli ½ c cooked (22 kcal)
Carrots ½ c shredded raw (24 kcal)
Green peas ½ c cooked (62 kcal)
Corn ½ c cooked (66 kcal)
Green beans ½ c cooked (22 kcal)
Sweet potatoes ½ c cooked (117 kcal)
Potato 1 baked w/skin (220 kcal)
Tomato juice ¾ c (31 kcal)
Apple 1 medium raw (81 kcal)
Banana 1 medium raw (104 kcal)
Orange 1 medium raw (62 kcal)
Strawberries ½ c fresh (23 kcal)
Raisins ¼ c (109 kcal)
Watermelon 1 slice (154 kcal)
Grapefruit juice ¾ c fresh (72 kcal)
Avocado ¼ (85 kcal)
Milk 1 c low-fat 2% (121 kcal)
Yogurt, plain[a] 1 c low fat (143 kcal)
Cheddar cheese 1½ oz (171 kcal)
Cottage cheese ½ c low-fat 2% (101 kcal)
Swiss cheese 1½ oz (159 kcal)
Ice cream ½ c, 10% fat (134 kcal)
Navy beans ½ c cooked (129 kcal)
Pinto beans ½ c cooked (117 kcal)
Kidney beans ½ c cooked (109 kcal)
Garbanzo beans ½ c cooked (134 kcal)
Peanut butter 2 tbs (190 kcal)
Sunflower seeds 1 oz dry (159 kcal)
Tofu (soybean curd) ½ c (94 kcal)
Shrimp 3 oz boiled (85 kcal)
Ground beef, lean 3 oz broiled (239 kcal)
Chicken breast 3 oz roasted (141 kcal)
Cod 3 oz poached (88 kcal)
Ham, lean 3 oz roasted (123 kcal)
Sirloin steak, lean 3 oz broiled (171 kcal)
Tuna, canned in water 3 oz (99 kcal)
Bologna, beef 2 slices (144 kcal)
Egg 1 hard cooked (77 kcal)
Additional 5 foods:
Wheat germ oil 1 tbs (120 kcal)
Soybean oil 1 tbs (120 kcal)
Corn oil 1 tbs (120 kcal)
Canola oil 1 tbs (120 kcal)
Cashews 1 oz (163 kcal)
RDA for women
RDA for men
VITAMIN E
Fat-soluble vitamin E is found predominately in vegetable oils and nuts.
[a]Data not available
= Breads and cereals
= Vegetables
= Fruits
= Milks and milk products
= Legumes, nuts, seeds
= Meats
= Miscellaneous
Best sources per kcalorie
Note: See p. 350 for more information on using this figure.

VITAMIN E IN FOODS

Vitamin E is widespread in foods (see Figure 11–9 on p. 414). About 20 percent of the vitamin E in the diet comes from vegetable oils and products made from them, such as margarine, salad dressings, and shortenings. Another 20 percent comes from fruits and vegetables. Fortified cereals and other grain products contribute about 15 percent of the vitamin E in the diet, and smaller percentages come from meats, poultry, fish, eggs, nuts, and seeds.[33] Wheat germ oil is especially rich in vitamin E; corn and soybean oils rank second, with a tablespoon of either of these supplying more than 10 milligrams (more than the RDA) of the vitamin. Other oils contain less (for example, peanut oil supplies about a third as much per tablespoon). Animal fats such as meat and milk fat contain little or no vitamin E.

Vitamin E is readily destroyed by heat processing (such as deep-fat frying) and oxidation, so fresh or lightly processed foods are preferable sources. Most processed and convenience foods do not contribute enough vitamin E to ensure an adequate intake.

To review, vitamin E acts as an antioxidant, defending lipids and other components of the cells against oxidative damage. Deficiencies are rare, but do occur in premature infants, the primary symptom being erythrocyte hemolysis. Vitamin E is found predominantly in vegetable oils and appears to be one of the least toxic of the fat-soluble vitamins.

Vitamin K

Blood has a remarkable ability to remain a liquid even though it carries many large molecules and cells through the circulatory system. But blood can also turn solid within seconds when the integrity of that system is disturbed. (If blood did not clot, a single pinprick could drain the entire body of all its blood, just as a tiny hole in a bucket makes the bucket forever useless for holding water.) Vitamin K acts primarily in blood clotting, where its presence can make the difference between life and death. At least 13 different proteins and the mineral calcium are involved in making a blood clot. Vitamin K is essential for the synthesis of at least four of these proteins, among them prothrombin, made by the liver as a precursor of the protein thrombin (see Figure 11–10 on p. 415). When any of the blood-clotting factors is lacking, hemorrhagic disease results. If an artery or vein is cut or broken, bleeding goes unchecked. (Of course, this is not to say that hemorrhaging is always caused by vitamin K deficiency. Another cause is hemophilia, which is not curable by vitamin K.)

K stands for the Danish word *koagulation* ("coagulation" or "clotting").

hemorrhagic (hem-o-RAJ-ik) **disease:** a disease characterized by excessive bleeding.

hemophilia: a hereditary disease that has no relation to vitamin K, but is caused by a genetic defect; the blood is unable to clot because it lacks the ability to synthesize certain clotting factors.

Vitamin K also participates in the synthesis of a bone protein. The rate of synthesis of this protein is regulated by the more famous bone vitamin—vitamin D. Without vitamin K, the bones produce an abnormal protein that cannot bind to the minerals that normally form bones.

Like vitamin D, vitamin K can be obtained from a nonfood source. Bacteria in the GI tract synthesize vitamin K that the body can absorb, but bacterial synthesis alone is insufficient to meet all of a person's needs.

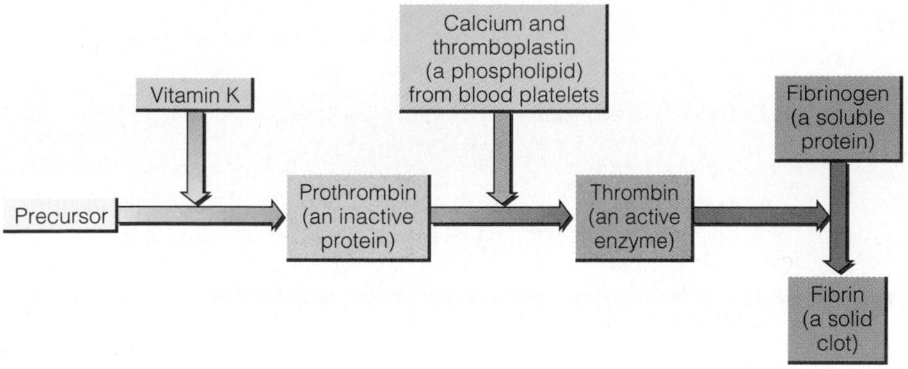

Figure 11–10

Blood-Clotting Process
When blood is exposed to air, foreign substances, or secretions from injured tissues, platelets (small, cell-like structures in the blood) release a phospholipid known as thromboplastin. Thromboplastin catalyzes the conversion of the inactive protein prothrombin to the active enzyme thrombin. Thrombin then catalyzes the conversion of the precursor protein fibrinogen to the active protein fibrin that forms the clot.

VITAMIN K DEFICIENCY

A deficiency of vitamin K may occur whenever absorption of fat is impaired—for example, when bile production is faulty or in diarrhea. The vitamin is sometimes administered before operations to reduce bleeding in surgery, but is only of value at this time if a vitamin K deficiency exists. Table 11–4 (on p. 416) summarizes vitamin K information.

Vitamin K deficiency is seldom seen except when an unusual combination of circumstances conspires to bring it about. When it does occur, however, it can be fatal. The scenario goes like this. A hospital client with marginal vitamin K stores is given antibiotics to prevent or overcome infection and is fed a formula diet that does not include vitamin K. The antibiotics kill the intestinal bacteria, and the vitamin K stores become depleted. During surgery, the blood fails to clot normally, and the client bleeds to death. The combination of antibiotics, inadequate intake, and surgery raises a warning flag that clotting time should be checked before surgery is performed. People taking sulfa drugs, which destroy intestinal bacteria, may also become deficient in vitamin K.

Newborn babies present a unique case of vitamin K nutrition. A baby is born with a sterile digestive tract, and the vitamin K–producing bacteria take weeks to establish themselves in the baby's intestines. At the same time, plasma prothrombin concentrations are low (this makes fatal blood clotting unlikely during the stress of birth). To prevent hemorrhagic disease in the newborn, a single dose of vitamin K (usually as the naturally occurring form, phylloquinone) is given at birth either orally or by intramuscular injection. Concerns that vitamin K given at birth raises the risks of childhood cancer are uproven and unlikely.[34]

sterile: free of microorganisms, such as bacteria.

A synthetic form of vitamin K is **menadione** (men-uh-DYE-own); see Appendix C.

VITAMIN K TOXICITY

Toxicity is not common but can result when vitamin K supplements are prescribed, especially to infants or to pregnant women. High doses of vitamin K can reduce the effectiveness of anticoagulant drugs used to prevent blood clotting. People taking these drugs should eat vitamin K–rich foods in moderation and keep their intakes consistent from day to day. Toxicity symptoms include red blood cell hemolysis, jaundice, and brain damage.

jaundice: yellowing of the skin, due to spillover of the bile pigments **bilirubin** (bill-ee-ROO-bin) from the liver into the general circulation; also known as **hyperbilirubinemia** (HIGH-per-BILL-eh-roo-bin-EE-me-ah). When these pigments invade the brain, the condition is **kernicterus** (ker-NICK-ter-us). Jaundice may be caused by obstruction of bile passageways, hemolysis, or dysfunctional liver cells.

Table 11–4

Vitamin K—A Summary

Other Names	Deficiency Symptoms	Toxicity Symptoms
Menadione, menaquinone, phylloquinone, naphthoquinone	BLOOD/CIRCULATORY SYSTEM	
	Hemorrhaging	Interference with anticlotting medication; vitamin K analogues may cause jaundice, red blood cell hemolysis, and brain damage
Adult RDA	**Chief Functions in the Body**	
1 μg/kg body weight/day Men: 70 μg/day (19–24 yr) 80 μg/day (25 and over) Women: 60 μg/day (19–24 yr) 65 μg/day (25 and over)	Participates in the synthesis of blood-clotting proteins and a bone protein that regulates blood calcium	
	Significant Sources	
	Bacterial synthesis in the digestive tract; liver; leafy green vegetables, cabbage-type vegetables; milk	

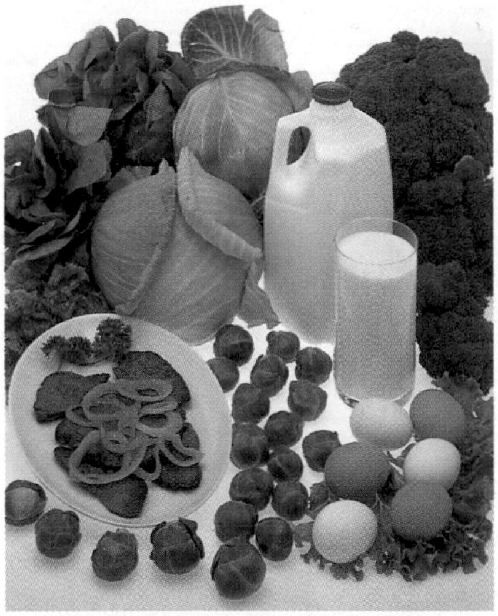

Notable food sources of vitamin K include milk, eggs, brussels sprouts, liver, cabbage, spinach, and broccoli.

VITAMIN K RECOMMENDATIONS AND SOURCES

As mentioned earlier, vitamin K is made in the GI tract by the billions of bacteria that normally reside there. Once synthesized, vitamin K is absorbed and stored in the liver. The total need for vitamin K cannot be met by bacterial synthesis alone. People eating vitamin K–rich foods such as liver, leafy green vegetables, and members of the cabbage family can easily meet their needs. Milk, meats, eggs, cereals, fruits, and vegetables provide smaller, but still significant, amounts.

To sum up, vitamin K helps with blood clotting, and its deficiency causes uncontrolled bleeding. Bacteria in the GI tract can make the vitamin; people typically receive about half of their requirements from bacterial synthesis and half from foods such as liver, leafy green vegetables, and members of the cabbage family. Because people depend on bacterial synthesis for vitamin K, deficiency is most likely in newborn infants and in people taking antibiotics.

The Fat-Soluble Vitamins—In Summary

The four fat-soluble vitamins play many specific roles in the growth and maintenance of the body. Their presence affects the health and function of the eyes, skin, GI tract, lungs, bones, teeth, nervous system, and blood; their deficiencies become apparent in these same areas. Toxicities of the fat-soluble vitamins are possible, especially when people use supplements because the body stores excesses.

As with the water-soluble vitamins, the function of one fat-soluble vitamin often depends on the presence of another. Recall that vitamin E protects vitamin

A from oxidation. In vitamin E deficiency, vitamin A absorption and storage are impaired. Three of the four fat-soluble vitamins—A, D, and K—play important roles in bone growth and remodeling. As mentioned, vitamin K helps synthesize a specific bone protein, and vitamin D regulates that synthesis. Vitamin A, in turn, may control which bone-building genes respond to vitamin D.[35]

Fat-soluble vitamins also interact with minerals: vitamin D and calcium cooperate in bone formation; and zinc is required for the synthesis of vitamin A's transport protein, retinol-binding protein. Zinc also assists the enzyme that regenerates retinal from retinol in the eye.

The roles the fat-soluble vitamins play differ from those of the water-soluble vitamins, and they appear in different foods, yet they are just as essential to life. The need for them underlines the importance of eating a wide variety of nourishing foods daily.

Study Questions

1. List the fat-soluble vitamins. What characteristics do they have in common? How do they differ from the water-soluble vitamins?
2. Summarize the roles of vitamin A and the symptoms of its deficiency.
3. What is meant by vitamin precursors? Name the precursors of vitamin A, and tell in what classes of foods they are located. Give examples of foods with high vitamin A activity.
4. How is vitamin D unique among the vitamins? What is its chief function? What are the richest sources of this vitamin?
5. Describe vitamin E's role as an antioxidant. What are the chief symptoms of vitamin E deficiency?
6. What is vitamin K's primary role in the body? What conditions may lead to vitamin K deficiency?

Problem Set appears on pp. 419–420

Notes

1. A. C. Ross and M. E. Ternus, Vitamin A as a hormone: Recent advances in understanding the actions of retinol, retinoic acid, and beta carotene, *Journal of the American Dietetic Association* 93 (1993): 1285–1290.
2. J. E. Dowling and G. Wald, The biological function of vitamin A acid, *Proceedings of the National Academy of Sciences, USA* 46 (1960): 587–608, as cited in A. C. Ross, Vitamin A: Current understanding of the mechanisms of action, *Nutrition Today*, January/February 1991, pp. 6–12.
3. L. M. DeLuca, Vitamin A in epithelial differentiation and skin carcinogenesis, *Nutrition Reviews* (supplement) 52 (1994): S45–S52.
4. J. H. Humphrey and K. P. West, Jr., Vitamin A deficiency: Role in childhood infection and mortality, in *Micronutrients in Health and Disease*, eds. A. Bendich and C. E. Butterworth, Jr. (New York: Marcel Dekker, 1991), pp. 307–329.
5. J. N. Hathcock and coauthors, Evaluation of vitamin A toxicity, *American Journal of Clinical Nutrition* 52 (1990): 183–202.
6. J. A Olson, 1992 Atwater Lecture: The irresistible fascination of carotenoids and vitamin A, *American Journal of Clinical Nutrition* 57 (1993): 833–839.
7. Hathcock and coauthors, 1990.
8. J. H. Humphrey, K. P. West, Jr., and A. Sommer, Vitamin A deficiency and attributable mortality among under-5-year-olds, *Bulletin of the World Health Organization* 70 (1992): 225–232.
9. Muhilal and coauthors, Vitamin A–fortified monosodium glutamate and health, growth, and survival of children: A controlled field trial, *American Journal of Clinical Nutrition* 48 (1988): 1271–1276; L. Rahmathullah and coauthors, Reduced mortality among children in southern India receiving a small weekly dose of vitamin A, *New England Journal of Medicine* 323 (1990): 929–935; K. P. West, Jr., and coauthors, Efficacy of vitamin A in reducing preschool child mortality in Nepal, *Lancet* 338 (1991): 67–71; N. M. P. Daulaire and coauthors, Childhood mortality after a high dose of vitamin A in high risk populations, *British Medical Journal* 304 (1992): 207–210; W. W. Fawzi and coauthors, Dietary vitamin A intake and risk

of mortality among children, *American Journal of Clinical Nutrition* 59 (1994): 401–408.
10. J. P. Grant, *The State of the World's Children* (Oxford: Oxford University Press, 1988), p. 3, as cited in G. D. Hussey and M. Klein, A randomized, controlled trial of vitamin A in children with severe measles, *New England Journal of Medicine* 323 (1990): 160–164.
11. J. C. Butler and coauthors, Measles severity and serum retinol (vitamin A) concentration among children in the United States, *Pediatrics* 91 (1993): 1176–1181.
12. A. Coutsoudis, M. Broughton, and H. M. Coovadia, Vitamin A supplementation reduces measles morbidity in young African children: A randomized, placebo-controlled, double-blind trial, *American Journal of Clinical Nutrition* 54 (1990): 890–895; Vitamin A administration reduces mortality and morbidity from severe measles in populations nonendemic for hypovitaminosis A, *Nutrition Reviews* 49 (1991): 89–91; W. W. Fawzi and coauthors, Vitamin A supplementation and child mortality: A meta-analysis, *Journal of the American Medical Association* 269 (1993): 898–903; L. J. Machlin and H. E. Sauberlich, New views on the function and health effects of vitamins, *Nutrition Today*, January/February 1994, pp. 25–29.
13. A. J. G. Barclay, A. Foster, and A. Sommer, Vitamin A supplements and mortality related to measles: A randomized clinical trial, *British Medical Journal* 294 (1987): 294–296; Hussey and Klein, 1990.
14. J. B. Ellison, Intensive vitamin therapy in measles, *British Medical Journal* 2 (1932): 708–711.
15. The joint WHO/UNICEF statement on vitamin A for measles, *Lancet* 1 (1987): 1067–1068.
16. American Academy of Pediatrics, Committee on Infectious Diseases, Vitamin A treatment of measles, *Pediatrics* 91 (1993): 1014–1015.
17. W. W. Fawzi and coauthors, Vitamin A supplementation and dietary vitamin A in relation to the risk of xerophthalmia, *American Journal of Clinical Nutrition* 58 (1993): 385–391.
18. Hathcock and coauthors, 1990.
19. Hathcock and coauthors, 1990.
20. S. M. Bulengo-Ransby and coauthors, Topical tretinoin (retinoic acid) therapy for hyperpigmented lesions caused by inflammation of the skin in black patients, *New England Journal of Medicine* 328 (1993):1438–1443.
21. H. S. Garewal, Potential role of β-carotene in prevention of oral cancer, *American Journal of Clinical Nutrition* 53 (1991): 294S–297S.
22. T. O. Carpenter and coauthors, Severe hypervitaminosis A in siblings: Evidence of variable tolerance to retinol intake, *Journal of Pediatrics* 111 (1987): 507–512.
23. T. Suda, T. Shinki, and N. Takahashi, The role of vitamin D in bone and intestinal cell differentiation, *Annual Review of Nutrition* 10 (1990): 195–211.
24. S. S. Hannah and A. W. Norman, $1\alpha,25(OH)_2$ Vitamin D_3-regulated expression of the eukaryotic genome, *Nutrition Reviews* 52 (1994): 376–382; H. F. DeLuca, Vitamin D: 1993, *Nutrition Today*, November/December 1993, pp. 6–11; Machlin and Sauberlich, 1994.
25. H. F. DeLuca, New concepts of vitamin D functions, *Annals of the New York Academy of Sciences* 669 (1992): 59–68.
26. American Academy of Pediatrics, The prophylactic requirement and the toxicity of vitamin D, *Pediatrics* 31 (1963): 512–525, as cited in Committee on Dietary Allowances, *Recommended Dietary Allowances*, 10th ed. (Washington, D.C.: National Academy Press, 1989), pp. 92–97.
27. C. H. Jacobus and coauthors, Hypervitaminosis D associated with drinking milk, *New England Journal of Medicine* 326 (1992): 1173–1177.
28. C. Lamberg-Allardt and coauthors, Low serum 25-hydroxyvitamin D concentrations and secondary hyperparathyroidism in middle-aged white strict vegetarians, *American Journal of Clinical Nutrition* 58 (1993): 684–689.
29. A. Greely, Dodging the rays, *FDA Consumer*, July/August 1993, pp. 30–33.
30. M. C. Linder, Nutrition and metabolism of vitamins, in *Nutritional Biochemistry and Metabolism with Clinical Applications*, 2nd ed., ed. M. C. Linder (New York: Elsevier, 1991), pp. 111–189.
31. S. N. Meydani, M. Hayek, and L. Coleman, Influence of vitamin E and B_6 on immune response, *Annals of the New York Academy of Science* 669 (1992): 125–139; S. N. Meydani and coauthors, Vitamin E supplementation enhances cell-mediated immunity in healthy elderly subjects, *American Journal of Clinical Nutrition* 52 (1990): 557–563.
32. W. Koller (and other members of the Parkinson Study Group), Effects of tocopherol and deprenyl on the progression of disability in early Parkinson's disease, *New England Journal of Medicine* 328 (1993): 176–183.
33. S. P. Murphy, A. F. Subar, and G. Block, Vitamin E intakes and sources in the United States, *American Journal of Clinical Nutrition* 52 (1990): 361–367.
34. American Academy of Pediatrics, Vitamin K Ad Hoc Task Force, Controversies concerning vitamin K and the newborn, *Pediatrics* 91 (1993): 1001–1003; M. A. Klebanoff and coauthors, The risk of childhood cancer after neonatal exposure to vitamin K, *New England Journal of Medicine* 329 (1993): 905–908.
35. R. T. Franceschi, Nuclear signaling pathways for 1,25-dihydroxyvitamin D_3 are controlled by the vitamin A metabolite, 9-*cis*-retinoic acid, *Nutrition Reviews* 51 (1993): 303–305.

Problem Set

1. Review the units in which vitamins are measured (a spot check). For each of these vitamins, note the unit of measure:

Vitamin A: ______________________ Vitamin D: ______________________

Vitamin E: ______________________ Vitamin K: ______________________

2. Analyze the fat-soluble vitamin contents of a day's meals. Vitamin A is the only fat-soluble vitamin for which data are available, but it is an interesting vitamin and well worth study.

   a. Record the vitamin A contributions of the meals presented in Chapter 10 problem 2:

Item No./Food	Energy (kcal)	Vitamin A (RE)
• Grains (6)		
# 357 Wheat bread, 6 slices	______	______
Total in grains:	______	______
• Vegetables (3)		
# 929 Spinach cooked from fresh, ½ c	______	______
# 891 Green peas, cooked from frozen, ½ c	______	______
# 834 Carrots, cooked from fresh, ½ c	______	______
Total in vegetables:	______	______
• Fruits (2)		
# 269 Orange juice, fresh, 1 c	______	______
# 264 Cantaloupe melon, ½	______	______
Total in fruits:	______	______
• Meats (2 to 3)		
# 1045 Bass fish, baked, 4 oz	______	______
# 598 Hamburger, lean, 4 oz	______	______
Total in meats:	______	______
• Milks (2)		
# 98 Milk, nonfat, 2 c	______	______
Total in milks:	______	______

   b. Which group(s) of foods offered the most vitamin A? ______________________

   c. Which groups of foods offered no or very little vitamin A? ______________________

   d. Which foods offered preformed vitamin A? ______________________

   e. Which foods offered the vitamin A precursor beta-carotene? ______________________

   f. Speculate on the reason why fast-food meals are so often short in vitamin A: ______________________

(continued on the next page)

Problem Set (continued)

3. Learn how to ensure that you get enough vitamin A every day. Following is a list of foods ranked in order of their vitamin A contents per serving.

   a. How many servings (and kcalories) of any one of these foods would you have to eat to get 100% of the Daily Value of 875 μg RE? Calculate your answer in the last two columns of the table (round off your answers); the first one is done for you.

Item No./Food		Energy (kcal)	Vitamin A (RE)	Servings	kCalories
# 939	Sweet potato, baked in skin, 1 ea	117	2486	875 ÷ 2486 = 0.4 potato	½ potato = 58.5 kcal
# 834	Carrots, from fresh, ½ c	______	______	______	______
# 264	Cantaloupe melon, ½	______	______	______	______
# 820	Broccoli, cooked from fresh, 1 c	______	______	______	______
# 98	Milk, nonfat, 1 c	______	______	______	______
# 37	Cheddar cheese, 1 oz	______	______	______	______
# 891	Green peas, cooked from frozen, ½ c	______	______	______	______
# 206	Apple, fresh, 3¾″	______	______	______	______
# 623	Pork chop, lean broiled, 1 ea	______	______	______	______
# 606	Sirloin steak, lean, 4 oz	______	______	______	______
# 357	Whole-wheat bread, 1 slice	______	______	______	______

   b. Suppose you wanted to eat one serving of one of these foods and get all of the vitamin A you needed in a day in less than 100 kcal. Which foods could provide this much vitamin A in a serving? ____________

   c. Of course you don't have to rely on just one food to get all of your vitamin A. You can get ¼ of your RDA from each of 4 foods, ⅛ of your RDA from each of 8 foods, etc. Suppose that limiting kcalories is a high priority for you. Which are the four best sources of vitamin A per kcalorie? ________ Is this rank order different from the four best sources per serving? ____

This exercise just hints at a finding that the next chapter's exercises will make clearer—that vegetables are often the most nutrient-dense foods for many nutrients.

Antioxidant Nutrients and Nonnutrients in Disease Prevention

Count on supplement manufacturers to proclaim the day's hot topics in nutrition. The moment bits of research news surface, new supplements appear—and terms like "antioxidants" become household words. Friendly faces in TV commercials begin to persuade us that these antioxidants are new magic bullets in the fight against aging, disease, and death. Then the antioxidants hit the market and cash registers ring. Vitamin C, long the leading single nutrient supplement, gains new popularity, and sales of beta-carotene and vitamin E supplements soar as well.

In the meantime, scientists and medical experts around the world continue their work to clarify and confirm the roles of these antioxidant nutrients in preventing chronic diseases.[1] This highlight summarizes some of the accumulating evidence on nutrients, *non*nutrients, and their antioxidant actions. It also revisits the advantages of foods over supplements.

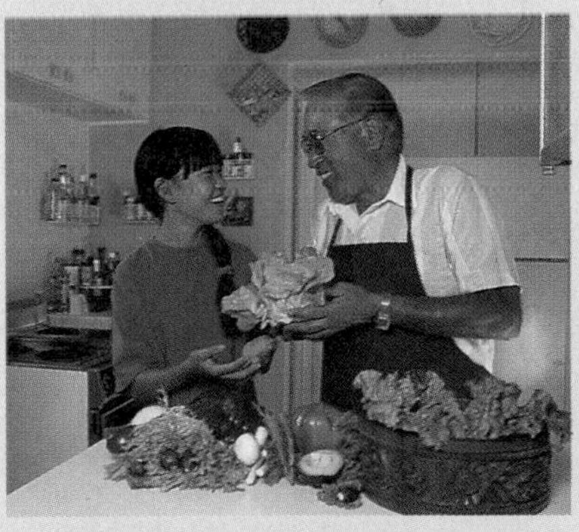

People who eat generous amounts of fruits and vegetables daily are helping their bodies to fight disease.

FREE RADICAL FORMATION AND THE BODY'S DEFENSES

All of the body's cells use oxygen to produce energy for their work. During these normal metabolic processes, oxygen sometimes reacts with body compounds to produce highly unstable molecules known as free radicals—molecules with unpaired electrons (the glossary on p. 423 defines free radicals and related terms).* An electron without a partner is unstable and highly reactive; it needs to pair up with another electron in order to return to a stable state. Free radicals quickly react with other compounds in an attempt to capture that needed electron (see Figure H11–1).

When two free radicals react with each other, their unpaired electrons form a bond. In some cases, this is fine, but in others, the product is toxic. Generally, though, free radicals simply attack the nearest stable molecule in the body, "stealing" an electron. With the loss of an electron, the stable molecule becomes a free radical itself, and a chain reaction is under way. Antioxidants neutralize free radicals by donating one of their own electrons, thus ending the electron-snatching reactions. (Review Figure 10–12 on p. 376 to see how ascorbic acid can give up two hydrogens with their electrons and become dehydroascorbic acid; antioxidants do not become free radicals when they lose electrons because they are stable in either form.)

Free radicals not only arise spontaneously during metabolism, but also are made on purpose by cells of the immune system to help them inactivate viruses and bacteria. In addition to these normal body processes, environmental factors such as radiation, pollution, and herbicides can generate free radicals. Free radicals are also involved in the oxidative damage caused by cigarette smoking.[2]

The body's natural defense and repair systems try to handle all free radicals, but these systems are not 100 percent effective. If antioxidants are unavailable, or if free-radical production becomes excessive, problems develop.[3] Unrepaired damage accumulates with age.

Free radicals are like tornadoes, causing damage wherever they go. They commonly attack lipoproteins and unsaturated fatty acids in cell membranes, starting chain reactions called lipid peroxidation.[4] Left uncontrolled, lipid peroxidation

*Many free radicals exist, but the oxygen-derived ones are most common in the human body. Examples of oxygen-derived free radicals include superoxide radical ($O_2^{\cdot -}$), hydroxyl radical ($OH^{\cdot}$), and nitric oxide ($NO^{\cdot}$). (The dots in the symbols represent the unpaired electrons.) Technically, hydrogen peroxide (H_2O_2) and singlet oxygen are not free radicals because they contain paired electrons, but their unstable conformation of electrons makes radical-producing reactions likely. Scientists sometimes use the term *reactive oxygen species* to describe all of these compounds.

Figure H11–1

The Actions of Free Radicals and Antioxidants

1 FREE RADICAL FORMATION

During normal energy metabolism, hydrogens and electrons are added to oxygen in a series of reactions known as the electron transport chain (introduced in Chapter 7). This sequence eventually produces water, but some of the intermediate compounds inevitably created during the process are free radicals. Reminder: the dot in the symbols represents the unpaired electrons.

$$O_2 \text{ (Oxygen)} \xrightarrow{e^-} O_2^{\bullet -} \text{ (Superoxide radical)} \xrightarrow{e^-} \xrightarrow{H^+} \xrightarrow{H^+} H_2O_2 \text{ (Hydrogen peroxide)} \xrightarrow{e^-} \xrightarrow{H^+} OH^{\bullet} \text{ (Hydroxyl radical)} + H_2O \text{ (Water)}$$

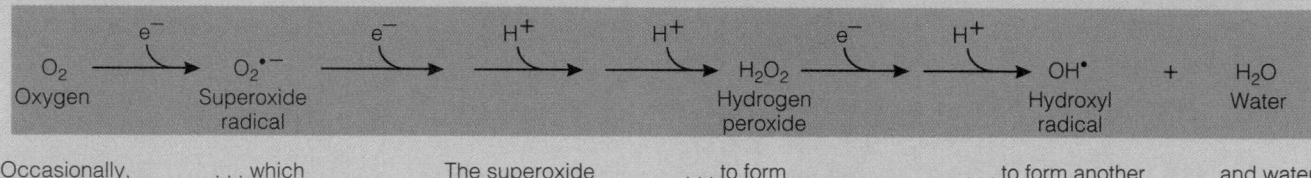

Occasionally, oxygen gains an extra electron from the electron transport chain . . . . . . which generates the free radical called superoxide radical (a molecule of oxygen with an extra, unpaired electron). The superoxide radical can gain another electron (again, from the electron transport chain) and react with two hydrogen ions . . . . . . to form hydrogen peroxide. Hydrogen peroxide can react with an electron and hydrogen . . . . . . to form another free radical called a hydroxyl radical . . . . . . and water.

2 FREE RADICAL CHAIN REACTION AND DAMAGE

Hydroxyl radicals are highly reactive, wanting to match their unpaired electrons. For example, they might take electrons from the lipids in a cell membrane, which causes damage that gives rise to degenerative diseases.

$$\text{Lipid} + OH^{\bullet} \longrightarrow \text{Lipid}^{\bullet} + H_2O$$

When a hydroxyl radical takes a hydrogen atom from a lipid (such as a polyunsaturated fatty acid) . . . . . . it generates a lipid radical . . . . . . and water.

The lipid radical can, in turn, react with oxygen to form another lipid radical, which can, in turn, remove hydrogen atoms from other lipids, producing new radicals, thereby initiating a chain reaction.

3 ANTIOXIDANT PROTECTION

Antioxidants interact with free radicals and break the destructive chain reaction that damages tissues.

$$\text{Active vitamin E} + \text{Lipid}^{\bullet} \longrightarrow \text{Inactive vitamin E}^{\bullet} + \text{Lipid}$$

$$\text{Inactive vitamin E}^{\bullet} + \text{Vitamin C (ascorbic acid with its H atoms)} = \text{Active vitamin E (with its H atom)} + \text{Vitamin C (dehydroascorbic acid without its H atoms)}$$

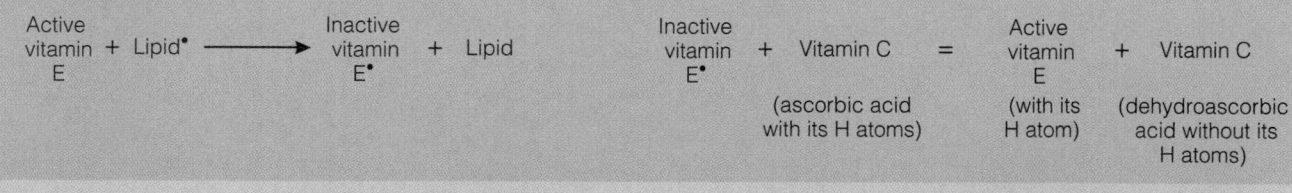

Vitamin E gives up one of its hydrogens to a lipid radical.*

The result is that vitamin E is no longer active, but it has successfully stopped the radicals from causing more damage and generating more radicals.

Vitamin E can be reactivated by accepting a hydrogen atom from fellow antioxidant vitamin C. Vitamin C's two structures are presented in Figure 10-12 on page 376.

*The compound is actually a lipid peroxyl radical.

Glossary

free radical: an atom or molecule that has one or more unpaired electron(s) in the outer orbital (see Appendix B for a review of basic chemistry concepts). This electron imbalance makes free radicals unstable and highly reactive. Radicals typically arise during oxidation reactions and readily attack other molecules with which they come in contact.

oxidant: a compound (such as oxygen itself) that oxidizes other compounds. Compounds that prevent oxidation are called *anti*oxidants, whereas those that encourage it are called *pro*oxidants.
anti = against
pro = for

oxidative stress: damage to biological systems caused by free-radical formation.

peroxidation: the production of unstable molecules containing more than the usual amount of oxygen. Hydrogen peroxide, H_2O_2, for example, may be produced from water, H_2O.

phytochemicals: nonnutrient compounds in plant-derived foods that have biological activity in the body.
phyto = plant

Reminder: *Nonnutrients* are compounds in foods with no known nutritional value.

damages cell structures and impairs their functions. Free radicals also damage proteins and DNA.

Rampant free-radical formation and the resulting damage together are called oxidative stress. This stress has been implicated in the aging process and in the development of diseases such as cancer, arthritis, cataracts, and heart disease.[5] Not unreasonably, researchers have predicted, and to some extent confirmed, that dietary antioxidants help the body fight oxidative stress. Vitamin E, for example, has been credited with reducing the oxidative stresses that accompany diabetes.[6] Daily supplements of vitamin E enhance the action of insulin, perhaps by stabilizing the membranes of responding cells. The result is to improve glucose control in diabetes.[7]

THE ANTIOXIDANT NUTRIENTS

Much research has focused on the theory that antioxidant nutrients act as scavengers of oxygen-derived free radicals, thereby helping to prevent cell and tissue damage that otherwise would give rise to degenerative diseases. The beneficial effects of fruits, vegetables, and grains in fighting degenerative diseases have been attributed, in part, to the antioxidants they provide. The antioxidant roles of several vitamins that these plant foods are famous for—beta-carotene, vitamin C, and vitamin E—are under especially extensive study.

Beta-Carotene

For many years scientists believed beta-carotene's sole function was to serve as a vitamin A precursor. Now they recognize that beta-carotene also serves as an antioxidant, important in human health.

Vitamin C

Vitamin C is the most abundant water-soluble antioxidant in the body and is active primarily in extracellular fluid. Its actions are most notable in combating the free radicals of polluted air and cigarette smoke. Not only does vitamin C scavenge many free radicals, but it helps return vitamin E to its active form.

Vitamin E

Vitamin E is the most abundant fat-soluble antioxidant and one of the body's primary defenders against oxidation. It protects the polyunsaturated fatty acids, all other lipids, and related fat-soluble compounds such as vitamin A.

Vitamin E serves as the body's first line of defense against lipid peroxidation by effectively breaking the chain reaction. In fact, vitamin E is one of the most efficient chain-breaking antioxidants available, reacting 200 times faster than the antioxidant BHT (butylated hydroxytoluene) commonly used in commercial bakery products. For this reason, a small amount of vitamin E can protect a large amount of lipid. Of course, in protecting other substances, vitamin E is used up and so needs to be replenished from dietary sources.

Other vitamins may serve not as antioxidants, but in supporting roles. For example, riboflavin forms part of the coenzymes that are required by several enzymes active in oxidative metabolism.[8]

ANTIOXIDANT NUTRIENTS AND CANCER

Cancers arise when cellular DNA is damaged—perhaps by free-radical attacks.[9] Antioxidant nutrients may reduce cancer risks by protecting DNA from this damage. Epidemiological reports indicate a correlation between low intakes of foods rich in antioxidant nutrients and high cancer rates. Laboratory studies with animals and cells in tissue culture seem to support such findings.

Many studies using animals as subjects have shown that beta-carotene protects against cancer.[10] The protective effects vary, depending on the experimental conditions, the types of animals tested, and the cancer types and sites.[11]

Research on human beings also produces diverse results. Researchers have compared groups of people with high cancer rates with groups that have low cancer rates, but are similar in other characteristics—for example, smoking history and age. They report a consistent relationship between low intakes of vegetables and fruits (specifically of those containing beta-carotene and its relatives) and high rates of lung cancer.[12] Such findings suggest that beta-carotene is protective, but researchers are quick to add that other constituents of fruits and vegetables may be responsible for the effect. When researchers collect blood samples, though, they find that low concentrations of beta-carotene consistently correlate with the development of both lung and breast cancers.[13]

Research has not always made it clear whether preformed vitamin A, beta-carotene, or both are protective against cancer.[14] Some research indicates that dietary vitamin A—from whatever source—seems to play a role in inhibiting the development of breast cancer.[15] Evidence of protection against cancers of the colon or prostate is less convincing.

Large-scale studies of populations suggest that vitamin C also helps protect against certain types of cancers, especially those of the mouth, larynx, and esophagus.[16] A dozen or so different studies have correlated high vitamin C intakes with low rates of cancer. Such a correlation may reflect the benefits of a diet rich in fruits and vegetables and low in fat and does not necessarily support the taking of vitamin C supplements to treat or prevent cancer.

Some research suggests that vitamin C protects against stomach cancer specifically, by preventing the formation of carcinogenic nitrite compounds in the stomach.[17] More research is needed, but the results so far are promising.

Evidence that vitamin E helps guard against cancer is less consistent than for beta-carotene and vitamin C. One large population study showed the highest risks of certain cancers in the people with lowest blood vitamin E.[18] The association was strongest for some gastrointestinal cancers and for cancers not related to smoking.

ANTIOXIDANTS AND HEART DISEASE

Much of the research on antioxidant nutrients has focused on cancer prevention, but antioxidants, especially vitamin E, may protect against cardiovascular disease as well.[19] Research confirms that high blood cholesterol carried in low-density lipoproteins (LDL) correlates directly with cardiovascular disease. Researchers are now asking how high LDL exert their damage. Some of the most promising research suggests that LDL first undergo oxidation by free radicals inside the artery wall and then promote the formation of artery-clogging plaques.[20] Evidence thus far is persuasive but not conclusive.

If oxidized LDL are a factor in heart disease, might antioxidant nutrients offer some protection? Some research suggests that they do. Findings from an epidemiological study suggest a negative correlation between vitamin E status and death rates from heart disease.[21] Researchers selected groups of men in 16 European regions where rates of death from heart disease varied sixfold. The researchers measured plasma vitamin E, cholesterol, and blood pressure in men from each region. When the groups were compared, high death rates from heart disease correlated more strongly with low vitamin E concentrations than with either cholesterol or blood pressure. The authors cautioned that the evidence for the "antioxidant hypothesis" of heart disease was suggestive, but indirect.

Two other large epidemiological studies found that large doses of vitamin E supplements were associated with a significantly reduced risk of heart disease.[22] This correlation remaining strong after the researchers analyzed for coronary risk factors and other dietary antioxidants.

Vitamin C may also affect the susceptibility of LDL to oxidation. Some epidemiological studies have found an association between vitamin C and cardiovascular disease; others have not.[23] Research suggests a synergism between vitamin C and vitamin E in defending LDL against oxidation; vitamin C defends against free radicals in the water compartments of cells, and vitamin E acts in lipid environments. Together, they effectively protect LDL against oxidation. In addition, vitamin C may regenerate vitamin E from its oxidized form, making it available to act as an antioxidant once again.[24] Some studies also suggest that vitamin C may raise HDL, lower total cholesterol, and improve blood pressure.[25]

SUPPLEMENTS VERSUS FOODS

Of course, researchers are genuinely excited to learn that the antioxidant nutrients might help prevent such life-threatening diseases as cancer and cardiovascular disease, but their findings have sparked new controversies.[26] Some research suggests a protective effect from as little as a daily glass of orange juice and carrot juice (rich sources of vitamin C and beta-carotene, respectively). [27] Other current intervention studies, however, are using levels of nutrients that far exceed the RDA and can only be achieved by taking supplements. What if research finds a true benefit in taking vitamin pills as opposed to eating a healthy diet alone? Members of the Food and Nutrition Board of the National Research Council are reconsidering their long-held bias against vitamin supplements. They realize that it may be necessary to broaden the concept of the RDA to include both a recommended daily intake to prevent classic deficiency diseases and another substantially higher intake to help protect against chronic diseases.[28]

While awaiting final answers, should people anticipate the go-ahead and start taking vitamin E or other antioxidant supplements now?[29] Most scientists agree that it is too early to make such a recommendation. While fruits and vegetables that contain many antioxidant nutrients have been associated with a diminished risk of many cancers, supplements of beta-carotene and vitamins C and E have not always proven beneficial.[30] Clinical studies will take several years to complete, and until they prove a clear benefit from taking antioxidant supplements, it would be irresponsible for health care professionals to make such recommendations. We do not know the consequences of taking large doses of antioxidants, even naturally occurring ones, over the long term, much less over a lifetime. Without data to confirm the benefits, we cannot accept the potential risks. And the risks are real.

Consider the findings from a study to determine whether daily supplements of vitamin E, beta-carotene, or both would reduce the incidence of lung cancer among smokers.[31] After five to eight years of supplementation, there was no reduction in the incidence of lung cancer; in fact, there was a higher incidence of lung cancer among those receiving the beta-carotene. Such findings were surprising, to say the least, especially given the association between high beta-carotene intakes and low rates of lung cancer reported in earlier epidemiological studies. These discrepancies highlight the importance of considering research findings from a variety of studies and the need for replication, already emphasized in Chapter 1. The findings also suggest that remedies to life-threatening diseases such as lung cancer may not be as simple as taking daily pills. Smokers are much wiser to stop smoking than to rely on vitamin supplements to protect them from lung cancer. Much more research is needed to define optimal and dangerous levels of intake. The Food and Drug Administration (FDA) is now in the process of establishing guidelines for the safe use of nutrient supplements in quantities greater than those needed to meet basic nutrient requirements.

This much we know: antioxidant nutrients behave differently at various levels of intake. At physiological levels typical of a healthy diet, they act as antioxidants, but at pharmacological doses typical of supplements, they may act as *prooxidants, stimulating* the production of free radicals, especially when metal ions such as iron are present.[32] As long as the risks of supplement use remain unclear, the best way to supplement antioxidant nutrients is to eat generous servings of fruits and vegetables, especially citrus fruits and green and yellow vegetables.

FOODS MAKING HEALTH CLAIMS

Results of clinical studies may one day support the use of selected supplements to prevent disease, but until then, people will want to select foods rich in all of the vitamins and minerals—particularly the antioxidants. Which foods to select?

The FDA examined the available scientific evidence concerning antioxidant vitamins and cancer to determine whether a health claim on food labels was appropriate. The agency concluded that *diets* high in fruits and vegetables, which are good sources of two antioxidant vitamins (vitamin A as beta-carotene and vitamin C), are strongly associated with reduced risks of several types of cancer. Still, the FDA rejected the antioxidant health claim, stating that the reduction in risk could not be attributed directly and solely to the antioxidant effect of the vitamins. Therefore labels may not claim an association between antioxidant vitamins and cancer; the health claim must be stated in terms of "fruits and vegetables and cancer."

NONNUTRIENTS IN DISEASE PREVENTION

What do fruits and vegetables have in them besides nutrients? They must have something, for as research has shown, the nutrients alone are not fully responsible for the beneficial effects fruits and vegetables have on disease prevention. Other, nonnutrient compounds must also be involved.

The nonnutrient compounds found in plants are called phytochemicals, and they have been the topic of much recent research. In foods, these compounds may impart flavors and colors, but in the body, they can have profound physiological effects, including suppression of the development of cancer.[33] Table H11–1 summarizes the common food sources and actions of selected phytochemicals.

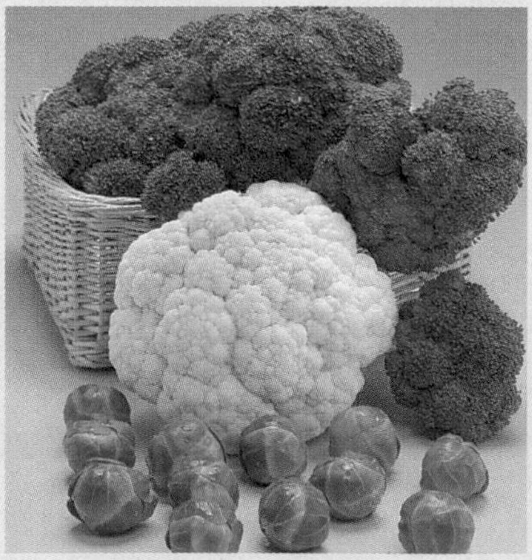

Cruciferous vegetables, such as cauliflower, broccoli, and brussels sprouts contain nutrients and nonnutrients that may inhibit cancer development.

This book has focused primarily on the nutrients, but foods deliver thousands of other chemicals. For this reason, researchers must be careful in giving credit for particular health benefits to any one nutrient. Diets rich in whole grains, legumes, vegetables, and fruits seem to be protective against cancer, but identifying *the* specific foods or components of foods that are responsible is difficult. Green leafy vegetables such as spinach and kale, for example, contain lutein, an antioxidant more active than beta-carotene. The anticancer benefits of green leafy vegetables may be due to beta-carotene, but they may be due to lutein—or to another as yet unnamed character. Perhaps credit even belongs to the unique *combination* of chemicals found in leafy greens. Similarly, soybeans contain several compounds that appear to have anticancer activity.[34] We simply do not have all the answers.

Other nonnutrients with antioxidant activity are the flavonoids commonly found in vegetables, fruits, beverages such as tea and wine, and spices such as oregano. These compounds may offer important health benefits and explain, in part, why people who drink wine and others who have high intakes of flavonoids have reduced risks of heart diseases.[35]

Everyone eats a variety of phytochemicals in small quantities every day. This approach may be more beneficial than taking large doses of any one phytochemical.[36] In large doses, some phytochemicals can be toxic. The regulation of phytochemicals depends on how they are used.[37] Consider garlic, for example. A clove of garlic is a food. The FDA classifies dehydrated garlic and garlic extracts as generally recognized as safe (GRAS) substances. A product derived from garlic that makes a special health claim, on the other hand, is classified as a drug.

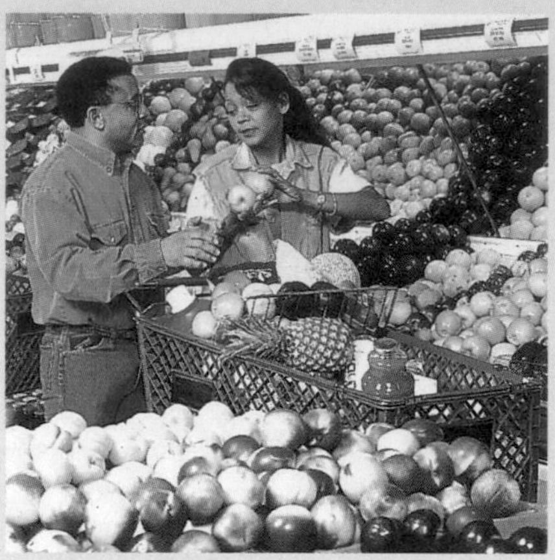

Many cancer-fighting products are available now at your local produce counter.

Of course, as soon as science discovers a role for phytochemicals in disease prevention, manufacturers will begin marketing supplements. (Highlight 10 explained how some manufacturers have already tried to sell antioxidant supplements marketed as "nutraceuticals.") It should be clear by now, though, that we cannot know the identity and action of every chemical in every food. Even if we did, why create a supplement to replicate a food? Why not eat foods and enjoy the pleasure, nourishment, and health benefits they provide? The beneficial constituents in foods are widespread among plants.[38] Don't try to single out one particular food for its magic phytochemical. Instead, eat a wide variety of fruits and vegetables in generous quantities every day—and get *all* the magic compounds these foods have to offer.

Table H11–1

Phytochemicals—Their Food Sources and Actions

Food Source	Name	Action in the Body
Deeply pigmented fruits and vegetables (carrots, sweet potatoes, tomatoes, spinach, broccoli, cantaloupe, pumpkin, apricots)	Carotenoids[a] (including beta-carotene)	Act as antioxidants, reducing the risk of cancer.
Citrus fruits	Limonene	Triggers enzyme production to facilitate carcinogen excretion.
	Phenols	Inhibit lipid oxidation; block formation of carcinogenic nitrosamines in the body.
Garlic/onions	Allyl sulfides	Trigger enzyme production to facilitate carcinogen excretion.
Broccoli and other cruciferous vegetables (cauliflower and brussels sprouts)	Sulforaphane	Protects against cancer.
	Dithiolthiones	Trigger enzyme production to block carcinogen damage to cells' DNA.
	Indoles	Trigger enzymes to inhibit estrogen action, reducing the risk of breast cancer.
	Isothiocyanates	Trigger enzyme production to block carcinogen damage of cells' DNA.
Grapes	Ellagic acid	Scavenges carcinogens.
Soy/legumes	Protease inhibitors	Suppress enzyme production in cancer cells, slowing tumor growth.
	Phytosterols	Inhibit cell reproduction in GI tract, preventing colon cancer.
	Isoflavones[b]	Block estrogen activity in cells, reducing the risk of breast and ovarian cancer.
	Saponins	Interfere with DNA reproduction, preventing cancer cell multiplication.
Flaxseed	Lignans[b]	Block estrogen activity in cells, reducing the risk of breast and ovarian cancer.
Fruits (blueberries, prunes, grapes), oats, soybeans	Caffeic acid	Triggers enzyme production to make carcinogens water-soluble, facilitating excretion.
	Ferulic acid	Binds to nitrates in stomach, preventing the conversion to nitrosamines.
Grains	Phytic acid	Binds to minerals, preventing cancer-causing free-radical formation.
Fruits, vegetables, tea, wine, oregano	Flavonoids	Act as antioxidants, reducing the risk of cancer.

[a]In addition to beta-carotene, other carotenoids include alpha-carotene, beta-cryptoxanthin, lectein, zeaxanthin, and lycopene.
[b]Isoflavones and lignans are types of phytoestrogens—compounds that bind to estrogen receptors and reduce estrogen activity.

NOTES

1. Health promotion and disease prevention: The role of antioxidant vitamins, *American Journal of Medicine* 97 (supplement 3A) (1994): 1S–28S; B. Halliwell, J. M. C. Gutteridge, and C. E. Cross, Free radicals, antioxidants, and human disease: Where are we now? *Journal of Laboratory and Clinical Medicine* 119 (1992): 598–620; A. T. Diplock, Antioxidant nutrients and disease prevention: An overview, *American Journal of Clinical Nutrition* 53 (1991): 189S–193S.

2. J. D. Morrow and coauthors, Increase in circulating products of lipid peroxidation (F_2-

isoprostanes) in smokers—Smoking as a cause of oxidative damage, *New England Journal of Medicine* 332 (1995): 1198–1203.
3. B. Halliwell, Free radicals and antioxidants: A personal view, *Nutritional Reviews* 52 (1994): 253–265.
4. G. W. Burton and M. G. Traber, Vitamin E: Antioxidant activity, biokinetics, and bioavailability, *Annual Review of Nutrition* 10 (1990): 357–382.
5. Diplock, 1991; L. Packer, Protective role of vitamin E in biological systems, *American Journal of Clinical Nutrition* 53 (1991): 1050S–1055S.
6. B. Caballero, Vitamin E improves the action of insulin, *Nutrition Reviews* 51 (1993): 339–340.
7. G. Paolisso and coauthors, Pharmacologic doses of vitamin E improve insulin action in healthy subjects and non-insulin-dependent diabetic subjects, *American Journal of Clinical Nutrition* 57 (1993): 650–656.
8. R. S. Rivlin and P. Dutta, Vitamin B2 (riboflavin)—Relevance to malaria and antioxidant activity, *Nutrition Today* 30 (1995): 62–67.
9. I. T. Johnson, G. Williamson, and S. R. R. Musk, Anticarcinogenic factors in plant foods: A new class of nutrients? *Nutrition Research Reviews* 7 (1994): 175–204; B. N. Ames, M. K. Shigenaga, and T. M. Hagen, Oxidants, antioxidants, and the degenerative diseases of aging, *Proceedings of the National Academy of Sciences* 90 (1993): 7915–7922.
10. N. I. Krinsky, Effects of carotenoids in cellular and animal systems, *American Journal of Clinical Nutrition* 52 (1991): 238S–246S.
11. T. Byers and G. Perry, Dietary carotenes, vitamin C, and vitamin E as protective antioxidants in human cancers, *Annual Review of Nutrition* 12 (1992): 139–159.
12. R. G. Ziegler, Vegetables, fruits, and carotenoids and the risk of cancer, *American Journal of Clinical Nutrition* 53 (1991): 251S–259S.
13. H. B. Stahalein and coauthors, Beta-carotene and cancer prevention: The Basel Study, *American Journal of Clinical Nutrition* 53 (1991): 265S–269S; N. Potischman and coauthors, Breast cancer and dietary and plasma concentrations of carotenoids and vitamin A, *American Journal of Clinical Nutrition* 52 (1990): 909–915.
14. W. C. Willett and D. J. Hunter, Vitamin A and cancers of the breast, large bowel, and prostate: Epidemiologic evidence, *Nutrition Review* (supplement) 52 (1994): S53–S59.
15. D. J. Hunter and coauthors, A prospective study of the intake of vitamins C, E, and A and the risk of breast cancer, *New England Journal of Medicine* 329 (1993): 234–240.
16. G. Block, Vitamin C and cancer prevention: The epidemiologic evidence, *American Journal of Clinical Nutrition* 53 (1991): 270S–282S.
17. S. R. Tannenbaum, J. S. Wishnok, and C. D. Leaf, Inhibition of nitrosamine formation by ascorbic acid, *American Journal of Clinical Nutrition* 53 (1991): 247S–250S.
18. P. Knekt and coauthors, Vitamin E and cancer prevention, *American Journal of Clinical Nutrition* 53 (1991): 283S–286S.
19. T. Byers, Vitamin E supplements and coronary heart disease, *Nutrition Reviews* 51 (1993): 333–336; K. F. Gey and coauthors, Increased risk of cardiovascular disease at suboptimal plasma concentrations of essential antioxidants: An epidemiological update with special attention to carotene and vitamin C, *American Journal of Clinical Nutrition* 57 (1993): 787S–797S.
20. B. Halliwell, Oxidation of low-density lipoproteins: Questions of initiation, propagation, and the effect of antioxidants, *American Journal of Clinical Nutrition* 61 (1995): 670S–677S.
21. K. F. Gey and coauthors, Inverse correlation between plasma vitamin E and mortality from ischemic heart disease in cross-cultural epidemiology, *American Journal of Clinical Nutrition* 53 (1991): 326S–334S; Gey and coauthors, 1993.
22. M. J. Stampfer and coauthors, Vitamin E consumption and the risk of coronary disease in women, *New England Journal of Medicine* 328 (1993): 1444–1449; E. B. Rimm and coauthors, Vitamin E consumption and the risk of coronary disease in men, *New England Journal of Medicine* 328 (1993): 1450–1456.
23. Gey and coauthors, 1993; D. L. Trout, Vitamin C and cardiovascular risk factors, *American Journal of Clinical Nutrition* 53 (1991): 322S–325S; Stampfer and coauthors, 1993; Rimm and coauthors, 1993.
24. D. Kritchevsky, Antioxidant vitamins in the prevention of cardiovascular disease, *Nutrition Today*, January/February 1992, pp. 30–33.
25. Trout, 1991; J. P. Moran and coauthors, Plasma ascorbic acid concentrations relate inversely to blood pressure in human subjects, *American Journal of Clinical Nutrition* 57 (1993): 213–217.
26. J. Blumberg, Are antioxidants at an awkward age? *Journal of the American College of Nutrition* 13 (1994): 218–219.
27. M. Abbey, M. Noakes, and P. J. Nestel, Dietary supplementation with orange and carrot juice in cigarette smokers lowers oxidation products in copper-oxidized low-density lipoproteins, *Journal of the American Dietetic Association* 95 (1995): 671–675.
28. W. A. Pryor, The antioxidant nutrients and disease prevention—What do we know and what do we need to find out? *American Journal of Clinical Nutrition* 53 (1991): 391S–393S.
29. D. Steinberg, Antioxidant vitamins and coronary heart disease, *New England Journal of Medicine* 328 (1993): 1487–1489.
30. E. R. Greenberg and coauthors, A clinical trial of antioxidant vitamins to prevent colorectal adenoma, *New England Journal of Medicine* 331 (1994): 141–147.
31. O. P. Heinonen, J. K. Huttunen, and D. Albanes (and other participants in the alpha-tocopherol, beta carotene cancer prevention study group), The effect of vitamin E and beta carotene on the incidence of lung cancer and other cancers in male smokers, *New England Journal of Medicine* 330 (1994): 1029–1035.
32. T. Repka and R. P. Hebbel, Hydroxyl radical formation by sickle erythrocyte membranes: Role of pathological iron deposits and cytoplasmic reducing agents, *Blood* 78 (1991): 2753–2758; V. Herbert, The antioxidant supplement myth, *American Journal of Clinical Nutrition* 60 (1994): 157–158; B. Halliwell, Antioxidants: Sense or speculation? *Nutrition Today*, November/December 1994, pp. 15–19.
33. L. W. Wattenberg, Inhibition of carcinogenesis by minor dietary constituents, *Cancer Research* 52 (1992): 2085s–2091s.
34. M. Messina and S. Barnes, The role of soy products in reducing risk of cancer, *Journal of the National Cancer Institute* 83 (1991): 541–546.
35. Dietary flavonoids and risk of coronary heart disease, *Nutrition Reviews* 52 (1994): 59–61.
36. L. U. Thompson, Antioxidants and hormone-mediated health benefits of whole grains, *Critical Reviews in Food Science and Nutrition* 34 (1994): 473–497.
37. J. N. Hathcock, Safety and regulatory issues for phytochemical sources: "Designer foods," *Nutrition Today*, November/December 1993, pp. 23–25.
38. Position of the American Dietetic Association: Phytochemicals and functional foods, *Journal of the American Dietetic Association* 95 (1995): 493–496; E. A. Decker, The role of phenolics, conjugated linoleic acid, carnosine, and pyrroloquinoline quinone as nonessential dietary antioxidants, *Nutrition Reviews* 53 (1995): 19–58.

Chapter 12

Water and the Major Minerals

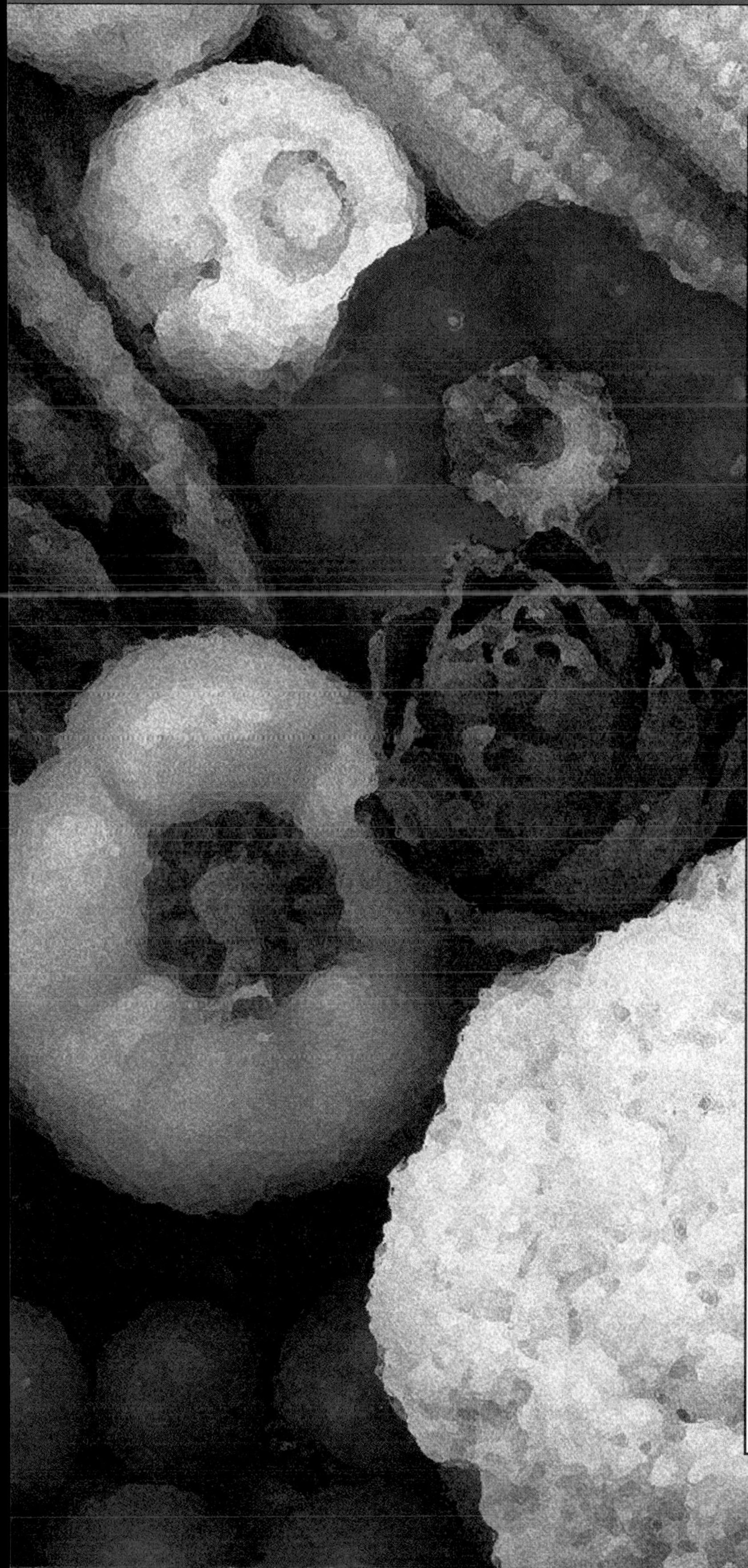

CONTENTS

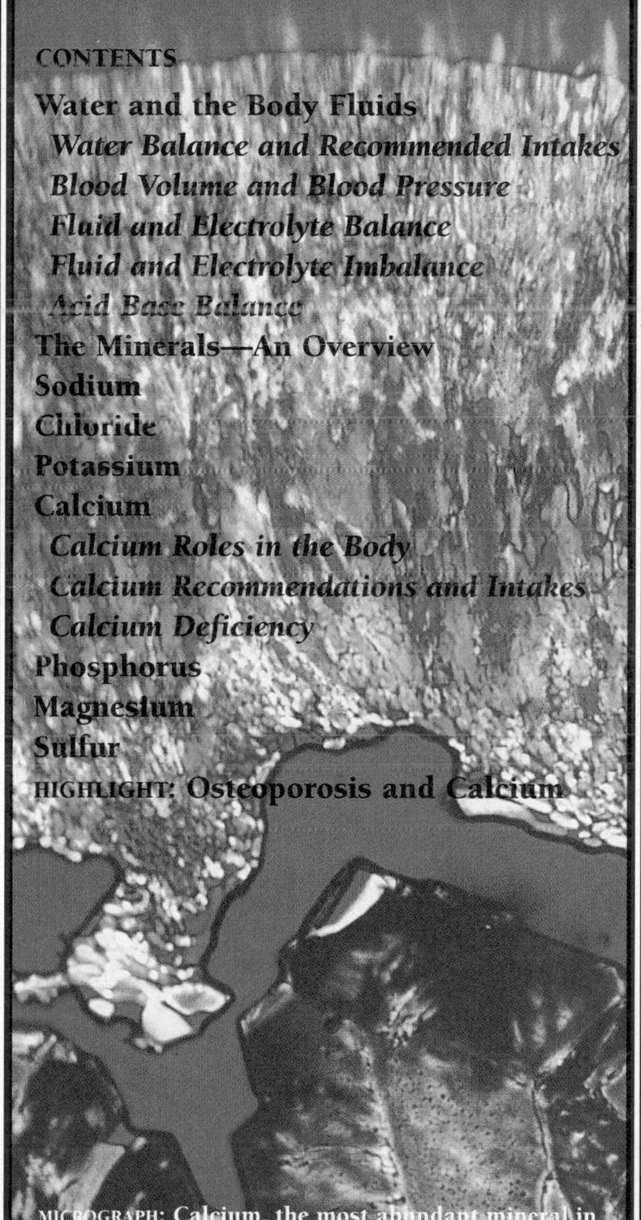

MICROGRAPH: Calcium, the most abundant mineral in the body

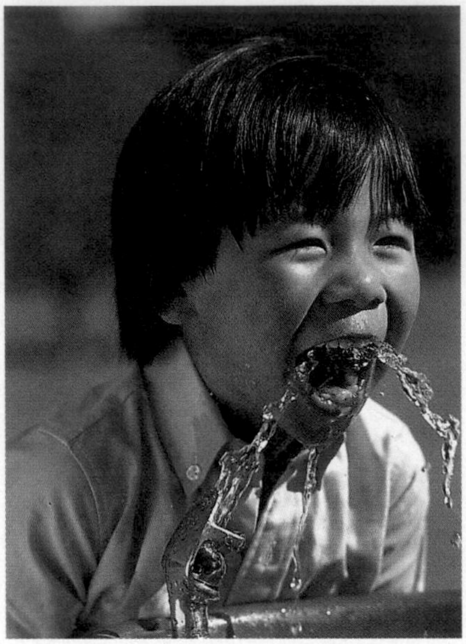

Water is the most indispensable nutrient.

Water is an essential nutrient, as important to life as any of the others. In fact, you can survive only a few days without water, whereas a deficiency of the other nutrients may take weeks, months, or even years to develop.

This chapter begins with a look at water and the body's fluids. The body maintains an appropriate balance and distribution of water with the help of another class of nutrients—the minerals. In addition to introducing the minerals that help regulate body fluids, the chapter describes many of the other important functions minerals perform in the body.

Water and the Body Fluids

In the body, water becomes the fluid in which all life processes occur. Every cell contains intracellular fluid of the exact composition that is best for that cell and is bathed externally in another such fluid (interstitial fluids.) (Figure 6–9 on p. 208 illustrates a cell and its associated fluids.) The interstitial fluid provides each cell with the ingredients it requires and receives the end products of the chemical reactions that take place within the cells' boundaries. The water molecules of the intracellular fluid nestle around the cell's giant proteins, glycogen, and other large molecules, helping to maintain their structures and participating in many chemical reactions.

These fluids are constantly losing and replacing their constituent parts, yet the composition in each compartment remains remarkably constant at all times. The entire system of cells and fluids remains in a delicate but firmly maintained state of homeostasis. The water in the body fluids:

- Carries nutrients and waste products throughout the body.
- Helps to form the structure of large molecules.
- Actively participates in many chemical reactions.
- Serves as the solvent for minerals, vitamins, amino acids, glucose, and a multitude of other small molecules.
- Acts as a lubricant and cushion around joints.
- Serves as a shock absorber inside the eyes, spinal cord, and, in pregnancy, the amniotic sac surrounding the fetus in the womb.
- Aids in the body's temperature regulation.
- Maintains blood volume.

Because water is so vital to these and other functions, the body directs many of its activities toward maintaining an appropriate balance.

intracellular fluid: fluid within the cells, usually high in potassium and phosphate. Intracellular fluid accounts for approximately two-thirds of the body's water.
intra = within

interstitial fluid (IN-ter-STISH-al)**:** fluid between the cells, usually high in sodium and chloride. Interstitial fluid is a large component of **extracellular fluid** (fluid outside the cells), which also includes plasma and the water of structures such as the skin and bones. Extracellular fluid accounts for approximately one-third of the body's water.
inter = in the midst, between
extra = outside

Reminder: *Homeostasis* is the maintenance of relatively constant conditions within the body's systems.

WATER BALANCE AND RECOMMENDED INTAKES

Water constitutes about 60 percent of an adult's body weight and a higher percentage of a child's. The proportion of water is generally lower in females, obese people, and the elderly. The amount of fluid in the body is tightly controlled because imbalances can be devastating. The body attempts to restore homeostasis as promptly as possible, adjusting both water intake and excretion as needed.

water balance: the balance between water intake and output (losses).
Water balance = intake − output.

Water Intake Thirst and satiety influence water intake, apparently in response to changes sensed by the mouth, hypothalamus, and nerves. When the blood is too concentrated (having lost water, but not the dissolved substances within it), the mouth becomes dry, and the person responds by drinking. When the hypothalamus detects that the blood is too concentrated, it also initiates drinking behavior. The nerves also play a role: thirsty animals drink until stretch receptors in the stomach turn off the drinking. Similarly, receptors in the heart monitor blood volume and suppress thirst when the volume is elevated.

thirst: a conscious desire to drink.

hypothalamus (high-po-THAL-ah-mus)**:** a brain center that controls activities such as maintenance of water balance and regulation of body temperature.

Thirst drives a person to seek water, but it lags behind the body's need. A water deficiency that develops slowly can switch on drinking behavior in time to prevent serious dehydration, but a deficiency that develops quickly may not. Also, thirst itself does not remedy a water deficiency; a person must notice the thirst signal, pay attention, and take the time to get a drink. The long-distance runner, the gardener in hot weather, the child busy playing, and the elderly person whose thirst sensation may be blunted can experience serious dehydration if they fail to drink promptly in response to their need for water.

dehydration: the condition in which body water output exceeds water input.

Dehydration may easily develop with either water deprivation or excessive water losses. The symptoms progress rapidly from thirst, to weakness, to exhaustion and delirium and end in death if not corrected. Water intoxication, on the other hand, is rare but can occur with excessive water ingestion and kidney disorders that reduce urine output. The symptoms may include confusion, convulsion, and even death in extreme cases.

water intoxication: the condition in which body water contents are too high.

Water Sources The obvious dietary sources of water are water itself and other beverages, but nearly all foods also contain water. Most fruits and vegetables contain up to 95 percent water; many meats and cheeses contain at least 50 percent (see Appendix H). Water is also generated during metabolism. Recall that when the energy-yielding nutrients break down, their carbons and hydrogens combine with oxygen to yield carbon dioxide (CO_2)—and water (H_2O). The water derived daily from these three sources totals, on the average, about 2½ liters (about 2½ quarts), as Table 12–1 shows.

Table 12–1

Water Balance

Water Sources	Amount (ml)	Water Excretion	Amount (ml)
Liquids	550 to 1500	Kidneys	500 to 1400
Foods	700 to 1000	Skin	450 to 900
Metabolic water	200 to 300	Lungs	350
		Feces	150
	1450 to 2800		1450 to 2800

Note: These values reflect data from several sources and are compatible with those cited in many other references. For further information, see L. Sherwood, *Fundamentals of Physiology: A Human Perspective* (St. Paul, Minn.: West Publishing, 1995), pp. 396–417; Committee on Dietary Allowances, *Recommended Dietary Allowances* (Washington, D.C.: National Academy Press, 1989), pp. 247–261; J. L. Groff, S. S. Gropper, and S. M. Hunt, *Advanced Nutrition and Human Metabolism* (St. Paul, Minn.: West Publishing, 1995), pp. 423–438.

The amount of water the body has to excrete each day to dispose of its wastes is the **obligatory** (ah-BLIG-ah-TORE-ee) **water excretion**—about 500 ml, or a pint.

Water Losses The body must excrete a minimum of about 500 milliliters of water each day as urine—enough to carry away the waste products generated by a day's metabolic activities. Above this amount, excretion adjusts to balance intake. If a person drinks more water, the urine becomes more dilute. In addition, water is lost from the lungs as vapor and from the skin as sweat; some is also lost in feces.* The losses from all of these sources total about 2½ liters a day on the average. Table 12–1 shows how water excretion balances intake.

Fluid needs before, during, and after exercise are addressed in Chapter 14.

Water recommendation for adults:
- 1.0 to 1.5 ml/kcal expended.
- 4.2 to 6.3 ml/kJ expended.

Water recommendation for infants:
- 1.5 ml/kcal expended.

Note: 1 ml = 0.03 fluid oz.
125 ml ≈ ½ c.

Easy estimation: ½ c per 100 kcal expended.

Water Recommendations Water needs vary, depending primarily on diet, activity, environmental temperature, and humidity. Accordingly, a general water requirement is difficult to establish. Recommendations for adults are expressed in proportion to the amount of energy expended under average environmental conditions.[1] A person who expends 2000 kcalories a day needs about 2 to 3 liters of water (about 7 to 11 cups).

Fluid needs are best met by water, but milk and juices can account for part of the day's recommended intake.[2] In addition to their high water content, these beverages deliver valuable nutrients. Alcoholic beverages and those containing caffeine, such as coffee, tea, and sodas, however, are not good substitutes for water. Both alcohol and caffeine act as diuretics, causing the body to lose fluids.

BLOOD VOLUME AND BLOOD PRESSURE

ADH (antidiuretic hormone): a hormone released by the pituitary gland in response to highly concentrated blood. The kidneys respond by reabsorbing water, thus preventing water loss. In addition to its antidiuretic effect, ADH also elevates blood pressure and is called **vasopressin**.
- *anti* = against
- *di* = through
- *ure* = urine
- *vaso* = vessel
- *press* = pressure

Recall from Highlight 7 how alcohol depresses ADH activity, thus promoting fluid losses and dehydration.

renin: an enzyme from the kidneys that works by activating angiotensin.

angiotensin: a blood protein that helps to raise blood pressure. Its precursor protein is called **angiotensinogen.**

vasoconstrictor: a substance that constricts or narrows the blood vessels.

aldosterone (al-DOS-ter-own)**:** a hormone secreted by the adrenal glands that stimulates the reabsorption of sodium by the kidneys; aldosterone also regulates chloride and potassium concentrations.

adrenal glands: glands adjacent to, and just above, each kidney.

Water balance is critical to maintaining the blood volume, which in turn influences blood pressure. If too much water is lost from the body, blood volume and blood pressure fall.

ADH and Water Retention The hypothalamus stimulates the pituitary gland to release the antidiuretic hormone (ADH) whenever the blood becomes too concentrated, or whenever blood volume or blood pressure falls too low. ADH stimulates the kidneys to reabsorb water, so they recirculate it, rather than excrete it. Consequently, the more water you need, the less you excrete.

Angiotensin and Blood Vessel Constriction Cells in the kidneys respond to low blood pressure by releasing an enzyme called renin. Through a complex series of events, renin causes the kidneys to reabsorb sodium. Sodium reabsorption, in turn, is always accompanied by water retention, which helps to restore blood volume and blood pressure. Renin activates a protein in the blood called angiotensinogen to its active form, angiotensin. Angiotensin is a powerful vasoconstrictor: it narrows blood vessel diameters, thereby raising the blood pressure.

Aldosterone and Sodium Retention Angiotensin also mediates the release of the hormone aldosterone from the adrenal glands. Aldosterone causes the kidneys to retain more sodium (and thus more water). Again, the effect is that when more water is needed, less is excreted.

In summary, in response to low blood volume or highly concentrated blood, these three actions effectively restore homeostasis (see Figure 12–1):

---

*Water lost from the lungs and skin accounts for almost one-half of the daily losses even when a person is not visibly perspiring; these losses are commonly referred to as *insensible water losses*.

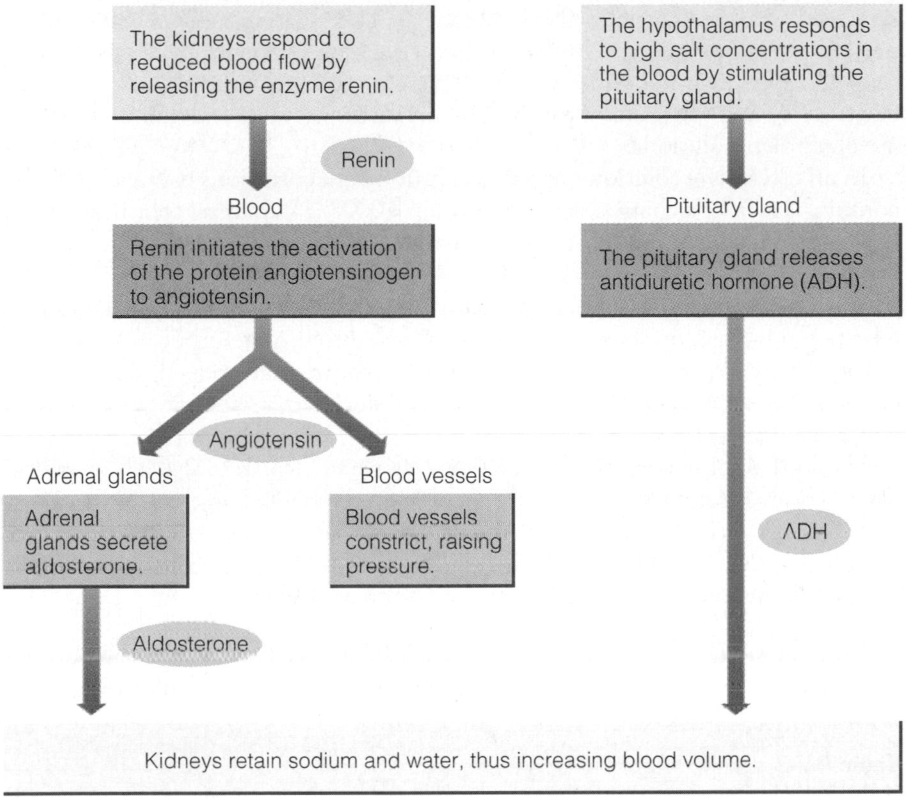

Figure 12–1

How the Body Regulates Water Excretion

- ADH causes water retention.
- Angiotensin constricts blood vessels.
- Aldosterone causes sodium retention.

These mechanisms cannot maintain water balance by themselves, however; they work only if a person drinks enough water.

FLUID AND ELECTROLYTE BALANCE

The body cells, with only a few exceptions, cannot move water from place to place; they need to use minerals and other constituents to regulate the distribution of body fluids. About two-thirds of the body fluids reside inside the cells and one-third outside. This balance is vital to the life of the cells. If too much water entered the cells, it might rupture them; if too much water were to leave, they would collapse. To control the movement of water, the body uses its major minerals, which form salts that dissolve in the body fluids. The cells direct the movement of these salts, and this determines where the fluids flow because *water follows salt*. (This simple statement sums up how osmotic pressure works; a later section describes osmosis in more detail.)

Dissociation of Salt in Water When a mineral salt much as sodium chloride (NaCl) dissolves in water, it separates (dissociates) into ions—positively and

Reminder: *Fluid and electrolyte balance* is the maintenance of the proper amounts and kinds of fluid and minerals in each compartment of the body fluids.

The cell membrane is **selectively permeable**; that is, it permits some, but not all, substances to pass freely.

salts: compounds composed of a positive ion other than H^+ and a negative ion other than OH^-. An example is sodium chloride (Na^+Cl^-).
Na = sodium.
Cl = chloride.

dissociation: the physical separation of a compound into ions.

ions (EYE-uns)**:** atoms or molecules that have gained or lost electrons and therefore have electrical charges. Examples include the positively charged sodium ion (Na^+) and the negatively charged chloride ion (Cl^-). For a closer look at ions, see Appendix B.

cations (CAT-eye-uns): positively charged ions.

anions (AN-eye-uns): negatively charged ions.

electrolytes: salts that dissolve in water and dissociate.

electrolyte solutions: solutions that can conduct electricity due to the presence of ions.

milliequivalents (mEq): the concentration of electrolytes in a volume of solution. The number of milliequivalents is a useful measure when considering ions, because the number of charges reveals characteristics about the solution that are not evident when expressed in terms of weight.

polar: describes a neutral molecule that has opposite charges spatially separated within the molecule; see Appendix B for more details.

negatively charged particles (Na^+ and Cl^-). The positive ions are cations; the negative ones are anions. Unlike pure water, which conducts electricity poorly, ions dissolved in water carry electrical current. For this reason, ions are called electrolytes, and the fluids of the body, which contain water and dissociated salts, are electrolyte solutions.

In all electrolyte solutions, anion and cation concentrations balance. If a fluid contains 1000 "−" charges, it must contain 1000 "+" charges, too. If an anion enters the fluid, a cation must accompany it or another anion must leave so that electroneutrality will be maintained.

It is not necessary, though, to have the same number of Na^+ and Cl^- ions in a body fluid. Na^+ ions can leave a cell, provided that some other + ions enter: potassium (K^+) ions, for example. Table 12–2 shows that, indeed, the numbers of each kind of ion inside and outside cells differ over a wide range, but the + and − charges are perfectly balanced.

Inside the cells, in each liter of fluid, there are 150 K^+, 2 Ca^{++}, and 40 Mg^{++} charges for each 10 Na^+. (Chemists count these charges in milliequivalents, mEq.) The + charges total 202. The − charges inside the cells balance these perfectly. Outside the cells, the amounts of ions and their proportions differ from those inside, but again the + and − charges balance.

Electrolytes Attract Water Because electrolytes are charged, they attract water molecules, which are polar. Although each water molecule bears a net

Table 12–2

Important Body Electrolytes

Electrolyte	Extracelluar Concentration (mEq/L)	Intracellular Concentration (mEq/L)
Cations		
Sodium (Na^+)	142	10
Potassium (K^+)	5	150
Calcium (Ca^{++})	5	2
Magnesium (Mg^{++})	3	40
	155	202
Anions		
Chloride (Cl^-)	103	2
Bicarbonate (HCO_3^-)	27	10
Phosphate ($HPO_4^{=}$)	2	103
Sulfate ($SO_4^{=}$)	1	20
Organic acids (lactate, pyruvate)	6	10
Proteins	16	57
	155	202

Note: The number of positive and negative charges in a given fluid is the same. For example, in extracellular fluid, the cations and anions both equal 155 milliequivalents per liter (mEq/L). Of the cations, sodium ions make up 142 mEq/L; and potassium, calcium, and magnesium ions make up the remainder. Of the anions, chloride ions number 103 mEq/L; bicarbonate ions number 27; and the rest are provided by phosphate ions, sulfate ions, organic acids, and protein.

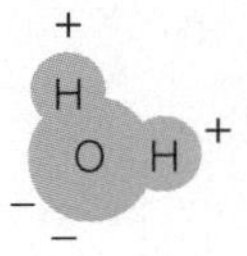

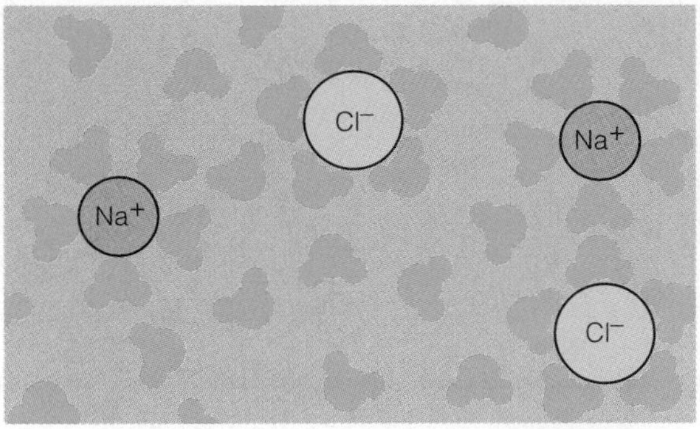

Water is polar, because the negatively charged electrons that bond the hydrogens to the oxygen spend most of their time near the oxygen atom. As a result, the oxygen is slightly negative, and the hydrogen is slightly positive (see Appendix B).

In an electrolyte solution, therefore, water molecules are attracted to both anions and cations. Notice that the negative oxygen atoms of the water molecules are drawn to the sodium cation (Na^+) here, while the positive sides of the water molecules are drawn to the chloride ions (Cl^-).

Figure 12–2

Water Dissolves Salts and Follows Electrolytes

The structural arrangement of the two hydrogen atoms and one oxygen atom enables water to dissolve solutes. Water's role as a solvent is one of its most valuable characteristics.

charge of zero, the oxygen side of the molecule is slightly negatively charged, and the hydrogens are slightly positively charged. Figure 12–2 shows the result in an electrolyte solution: both positive and negative ions attract clusters of water molecules around them. It is this attraction that dissolves salts in water and enables the body to move fluids into appropriate compartments.

Water Follows Electrolytes Some electrolytes reside primarily outside the cells (notably, sodium and chloride), and some predominate inside the cells (notably, potassium, magnesium, phosphate, and sulfate). Cells can move the electrolytes in and out, and water will follow them.

The statement that water follows salt means that a force moves water toward concentrated solutes. This force, known as osmotic pressure, moves water across a membrane whenever the solute concentrations on the two sides are not equal—the solutes themselves cannot cross the membrane. Figure 12–3 (on p. 436) shows this principle in operation.

Proteins Regulate Flow of Fluids and Ions Transport proteins in the cell membranes also regulate the passage of positive ions and other substances from one side of the membrane to the other. Negative ions follow positive ions, and water flows toward the more concentrated solution.

A well-understood member of this class of proteins is the sodium pump, an enzyme that pumps sodium out of cells faster than it can diffuse back in. Simultaneously, the enzyme pumps potassium ions the other way, into the cell. Figure 6–10 on p. 209 illustrates this action.

Maintenance of Fluid and Electrolyte Balance The amounts of various salts in the body must remain nearly constant. If salts are lost, they must be replaced from external sources—meaning foods and beverages. The body has discrete regulatory mechanisms to help ensure that the concentrations of all minerals stay within bounds. Regulation occurs chiefly at two sites: the GI tract and the kidneys.

The word ending **-ate** denotes a salt of the mineral.

solutes (SOLL-yutes)**:** the substances that are dissolved in a solution.

osmotic pressure: the pressure that develops when two solutions of different concentrations are separated by a membrane that permits water, but not the solutes, to cross. Water flows *toward* the side of the membrane on which the solutes are more concentrated.

The pump activity exchanges sodium for potassium across the cell membrane, maintaining a strong *concentration gradient* of each. Known as the **sodium-potassium pump**, it uses ATP (Chapter 7) as an energy source and the enzyme **sodium-potassium ATPase** (A-T-P-ace) to release that energy from ATP.

Figure 12–3

Osmotic Pressure

Water flows in the direction of the higher concentration of solute.

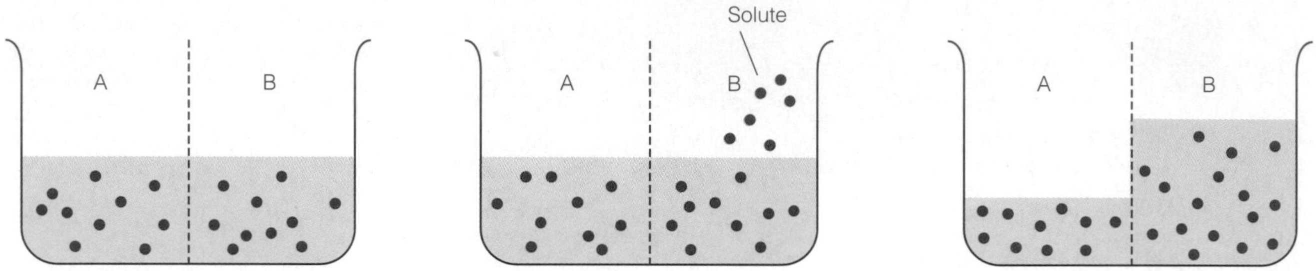

1. With equal numbers of solute particles on both sides, the concentrations are equal, and the tendency of water to move in either direction is about the same.
2. Now additional solute is added to side B. Solute cannot flow across the divider (in the case of a cell, its membrane).
3. Water can flow both ways across the divider, but has a greater tendency to move from side A to side B, where there is a greater concentration of solute. The volume of water becomes greater on side B, and the concentrations on sides A and B become equal.

Regulation by the GI Tract The GI tract continuously pours minerals out into its upper portions (stomach and small intestine) in the digestive juices and bile it secretes. It then reabsorbs these minerals and those from foods in its lower segment (the colon) as needed. In a day, 8 liters of fluids and associated minerals are recycled this way, providing ample opportunity for the regulation of electrolyte balance.

Regulation by the Kidneys The kidneys' control of the body's *water* content has already been described; the hormone ADH determines how much water the kidneys will release in urine and how much they will reabsorb into the bloodstream. To regulate the *electrolyte* contents, the kidneys depend on the adrenal glands, which send out the hormone aldosterone to convey messages. If the body's sodium is low, aldosterone promotes sodium reabsorption from the kidney tubules. As sodium is reabsorbed, potassium is excreted, obeying the rule that total positive charges must remain the same. (A review of kidney function may be helpful: see Figure 3–8 on p. 98.)

FLUID AND ELECTROLYTE IMBALANCE

Normally, the body defends itself successfully against fluid and electrolyte imbalances. However, a person may encounter situations of imbalance for which the cell membranes, kidneys, and thirst instinct cannot compensate. Vomiting, diarrhea, heavy sweating, burns, wounds, and the like may incur great fluid and electrolyte losses, precipitating a medical emergency.

The details of electrolyte balances are among the most important concepts that health care professionals must learn. They are emphasized in physiology courses and in medical and nursing curricula. Everyone, however, should appreciate the importance of the balance and the principles by which it is maintained. Knowledge of the situations that threaten fluid and electrolyte balance enables a person to take the appropriate action and seek medical help. People usually take water and salts for granted and ignore them, but the rapid loss of fluid and electrolytes can threaten life.

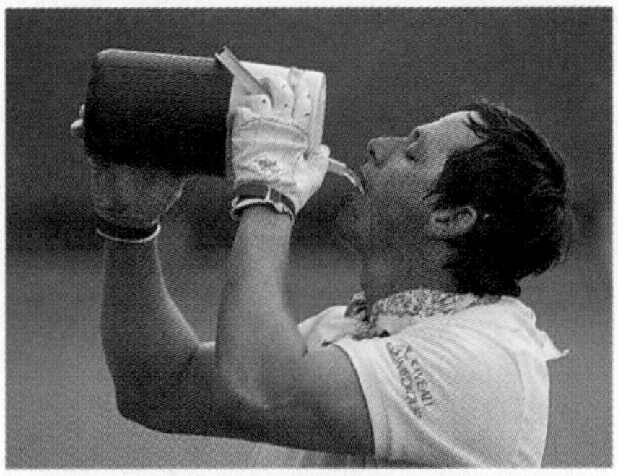

Physically active people must remember to replace their body fluids.

Sodium and Chloride Most Easily Lost Because sodium and chloride are the body's principal extracellular cation and anion, they are first to be lost when fluid is lost by sweating, bleeding, or renal or fecal excretion. It is no accident that after sweating excessively or losing fluid in other ways, a person craves salty foods and refreshing drinks.

Different Solutes Lost by Different Routes If fluid is lost by vomiting or diarrhea, sodium is lost indiscriminately. If the adrenal glands oversecrete aldosterone, as occurs when a tumor develops, the kidneys may excrete too much potassium. And the person with uncontrolled diabetes may lose a solute not normally excreted: glucose, and with it, large amounts of water. All three situations bring on dehydration, but just drinking water cannot restore balance. In each case, medical intervention is required.

Replacing Lost Fluids and Electrolytes In many cases, people can replace the fluids and minerals lost in sweat or in a temporary bout of diarrhea by drinking plain cool water and eating regular foods. (Chapter 14 presents the advantages and disadvantages of sport drinks, and Highlight 3 discusses diarrhea.) Some cases, however, demand rapid replacement of fluids and electrolytes—for example, when diarrhea threatens the life of a malnourished child.

Caretakers around the world have learned to use simple formulas to treat mild-to-moderate cases of diarrhea. These lifesaving formulas do not require hospitalization and can be prepared from ingredients available locally. Caretakers must only learn to measure ingredients carefully and use sanitary water. Once rehydrated, children can begin eating foods.

The administration of a simple solution of sugar, salt, and water, taken by mouth, to treat dehydration caused by diarrhea is called **oral rehydration therapy (ORT)**. A simple ORT recipe: 1 c boiling water.
2 tsp sugar.
A pinch of salt.

ACID-BASE BALANCE

The body uses its ions not only to help maintain water balance, but also to help regulate the acidity (pH) of its fluids. The pH scale of Chapter 3 is repeated here, in Figure 12–4, with the normal and abnormal pH ranges of body fluids added.

pH: a measure of the concentration of H^+ ions (see Appendix B). The lower the pH, the stronger the acid. Thus at pH 2, a solution is a strong acid, and at pH 6, a solution is a weak acid (pH 7 is neutral). A pH above 7 is alkaline, or base (a solution in which OH^- ions predominate).

Regulation by Buffers Some of the electrolyte mixtures in the body fluids, as well as some of the proteins, protect the body against changes in acidity by acting as buffers—substances that can neutralize acids or bases. The body's buffer systems serve as a first line of defense against changes in the fluids' acid-base balance.

Reminder: *Buffers* are compounds that help keep a solution's acidity or alkalinity constant. The buffering action of proteins is described in Chapter 6.

Regulation by Excretion The lungs, skin, GI tract, and kidneys provide other defenses. Carbon dioxide, which is formed all the time by cellular respiration, forms carbonic acid in the blood, pushing the balance toward acid. If too much acid builds up, the respiration rate speeds up, and more carbon dioxide is exhaled. If base builds up, the respiration rate slows; more carbon dioxide is retained and forms more carbonic acid. The skin can excrete acid in sweat, and

carbonic acid: a compound with the formula H_2CO_3 that results from the combination of carbon dioxide (CO_2) and water (H_2O), of particular importance in the body's buffer system.

Figure 12–4

The pH Scale
Note: Each step is ten times as concentrated in base (1/10 as much acid, or H^+) as the one below it.

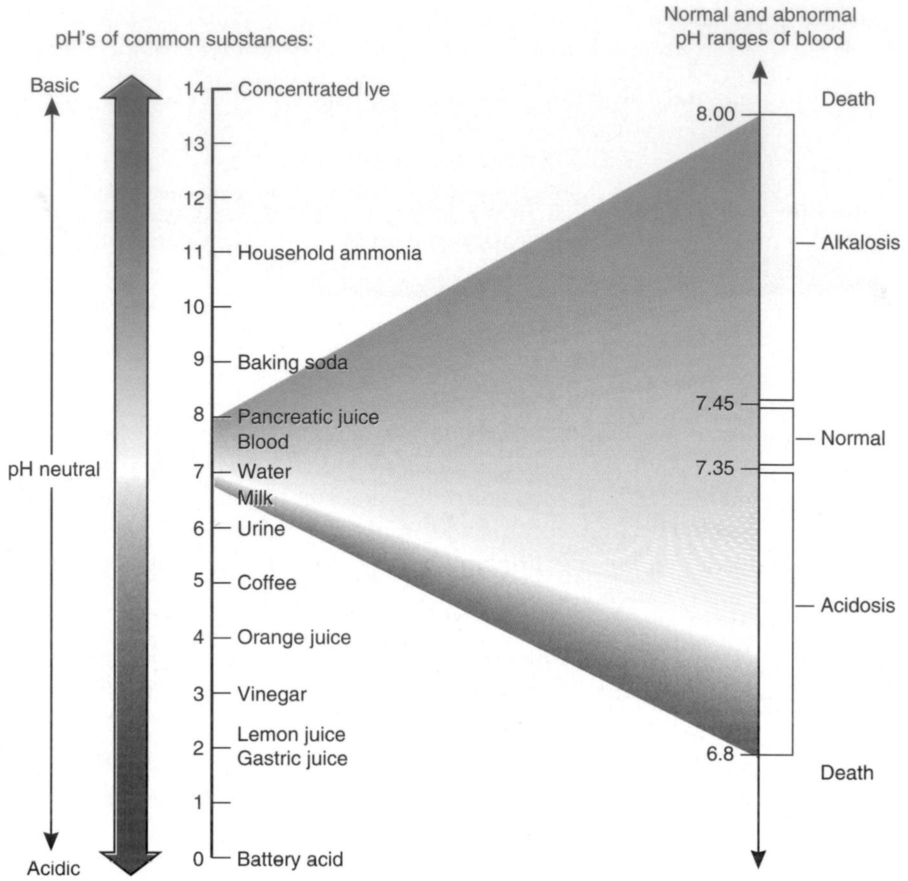

the specialized tear ducts can alter the composition of tears. These are of minor, although not negligible, importance; the kidneys play the primary role in maintaining acid-base balance.

Regulation by the Kidneys The kidneys adjust the acid-base balance by selecting which ions to retain and which to excrete. Their work is complex, but their net effect is easy to sum up. The *body's* total acid burden remains nearly constant; to a great extent, what a person ingests affects the acidity, not of the body, but of the *urine*.

In summary, water makes up about 60 percent of the body's weight. It assists with transportation of nutrients and waste products throughout the body, participates in chemical reactions, acts as a solvent, serves as a shock absorber, and regulates body temperature. To maintain water balance, intake from liquids, foods, and metabolism must equal losses from kidneys, skin, lungs, and feces. The antidiuretic hormone (ADH) signals the kidneys to retain water, and the hormone aldosterone causes the kidneys to retain sodium; together, they increase blood volume and restore normal blood pressure. Because water follows salt, electrolytes (charged minerals) in the fluids help distribute the fluids inside and outside of cells, thus ensuring the appropriate balance to support all life processes.

The Minerals—An Overview

Figure 12–5 shows the amounts of the major minerals and, for comparison, some of the trace minerals found in the body. The distinction between the major and trace minerals does not mean that one group is more important than the other—all are vital. The major minerals are so named because they are the minerals present, and needed, in the largest amounts in the body. The major minerals, sometimes referred to as macrominerals, are shown at the top of the figure and are discussed in this chapter. The trace minerals (shown at the bottom), sometimes referred to as microminerals, are discussed in Chapter 13.

A few generalizations pertain to all of the minerals and distinguish them from the vitamins. Especially notable is their chemical nature.

Reminder: *Minerals* are inorganic elements; some minerals are required in small amounts and are therefore essential nutrients.

major minerals: essential mineral nutrients found in the human body in amounts larger than 5 grams.

trace minerals: essential mineral nutrients found in the human body in amounts less than 5 grams.

Inorganic Elements Unlike the vitamins, which are organic compounds, minerals are inorganic elements that always retain their chemical identity. For example, iron may reversibly combine with other charged elements in salts, but it is always iron. Once minerals enter the body proper, they remain there until excreted; they cannot be changed into anything else. Neither can minerals be destroyed by heat, air, acid, or mixing; only a little care is needed to preserve minerals during food preparation. In fact, the ash that remains when a food is burned contains all the minerals that were in the food originally. Minerals can be lost from food only when they leach into water that is then thrown away.

The Body's Handling of Minerals The minerals also differ from the vitamins in the amounts the body can absorb and in the extent to which they must be specially handled. Some minerals are easily absorbed into the blood, transported freely, and readily excreted by the kidneys, much like the water-soluble vitamins. Some minerals are more like fat-soluble vitamins in that they must have carriers to be absorbed and transported. And, like the fat-soluble vitamins, minerals taken in excess can be toxic.

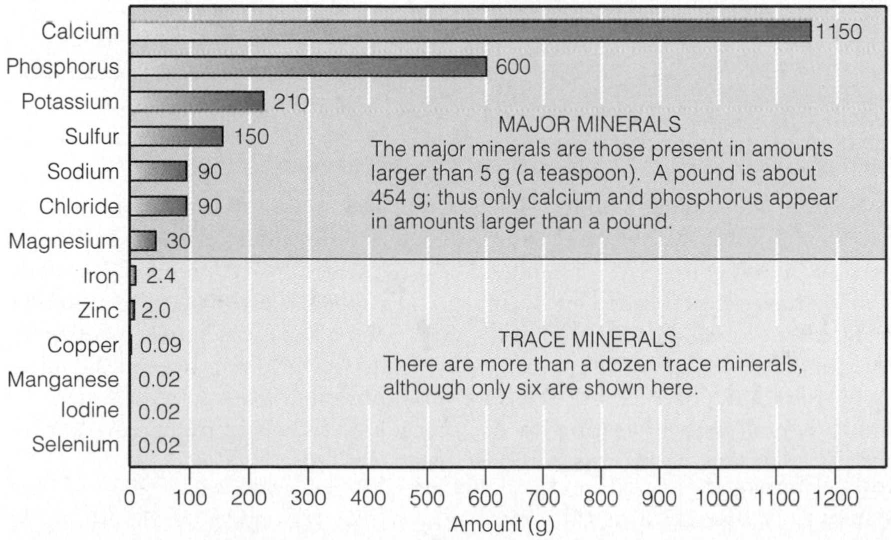

Figure 12–5

The Amounts of Minerals in a 60-kilogram (132-pound) Human Body

Reminder: *Bioavailability* refers to the rate and extent to which a nutrient is absorbed. Some nutrients are not readily released from foods during digestion or are not efficiently absorbed, which reduces their bioavailability.

binders: chemical compounds occurring in foods that can combine with nutrients (especially minerals) to form complexes the body cannot absorb. Examples of such binders include **phytic** (FIGHT-ic) **acid** and **oxalic** (ox-AL-ic) **acid**.

Variable Bioavailability Some foods contain binders that combine chemically with minerals, preventing their absorption and carrying them out of the body with other wastes. For example, phytic acid makes the calcium (as well as iron and zinc) in certain foods less available than it might be otherwise; oxalic acid also binds calcium and iron. Phytic acid is found primarily in legumes and grains; oxalic acid is present in rhubarb and spinach, among other foods.

To quickly review, the major minerals are found in larger quantities in the body, whereas the trace minerals occur in smaller amounts. Minerals are inorganic elements that retain their chemical identities; they usually receive special handling and regulation in the body; and they may bind with other substances, thus limiting their absorption.

While all the major minerals help to maintain the body's fluid balance described earlier, sodium, chloride, and potassium are most noted for that role. For this reason, these three minerals are discussed first here. Later sections describe the minerals most noted for their roles in bone growth and maintenance—calcium, phosphorus, and magnesium.

Sodium

People have held salt (sodium chloride) in high regard throughout recorded history. We say "you are the salt of the earth" to someone we admire and "you are not worth your salt" to someone we consider worthless. Even the word *salary* comes from the word salt.

sodium: the principal cation in the extracellular fluids of the body, critical to the maintenance of fluid balance, nerve transmissions, and muscle contractions.

Sodium Roles in the Body Sodium is the principal cation of the extracellular fluid and the primary regulator of its volume. Sodium also helps maintain acid-base balance and is essential to nerve transmission and muscle contraction.* Table 12–3 summarizes information about sodium.

Foods usually provide more sodium than the body needs. The intestinal tract absorbs sodium readily, and it travels freely in the blood, but the kidneys filter all the sodium out of the blood; then with great precision, they return to the bloodstream the exact amount the body needs. Normally, the amount excreted is approximately equal to the amount ingested on a given day. When blood sodium rises, as when a person eats salted foods, thirst signals the person to drink until the appropriate sodium-to-water ratio is restored. Then the kidneys secrete the extra water and the extra sodium together.

Sodium Recommendations Diets rarely lack sodium. For this reason, no RDA is set; instead, the Committee on Dietary Allowances estimated the *minimum* sodium requirement for adults to be 500 milligrams (0.5 grams). Similarly, Canada has not established an RNI for sodium, but has estimated the minimum requirement for adults to be 115 milligrams. Such differences between countries' recommendations are not unusual and typically reflect differences in judgment more than differences in research data. The minimum average requirement for adults without active sweating has been estimated to be 115 milligrams, but the

*One of the ways the kidneys regulate acid-base balance is by excreting hydrogen ions in exchange for sodium ions.

Table 12–3

Sodium—A Summary

Estimated Minimum Requirement	Chief Functions in the Body	Deficiency Symptoms	Toxicity Symptoms	Significant Sources
Adults: 500 mg/day	An electrolyte that maintains normal fluid and electrolyte balance; assists in nerve impulse transmission and muscle contraction	Muscle cramps, mental apathy, loss of appetite	Edema, acute hypertension	Table salt, soy sauce; moderate amounts in meats, milks, breads, and vegetables; large amounts in processed foods

U.S. Committee on Dietary Allowances set its recommendation slightly higher to accommodate a wide variety of physical activities and climates.

The *Diet and Health* recommendations, which emphasize moderation, not adequacy, advise limiting daily *salt* intake to less than 6 grams (the equivalent of 2.4 grams or 2400 milligrams *sodium*). Similarly, the American Heart Association recommends limiting sodium intake to 3 grams daily; people with mild-to-moderate hypertension may benefit from restriction to 2 grams of sodium daily.[3]

Salt (sodium chloride) is about 40% sodium.
1 g salt contributes 400 mg sodium.
5 g salt = 1 tsp.
1 tsp salt contributes 2000 mg sodium.

HEALTHY PEOPLE 2000: Decrease salt and sodium intake so at least 65% of home meal preparers prepare foods without adding salt, at least 80% of people avoid using salt at the table, and at least 40% of adults regularly purchase foods modified or lower in sodium.

Sodium and Hypertension For years, a high *sodium* intake was considered *the* primary factor responsible for high blood pressure. Then research pointed to *salt* (sodium chloride) as the dietary culprit. Salt has a greater effect on blood pressure than either sodium or chloride alone or in combination with other ions.[4]

Some individuals are genetically sensitive and experience high blood pressure from excesses in salt intake. People with chronic renal disease, those who have one or two parents with hypertension, blacks, and people over 50 years of age are most likely to be salt sensitive.* Salt avoidance promises to help prevent hypertension in salt-sensitive individuals, but for the majority of people with hypertension, salt restriction does not lower blood pressure. The most effective dietary treatment for hypertension is weight loss.

Sodium Intakes Cultures vary in their use of salt. The most recent food intake survey in the United States estimates that men consume an average of 3300 milligrams of sodium (equivalent to 8 grams of salt) a day, which is slightly more than the American Heart Association recommends.[5] Asian people, whose staple sauces and flavorings are based on soy sauce and monosodium glutamate (MSG), consume the equivalent of about 30 to 40 grams of salt per day. In

*Salt-sensitive individuals have elevated concentrations of renin in their blood, compared with others.

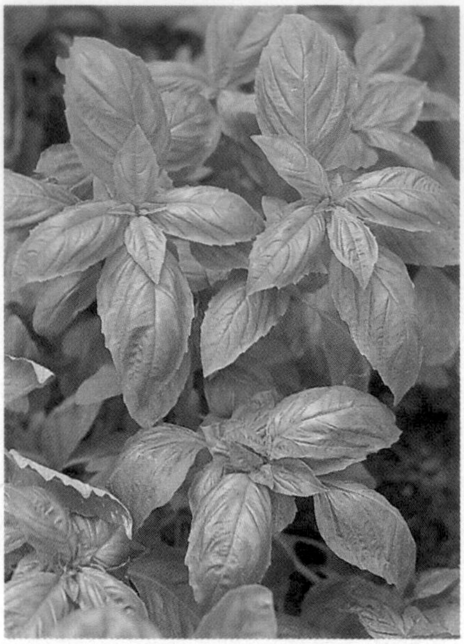

Fresh herbs add flavor to a recipe without adding salt.

China, Japan, and Korea, the prevalence of high blood pressure is equal to or greater than that of the United States.[6]

Sodium in Foods In general, processed foods have the most sodium, while unprocessed foods such as fresh fruits and vegetables have the least. In fact, as much as 75 percent of the sodium in people's diets comes from salt added to foods by manufacturers; about 15 percent comes from salt added during cooking and at the table; and only 10 percent comes from the natural salt in foods.[7]

Because processed foods may contain sodium without chloride, as in additives such as sodium bicarbonate or sodium saccharin, they do not always taste salty. Most people are surprised to learn that 1 ounce of cornflakes (a 1¼-cup serving) contains more sodium than 1 ounce of salted peanuts—and that ½ cup of instant chocolate pudding contains still more. (A reason the peanuts taste saltier is that the salt is all on the surface, where the tongue's sensors immediately pick it up.)

Figure 12–6 shows that processed foods contain not only more sodium but also less potassium than their less-processed counterparts. Low potassium may be as significant as excess sodium when it comes to blood pressure regulation, so these foods have two strikes against them. The accompanying box offers strategies for

How to Cut Salt Intake

Most people eat more salt and sodium than they need, and some people can lower their blood pressure by avoiding highly salted foods and removing the saltshaker from the table. Foods eaten without salt may seem less tasty at first, but with repetition, people can learn to enjoy the natural flavors of many unsalted foods. Strategies to cut salt intake include:

- Cook with only small amounts of added salt.
- Prepare foods with sodium-free spices such as basil, bay leaves, curry, garlic, ginger, lemon, mint, oregano, pepper, rosemary, and thyme.
- Add little or no salt at the table.
- Read labels with an eye open for salt. (See Table 2–11 on p. 68 for terms used to describe the sodium contents of foods on labels.)
- Eat high-salt foods in moderation and use low-salt or salt-free products regularly.

Use these foods sparingly:

- Foods prepared in brine, such as pickles, olives, and sauerkraut.
- Salty or smoked meats, such as bologna, corned or chipped beef, frankfurters, ham, lunch meats, salt pork, sausage, and smoked tongue.
- Salty or smoked fish, such as anchovies, caviar, salted and dried cod, herring, sardines, and smoked salmon.
- Snack items such as potato chips, pretzels, salted popcorn, salted nuts, and crackers.
- Bouillon cubes; seasoned salts; soy, Worcestershire, and barbeque sauces.
- Cheeses, especially processed types.
- Canned and instant soups.
- Prepared horseradish, catsup, and mustard.

cutting sodium/salt intake. Chapter 18 reviews the research on sodium, potassium, and hypertension in relation to heart disease.

Sodium Deficiency Overly strict use of low-sodium diets in the treatment of hypertension, kidney disease, or heart disease can deplete the body of needed

Note how potassium is lost and sodium is gained as foods become more processed.

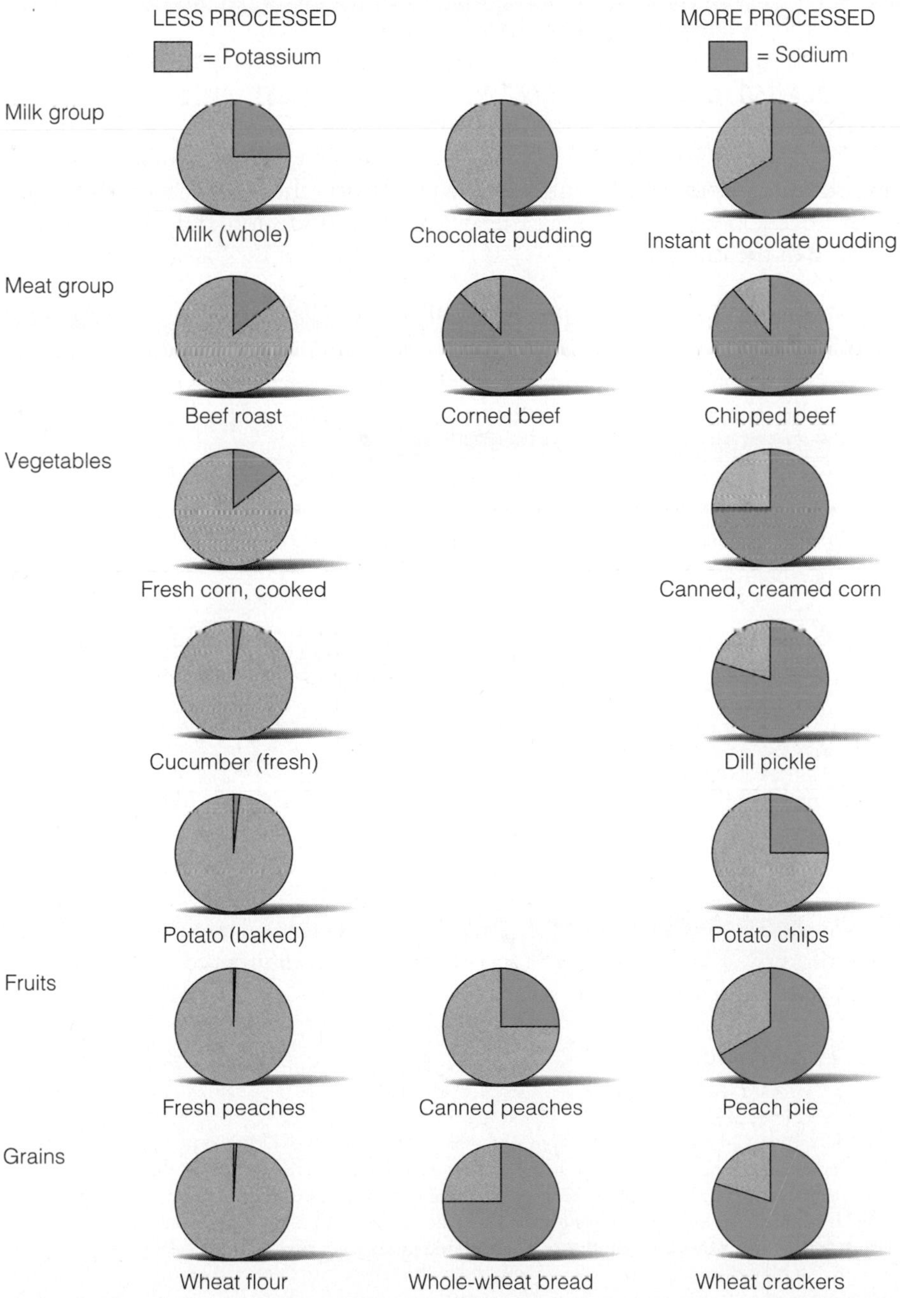

Figure 12–6

What Processing Does to the Sodium and Potassium Contents of Foods

People who eat foods high in salt often happen to be eating fewer potassium-containing foods at the same time. Note how the *same* food loses potassium and gains sodium as it goes through processing, so that its potassium-to-sodium ratio falls dramatically. Limiting sodium intake may help in two ways, then—by lowering blood pressure in salt-sensitive individuals and by indirectly raising potassium intakes in all individuals.

sodium. Vomiting, diarrhea, or heavy sweating can, too. If blood sodium drops, both sodium and water must be replenished. Under normal conditions of sweating due to exercise, salt losses can easily be replaced later in the day with ordinary foods. Salt tablets are not recommended because too much salt, especially if taken with too little water, can induce dehydration.

Sodium Toxicity The immediate symptoms of acute sodium toxicity are edema and hypertension, but such toxicity is not a problem as long as water needs are met. Prolonged excessive sodium intake, especially when the sodium is derived from salt, may be related to the development of hypertension in sensitive people, as explained earlier.

Chloride

The element *chlorine* (Cl_2), is a poisonous gas. When chlorine reacts with sodium or hydrogen, however, it forms the negative chloride ion (Cl^-). *Chloride* is required in the diet.

chloride: the major anion in the extracellular fluids of the body. Chloride is the ionic form of chlorine, Cl^-; see Appendix B for a description of the chlorine-to-chloride conversion.

Chloride Roles in the Body Chloride is the major anion of the extracellular fluids, where it occurs mostly in association with sodium (Table 12–4 summarizes information on chloride). Chloride can move freely across membranes and so also associates with potassium inside cells. Like sodium, chloride is critical to maintaining fluid and electrolyte balance.

In the stomach, the chloride ion is part of hydrochloric acid, which maintains the strong acidity of the gastric juice. One of the most serious consequences of vomiting is the loss of this acid from the stomach, which upsets the acid-base balance.*

Reminder: The loss of acid can lead to *alkalosis*, an above-normal alkalinity in the blood and body fluids.

Chloride Recommendations and Intakes Chloride is abundant in foods (especially processed foods) as part of sodium chloride and other salts. The Committee on Dietary Allowances has not set an RDA for chloride, but has estimated a minimum requirement for adults.

Chloride Deficiency and Toxicity Diets rarely lack chloride. A case is on record in which chloride was omitted from an infant formula and the deficiency caused illness and death before it was discovered. Chloride losses may occur in sodium-depleting conditions such as heavy sweating or chronic diarrhea and vomiting. The only known cause of high blood chloride concentrations is dehydration due to water deficiency.[8] In both cases, consuming ordinary foods and beverages can restore chloride balance.

---

*Hydrochloric acid secretion into the stomach involves the addition of bicarbonate ions to the plasma. These bicarbonate ions are neutralized by hydrogen ions from the gastric secretions that are reabsorbed into the plasma. When hydrochloric acid is lost during vomiting, these hydrogen ions are no longer available for reabsorption, which in effect increases the concentration of bicarbonate ions in the plasma. In this way, excessive vomiting of acidic gastric juices leads to *metabolic alkalosis*.

Table 12–4
Chloride—A Summary

Estimated Minimum Requirement	Chief Functions in the Body	Deficiency Symptoms	Toxicity Symptoms	Significant Sources
Adults: 750 mg/day	An electrolyte that maintains normal fluid and electrolyte balance; part of hydrochloric acid found in the stomach, necessary for proper digestion	Do not occur under normal circumstances	Vomiting	Table salt, soy sauce; moderate amounts in meats, milks, eggs; large amounts in processed foods

Potassium

Like sodium, potassium is a positively charged ion. In contrast to sodium, potassium is the body's principal cation *inside* the body cells.

potassium: the principal cation within the body's cells, critical to the maintenance of fluid balance, nerve transmissions, and muscle contractions.

Potassium Roles in the Body Potassium plays a major role in maintaining fluid and electrolyte balance and cell integrity. During nerve transmission and muscle contraction, potassium and sodium briefly trade places across the cell membrane. The cell then quickly pumps them back into place. The control of potassium distribution is a high priority for the body because it affects many aspects of homeostasis, including a steady heartbeat.

Potassium Recommendations and Intakes As for sodium and chloride, the Committee on Dietary Allowances has estimated a minimum potassium requirement for adults. Potassium is abundant inside all living cells, both plant and animal. Because cells remain intact unless foods are processed, the richest sources of potassium are *fresh* foods of all kinds, as Figure 12–7 shows. People who emphasize fresh fruits and vegetables in their diets have intakes as high as 11 grams per day, but toxicity is normally not a concern when the source is foods.[9]

Fresh foods, especially fruits, contain much more potassium than sodium. In contrast, most processed foods such as canned vegetables, ready-to-eat cereals, and luncheon meats contain more sodium and less potassium (recall Figure 12–6).

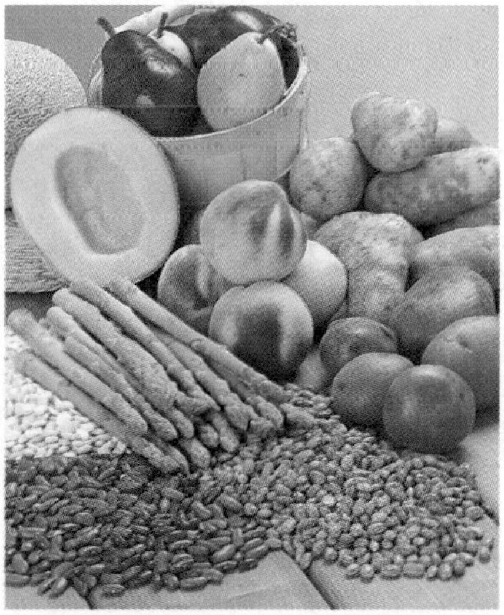

Fresh fruits and vegetables provide potassium in abundance.

Potassium and Hypertension Some authorities believe that potassium might both prevent and help to correct hypertension. Low-potassium-diets raise blood pressure in men with normal blood pressure and in those who are hypertensive, whereas a high potassium intake seems to protect against stroke.

Potassium Deficiency A dietary deficiency of potassium is unlikely, but with a regular diet low in fresh fruits and vegetables, it is possible. Potassium deficiency occurs more often due to excessive losses than to deficient intakes. Conditions such as diabetic acidosis, dehydration, or prolonged vomiting or diarrhea can create a potassium deficiency, as can the regular use of certain drugs, includ-

Figure 12–7 Potassium in Selected Foods

Food	Serving size (kcalories)
Bread, whole wheat	1 slice (64 kcal)
Corn flakes, fortified	1 oz (108 kcal)
White rice	1/2 c cooked (134 kcal)
Spaghetti pasta	1/2 c cooked (99 kcal)
Oatmeal	1/2 c cooked (73 kcal)
Tortilla, flour	1 8"-round (115 kcal)
Spinach	1 c raw (12 kcal)
Broccoli	1/2 c cooked (22 kcal)
Carrots	1/2 c shredded raw (24 kcal)
Green peas	1/2 c cooked (62 kcal)
Corn	1/2 c cooked (66 kcal)
Green beans	1/2 c cooked (22 kcal)
Sweet potatoes	1/2 c cooked (117 kcal)
Potato	1 baked w/skin (220 kcal)
Tomato juice	3/4 c (31 kcal)
Apple	1 medium raw (81 kcal)
Banana	1 medium raw (104 kcal)
Orange	1 medium raw (62 kcal)
Strawberries	1/2 c fresh (23 kcal)
Raisins	1/4 c (109 kcal)
Watermelon	1 slice (154 kcal)
Grapefruit juice	3/4 c fresh (72 kcal)
Avocado	1/4 (85 kcal)
Milk	1 c low-fat 2% (121 kcal)
Yogurt, plain	1 c low-fat (143 kcal)
Cheddar cheese	1 1/2 oz (171 kcal)
Cottage cheese	1/2 c low-fat 2% (101 kcal)
Swiss cheese	1 1/2 oz (159 kcal)
Ice cream	1/2 c, 10% fat (134 kcal)
Navy beans	1/2 c cooked (129 kcal)
Pinto beans	1/2 c cooked (117 kcal)
Kidney beans	1/2 c cooked (109 kcal)
Garbanzo beans	1/2 c cooked (134 kcal)
Peanut butter	2 tbs (190 kcal)
Sunflower seeds	1 oz dry (159 kcal)
Tofu (soybean curd)	1/2 c (94 kcal)
Shrimp	3 oz boiled (85 kcal)
Ground beef, lean	3 oz broiled (239 kcal)
Chicken breast	3 oz roasted (141 kcal)
Cod	3 oz poached (88 kcal)
Ham, lean	3 oz roasted (123 kcal)
Sirloin steak, lean	3 oz broiled (171 kcal)
Tuna, canned in water	3 oz (99 kcal)
Bologna, beef	2 slices (144 kcal)
Egg	1 hard cooked (77 kcal)
Additional 5 foods:	
Acorn squash	1/2 c baked (68 kcal)
Soybeans	1/2 c cooked (149 kcal)
Artichoke	1 (60 kcal)
Pomegranate	1 (105 kcal)
Buttermilk, nonfat	1 c (99 kcal)

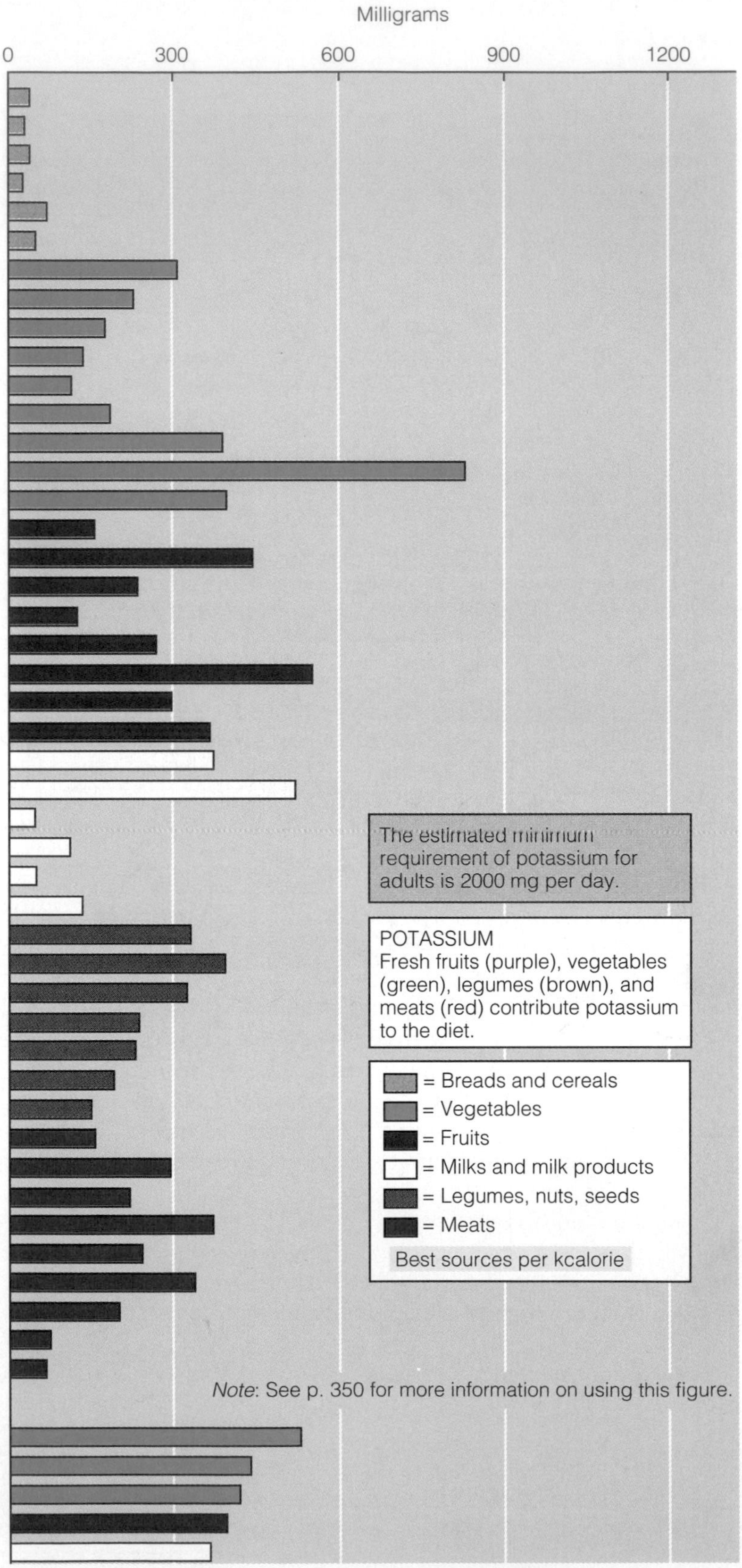

Note: See p. 350 for more information on using this figure.

Table 12–5

Potassium—A Summary

Adult Estimated Minimum Requirement	Chief Functions in the Body	Deficiency Symptoms[a]	Toxicity Symptoms	Significant Sources
2000 mg/day	An electrolyte that maintains normal fluid and electrolyte balance; facilitates many reactions; supports cell integrity; assists in nerve impulse transmission and muscle contractions	Muscular weakness, paralysis, confusion	Muscular weakness; vomiting; if given into a vein, can stop the heart	All whole foods: meats, milks, fruits, vegetables, grains, legumes

[a]Deficiency accompanies dehydration.

ing diuretics, steroids, and strong laxatives.* For this reason, many physicians prescribe potassium supplements along with drugs. One of the earliest symptoms of deficiency is muscle weakness. Table 12–5 summarizes facts about potassium.

Potassium Toxicity Potassium toxicity can result from the overuse of potassium salt, especially in an infant or a person with heart disease; it does not result from overeating foods high in potassium. Given more potassium than the body needs, the kidneys accelerate excretion. If the GI tract is bypassed, however, and potassium is injected rapidly into a vein, it can stop the heart.

To summarize, the electrolytes primarily responsible for maintaining fluid balance are sodium, chloride, and potassium. Sodium is the main cation outside cells; dietary deficiency is rare, and excesses may aggravate hypertension in some people. The kidneys regulate blood sodium in response to hormonal signals from ADH and aldosterone. Chloride is the major anion outside cells, and it associates closely with sodium. In addition to its role in fluid balance, chloride is part of the stomach's hydrochloric acid, which facilitates protein digestion and iron absorption. Potassium is the primary cation inside cells; fresh fruits and vegetables are its best sources.

Calcium

Calcium is the most abundant mineral in the body. It receives much emphasis in this chapter and in the highlight that follows because an adequate intake early in life helps grow a healthy skeleton and minimize bone loss in later life. Calcium's roles, deficiency symptoms, and food sources appear in Table 12–6.

calcium: the most abundant mineral in the body, found primarily in the body's bones and teeth.

*People using diuretics to control hypertension should know that some cause potassium excretion and can induce a deficiency. Those using these drugs must be particularly careful to include rich sources of potassium in their daily diets. (Some diuretics are designed to spare potassium.)

Table 12–6

Calcium—A Summary

Adult RDA	Chief Functions in the Body	Deficiency Symptoms	Toxicity Symptoms	Significant Sources
1200 mg/day (19–24 yr) 800 mg/day (25 and older)	The principal mineral of bones and teeth; also involved in muscle contraction and relaxation, nerve functioning, blood clotting, blood pressure, and immune defenses	Stunted growth in children; bone loss (osteoporosis) in adults	Constipation; increased risk of urinary stone formation and kidney dysfunction; interference with absorption of other minerals	Milk and milk products, small fish (with bones), tofu (bean curd), greens (broccoli, chard), legumes

Figure 12–8

A Tooth

The inner layer of dentin is a bonelike material that forms on a protein (collagen) matrix, which requires a variety of substances, including vitamin C, for proper formation. The outer layer of enamel is harder than bone and forms on a protein (keratin) matrix, which depends in part on vitamin A for its synthesis. Both dentin and enamel contain **hydroxyapatite** (high-drox-ee-APP-ah-tite), crystals made of calcium and phosphorus. The crystals of enamel may become even harder when exposed to the trace mineral fluoride.

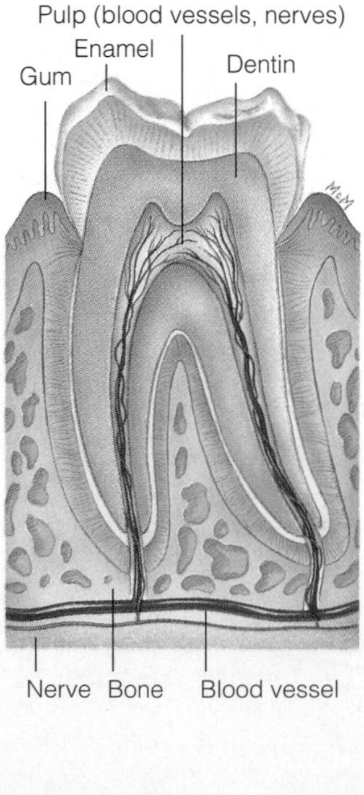

CALCIUM ROLES IN THE BODY

Ninety-nine percent of the body's calcium is in the bones, where it plays two roles. First, it is an integral part of bone structure, providing a rigid frame that holds the body upright and serves as attachment points for muscles, making motion possible. Second, it serves as a calcium bank, offering a readily available source of the mineral to the body fluids should a drop in blood calcium occur.

Calcium in Bones Many people have the idea that once a bone is built, it is inert like a rock. Actually, the bones are in a state of constant flux, with formation and dissolution simultaneously taking place. As bones begin to form, calcium salts form crystals on a matrix of the protein collagen. These crystals, called hydroxyapatite, invade the collagen and gradually lend more and more strength and rigidity to the maturing bones until they are able to support the weight they will have to carry. Thus the long leg bones of children can support their weight by the time they have learned to walk.

The formation of teeth follows a pattern similar to that of bones. Hydroxyapatite crystals form on a collagen matrix to create the dentin that gives strength to the teeth (see Figure 12–8). The turnover of minerals in teeth is not as rapid as in bone, but some withdrawal and redepositing does take place throughout life. Fluoride hardens and stabilizes the crystals of teeth, opposing the withdrawal of minerals from them.

Calcium in Body Fluids The 1 percent of the body's calcium that circulates in the fluids as ionized calcium is vital to life. The calcium ion participates in the regulation of muscle contraction, the clotting of blood, the transmission of nerve impulses, the secretion of hormones, and the activation of some enzyme reactions.

Calcium also serves as a cofactor in a protein that helps convey signals, received at the cell surface, to the inside of the cell. The protein that relays these messages is calmodulin. Several of the messages it delivers help to maintain normal blood pressure.

Calcium and Disease Prevention Calcium may be useful in both preventing and treating hypertension. Epidemiological studies show that low dietary calcium correlates with a high prevalence of hypertension.[10] Reports that an increase in calcium intake can lower blood pressure in people with and without hypertension further support this hypothesis. Some evidence also suggests relationships between dietary calcium and blood cholesterol, diabetes, and cancer.[11]

calmodulin (cal-MOD-you-lin): an inactive protein that becomes active when bound to calcium; then it becomes a messenger that tells other proteins what to do. The system serves as interpreter for hormone- and nerve-mediated messages arriving at cells.

Calcium Balance Calcium homeostasis is one of the body's highest priorities and involves a system of hormones and vitamin D that promotes calcium deposits into bone whenever blood calcium rises too high. Whenever blood calcium falls too low, three organ systems may raise it:

- Intestines: absorb more calcium.
- Bones: release more calcium.
- Kidneys: excrete less calcium.

Thus blood calcium can return to normal. Figure 12–9 illustrates how hormones regulate blood calcium.

The calcium in bone provides a nearly inexhaustible bank of calcium for the blood. The blood borrows and returns calcium as needed, so that even with a dietary deficiency, blood calcium remains normal—even as bone calcium diminishes. Blood calcium changes only in response to abnormal regulatory control, not to diet. This makes a developing calcium deficiency completely silent. A per-

The hormones **parathormone** (PAIR-ah-THOR-moan) from the parathyroid and **calcitonin** (KAL-see-TOE-nin) from the thyroid glands, as well as vitamin D, regulate calcium balance. Parathormone raises blood calcium, while calcitonin lowers it by inhibiting release of calcium from bone. **Vitamin D** raises blood calcium by acting at the three sites listed.

Figure 12–9

Calcium Balance in Bone

Blood calcium is regulated in part by vitamin D and two hormones—calcitonin and parathormone. Bone serves as a source of calcium when blood calcium is low and as a reservoir when blood calcium is high. Osteoclasts break down bone and release calcium into the blood; osteoblasts build new bone using calcium from the blood.

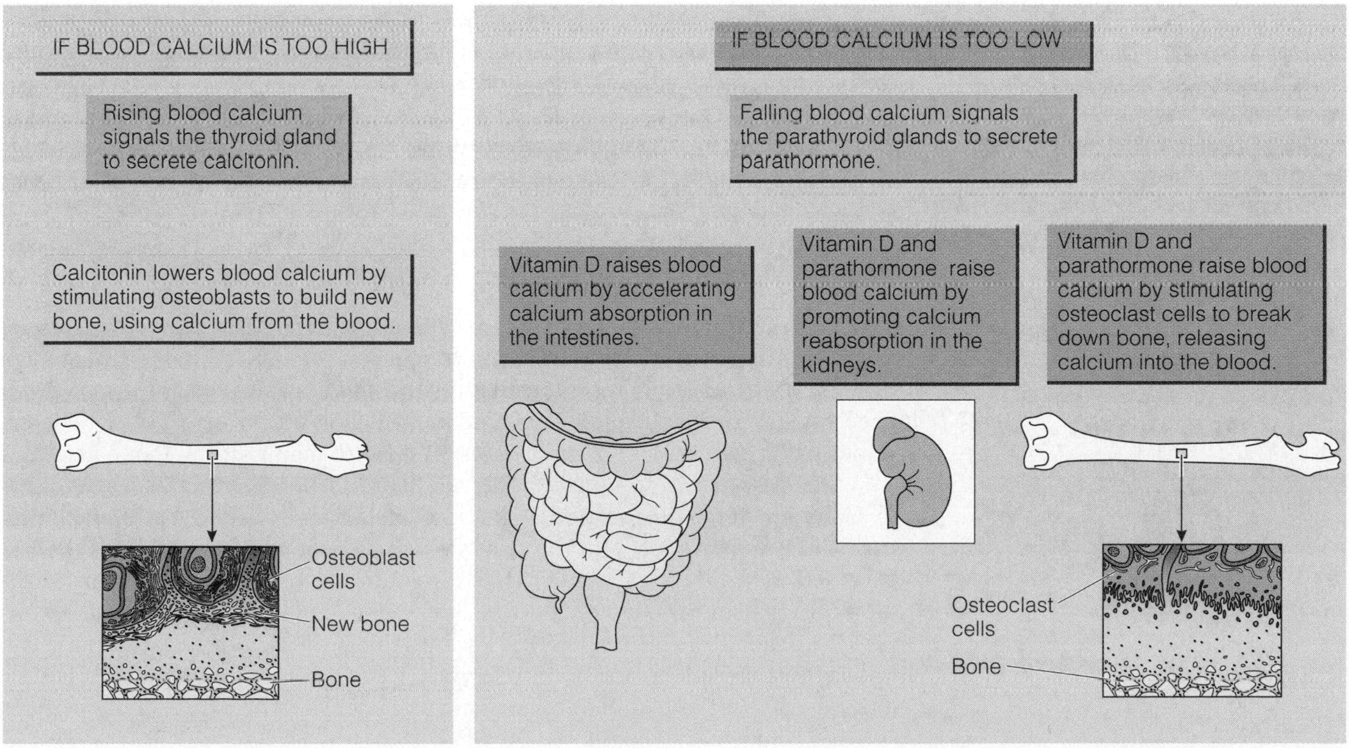

IF BLOOD CALCIUM IS TOO HIGH
Rising blood calcium signals the thyroid gland to secrete calcitonin.
Calcitonin lowers blood calcium by stimulating osteoblasts to build new bone, using calcium from the blood.
Osteoblast cells
New bone
Bone
IF BLOOD CALCIUM IS TOO LOW
Falling blood calcium signals the parathyroid glands to secrete parathormone.
Vitamin D raises blood calcium by accelerating calcium absorption in the intestines.
Vitamin D and parathormone raise blood calcium by promoting calcium reabsorption in the kidneys.
Vitamin D and parathormone raise blood calcium by stimulating osteoclast cells to break down bone, releasing calcium into the blood.
Osteoclast cells
Bone

son can have an inadequate calcium intake for years and suffer no noticeable symptoms. Only late in life does it become apparent that the integrity of the bones has been compromised.

calcium rigor: hardness or stiffness of the muscles caused by high blood calcium concentrations.

calcium tetany (TET-ah-nee): intermittent spasm of the extremities due to nervous and muscular excitability caused by low blood calcium concentrations.

Blood calcium above normal results in calcium rigor; the muscles contract and cannot relax. Similarly, blood calcium below normal causes calcium tetany—also characterized by uncontrolled muscle contraction. These conditions do *not* reflect a *dietary* excess or lack of calcium; they are caused by a lack of vitamin D or by abnormal secretion of the regulatory hormones. A chronic *dietary* deficiency of calcium, or a chronic deficiency due to poor absorption over the years, depletes the savings account in the bones. Again: it is the *bones*, not the blood, that are robbed by calcium deficiency.

calcium-binding protein: a protein in the intestinal cells, made with the help of vitamin D, that facilitates calcium absorption.

Calcium Absorption Many factors affect calcium absorption, but on the average, adults absorb about 30 percent of the calcium they ingest. The stomach's acidity helps to keep calcium soluble, and absorption is enhanced when calcium is consumed with a meal. Vitamin D helps the absorptive cells of the GI tract to make the necessary calcium-binding protein. It is no accident that calcium-rich milk is the chosen vehicle for fortification with vitamin D. The lactose in milk also enhances calcium absorption. Also, calcium seems to be better absorbed if accompanied by an approximately equal amount of phosphorus.

The body regulates calcium absorption by altering its production of the calcium-binding protein, making more if more calcium is needed. The result is obvious in the case of a pregnant woman, who absorbs 50 percent of the calcium from the milk she drinks. Similarly, growing children absorb 50 to 60 percent of ingested calcium. Then, when their bones' growth slows or stops, their absorption falls to the adult level of about 30 percent. In addition, calcium absorption is more efficient at low intakes than at high intakes.

Reminder: Phytate and oxalate are *binders* that combine with minerals to form complexes that the body cannot absorb. Phytates are common in cereal grain husks; oxalates occur in beets, rhubarb, spinach, and peanuts.

Many of the conditions that enhance calcium absorption hinder its absorption when they are absent. For example, sufficient vitamin D supports absorption, while a deficiency impairs it. In addition, fiber, in general, and phytate and oxalate, in particular, interfere with calcium absorption, but their effects are relatively minor at intakes typical of U.S. diets. Vegetables with oxalates and whole grains with phytates are nutritious foods, of course, but they are not useful calcium sources. Table 12–7 summarizes the factors influencing calcium absorption.

CALCIUM RECOMMENDATIONS AND INTAKES

The ideal calcium intake for people is difficult to determine. Calcium is unlike most other nutrients, in that its blood concentration does not reflect the body's calcium status. Calcium recommendations are therefore arrived at by way of balance studies. These studies, which measure daily absorption and excretion, determine how much calcium must be ingested daily to maintain calcium balance.

Calcium Recommendations Because obtaining enough calcium during early life helps to ensure that the skeleton will be strong and dense, the RDA has been set high at 1200 milligrams daily for adults up to the age of 24 years. Such an intake is hard to achieve, since the best source, milk, has only 300 milligrams per cup. After 24 years, the RDA is lowered to 800 milligrams a day because the opportunity to build strong bones may have passed and the lower amount is considered sufficient to maintain bone tissue. For later life, the RDA should perhaps

Table 12–7

Factors Influencing Calcium Absorption

Calcium absorption is a complex process that is influenced to various degrees by several dietary and physiological factors.

Factors That Promote Calcium Absorption	Factors That Interfere with Calcium Absorption
• Hormones that promote growth.	• Diminished absorption with aging.
• Ingestion with a meal; stomach acid.	• Lack of stomach acid.
• Vitamin D.	• Vitamin D deficiency.
• Lactose.	• High phosphorus intake.
• Phosphorus in an optimal ratio.	• High-fiber diet.
	• Phytates and oxalates.
	• High protein intake.

be raised again to minimize the bone loss that tends to occur late in life. Some authorities advocate as much as 1500 milligrams a day for women over 50. Many people in the United States and Canada, particularly women, have calcium intakes below current recommendations.

Unfortunately, many people perceive milk as fattening and omit it from their diets in their attempts to lose weight. Whole milk and many cheeses are high in fat, but low-fat options are available and many people have switched from whole milk to nonfat or low-fat milk and milk products.[12] Such choices help a person both meet calcium needs and stay within a reasonable energy and fat allowance.

Recommended daily milk servings:

- Children: 2 c
- Teenagers: 3 c
- Adults: 2 c
- Pregnant or lactating women: 3 c
- Pregnant or lactating teens: 4 c

Internationally, calcium recommendations vary widely. Calcium intakes are low in most of the world, but given long times to adjust, adults can adapt to very low intakes. The World Health Organization recommends only 400 to 500 milligrams per day for adults. Protein intakes are also low in most of the world. As Chapter 6 mentioned, high protein intakes seem to accelerate calcium excretion, and so perhaps the higher intakes of protein by North Americans warrant the setting of higher calcium allowances.

HEALTHY PEOPLE 2000: Increase calcium intake so that at least 50% of people aged 25 years and older consume two or more servings of calcium-rich foods daily.

Calcium Sources Figure 12–10 shows that calcium is found most abundantly in a single class of foods—milk and milk products. For this reason, dietary recommendations advise daily consumption of low- or nonfat milk products. Milk offers about 300 milligrams of calcium per cup, so an adult who drinks 2 to 3 cups of milk a day should have no problem meeting calcium needs, given the additional contributions from other foods; teenagers and young adults need 3 to 4 cups of milk daily. The word *daily* should be stressed because the body has a limited ability to absorb calcium, and so needs frequent opportunities to take in small amounts. The consumption of *milk* products, not just *dairy* products, should also be stressed. Dairy products such as butter and cream are milk fats that contain negligible calcium because calcium is not soluble in fat.

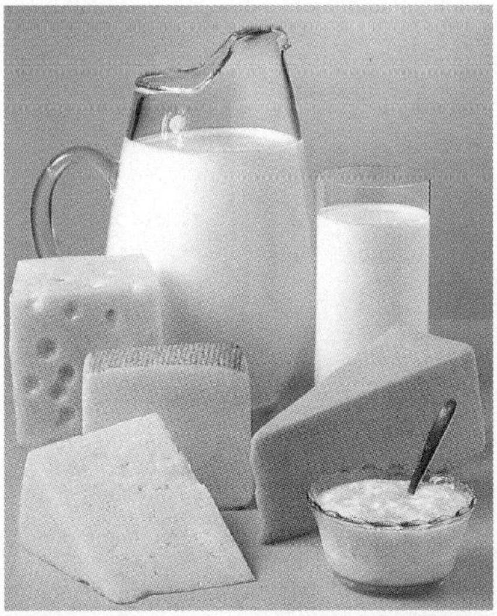

Milk and milk products are rightly famous for their calcium contents.

Figure 12–10 Calcium in Selected Foods

Food	Serving size (kcalories)
Bread, whole wheat	1 slice (64 kcal)
Corn flakes, fortified	1 oz (108 kcal)
White rice	1/2 c cooked (134 kcal)
Spaghetti pasta	1/2 c cooked (99 kcal)
Oatmeal	1/2 c cooked (73 kcal)
Tortilla, flour	1 8"-round (115 kcal)
Spinach[a]	1 c raw (12 kcal)
Broccoli	1/2 c cooked (22 kcal)
Carrots	1/2 c shredded raw (24 kcal)
Green peas	1/2 c cooked (62 kcal)
Corn	1/2 c cooked (66 kcal)
Green beans	1/2 c cooked (22 kcal)
Sweet potatoes	1/2 c cooked (117 kcal)
Potato	1 baked w/skin (220 kcal)
Tomato juice	3/4 c (31 kcal)
Apple	1 medium raw (81 kcal)
Banana	1 medium raw (104 kcal)
Orange	1 medium raw (62 kcal)
Strawberries	1/2 c fresh (23 kcal)
Raisins	1/4 c (109 kcal)
Watermelon	1 slice (154 kcal)
Grapefruit juice	3/4 c fresh (72 kcal)
Avocado	1/4 (85 kcal)
Milk	1 c low-fat 2% (121 kcal)
Yogurt, plain	1 c low-fat (143 kcal)
Cheddar cheese	1½ oz (171 kcal)
Cottage cheese	1/2 c low-fat 2% (101 kcal)
Swiss cheese	1 1/2 oz (159 kcal)
Ice cream	1/2 c, 10% fat (134 kcal)
Navy beans	1/2 c cooked (129 kcal)
Pinto beans	1/2 c cooked (117 kcal)
Kidney beans	1/2 c cooked (109 kcal)
Garbanzo beans	1/2 c cooked (134 kcal)
Peanut butter	2 tbs (190 kcal)
Sunflower seeds	1 oz dry (159 kcal)
Tofu (soybean curd)[b]	1/2 c (94 kcal)
Shrimp	3 oz boiled (85 kcal)
Ground beef, lean	3 oz broiled (239 kcal)
Chicken breast	3 oz roasted (141 kcal)
Cod	3 oz poached (88 kcal)
Ham, lean	3 oz roasted (123 kcal)
Sirloin steak, lean	3 oz broiled (171 kcal)
Tuna, canned in water	3 oz (99 kcal)
Bologna, beef	2 slices (144 kcal)
Egg	1 hard cooked (77 kcal)
Additional 5 foods:	
Sardines, with bones[c]	3 oz canned (117 kcal)
Molasses, blackstrap[d]	1 tbs (47 kcal)
Pudding	1/2 c (148 kcal)
Bok choy (Chinese cabbage)	1/2 c cooked (10 kcal)
Almonds	1 oz (167 kcal)

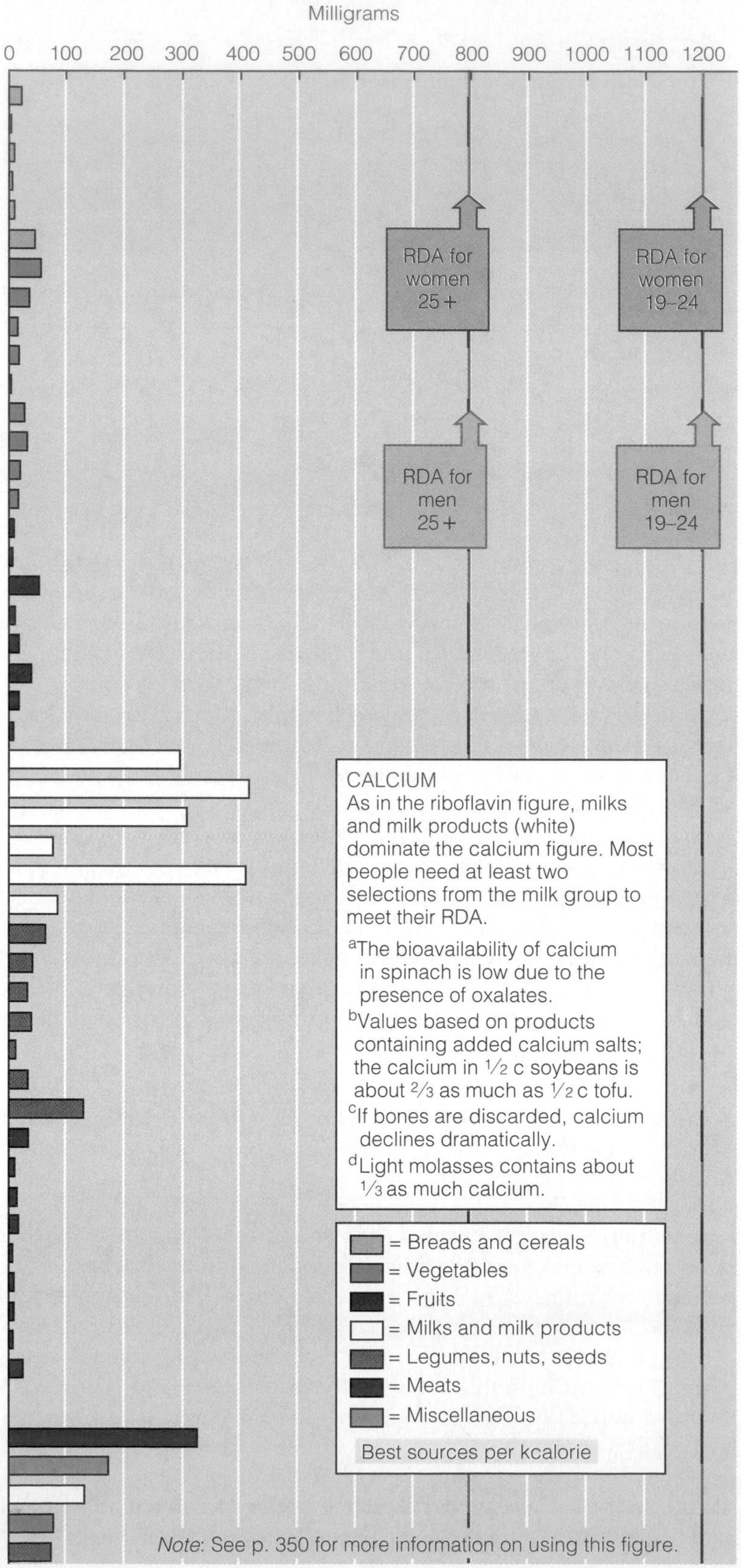

Milligrams
0 100 200 300 400 500 600 700 800 900 1000 1100 1200
RDA for women 25+
RDA for women 19–24
RDA for men 25+
RDA for men 19–24
CALCIUM
As in the riboflavin figure, milks and milk products (white) dominate the calcium figure. Most people need at least two selections from the milk group to meet their RDA.
[a]The bioavailability of calcium in spinach is low due to the presence of oxalates.
[b]Values based on products containing added calcium salts; the calcium in 1/2 c soybeans is about 2/3 as much as 1/2 c tofu.
[c]If bones are discarded, calcium declines dramatically.
[d]Light molasses contains about 1/3 as much calcium.
= Breads and cereals
= Vegetables
= Fruits
= Milks and milk products
= Legumes, nuts, seeds
= Meats
= Miscellaneous
Best sources per kcalorie
Note: See p. 350 for more information on using this figure.

For the person who doesn't like to drink milk, milk and milk products can be concealed in foods. Powdered nonfat milk, which is an excellent and inexpensive source of protein, calcium, and other nutrients, can be added to casseroles, meatloaf, and other mixed dishes in preparation; 5 heaping tablespoons offer the equivalent of a cup of milk. This simple step is probably the best way for older women to obtain added calcium beyond what they can get from liquid milk.

Figure 12–11

Foods Ranked According to Absorbability of Calcium

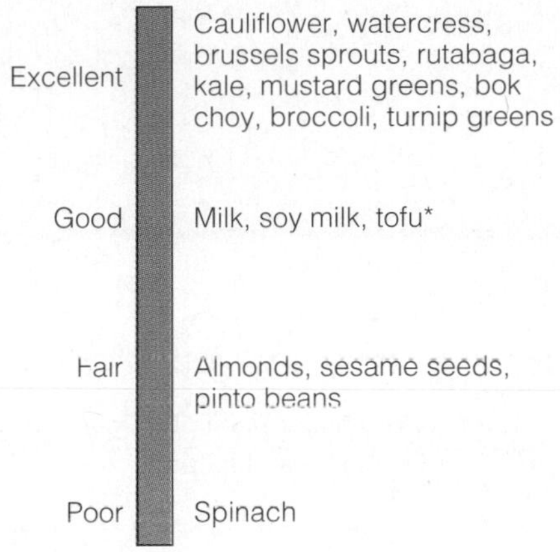

*Calcium–set tofu

Note: For reference, calcium absorption for foods categorized as excellent was greater than 50%; for those considered good, it was about 30%; for those listed as fair, it was about 20%; and for poor, it was 5%.

Source: Figure created based on data from C. M. Weaver and K. L. Plawecki, Dietary calcium: Adequacy of a vegetarian diet, *American Journal of Clinical Nutrition* 59 (1994): 1238S–1241S.

Nonmilk Sources Some cultures do not use milk in their cuisines; some vegetarians exclude milk as well as meat; and some people are allergic to milk protein or are lactose intolerant. These people need to find nonmilk sources of calcium to help meet their calcium needs. Some brands of tofu, corn tortillas, some nuts (such as almonds), and some seeds (such as sesame seeds) can supply calcium for the person who doesn't use milk products. Wheat bread contains only about 1/10 of the calcium found in milk, but can be a major source for people who eat a lot of it because the calcium is well absorbed. Among the vegetables, mustard and turnip greens, bok choy, kale, parsley, watercress, and broccoli are good sources of available calcium. So are some seaweeds such as the nori popular in Japanese cooking. Some dark green, leafy vegetables—notably spinach, rhubarb, and Swiss chard—appear to be calcium-rich but actually provide little, if any, calcium to the body because of the binders they contain. Figure 12–11 ranks selected foods according to the absorbability of their calcium.

Oysters are also a rich source of calcium, as are small canned fish prepared with their bones, such as canned sardines. Many Asians prepare a stock from bones that helps account for their adequate calcium intake without the use of milk. To make a high-calcium extract, they soak the cracked bones from chicken, turkey, pork, or fish in vinegar and then slowly boil the bones until they become soft. The bones release calcium into the acid medium, and most of the vinegar taste boils off. Then the cooks use the stock in place of water to prepare soup, vegetables, rice, or stew. One tablespoon of such stock may contain over 100 milligrams of calcium.

Some foods offer large amounts of calcium because they are fortified. Calcium-fortified orange juice, for example, provides as much calcium as regular milk. High-calcium milk (milk with extra calcium added) and calcium-fortified bread are other examples of calcium-fortified foods.

Calcium supplements are discussed in Highlight 12.

A generalization that has been gaining strength throughout this book is supported by the information given here about calcium. A balanced diet that supplies a variety of foods is the best assurance of adequacy for all essential nutrients. All food groups should be included, and none should be overused. In our culture, calcium is usually lacking wherever milk is underemphasized in the diet—whether through ignorance, poverty, simple dislike, fad dieting, lactose intolerance, or allergy. By contrast, iron is usually lacking whenever milk is overemphasized, as Chapter 13 will show.

CALCIUM DEFICIENCY

Bone mass peaks at the time of skeletal maturity (about age 30), and a dense bone mass is the best protection against later age-related bone loss and fracture. A low calcium intake during the growing years impairs acquisition of an optimal bone mass and density.[13] All adults lose bone as they grow older, beginning before they are 40. When bone loss reaches the point at which bones fracture

peak bone mass: the highest attainable bone density for an individual, developed during the first three decades of life.

osteoporosis (OSS-tee-oh-pore-OH-sis): a condition of older persons in which the bones become porous and fragile due to a loss of minerals; also called **adult bone loss**.
osteo = bone
porosis = porous

under common, everyday stresses, the condition is known as osteoporosis. Osteoporosis afflicts over 25 million people in the United States, mostly older women.

The urgency of protecting oneself against osteoporosis has to be learned through education because the body sends no signals saying bone loss is occurring. Many diseases make themselves known by symptoms that can be felt or seen, such as pain, shortness of breath, skin lesions, tiredness, and the like, but bone loss is silent. No evidence can be found in a blood sample because blood calcium remains normal no matter what the bone content may be. Measures of bone density are not often taken. Highlight 12 suggests strategies to protect against bone loss, of which obtaining enough calcium is only one.

Phosphorus

phosphorus: a major mineral found mostly in the body's bones and teeth.

Phosphorus is the second most abundant mineral in the body. About 85 percent of it is found combined with calcium in the hydroxapatite crystals of bones and teeth.

Phosphorus Roles in the Body The concentration of phosphorus salts (phosphates) in blood plasma is less than half that of calcium. Phosphates are in all body cells as part of a major buffer system (phosphoric acid and its salts). Phosphorus is also part of DNA and RNA, the genetic code material present in every cell, and therefore is necessary for all growth.

Phosphorus assists in energy transfers during cellular metabolism. Many enzymes and the B vitamins become active only when a phosphate group is attached. (Recall that the B vitamins play major roles in energy metabolism.) ATP itself, the energy carrier of the cells, uses three phosphate groups to do its work.

Lipids containing phosphorus as part of their structures (phospholipids) help to transport other lipids in the blood. Phospholipids are also the major structural components of cell membranes, where they affect transport of nutrients into and out of the cells. Some proteins, such as the casein in milk, contain phosphorus as part of their structures (phosphoproteins). Table 12–8 lists functions and food sources of phosphorus.

Table 12–8

Phosphorus—A Summary

Adult RDA	Chief Functions in the Body	Deficiency Symptoms	Toxicity Symptoms	Significant Sources
1200 mg/day (19–24 yr) 800 mg/day (25 and older)	A principal mineral of bones and teeth; part of every cell; important in genetic material, part of phospholipids, used in energy transfer and in buffer systems that maintain acid-base balance	Weakness, bone pain[a]	Low blood calcium levels	All animal tissues (meat, fish, poultry, eggs, milk)

[a]Dietary deficiency rarely occurs, but some drugs can bind with phosphorus making it unavailable and resulting in bone loss that is characterized by weakness and pain.

Phosphorus Recommendations Recommended intakes of phosphorus are the same as those for calcium, except during infancy. Diets that provide adequate energy and protein also supply adequate phosphorus.

Phosphorus Intakes Dietary deficiencies of phosphorus are unknown. Animal protein is the best source of phosphorus, because the mineral is so abundant in cells. In addition to foods from the milk and meat groups, processed foods (including soft drinks) are usually high in phosphorus. Phosphorus from additives in processed foods can add significantly to people's intakes.

Magnesium

Magnesium barely qualifies as a major mineral: only about 1 ounce of magnesium is present in the body of a 130-pound person. Over half of the body's magnesium is in the bones. Most of the rest is in the muscles and soft tissues, with only 1 percent in the extracellular fluid. Bone magnesium seems to be a reservoir to ensure that some will be on hand for vital reactions, regardless of recent dietary intake.

magnesium: a cation within the body's cells, active in many enzyme systems.

Magnesium Roles in the Body Magnesium is important to more than 300 of the body's enzyme systems. Magnesium acts in all the cells of the soft tissues, where it forms part of the protein-making machinery and is necessary for energy metabolism. A major role seems to be as a catalyst in the reaction that adds the last phosphate to the high-energy compound ATP. As a required component for ATP metabolism, magnesium is essential to the body's use of glucose; the synthesis of protein, fat, and nucleic acids; and the cells' membrane transport systems. Together with calcium, magnesium is involved in muscle contraction and blood clotting: calcium promotes the processes, whereas magnesium inhibits them. This dynamic interaction between the two minerals helps regulate the functioning of the lungs.[14] Magnesium also helps prevent dental caries by holding calcium in tooth enamel. Like many other nutrients, magnesium supports the normal functioning of the immune system.[15] Table 12–9 offers a summary.

Table 12–9

Magnesium—A Summary

Adult RDA	Chief Functions in the Body	Deficiency Symptoms	Toxicity Symptoms	Significant Sources
Men: 350 mg/day Women: 280 mg/day	Involved in bone mineralization, the building of protein, enzyme action, normal muscular contraction, nerve impulse transmission, maintenance of teeth, and functioning of immune system	Weakness; confusion; if extreme, convulsions, bizarre muscle movements (especially of eye and face muscles), hallucinations, and difficulty in swallowing; in children, growth failure[a]	Not known; large doses have been taken in the form of the laxative Epsom salts without ill effects except diarrhea	Nuts, legumes, whole grains, dark green vegetables, seafood, chocolate, cocoa

[a]A still more severe deficiency causes tetany, an extreme, prolonged contraction of the muscles similar to that caused by low blood calcium.

Magnesium Intakes Dietary magnesium intakes average about three-quarters of the RDA for U.S. adults.[16] Dietary intake data, however, do not include the contribution made by water. In some parts of the country, the water contains both calcium and magnesium ("hard" water) and contributes significantly to intakes.

The brown bars in Figure 12–12 indicate that legumes, seeds, and nuts make significant magnesium contributions. Magnesium is part of the chlorophyll molecule, so leafy green vegetables are magnesium-rich.

Magnesium Deficiency Even when average magnesium intakes are below the RDA, deficiency symptoms are not apparent except with disease.[17] Magnesium deficiency develops in alcohol abuse, protein malnutrition, renal or endocrine disorders, or diseases that cause prolonged vomiting or diarrhea. People using diuretics may also show symptoms. A severe magnesium deficiency causes a tetany similar to the calcium tetany described earlier. Magnesium deficiencies also impair central nervous system activity and are thought to cause the hallucinations experienced by people withdrawing from alcohol intoxication.

Magnesium and Hypertension The magnesium ion appears critical to heart function and seems to protect against hypertension and heart disease. With magnesium deficiency, the walls of arteries and capillaries undergo visible changes and tend to constrict, a possible mechanism for the hypertensive effect. Studies have reported that magnesium intakes are lower in men who have heart attacks and that injections of magnesium can be used successfully in the treatment of heart attack victims.[18]

To sum up, most of the body's calcium is in the bones where it provides a rigid structure and reservoir of calcium for the blood. Blood calcium participates in muscle contraction, blood clotting, and nerve impulses and is closely regulated by a system of hormones and vitamin D. Phosphorus accompanies calcium both in the crystals of bone and in many foods such as milk. Magnesium also supports bone mineralization and is involved in numerous enzyme systems.

Sulfur

The body does not use sulfur by itself as a nutrient (see Table 12–10). The reason sulfur is mentioned here is that it occurs in essential nutrients that the body does use, such as thiamin and the amino acids methionine and cysteine. Sulfur plays a well-known role in determining the contour of protein molecules. The sulfur-containing side chains in cysteine molecules can link to each other, forming disulfide bridges, which stabilize the protein structure. Skin, hair, and nails contain some of the body's more rigid proteins, which have a high sulfur content.

sulfur: a mineral present in the body as part of some amino acids.

Cysteine in one part of a protein chain can bind to cysteine in another part of the chain by way of a disulfide bridge (see the drawing of insulin with its disulfide bridge on p. 199). Two cysteine molecules linked this way are called cysteine (see Appendix C).

There is no recommended intake for sulfur, and no deficiencies are known. Only when people lack protein to the point of severe deficiency will they lack the sulfur-containing amino acids.

Like the other nutrients, the minerals' actions are coordinated to get the body's work done. The major minerals, especially sodium, chloride, and potassium, influence the body's fluid balance; whenever an anion moves, a cation moves—always maintaining homeostasis. Sodium, chloride, potassium, calcium, and magnesium

Figure 12–12 Magnesium in Selected Foods

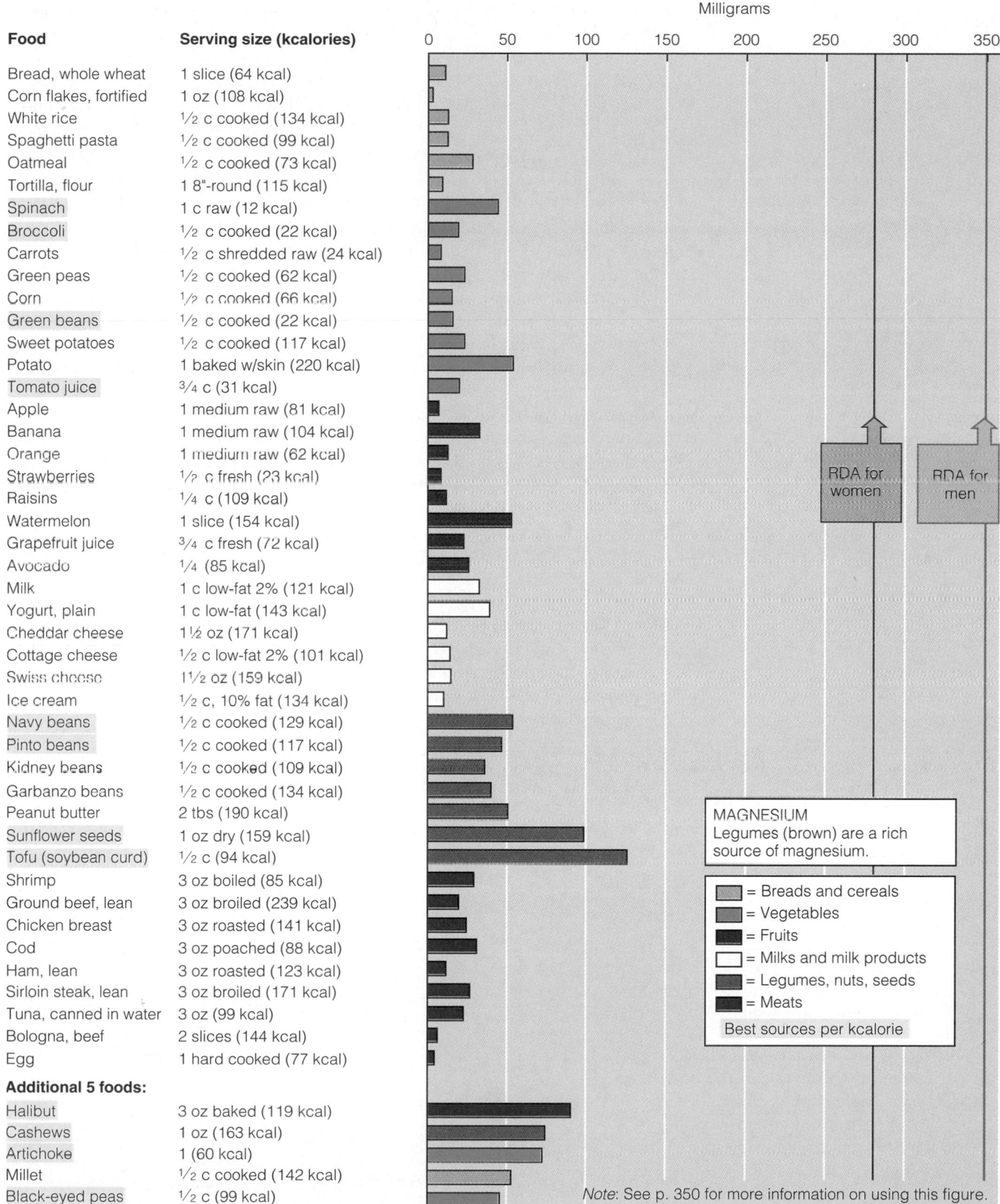

Food	Serving size (kcalories)
Bread, whole wheat	1 slice (64 kcal)
Corn flakes, fortified	1 oz (108 kcal)
White rice	1/2 c cooked (134 kcal)
Spaghetti pasta	1/2 c cooked (99 kcal)
Oatmeal	1/2 c cooked (73 kcal)
Tortilla, flour	1 8"-round (115 kcal)
Spinach	1 c raw (12 kcal)
Broccoli	1/2 c cooked (22 kcal)
Carrots	1/2 c shredded raw (24 kcal)
Green peas	1/2 c cooked (62 kcal)
Corn	1/2 c cooked (66 kcal)
Green beans	1/2 c cooked (22 kcal)
Sweet potatoes	1/2 c cooked (117 kcal)
Potato	1 baked w/skin (220 kcal)
Tomato juice	3/4 c (31 kcal)
Apple	1 medium raw (81 kcal)
Banana	1 medium raw (104 kcal)
Orange	1 medium raw (62 kcal)
Strawberries	1/2 c fresh (23 kcal)
Raisins	1/4 c (109 kcal)
Watermelon	1 slice (154 kcal)
Grapefruit juice	3/4 c fresh (72 kcal)
Avocado	1/4 (85 kcal)
Milk	1 c low-fat 2% (121 kcal)
Yogurt, plain	1 c low-fat (143 kcal)
Cheddar cheese	1 1/2 oz (171 kcal)
Cottage cheese	1/2 c low-fat 2% (101 kcal)
Swiss cheese	1 1/2 oz (159 kcal)
Ice cream	1/2 c, 10% fat (134 kcal)
Navy beans	1/2 c cooked (129 kcal)
Pinto beans	1/2 c cooked (117 kcal)
Kidney beans	1/2 c cooked (109 kcal)
Garbanzo beans	1/2 c cooked (134 kcal)
Peanut butter	2 tbs (190 kcal)
Sunflower seeds	1 oz dry (159 kcal)
Tofu (soybean curd)	1/2 c (94 kcal)
Shrimp	3 oz boiled (85 kcal)
Ground beef, lean	3 oz broiled (239 kcal)
Chicken breast	3 oz roasted (141 kcal)
Cod	3 oz poached (88 kcal)
Ham, lean	3 oz roasted (123 kcal)
Sirloin steak, lean	3 oz broiled (171 kcal)
Tuna, canned in water	3 oz (99 kcal)
Bologna, beef	2 slices (144 kcal)
Egg	1 hard cooked (77 kcal)
Additional 5 foods:	
Halibut	3 oz baked (119 kcal)
Cashews	1 oz (163 kcal)
Artichoke	1 (60 kcal)
Millet	1/2 c cooked (142 kcal)
Black-eyed peas	1/2 c (99 kcal)

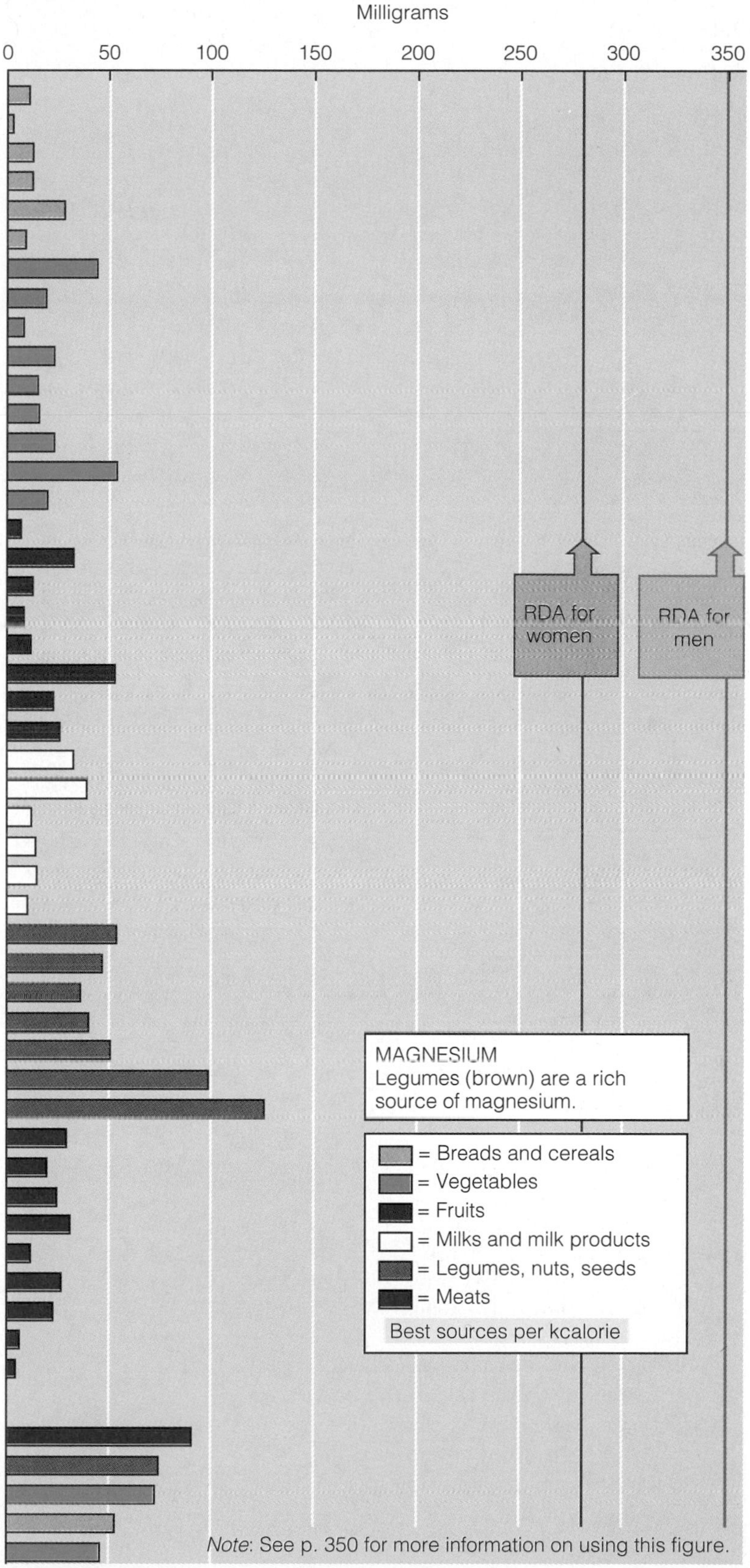

Note: See p. 350 for more information on using this figure.

Table 12–10

Sulfur—A Summary

Chief Functions in the Body	Deficiency Symptoms	Toxicity Symptoms	Significant Sources
As part of proteins, stabilizes their shape by forming disulfide bridges; part of the vitamins biotin and thiamin and the hormone insulin	None known; protein deficiency would occur first	Toxicity would occur only if sulfur-containing amino acids were eaten in excess; this (in animals) depresses growth	All protein-containing foods (meats, fish, poultry, eggs, milk, legumes, nuts)

are key members of the team of nutrients that direct nerve transmission and muscle contraction; they are also the primary nutrients involved in regulating blood pressure.[19] Phosphorus and magnesium participate in many reactions involving glucose, fatty acids, amino acids, and the vitamins. Calcium, phosphorus, and magnesium combine to form the structure of the bones and teeth. Each major mineral also plays other specific roles in the body. With all of the tasks these minerals perform, they are of great importance to life. Consuming enough of each of them every day is not difficult, given a variety of food choices from each of the food groups. Whole-grain breads supply magnesium; fruits, vegetables, and legumes also provide magnesium and potassium, too; milks offer calcium and phosphorus; meats also offer phosphorus and sulfur as well; all foods provide sodium and chloride, excesses being more problematic than inadequacies. The message is quite simple and has been repeated throughout this text: for an adequate intake of all the nutrients, including the major minerals, choose different foods from each of the five food groups. And drink plenty of water.

Study Questions

1. List the roles of water in the body.
2. List the sources of water intake and routes of water excretion.
3. What is ADH? Where does it exert its action? What is aldosterone? How does it work?
4. How does the body use electrolytes to regulate fluid balance?
5. What do the terms *major* and *trace* mean when describing the minerals in the body?
6. Describe some characteristics of minerals that distinguish them from vitamins.
7. What is the major function of sodium in the body? Describe how the kidneys regulate blood sodium. Is a dietary deficiency of sodium unlikely? Why?
8. List calcium's roles in the body. How does the body keep blood calcium constant regardless of intake?
9. Name significant food sources of calcium. What are the consequences of inadequate intakes?
10. List the roles of phosphorus in the body. Discuss the relationships between calcium and phosphorus. Is a dietary deficiency of phosphorus likely? Why?
11. State the major functions of chloride, potassium, magnesium, and sulfur in the body. Are deficiencies of these nutrients likely to occur in your own diet. Why?

Notes

1. Committee on Dietary Allowances, *Recommended Dietary Allowances*, 10th ed. (Washington, D.C.: National Academy Press, 1989), pp. 247–261.
2. Pamphlet from The American Dietetic Association, Water: The beverage of life, 1994.
3. Nutrition Committee, American Heart Association, *Dietary Guidelines for Healthy American Adults: A Statement for Physicians and Health Professionals* (Dallas, Tex.: American Heart Association, 1988).
4. T. A. Kotchen and J. M. Kotchen, Nutrition, diet, and hypertension, in *Modern Nutrition in Health and Disease*, 8th ed., eds. M. E. Shils, J. A. Olson, and M. Shike (Philadelphia; Lea & Febiger, 1994), pp. 1287–1297.
5. H. S. Wright and coauthors, The 1978–88 Nationwide Food Consumption Survey: An update on the nutrient intake of respondents, *Nutrition Today*, May/June 1991, pp. 21–27.
6. Committee on Diet and Health, *Diet and Health: Implications for Reducing Chronic Disease Risk* (Washington, D.C.: National Academy Press, 1989), pp. 99–135.
7. R. D. Mattess, Discretionary salt use, *American Journal of Clinical Nutrition* (1990 ASCN Annual Meeting) 51 (1990): 519.
8. Committee on Dietary Allowances, 1989, pp. 247–261.
9. Committee on Dietary Allowances, 1989, pp. 247–261.
10. D. A. McCarron and coauthors, Dietary calcium and blood pressure: Modifying factors in specific populations, *American Journal of Clinical Nutrition* (supplement) 54 (1991): 215–219.
11. J. Sharlin and coauthors, Nutrition and behavioral characteristics and determinants of plasma cholesterol levels in men and women, *Journal of the American Dietetic Association* 92 (1992): 434–440; G. A. Golditz and coauthors, Diet and risk of clinical diabetes in women, *American Journal of Clinical Nutrition* 55 (1992): 1018–1023; C. F. Garland, F. C. Garland, and E. D. Gorham, Can colon cancer incidence and death rates be reduced with calcium and vitamin D? *American Journal of Clinical Nutrition* 54 (1991): 193S–201S; K. K. Carroll and coauthors, Calcium and carcinogenesis of the mammary gland, *American Journal of Clinical Nutrition* 54 (1991): 206S–208S.
12. *Nutrition Monitoring in the United States: Selected Findings from the National Nutrition Monitoring and Related Research Program* (Hyattsville, Md.: Public Health Service, 1993), pp. 29, 31.
13. V. Matkovic, Calcium metabolism and calcium requirements during skeletal modeling and consolidation of bone mass, *American Journal of Clinical Nutrition* 54 (1991): 245–260.
14. R. A. Landon and E. A. Young, Role of magnesium in regulation of lung function, *Journal of the American Dietetic Association* 93 (1993): 674–677.
15. H. McCoy and M. A. Kenney, Magnesium and immune function: Recent findings, *Magnesium Research* 5 (1992): 281–293.
16. Wright and coauthors, 1991.
17. Committee on Dietary Allowances, 1989, pp. 190–191.
18. P. C. Elwood and coauthors, Dietary magnesium and prediction of heart disease, *The Lancet* 340 (1992): 483; K. L. Woods and coauthors, Intravenous magnesium sulphate in suspected acute myocardial infarction: Results of the second Leicester Intravenous Magnesium Intervention Trial (LIMIT-2), *The Lancet* 339 (1992): 1553–1558.
19. M. E. Reusser and D. A. McCarron, Micronutrient effects on blood pressure regulation, *Nutrition Reviews* 52 (1994): 367–375.

Problem Set

1. For each of these minerals, note the unit of measure:

Calcium: ______ Magnesium: ______ Phosphorus: ______ Potassium: ______ Sodium: ______

2. Analyze the mineral contents of a day's meals.

a. Record mineral contributions of the meals presented in Chapter 10 problem 2:

Item No./Food	Ener (kcal)	Calc (mg)	Magn (mg)	Phos (mg)	Potas (mg)	Sod (mg)
• Grains (6)						
# 357 Wheat bread, 6 slices	_______	_______	_______	_______	_______	_______
Total in grains:	_______	_______	_______	_______	_______	_______

(continued on the next page)

Problem Set (continued)

Item No./Food	Ener (kcal)	Calc (mg)	Magn (mg)	Phos (mg)	Potas (mg)	Sod (mg)
• Vegetables (3)						
# 929 Spinach, cooked from fresh, ½ c	______	______	______	______	______	______
# 891 Green peas, cooked from frozen, ½ c	______	______	______	______	______	______
# 834 Carrots, cooked from fresh, ½ c	______	______	______	______	______	______
Total in vegetables:	______	______	______	______	______	______
• Fruits (2)						
# 269 Orange juice, fresh, 1 c	______	______	______	______	______	______
# 264 Cantaloupe melon, ½	______	______	______	______	______	______
Total in fruits:	______	______	______	______	______	______
• Meats (2 to 3)						
# 1045 Bass fish, 4 oz	______	______	______	______	______	______
# 598 Hamburger, lean, 4 oz	______	______	______	______	______	______
Total in meats:	______	______	______	______	______	______
• Milks (2)						
# 98 Milk, nonfat, 2 c	______	______	______	______	______	______
Total in milks:	______	______	______	______	______	______

b. Which group of foods offered the most calcium? ______________ The least? ______________

c. Which group of foods offered the most magnesium? ______________ The least? ______________

d. Which group of foods offered the most phosphorus? ______________ The least? ______________

e. Which group of foods offered the most potassium? ______________ The least? ______________

f. Which group of foods offered the most sodium? ______________ The least? ______________

g. List each of the groups that provided "the most" for each of the major minerals: ______________

This exercise should provide further evidence that people need to eat foods from each of the food groups daily.

3. Appreciate milk products as calcium-dense foods. Following is a list of foods ranked in order of their calcium contents per serving. Those listed first offer the most calcium per serving.

   a. How many servings (and kcalories) of any one of these foods would you have to eat to get 100% of the Daily Value of 1000 mg? Calculate your answer in the last two columns of the table (round your answers up); the first one is done for you.

Item No./Food	Energy (kcal)	Calcium (mg)	Servings	kCalories
# 98 Milk, nonfat, 1 c	85	301	1000 ÷ 301 = 3.3 c	3 c = 255 kcal
# 37 Cheddar cheese, 1 oz	______	______	______________	___________
# 820 Broccoli, cooked from fresh, chopped, 1 c	______	______	______________	___________
# 939 Sweet potato, baked in skin, 1 ea	______	______	______________	___________

Problem Set (continued)

Item No./Food	Energy (kcal)	Calcium (mg)	Servings	kCalories
# 264 Cantaloupe melon, ½	______	______	______	______
# 834 Carrots, from fresh, ½ c	______	______	______	______
# 357 Whole-wheat bread, 1 slice	______	______	______	______
# 891 Green peas, cooked from frozen, ½ c	______	______	______	______
# 206 Apple, fresh 3¼″	______	______	______	______
# 606 Sirloin steak, lean, 4 oz	______	______	______	______
# 623 Pork chop, lean broiled, 1 ea	______	______	______	______

b. The top three items ranked in order of calcium contents per serving are milk > cheese > broccoli. What are the top three items in order of calcium contents per kcalorie? ______________________

Based on this information, it is true that milk, milk products, and dark green vegetables are the foods richest in calcium? ______________________

Osteoporosis and Calcium

Osteoporosis is one of the most prevalent diseases of aging, affecting more than 25 million people in the United States—most of them women. Each year more than 1.5 million people suffer bone breaks in their hips, backs, and wrists due to osteoporosis.

Osteoporosis develops without warning. People cannot tell that they are losing bone tissue until late in life: Then dramatic symptoms suddenly emerge. The causes are tangled, and it is not yet clear whether abundant dietary calcium can prevent or forestall osteoporosis. This highlight addresses several questions: What is osteoporosis? What factors contribute to it? What, if anything, can people do to reduce their risks? And where does calcium fit into the picture?

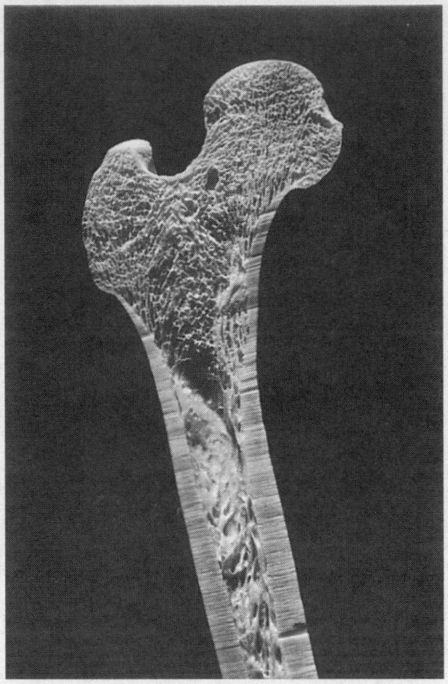

Trabecular bone is the lacy network of calcium-containing crystals that fills the interior. Cortical bone is the dense, ivorylike bone that forms the exterior shell.

THE PROBLEM OF OSTEOPOROSIS

Osteoporosis often first becomes apparent when someone's hip suddenly gives way. People say, "She fell and broke her hip," but in fact the hip may have been so fragile that it broke *before* she fell. Even stepping down off a curb may be enough to shatter a porous bone into fragments so numerous and scattered that they cannot be reassembled. Removing them and replacing them with an artificial joint requires major surgery. About a fifth die of complications within a year. Half of those who survive will never walk independently again.

Bone has two compartments: the outer, hard shell of cortical bone, and the inner, lacy structural matrix of trabecular bone. Both can lose minerals, but in different ways and at different rates. (The accompanying glossary defines relevant terms.) The opening photograph shows a human leg bone sliced lengthwise, exposing the lacy, calcium-containing crystals inside the bone. These crystals give up calcium to the blood when the day's supply from the diet runs short, and they take up calcium again when the dietary supply is plentiful. For people who have invested in their body's calcium bank during the bone-forming years of their childhood and young adulthood, these deposits provide a nearly inexhaustible fund of calcium.

In contrast to trabecular bone, cortical bone forms the dense, ivorylike exterior shell that surrounds and protects each bone. Cortical bone composes the shafts of the long bones, and a thin cortical shell caps the end of the bone, too. Both compartments confer strength on bone: cortical bone provides the sturdy outer wall, while trabecular bone provides support along the lines of stress.

The two types of bone play different roles in calcium balance and osteoporosis. Trabecular bone is generally supplied with blood vessels and is metabolically active. It is sensitive to hormones that govern day-to-day deposits and withdrawals of calcium,

Glossary

bone density: a measure of bone strength. When minerals fill the bone matrix, they give it strength.

cortical bone: the ivorylike outer bone layer that forms a shell surrounding trabecular bone and comprises the shaft of a long bone.

trabecular (tra-BECK-you-lar) **bone:** the lacy inner structure of calcium crystals that supports the bone's structure and provides a calcium storage bank.

type I osteoporosis: osteoporosis characterized by rapid bone losses, primarily of trabecular bone.

type II osteoporosis: osteoporosis characterized by gradual losses of both trabecular and cortical bone.

and it readily gives up minerals whenever blood calcium needs replenishing. Losses of trabecular bone start becoming significant for men and women in their 30s, although losses can occur whenever calcium withdrawals exceed deposits.

Cortical bone also gives up calcium, but slowly and at a steady pace. Cortical bone losses typically begin at about 40 years of age and continue slowly but surely thereafter.

Researchers have associated losses of trabecular and cortical bone with two types of osteoporosis, which cause two types of bone breaks. Type I osteoporosis involves losses of trabecular bone (see Figure H12–1). These losses sometimes exceed three times the expected rate, and bone breaks may occur suddenly. Trabecular bones become so fragile that even the body's own weight can overburden the spine—vertebrae may suddenly disintegrate and crush down, painfully pinching major nerves. Wrists may break as bone ends weaken, and teeth may loosen or fall out as the trabecular bone of the jaw recedes. Women are most often the victims of this type of osteoporosis, six to one over men. Taking estrogen for at least seven years after menopause is the most effective preventive measure against this type of osteoporosis.[1]

In type II osteoporosis, the calcium of both cortical and trabecular bone is drawn out of storage, but slowly over the years. As old age approaches, the vertebrae may compress into wedge shapes, forming what is often called "dowager's hump," the posture many older people assume as they "grow shorter." Figure H12–2 (on p. 464) shows the effect of compressed spinal bone on a woman's height and posture. Because both the cortical shell and the trabecular interior weaken, breaks most often occur in the hip, as in the opening example. A woman is twice as likely as a man to suffer type II osteoporosis. Table H12–1 summarizes the differences between the two types of osteoporosis.

Figure H12–1

Healthy and Osteoporotic Trabecular Bones

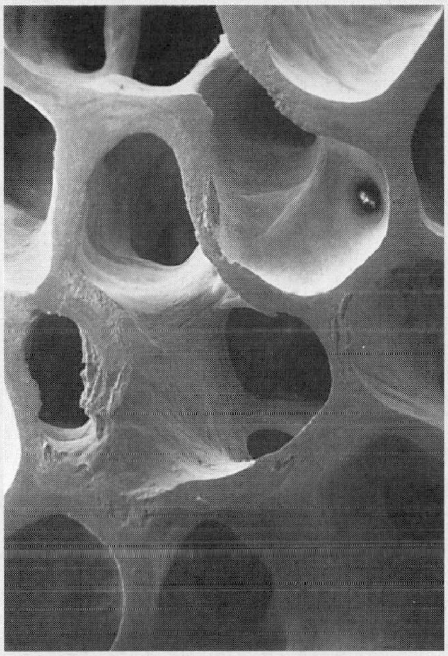

Electron micrograph of healthy trabecular bone.

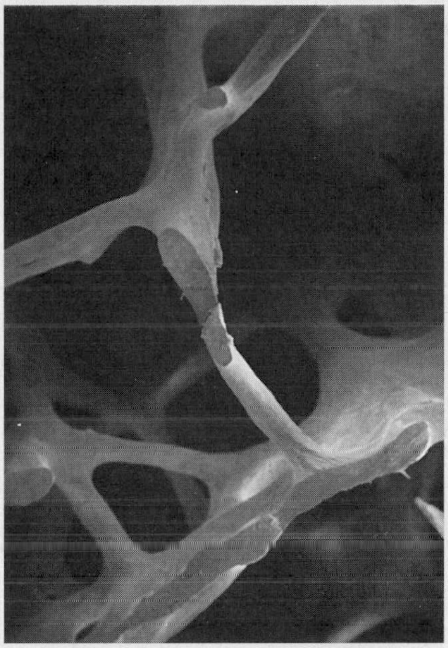

Electron micrograph of trabecular bone affected by osteoporosis.

Table H12–1

Types of Osteoporosis Compared

	Type I	Type II
Other name	Postmenopausal osteoporosis	Senile osteoporosis
Age of onset	50 to 70 years old	70 years and older
Bone loss	Trabecular bone	Both trabecular and cortical bone
Fracture sites	Wrist and spine	Hip
Gender incidence	6 women to 1 man	2 women to 1 man
Primary causes	Rapid loss of estrogen in women following menopause; loss of testosterone in men with advancing age	Reduced calcium absorption, increased bone mineral loss, increased propensity to fall

Source: Adapted from C. Niewoehner, Calcium and osteoporosis, *Cereal Foods World* 33 (1988): 784–787.

Figure H12–2

Loss of Height in a Woman Caused by Osteoporosis

The woman on the left is about 50 years old. On the right, she is 80 years old. Her legs have not grown shorter: only her back has lost length, due to collapse of her spinal bones (vertebrae). Collapsed vertebrae cannot protect the spinal nerves from pressure that causes excruciating pain.

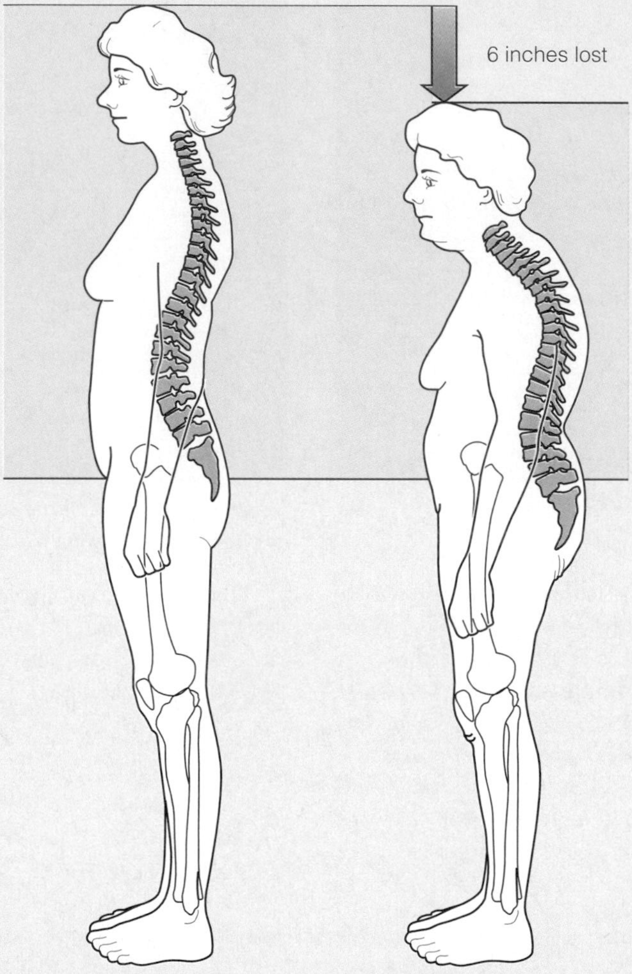

Whether a person develops osteoporosis seems to depend partly on heredity and partly on other factors, including nutrition. The strongest predictor of bone density is age, followed by sex. Other predictors, whose order of importance is not known, are hormonal status, racial inheritance, physical activity, body weight, smoking, alcohol, drugs, and nutrition.

AGE AND BONE CALCIUM

During the first two decades of life, the skeleton grows stronger and denser as it accumulates minerals. Then, in the late 20s to early 30s, the bones stop growing. As the years pass, the cells that build bone gradually become less active, while those that dismantle bone continue working. Thus, with advancing age, bones lose strength and density (see Figure H12–3).

Calcium intakes of older adults are typically low, and calcium absorption declines after about the age of 65 years. The kidneys do not activate vitamin D as well as they did earlier (recall that active vitamin D promotes calcium absorption). Also, sunlight is needed to form vitamin D, and many older people spend little or no time outdoors in the sunshine. For these reasons, and because intakes of vitamin D are typically low anyway, blood vitamin D decreases. A recent study found the rate of fractures was significantly reduced in women with osteoporosis who received a regular vitamin D supplement (0.25 μg twice daily for three years).[2]

Some of the hormones that regulate bone and calcium metabolism also change with age and accelerate bone mineral withdrawal.* Together, these age-related factors probably contribute to bone loss: inefficient bone remodeling, reduced calcium intakes, impaired calcium absorption, poor vitamin D status, physical inactivity, and hormonal changes that favor bone mineral withdrawal.

SEX AND HORMONES

After age, sex is the next strongest predictor of loss of bone density with aging: women have much more

*Among the hormones suggested as influential are parathormone, calcitonin, and estrogen.

substantial losses than men in later life. Menopause imposes special perils on women's bones. Bone dwindles rapidly when the hormone estrogen diminishes and menstruation ceases. Accelerated losses last for 6 to 8 years following menopause, then taper off, so that women again lose bone at the same rate as men their age (see Figure H12–4). Losses of bone minerals continue throughout the remainder of a woman's lifetime, but not at the free-fall pace of the menopause years.

When *young* women experience reduced estrogen secretion and cease menstruating, they, too, lose bone rapidly. Chapter 14 describes how women who overexercise and unreasonably restrict their body weights develop athletic amenorrhea and become susceptible to bone fractures. The combination of irregular or absent menstrual periods and low body weights explains much of the bone loss seen in young athletes.[3] Estrogen taken as a prescription drug can help nonmenstruating women prevent further bone loss and reduce the incidence of fractures.[4]

If estrogen deficiency is a major cause of osteoporosis in women, what is the cause of bone loss in men? Men produce only a little estrogen, yet they resist osteoporosis better than women. Male hormones must also play a role because men suffer more fractures after removal of the testes (in cases of disease) or when their testes lose functional ability with aging. Men who have delayed puberty also appear to have more fractures, suggesting that timing of puberty influences peak bone density.[5] Thus both male and female sex hormones appear to play roles in the development of osteoporosis.

Figure H12–3

Phases of Bone Development throughout Life

The active growth phase occurs from birth to approximately age 20. The next phase of peak bone mass development occurs between the ages of 12 and 40. The final phase, when bone resorption exceeds formation, begins between age 30 and 40 and continues throughout the remainder of life.

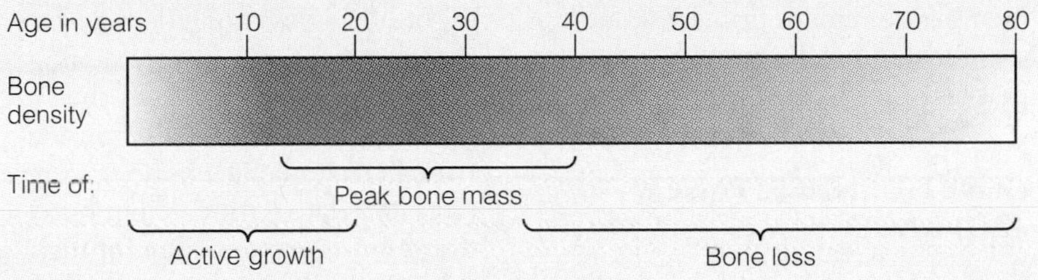

Figure H12–4

High Peak Bone Mass Early in Life Postpones Osteoporosis

Over a lifetime, women lose 30 to 40 percent of their bone mass and men, 20 to 30 percent. Can you see why it is so important for young people to consume enough calcium to attain a maximum bone mass?

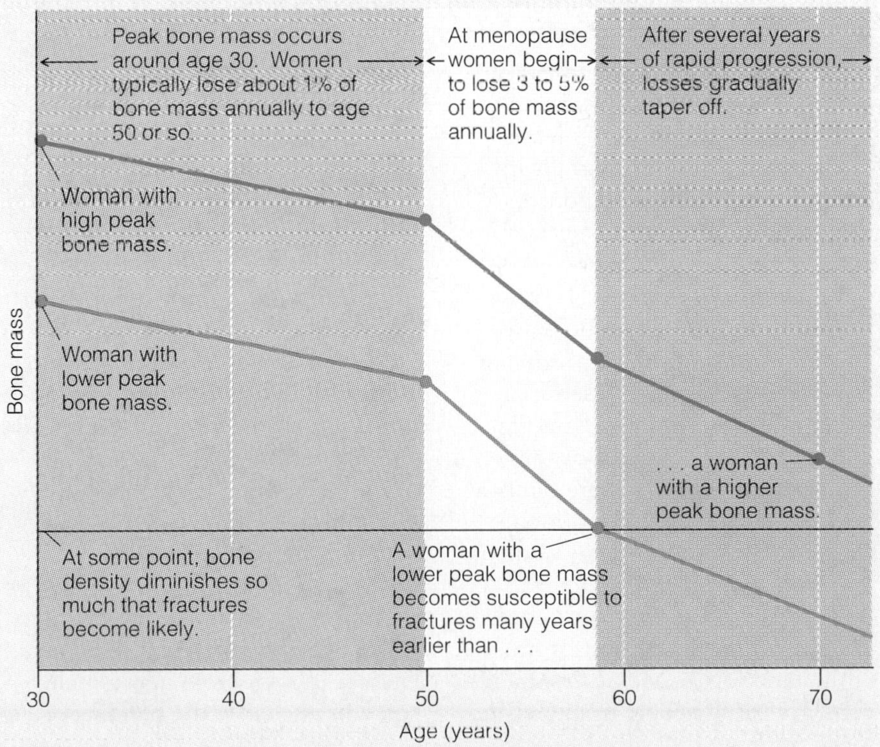

One more complication of the estrogen theory is that some women lose bone tissue in middle age before they reach menopause, as though they were predisposed to do so. Clearly, hormones are only one of several factors affecting bones. Still, being female and experiencing menopause remain prime risk factors for the development of osteoporosis.

GENETIC INHERITANCE AND RACE

Studies of mothers and daughters confirm that heredity plays an influential role in bone density.[6] Most likely, inheritance influences both peak bone mass achieved during growth and the extent of bone loss during menopause. The extent to which a given genetic potential is realized, however, depends on many outside factors. Nutrition and physical activity, for example, can maximize peak bone density during growth, whereas alcohol and tobacco abuse can accelerate bone losses later in life.

Risks of osteoporosis appear to run along racial lines. Significant differences in bone metabolism divide elderly African Americans from Caucasians.[7] Black people have denser bones than do white people, and these differences are evident even before birth.[8] Greater bone density expresses itself in a lower rate of osteoporosis among blacks. Hip fractures, for example, are about three times more likely at 80 years of age in white women than in African-American women.

Other ethnic groups have *less* dense bones than do many people of European heritage. Asians from China and Japan, Mexican Americans, Hispanic people from Central and South America, and Inuit people from St. Lawrence Island all have lower bone density than do people with a northern European background. One might predict that these groups would suffer more bone fractures, but this is not always the case. Chinese people living in Singapore have low bone density, but their hip fracture rates are among the lowest in the world. In the countries of the Balkan peninsula (former Yugoslavia), bone fracture rates correlate with calcium nutrition—lower rates in areas of high calcium intake, higher rates in areas of low calcium intake—despite racial similarities. These findings demonstrate that although a person's genes may lay the groundwork for a likely outcome, environmental factors influence the genes' ultimate expression. From the findings reported in the Balkans, calcium nutrition appears to be one of those environmental factors. Others include physical activity, body weight, smoking, alcohol, and protein intake—all factors within a person's control.

PHYSICAL ACTIVITY AND BODY WEIGHT

When people are idle—for example, when they are confined to bed—their bones lose strength just as their muscles do. Astronauts who live with reduced gravity for days or weeks at a time also lose bone and muscle strength.

Muscle strength and bone strength tend to go together. When muscles work, they pull on the bones, stimulating them to lay down more trabeculae and grow stronger. Also, when muscles work, the hormones that promote new muscle growth also favor the building of bone. As a result, active bones are denser than sedentary bones.[9] Even modest increases in physical activity and calcium intake help to maximize bone gains in young adulthood and minimize further losses that occur with inactivity.[10]

To keep the bones healthy, weight-bearing physical activity, such as walking, dancing, or jogging, are especially effective. Even swimming may be beneficial, perhaps because it increases muscle strength. Dr. Robert Heaney of Omaha's Creighton University stated the case for taking an active (quite literally) stand against osteoporosis: "Osteoporosis is a total life-style problem. You can't cure a bad life-style with a pill, and it's a terrible strategic mistake to encourage people to think you can. If I'm sitting all day, don't walk to work, don't carry loads or work in the garden on the weekend, I'm going to lose bone. You can give me all the calcium in the world, and it's not going to stop it."[11] Cells do not helplessly accept what is given to them; instead they respond, with the help of the necessary regulators, to the demands put upon them. Then they select the nutrients they need from what is offered. The way to increase bone density is to put a demand on the bones, make them work, and then provide the raw materials from which they can grow strong: calcium, other minerals, all the nutrients in the right balance.

Heavier body weights also place stress on the bones and promote their maintenance. In fact, body weight (and to some extent, body fatness) is a significant and consistent predictor of bone density and risk of fractures.[12] As mentioned earlier, the combination of a too-slender body, severely restricted energy intake, extreme daily exercise, and the absence of menstruation reliably predict bone loss.[13] Chapter 14 describes the bone loss that accompanies eating disorders in competitive athletes.

SMOKING, ALCOHOL, AND CAFFEINE

Smokers experience more fractures from slight injury than do nonsmokers. A study of twins reports that women who smoke a pack of cigarettes a day throughout adulthood lose an extra 5 to 10 percent of their bone density by menopause.[14] Although the mechanism of action remains undefined, both the lower body weights of smokers and the earlier menopause of female smokers may be factors.[15]

People who abuse alcohol often suffer from osteoporosis and experience more bone breaks than others. Several factors appear to be involved: alcohol promotes fluid excretion that leads to excessive calcium losses in the urine; alcohol may upset the hormonal balance required for healthy bones; alcohol may slow bone formation, leading to lower bone density; and alcohol abuse increases the risk of falling.

Caffeine has been considered a possible risk factor for the development of osteoporosis, but evidence is inconclusive.[16] Some studies indicate that caffeine accelerates calcium excretion; other studies have found no significant effects.[17] The effects of caffeine on calcium balance may be deleterious only when calcium intake is low.

Table H12–2 summarizes the risk factors and protective factors covered so far and includes some others, among them nutrition factors, discussed next. The more risk factors that apply to a person, the greater the chances of bone loss. Notice that several factors are more influential than diet in the development of osteoporosis.

Table H12–2

Risk and Protective Factors That Correlate with Osteoporosis

Risk Factors	Protective Factors
HIGH CORRELATION	
Advanced age	African American
Alcohol abuse	Estrogens, long-term use
Anorexia nervosa	
Caucasian	
Chronic steroid use	
Female sex	
Rheumatoid arthritis	
Surgical removal of ovaries	
Thinness	
MODERATE CORRELATION	
Chronic thyroid hormone use	Having given birth
Cigarette smoking	High body weight
Diabetes (insulin-dependent type)	
Early menopause	
Excessive antacid use	
Low-calcium diet	
Sedentary lifestyle	
Vitamin D deficiency	
PROBABLY IMPORTANT BUT NOT YET PROVED	
Alcohol taken in moderation	High-calcium diet
Caffeine use	Regular physical activity
Family history of osteoporosis	
High-fiber diet	
High-protein diet	

Source: Adapted from C. D. Arnaud and S. D. Sanchez, The role of calcium in osteoporosis, *Annual Review of Nutrition* 10 (1990): 397–414.

PROTEIN NUTRITION

Extra dietary protein seems to promote calcium excretion in the urine. A lifetime of consuming excess dietary protein may well accelerate bone loss.[18] Many women in the United States may have protein intakes high enough and calcium intakes low enough to compromise bone integrity.[19]

The converse is also true: diets low in protein help to conserve bone density. This is seen both in laboratory animals and in strict vegetarians, who consume a lower-than-average amount of protein. Vegetarians who center meals on eggs and dairy products, however, can consume as much protein and lose bone just as rapidly as do meat eaters.[20] A tentative link has been suggested between the hormone insulin, released in response to dietary protein, and calcium losses in the urine.[21] Diabetes (IDDM) also seems to alter the body's handling of calcium and magnesium with possible harmful effects on the health of the bones.[22]

Too little protein can be as harmful as too much, of course. Protein deprivation also stimulates calcium losses.[23] These facts seem to conflict at first glance, but they really just demonstrate a sound nutrition principle—that moderation is best.

CALCIUM NUTRITION

As stated earlier, a low calcium uptake into bones during the growing years make a person susceptible to osteoporosis later. Nutritional causes of poor calcium status early in life include deficiencies of vitamin D and calcium and possibly of fluoride. Fluoride taken during the bone-building years seems to increase bone density, but supplementation has not been effective in treating osteoporosis. When women with osteoporosis were given fluoride supplements for four years, their spinal bone mass increased, but their other bones fractured more, as compared with the control group.[24] Fluoride-treated women also experienced side effects such as stomach irritation and pain in the lower extremities.

As important as calcium may be to bone health, osteoporosis is not a calcium-deficiency disease comparable to iron-deficiency anemia. In iron-deficiency anemia, high iron intakes reliably reverse the condition; in osteoporosis, though, high calcium intakes alone during adulthood may do little or nothing to reverse bone loss.

Most experts agree that there must be a lower limit for calcium intakes, below which bone loss accelerates. Recommendations for adults in the United States and Canada are set well above this minimum, although exactly how much calcium is minimal is a point of disagreement. Defining an exact minimum is complicated because people who consume less calcium absorb more, and vice versa.

Some people question how certain ethnic groups can use no dairy products and have low calcium intakes, yet still maintain calcium balance. Part of the answer is the body's adaptation to low calcium intakes. Another part of the answer is that bone loss is not always apparent. Women in regions of China who have high calcium intakes have greater bone densities than women in other areas.[25]

CALCIUM RECOMMENDATIONS

Scientists agree that bone strength later in life depends on how well the bones are developed and maintained during youth, and that adequate calcium nutrition during the growing years is essential to achieving optimal peak bone mass.[26] On the basis of this agreement, the Committee on Dietary Allowances recommends 1200 milligrams of calcium per day for everyone 11 through 24 years of age. After age 24, throughout life, other factors can either hasten or slow the bone loss that occurs in everyone. Once a person reaches the bone-losing years of middle age, however, those who formed dense bones during youth have the advantage: they can afford to lose more bone tissue before beginning to suffer ill effects. After bone loss has begun, a person can still do a few things to maintain the bones, as discussed earlier.

Unfortunately, few girls meet the RDA for calcium during their bone-forming years. (Boys generally obtain intakes close to those recommended because they eat more food.) Even if girls do meet the RDA, it may not be high enough to achieve the maximum bone mass.[27] This may mean that most girls start their adult lives with less than optimal bone density. As for adults, women rarely meet the RDA of 800 to 1200 milligrams from food within their energy allowances. Furthermore, evidence is accumulating that calcium recommendations should be higher still, especially for postmenopausal women.[28] Some authorities suggest 1500 milligrams of calcium for postmenopausal women who are not receiving estrogen.

A PERSPECTIVE ON SUPPLEMENTS

People who do not consume milk products or other calcium-rich foods in amounts that provide even half the recommended calcium may benefit from calcium supplements.[29] During the menopausal years, calcium supplements of 1 gram may slow, but cannot fully prevent, the inevitable bone loss.[30] Supplements are commonly used as a part of therapy for osteoporosis, along with gentle exercise and, for women, estrogen replacement, but supplements should not be used as a substitute for estrogen.[31] As a rule, women taking estrogen need no more calcium than the RDA.

Regular vitamin-mineral pills contain little or no calcium. The label may list a few milligrams of calcium, but remember that the RDA is close to a gram for adults.

Anyone contemplating the use of calcium supplements should do so only on a physician's advice. Taking calcium supplements may present risks, as described in Table H12–3. If these risks are deemed acceptable, the consumer still has several decisions to make when selecting a calcium supplement.[32] Supplements are available in three forms. Simplest are the purified calcium compounds, such as calcium carbonate, citrate, gluconate, lactate, malate, or phosphate, and compounds of calcium with amino acids (called amino acid chelates). Then there are mixtures of calcium with other compounds, such as calcium carbonate with magnesium carbonate, with aluminum salts (as in some antacids), or with vitamin D. Then there are powdered, calcium-rich materials such as bone meal, powdered bone, oyster shell, or dolomite (limestone). (See Table H12–4's description of supplement terms.)

Table H12–3

Problems Arising from Calcium Supplementation

People who take calcium supplements risk:

- Impaired iron status. (This is due to the change in stomach pH caused by calcium, which interferes with iron absorption. Calcium citrate, calcium phosphate, calcium carbonate, and calcium chloride taken with meals interfere with iron absorption. Taking calcium supplements between meals limits calcium absorption.)
- Accelerated calcium loss. (Calcium-containing antacids that also contain aluminum and magnesium hydroxide cause a net calcium loss.)
- Urinary tract stones or kidney damage in susceptible individuals. (People who have a history of kidney stones need to be monitored by a physician and to use calcium citrate supplements, which are most soluble.)
- Exposure to contaminants. (Some preparations of bone meal and dolomites are contaminated with hazardous amounts of arsenic, cadmium, mercury, and lead.)
- Vitamin D toxicity. (Vitamin D is needed to enhance calcium absorption, but continued high intakes of vitamin D, which is present in many calcium supplements, can be toxic. Users must eliminate other concentrated vitamin D sources and take enough, but not too much, vitamin D to normalize calcium absorption.)
- Excess blood calcium. (This complication is seen only with doses of calcium fourfold or more greater than customarily prescribed.)
- Milk alkali syndrome. (This alkalosis is also only seen with doses of calcium of 4 to 10 grams/day. This condition disappears when supplementation is discontinued.)
- Other nutrient interactions. (Calcium phosphate dibasic inhibits magnesium absorption.)
- Drug interactions. (Calcium and tetracycline form an insoluble complex that impairs both mineral and drug absorption.)
- Constipation, intestinal bloating, and excess gas; confusion. (Older people are especially prone to these conditions.)

The first question to ask is how well the body absorbs and uses the calcium from various supplements. Based on limited research to date, it seems that most healthy people absorb calcium equally well—and as well as from milk—from any of these supplements: amino acids chelated with calcium; calcium phosphate dibasic; or calcium acetate, carbonate, citrate, gluconate, or lactate. People absorb calcium less well from a mixture of calcium and magnesium carbonates, from oyster shell calcium fortified with inorganic magnesium, from a chelated calcium-magnesium combination, or from calcium carbonate fortified with vitamins and iron.

A way to circumvent adverse nutrient interactions may be to take calcium supplements between, not with, meals. But for anyone with reduced stomach acid secretion, this is not a satisfactory solution because only a meal stimulates sufficient acid secretion to permit the absorption of the calcium. (Score a point here for food sources of calcium.)

Consider another point for food. Some people absorb calcium better from milk and milk products than from even the most absorbable supplements named above.

The next question to ask is how much calcium the supplement provides. Healthy people have consumed up to 2500 milligrams of calcium per day without problems.[33] To be safe, though, supplements should provide less than this, since foods also provide calcium. Read the label to find out how much a dose supplies. Calcium carbonate is 40 percent calcium, whereas calcium gluconate is only 9 percent. The user should select a low-dose supplement and take it several times a day rather than taking a large-dose supplement all at once. Divided doses can improve a day's total absorption by up to 20 percent.

Then consider that when manufacturers compress large quantities

Table H12–4

Calcium Supplements

- **Amino acid chelates** (KEY-lates) are compounds of minerals (such as calcium) combined with amino acids in a form that favors their absorption. A *chelating agent* is a molecule that surrounds another molecule and can then either promote or prevent its movement from place to place; *chele* means claw.
- **Antacids** are acid-buffering agents used to counter excess acidity in the stomach. Calcium-containing preparations (such as Tums) contain available calcium. Antacids with aluminum or magnesium hydroxides (such as Rolaids) can accelerate calcium losses.
- **Bone meal** or **powdered bones** are crushed or ground bone preparations intended to supply calcium to the diet. Calcium from bone is not well absorbed and is often contaminated with toxic materials such as arsenic, mercury, lead, and cadmium.
- **Dolomite** is a compound of minerals (calcium magnesium carbonate) found in limestone and marble. Dolomite is powdered and is sold as a calcium-magnesium supplement, but may be contaminated with toxic minerals, is not well absorbed, and interacts adversely with absorption of other essential minerals.
- **Oyster shell** is a product made from the powdered shells of oysters that is sold as a calcium supplement, but is not well absorbed by the digestive system.

of calcium into small pills, the stomach acid has difficulty penetrating the pill. To test a supplement's absorbability, drop it into a 6-ounce cup of vinegar, and stir occasionally. A high-quality formulation will dissolve within half an hour.

Finally, having chosen a supplement, a person must take it regularly. Clearly, taking supplements for calcium can be a burdensome choice.

Experts agree that it remains highly desirable to adjust food and beverage intakes to provide calcium. The Consensus Conference on Osteoporosis recommends milk. The American Society for Bone and Mineral Research recommends foods as a source of calcium in preference to supplements. The *Diet and Health* report urges people to eat low- or nonfat dairy products and dark green vegetables to meet their calcium needs and concludes that current research does not justify the use of calcium supplements.[34] Seldom is such a consensus seen among nutritionists.

SOME CLOSING THOUGHTS

Unfortunately, many of the strongest risk factors for osteoporosis are beyond people's control: age, sex, genetics, and race. But several factors within people's control can help to reduce the risk: a calcium-rich diet, a moderate protein intake, daily physical activity, abstinence from cigarette smoking, and moderation in, or abstinence from, alcohol use. Women should be evaluated for possible estrogen replacement therapy at menopause. The reward for taking these steps is the best possible chance of preserving bone health throughout life.

NOTES

1. D. T. Felson and coauthors, The effect of postmenopausal estrogen therapy on bone density in elderly women, *New England Journal of Medicine* 329 (1993): 1141–1146; L. G. Tolstoi and R. M. Levin, Osteoporosis—The treatment controversy, *Nutrition Today*, July/August 1992, pp. 6–12.
2. M. W. Tilyard and coauthors, Treatment of postmenopausal osteoporosis with calcitriol or calcium, *New England Journal of Medicine* 326 (1992): 357–362.
3. B. L. Drinkwater, B. Bruemner, and C. H. Chestnut III, Menstrual history as a determinant of current bone density in young athletes, *Journal of the American Medical Association* 263 (1990): 545–548.
4. B. L. Riggs and L. J. Melton, The prevention and treatment of osteoporosis, *New England Journal of Medicine* (1992): 620–627; C. D. Arnaud and S. D. Sanchez, The role of calcium in osteoporosis, *Annual Review of Nutrition* 10 (1990): 397–414.
5. J. S. Finkelstein and coauthors, Osteopenia in men with a history of delayed puberty, *New England Journal of Medicine* 326 (1992): 600–604.
6. S. R. Cummings and coauthors, Risk factors for hip fractures in white women, *New England Journal of Medicine* 332 (1995): 767–773; J. Lutz and R. Tesar, Mother-daughter pairs: Spinal and femoral bone densities and dietary intakes, *American Journal of Clinical Nutrition* 52 (1990): 878–888.
7. H. M. Perry and coauthors, A preliminary report of vitamin D and calcium metabolism in older African Americans, *Journal of the American Geriatric Society* 41 (1993): 612–616.
8. A history of racial and ethnic differences in regard to bone health is found in W. S. Pollitzer and J. J. B. Anderson, Ethnic and genetic differences in bone mass: A review with a hereditary vs environmental perspective, *American Journal of Clinical Nutrition* 50 (1989): 1244–1259.
9. J. A. Metz, J. J. B. Anderson, and P. N. Gallagher, Jr., Intakes of calcium, phosphorus, and protein, and physical activity are related to radial bone mass in young adult women, *American Journal of Clinical Nutrition* 58 (1993): 537–542; C. N. Meridith, Exercise in the prevention of osteoporosis, in *Nutrition of the Elderly* (New York: Raven, 1992), pp. 169–175.
10. ACSM Position stand on osteoporosis and exercise, *Medicine and Science in Sports and Exercise* 27 (1995): i–vii; R. R. Recker and coauthors, Bone gain in young adult women,

Journal of the American Medical Association 268 (1992): 2403–2408.
11. Health & Fitness: Going crazy over calcium—It sells a rainbow of products, but does it work? *Time*, February 23, 1987.
12. J. F. Aloia and coauthors, To what extent is bone mass determined by fat-free or fat mass? *American Journal of Clinical Nutrition* 61 (1995): 1110–1114; Cummings and coauthors, 1995; S. L. Edelstein and E. Barrett-Connor, Relation between body size and bone mineral density in elderly men and women, *American Journal of Epidemiology* 138 (1993): 160–169; I. R. Reid and coauthors, Determinants of total body and regional bone mineral density in normal postmenopausal women—A key role for fat mass, *Journal of Clinical Endocrinology and Metabolism* 75 (1992): 45–51.
13. Drinkwater, Bruemner, and Chestnut III, 1990; J. H. Wilson, Nutrition, physical activity and bone health in women, *Nutrition Research Reviews* 7 (1994): 67–91.
14. J. L. Hopper and E. Seeman, The bone density of female twins discordant for tobacco use, *New England Journal of Medicine* 330 (1994): 387–392.
15. C. W. Slemenda, Cigarettes and the skeleton, *New England Journal of Medicine* 330 (1994): 430–431.
16. Arnaud and Sanchez, 1990; Cummings and coauthors, 1995.
17. M. J. Barger-Lux, R. P. Heaney, and M. R. Stegman, Effects of moderate caffeine intake on the calcium economy of premenopausal women, *American Journal of Clinical Nutrition* 52 (1990): 722–725.
18. Committee on Dietary Allowance, *Recommended Dietary Allowances*, 10th ed. (Washington, D.C.: National Academy Press, 1989); Arnaud and Sanchez, 1990; R. P. Heaney, Protein intake and the calcium economy, *Journal of the American Dietetic Association* 93 (1993): 1259–1260;
J. C. Howe, Postprandial response of calcium metabolism in post menopausal women to meals varying in protein level/source, *Metabolism Clinical and Experimental* 39 (1990): 1246–1252.
19. Heaney, 1993.
20. R. Tesar and coauthors, Axial peripheral bone density and nutrient intakes of post menopausal vegetarian and omnivorous women, *American Journal of Clinical Nutrition* 56 (1992): 699–704.
21. Howe, 1990.
22. G. Saggese and coauthors, Hypomagnesemia and the parathyroid hormone–vitamin D endocrine system in children with insulin-dependent diabetes mellitus, *Journal of Pediatrics* 118 (1991): 220–225.
23. J. Bonjour and coauthors, Hip fracture, femoral bone mineral density, and protein supply in elderly patients, in *Nutrition of the Elderly* (New York: Raven, 1992), pp. 151–159.
24. B. L. Riggs and coauthors, Effect of fluoride treatment on the fracture rate in postmenopausal women with osteoporosis, *New England Journal of Medicine* 322 (1990): 802–809.
25. J. F. Hu and coauthors, Dietary calcium and bone density among middle-aged and elderly women in China, *American Journal of Clinical Nutrition* 58 (1993): 219–227.
26. R. P. Heaney, Nutritional factors in osteoporosis, *Annual Review of Nutrition* 13 (1993): 287–316; F. Bronner, Calcium and osteoporosis, *American Journal of Clinical Nutrition* 60 (1994): 831–836.
27. V. Matkovic and J. Z. Ilich, Calcium requirements for growth: Are current recommendations adequate? *Nutrition Reviews* 51 (1993): 171–180.
28. D. V. Porter, Washington update: NIH consensus Development Conference Statement Optimal Calcium Intake, *Nutrition Today*, September/October 1994, pp. 37–40; R. P. Heaney, Thinking straight about calcium, *New England Journal of Medicine* 328 (1993): 503–505.
29. B. Dawson-Hughes and coauthors, A controlled trial of the effect of calcium supplementation on bone density in postmenopausal women, *New England Journal of Medicine* 323 (1990): 878–883.
30. B. Dawson-Hughes, Calcium supplementation and bone loss: A review of controlled clinical trials, *American Journal of Clinical Nutrition* 54 (1991): 2745–2805; I. R. Reid and coauthors, Effect of calcium supplementation on bone loss in postmenopausal women, *New England Journal of Medicine* 328 (1993): 460–464.
31. Arnaud and Sanchez, 1990; B. Ettinger, H. K. Genant, and C. E. Cann, Long-term estrogen replacement therapy prevents bone loss and fractures, *Annals of Internal Medicine* 102 (1985): 319–324.
32. D. I. Levenson and R. S. Bockman, A review of calcium preparations, *Nutrition Reviews* 52 (1994): 221–232.
33. Committee on Dietary Allowances, 1989, pp. 174–184.
34. Committee on Diet and Health, *Diet and Health: Implications for Reducing Chronic Disease Risk* (Washington, D.C.: National Academy Press, 1989), p. 17.

Chapter 13

The Trace Minerals

CONTENTS

MICROGRAPH: Selenium, an essential trace mineral

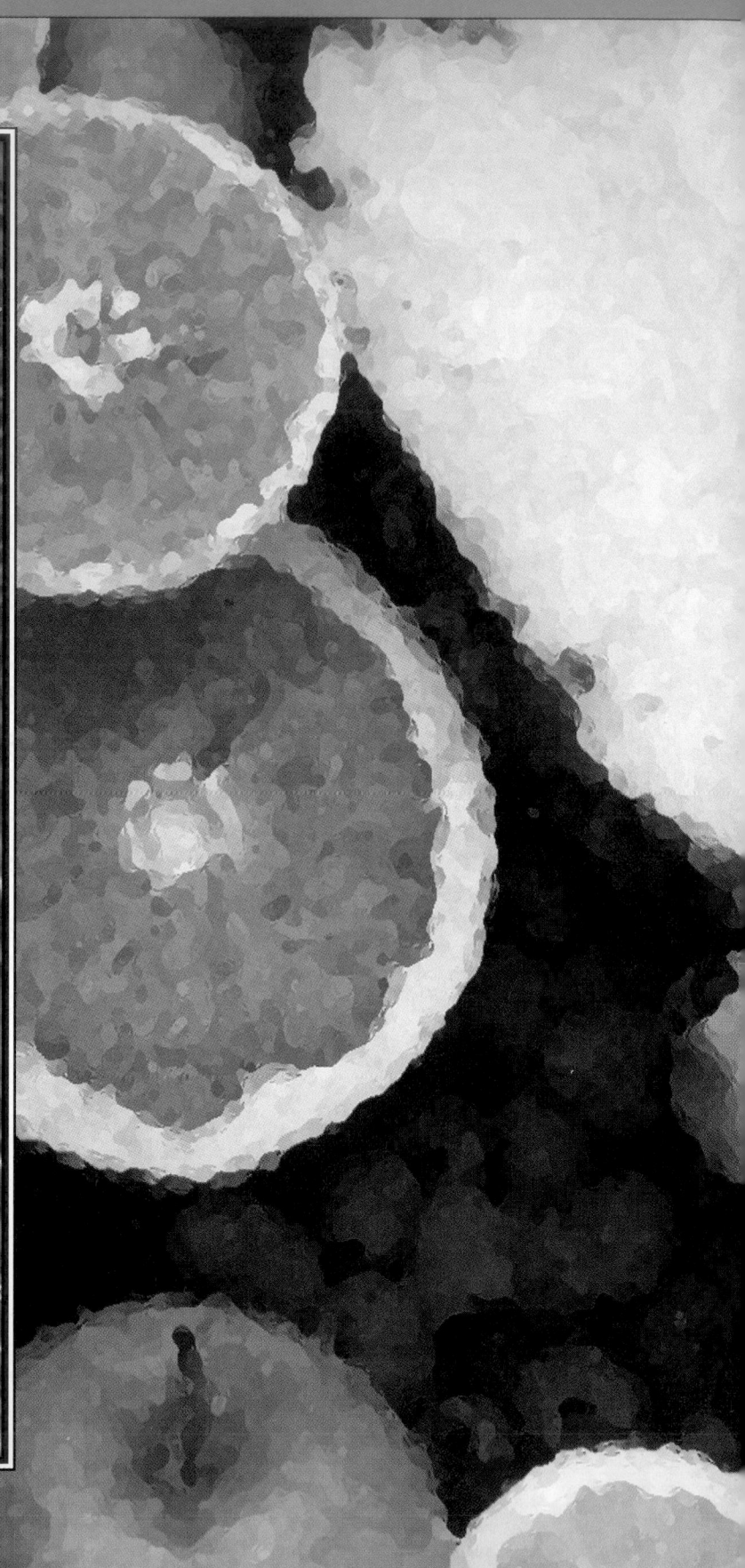

Figure 12–5 in the last chapter (p. 439) showed how tiny the quantities of trace minerals in the human body are. Taken all together, they are only a bit of dust, hardly enough to fill a teaspoon. Yet each of the trace minerals performs some vital role. A deficiency of any of them may be fatal, and an excess of many is equally deadly. Remarkably, people's diets normally supply just enough of these minerals to maintain health.

The best-known trace elements—iron, zinc, iodine, and selenium—have been extensively studied, and the Committee on Dietary Allowances has established RDA for them. For five others, the committee has published tentative ranges for safe and adequate daily intakes. Still others are recognized as essential for some animals, but data from which to estimate human requirements are lacking.[1] Many other trace elements are currently under study as possible nutrients.

The trace elements (minerals):

- Iron
- Zinc
- Iodine
- Selenium

RDA nutrients

- Copper
- Manganese
- Fluoride
- Chromium
- Molybdenum

Safe and adequate daily dietary intakes established

- Arsenic
- Nickel
- Silicon
- Boron

Known essential for animals; human requirements under study

The Trace Minerals—An Overview

A few statements apply to the trace minerals as a group. The body requires them in minuscule quantities, and they function in some similar ways, assisting enzymes in diverse tasks all over the body. In addition, each one has special duties that only it can perform.

Food Sources The trace mineral contents of foods are unpredictable, because they depend on soil and water quality and on how foods are processed. Furthermore, many factors in the diet and within the body affect bioavailability and absorption. Still, it is probably safe to say that a list of outstanding food sources for each of the trace minerals, just like the lists of outstanding foods for the other nutrients, would include a wide variety of foods, especially whole foods.

Deficiencies Severe deficiencies of the better-known minerals are easy to recognize. Deficiencies of less well-known minerals are harder to diagnose, and for all minerals, mild deficiencies are easy to overlook. In general, the most common result of a deficiency is failure of children to grow and thrive, for the minerals are active in all the body systems—the GI tract, cardiovascular system, blood, muscles, bones, and central nervous system.

Toxicities The trace elements are toxic at an intake not far above the estimated requirements. Thus it is important not to overdose. The Committee on Dietary Allowances places a special warning on its trace mineral table not to habitually exceed the upper end of the range of recommended intakes.

Supplements Many vitamin-mineral pills contain trace minerals, making it easy for pill takers to have excessive intakes. The Food and Drug Administration (FDA) is not permitted to limit the amounts of trace minerals in supplements; consumers have demanded the freedom to choose their own doses of nutrients. Individuals who take vitamin-mineral pills must therefore be aware of the possible dangers and avoid supplements that contain more than the RDA. They would be wiser to select foods from a variety of sources than to try to put together a combination of pills to meet all their needs without causing toxicity.

Interactions As research on the trace minerals unfolds, many interactions among them have come to light. An excess of one may cause a deficiency of another. (A slight manganese overload, for example, may aggravate an iron deficiency.) A deficiency of one may open the way for another to cause a toxic reaction. (Iron deficiency, for example, makes the body much more susceptible than normal to lead poisoning.) A deficiency of one may exacerbate the problems associated with the deficiency of another. (A combined iodine and selenium deficiency, for example, reduces thyroid hormone production more than an iodine deficiency alone.)[2] These examples point out the need to balance intakes and to steer clear of supplement use. A good food source of one nutrient may be a poor food source of another; and factors that cooperate with some trace elements may oppose others. (Vitamin C, for example, enhances the absorption of iron but depresses that of copper.) The continuous outpouring of new information about the trace minerals is a sign that we have much more to learn about them.

Iron

Iron is an essential nutrient that is vital to the processes by which cells generate energy. Iron can also be damaging when it accumulates in the body. In fact, iron is a problem nutrient for millions of people: some people simply don't eat enough iron-containing foods to support their health optimally, while others have so much iron that it threatens their well-being. The principle that too little or too much of a nutrient is harmful seems particularly apropos for iron.

IRON ROLES IN THE BODY

Iron's two ionic states:

- **Ferrous iron** (reduced): Fe^{++}.
- **Ferric iron** (oxidized): Fe^{+++}.

For details about these ions, oxidation, and reduction, see Appendix B.

Reminder: A *cofactor* is a mineral element that works with an enzyme to facilitate a chemical reaction.

Reminder: *Hemoglobin* is the oxygen-carrying protein of the red blood cells that transports oxygen from the lungs to tissues throughout the body; hemoglobin accounts for 80% of the body's iron.

myoglobin: the oxygen-holding protein of the muscle cells.
myo = muscle

Iron has a knack of switching back and forth between two ionic states. In the reduced state, iron has lost two electrons and therefore has a net positive charge of two. Iron in the reduced state is known as ferrous iron. In the oxidized state, iron has lost a third electron, has a net positive charge of three, and is known as ferric iron. Because it can exist in different ionic states, iron can serve as a cofactor to enzymes involved in oxidation-reduction reactions. In every cell, iron works with several of the electron-transport-chain proteins that perform the final steps of the energy-yielding metabolic pathways.* These proteins transfer hydrogens and electrons from energy-yielding nutrients to oxygen, forming water, and in the process make ATP for the cell's use.

Most of the body's iron is found in two proteins: hemoglobin in the red blood cells and myoglobin in the muscle cells. In both, iron helps accept, carry, and then release oxygen. Iron is also found in many enzymes that oxidize compounds—reactions so widespread in metabolism that they occur in all cells. Iron is required by enzymes involved in the making of amino acids, hormones, and neurotransmitters.

*The iron-containing proteins at the end of the metabolic pathway include several TCA cycle enzymes and the electron carriers of the electron transport chain—known as *cytochromes*. See Appendix C for these pathways.

IRON ABSORPTION AND METABOLISM

The body conserves iron zealously and has devised many special provisions for its handling, depicted in Figure 13–1. Because iron losses are usually limited, balance is maintained primarily through absorption.

Iron Absorption Two special proteins in the intestinal mucosal cells help the body absorb iron from food. One protein, called *mucosal ferritin,* receives iron from the GI tract and stores it in the mucosal cell. When the body needs iron, mucosal ferritin releases some iron to another protein, called *mucosal transferrin.* Mucosal transferrin transfers the iron to a carrier in the blood called *blood transferrin,* which transports iron to the rest of the body. Intestinal mucosal cells are

Mucosal ferritin (FERR-ih-tin), holds iron in the cell, and mucosal transferrin (trans-FERR-in) passes the iron on to blood transferrin.

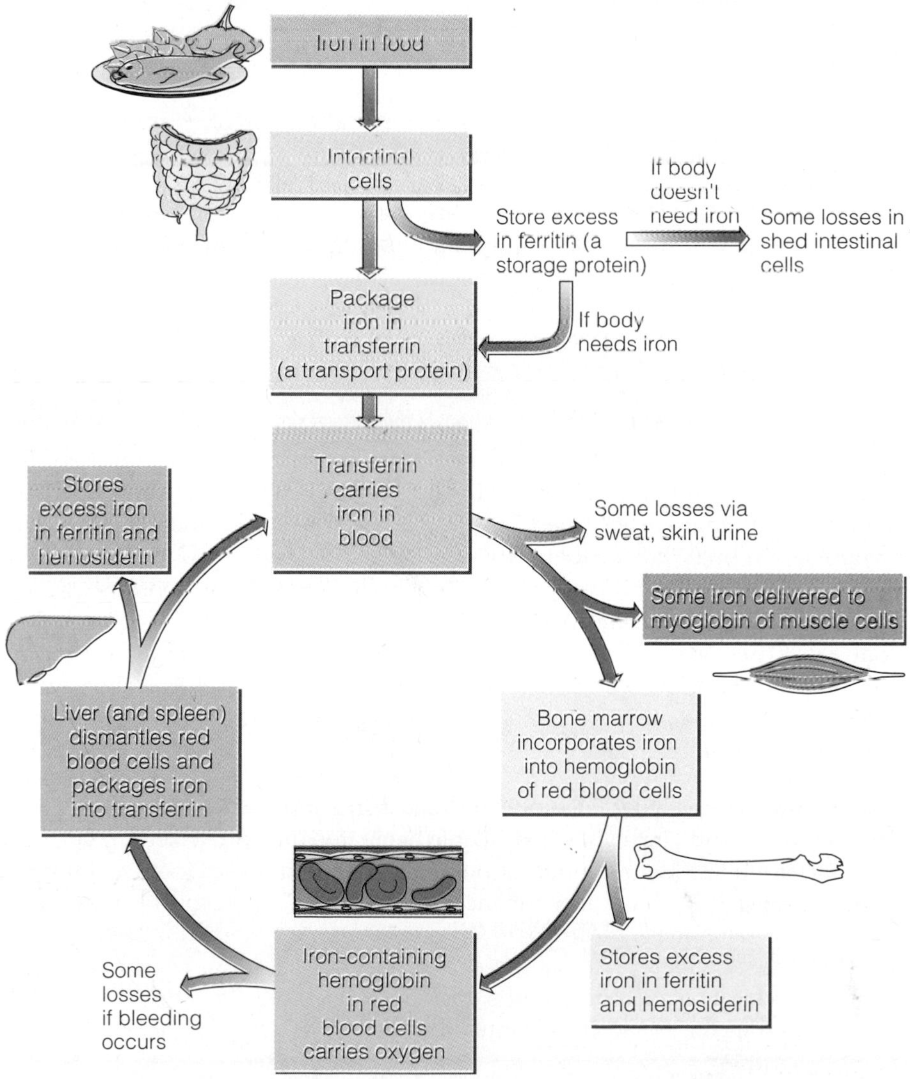

Figure 13–1

Iron Routes in the Body

Most iron is recycled. Some is lost with body tissues and must be replaced by eating iron-containing food.

Figure 13–2

Heme and Nonheme Iron in Foods

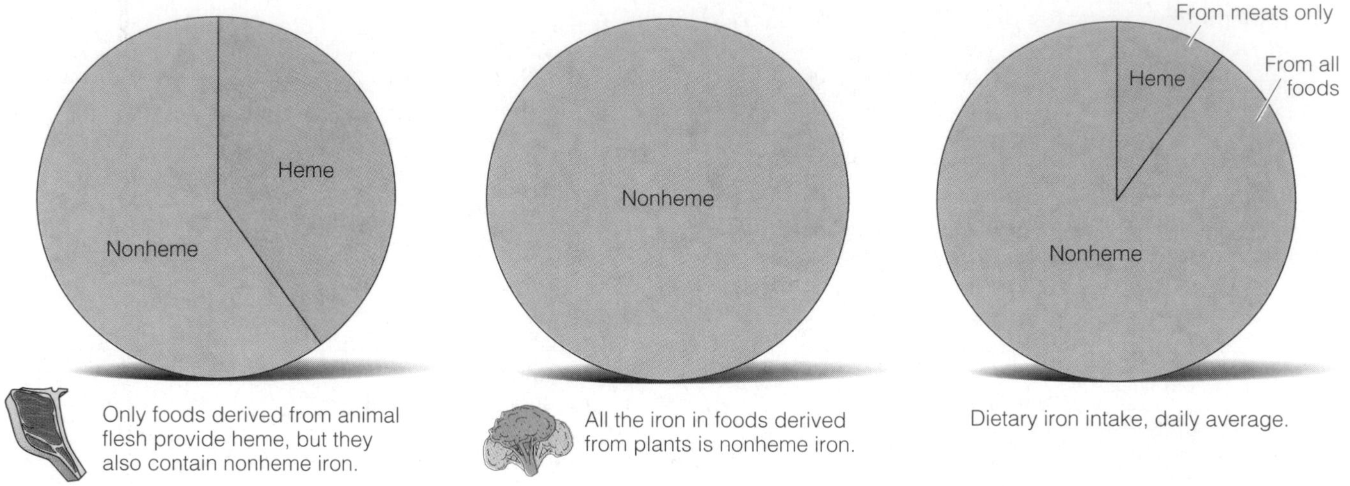

Only foods derived from animal flesh provide heme, but they also contain nonheme iron.

All the iron in foods derived from plants is nonheme iron.

Dietary iron intake, daily average.

replaced about every three days; when the cells are shed from the intestinal mucosa and excreted in the feces, they carry some iron out with them. The iron-holding capacity of these cells provides a buffer against short-term changes in iron need or supply.

heme (HEEM): the iron-holding part of the hemoglobin and myoglobin proteins. About 40% of the iron in meat, fish, and poultry is bound into heme; the other 60% is nonheme iron.

Heme and Nonheme Iron How much iron is absorbed depends in part on its source. Iron occurs in two forms in foods: as heme iron, which is found only in foods derived from the flesh of animals, such as meats, poultry, and fish; and as nonheme iron, which is found in both plant-derived and animal-derived foods (see Figure 13–2). Heme iron contributes only about 10 percent of the iron the average person consumes in a day; most of the rest is nonheme iron from vegetables, fruits, grains, eggs, meat, fish, and poultry. Even though heme iron accounts for a small proportion of the intake, it is so well absorbed that it contributes significant iron: heme iron is absorbed at a relatively constant rate of about 23 percent. The rates of absorption of nonheme iron are lower, ranging from 2 to 20 percent, and are strongly influenced by dietary factors and body iron stores. People with severe iron deficiencies absorb both heme and nonheme iron more efficiently and are more sensitive to dietary enhancing factors than people with better iron status.

MFP factor: a factor associated with the digestion of meat, fish, and poultry that enhances iron absorption.

Factors that enhance nonheme iron absorption:
- Vitamin C (ascorbic acid).
- MFP factor.
- Citric acid and lactic acid from foods and HCl acid from the stomach.
- Sugars (including the sugars in wine).

Factors that reduce iron absorption:
- Phytates and fibers.
- EDTA (in food additives).
- Calcium and phosphorus (milk).
- Tannic acid (and other polyphenols).

Absorption-Enhancing Factors: MFP and Vitamin C Meat, fish, and poultry contain not only the highly bioavailable heme iron, but also a factor (MFP factor) that promotes the absorption of nonheme iron from other foods eaten with them.[3] Vitamin C, which also enhances nonheme iron absorption from foods eaten in the same meal, is the most potent promoter of nonheme iron absorption.[4] Vitamin C captures iron and keeps it in the ferrous form, ready for absorption. A system of calculating the iron absorbed from a meal has been developed and reveals some factors worthy of attention (see the accompanying box).[5]

Absorption Inhibitors Some dietary factors bind with nonheme iron, inhibiting absorption. These include the phytates and fibers in whole-grain cere-

How to Calculate Iron Absorbed from Meals

Three factors go into the calculation of the amount of iron absorbed from a meal: first, how much of the iron in the meal was heme and how much was nonheme iron; second, how much vitamin C was in the meal; and third, how much total meat, fish, and poultry (MFP) was consumed. Iron stores are assumed to be moderate and are not taken into consideration. Write down the foods you eat at a typical meal, look up their iron content in Appendix H, and then answer these questions:

1. How much iron was from meat, fish, and poultry? ____ mg.
2. On average, 40% of the amount in step 1 is heme iron:

   ____ mg (step 1) × 0.40 = ____ mg heme iron.
3. How much iron was from other sources? ____ mg.
4. The amount in step 3 plus 60% of step 1 is nonheme iron:

   ____ mg (step 3) + 0.60 × ____ mg (step 1)
   = ____ mg nonheme iron.
5. How much vitamin C was in the meal? ____ mg. Less than 25 milligrams is low; 25 to 75 milligrams is medium; more than 75 milligrams is high.
6. How much MFP was in the meal? ____ oz. Less than 1 ounce lean MFP is low; 1 to 3 ounces is medium, more than 3 ounces is high.*

Now calculate: You absorbed 23% of the heme iron, or:

____ mg (step 2) × 0.23 =
____ mg heme iron absorbed.

Now, take your best score from steps 5 and 6. If either vitamin C or MFP was high or if both were medium, the availability of your nonheme iron was high. If neither was high, but one was medium, the availability of your nonheme iron was medium. If both were low, your nonheme iron had poor availability. You absorbed:

- High availability: 8% of the nonheme iron.
- Medium availability: 5% of the nonheme iron.
- Poor availability: 3% of the nonheme iron.

Now calculate: You absorbed ____ % of the nonheme iron, or:

____ mg (step 4) × ____ =
____ mg nonheme iron absorbed.

Your total: ____ mg nonheme iron absorbed.

Add the two together:

- ____ mg heme iron absorbed.
- ____ mg nonheme iron absorbed.

Total = ____ mg iron absorbed.

The RDA assumes you will absorb 10 percent of the iron you ingest. Thus, if you are a man of any age or a woman over 50 years old (RDA 10 milligrams), you need to absorb 1 milligram per day; if you are a woman 11 to 50 years old (RDA 15 milligrams), you need to absorb 1.5 milligrams per day. If you have higher menstrual losses than the average woman, you may need still more.

---

*In question 6, we adapted the calculation of Monsen and coauthors, stating it in ounces. Actual numbers are less than 23 grams cooked meat, low; 23 to 46 grams, medium; and 69 grams or more, high.

Source: E. R. Monsen and coauthors, Estimation of available dietary iron, *American Journal of Clinical Nutrition* 31 (1978): 134–141.

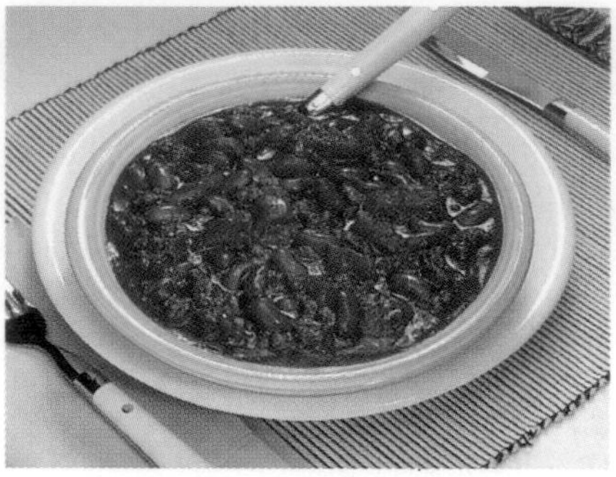

This chili dinner provides heme and nonheme iron and MFP from meat, nonheme iron from legumes, and vitamin C from tomatoes. The combination of heme iron, nonheme iron, MFP, and vitamin C helps to achieve maximum iron absorption.

The iron storage proteins are ferritin (FERR-ih-tin) and hemosiderin (heem-oh-SID-er-in).

als and nuts, the calcium and phosphorus in milk, the EDTA in food additives,* and tannic acid. Tannic acid is present in tea, coffee, nuts, and some fruits and vegetables.[6] The effect of soy on iron absorption is inconclusive; several studies have found that soy inhibits iron absorption while others indicate no effect.[7]

Adaptability of Absorption Overall, only about 10 to 15 percent of dietary iron is absorbed, although this amount varies widely from person to person and from time to time in the same person. Absorption can be as low as 2 percent in a person with GI disease or as high as 35 percent in a rapidly growing, healthy child. Absorption also adjusts to supply and to need: if a person's iron intake diminishes, or if the need increases for any reason (such as pregnancy), absorption increases. More mucosal transferrin and blood transferrin are produced to absorb more iron from the intestines and carry more into the body.

Iron Transport and Storage Blood transferrin captures absorbed iron and carries it to the bone marrow and other tissues. The bone marrow takes up large quantities for use in making new red blood cells; other tissues take less. Surplus iron is stored in proteins (ferritin and hemosiderin), primarily in the liver, but also in the bone marrow and spleen. When dietary iron has been plentiful, ferritin is constantly and rapidly made and broken down, providing an ever-ready supply of iron. When iron concentrations become abnormally high, the liver converts some ferritin into another storage protein called hemosiderin. Hemosiderin releases iron more slowly than ferritin does. By storing excess iron, the body protects itself: free iron would attack cell lipids, DNA, and protein.[8]

Iron Recycling The average red blood cell lives about four months; then the spleen and liver cells remove it from the blood, take it apart, and prepare the degradation products for excretion or recycling. The iron is salvaged: the liver attaches it to blood transferrin, which transports it back to the bone marrow to be reused in making new red blood cells. Thus, although red blood cells live for only about four months, the iron recycles through each new generation of cells. The body loses some iron daily via the GI tract and, if bleeding occurs, in blood; only tiny amounts of iron are lost in urine, sweat, and shed skin.†

IRON DEFICIENCY

If absorption cannot compensate for losses or low dietary intakes, and body stores are used up, then iron deficiency sets in. Because so much of the body's iron is in the blood, iron losses are greatest whenever blood is lost.

Blood Losses Bleeding from any site incurs iron losses. In some cases, as in an active ulcer, the bleeding may not be obvious, but even small chronic blood losses significantly deplete iron reserves.[9] In developing countries, blood loss is

---

*EDTA is ethylenediamine tetra acetate, a chelating agent that is used in food processing to retard crystal formation and promote color retention.

†Daily iron losses in the adult male are about 0.9 to 1.0 milligrams per day. Because of their smaller surface area, women's basal losses are 0.7 to 0.8 milligrams per day, but women lose additional iron in menses. Menstrual losses vary considerably, but over a month, they average about 0.5 milligrams per day.

often brought on by parasitic infections of the GI tract. Regular blood donations incur similar losses and necessitate increased iron intakes. Regular menstrual losses make women's iron needs much greater than men's.

The iron content of blood is about 0.5 mg/100 mL blood. A person donating a pint of blood (approximately 500 mL) loses about 2.5 mg iron.

Vulnerable Stages of Life Some stages of life both demand more iron and provide less, making deficiency likely. As mentioned, women are especially prone to iron deficiency during their reproductive years because of repeated blood losses during menstruation. Pregnancy places iron demands on women as well; iron is needed to support the added blood volume, the growth of the fetus, and blood loss during childbirth. Infants and young children receive little iron from their high-milk diets, yet need extra iron to support their rapid growth. The rapid growth of adolescence, especially for males, and the menstrual losses of females also demand extra iron that a typical teen diet may not provide. The information about iron in foods, which appears later in this chapter, is especially important during these stages of life.

High risk for iron deficiency:

- Women in their reproductive years.
- Pregnant women.
- Infants and young children.
- Teenagers.

HEALTHY PEOPLE 2000: Reduce iron deficiency to less than 3% among children aged 1 to 4 and women of childbearing age.

Assessment of Iron Deficiency Iron deficiency develops in stages.[10] This section provides a brief overview of how assessors detect these stages, and Appendix E provides more details. In the first stage of iron deficiency, iron stores diminish. Measures of serum ferritin reflect iron stores and are most valuable in assessing iron status.

iron deficiency: the state of having depleted iron stores.

Stages of iron deficiency:

- Iron stores diminish.
- Transport iron decreases.
- Hemoglobin production falls.

The second stage of iron deficiency is characterized by a decrease in iron being transported within the body: serum iron falls, and the iron-carrying protein transferrin *increases* (an adaptation that enhances iron absorption). Together, these two measures can determine the severity of the deficiency—the more transferrin and the less iron in the blood, the more advanced the deficiency is.

The third stage of iron deficiency occurs when the supply of transport iron diminishes to the point that it limits hemoglobin production. Now the hemoglobin precursor, erythrocyte protoporphyrin, begins to accumulate as hemoglobin and hematocrit values decline.

Hemoglobin and hematocrit tests are easy, quick, and inexpensive, so they are the tests most commonly used in evaluating iron status; their usefulness is limited, however, because they are late indicators of iron deficiency. Furthermore, other nutrient deficiencies and medical conditions can influence their values. Table 13–1 includes a list of the symptoms of iron deficiency.

erythrocyte protoporphyrin (PRO-toe-PORE-fe-rin): a precursor to hemoglobin.

hematocrit: measurement of the volume of the red blood cells packed by centrifuge in a given volume of blood; the volume reflects red blood cell size.

Iron Deficiency and Anemia Iron deficiency and anemia are not the same: people may be iron deficient without being anemic. The term *iron deficiency* refers to depleted body iron stores without regard to the degree of depletion or to the presence of anemia. The term *anemia* refers to the severe depletion of iron stores that results in a low hemoglobin concentration. The red blood cells in a person with iron-deficiency anemia are pale and small (Figure 13–3). They can't carry enough oxygen from the lungs to the tissues, so energy metabolism in the cells falters. The result is fatigue, weakness, headaches, apathy, pallor, and poor resistance to cold temperatures. Since hemoglobin is the bright red pigment of

iron-deficiency anemia: a blood iron deficiency that results in small, pale, red blood cells. Iron-deficiency anemia is a **microcytic** (my-cro-SIT-ic) **hypochromic** (high-po-KROME-ic) **anemia.**

micro = small
cytic = cells
hypo = too little
chrom = color

Table 13–1

Iron—A Summary

Adult RDA
Men: 10 mg/day
Women: 15 mg/day (19–50 yr) 10 mg/day (51+)
Chief Functions in the Body
Part of the protein hemoglobin, which carries oxygen from place to place in the body; part of the protein myoglobin in muscles, which makes oxygen available for muscle contraction; necessary for the utilization of energy as part of the cells' metabolic machinery
Significant Sources
Red meats, fish, poultry, shellfish, eggs, legumes, dried fruits

Deficiency Symptoms	Toxicity Symptoms
EYES	
Blue sclera[a]	
IMMUNE SYSTEM	
Reduced resistance to infection (lowered immunity)	Infections
NERVOUS/MUSCULAR SYSTEMS	
Reduced work productivity, tolerance to work, and voluntary work; reduced physical fitness; weakness; fatigue; impaired cognitive function (children); reduced learning ability; increased distractibility (inability to pay attention); impaired visual discrimination; impaired reactivity and coordination (infants)	Lethargy, joint disease
SKIN	
Itching; pale nailbeds, eye membranes, and palm creases; concave nails; impaired wound healing	Pigmentation, loss of hair
GENERAL	
Reduced resistance to cold, inability to regulate body temperature, pica (clay eating, ice eating)	Death by accidental poisoning in children; organ damage, enlarged liver, amenorrhea, impotence

[a]*Sclera* is a tough fibrous tissue that covers the "white" of the eye; *blue sclera* has an abnormal degree of blueness.

the blood, the skin of a fair person who is anemic may become noticeably pale. In a dark-skinned person, the eye lining, normally pink, will be very pale.

Prevalence of Iron Deficiency Worldwide, iron deficiency is the most common nutrient deficiency.[11] Iron-deficiency anemia affects an estimated 15 percent of the world's population, with the highest prevalence in developing countries.[12] Young children and pregnant women are especially vulnerable. In the United States, the prevalence of iron-deficiency anemia has declined considerably in the last decade or so. Among adult women, more adequate iron status may be attributed to such factors as improved socioeconomic status, iron and vitamin C fortification, increased use of vitamin C and iron supplements, and reduced menstrual blood loss thanks to birth control pills.[13] The iron status of infants and young children in the United States has also improved in the last decade thanks to more widespread breastfeeding and greater use of iron-fortified infant formulas and cereals.[14] For children from low-income families, the Special Supplemental Food Pro-

Figure 13–3

Normal and Anemic Blood Cells

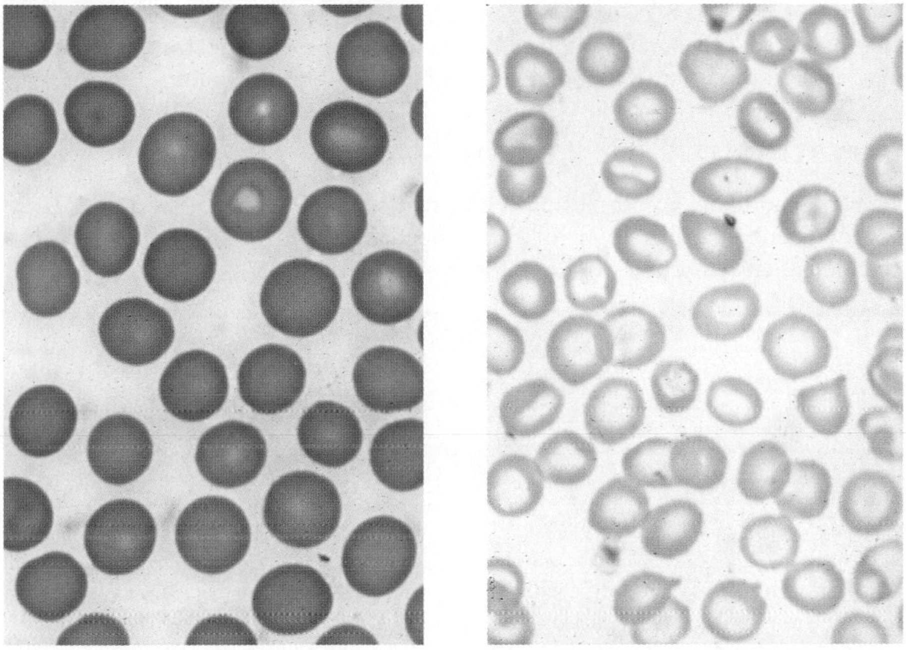

Normal blood cells. Both size and color are normal.

Blood cells in iron-deficiency anemia. These cells are small (microcytic) and pale (hypochromic) because they contain less hemoglobin.

---

gram for Women, Infants, and Children (WIC), which provides foods high in iron to low-income families, appears also to have helped.

Iron Deficiency and Behavior Long before the red blood cells are affected and anemia is diagnosed, a developing iron deficiency affects behavior. Even at slightly lowered iron levels, the complete oxidation of pyruvate is impaired, reducing physical work capacity and productivity. With reduced energy available to work, plan, think, play, sing, or learn, people simply do these things less. They have no obvious deficiency symptoms; they just appear unmotivated, apathetic, and less physically fit.

The effects of iron deficiency on children's behavior are discussed in Chapter 16.

The iron needs of physically active people and the special iron deficiency known as runner's anemia are discussed in Chapter 14.

Many of the symptoms associated with iron deficiency are easily mistaken for behavioral or motivational problems. A restless child who fails to pay attention in class might be thought contrary. An apathetic homemaker who has let housework pile up might be thought lazy. No responsible nutritionist would ever claim that all behavioral problems are caused by nutrient deficiencies, but poor nutrition is always a possible contributor to problems like these. When investigating a behavioral problem, it makes sense to check the adequacy of the diet and to seek a routine physical examination before undertaking more expensive, and possibly harmful, treatment options.

Iron Deficiency and Pica A curious behavior seen in some iron-deficient people, especially in women and children of low-income groups, is pica—an appetite for ice, clay, paste, and other nonfood substances. It is not clear whether

pica (PIE-ka): a craving for nonfood substances. Also known as **geophagia** (gee-oh-FAY-gee-uh) when referring to clay eating and **pagophagia** (pag-oh-FAY-gee-uh) when referring to ice craving.
- *picus* = woodpecker or magpie
- *geo* = earth
- *phagein* = to eat
- *pago* = frost

iron deficiency precedes or follows pica. These substances contain no iron and cannot remedy a deficiency; in fact, clay actually inhibits iron absorption, which may explain the iron deficiency that accompanies such behavior.

IRON TOXICITY

iron overload: toxicity from excess iron.

The body normally absorbs less iron if its stores are full, but some individuals are poorly defended against iron toxicity. Once considered rare, iron overload has emerged as an important disorder of iron metabolism.

hemochromatosis (heem-oh-crome-a-TOCE-iss): a hereditary defect in iron metabolism characterized by deposits of iron-containing pigment in many tissues, with tissue damage.

hemosiderosis (heem-oh-sid-er-OH-sis): a condition characterized by the deposition of hemosiderin in the liver and other tissues.

Iron Overload Iron overload is known as hemochromatosis and is usually caused by a gene that enhances iron absorption. Other causes of iron overload include repeated blood transfusions, massive doses of dietary iron, and rare metabolic disorders. Long-term overconsumption of iron may cause hemosiderosis, a condition characterized by large deposits of the iron storage protein hemosiderin in the liver and other tissues.

Some of the signs and symptoms of iron overload are similar to those of iron deficiency: fatigue, headache, irritability, lowered work performance, and anemia. Therefore, taking iron supplements before measuring iron status is clearly unwise; hemoglobin tests alone would fail to make the distinction.[15]

Iron overload is most often diagnosed when tissue damage occurs, especially in iron-storing organs such as the liver. Infections are likely to develop because bacteria thrive on iron-rich blood. Other common symptoms include enlarged liver, skin pigmentation, lethargy, joint diseases, loss of body hair, amenorrhea, and impotence. These effects are most severe in people who drink large quantities of alcohol because alcohol damages the intestine, further impairing its defenses against absorbing excess iron. Untreated hemochromatosis aggravates the risks of diabetes, liver cancer, heart disease, and arthritis.

In the United States, an estimated 10 percent of the population is in positive iron balance, with 1 percent having iron overload. Iron overload is more common in men than in women and is twice as prevalent among men as is iron deficiency. Some people have expressed concerns about the widespread iron fortification of foods.[16] Widespread fortification does make it hard for people with hemochromatosis to follow a low-iron diet, but greater dangers lie in the indiscriminate use of iron and vitamin C supplements.

Iron and Heart Disease Recent research has found that the risk of heart disease is markedly higher for the small proportion of people who have both high blood iron and high LDL cholesterol.[17] For every 1 percent rise in blood iron, there was a 4 percent rise in the risk; only smoking predicted heart attacks better than iron status. High LDL alone was not a major risk factor in this study; it only became a risk factor when accompanied by high iron. Free iron oxidizes LDL, and oxidized LDL is most damaging to the cardiovascular system. This is an important finding in light of this nation's extensive use of vitamin C supplements: vitamin C not only enhances iron absorption, but releases iron from ferritin, allowing free iron to wreak the damage typical of free radicals.[18] This is an example of how vitamin C acts as a *pro*oxidant when taken in high doses (see Highlight 11).

Prior to these findings, scientists had speculated that premenopausal women were protected against heart disease by their estrogen (women's rate of heart disease is lower and begins to approach that of men only after menopause). Now scientists are asking whether low iron stores from repeated menstrual losses might be the protective factor. (Women's iron stores tend to catch up with men's after menopause.)

Iron and Cancer There also appears to be a positive association between iron and cancer.[19] Explanations for how iron might be involved in causing cancer focus on its involvement in lipid peroxidation (see Highlight 11). These reactions generate free radicals that can damage DNA, possibly causing cancer. One of the beneficial effects of a high-fiber diet may be that its phytate binds iron, making it less available for such reactions.

Iron Poisoning The most common cause of accidental poisoning in small children is ingestion of iron supplements or multivitamin supplements with iron. Symptoms of intoxication include nausea, vomiting, diarrhea, a rapid heartbeat, a weak pulse, dizziness, shock, and confusion. As few as 6 to 12 iron tablets have caused death in a child within four hours. A child suspected of iron poisoning should be rushed to the hospital to have the stomach pumped; 30 minutes may make a crucial difference.

IRON RECOMMENDATIONS AND INTAKES

To obtain enough iron, people must first select iron-rich foods and then eat so as to maximize iron absorption. This discussion begins by identifying iron-rich foods, then reviews factors affecting absorption.

Recommended Iron Intakes The usual Western mixed diet provides only about 6 to 7 milligrams of iron in every 1000 kcalories. The RDA for an adult man is 10 milligrams and most men eat more than 2000 kcalories a day, so men can meet their iron needs without special effort. The RDA for a woman during her childbearing years, however, is 15 milligrams.[20] (The box on p. 484 explains how the recommended intake is calculated.) Because women have higher iron needs and typically need fewer than 2000 kcalories per day, they have trouble obtaining sufficient iron. On the average, women receive only 10 to 11 milligrams iron per day, not enough until after menopause. To meet their iron needs from foods, premenopausal women must emphasize the most iron-rich foods in every food group at every meal.

Iron in Foods Figure 13–4 shows the amounts of iron in selected foods. Meats, fish, and poultry contribute the most iron; other protein-rich foods such as legumes and eggs provide less. Foods in the milk group are as poor in iron as they are rich in calcium. Although an indispensable part of the diet, milk products should not be overemphasized. Grain foods vary; whole-grain and enriched breads and cereals are the richest in iron. Finally, among other plant foods, legumes, dark greens, and some fruits (especially when dried) contribute iron.

Iron-Enriched Foods Iron is one of the enrichment nutrients for breads and cereals. One serving of enriched bread or cereal provides only a little iron, but because people eat many servings of these foods, the contribution can be significant. Iron added to foods is not absorbed as well as iron occurring naturally in

How to Estimate the Recommended Daily Intake for Iron

To calculate the recommended daily iron intake, a number of factors need to be considered. For example, for an adult woman:

- Losses from shed skin: 1.0 milligram.
- Losses through menstruation (about 15 milligrams total averaged over 30 days): 0.5 milligram.
- Average daily need (total): 1.5 milligrams.
- Average iron intake: 10 to 11 milligrams per day (provides adequate stores for most women).
- Added margin of safety to cover the needs of essentially all adult women.

Assuming that an average of 10 to 15 percent of ingested iron is absorbed, the RDA is set at 15 milligrams.

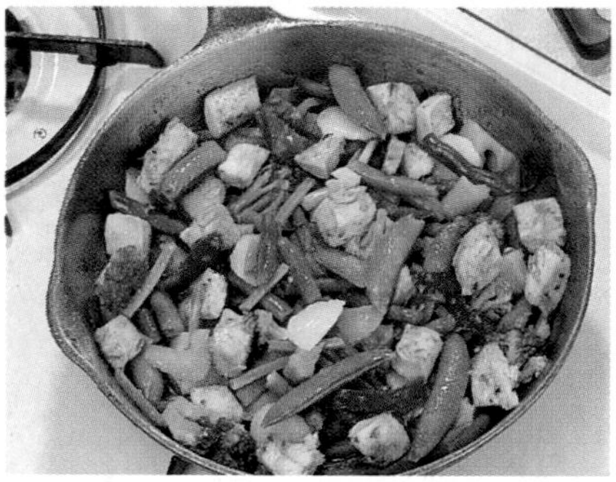

An old-fashioned iron skillet adds iron to foods.

foods, but eaten with absorption-enhancing foods, enrichment iron can make a difference. In some cases, enrichment may even contribute to iron overload, at least in men. At present, 25 percent of all the iron consumed in the United States derives from enriched breads, fortified breakfast cereals, and the like.

Maximizing Iron Absorption In general, the bioavailability of iron in meats, fish, and poultry is high; in grains and legumes, intermediate; and in most vegetables, especially those high in oxalate such as spinach, low. The amount of iron ultimately absorbed from a meal depends on the interplay between enhancing and inhibiting factors. For maximum absorption of nonheme iron, eat meat for MFP and fruits or vegetables for vitamin C. The iron of baked beans, for example, will be enhanced by the MFP in a piece of ham served with them; the iron of bread will be enhanced by vitamin C in a slice of tomato on a sandwich.

CONTAMINATION AND SUPPLEMENTAL IRON

In addition to the iron from foods, contamination iron from nonfood sources of inorganic iron salts can contribute to the day's intakes. People can also ingest iron in supplement form.

contamination iron: iron found in foods as the result of contamination by inorganic iron salts from iron cookware, iron-containing soils, and the like.

Contamination Iron Foods cooked in iron cookware take up iron salts. A half cup of spaghetti sauce simmered in a glass dish provides 3 milligrams of iron, but the iron increases to 87 milligrams when the sauce is simmered for three hours in an iron skillet. The more acidic the food, and the longer it is cooked in iron cookware, the higher the iron content. Even in the short time it takes to scramble eggs, the cook can triple their iron content by cooking them in an iron pan. Similarly, dried peaches or raisins contain more iron than the fresh fruits do, because they are dried in iron pans. Admittedly, the absorption of this iron may be poor (perhaps only 1 to 2 percent, depending on what else is eaten with the meal), but every little bit counts.

Figure 13–4 Iron in Selected Foods

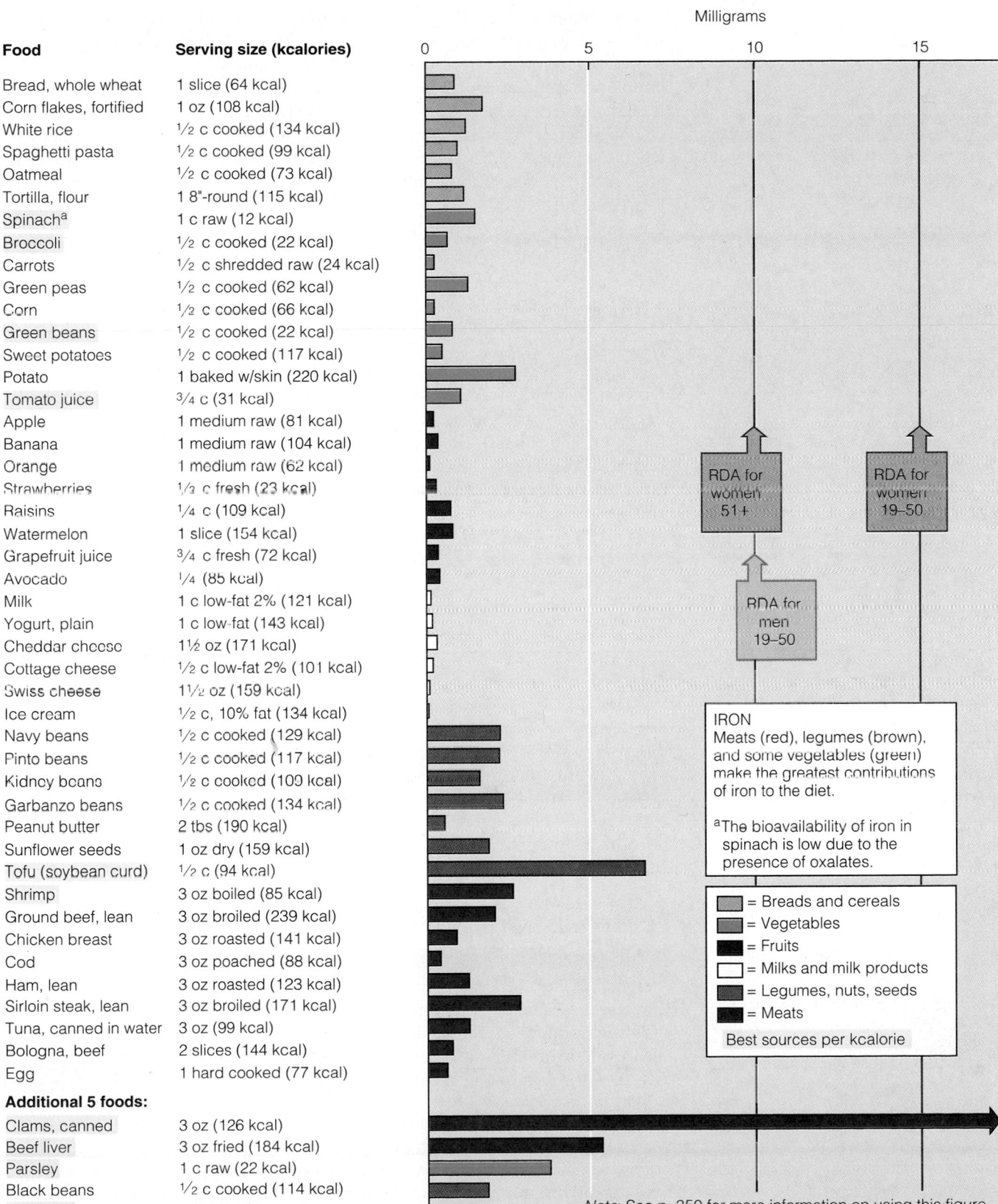

Food	Serving size (kcalories)
Bread, whole wheat	1 slice (64 kcal)
Corn flakes, fortified	1 oz (108 kcal)
White rice	1/2 c cooked (134 kcal)
Spaghetti pasta	1/2 c cooked (99 kcal)
Oatmeal	1/2 c cooked (73 kcal)
Tortilla, flour	1 8"-round (115 kcal)
Spinach[a]	1 c raw (12 kcal)
Broccoli	1/2 c cooked (22 kcal)
Carrots	1/2 c shredded raw (24 kcal)
Green peas	1/2 c cooked (62 kcal)
Corn	1/2 c cooked (66 kcal)
Green beans	1/2 c cooked (22 kcal)
Sweet potatoes	1/2 c cooked (117 kcal)
Potato	1 baked w/skin (220 kcal)
Tomato juice	3/4 c (31 kcal)
Apple	1 medium raw (81 kcal)
Banana	1 medium raw (104 kcal)
Orange	1 medium raw (62 kcal)
Strawberries	1/2 c fresh (23 kcal)
Raisins	1/4 c (109 kcal)
Watermelon	1 slice (154 kcal)
Grapefruit juice	3/4 c fresh (72 kcal)
Avocado	1/4 (85 kcal)
Milk	1 c low-fat 2% (121 kcal)
Yogurt, plain	1 c low-fat (143 kcal)
Cheddar cheese	1½ oz (171 kcal)
Cottage cheese	1/2 c low-fat 2% (101 kcal)
Swiss cheese	1½ oz (159 kcal)
Ice cream	1/2 c, 10% fat (134 kcal)
Navy beans	1/2 c cooked (129 kcal)
Pinto beans	1/2 c cooked (117 kcal)
Kidney beans	1/2 c cooked (109 kcal)
Garbanzo beans	1/2 c cooked (134 kcal)
Peanut butter	2 tbs (190 kcal)
Sunflower seeds	1 oz dry (159 kcal)
Tofu (soybean curd)	1/2 c (94 kcal)
Shrimp	3 oz boiled (85 kcal)
Ground beef, lean	3 oz broiled (239 kcal)
Chicken breast	3 oz roasted (141 kcal)
Cod	3 oz poached (88 kcal)
Ham, lean	3 oz roasted (123 kcal)
Sirloin steak, lean	3 oz broiled (171 kcal)
Tuna, canned in water	3 oz (99 kcal)
Bologna, beef	2 slices (144 kcal)
Egg	1 hard cooked (77 kcal)
Additional 5 foods:	
Clams, canned	3 oz (126 kcal)
Beef liver	3 oz fried (184 kcal)
Parsley	1 c raw (22 kcal)
Black beans	1/2 c cooked (114 kcal)
Artichoke	1 (60 kcal)

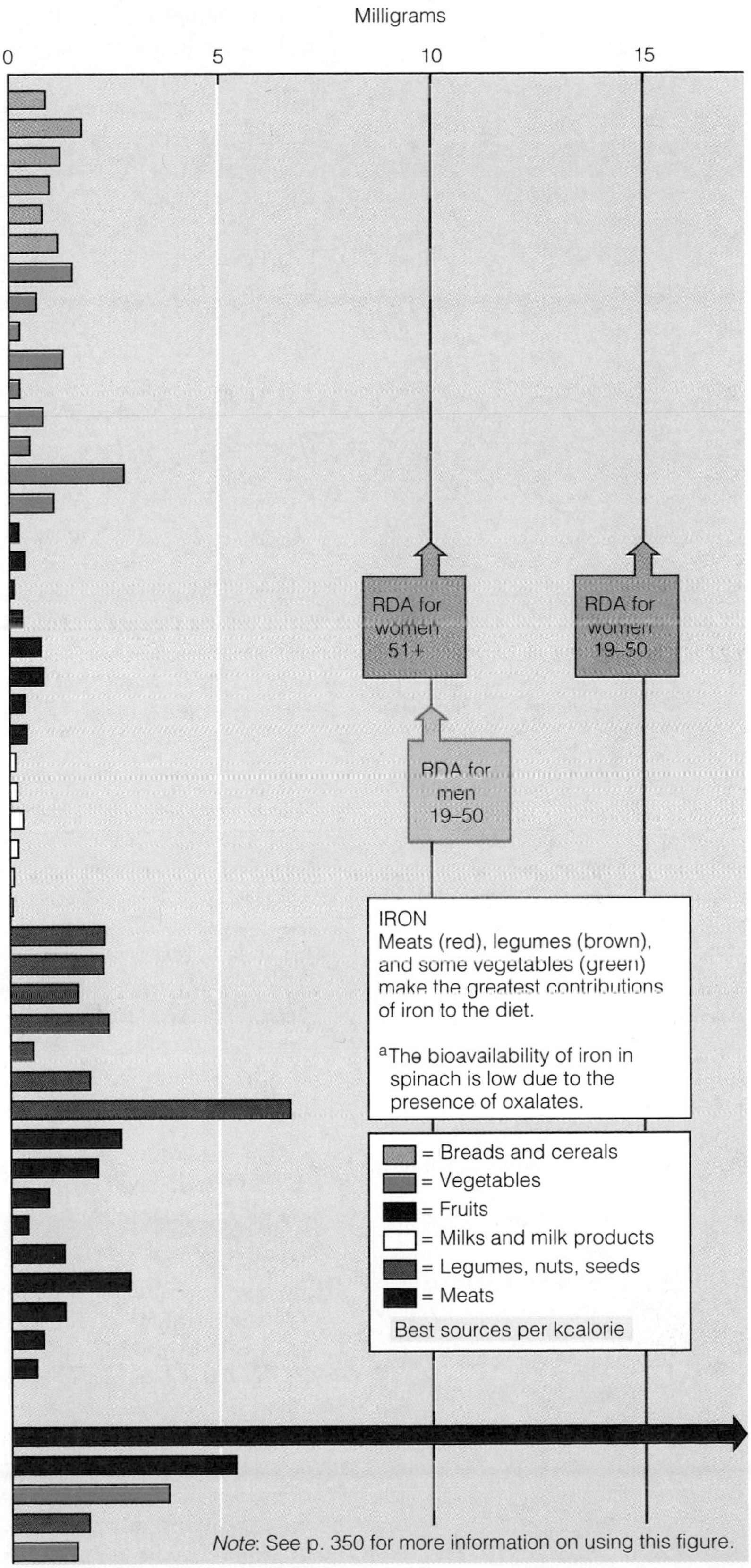

Note: See p. 350 for more information on using this figure.

Iron Supplements People who are iron deficient may need supplements as well as an iron-rich, absorption-enhancing diet. In addition, many physicians routinely recommend iron supplements to pregnant women, infants, and young children. Iron from supplements is less well absorbed than that from food, so the doses have to be high. The absorption of iron taken as ferrous sulfate or as an iron chelate is better than that from other iron supplements. Absorption also improves when supplements are taken between meals or at bedtime on an empty stomach, and with liquids other than milk, tea, or coffee, which inhibit absorption. There is no benefit to taking iron supplements with orange juice because vitamin C does not enhance absorption from supplements as it does for dietary iron. (Vitamin C helps iron absorption by converting insoluble ferric iron in foods to the more soluble ferrous iron, and supplemental iron is already in the ferrous form.) Constipation is a common side effect of iron supplementation; a plentiful fluid intake may help to relieve this problem.

A chelate (KEY-late) is a substance that can grasp the positive ions of a metal.
chele = claw

In summary, most of the body's iron is in hemoglobin and myoglobin where it carries oxygen for use in energy metabolism; some iron is also a cofactor for enzymes involved in a variety of reactions. Special proteins assist with iron absorption, transport, and storage—all helping to maintain an appropriate balance, because both too little and too much iron can be damaging. Iron deficiency is most common among infants and young children, teenagers, women of childbearing age, and pregnant women; symptoms include fatigue and anemia. Iron overload is most common in men and has been linked with heart disease. Heme iron, which is found only in meat, fish, and poultry, is better absorbed than nonheme iron, which occurs in most foods. Nonheme iron absorption is improved by eating iron-containing foods with foods containing the MFP factor and vitamin C.

Zinc

Zinc is a versatile trace element required as a cofactor by more than 100 enzymes in every organ in the body. Wherever protein is, zinc is. Virtually all cells contain zinc, but the highest concentrations are in bone, the prostate gland, and the eyes.[21] Muscle contains the highest proportion of total body zinc (60 percent), however, because it accounts for most of the body's mass. Tissues do not readily give up their zinc when blood levels fall, so frequent dietary intakes are necessary.[22]

Reminder: A *cofactor* is a mineral element that works with an enzyme to facilitate a chemical reaction.

metalloenzyme (MEH-tal-oh-EN-zime): an enzyme that contains one or more minerals as part of its structure.

A sampling of enzymes that zinc assists:
- Enzymes that help make parts of the genetic materials DNA and RNA.
- An enzyme that manufactures heme for hemoglobin.
- An enzyme involved in essential fatty acid metabolism.
- An enzyme that releases vitamin A from liver stores.
- Enzymes that metabolize carbohydrates.
- Enzymes that synthesize proteins.
- An enzyme that metabolizes alcohol in the liver.
- An eyzyme that disposes of damaging free radicals.

ZINC ROLES IN THE BODY

Zinc supports the work of numerous proteins in the body—among them are the metalloenzymes, which are involved in a variety of metabolic processes.* Zinc also assists in immune function and in growth and development. Zinc associates with the hormone insulin in the pancreas, although it does not appear to play a direct role in insulin's action.[23] Zinc interacts with platelets in blood clotting, affects thyroid hormone function, and influences behavior and learning per-

*Among the metalloenzymes requiring zinc are carbonic anhydrase, deoxythymidine kinase, DNA and RNA polymerase, and alkaline phosphatase.

formance. It is necessary to produce the active form of vitamin A (retinal) in visual pigments and the retinol-binding protein that transports vitamin A. It is essential to normal taste perception, wound healing, the making of sperm, and fetal development. A zinc deficiency impairs all these and other functions, underlining the vast importance of proteins as the body's working machines.

Zinc, like iron, helps protect the body from heavy metal poisoning—for example, poisoning by lead. This is especially important during fetal development and early childhood. Highlight 19 reveals the damage heavy metals can do and shows how iron and zinc help ward it off.

ZINC ABSORPTION AND METABOLISM

The body's handling of zinc resembles that of iron in some ways and differs in others. A key difference is that the mucosal cells in the intestine provide a two-way passage for zinc from the intestine to the blood and back again.

Zinc Absorption Upon absorption into an intestinal cell, zinc has several options. It may become involved in the metabolic functions of the cell itself. Alternatively, it may be retained within the cell by metallothionein, a special binding protein that is similar to the iron storage protein ferritin.

metallothionein (meh-TAL-oh-THIGH-oh-neen): a sulfur-rich protein that avidly binds with metals such as zinc.
metallo = containing a metal
thio = containing sulfur
ein = a protein

Metallothionein, the Zinc-Binding Protein The synthesis of metallothionein in the intestinal cells helps to regulate zinc absorption. When zinc intakes are high, more metallothionein is made; it holds zinc in reserve, thus inhibiting absorption.[24] (Similarly, metallothionein in the liver binds zinc until other body tissues signal a need for it.) When the body needs zinc, intestinal metallothionein releases it into the blood where it can be transported around the body. Some zinc eventually reaches the pancreas.

Enteropancreatic Circulation of Zinc Many of the digestive enzymes released from the pancreas into the intestine at mealtimes contain zinc. The intestine thus receives two doses of zinc with each meal—one from ingested foods and the other from the zinc-rich pancreatic secretions. The circulation of zinc in the body from the pancreas to the intestines and back to the pancreas is referred to as the enteropancreatic circulation of zinc. Thus even zinc that has already entered the body is rescreened periodically by the intestine and can be refused entry or tied up in intestinal cells on any of its times around (see Figure 13-5).

enteropancreatic (EN-ter-oh-PAN-kree-AT-ik) circulation: the circulatory route from the pancreas to the intestine and back to the pancreas.

Factors Affecting Absorption The rate of zinc absorption varies from about 15 to 40 percent, depending on a person's zinc status: if more is needed, more is absorbed. Also, dietary constituents influence zinc absorption. Zinc bioavailability from beef is about four times greater than from high-fiber cereals.[25] Fiber and phytates bind zinc, thus limiting its bioavailability. Cow's milk protein (casein) also binds zinc avidly and seems to hinder absorption somewhat; infants absorb zinc better from breast milk. Milk does not inhibit adults' zinc absorption, however, so long as they ingest adequate animal protein.

Zinc Transport by Albumin Zinc's main transport vehicle in the blood is the protein albumin, which is a major determinant of zinc absorption. This may

Figure 13–5

Zinc's Routes in the Body
Notice the enteropancreatic circulation of zinc from the intestines to the pancreas and back to the intestines.

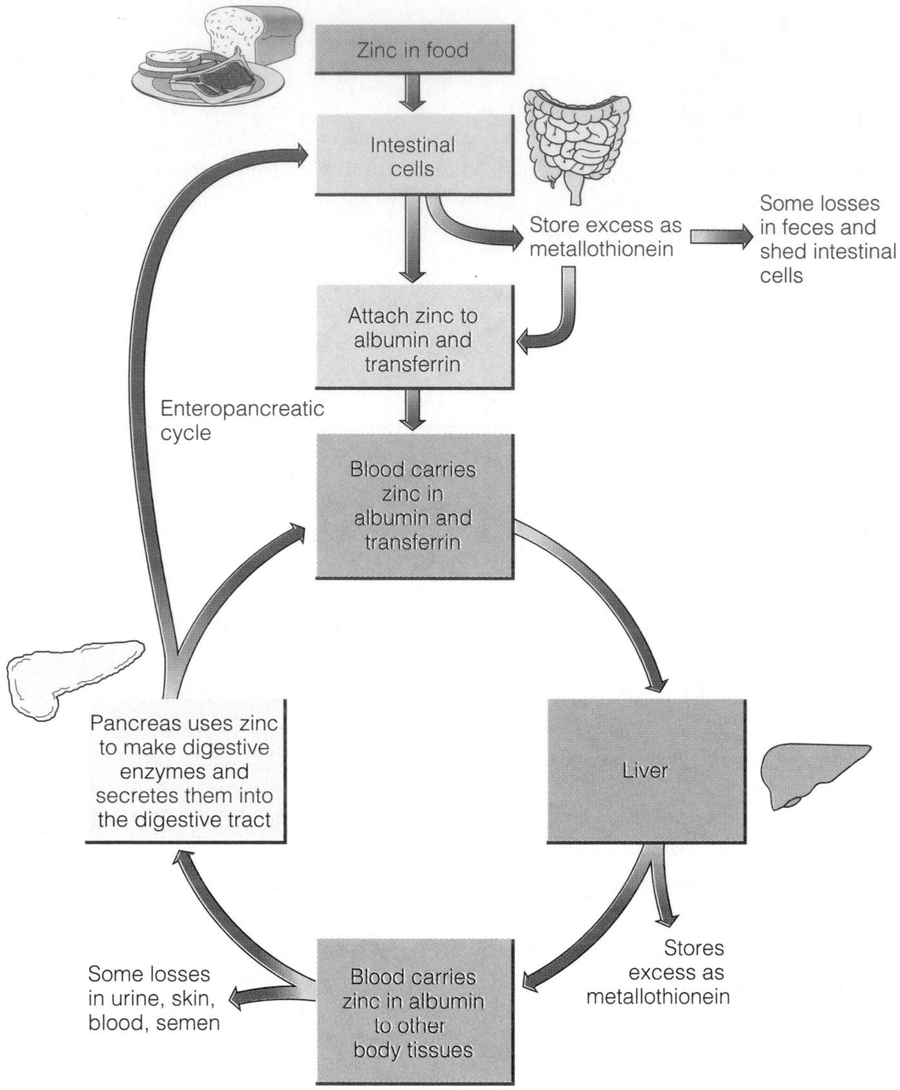

account for observations that zinc absorption declines in conditions that lower albumin concentrations—for example, pregnancy and malnutrition.

Zinc Interactions with Iron and Copper Some plasma zinc also binds to transferrin—the same transferrin that carries iron in the blood. In healthy individuals, transferrin is usually less than 50 percent saturated with iron, but in iron overload, it is more saturated. Dietary iron-to-zinc ratios of greater than 2 to 1 leave too few transferrin-binding sites available for zinc and thereby impair zinc absorption. The converse is also true: large doses of zinc inhibit iron absorption.

Large doses of zinc create a similar problem with another essential mineral, copper. Recall that when zinc intakes are high, the intestinal cells synthesize large amounts of the binding protein metallothionein. This protein binds copper more strongly than zinc and captures copper in a nonabsorbable form.[26] This binding impairs copper absorption and may result in a copper deficiency. These nutrient interactions highlight one of the many reasons why people should use supplements conservatively: supplementation can easily create imbalances.

Zinc Losses Zinc exits the body primarily in feces. Smaller losses occur in urine, shed skin, hair, sweat, menstrual fluids, and semen.

ZINC DEFICIENCY

Human zinc deficiency was first reported in the 1960s in children and adolescent boys in Egypt, Iran, and Turkey. Children have especially high zinc needs because they are growing rapidly and synthesizing many zinc-containing proteins; the native diets among those populations were not meeting these needs. Middle Eastern diets are typically low in the richest zinc source, meats, and the staple foods are beans, unleavened breads, and other whole-grain foods—all high in fiber and phytates, which inhibit zinc absorption.*

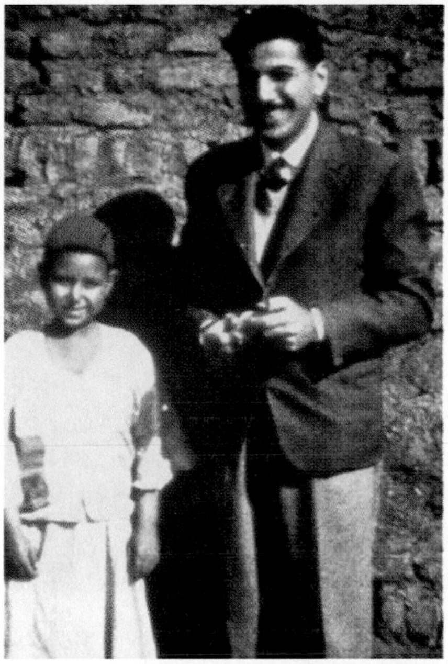

The Egyptian man on the right is an adult of average height. The Egyptian boy on the left is 17 years old but is only 4 feet tall, like a 7-year-old in the United States. His genitalia are like those of a 6-year-old. The retardation, known as *dwarfism*, is rightly ascribed to zinc deficiency because it is partially reversible when zinc is restored to the diet.

Zinc-Deficiency Symptoms The zinc deficiency seen in the 1960s was marked by severe growth retardation and arrested sexual maturation—symptoms that responded to zinc supplementation. Since the 1960s, zinc deficiency has been recognized elsewhere, and it is now known to affect much more than just growth. It alters digestive function by impairing pancreatic function, chylomicron formation, and GI tract function. It causes diarrhea, which worsens malnutrition not only for zinc, but for all nutrients. It impairs the immune response, making infections likely—among them, infections of the intestinal tract, which worsen malnutrition, including zinc malnutrition (a classic downward spiral of events).[27] Chronic zinc deficiency hinders central nervous system and brain functioning. Because zinc deficiency directly impairs vitamin A metabolism, vitamin A–deficiency symptoms often appear. Zinc deficiency also disturbs thyroid function and the metabolic rate. It alters taste, causes anorexia, and slows wound healing—in fact, its symptoms are so all-pervasive that generalized malnutrition and sickness are more likely to be the diagnosis than simple zinc deficiency. Table 13–2 (on p. 490) includes a list of zinc-deficiency symptoms.

Vulnerable Stages of Life Severe zinc deficiencies are not widespread in developed countries, but they do occur in vulnerable groups—pregnant women, young children, the elderly, and the poor. Research shows that even a mild zinc deficiency can result in poor growth, poor appetite, impaired immune response, abnormal taste, and abnormal vision in darkness.[28]

ZINC TOXICITY

Accidental high doses (2 grams or more) of zinc may cause vomiting, diarrhea, fever, exhaustion, and other symptoms (see Table 13–2). A dose of just a few milligrams above the RDA, especially when taken regularly over time, lowers the

*Unleavened bread contains no yeast, which normally breaks down phytates during fermentation.

Table 13–2

Zinc—A Summary

Adult RDA	Deficiency Symptoms[a]	Toxicity Symptoms
Men: 15 mg/day Women: 12 mg/day	BLOOD	
	High ammonia, low alkaline phosphatase, low insulin	Anemia: reduced hemoglobin production
Chief Functions in the Body	BONES	
Part of many enzymes; associated with the hormone insulin; involved in making genetic material and proteins, immune reactions, transport of vitamin A, taste perception, wound healing, the making of sperm, and the normal development of the fetus	Growth retardation, abnormal collagen synthesis	Growth in length, but without normal zinc content
	CELLS/METABOLISM	
	Slow DNA synthesis, impaired cell division and protein synthesis	Raised LDL, lowered HDL
	DIGESTIVE SYSTEM	
	Weak sense of smell, poor sensitivity to the taste of salt, weight loss, delayed glucose absorption, diarrhea, nausea, impaired folate absorption	Diarrhea, vomiting, decreased calcium and copper absorption
Significant Sources	EYES	
Protein-containing foods: meats, fish, poultry, whole grains, vegetables	Night blindness	
	GLANDULAR SYSTEM	
	Delayed onset of puberty, small gonads in males, decreased synthesis and release of testosterone, abnormal glucose tolerance, reduced synthesis of adrenocortical hormones, altered thyroid function	
	IMMUNE SYSTEM	
	Altered skin test responses, low white blood cell count, few antibody-forming cells, thymus atrophy, susceptibility to infection	Fever, elevated white blood cell count
	KIDNEY	
		Renal failure
	LIVER/SPLEEN	
	Enlargement	
	NERVOUS/MUSCULAR SYSTEMS	
	Anorexia (poor appetite), mental lethargy, irritability	Muscular pain and incoordination, heart muscle degeneration, exhaustion, dizziness, drowsiness
	REPRODUCTIVE SYSTEM	
	Impaired reproductive function (rats), low sperm counts	Reproductive failure
	SKIN	
	Generalized hair loss; lesions; rough, dry appearance; slow healing of wounds and burns	

[a]A rare inherited disease, *acrodermatitis enteropathica,* causes additional and more severe symptoms.

body's copper content—an effect that, in animals, leads to degeneration of the heart muscle. High doses also affect cholesterol metabolism, alter lipoprotein levels, and appear to accelerate the development of atherosclerosis.

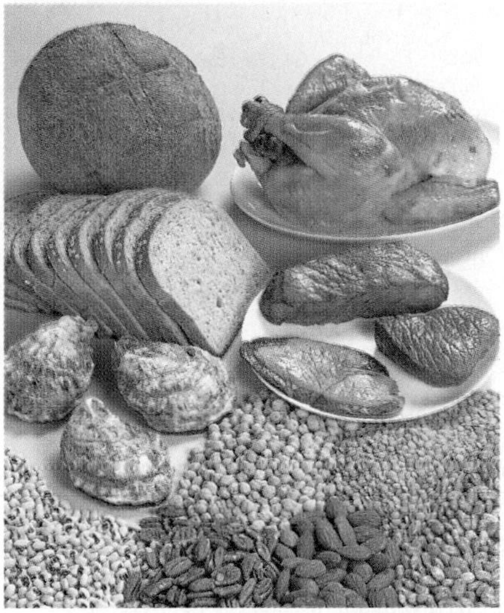

Zinc-rich foods include oysters, meat, and poultry; whole-grain breads; and legumes and nuts.

ZINC RECOMMENDATIONS AND INTAKES

In setting the zinc RDA, the Committee on Dietary Allowances assumed that 20 percent of dietary zinc is available to the body.[29] Average intakes in the United States are about 10 milligrams per day, so most people are probably not meeting the RDA. Requirements for infants and children are relatively higher than for adults due to zinc's role in normal growth and development.

Figure 13–6 (on p. 492) shows zinc amounts in foods per serving. Zinc is highest in protein-rich foods such as shellfish (especially oysters), meats, poultry, and liver. Legumes and whole-grain products are good sources of zinc if large quantities are eaten; in typical U.S. diets, phytate intake from grains is not high enough to impair zinc absorption. Vegetables vary in zinc content depending on the soil in which they are grown.

CONTAMINATION AND SUPPLEMENTAL ZINC

In earlier times, galvanized cooking pots and storage vessels, contributed zinc to foods, especially to acid foods. Galvanized pipes, used in plumbing in earlier times, may also have contributed zinc to people's intakes. With today's use of stainless steel and plastic, these sources of zinc have been largely eliminated.

galvanized: a term referring to metals that have been treated with a zinc-containing coating to prevent rust.

Zinc supplements are seldom appropriate. A decade ago, much excitement surrounded the publication of a research study that showed that zinc lozenges shortened the duration of the common cold.[30] However, results from many other studies attempting to confirm this finding have contradicted it.[31]

Zinc supplements are known to be useful in two instances: to remedy an accurately diagnosed zinc deficiency and to displace other ions in unusual medical circumstances. Otherwise, it should be possible to obtain enough zinc from the diet without resorting to supplements.

To summarize, zinc assists enzymes in a multitude of reactions affecting growth, vitamin A activity, and pancreatic digestive enzyme synthesis, among others. Both dietary zinc and zinc-rich pancreatic secretions (via enteropancreatic circulation) are available for absorption. Absorption is monitored by a special binding protein (metallothionein) in the intestine. High-protein foods derived from animals are the best sources of zinc of high bioavailability. Fiber and phytates in cereals bind zinc, limiting absorption. Growth retardation and sexual immaturity are hallmark symptoms of zinc deficiency.

Iodine

Like chlorine gas, iodine gas is poisonous; however, the iodine ion that occurs in foods is far less toxic, and traces of it are indispensable to life. Any iodine ingested in foods is converted to the iodide ion in the GI tract; this chapter uses *iodine* when referring to the nutrient in foods and *iodide* when referring to it in

Figure 13–6 Zinc in Selected Foods

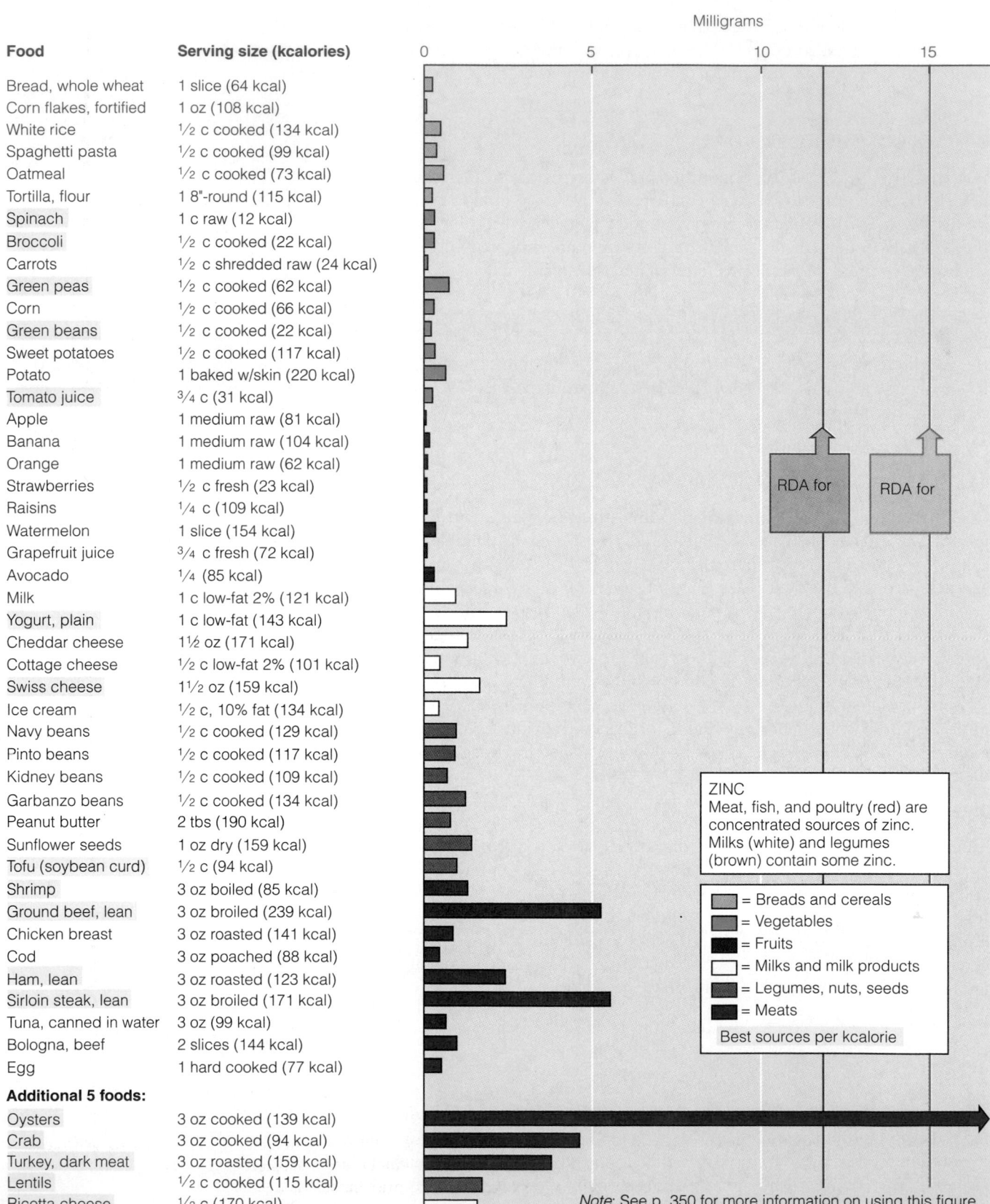

Food	Serving size (kcalories)
Bread, whole wheat	1 slice (64 kcal)
Corn flakes, fortified	1 oz (108 kcal)
White rice	1/2 c cooked (134 kcal)
Spaghetti pasta	1/2 c cooked (99 kcal)
Oatmeal	1/2 c cooked (73 kcal)
Tortilla, flour	1 8"-round (115 kcal)
Spinach	1 c raw (12 kcal)
Broccoli	1/2 c cooked (22 kcal)
Carrots	1/2 c shredded raw (24 kcal)
Green peas	1/2 c cooked (62 kcal)
Corn	1/2 c cooked (66 kcal)
Green beans	1/2 c cooked (22 kcal)
Sweet potatoes	1/2 c cooked (117 kcal)
Potato	1 baked w/skin (220 kcal)
Tomato juice	3/4 c (31 kcal)
Apple	1 medium raw (81 kcal)
Banana	1 medium raw (104 kcal)
Orange	1 medium raw (62 kcal)
Strawberries	1/2 c fresh (23 kcal)
Raisins	1/4 c (109 kcal)
Watermelon	1 slice (154 kcal)
Grapefruit juice	3/4 c fresh (72 kcal)
Avocado	1/4 (85 kcal)
Milk	1 c low-fat 2% (121 kcal)
Yogurt, plain	1 c low-fat (143 kcal)
Cheddar cheese	1½ oz (171 kcal)
Cottage cheese	1/2 c low-fat 2% (101 kcal)
Swiss cheese	1 1/2 oz (159 kcal)
Ice cream	1/2 c, 10% fat (134 kcal)
Navy beans	1/2 c cooked (129 kcal)
Pinto beans	1/2 c cooked (117 kcal)
Kidney beans	1/2 c cooked (109 kcal)
Garbanzo beans	1/2 c cooked (134 kcal)
Peanut butter	2 tbs (190 kcal)
Sunflower seeds	1 oz dry (159 kcal)
Tofu (soybean curd)	1/2 c (94 kcal)
Shrimp	3 oz boiled (85 kcal)
Ground beef, lean	3 oz broiled (239 kcal)
Chicken breast	3 oz roasted (141 kcal)
Cod	3 oz poached (88 kcal)
Ham, lean	3 oz roasted (123 kcal)
Sirloin steak, lean	3 oz broiled (171 kcal)
Tuna, canned in water	3 oz (99 kcal)
Bologna, beef	2 slices (144 kcal)
Egg	1 hard cooked (77 kcal)
Additional 5 foods:	
Oysters	3 oz cooked (139 kcal)
Crab	3 oz cooked (94 kcal)
Turkey, dark meat	3 oz roasted (159 kcal)
Lentils	1/2 c cooked (115 kcal)
Ricotta cheese	1/2 c (170 kcal)

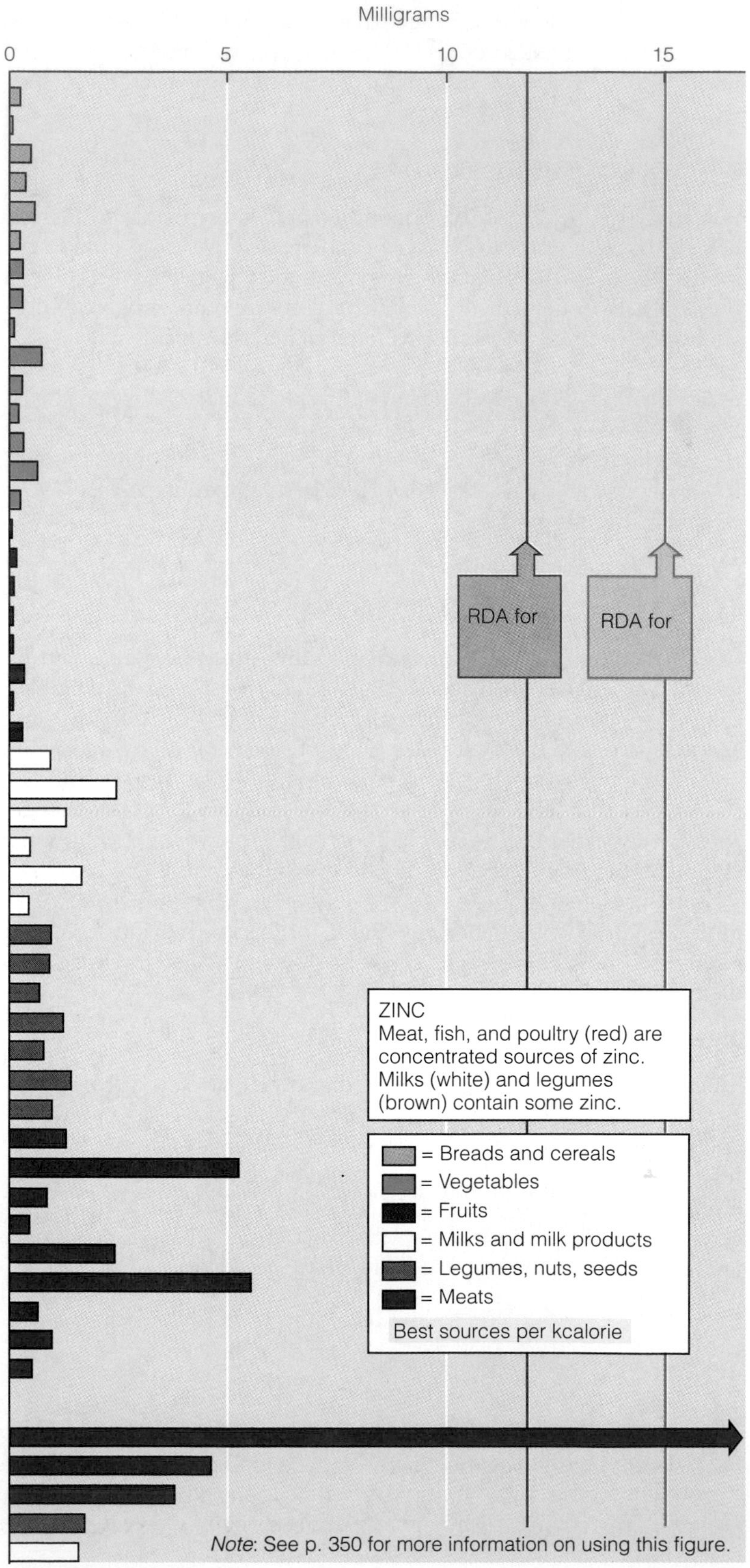

Note: See p. 350 for more information on using this figure.

the body. Iodide occurs in the body in a tiny quantity, but its principal role in human nutrition is well known, and the amount needed is well established.

Iodide Roles in the Body Iodide is an integral part of two hormones released by the thyroid gland that regulate body temperature, metabolic rate, reproduction, growth, the making of blood cells, nerve and muscle function, and more. These hormones control the rate at which the cells use oxygen; that is to say, these hormones control the rate at which energy is released during metabolism.

The two hormones from the thyroid gland are triiodothyronine (T_3), which is the active form, and tetraiodothyronine (T_4), which is more commonly known as *thyroxin*.

Iodine Deficiency The hypothalamus regulates the plasma concentrations of thyroid hormones by controlling the release of the pituitary's thyroid-stimulating hormone (TSH). With iodine deficiency, thyroid hormone declines, and the body responds by secreting more TSH in a futile attempt to accelerate iodide uptake by the thyroid gland. If a deficiency persists, the cells of the thyroid gland enlarge, so as to trap as much iodide as possible. Sometimes the gland enlarges until it makes a visible lump in the neck, a simple goiter. Goiter afflicts about 200 million people the world over, many of them in Africa. In all but 4 percent of these cases, the cause is iodine deficiency. As for the 4 percent (8 million), most have goiter because they overconsume plants of the cabbage family and other foods that contain an antithyroid substance (goitrogen) whose effect is not counteracted by dietary iodine. The goitrogens present in plants serve notice that even natural components of foods can cause harm when eaten in excess.

An iodine deficiency causes sluggishness and weight gain. During pregnancy, it may impair development of the fetus, causing the extreme and irreversible mental and physical retardation known as cretinism. An infant with cretinism may have a mental deficiency and a face and body with many physical abnormalities. Much of the mental retardation of cretinism can be averted by diagnosis of iodine deficiency and treatment early in pregnancy. Iodine deficiency in young children is typically associated with goiter and poor school performance.

goiter (GOY-ter): an enlargement of the thyroid gland due to an iodine deficiency, malfunction of the gland, or overconsumption of a goitrogen. Goiter caused by iodine deficiency is **simple goiter**.

goitrogen (GOY-troh-jen): a thyroid antagonist found in food; causes **toxic goiter**. Goitrogens are found in such foods as cabbage, kale, brussels sprouts, cauliflower, broccoli, and kohlrabi.

cretinism (CREE-tin-ism): an iodine-deficiency disease characterized by mental and physical retardation.

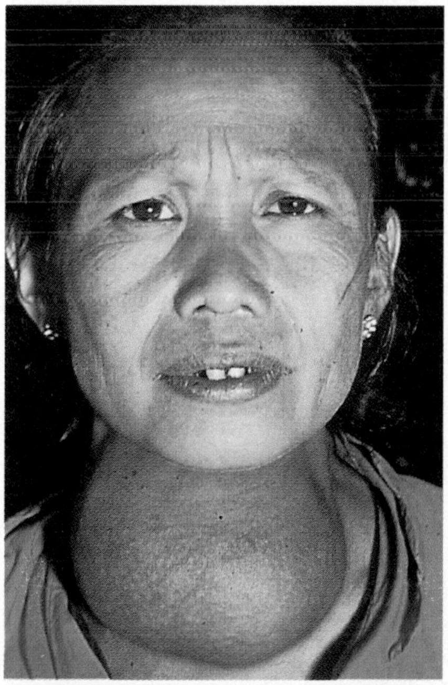

In iodine deficiency, the thyroid gland enlarges—a condition known as simple goiter.

Iodine Toxicity Excessive intakes of iodine can enlarge the thyroid gland, just as deficiency can. This goiterlike condition can be so severe as to block the airways in infants and cause suffocation. The toxic dose is thought to be over 2000 micrograms per day for an adult—several times higher than average intakes.

Iodine Sources The ocean is the world's major source of iodine. In coastal areas, seafood, water, and even iodine-containing sea mist are dependable iodine sources. Further inland, the amount of iodine in foods is variable and generally reflects the amount present in the soil in which plants are grown or on which animals graze. Landmasses that were once under the ocean have soils rich in iodine; those that were not have iodine-poor soils. In the United States and Canada, the soil around the Great Lakes and the inland valleys of Oregon is iodine-poor. The iodization of salt eliminated widespread misery caused by iodine deficiency in the people of these regions during the 1930s.

Iodine Intakes Average consumption of iodine in the United States is about 200 to 500 micrograms—more than the RDA, but below toxic levels as well. Some of the excess iodine in the U.S. diet seems to be coming from fast foods, which use iodized salt liberally. Some comes from bakery products and from milk. The baking industry uses iodates as dough conditioners, and most

Table 13–3

Iodine—A Summary

Adult RDA	Deficiency Disease Name	
150 µg/day	Simple goiter, cretinism	
Chief Functions in the Body	**Deficiency Symptoms**	**Toxicity Symptoms**
A component of two thyroid hormones that help to regulate growth, development, and metabolic rate	Enlargement of the thyroid gland, weight gain, mental and physical retardation of an infant	Enlargement of the thyroid gland, depressed thyroid activity
Significant Sources		
Iodized salt, seafood, bread, dairy products, plants grown in iodine-rich soil and animals fed those plants		

dairies feed cows iodine-containing medications and use iodine to disinfect milking equipment. Now that these sources have been identified, food industries have reduced their use of these compounds, but the sudden emergence of this problem points to a need for continued surveillance of the food supply. Table 13–3 provides a summary of iodine.

2 g iodized salt (less than ½ tsp) contains the RDA for iodine.

Iodine Recommendation The recommended intake of iodine for adults is a minuscule amount. The need for iodine is easily met by consuming seafood, vegetables grown in iodine-rich soil, and iodized salt. In the United States, labels state whether salt is iodized; in Canada, all table salt is iodized.

Selenium

selenium (se-LEEN-ee-um): a trace element.

The essential mineral selenium is one of the body's antioxidants, working closely with the enzyme glutathione peroxidase. Glutathione peroxidase prevents free-radical formation, thus blocking the chain reaction before it begins. (Highlight 11 describes free-radical formation, chain reactions, and antioxidant action in detail.) Glutathione peroxidase and vitamin E work in concert: if free radicals do form and a chain reaction starts, vitamin E halts it. Selenium also works closely with the enzyme that converts thyroid hormone to its active form.

The heart disease associated with selenium deficiency is named Keshan disease for one of the provinces of China where it was studied. Keshan disease is characterized by heart enlargement and insufficiency; the middle layer of the walls of the heart, which are normally composed of muscle tissue, are replaced with fibrous tissue.

Selenium Deficiency At first, selenium's antioxidant function was the only evidence that it was essential for human beings. Then, in the 1970s, the discovery that selenium deficiency was associated with a heart disease in hundreds of thousands of children in China intensified research efforts to learn more about this mineral. The heart disease is prevalent in regions of China where the soil and foods are selenium-poor. The primary cause of this heart disease is probably a virus, but selenium deficiency appears to predispose people to it, and adequate selenium seems to prevent it.

Selenium and Cancer In other parts of the world, selenium-poor soil correlates with a high incidence of certain kinds of cancer. This finding has stimulated research with both animal and human subjects seeking to find out whether

Table 13–4

Selenium—A Summary

Adult RDA	Chief Functions in the Body	Deficiency Symptoms	Toxicity Symptoms	Significant Sources
Men: 70 μg/day Women: 55 μg/day	Part of an enzyme system that works with vitamin E to protect body compounds from oxidation	Predisposition to heart disease characterized by cardiac tissue becoming fibrous	Digestive system disorders, loss of hair and nails, skin lesions, nervous system disorders, tooth damage	Seafood, meat, grains

dietary selenium adequacy is one of the many factors that may protect against cancer. So far, research results are inconclusive.

Selenium Intakes Some regions in the United States and Canada produce crops on selenium-poor soil, but the people are protected from deficiency, partly because they eat supermarket foods transported from other regions, and partly because of their high intakes of selenium-rich meats. Meats and other animal products are reliable sources of selenium because selenium is associated with the protein parts of foods.

Selenium Toxicity High doses (a milligram or more daily) of selenium are toxic. Selenium toxicity causes vomiting, diarrhea, loss of hair and nails, and lesions of the skin and nervous system. The inappropriate use of selenium supplements as an anticancer agent poses the possibility of selenium overdose.[32] See Table 13–4 for a summary of selenium.

Copper

The body contains about 100 milligrams of copper.[33] About one-third is in the muscles, one-third is in the liver and brain, and the rest is in the bones, kidneys, blood, and other tissues.

Copper Roles in the Body Copper serves as a constituent of enzymes. The copper-containing enzymes have diverse metabolic roles with one common characteristic: all involve reactions that consume oxygen or oxygen radicals. For example, copper-containing enzymes catalyze the oxidation of ferrous iron to ferric iron.* Copper's role in iron metabolism makes it a key factor in hemoglobin synthesis. Another copper- and zinc-containing enzyme functions as an antioxidant.† Still another copper enzyme helps to manufacture collagen and heal wounds.†† Copper, like iron, is needed in many of the reactions related to respiration and the release of energy.**

---

*The copper-requiring enzymes ceruloplasmin and ferroxidase II participate in the oxidation of ferrous iron to ferric iron.

†The copper-requiring enzyme superoxide dismutase protects cell membranes against free-radical damage.

‡The copper-requiring enzyme lysyl oxidase helps synthesize connective tissues.

**The copper-requiring enzyme cytochrome C oxidase is part of the electron transport chain.

Table 13–5

Copper—A Summary

Estimated Safe and Adequate Intake	Chief Functions in the Body	Deficiency Symptoms	Toxicity Symptoms	Significant Sources
Adults: 1.5–3.0 mg/day	Necessary for the absorption and use of iron in the formation of hemoglobin; part of several enzymes	Anemia, bone abnormalities (rare in human beings)	Vomiting, diarrhea	Meat, drinking water

Copper Deficiency and Toxicity Copper deficiency is rare, but not unknown. It has been seen in malnourished children, and it can severely disturb growth and metabolism. Excess zinc, as mentioned, interferes with copper absorption and can cause deficiency. Copper deficiency in animals raises blood cholesterol and damages blood vessels, leading researchers to explore whether low dietary copper might contribute to cardiovascular disease.[34] Copper toxicity from foods is unlikely, but supplements can cause it.

Copper Recommendations and Intakes The richest food sources of copper are legumes, grains, nuts, organ meats, and seeds. About a third of the copper taken in food is absorbed, and the rest is eliminated in the feces. Water also provides copper; its content varies with the type of plumbing pipe and hardness of the water. See Table 13–5 for a summary of copper facts.

Manganese

The human body contains a tiny 20 milligrams of manganese, mostly in the bones and metabolically active organs such as the liver, kidneys, and pancreas. Manganese acts as cofactor for many enzymes that facilitate dozens of different metabolic processes. For example, manganese metalloenzymes assist in urea synthesis, the conversion of pyruvate to a TCA cycle compound, and the prevention of lipid peroxidation by free radicals.

Manganese Deficiency Deficiencies of manganese have not been seen in human beings. In animals, manganese deficiency alters fat metabolism and deranges many systems, including the skeletal, reproductive, and nervous systems. Manganese requirements are low, and many plant foods contain significant amounts of this trace mineral, so deficiencies are unlikely. As is true of other trace minerals, however, dietary factors influence manganese absorption: both iron and calcium inhibit manganese absorption. This interaction may depress the manganese status of people who use iron and calcium supplements regularly.

Manganese Toxicity Toxicity is more likely to occur when the environment is contaminated with manganese than from dietary intake. Miners who inhale large quantities of manganese dust on the job over prolonged periods show symptoms of a brain disease, along with abnormalities of appearance and behavior. A summary of manganese appears in Table 13–6.

Table 13–6

Manganese—A Summary

Estimated Safe and Adequate Intake	Chief Functions in the Body	Deficiency Symptoms	Toxicity Symptoms	Significant Sources
Adults: 2–5 mg/day	Facilitator, with enzymes, of many cell processes	(In experimental animals): poor growth, nervous system disorders, reproductive abnormalities	Nervous system disorders	Widely distributed in foods

Fluoride

Fluoride is present in virtually all soils, water supplies, plants, and animals. Only a trace of fluoride occurs in the human body, but with this amount, the crystalline deposits in bones and teeth are larger and more perfectly formed. Table 13–7 summarizes fluoride information.

Fluoride Roles in the Body When bones and teeth become mineralized, a crystal called hydroxyapatite forms from calcium and phosphorus. Then fluoride replaces the hydroxyl (OH) portions of the hydroxyapatite crystal, forming fluorapatite, which makes the bones stronger and the teeth more resistant to decay.

Reminder: *Hydroxyapatite* is the major calcium-containing crystal of bones and teeth.

fluorapatite (floor-APP-uh-tite): the stabilized form of bone and tooth crystal, in which fluoride has replaced the hydroxyl groups of hydroxyapatite.

Fluoridation and Dental Caries Dental caries ranks as the nation's most widespread health problem: an estimated 95 percent of the population have decayed, missing, or filled teeth. Dental problems interfere with a person's ability to chew and eat a wide variety of foods, and this can lead to a multitude of nutrition problems. Where fluoride is lacking, dental decay is common. By fluoridating the drinking water, a community offers its residents, particularly the children, a safe, economical, practical, and effective way to defend against dental caries.[35]

All normal diets contain some fluoride, but drinking water is usually the most significant source. The National Research Council of the National Academy of Sciences recommends fluoridation of drinking water to raise the concentration

Table 13–7

Fluoride—A Summary

Estimated Safe and Adequate Intake	Chief Functions in the Body	Deficiency Symptoms	Toxicity Symptoms	Significant Sources
Adults: 1.5–4.0 mg/day	An element involved in the formation of bones and teeth; helps to make teeth resistant to decay	Susceptibility to tooth decay	Fluorosis (discoloration of teeth), nausea, diarrhea, chest pain, itching, vomiting	Drinking water (if fluoride containing or fluoridated), tea, seafood

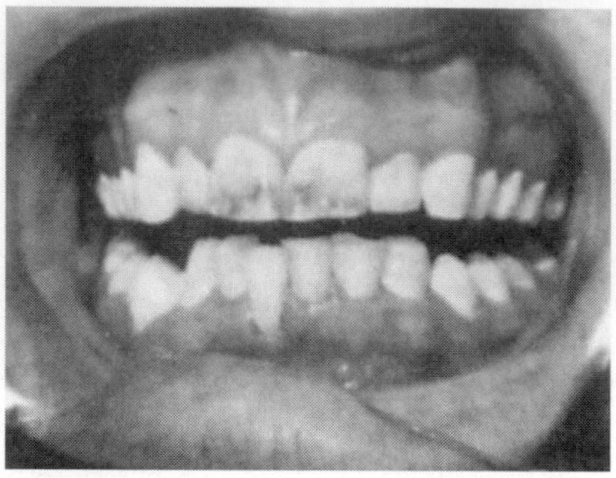

Fluorosis.

1 ppm = 1 mg per liter.

fluorosis: discoloration of tooth enamel caused by excess fluoride.

to about 1 part fluoride per 1 million parts water. Water with 1 part per million (1 ppm) fluoride offers the greatest protection against dental caries at virtually no risk of toxicity.

Fluoride and Osteoporosis The role of fluoride in protecting against adult bone loss (osteoporosis) is less clear than its role in protecting against tooth decay. Early studies reported that osteoporosis was more common in areas where the water was low in fluoride than in high-fluoride areas. Subsequent research shows that fluoride (administered as sodium fluoride) clearly affects bone, but the effects may be detrimental.[36] Highlight 12 mentions research findings on the use of fluoride in osteoporosis treatment.

Fluorosis and Other Toxic Effects In communities where the water naturally contains elevated levels of fluoride (2 to 8 parts per million), fluorosis, or discoloration of the teeth, may occur. More serious cases of fluoride poisoning have been reported in communities where the public water system failed and allowed fluoride concentrations to reach 150 parts per million.[37] Symptoms of fluoride poisoning include nausea, vomiting, diarrhea, abdominal pain, and numbness or tingling of the face and extremities.

Fluoride Intakes About half of the U.S. population has access to water with an optimal fluoride concentration, which typically delivers about 1 milligram per person per day. Fish and most teas contain appreciable amounts of natural fluoride.

Chromium

Chromium is an essential mineral that participates in carbohydrate and lipid metabolism. Like iron, chromium can have different charges. In the case of chromium, the Cr^{+++} ion seems to be the best absorbed and most effective in living systems. The percentage of chromium absorbed rises with low dietary intake and falls with high dietary intake.

Chromium Roles in the Body Chromium helps maintain glucose homeostasis. Experiments on animals have shown that chromium works closely with the hormone insulin to facilitate glucose uptake into cells and energy release. When chromium is lacking, a diabeteslike condition of high blood glucose results. Research on human beings suggests that diets low in chromium may impair glucose tolerance, insulin response, and glucagon response.[38]

glucose tolerance factor (GTF): a small organic compound that enhances insulin's action.

Early research identified chromium as a part of a small organic compound called the glucose tolerance factor (GTF) that enhances insulin's action. Recent studies have identified other glucose tolerance factors that do not contain chromium. Because nonchromium factors may also enhance insulin's action, "biologically active chromium" may better describe the chromium-containing compounds. Although the details remain somewhat unclear, most researchers agree that chromium participates in insulin's action.

Chromium Recommendations and Intakes Chromium is present in a variety of foods.[39] Still, an estimated 90 percent of U.S. adults consume less than the suggested minimum intake of 50 micrograms a day.[40] Unrefined foods are the

Table 13–8

Chromium—A Summary

Estimated Safe and Adequate Intake	Chief Functions in the Body	Deficiency Symptoms	Toxicity Symptoms	Significant Sources
Adults: 50–200 μg/day	Associated with insulin and required for the release of energy from glucose	Diabetes-like condition marked by an inability to use glucose normally	Unknown as a nutrition disorder; occupational exposures damage skin and kidneys	Meat, unrefined foods, fats, vegetable oils

best sources, particularly liver, brewer's yeast, whole grains, nuts, and cheeses. The more refined foods people eat, the less chromium they ingest. Older people are most susceptible to marginal intakes because many lack appetite or the desire to prepare and eat meals. Table 13–8 provides a summary of chromium.

Molybdenum

Molybdenum is an important mineral in human and animal physiology. It acts as a working part of several metalloenzymes. Deficiencies of molybdenum are unknown in animals and human beings because the amounts needed are minuscule—as little as 0.1 part per million parts of body tissue. Legumes, breads and other grains, leafy green vegetables, milk, and liver are molybdenum-rich foods.[41] Average daily intakes fall within the suggested range of intakes.

molybdenum (mo-LIB-duh-num): a trace element.

Molybdenum toxicity is rare, but has been reported in workers exposed to its dust. Characteristics include goutlike symptoms in human beings. For a summary of molybdenum facts, see Table 13–9.

Other Trace Minerals

Several trace minerals have been known for decades, and understanding their roles in the body has become a rapidly growing research area. Research to determine whether other trace minerals are essential is difficult, both because their

Table 13–9

Molybdenum—A Summary

Estimated Safe and Adequate Intake	Chief Functions in the Body	Deficiency Symptoms	Toxicity Symptoms	Significant Sources
Adults: 75–250 μg/day	Facilitator, with enzymes, of many cell processes	Unknown	Enzyme inhibition, gout-like symptoms	Legumes, cereals, organ meats

Figure 13–7

Cobalt with Vitamin B_{12}
The intricate vitamin B_{12} molecule contains one atom of cobalt. The alternative name for vitamin B_{12}, cobalamin, reflects the presence of cobalt in its structure.

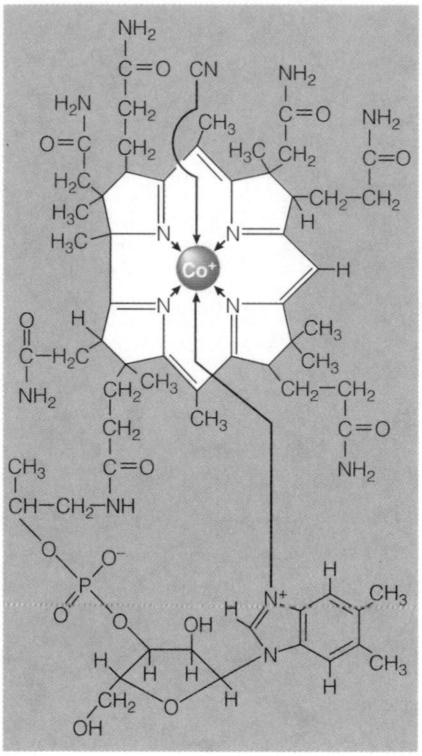

quantities in the body are so small and because human deficiencies are unknown. Much of the available knowledge comes from research using animals.

Nickel is now recognized as important for the health of many body tissues; deficiencies harm the liver and other organs. Silicon is needed for healthy bones, brains, and blood vessels in animals; some researchers believe it may be essential for human beings as well.[42] Tin is necessary for growth in animals. Vanadium, too, is necessary for growth and bone development and also for normal reproduction; human intakes of vanadium may barely exceed the minimum needed for health. Cobalt is a key mineral in the large vitamin B_{12} molecule (see Figure 13–7), but it is not an essential nutrient and no RDA has been established. Boron may play a key role in bone development and oppose demineralization in osteoporosis.[43] In the future many other trace minerals may turn out to play key nutritional roles: silver, mercury, lead, barium, and cadmium. Even arsenic—famous as a poison used by murderers and known to be a carcinogen—may turn out to be essential for human beings in tiny quantities.

Closing Thoughts on the Nutrients

This chapter completes the introductory lessons on the nutrients. Each nutrient from the amino acids to zinc has been described rather thoroughly—its chemistry, roles in the body, sources in the diet, symptoms of deficiency and toxicity, and influences on health and disease. Such a detailed examination is informative, but it can also be misleading. It is important to step back from the myopic study of the individual nutrients to look at them as a whole. After all, people eat foods, not nutrients, and most foods deliver several nutrients. Furthermore, nutrients work cooperatively with each other in the body; their actions are most often *inter*actions. This chapter alone mentioned how iron needs vitamin C to keep it in its active form and copper to incorporate it into hemoglobin; how zinc is needed to activate and transport vitamin A; and how both iodine and selenium are needed in the synthesis of thyroid hormones.

Estimates of how much of each particular nutrient the body needs are based on principles that are changing.[44] Nutrient needs fall into the broad area between intakes that are inadequate and cause illness and intakes that are excessive and cause illness. Between deficiency and toxicity lies a wide range of intakes that support health—to varying degrees. In the past, nutrient needs were determined by how much was needed to cure deficiency symptoms. If lack of a nutrient caused illness, it was defined as essential.

Today's research is rethinking nutrient needs based on how much is needed to support optimal health. The amount of vitamin C needed to prevent scurvy is much less than the amount correlated with reducing the risk of cancer, for example. Furthermore, nutrients are being examined within the context of the whole diet. Health benefits are not credited to vitamin C alone, but to the vitamin C–rich fruits and vegetables that also provide many other nutrients—and nonnutrients—important to health. With these thoughts in mind, the following highlight will review the nutrient contributions of two days' meals, identifying their strengths and shortcomings in support of good health.

People can also improve their health with physical activity. Energy expenditure is the opposite of money expenditure: it is desirable to *spend* energy, not to save it (within reason, of course). The more energy people spend, the more food they can afford to eat—food delivering both nutrients and pleasure. The next chapter describes nutrition and physical activity.

Study Questions

1. Distinguish between heme and nonheme iron. Discuss the factors that enhance iron absorption.
2. Distinguish between iron deficiency and iron-deficiency anemia. What are the symptoms of iron-deficiency anemia?
3. What causes iron overload? What are its symptoms?
4. Discuss possible reasons for a low intake of zinc. What factors affect the bioavailability of zinc?
5. Describe the similarities and differences in the absorption and regulation of iron and zinc.
6. Describe the principal functions of iodide, selenium, copper, fluoride, and chromium in the body.
7. What public health measure has been used in preventing simple goiter? What measure has been recommended for protection against tooth decay?
8. Discuss the importance of balanced and varied diets in obtaining the essential minerals and avoiding toxicities.
9. Describe some of the ways trace minerals interact with each other and with other nutrients.

Notes

1. Committee on Dietary Allowances, *Recommended Dietary Allowances*, 10th ed. (Washington, D.C.: National Academy Press, 1989), pp. 262–271.
2. G. J. Beckett and coauthors, Effects of combined iodine and selenium deficiency on thyroid hormone metabolism in rats, *American Journal of Clinical Nutrition* 57 (1993): 240S–243S.
3. R. D. Baynes and T. H. Bothwell, Iron deficiency, *Annual Review of Nutrition* 10 (1990): 133–148.
4. Baynes and Bothwell, 1990.
5. E. R. Monsen and coauthors, Estimation of available dietary iron, *American Journal of Clinical Nutrition* 31 (1978): 134–141.
6. M. Tuntawiroon and coauthors, Dose-dependent inhibitory effect of phenolic compounds in foods on nonheme iron absorption in men, *American Journal of Clinical Nutrition* 53 (1991): 554–557.
7. E. R. Monsen, Iron nutrition and absorption: Dietary factors which impact iron bioavailability, *Journal of the American Dietetic Association* 88 (1988): 786–790.
8. H. Munro, The ferritin genes: Their response to iron status, *Nutrition Reviews* 51 (1993): 65–73.
9. D. C. Rockey and J. P. Cello, Evaluation of the gastrointestinal tract in patients with iron-deficiency anemia, *New England Journal of Medicine* 329 (1993): 1691–1695.
10. V. Herbert, Everyone should be tested for iron disorders, *Journal of the American Dietetic Association* 92 (1992): 1502–1509.
11. P. R. Dallman, Iron, in *Present Knowledge in Nutrition*, 6th ed., ed. M. L. Brown (Washington, D.C.: International Life Sciences Institute, Nutrition Foundation, 1990), pp. 241–250.
12. Baynes and Bothwell, 1990.
13. Baynes and Bothwell, 1990.
14. F. A. Oski, Iron deficiency in infancy and childhood, *New England Journal of Medicine* 329 (1993): 190–193.
15. Herbert, 1992.
16. C. B. Gable, Hemochromatosis and dietary iron supplementation: Implications from U.S. mortality, morbidity, and health survey data, *Journal of the American Dietetic Association* 92 (1992): 208–212.
17. J. T. Salonen and coauthors, High stored iron levels are associated with excess risk of myocardial infarction in Eastern Finnish men, *Circulation* 86 (1992): 803–811.
18. V. Herbert, S. Shaw, and E. Jayatilleke, Vitamin C supplements are harmful to lethal for the over 10% of Americans with high iron stores, *FASEB Journal* 8 (1994): A678.
19. R. L. Nelson and coauthors, Body iron stores and risk of colonic neoplasia, *Journal of the National Cancer Institute* 86 (1994): 455–460.
20. Committee on Dietary Allowances, 1989.
21. R. J. Cousins and J. M. Hempe, Zinc, in *Present Knowledge in Nutrition*, 6th ed., ed. M. L. Brown (Washington, D.C.: International Life Sciences Institute, Nutrition Foundation, 1990), pp. 251–260.
22. C. L. Keen, Zinc deficiency and immune function, *Annual Review of Nutrition* 10 (1990): 415–431.
23. M. C. Linder, Nutrition and the metabolism of trace elements, in *Nutritional Biochemistry and Metabolism with Clinical Implications*, ed. M. C. Linder (New York: Elsevier, 1991), pp. 215–276.
24. Cousins and Hempe, 1990.
25. J. Zheng and coauthors, Measurement of zinc bioavailability from beef and a ready-to-eat high-fiber breakfast cereal in humans: Application of a whole-gut lavage technique, *Amer-*

ican Journal of Clinical Nutrition 58 (1993): 902–907.
26. Cousins and Hempe, 1990; B. L. O'Dell, Copper, in *Present Knowledge in Nutrition*, 6th ed., ed. M. L. Brown (Washington, D.C.: International Life Sciences Institute, Nutrition Foundation, 1990), pp. 261–267.
27. Keen, 1990.
28. A. S. Prasad, Discovery of human zinc deficiency and studies in an experimental human model, *American Journal of Clinical Nutrition* 53 (1991): 403–412.
29. Committee on Dietary Allowances, 1989, pp. 205–213.
30. G. A. Eby, D. R. David, and W. W. Halcomb, Reduction in duration of common colds by zinc gluconate lozenges in a double-blind study, *Antimicrobial Agents and Chemotherapy* 25 (1984): 20–24.
31. J. C. Godfrey, Zinc for the common cold: Antimicrobial prophylaxis and treatment of rhinovirus colds with zinc gluconate lozenges, *Journal of Antimicrobial Chemotherapy* 20 (1987): 893–901; B. M. Farr and coauthors, Two randomized controlled trials of zinc gluconate lozenge therapy of experimentally induced rhinovirus colds, *Antimicrobial Agents and Chemotherapy* 31 (1987): 1183–1187.
32. A. M. Fan and K. W. Kizer, Selenium—Nutritional, toxicologic, and clinical aspects, *The Western Journal of Medicine* 153 (1990): 160–167.
33. M. A. Johnson and S. E. Kays, Copper: Its role in human nutrition, *Nutrition Today*, January/February 1990, pp. 6–14.
34. G. E. Bunce, Hypercholesterolemia of copper deficiency is linked to glutathione metabolism and regulation of hepatic HMG-CoA reductase, *Nutrition Reviews* 51 (1993): 305–307; Decreased dietary copper impairs vascular function, *Nutrition Reviews* 51 (1993): 188–189; Low-copper diets increase aortic lipid peroxides in rats, *Nutrition Reviews* 51 (1993): 88–89.
35. Position of The American Dietetic Association: The impact of fluoride on dental health, *Journal of the American Dietetic Association* 94 (1994): 1428–1431.
36. M. Kleerekoper and R. Balena, Fluorides and osteoporosis, *Annual Review of Nutrition* 11 (1991): 309–324.
37. B. D. Gessner and coauthors, Acute fluoride poisoning from a public water system, *New England Journal of Medicine* 330 (1994): 95–99; D. E. Leland, K. E. Powell, and R. S. Anderson, Jr., A fluoride overfeed incident at Harbor Springs, Mich., *Journal of the American Water Works Association* 72 (1980): 238–243; L. R. Petersen and coauthors, Community health effects of a municipal water supply hyperfluoridation accident, *American Journal of Public Health* 78 (1988): 711–713; Acute fluoride poisoning—North Carolina, *Morbidity and Mortality Weekly Report* 23 (1974): 199.
38. R. A. Anderson and coauthors, Supplemental-chromium effects on glucose, insulin, glucagon, and urinary chromium losses in subjects consuming controlled low-chromium diets, *American Journal of Clinical Nutrition* 54 (1991): 909–916.
39. E. G. Offenbacher and F. X. Pi-Sunyer, Chromium in human nutrition, *Annual Review of Nutrition* 8 (1988): 543–563.
40. J. McBride, Chromium supplementation helps keep blood glucose levels in check (Of Interest to You), *Journal of the American Dietetic Association* 91 (1991): 178.
41. K. V. Rajagopalan, Molybdenum: An essential trace element in human nutrition, *Annual Review of Nutrition* 8 (1988): 401–427.
42. C. D. Seaborn and F. H. Nielsen, Silicon: A nutritional beneficence for bones, brains, and blood vessels? *Nutrition Today*, July/August 1993, pp. 13–18.
43. H. McCoy and coauthors, Relation of boron to the composition and mechanical properties of bone, *Environmental Health Perspectives* (supplement) 102 (1994): 49–53.
44. W. Mertz, Essential trace metals: New definitions based on new paradigms, *Nutrition Today* 51 (1993): 287–295.

Problem Set

1. For each of these minerals, make note of the unit of measure:

Iron: ________ Zinc: ________

2. Analyze the energy and trace mineral contents of the meals presented in Chapter 10 problem 2.

a. Record their iron and zinc contributions:

Item No./Food	Energy (kcal)	Iron (mg)	Zinc (mg)
• Grains (6)			
# 357 Wheat breads, 6 slices	________	________	________
Total in grains:	________	________	________

Problem Set (continued)

Item No./Food		Energy (kcal)	Iron (mg)	Zinc (mg)
• Vegetables (3)				
# 929	Spinach, cooked from fresh, ½ c	______	______	______
# 891	Green peas, cooked from frozen, ½ c	______	______	______
# 834	Carrots, cooked from fresh, ½ c	______	______	______
Total in vegetables:		______	______	______
• Fruits (2)				
# 269	Orange juice, fresh, 1 c	______	______	______
# 264	Cantaloupe melon, ½	______	______	______
Total in fruits:		______	______	______
• Meats (2 to 3)				
#1045	Bass fish, 4 oz	______	______	______
# 598	Hamburger, lean, 4 oz	______	______	______
Total in meats:		______	______	______
• Milks (2)				
# 98	Milk, nonfat, 2 c	______	______	______
Total in milks:		______	______	______

b. Which group(s) of foods offered the most iron? ____________ No or very little iron? ____________

c. Which group(s) of foods offered the most zinc? ____________ No or very little zinc? ____________

3. Appreciate foods for their iron density. Following is a list of foods shown with their iron contents per serving, the energy amounts in each, and the serving sizes that would deliver a woman's RDA of 15 mg a day.

Item No./Food		Energy (kcal)	Iron (mg)	Iron Density (mg/kcal)	Servings and kcalories to Deliver 15 mg
# 98	Milk, nonfat, 1 c	85	0.1	______	150 c (12,750 kcal)
# 37	Cheddar cheese, 1 oz	114	0.19	______	79 oz (9006 kcal)
# 820	Broccoli, cooked from fresh, chopped, 1 c	44	1.31	______	11.5 c (506 kcal)
# 939	Sweet potato, baked in skin, 1 ea	117	0.51	______	29 potatoes (3393 kcal)
# 264	Cantaloupe melon, ½	93	0.56	______	27 (½ melon svgs) (2511 kcal)
# 834	Carrots, from fresh, ½ c	35	0.48	______	31 (½ c svgs) (1085 kcal)
# 357	Whole-wheat bread, 1 slice	64	0.87	______	17 slices (1088 kcal)
# 891	Green peas, cooked from frozen, ½ c	62	1.26	______	12 (½ c svgs) (744 kcal)
# 206	Apple, fresh, 3¼″	125	0.38	______	40 apples (5000 kcal)
# 606	Sirloin steak, lean, 4 oz	228	3.81	______	4 (4 oz) steaks (912 kcal)
# 623	Pork chop, lean, broiled, 1 ea	166	0.66	______	23 chops (3818 kcal)

a. First rank these foods by iron per serving: ____________________

b. Calculate the iron density for these foods and rank them by their iron per kcalorie: ____________

c. Name three foods that are higher on the second list: ____________________

d. What do these foods have in common? ____________________

(continued on the next page)

Problem Set (continued)

Although vegetables may not offer very much of a nutrient per serving, they may still be significant sources of nutrients if you eat a lot of them, and you can, because vegetables are so low in kcalories.

4. Because some people find it very hard to eat enough iron-rich foods and absorb enough iron to meet their needs, focus on this problem for a woman of childbearing age.

a. Calculate the iron that this person might absorb from the following meal. Start by filling in the following data:

Item No./Food	Iron (mg)	Vitamin C (mg)
# 606 Sirloin steak, lean, 4 oz	______	______
# 891 Green peas, cooked from frozen, ½ c	______	______
# 542 Brown rice, cooked, 1 c	______	______
# 32 Iced tea, instant, sweetened, 1 c	______	______
Totals	______	______

b. Use the box on p. 477 to calculate the iron the person received from the meal. Show your calculations. Total iron absorbed = ______________________________

c. The RDA assumes that a person absorbs 10% of the iron eaten. Was that true in this case? What percentage of iron did this person absorb? Show your calculations: ______________________________

d. Is there any factor in the meal that might reduce the absorption of iron as calculated here? ______________

e. Setting this factor aside for the moment, and assuming the person eats three meals similar to this one, is a woman of childbearing age likely to meet her iron RDA for the day? Show your calculations: ______________

____

5. Read Highlight 13 and calculate a Healthy Eating Index score for Tuesday's meals. Show your calculations:

____

What suggestions do you have for improving this day's meals? ______________________________

Putting It All Together—Appraising Two Days' Meals

Glossary

Healthy Eating Index: a standard developed by USDA for assessing overall dietary quality; a single numerical summary of degree of adherence to the recommendations of the *Food Guide Pyramid* and the *Dietary Guidelines for Americans*.

Chapter 2 introduced the Food Guide Pyramid and the *Dietary Guidelines for Americans* and the intervening chapters provided in-depth information on the nutrients. This highlight presents two days' meals and appraises them in light of all that knowledge—using a combination of two different methods. One method, a computer diet analysis, gives specific details of nutrient intake, whereas the other, the Healthy Eating Index, shows an overall view of the diet. Together, they offer an abundance of information about how well these meals meet recommended eating patterns.

The first set, labeled "Monday's Meals," shows selections made by following the suggested number of servings from the Daily Food Guide. The second set of meals, labeled "Tuesday's Meals," represents selections made without a plan (but not unlike real-life choices). Before reading further, inspect the photos of the meals shown in Figure H13–1 (on p. 506). Which might you have chosen for yourself? Just by eyeballing the pictures, can you suggest food choices that might improve either day's nutrient intakes? Now read the following paragraphs and see how well your evaluation compares with ours.

COMPARING MONDAY'S MEALS WITH TUESDAY'S

A computer analysis reveals that both days' meals provide almost 1900 kcalories, somewhat less than the RDA for young adults. Figure H13–2 (on p. 507) presents the computer analysis results, comparing the two days' selections with each other and with the RDA for selected vitamins and minerals.

For the same food energy, both sets of meals provide more than adequate protein. Because Monday's meals included plenty of grain products, vegetables, and fruits, carbohydrates dominated the day's energy intake (57 percent of total kcalories). Furthermore, Monday's meals provided over 30 grams of fiber (20 to 35 grams of fiber daily is desirable). In contrast, Tuesday's meals provided only 34 percent kcalories from carbohydrates and less than 10 grams of fiber.

On Tuesday, fat dominated the energy intake, contributing 46 percent of the total kcalories. Almost 20 percent of the kcalories derived from saturated fat, whereas less than 10 percent is recommended. There were 450 milligrams of cholesterol—more than twice as much as in Monday's meals. In contrast, Monday's meals met the goal of having less than 30 percent of the kcalories from fat; they were also low in saturated fat and cholesterol. Notice (from Tuesday) that a person can eat a lot of fat without consuming much food and, conversely (from Monday), that a person can eat a lot of food without having to consume too much food energy or fat.

Tuesday's meals were lower in sodium than Monday's meals. While Tuesday met guidelines to limit sodium to less than 2400 milligrams, Monday exceeded these recommendations by about 25 percent (luncheon meats and canned tomato sauces are high in sodium).

Monday's meals consisted of a variety of foods, which helped to provide an array of vitamins and minerals. As you can see, the nutrients most notably lacking from Tuesday's meals are those that fruits, vegetables, and milk are famous for: vitamin A, vitamin C, and calcium. On a day like Monday, when nutrient intakes meet or exceed most recommendations, the person might add other foods for sheer pleasure. On a day like Tuesday, though, when several nutrient intakes fall short of recommendations, added foods, selected wisely, would help a lot to meet nutrient needs.

SCORING MONDAY'S MEALS

Overall, Monday's meals seem to outshine Tuesday's meals, but were they truly excellent choices? (Just because you make a better grade than your roommate, doesn't necessarily mean that you got an "A".) To give Monday's meals a grade requires using an assessment tool developed by the USDA—The Healthy Eating Index. This index appraises a diet according to the Food Guide Pyramid and the

Figure H13–1

Monday's and Tuesday's Meals

Monday's meals were based on the sample plan developed in Tables 2–5 and 2–6. Tuesday's meals followed no plan.

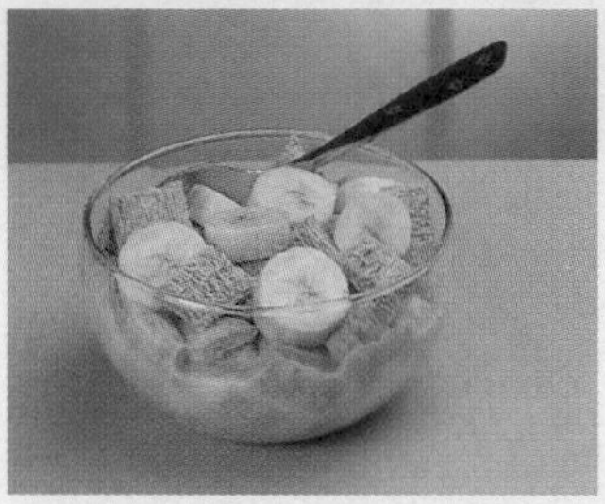

Monday's Meals

1 c shredded wheat
1 c 1% low-fat milk
½ small banana (sliced)

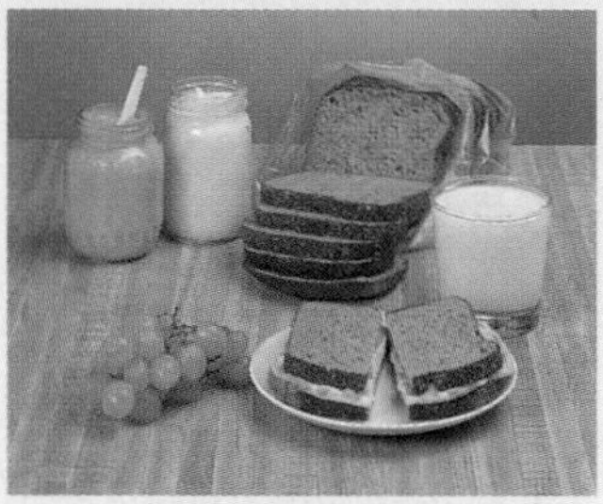

1 turkey sandwich on whole-wheat bread with mayonnaise and mustard
1 c 1% low-fat milk
small bunch of grapes

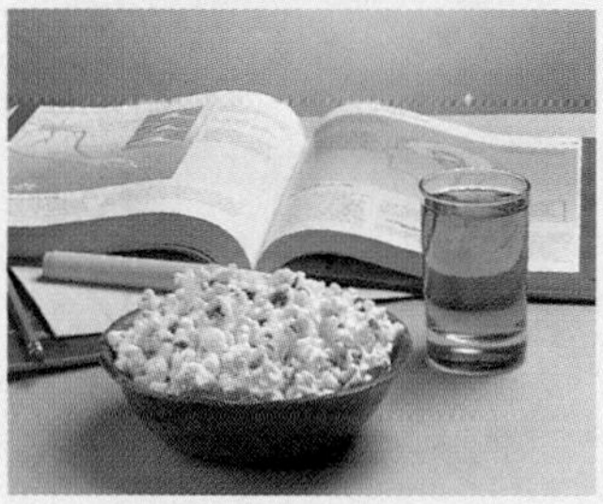

3 c plain popcorn
½ c apple juice

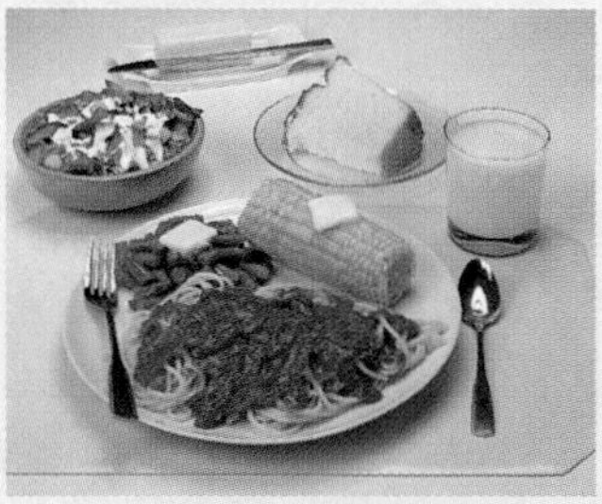

A salad made with:
- 1 c raw spinach leaves, shredded carrots, and sliced mushrooms
- ½ c garbanzo beans
- 1 tbs sunflower seeds
- 1 tbs ranch salad dressing

1 c spaghetti with meat sauce
½ c green beans
1 corn on cob
2 tsp butter
1 c 1% low-fat milk
1 piece angel food cake

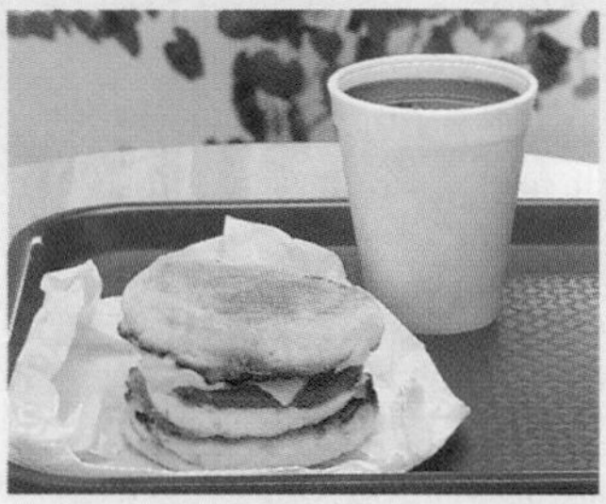

Tuesday's Meals

1 c coffee
1 English muffin with an egg, cheese, and bacon

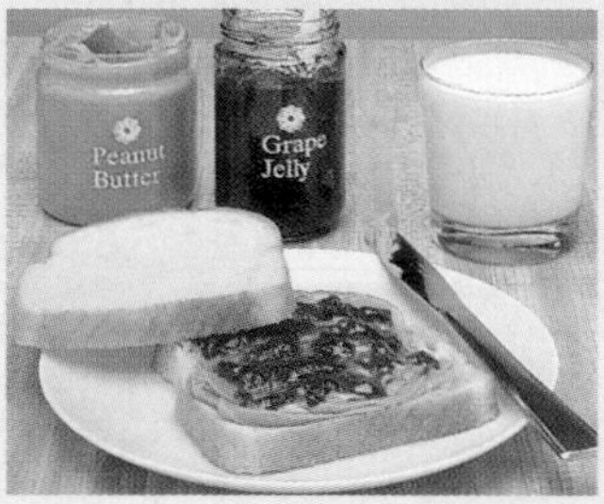

1 peanut butter and jelly sandwich on white bread
1 c whole milk

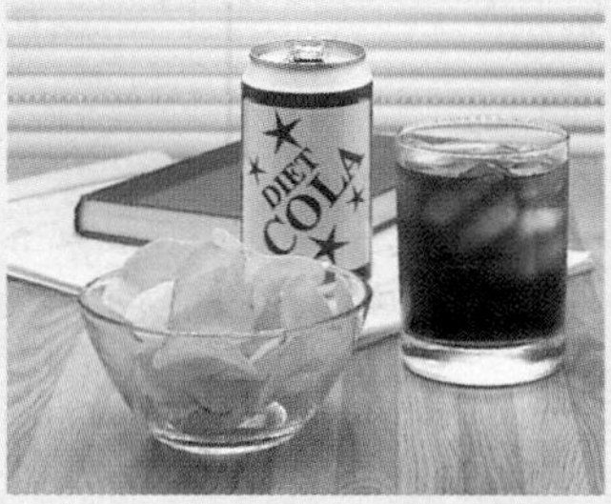

12 oz diet cola
a few potato chips

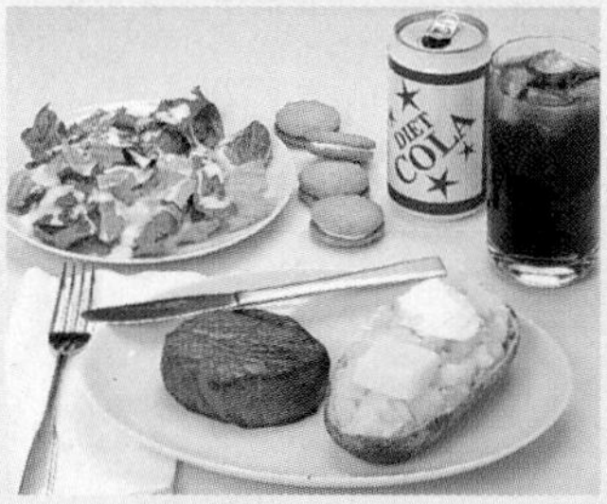

A salad made with:
- 1 c lettuce
- 1 tbs blue cheese dressing

6 oz steak
½ baked potato (large) with 1 tbs butter and 1 tbs sour cream
12 oz diet cola
4 sandwich-type cookies

Figure H13–2

Meal Selections Compared

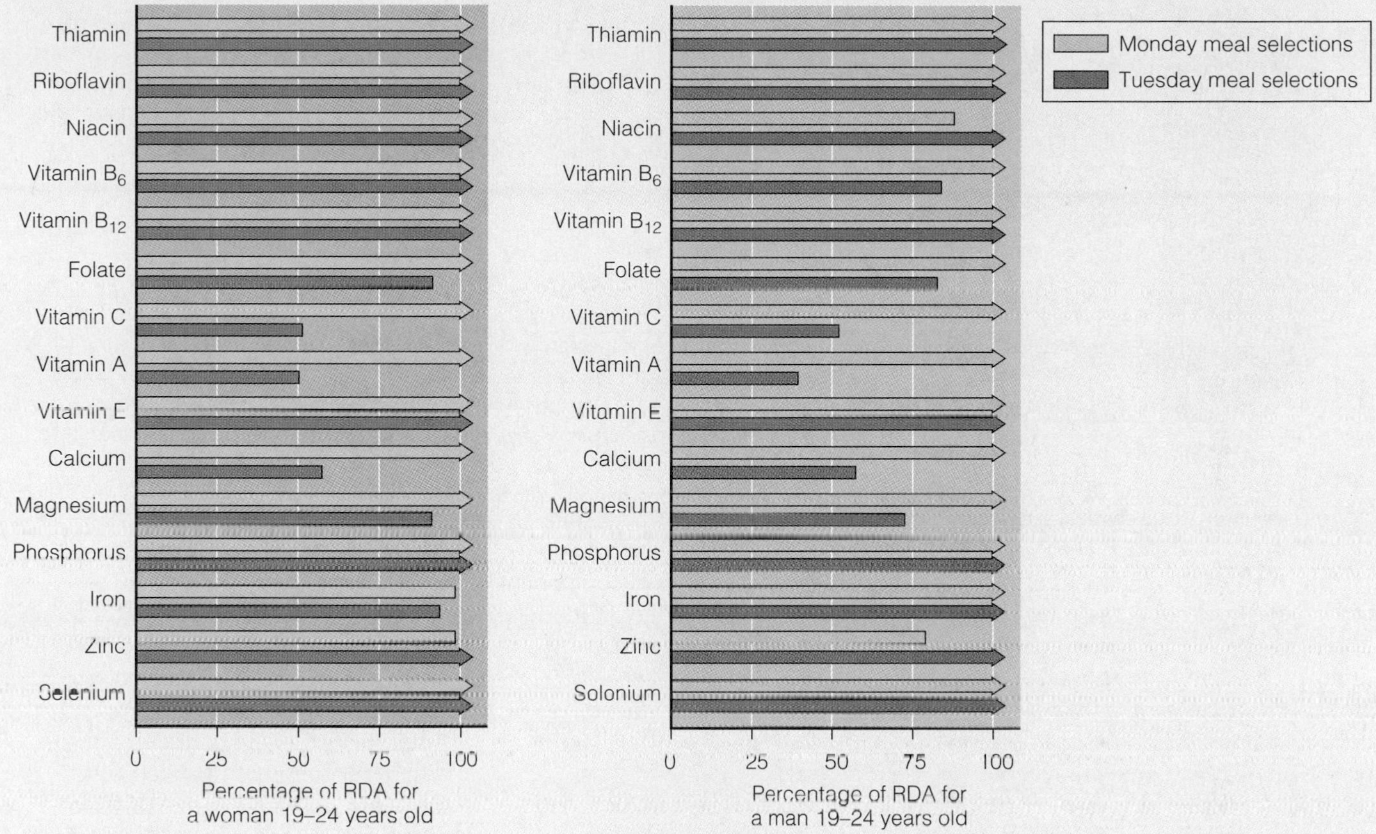

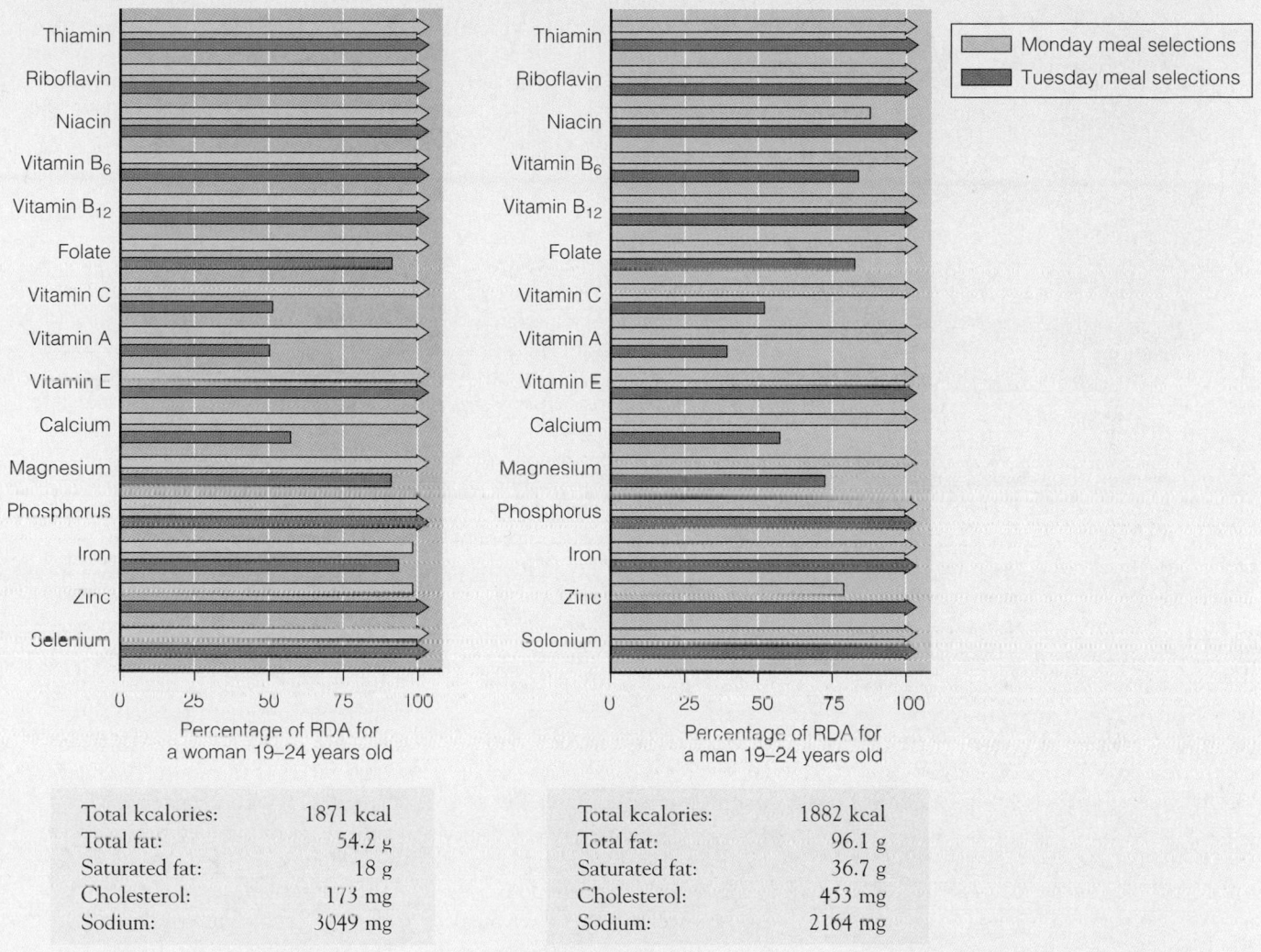

Total kcalories:	1871 kcal
Total fat:	54.2 g
Saturated fat:	18 g
Cholesterol:	173 mg
Sodium:	3049 mg

Total kcalories:	1882 kcal
Total fat:	96.1 g
Saturated fat:	36.7 g
Cholesterol:	453 mg
Sodium:	2164 mg

dietary guidelines.*[1] Ten different elements of the diet are given scores from 0 to 10 each—thus 100 is a perfect score.

The first five scores come from the Food Guide Pyramid. Each of the five food groups can contribute up to 10 points, if it meets at least the recommended minimum number of servings for a given energy intake (see Table 2–3 on p. 43). Thus a diet could receive 10 points for providing six or more grains, 10 points for three or more vegetables, 10 points for two or more fruits, 10 points for two or more milks, and 10 points for two or more meats. If no servings from a particular group were eaten, score 0; if fewer than the recommended number of servings were eaten, give a partial score (such as 5 points for eating one of the two recommended fruits, for example). Extra foods in any group receive no extra points (seven grains receive 10 points, just as six grains do). Extra foods do not receive penal-

*The Healthy Eating Index has proved reliable and valid in assessing dietary quality in over 7000 diets obtained in the 1989 and 1990 Continuing Survey of Food Intake by Individuals. Results from three-day records vary only slightly from those of one-day records.

Figure H13–3

Healthy Eating Index Components

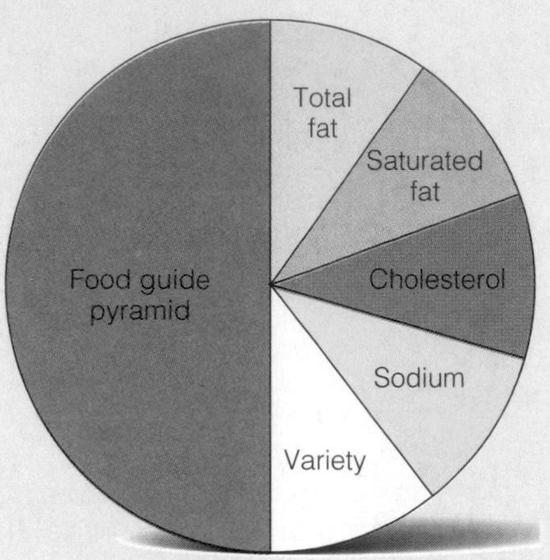

Table H13–1

Scoring Guide for Dietary Guidelines Portion of Healthy Eating Index

Points	Total fat (% of kcal)	Saturated fat (% of kcal)	Cholesterol (mg)	Sodium (mg)	Variety[a]
10	30 or less	10 or less	300 or less	2400 or less	8 or more
9	31.5	10.5	315	2640	7.5
8	33	11	330	2880	7.0
7	34.5	11.5	345	3120	6.5
6	36	12	360	3360	6.0
5	37.5	12.5	375	3600	5.5
4	39	13	390	3840	5.0
3	40.5	13.5	405	4080	4.5
2	42	14	420	4320	4.0
1	43.5	14.5	435	4560	3.5
0	45 or more	15 or more	450 or more	4800 or more	3.0 or less

[a] Values for variety are based on a one-day period; for a three-day period, the values range from 16 to 6.

ties either, even though they might contribute to an excessively high energy intake. The Healthy Eating Index accounts for energy intake only in setting the *minimum* recommended number of servings from each food group, not in comparing energy intake with needs. Consequently a person can overeat and still receive an excellent score. Another apparent shortcoming of this index is the weight given to a food group. A person could score the maximum number of points in all areas except the milk group, for example, and still end up with an outstanding final score. Yet, if the person's diet consistently lacked foods from the milk group without careful substitutions, then calcium nutrition would suffer. Like many good tools, the Healthy Eating Index accomplishes much of what it sets out to do, but cannot complete the job alone. Common sense based on nutrition knowledge is needed to round out the evaluation.

The next four dietary components in the Healthy Eating Index reflect nutrients that must be limited—fat, saturated fat, cholesterol, and sodium—these can contribute up to 10 points each. The final component of a healthy diet—variety in food choices—also contributes up to 10 points. Figure H13–3 shows how these ten dietary components are combined to produce the Healthy Eating Index.

How do Monday's meals score? Monday's meals provided at least the recommended minimum number of servings in every food group, so they score 50 points for the pyramid portion of the Healthy Eating Index.

Now, how well do Monday's meals rate against the dietary guidelines? They score 10 points for providing each of the following: 30 percent or less of their energy from fat, less than 10 percent of their energy from saturated fat, and less than 300 milligrams of cholesterol. They don't do as well in meeting sodium recommendations. At just over 3000 milligrams, sodium receives a score of 7 (see Table H13–1 and the little tables that accompany Figure H13–2).

The Healthy Eating Index gives 10 points for including at least 8 different foods in a day. Monday met this goal before dinner. All in all, Monday's Healthy Eating Index score was 97: excellent. Scores above 80 are considered good; those between 50 and 80 need improvement; and those below 50 are considered poor. Higher scores are associated with greater likelihoods of meeting the RDA for most nutrients. A review of Figure H13–2 confirms that Monday's meals did indeed meet or exceed most of the RDA.

The problem set in Chapter 13 asks you to calculate the Healthy Eating Index score for Tuesday's meals and to suggest ways to improve the day's choices. A hint: cut the fat by selecting foods high in nutrient density.

NOTES

1. USDA Center for Nutrition Policy and Promotion, The Healthy Eating Index (Washington, D.C.: Government Printing Office, 1995).

Chapter 14

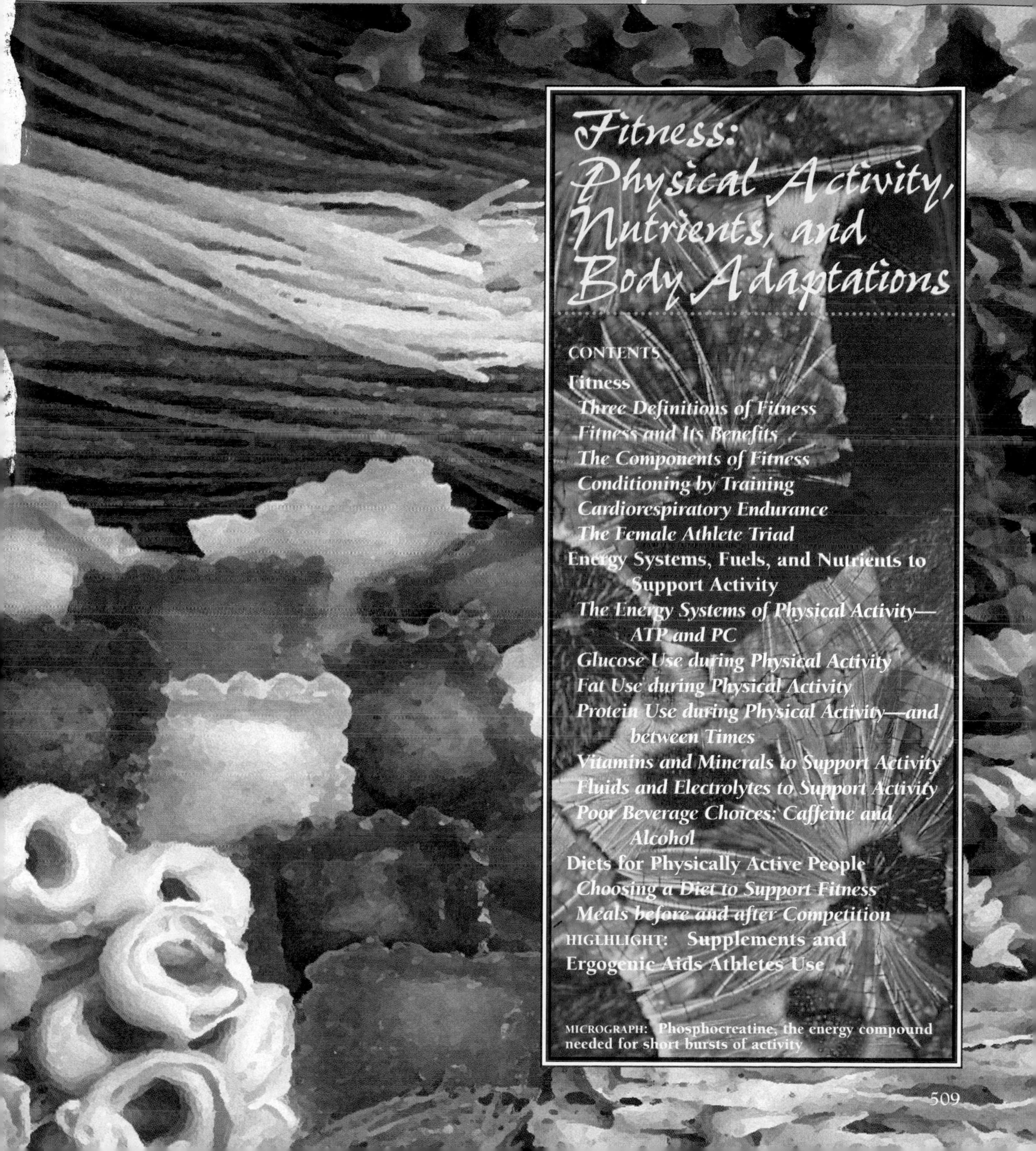

Fitness: Physical Activity, Nutrients, and Body Adaptations

CONTENTS

MICROGRAPH: Phosphocreatine, the energy compound needed for short bursts of activity

Physical activity, or its lack, exerts a significant and pervasive influence on everyone's nutrition and overall health. Therefore, this chapter is written for "you," whoever you are—an athlete, a health seeker, a future health counselor, a sports player, a weight-loss seeker, or a person who has yet to become physically active. Extensive evidence confirms that regular physical activity promotes health and prevents disease.[1] Still, despite an increasing awareness of the health benefits that physical activity confers, more than 75 percent of adults in the United States are either irregularly active or completely inactive.[2] Physical inactivity is linked to the major degenerative diseases—heart disease, cancer, stroke, diabetes, and hypertension—that are the primary killers of adults in developed countries.[3]

People don't have to run marathons to reap the health rewards of physical activity. Most experts agree that any physical activity, even moderate activity, provides health benefits. In fact, people who are extremely inactive stand to gain the greatest health benefits by engaging in regular moderate-intensity, endurance-type activity.[4] The authors of an extensive study on fitness and mortality concluded that "moderate levels of physical fitness that are attainable by most adults appear to be protective against early mortality."[5] It makes sense, then, to promote activities that can readily be performed by the least active people, since they may benefit most.

In 1990, the American College of Sports Medicine (ACSM) updated its position statement on the quantity and quality of exercise recommended for developing and maintaining fitness in healthy adults (see Table 14–1).[6] The main objective of these guidelines was to outline the types and amounts of physical activity needed to improve *physical fitness*. These familiar guidelines have helped adults develop programs to improve their cardiorespiratory endurance and body composition. The types and amounts of physical activity needed to promote *fit-*

Table 14–1

Physical Activity Guidelines

Guidelines for developing and maintaining *physical fitness:*

- **Frequency of activity:** three to five days per week.
- **Intensity of activity:** 50 to 90% of maximum heart rate.
- **Duration of activity:** 20 to 60 minutes of continuous activity.
- **Mode of activity:** any activity that uses large muscle groups.
- **Resistance activity:** strength training of moderate intensity at least two times per week.

Guidelines for obtaining *health* benefits:

- **Frequency of activity:** every day.
- **Intensity of activity:** any level (can be minimal).
- **Duration of activity:** at least 30 minutes total of activity (can be intermittent).
- **Mode of activity:** any activity.

Note: Duration and intensity are inversely related. To obtain similar fitness benefits, a person may exercise either at a low intensity for a long duration or at a high intensity for a short duration. For example, a person may choose to walk briskly for 40 to 50 minutes (lower intensity and longer duration) or to jog for 20 to 30 minutes (higher intensity and shorter duration).

ness, however, may differ from those needed to obtain *health* benefits. For health's sake, the ACSM specifies that people should spend an accumulated minimum of 30 minutes in some sort of physical activity on most days of each week.[7] The activity need not be sports. Eight minutes spent climbing up stairs, another 10 spent pulling weeds, and 12 more spent walking the dog all contribute to the day's total. The guidelines for developing fitness are still optimal, though, because improving fitness provides additional health benefits.

The recent findings of an extensive study of healthy men from Harvard University support the findings of previous studies: regular physical activity confers health benefits that can prolong life.[8] This same study also raises new questions, however, because the researchers concluded that only *vigorous* activity prolonged life. Men who expended more than 1500 kcalories per week in vigorous activities such as running, swimming, and cycling had as much as a 25 percent reduced risk of dying compared with others. Any benefits of moderate activity were not apparent, perhaps because this study lumped moderate and minimal exercisers together.

The following comparisons reflect similar differences in the risks associated with chronic disease and death:

- Vigorous exercise vs minimal exercise.
- Ideal weight vs 20% overweight.
- Nonsmoking vs smoking (one pack a day).

One of the coauthors of this study conducted an earlier study of the Harvard men that showed that moderate physical activity can prolong life.[9] This researcher, as well as many others, remains confident that moderate activity confers health benefits and has concluded that the more vigorous the activity, the greater the benefit—to a point. No one yet knows the minimal, optimal, or hazardous amount of activity, if there is one. For the vast majority of Americans, however, too much activity is not the problem.

This chapter begins by defining fitness and presenting its benefits. The chapter goes on to explain how the body uses energy nutrients to fuel physical activity and finally describes how nutrition supports fitness.

Fitness

Perhaps you are already physically fit. If so, the following description applies to you. You are graceful and move with ease. You are strong and meet physical challenges without strain. You have endurance, and your energy lasts for hours. You can meet normal physical challenges with ease and have plenty of energy in reserve to handle emergencies. What's more, you are likely to be well able to meet mental and emotional challenges, too—for physical fitness supports mental and emotional energy and resilience as well.

THREE DEFINITIONS OF FITNESS

Narrowly defined, fitness refers to *the characteristics that enable the body to perform physical activity*. These characteristics include flexibility of the joints; strength and endurance of the muscles, including the heart muscle; and a healthy body composition. A broader definition of fitness is *the ability to meet routine physical demands with enough reserve energy to rise to a sudden challenge*. This definition shows how fitness relates to everyday life. Ordinary tasks such as carrying heavy suitcases, opening a stuck window, or climbing four flights of stairs, which might strain an unfit person, are easy for a fit person. Still another definition is *the body's ability to withstand stress*, meaning both physical and psychological stresses.

fitness: the characteristics that enable the body to perform physical activity; more broadly, the ability to meet routine physical demands with enough reserve energy to rise to a sudden challenge; or the body's ability to withstand stress of all kinds.

These definitions do not contradict each other; they are three different descriptions of the same wonderful condition of the body.

sedentary: physically inactive (literally, "sitting down a lot").

The Lack of Fitness The opposite of a physically active life is a sedentary life, which means literally "sitting down a lot." Today's world fosters inactivity by providing people with escalators, cars, golf carts, and other labor-saving devices. As people go through life exerting minimal physical effort, they become weak and unfit and begin to feel unwell. The body responds to inactivity by losing muscle and skill, just as it responds to activity by gaining them.

Fitness and Physical Activity Fitness depends on a certain minimum daily or weekly amount of physical activity. In fact, a specific recommendation for energy *expenditure* might be useful, although no such recommendation has yet been made. Stretching the point, we might even speak of an "activity deficiency," just as we speak of a protein, vitamin, or mineral deficiency.

FITNESS AND ITS BENEFITS

Physical activity produces fitness, and fitness in turn makes activity easy, a beneficial cycle. Activity and fitness are so closely connected that this chapter makes no distinction between them. The benefits of fitness are the benefits of physical activity, and vice versa. In general, physically fit people enjoy:

- *Restful sleep.* Rest and sleep occur naturally after periods of physical activity. During rest, the body repairs injuries, disposes of wastes generated during activity, and builds new physical structures.
- *Nutritional health.* Physical activity spends energy and thus allows people to eat more food. If they choose wisely, active people will consume more nutrients and be less likely to develop nutrient deficiencies.
- *Optimal body composition.* A balanced program of physical activity limits body fat and maintains lean tissue. Physically active people have relatively less body fat than sedentary people at the same body weight.
- *Optimal bone density.* Weight-bearing physical activity builds bone strength and protects against osteoporosis.[10]
- *Resistance to colds and other infectious diseases.* Fitness enhances immunity.[11]
- *Low risks of some types of cancer.* Lifelong physical activity may help to protect against colon cancer, breast cancer, and others.[12]
- *Strong circulation and lung function.* Physical activity that challenges the heart and lungs slows the aging of the circulatory system.
- *Low risk of cardiovascular disease.* Physical activity lowers blood pressure, slows resting pulse rate, and lowers blood cholesterol, thus reducing the risks of heart attack and strokes.[13]
- *Low risk of diabetes.* Physical activity normalizes glucose tolerance, especially via the secretion of insulin.[14]
- *Low incidence and severity of anxiety and depression.* Compared with sedentary people, physically active people deal better with stress.
- *Strong self-image.* The sense of achievement that comes from meeting physical challenges promotes self-confidence.

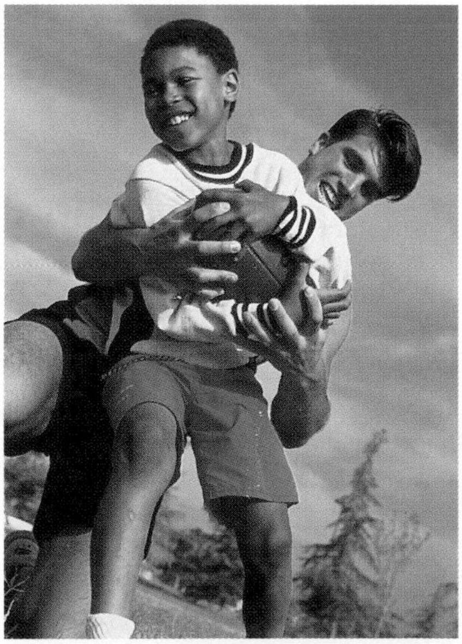

Physical activity helps you look good, feel good, and have fun, and it brings many long-term health benefits as well.

- *Long life and high quality of life in the later years*. Active people have a lower mortality rate than sedentary people. Just a brisk half-hour walk daily can add years to a person's life. In addition to extending longevity, physical activity supports independence and mobility in later life by reducing the risks of falls and minimizing the risk of injury should a fall occur.[15]

A person who practices a physical activity *adapts* by becoming better able to perform it after each session—more flexible, stronger, more enduring.

THE COMPONENTS OF FITNESS

To be physically fit, a person needs to develop enough flexibility, muscle strength, and endurance, and cardiorespiratory endurance to meet the everyday demands of life with some to spare and to achieve a reasonable body weight and body composition. Flexibility allows the joints to move with less chance of injury. Muscle strength and endurance enable muscles to work longer without fatigue. Cardiorespiratory endurance supports the ongoing action of the heart and lungs. Physical activity augments desirable lean body tissue and eliminates excess body fat. As a person becomes physically fit, the health of the entire body improves.

CONDITIONING BY TRAINING

Whatever component of fitness a person seeks to develop—flexibility, strength, or endurance—the principles of conditioning apply. During conditioning, the body adapts microscopically to perform the work asked of it. The way to achieve conditioning is by training, primarily by applying the progressive overload principle—that is, by asking a little more of the body in each training session.

The Overload Principle You can apply the progressive overload principle in several different ways. You can perform the activity more often—that is, increase its frequency; you can perform it more strenuously—that is, increase its intensity; or you can do it for longer times—that is, increase its duration. All three strategies work well, and combinations also work. The rate of progression depends on individual characteristics such as fitness level, health status, age, and preference. If you really love your workout, do it more often. If you do not have much time, increase intensity. If you hate hard work, take it easy and go longer. If you want continuous improvements, remember to overload progressively as you reach higher levels of fitness.

Applying Overload When you are increasing the frequency, intensity, or duration of your workout, exercise to a point that only *slightly* exceeds your comfortable capacity to work. It is better to progress too slowly than to risk serious injury by overexertion. Other pointers include:

- Be active all week. Don't be a weekend athlete.
- Use proper equipment and attire.
- Perform approved exercises using proper form.
- Within each activity session, include warm-up and cool-down activities. Warming up helps to prepare muscles, ligaments, and tendons for the upcoming activ-

flexibility: the capacity of the joints to move through a full range of motion; the ability to bend and recover without injury.

muscle strength: the ability of muscles to work against resistance.

muscle endurance: the ability of a muscle to contract repeatedly without becoming exhausted.

cardiorespiratory endurance: the ability to perform large-muscle, dynamic exercise of moderate-to-high intensity for prolonged periods.

Reminder: *Body composition* refers to the proportions of muscle, bone, fat, and other tissue that make up a person's total body weight.

conditioning: the physical effect of *training*; improved flexibility, strength, and endurance.

training: practicing an activity regularly, which leads to conditioning. (Training is what you do; conditioning is what you get.)

progressive overload principle: the training principle that a body system, in order to improve, must be worked at frequencies, durations, or intensities that gradually increase physical demands.

frequency: the number of occurrences per unit of time (for example, the number of exercise sessions per week).

intensity: the degree of exertion while exercising (for example, the amount of weight lifted or the speed of running).

duration: length of time (for example, the time spent in each exercise session).

warm-up: five to ten minutes of light activity, such as easy jogging or cycling, to warm up the body in preparation for more vigorous activity.

cool-down: five to ten minutes of light activity following a vigorous workout to gradually cool the body's core to near-normal temperature.

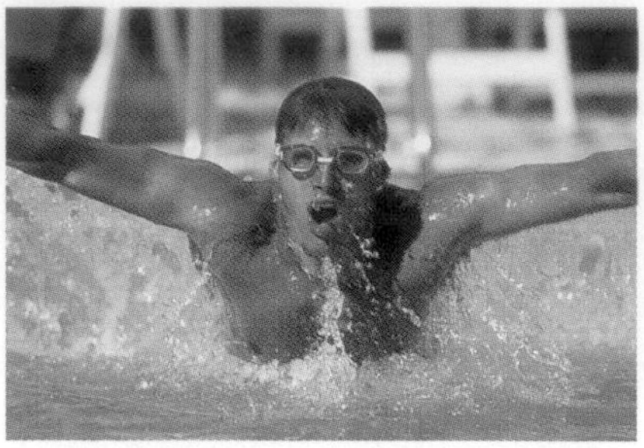

People's bodies are shaped by the activities they perform.

ity and mobilizes fuels to support strength and endurance activities; cooling down reduces muscle cramping and allows the heart rate to slow gradually.

- Train hard enough to challenge your strength or endurance once or twice a week, not every time you work out. Between times, do moderate workouts and include at least one day of rest each week.
- Pay attention to body signals. Symptoms such as abnormal heartbeats; pain or pressure in the middle of the chest, teeth, jaw, neck, or arm; dizziness; lightheadedness; cold sweat; or confusion demand immediate medical attention.

It does not make sense to start with activities so demanding that pain stops you within two days. Learn to enjoy small steps toward improvement. Fitness builds slowly.

Major coronary risk factors:

1. Hypertension.
2. Serum cholesterol ≥240 mg/dL.
3. Cigarette smoking.
4. Diabetes mellitus.
5. Family history of heart disease.

Cautions on Starting Before you begin any fitness program, make sure it is safe for you to do so. The ACSM classifies individuals into three groups based on major coronary risk factors: "apparently healthy" individuals have no more than one of the risk factors listed in the margin, "individuals at higher risk" have two or more of the risk factors and/or symptoms suggestive of disease, and "individuals with disease" are known to have cardiac, pulmonary, or metabolic disease.[16] Most apparently healthy people can begin moderate exercise programs such as walking or increasing daily activities without medical examination, but people in either of the other two classifications need medical advice.

moderate exercise: activity that can be sustained comfortably for 60 minutes or so.

The Body's Response to Physical Activity Fitness develops in response to demand and wanes when demand ceases. Muscles gain size and strength after being made to work repeatedly, a response called hypertrophy. Conversely, without activity, muscles diminish in size and lose strength, a response called atrophy.

hypertrophy (high-PER-tro-fee): of muscles, growing larger; an increase in size in response to use.

atrophy (AT-ro-fee): of muscles, a decrease in size because of disuse, undernutrition, or wasting diseases.

Both hypertrophy and atrophy are forms of adaptation, and they are closely matched to the muscles' greater and lesser work demands. Thus cyclists often have well-developed legs but little arm or chest strength; a tennis player may have one superbly strong arm, while the other is just average. For balanced muscular development, people should work different muscle groups from day to day. This strategy provides a day or two of rest for different muscle groups, giving them time to replenish nutrients and to repair any slight damage incurred by the activity.

muscle fibers: muscle cells.

Muscle fibers best suited to producing energy by aerobic processes for prolonged endurance activity are slow-twitch muscle fibers.

Muscle fibers best suited to producing energy by anaerobic processes for high-intensity, short-duration activity are fast-twitch muscle fibers.

Types of Muscle Fibers Muscles are largely made up of contractile cells called muscle fibers. Muscle fibers have a limited potential to adapt in size and work capacity to the kind of work the muscles are asked to do.

Heredity sets limits on the types of muscle fibers a person can develop and on the extent to which they can respond to training. A person's athletic potential is inborn, partly because every person is born with a set number of each type of fiber. In a sense, a person is born to be either a sprinter or a long-distance runner. A person born with tremendous capacity who chooses to develop it to the fullest can become a great athlete. But even if you were not born with the "right stuff" to be an elite athlete, you can still develop your muscles, within their limits, by choosing the right activities.

Reminder: *Anaerobic* refers to energy-producing processes that do not involve the immediate use of oxygen.

Anaerobic Work Anaerobic activity is associated with strength, agility, and split-second surges of power. The jump of the basketball player, the slam of the

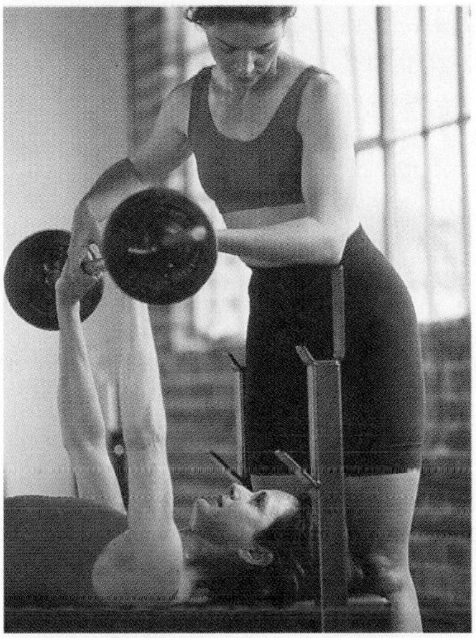

← Split-second surges of power as in the heave of a barbell or jump of a basketball player involve *anaerobic* work.

Sustained muscular efforts as in a long-distance bike ride or cross-country run involve *aerobic* work. ↓

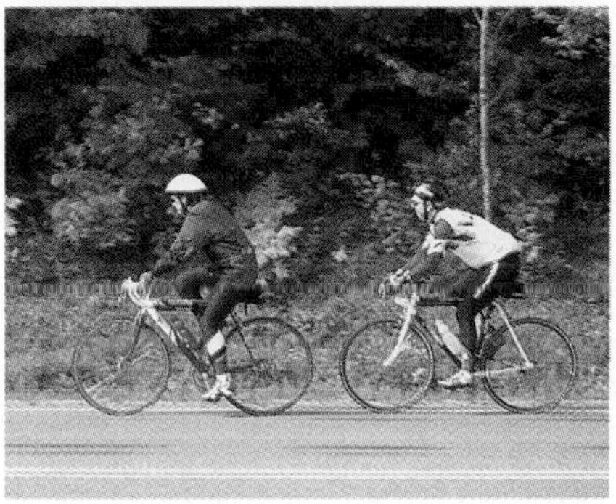

tennis serve, the heave of the weight lifter at the barbells, and the blast of the fullback through the opposing line are all anaerobic work. Such high-intensity, short-duration activities depend mostly on glucose breakdown without oxygen as the chief energy fuel.

Aerobic Work Endurance activities of low intensity and long duration depend more on fat to provide energy aerobically. The ability to continue swimming to the shore, to keep on hiking to the top of the mountain, or to continue pedaling all the way home reflects aerobic capacity. Aerobic capacity is also crucial to maintaining the health of the heart and circulatory system. The relationships among fuel use, energy production, and physical activity appear again later in this chapter, and they bear heavily on what foods best support your chosen activities.

Reminder: *Aerobic* refers to energy-producing processes involving the immediate use of oxygen.

CARDIORESPIRATORY ENDURANCE

The length of time a person can remain active with an elevated heart rate—that is, the ability of the heart, lungs, and blood to sustain a given demand—defines the person's cardiorespiratory endurance. Cardiorespiratory endurance training can improve ability to sustain a vigorous activity such as running, brisk walking, or swimming. Such training enhances the ability of the heart, lungs, and blood to deliver oxygen to, and remove waste from, the body's cells during such activity. The benefits of this training are not just physical, though, because all of the body's cells, including the brain cells, require oxygen to function. When the cells receive more oxygen more readily, both the body and the mind benefit.

Working muscles need large amounts of oxygen to produce energy. Cardiorespiratory endurance training requires the heart and lungs to work hard for a sustained period to deliver oxygen to the muscle cells. Cardiorespiratory endurance training, therefore, is *aerobic*. As the cardiorespiratory system gradually adapts to the demands of aerobic activity, the body delivers oxygen more efficiently.

Benefits of Aerobic Training: Cardiorespiratory Conditioning The changes brought about by aerobic workouts are called cardiorespiratory condi-

cardiorespiratory conditioning: improvements in the heart and lung function and increased blood volume, brought about by aerobic training.

cardiac output: the volume of blood discharged by the heart each minute.

Cardiorespiratory conditioning:
- Increases cardiac output and oxygen delivery.
- Increases stroke volume.
- Slows resting pulse.
- Increases breathing efficiency.
- Improves circulation.
- Reduces blood pressure.

stroke volume: the amount of oxygenated blood the heart ejects toward the tissues at each beat.

tioning. Among its benefits, cardiac output increases, so that the blood can carry more oxygen. The heart becomes larger and stronger, and each beat pumps more blood. Because the heart pumps more blood with each beat, fewer beats are necessary, and the resting heart rate slows down. The average resting pulse rate for adults is around 70 beats per minute, but people who have cultivated cardiorespiratory conditioning may have resting pulse rates of 50 or even lower. The muscles that work the lungs become stronger, too, so that breathing becomes more efficient. Circulation through the arteries and veins improves. Blood moves easily, and blood pressure falls.

Cardiorespiratory endurance is the physical achievement that many people appropriately prize the most highly because it reflects the health of the heart and circulatory system, on which all other body systems depend. Figure 14–1 shows the major relationships among the heart, circulatory system, and lungs.

Figure 14–1

Delivery of Oxygen by the Heart and Lungs to the Muscles

The cardiovascular system responds to the muscles' demand for oxygen by building up its capacity to deliver oxygen. Researchers can measure cardiovascular fitness by measuring the amount of oxygen a person consumes per minute while working out, a measure called **VO_2 max.**

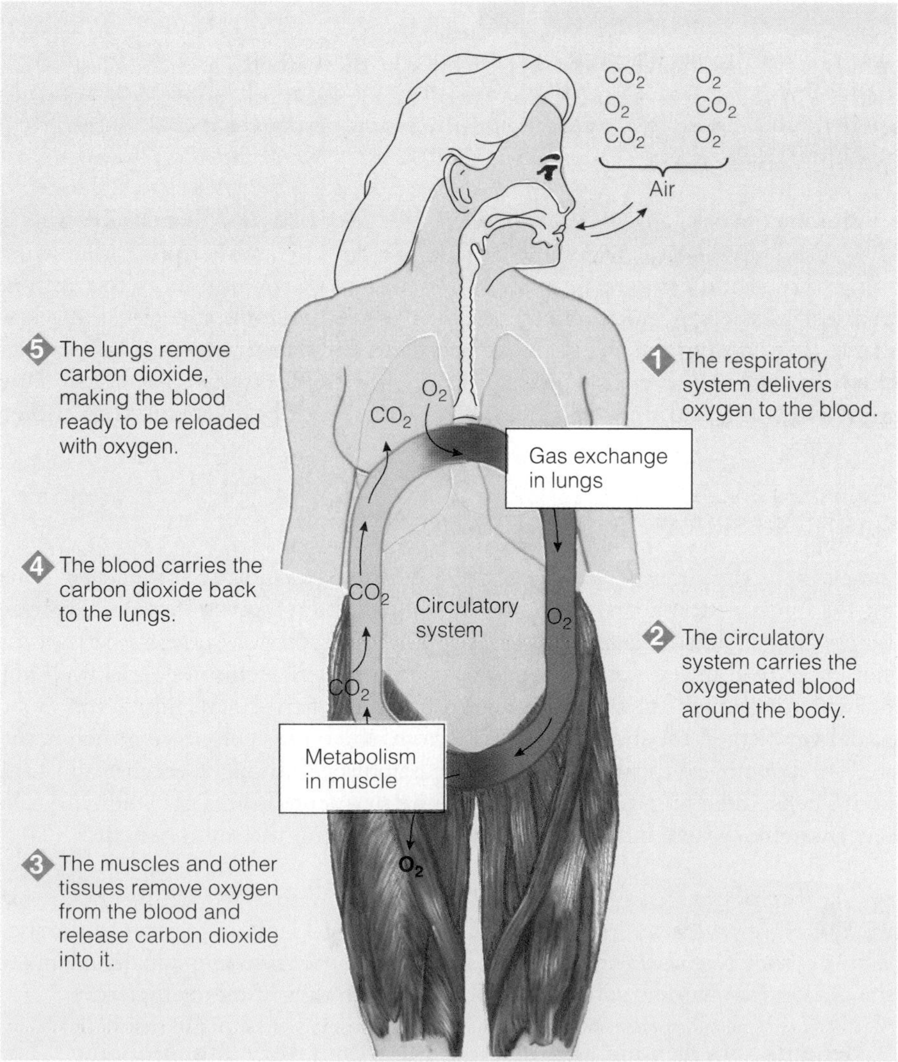

CO2 O2
O2 CO2
CO2 O2
Air
1 The respiratory system delivers oxygen to the blood.
Gas exchange in lungs
2 The circulatory system carries the oxygenated blood around the body.
Circulatory system
Metabolism in muscle
3 The muscles and other tissues remove oxygen from the blood and release carbon dioxide into it.
4 The blood carries the carbon dioxide back to the lungs.
5 The lungs remove carbon dioxide, making the blood ready to be reloaded with oxygen.
O2
CO2

To improve your cardiorespiratory endurance, you must train at an intensity that elevates your heart rate a certain percent above its resting rate. Although formulas based on maximal oxygen uptake (VO_2 max) or maximal heart rate are available, a person's own perceived effort is usually a reliable indicator of activity intensity. In general, when you're working out, do so at an intensity that raises your heart rate, but still leaves you able to talk comfortably. If you are more competitive and want to work to your limit on some days, a treadmill test can reveal your maximal heart rate. You can work out safely at up to 90 percent of that rate. The ACSM guidelines for developing and maintaining cardiorespiratory fitness were given in Table 14–1 on p. 510.[17]

VO_2 max: the maximum rate of oxygen consumption by an individual at sea level.

Benefits of Aerobic Training: Muscle Conditioning A fringe benefit of cardiorespiratory training is that fit muscles use oxygen more efficiently than less fit muscles, reducing the heart's workload. An added bonus is that muscles that can use more oxygen can burn fat longer—a plus for body composition and weight control.

Benefits of Anaerobic Training: Muscle Strength and Endurance In contrast to aerobic activity, anaerobic activity develops muscle strength and bulk, but generally does not bring about cardiorespiratory conditioning. Anaerobic activity involves short, all out exertions of muscles. Examples include sprinting, jumping a hurdle, doing push-ups, or lifting weights. In a balanced fitness program, aerobic activity improves cardiorespiratory fitness, stretching enhances flexibility, and weight training or calisthenics develops muscle strength and endurance. Table 14–2 provides an example of a balanced fitness program.

Table 14–2

A Sample Balanced Fitness Program (45 Minutes a Day)

Monday, Wednesday, Friday:
- 10 minutes of warm-up activity and stretching.
- 25 minutes of aerobic exercise.
- 10 minutes of cool-down activity.

Tuesday, Thursday:
- 10 minutes of warm-up activity and stretching.
- 25 minutes of weight training.
- 10 minutes of cool-down activity.

Saturday or Sunday:
- Softball, walking, hiking, biking, or swimming.

Physical activity, appropriately pursued, brings positive rewards: good health, long life, and freedom from disease. Pursued in excess, however, intensive physical activity combined with poor eating habits can undermine health, as the next section explains.

THE FEMALE ATHLETE TRIAD

Many young athletes severely restrict energy intakes to improve performance, to enhance the aesthetic appeal of their performance, or to meet the weight guidelines of their specific sports.[18] The increasing incidence of abnormal eating habits among athletes is causing concern, especially for women athletes.

Many women athletes appear healthy but are in fact at risk of developing a potentially fatal triad of medical problems: disordered eating, amenorrhea, and osteoporosis. These three associated disorders are called "the female athlete triad."[19] Male athletes and nonathletes of both sexes may be affected by these disorders as well, but research shows that female athletes, especially young ones, are most at risk.[20] Risk factors for this triad of disorders are listed in the margin.

Female athlete triad:
- Disordered eating.
- Amenorrhea.
- Osteoporosis.

Risk factors for the female athlete triad are:
- Young age (adolescence).
- Pressure to excel at a chosen sport.
- Focus on achieving or maintaining an "ideal" body weight or body fat percentage.
- Participation in endurance sports or competitions that judge performance on aesthetic appeal such as gymnastics, figure skating, or dance.

Eating Disorders in Athletes At the extreme, disordered eating includes both anorexia nervosa and bulimia nervosa (discussed in Highlight 9), but not all athletes with abnormal or pathological eating behaviors meet the official criteria for these disorders (provided in Tables H9–1 and H9–3 on pp. 337 and 339). Still, their eating behaviors are abnormal enough to incur the risk of developing the other two medical problems in the triad (see Figure 14–2).

Figure 14–2

The Female Athlete Triad

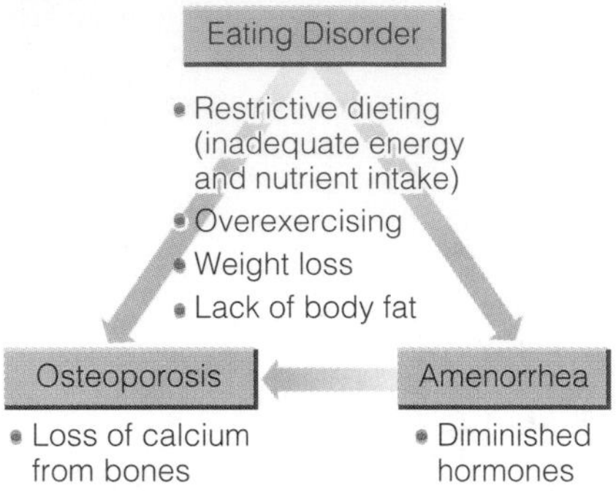

Some authorities have suggested that at least part of the reason many athletic women engage in self-destructive eating behaviors is because they and their coaches have adopted unsuitable weight standards. An athlete's body must be heavier than a nonathlete's body because the athlete's body is denser; it contains more healthy muscle and bone tissue and less fat than a nonathlete's body. Athletes consulting standard weight-for-height tables and seeing that they are on the heavy side for their heights can easily be misled into believing that they are too fat. Many problems are associated with the use of standard weight-for-height charts, as Chapter 8 explained, but they are particularly inappropriate for athletes. Body composition measures are better.

Researchers have identified some risk factors for eating disorders in young women athletes.[21] Dieting at an early age is one risk factor. Many young women begin dieting because their coaches recommend they lose weight. The women perceive weight loss to be a requirement for peak performance and are driven to lose as much weight as possible. Unsupervised dieting is another risk factor; the restrictive diets many athletes adopt fail to meet the high energy needs of physical training.

amenorrhea: the absence of or cessation of menstruation. *Primary amenorrhea* is menarche delayed beyond 16 years of age. *Secondary amenorrhea* is the absence of three to six consecutive menstrual cycles.

Amenorrhea The prevalence of amenorrhea among premenopausal women in the United States is about 2 to 5 percent overall, but among female athletes, it may be as high as 66 percent.[22] Contrary to previous notions, amenorrhea is *not* a normal adaptation to strenuous physical training: it is a symptom of something going wrong.[23] Amenorrhea is characterized by low blood estrogen, infertility, and often bone mineral losses. Amenorrheic athletes are more likely to suffer bone loss than other women.

stress fractures: bone damage or breaks caused by stress on bone surfaces during exercise.

Osteoporosis Osteoporosis, in which bone mass is reduced, increases susceptibility to stress fractures and bone breakage during physical activity. In general, weight-bearing physical activity, dietary calcium, and the hormone estrogen protect against bone loss (see Highlight 12), but in women with disordered eating and amenorrhea, strenuous activity may impair bone health. One study found that dancers with recent stress fractures had low body weights, had a high incidence of eating disorders, and ate diets low in fat and energy.[24] Vigorous training combined with low food energy intakes and other life stresses seems to trigger amenorrhea and promote bone loss. Low estrogen leads to diminished bone mass and increased bone fragility. Many amenorrheic athletes have bones like those of 50- to 60-year-old women when they should have dense, strong, bones. Amenorrheic athletes should be encouraged to consume at least 1500 milligrams of calcium each day and to modify activity so that they expend no more energy than they consume. Future research will focus on the question of hormone replacement therapy for these women.

To sum up, physical activity benefits a person's physical, psychological, and social well-being and improves resistance to disease. To develop fitness—whose components are flexibility, strength, muscle endurance, and cardiorespiratory endurance—a person must condition the body, through training, to adapt to the activity performed. Female athletes who overexercise and restrict their food intake risk developing a triad of problems: eating disorders, amenorrhea, and osteoporosis.

Energy Systems, Fuels, and Nutrients to Support Activity

Nutrition and physical activity go hand in hand. Activity demands carbohydrate and fat as fuel; protein to build and maintain lean tissues; vitamins and minerals to support both energy metabolism and tissue building; and water to help distribute the fuels and to dissipate the resulting heat and wastes. This section describes how nutrition supports a person who decides to get up and go.

THE ENERGY SYSTEMS OF PHYSICAL ACTIVITY—ATP AND PC

Muscles contract fast. When called upon, they respond quickly without taking time to metabolize fat or carbohydrate for energy. In the first fractions of a second, muscles starting to move depend on their supplies of quick-energy compounds to power their movements. Exercise physiologists know these compounds by their abbreviations, ATP and PC.

ATP As Chapter 7 described, all of the energy-yielding nutrients—glucose, fatty acids, and amino acids—can transfer energy to make the high-energy compound ATP (adenosine triphosphate). ATP is present in small amounts in all body tissues all the time, and it can deliver energy instantaneously. In the muscles, ATP provides the chemical driving force for contraction. When ATP is split, its energy is released, and the muscle cells channel some of that energy into mechanical movement and most of it into heat—heat the exerciser can feel building up. A tiny but essential pool of ATP is always ready to meet the cells' sudden demands for movement.

PC Unlike a single reflexive muscle jerk, prolonged activity involves sustained or repeated muscle contractions that require ongoing use of ATP. This creates a demand: more must be made.

Immediately after the onset of the demand, before muscle ATP pools dwindle, a muscle enzyme begins to break down another high-energy compound that is stored in the muscle, PC, or phosphocreatine. PC is made from creatine, a compound commonly found in muscles, with a phosphate group attached, and it can split (anaerobically) to release phosphate and replenish ATP supplies. Supplies of PC in a muscle last for only about 20 seconds, but can produce enough quick energy without oxygen for a 100-meter dash.

When activity ceases and the muscles are resting, ATP feeds energy back to PC by giving up one of its phosphate groups to creatine. Thus PC is produced during rest by reversing the process that occurs during muscular activity.

PC, phosphocreatine (also called **creatine phosphate**)**:** a high-energy compound in muscle cells that acts as a reservoir of energy that can maintain a steady supply of ATP; PC provides the energy for short bursts of activity.

During activity: PC → ATP + creatine.
During rest: ATP + creatine → PC.

The Energy-Yielding Nutrients To meet more prolonged demands, the muscles keep generating ATP from the more abundant fuels: glucose, fatty acids, and amino acids. The breakdown of these nutrients generates ATP all day every day, and so maintains the supply indefinitely.

During rest, the body derives slightly more than half of its ATP from fatty acids and most of the rest from carbohydrate, along with a small percentage from amino acids. During physical activity, the body adjusts its mixture of fuels. Muscles never use just one single fuel. How much of which fuels they use during

Fuel mixture during activity depends on:
- Diet.
- Intensity and duration of activity.
- Training.

physical activity depends on an interplay among the fuels available from the diet, the intensity and duration of the activity, and the degree to which the body is conditioned to perform that activity. The next sections explain these relationships by examining each of the energy-yielding nutrients individually, but keep in mind that fuel use is not an all-or-none process. One fuel may predominate at a given time, but the other two will still be active.

GLUCOSE USE DURING PHYSICAL ACTIVITY

Glucose, stored in the liver and muscles as glycogen, is vital to physical activity. During exertion, the liver releases its glucose into the bloodstream. The muscles use both this glucose and their own private glycogen stores to fuel their work. Glycogen supplies can easily support everyday activities, but are limited. The more glycogen the muscles store, the longer the stores will last during physical activity.

Diet Affects Glycogen Storage and Use The body constantly uses and replenishes its glycogen. How much carbohydrate a person eats influences how much glycogen is stored, which in turn influences how much will be used during activity. Thus dietary carbohydrate bears on performance because the more glycogen the muscles store, the longer the stores will last during activity. When glycogen is depleted, the muscles become fatigued.

A classic study compared fuel use during activity among three groups of runners on different diets. For several days before testing, one group consumed a normal mixed diet, a second group consumed a high-carbohydrate diet, and the third group consumed a no-carbohydrate diet. Figure 14–3 shows that the high-carbohydrate diet allowed the runners to keep going longer before exhaustion. This study and many others that followed have confirmed that high-carbohydrate diets enhance endurance by enlarging glycogen stores.[25]

Intensity of Activity Affects Glycogen Use How long an exercising person's glycogen will last depends not only on diet, but also on the intensity of the

Figure 14–3

The Effect of Diet on Physical Endurance

A high-carbohydrate diet can increase an athlete's endurance. In this study, the fat and protein diet provided 94 percent of kcalories from fat and 6 percent from protein; the normal mixed diet provided 55 percent of kcalories from carbohydrate; and the high-carbohydrate diet provided 83 percent of kcalories from carbohydrate.

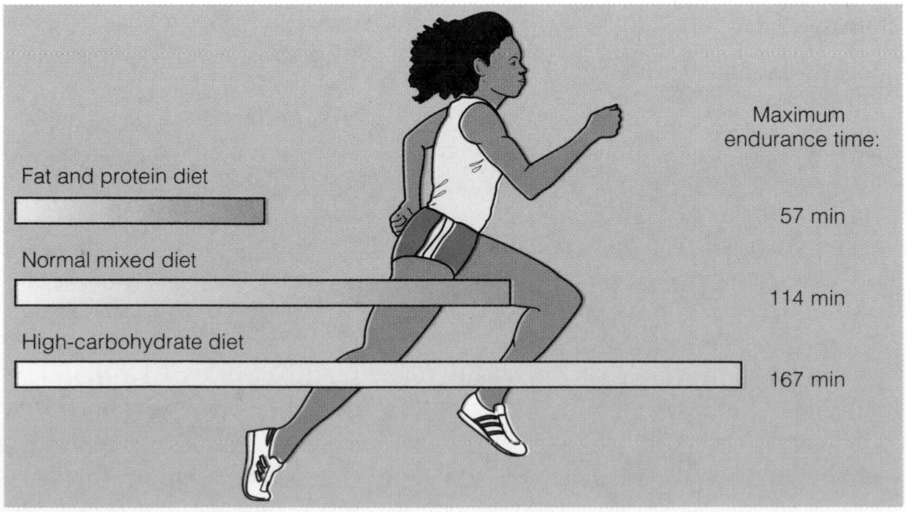
Maximum endurance time:
Fat and protein diet
57 min
Normal mixed diet
114 min
High-carbohydrate diet
167 min

Table 14–3

Fuels Used for Activities of Different Intensities and Durations

Activity Intensity	Activity Duration	Preferred Fuel Source	Oxygen Needed?	Activity Example
Extreme[a]	Less than 30 sec	ATP-PC (immediate availability)	No	100-yard dash, shot put
Very high	30 sec to 3 min	ATP from carbohydrate (lactic acid)	No (anaerobic)	¼-mile run at maximal speed
High	3 min to 20 min	ATP from carbohydrate	Yes (aerobic)	Cycling, swimming, or running
Moderate	More than 20 min	ATP from fat	Yes (aerobic)	Hiking

[a]All levels of exercise intensity use the ATP-PC system initially; extremely intense short-term exercises rely solely on the ATP-PC system.

activity. The most intense activities—the kind that make it difficult "to catch your breath," such as a quarter-mile run—use glycogen quickly. Other, less intense activities, such as jogging, during which breathing is steady and easy, use glycogen more slowly. Joggers still use glycogen, though, and if they jog long enough, they will eventually run out of it. Glycogen depletion usually occurs within two hours from the onset of intense activity.

The complete breakdown of glucose to carbon dioxide and water during intense activity depends on the availability of adequate oxygen. With ample oxygen, the breakdown of glucose need not stop at pyruvate, but can proceed to acetyl CoA and then on through the TCA cycle and electron transport chain. Figure 7–8 on p. 248 illustrates the breakdown of glucose when oxygen is available.

During *moderate* physical activity, the lungs and circulatory system have no trouble keeping up with the muscles' need for oxygen. The individual breathes easily, and the heart beats steadily—the activity is aerobic. The muscles derive their energy from both glucose and fatty acids. By depending partly on fatty acids, moderate aerobic activity conserves glycogen. Table 14–3 shows how fuel use changes according to the intensity of the activity.

Intense activity presents a different metabolic situation. Whenever a person exercises at a rate that exceeds the capacity of the heart and lungs to supply oxygen to the muscles, aerobic metabolism slows and cannot sufficiently meet energy needs. Instead, the muscles must draw more heavily on glucose, which they can use anaerobically, breaking it down to pyruvate and producing some energy (ATP) without requiring oxygen.

Lactic Acid When the rate of activity exceeds the ability to provide enough oxygen, the accumulating pyruvate molecules are converted to lactic acid in an anaerobic process (see the first part of Figure 14–4). Lactic acid can produce ATP during intense activity for only 1 to 3 minutes (as in a 400- to 800-meter race or a boxing match).

Reminder: *Lactic acid* is the anaerobic breakdown product of pyruvate. When energy production depends on anaerobic metabolism and lactic acid accumulates, exhaustion sets in and the exerciser cannot continue.

Lactic acid production increases with activity intensity. At low intensities, lactic acid is readily cleared from the blood, but at higher intensities, lactic acid accumulates. Just *prior to* the onset of lactic acid accumulation, exercisers may describe their activity as "somewhat hard"—an ideal degree of activity intensity. At that level a person is developing cardiorespiratory endurance. The person can

Figure 14–4

Incomplete Breakdown of Glucose during Anaerobic Metabolism

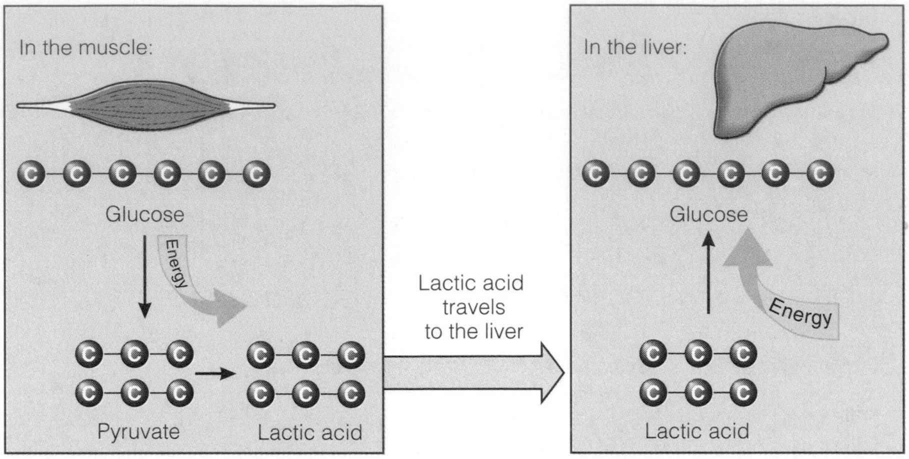

Without ample oxygen, working muscles break down most of their glucose molecules anaerobically to pyruvate, releasing a little energy. Pyruvate is then converted to lactic acid.

Liver enzymes can convert lactic acid to glucose, but this reaction requires a lot of energy.

Note: Lactic acid production serves the body's metabolic needs well during anaerobic times. When pyruvate is converted to lactic acid, an enzyme uses the niacin coenzyme NADH and produces NAD^+. NAD^+ can then be used to break down glucose to pyruvate, thus permitting glucose to continue producing energy anaerobically for a while.

---

think, converse, enjoy the activity and surroundings, and continue for a prolonged time.

Muscle cells cannot accommodate much lactic acid; they release it, and it travels in the blood to the liver. There, liver enzymes convert it back into glucose (as shown in the second part of Figure 14–4). Glucose can then return to the muscles to fuel additional activity. (This cycle, known as the Cori cycle, was first introduced in Chapter 7.)

Reminder: The recycling process that regenerates glucose from lactic acid is known as the *Cori cycle*.

Factors that influence glycogen use during physical activity:

- Amount of carbohydrate in the diet.
- Intensity and duration of the activity.
- Degree of training to perform the activity.

Duration of Activity Affects Glycogen Use Glycogen use depends not only on the intensity of an activity, but also on its duration. Within the first 20 minutes or so of moderate activity, a person uses mostly glycogen for fuel—about one-fifth of the available glycogen. As the muscles devour their own glycogen, they become ravenous for more glucose and increase their intake of blood glucose 20-fold or more. The person's blood glucose rises for a while—a signal that the liver is emptying out its glycogen stores for use by the exercising muscles. The muscles' accelerated uptake keeps blood glucose from rising too high, however, and it soon begins to decline.

After 20 minutes, a person who continues exercising moderately (mostly aerobically) begins to use less and less glycogen and more and more fat for fuel (review Table 14–3). Still, glycogen use continues, and if the activity lasts long enough and is intense enough, muscle and liver glycogen stores will be depleted. Physical activity can continue for a short time thereafter only because the liver scrambles to produce, from lactic acid and certain amino acids, the minimum amount of glucose needed to briefly forestall total depletion.

Glucose Depletion After a couple of hours of strenuous activity, glucose stores are depleted. When depletion hits, it brings nervous system function to a near halt, making continued exertion almost impossible. Marathon runners refer to this point of glucose exhaustion as "hitting the wall."

To avoid such debilitation, endurance athletes try to maintain their blood glucose for as long as they can. To maximize glucose supply, endurance athletes:

- Eat a high-carbohydrate diet (approximately 8 grams carbohydrate per kilogram body weight or about 70 percent of energy intake) regularly.*
- Take glucose (usually in diluted fruit juice or other sweet beverages) periodically during activity that lasts for an hour or more.
- Train the muscles to store as much glycogen as possible.

The last section of this chapter, "Diets for Physically Active People," discusses how to design a high-carbohydrate diet for performance, and the box on p. 524 describes how to maximize glycogen stores for long endurance competitions.

Glucose during Activity Muscles can obtain the carbohydrate they need, not only from glycogen stores but also from sugar taken during activity, which elevates blood glucose and enhances endurance. Normally, insulin stimulates all tissues of the body to drain glucose from the blood and stow it away—exactly the opposite of what is needed for performance. During physical activity, however, the body's release of the hormone epinephrine keeps insulin from rising in response to glucose entering the blood. Physical activity also enhances muscle sensitivity to insulin so that the muscles become the primary recipient of blood glucose. Consuming sugar is especially useful during exhausting endurance exercise (lasting more than an hour). Endurance athletes often run short of glucose by the end of competitive events, and they are wise to take light carbohydrate snacks or drinks (under 200 kcalories) periodically during activity.[26] During the last stages of an endurance competition, when glycogen is running low, glucose consumed during the event can make its way slowly from the digestive tract to the muscles and augment the body's supply of glucose enough to forestall exhaustion.

Reminder: *Epinephrine* is one of the stress hormones that is secreted whenever emergency action is called for; it readies body systems for fast action and mobilizes fuel to support that action.

Research indicates that eating high-carbohydrate food *after* physical activity also enlarges glycogen stores. A high-carbohydrate meal eaten within 15 minutes after physical activity accelerates the rate of glycogen storage by 300 percent. After two hours, the rate of glycogen storage declines by almost half. This is particularly important to athletes who train extensively more than once a day. A practical tip: after your next workout, enjoy a bagel or a glass of juice for your glycogen's sake.

Training Affects Glycogen Use Training, too, affects how much glycogen muscles will store. Muscle cells that repeatedly deplete their glycogen through hard work adapt to store greater amounts of glycogen to support that work.

To make glycogen, muscles need carbohydrate, but they also need rest, so vary daily exercise routines to work different muscles on different days.

---

*Percentage of energy intake is meaningful only when total energy intake is known. Consider that at high energy intakes (say, 5000 kcalories/day), even a moderate carbohydrate diet (40 percent of energy intake) supplies 500 grams of carbohydrate—enough for a 137-pound athlete in heavy training. By comparison, at a moderate energy intake (2000 kcalories/day), a high carbohydrate intake (70 percent of energy intake) supplies 350 grams—plenty of carbohydrate for most people, but not enough for athletes in heavy training.

How to Maximize Glycogen Stores: Carbohydrate Loading

When the facts about glycogen stores and endurance performance first became known, athletes naturally wanted to make sure they had plenty of glycogen. Some used a technique called carbohydrate loading to trick their muscles into storing extra glycogen before a competition. In the early days, athletes were taught to restrict carbohydrates and exercise heavily to empty their muscles of glycogen. About a week before the event, they cut back on exercise and then switched abruptly to an extremely high-carbohydrate diet a few days before the event. Muscle glycogen rebounded to as high as three to four times the normal amount.

Carbohydrate loading practiced this way can have side effects that outweigh any performance advantage, including abnormal heartbeat, hypoglycemia, ketosis, nausea, dizziness, and fatigue. Today athletes follow a safer plan. Ideally, the athlete in training eats a high-carbohydrate diet. During the first four days of the week before competition, the athlete trains moderately hard (1 to 2 hours per day) and eats a diet that is moderate in carbohydrate. During the 3 days before competition, the athlete gradually cuts back on activity and eats a very-high-carbohydrate diet. This "modified" plan for carbohydrate loading is as effective as the earlier plan and does not require severe carbohydrate restriction. Athletes manipulate activity levels and pack extra carbohydrate in at the end.

Extra glycogen gained this way can benefit an athlete who must keep going for 90 minutes or longer. Those who exercise for shorter times simply need a regular high-carbohydrate diet. In a hot climate, extra glycogen confers an additional advantage: as glycogen breaks down, it releases water, which helps to meet the athlete's fluid needs.

carbohydrate loading: a regimen of moderate exercise followed by consuming a high-carbohydrate diet that enables muscles to store glycogen beyond their normal capacity; also called glycogen loading or glycogen supercompensation.

Conditioned muscles also rely less on glycogen and more on fat for energy, so that glycogen breakdown occurs more slowly in trained than in untrained individuals at a given work intensity. A person attempting an activity for the first time uses much more glucose than an athlete who is trained to perform it. Oxygen delivery to the muscles by the heart and lungs plays a role in this effect, but equally importantly, trained muscles are better equipped to use the oxygen because their cells contain more mitochondria. Untrained muscles depend more heavily on anaerobic glucose breakdown, even when physical activity is just moderate.

Reminder: The *mitochondria* are the structures within a cell responsible for producing ATP aerobically (see Figure 7–3 on p. 242).

FAT USE DURING PHYSICAL ACTIVITY

An active person who eats a fat-rich diet with little carbohydrate will sacrifice athletic performance, as Figure 14–3 showed, and will needlessly degrade protein tissues as the body struggles to obtain the glucose it needs from amino acids. Furthermore, a high-fat diet is a major risk factor for cardiovascular disease. Since even physically active people can suffer heart attacks and strokes, every reliable source speaks out against high-fat diets for active people.

In contrast to *dietary* fat, *body* fat stores are of tremendous importance during physical activity, as long as the activity is not too intense. Unlike glycogen stores, fat stores can fuel hours of activity without running out.

The fat used in physical activity is liberated as fatty acids from the internal fat stores and from the fat under the skin. Areas that have the most fat to spare donate the greatest amounts of fatty acids to the blood (although they may not be the areas that appear most fatty). This is why "spot reducing" doesn't work—muscles do not own the fat that surrounds them. Fat cells release fatty acids into the blood, not into the underlying muscles. Then the blood gives to each muscle the amount of fat that it needs. Proof of this is found in a tennis player's arms—the fatfolds measure the same in both arms, even though the muscles of one arm work much harder and may be larger than those of the other. A balanced fitness program that includes strength training, however, will tighten muscles underneath the fat, improving the overall appearance. Keep in mind that some body fat is essential to good health.

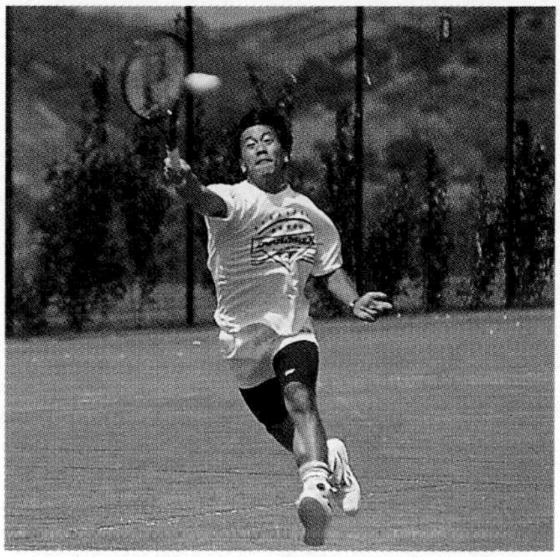

Abundant energy from the breakdown of fat can come only from aerobic metabolism.

Duration of Activity Affects Fat Use Early in an activity, as the muscles draw on fatty acids, blood levels fall. If the activity continues for more than a few minutes, the hormone epinephrine is released, and in response, the fat cells begin rapidly breaking down their stored triglycerides and liberating fatty acids into the blood. After about 20 minutes of physical activity, the blood fatty acid concentration surpasses the normal resting concentration. Thereafter, sustained, moderate activity uses body fat stores as its major fuel.

Intensity of Activity Affects Fat Use The intensity of physical activity also affects fat use. In general, as the intensity increases, fat makes less and less of a contribution to the mix of fuels used. Remember that fat can be broken down for energy in only one way—by aerobic metabolism. In fact, the use of fatty acids for energy requires more oxygen, even on a per-kcalorie basis, than does the use of glucose. This is because fatty acid oxidation generates so many acetyl CoA molecules that enter the TCA cycle, and because each turn of the cycle generates so many hydrogens that travel through the electron transport chain to oxygen. For fat to fuel activity, then, oxygen must be abundantly available. If a person is breathing easily during activity, the muscles are getting all the oxygen they need and are able to use more fat in the fuel mixture.

Training Affects Fat Use It is training—repeated aerobic activity—that produces the adaptations that permit the body to draw heavily on fat for fuel. Training stimulates the muscle cells to manufacture more and larger mitochondria, the cellular structures that conduct aerobic metabolism. Another adaptation: the heart and lungs become stronger and better able to deliver oxygen to muscles at high activity intensities. Still another: hormones in the body of a trained person slow glucose release from the liver and speed up fat use instead. These adaptations reward not only trained athletes but all active people: a person who exercises aerobically becomes well suited to the task.

Factors that influence fat use during physical activity:

- Amount of fat in the diet.
- Intensity and duration of the activity.
- Degree of training to perform the activity.

The first section of this chapter recommended aerobic activity to develop cardiorespiratory endurance. Just 20 minutes or more of aerobic activity, three or more times each week, stimulates even the untrained body to adapt by packing its cells with more fat-metabolizing enzymes and by improving the ability of the heart and lungs to deliver oxygen.

Recommended Intensities and Durations Health care professionals frequently advise people who want to control their body weight and lose fat to engage in activities of low-to-moderate intensity for a long duration, such as an hour-long fast-paced walk. The reasoning behind such advice is that people exercising at low-to-moderate intensity are likely to stick with their exercise pro-

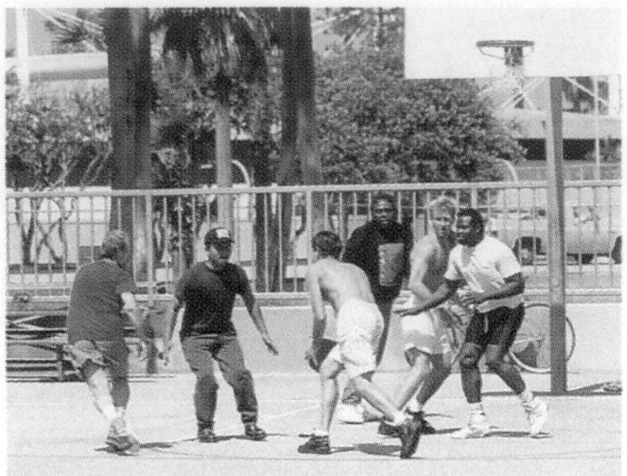

The key to regular physical activity is finding an activity that you enjoy.

grams for longer times and are less likely to injure themselves. In addition, some research suggests that the longer the duration of activity, the greater the contribution fat will make to the fuel mixture, and consequently, the more body fat will be lost—but this is controversial.[27] Some research refutes the notion that a person "burns more fat during low-intensity exercise" and suggests that weight-loss benefits are the same from either low- or high-intensity activity.[28] Regardless of the contribution fat makes to the fuel mix, people who engage in regular, vigorous physical activities have less body fat than those who engage in moderately intense activities.[29] Fat use may continue at an accelerated rate for some time after vigorous physical activity has ceased. The conditioned body that is adapted to strenuous and prolonged aerobic activity uses more fat all day long, not just during activity.[30] The bottom line on physical activity and weight and/or fat loss seems to be that total energy expenditure is the main factor, regardless of how you do it.

The intensity and type of physical activities that are best for one person may not be good for another. The intensity to choose depends on your present fitness: work so as to breathe fast, but not so fast as to incur an oxygen debt. A rule of thumb is that you should be breathing easily enough to talk but not sing. If you can sing, pick up the pace; if you have to huff and puff to talk, slow down. If you have been sedentary for the past few years, the activity intensity that will initially make you breathe slightly fast will differ dramatically from the intensity at which a fit person will breathe slightly fast.

The type of physical activity that is best for you depends, too, on what you want to achieve and what you enjoy doing. If you are looking for health benefits, such as reducing your disease risks and lowering your blood cholesterol, then you might want to spend at least 30 minutes each day doing some kind of physical activity. If you are looking to lose weight and improve body composition, then choose an activity that you can sustain for 45 minutes or more at least 3 days a week. Choose an activity you enjoy: some people love walking, others prefer to dance or ride a bike. If you want to be stronger and firmer, lift weights or do calisthenics. And remember, muscle is more metabolically active than body fat, so the more muscle you have, the more energy you'll burn.

Table 14–3 summarized the fuel uses discussed so far, but did not include the third energy-yielding nutrient, protein, because protein is not a major fuel for exercise. Protein does provide some energy, however, and more importantly, it provides the structural material of muscle tissue, so it is important to active people.

PROTEIN USE DURING PHYSICAL ACTIVITY—AND BETWEEN TIMES

If a high-fat diet is ill-advised for active people, what about a high-protein diet? Athletes may have slightly higher needs for protein than others do, but given the margin of safety used in establishing the RDA, no added allowance is made for work or physical training. The protein needs of most people, including athletes, are covered by a balanced diet of ordinary foods.

How do physical activity and training effect protein metabolism? Physically active people use protein just as other people do—to build muscle and other lean tissue structures and, to some extent, to fuel activity. The body does, however, handle protein differently during activity than during rest.

Protein Used in Muscle Building Synthesis of body proteins is suppressed during activity and for several hours afterward. In the hours following this period, though, protein synthesis accelerates beyond normal resting levels. Remember that the body adapts and builds the molecules, cells, and tissues it needs for the next period of activity. Whenever the body remodels a part of itself, it also tears down old structures to make way for new ones. Repeated activity, with just a slight overload, triggers the protein-dismantling and protein-synthesizing equipment of each muscle cell to make needed changes—that is, to adapt.

The physical work of each muscle cell acts as a signal to its DNA and RNA to begin producing the kinds of proteins that will best support that work. Take jogging, for example. In the first difficult sessions, the body is not yet equipped to perform aerobic work easily, but with each session, the cells' genetic material gets the message that an overhaul is needed. In the hours that follow the session, the genes send molecular messages to the protein-building equipment that tell it what old structures to break down and what new structures to build, and within the limits of its genetic potential, it responds. Among the new structures are more mitochondria to facilitate efficient aerobic metabolism. Over a few weeks' time, remodeling occurs and jogging becomes easier.

Such remodeling requires protein. During active muscle-building phases of training, an athlete may add between ¼ ounce and 1 ounce (between 7 and 28 grams) of body protein to existing muscle mass each day. This increase occurs only during periods of *building*—not times of maintenance—when the athlete exercises at high intensities.

Protein Used as Fuel Not only do athletes retain more protein in their muscles, they also use more protein as fuel: muscles speed up their use of amino acids for energy during physical activity, just as they speed up their use of fat and carbohydrate.[31] Still, protein contributes at most about 10 percent of the total fuel used, both during activity and during rest. The most active people of all, endurance athletes, use up enormous amounts of all energy fuels, including protein, during performance, but such athletes also eat more food and therefore usually consume enough protein.

Diet Affects Protein Use during Activity The factors that affect how much protein is used during activity seem to be the same three that influence the use of fat and carbohydrate—for one, diet. People who consume diets adequate in energy and rich in *carbohydrate* use less protein than those who eat protein- and fat-rich diets. Recall that carbohydrates spare proteins from being broken down to make glucose when needed. Since physical activity requires glucose, a diet lacking in carbohydrate necessitates the conversion of amino acids to glucose. So does a diet high in fat, because fatty acids can never provide glucose.

Factors that influence protein use during physical activity:

- Amount of energy and *carbohydrate* in the diet.
- Intensity and duration of the activity.
- Degree of training to perform the activity.

Intensity and Duration of Activity Affect Protein Use during Activity A second factor, the intensity and duration of activity, also modifies protein use.[32] Endurance athletes who train for over an hour a day, engaging in aerobic activity of moderate intensity and long duration, may deplete their glycogen stores by the end of their workouts and become somewhat more dependent on body protein for energy. The protein needs of bodybuilders and weight lifters are slightly higher than those of sedentary people, but not as high as some recommendations and certainly not as high as the protein intakes many bodybuilders consume.

Training Affects Protein Use A third factor that influences a person's use of protein during physical activity is the extent of training. Predictably, the higher the degree of training, the less protein a person uses during an activity.

Protein Recommendations for Active People As mentioned earlier, all active people, and especially those who work like athletes, probably need a little more protein than do sedentary people. Endurance athletes use more protein for fuel than power athletes do, and they retain some, especially in the muscles used for their sport. Power athletes use less protein for fuel but still use some, and retain much more. Therefore, *all* athletes in training should attend to protein needs, but should back up the protein with ample carbohydrate. Otherwise, they will burn off as fuel the very protein that they wish to retain in muscle.

How much protein, then, should an active person consume? A joint position paper from the American Dietetic Association (ADA) and the Canadian Dietetic Association (CDA) recommends 1.0 to 1.5 grams of protein per kilogram of body weight each day, an amount somewhat higher than the amount recommended for the general population.[33] Another authority suggests different protein intakes for athletes pursuing different activities.[34] Table 14–4 lists some recommendations and translates them into daily intakes for active people. Athletes who want to build muscle mass should first meet their energy needs with adequate carbohydrate intakes and then check that they have met protein needs as well. A later section translates protein recommendations into a diet plan and shows that no one needs protein supplements, or even large servings of meat, to obtain the highest recommended protein intakes.

Chapter 6 concluded that most people receive more than enough protein without supplements and reviewed the potential dangers of using protein and amino acid supplements.

Table 14–4

Recommended Protein Intakes for Athletes

	Recommendations (g/kg/day)	Protein Intakes (g/day)	
		MALES	FEMALES
RDA for adults	0.8	56	44
ADA/CDA recommended intake	1.0–1.5	70–105	55–83
Recommended intake for power (strength-speed) athletes	1.2–1.7	84–119	66–94
Recommended intake for endurance athletes	1.2–1.4	84–98	66–77
U.S. average intake		95	65

Note: Daily protein intakes are based on a 70-kilogram (154-pound) man and 55-kilogram (121-pound) woman.

Source: Committee on Dietary Allowances, *Recommended Dietary Allowances*, 10th ed. (Washington, D.C.: National Academy Press, 1989); Position of The American Dietetic Association and The Canadian Dietetic Association: Nutrition for physical fitness and athletic performance for adults, *Journal of the American Dietetic Association* 93 (1993): 691–695; P. W. R. Lemon, Effect of exercise on protein requirements, in *Foods, Nutrition, and Sports Performances: An International Scientific Consensus*, eds. C. Williams and J. T. Devlin (London: E & FN Spon, 1992), pp. 65–86.

VITAMINS AND MINERALS TO SUPPORT ACTIVITY

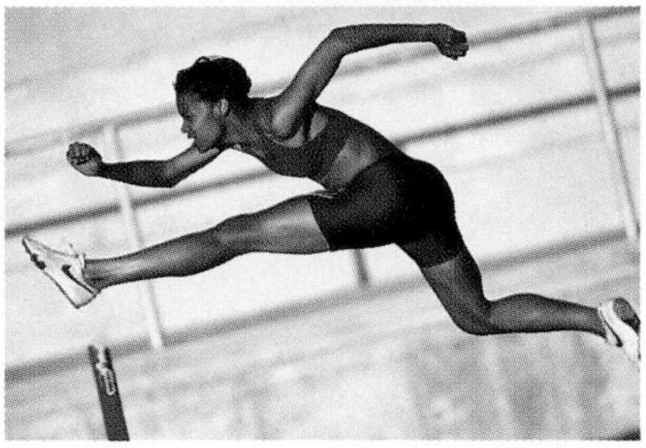

For perfect functioning, every nutrient is needed.

Many of the vitamins and minerals assist in releasing energy from fuels and in transporting oxygen. This knowledge has led many people to believe, mistakenly, that vitamin and mineral *supplements* offer physically active people both health benefits and athletic advantages. (Highlight 10 focuses on vitamin and mineral supplements, and Highlight 14 explores the many other tricks athletes use in the hope of enhancing performance.)

Supplements Research confirms that nutrient supplements do not enhance the performance of well-nourished people.[35] Studies do consistently find, though, that deficiencies of vitamins and minerals impede performance. In general, active people who eat enough nutrient-dense foods to meet energy needs also meet their vitamin and mineral needs. After all, active people eat more food; it stands to reason that with the right choices, they'll get more nutrients.

Some athletes mistakenly believe that taking vitamin or mineral supplements directly before competition will enhance performance. These beliefs are contrary to scientific reality. Most vitamins and minerals function as small parts of larger working units. After entering the blood, they have to wait for the tissues to combine them with their appropriate other parts so that they can do their work. This takes time—hours or days. Vitamins or minerals taken right before an event are useless for improving performance, even if the person actually is suffering deficiencies of them.

In general, then, active people need no vitamins or minerals in supplement form. Iron may be an exception to this rule, however, as a later section explains.

Vitamin E The antioxidant function of vitamin E deserves special mention here. Evidence for a relationship between physical activity and oxidative stress is accumulating rapidly.[36] Cells are equipped with many mechanisms, such as the antioxidant vitamins C and E, to defend against damage by free radicals, but in some situations, these defenses can be overwhelmed. Prolonged, high-intensity activity enhances production of damaging free radicals in the body. The consequences may be as minor as temporary inflammation or as extensive as damage to DNA.[37] In hopes of preventing oxidative damage to muscles, many athletes and active people are taking megadoses of vitamin E, even though studies examining vitamin E supplementation are lacking. One study showed that 300 milligrams of vitamin E daily reduced exercise-induced oxidative damage in cyclists.[38] Clearly, more research is needed, but in the meantime, active people can benefit by eating generous servings of antioxidant-rich fruits and vegetables.

Iron Physically active young women, especially those who engage in endurance activities such as distance running, are prone to iron deficiency. Physical activity can affect iron status in several ways. For one thing, iron losses in sweat can contribute to iron deficiency, even though the sweat of trained athletes contains less iron than the sweat of others (another adaptation of conditioning). For another, red blood cell destruction can lead to iron loss; blood cells are squashed when body tissues (such as the soles of the feet) make high-impact contact with an unyielding surface (such as the ground). Perhaps more significant than these losses are deficits caused by poor iron absorption in some athletes and the high demands of muscles for the iron-containing molecules of the mitochondria and the muscle protein, myoglobin. In addition, physical activity may cause small blood losses through the digestive tract, at least in some athletes.

Iron Deficiency Iron deficiency affects more young women than men, and physically active people are no exception. Habitually low intakes of iron-rich foods and high iron losses through menstruation, as well as through the other routes mentioned, cause iron deficiency in physically active young women. Even short-term moderate aerobic activity has been shown to compromise women's iron status.[39]

Iron-Deficiency Anemia Evidence is equivocal as to whether marginal iron deficiency impairs physical performance. Iron-deficiency anemia, however, clearly does dramatically impair physical performance because the hemoglobin in the red blood cells is indispensable for delivering oxygen for the energy processes that use it. Without adequate oxygen, an active person cannot use fat for fuel, cannot perform aerobic activities, and tires easily.

sports anemia: a transient condition of low hemoglobin in the blood, associated with the early stages of sports training or other strenuous activity.

Sports Anemia Early in training, athletes may develop low blood hemoglobin for a while. This condition, sometimes called "sports anemia," is not a true iron-deficiency condition. Strenuous aerobic activity promotes destruction of the more fragile, older red blood cells, and the resulting cleanup work reduces the blood's iron content temporarily. Strenuous activity also expands the blood's plasma volume, thereby reducing the red blood cell count per unit of blood, but the red blood cells do not diminish in size or number as in anemia, so oxygen-carrying capacity is not hindered. Most researchers view sports anemia as an *adaptive*, temporary response to endurance training. The increase in plasma volume may even help in training: it dilutes the blood and augments the amount of blood leaving the heart per minute. Iron-deficiency anemia requires iron supplementation, but sports anemia does not respond to it.

Iron Recommendations for Athletes The best strategy concerning iron depends on the individual. Many menstruating women probably border on iron deficiency even without the iron losses incurred by physical activity. Active teens of both sexes also have high iron needs because they are growing. Especially for women and teens, then, prescribed supplements may be needed to correct deficiencies of iron, but medical testing should guide decisions on supplementation. Chapter 13 provides many more details about iron and the tests used in assessing its status.

FLUIDS AND ELECTROLYTES TO SUPPORT ACTIVITY

The body relies on watery fluids as the medium for all of its life-supporting chemistry. Its need for water far surpasses its need for any other nutrient. If the body loses too much water, its chemistry becomes compromised.

Obviously, the body loses water via sweat. Breathing costs water, too, exhaled as vapor. During physical activity, both routes are significant, and dehydration becomes a threat. Dehydration's first symptom is fatigue: a water loss of even 1 to 2 percent of body weight can reduce a person's capacity to do muscular work. With a water loss of about 7 percent, a person is likely to collapse.[40]

Fluid Losses via Sweat Recall that working muscles produce heat as a by-product of ATP breakdown. The body cools itself by sweating. Each liter of sweat dissipates almost 600 kcalories of heat, preventing a rise in body temperature of almost 10°C. The body routes its blood supply through the capillaries just under the skin, and the skin secretes sweat to evaporate and cool the skin and the underlying blood. The blood then flows back to cool the deeper body chambers.

Hyperthermia In hot, humid weather, sweat doesn't evaporate well because the surrounding air is already laden with water. Body heat builds up and triggers maximum sweating, but without sweat evaporation, little cooling takes place. In such conditions, active people must take precautions to prevent heat stroke. The only way to prevent heat stroke is to drink enough fluid before and during the activity, rest in the shade when tired, and wear lightweight clothing that allows evaporation. (Hence the danger of rubber or heavy suits that supposedly promote weight loss during physical activity—they promote profuse sweating, prevent sweat evaporation, and invite heat stroke.) If you ever experience any of the symptoms of heat stroke listed in the margin, stop your activity, sip fluids, seek shade, and ask for help. Heat stroke can be fatal, young people often die of it, and these symptoms demand attention.

hyperthermia: an above-normal body temperature.

heat stroke: the dangerous accumulation of body heat with accompanying loss of body fluid.

Symptoms of heat stroke:
- Headache.
- Nausea.
- Dizziness.
- Clumsiness.
- Stumbling.
- Excessive or insufficient sweating.
- Confusion or other mental changes.

Hypothermia In cold weather, *hypothermia*, or low body temperature, can pose as serious a threat as heat stroke. Inexperienced, slow runners participating in long races on cold or wet, chilly days are especially vulnerable to hypothermia. Slow runners who produce little heat can become too cooled if clothing is inadequate. Early symptoms of hypothermia include shivering and euphoria. As body temperature continues to fall, shivering may stop, and weakness, disorientation, and apathy may occur. Each of these symptoms can impair a person's ability to act against a further drop in body temperature. Even in cold weather, however, the active body still sweats and still needs fluids. The fluids should be warm or at room temperature to help protect against hypothermia.

hypothermia: a below-normal body temperature.

Fluid Replacement via Hydration Endurance athletes can easily lose 1.5 liters or more of fluid during *each hour* of activity. To prepare for fluid losses, a person must hydrate before activity. To replace fluid losses, the person must rehydrate during and after activity. (Table 14–5 presents one schedule of hydration

Table 14–5

Hydration Schedule for Physical Activity

When to Drink	Approximate Amount of Fluid
2 hr before exercise	3 c
10 to 15 min before exercise	2 c
Every 15 min during exercise	1 c
After exercise	2 c

Source: D. C. Nieman, *Fitness and Sports Medicine: An Introduction* (Palo Alto, Calif.: Bull Publishing, 1990), p. 234.

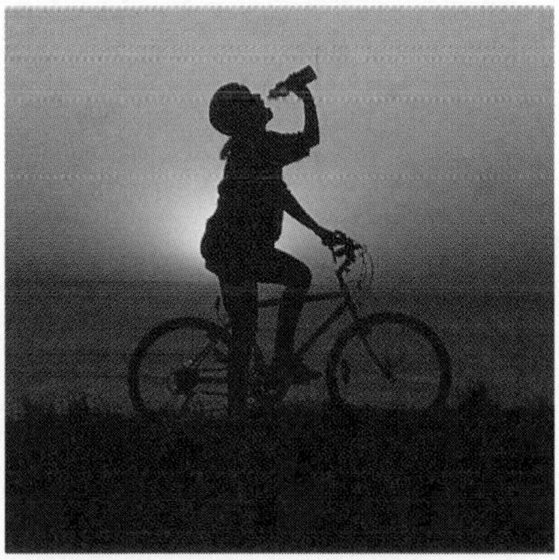

To prevent dehydration and the fatigue that accompanies it, drink plenty of liquids before, during, and after physical activity.

Water recommendation: 1.0 to 1.5 mL/kcal expended.
Note: 1 mL = 0.03 fluid oz.
Easy estimation: ≈ ½ c/100 kcal.

for physical activity.) Even then, in hot weather, the GI tract may not be able to absorb enough water fast enough to keep up with sweat losses, and some degree of dehydration may be inevitable.

Athletes who are preparing for competition are often advised to drink extra fluids in the *days* immediately beforehand, especially if they are still training. The extra water is not stored in the body, but drinking extra water ensures maximum hydration at the start of the event.

Some coaches and athletes withhold water during practice because they mistakenly believe the body adapts to use less water and that this will somehow be beneficial. This false and dangerous idea has cost some athletes their health, and some their lives. Full hydration is imperative for every athlete both in training and in competition. The athlete who arrives at an event even slightly dehydrated arrives with a disadvantage. Drinking extra water does no harm and may be protective.

What is the best fluid for an exercising body? For noncompetitive, everyday active people, plain, cool water is recommended, especially in warm weather, for two reasons: it rapidly leaves the digestive tract to enter the tissues where it is needed, and it cools the body from the inside out. For endurance athletes, other beverages may be appropriate. Fluid ingestion during the event has the dual purposes of replenishing water lost through sweating and providing a source of carbohydrate to supplement the body's limited glycogen stores. Carbohydrate depletion brings on fatigue in the athlete, but as already mentioned, fluid loss and the accompanying buildup of body heat can be life-threatening. Thus the first priority for endurance athletes should be to replace fluids.[41] Many good-tasting drinks are marketed for active people; the accompanying box compares them with water.

Electrolyte Losses and Replacement When a person sweats, small amounts of electrolytes—the electrically charged minerals sodium, potassium, chloride, and magnesium—are lost from the body along with water. Losses are greatest in beginners; training improves electrolyte retention.

To replenish lost electrolytes, a person ordinarily needs only to eat a regular diet that meets energy and nutrient needs. In extremely demanding endurance events lasting more than 3 hours, electrolyte replacements may be needed.[42] Electrolyte or salt tablets always cause water to flow out of the tissues into the GI tract; they also increase potassium losses, irritate the stomach, and cause vomiting. Thus these tablets can worsen dehydration and impair performance in several ways.

POOR BEVERAGE CHOICES: CAFFEINE AND ALCOHOL

Athletes, like others, sometimes drink beverages that contain caffeine or alcohol. Each of these substances can influence physical performance.

Caffeine Caffeine is a stimulant, and athletes sometimes use it to enhance performance as Highlight 14 explains. Caffeine is also a diuretic that induces fluid losses. It can be particularly hazardous when people competing in hot environments drink caffeine-containing beverages in place of other beverages.

Alcohol Some athletes mistakenly believe that they can replace fluids and load up on carbohydrates by drinking beer. A 12-ounce beer provides 16 grams

How to Evaluate Sports Drinks

Hydration is critical to optimal performance. Water best meets the fluid needs of most people, yet manufacturers market many good-tasting sports drinks for active people. More than 20 "power beverages" compete for their share of the $1 billion market. What do sports drinks have to offer?

- *Fluid.* Sports drinks offer fluids to help offset the loss of fluids during exercise, but plain water can do this, too. Alternatively, fruit juices can be diluted (by one-half to one-third), if preferred to plain water.
- *Glucose.* Sports drinks offer simple sugars or glucose polymers that help maintain hydration and blood glucose and enhance performance as effectively as, or maybe even better than, water.[a] Such measures are beneficial only for strenuous endurance activities lasting longer than an hour. Most sports drinks contain about 7 percent glucose (about half the sugar of ordinary soft drinks, or about 5 teapoons in each 12 ounces). Less than 6 percent may not enhance performance, and more than 10 percent may cause abdominal cramps, nausea, and diarrhea. Fluid transport to the tissues from beverages containing up to 10 percent glucose is rapid.[b]

  While glucose does enhance endurance performance in grueling competitive events, it is of no value to the moderate exerciser and is counterproductive if weight loss is the goal. Glucose is sugar, and like candy, it provides only empty kcalories—no vitamins or minerals. Most sports drinks provide between 50 and 100 kcalories per cup.
- *Sodium and other electrolytes.* Sports drinks offer sodium and other electrolytes to help replace those lost in exercise. Sodium in sports drinks also helps to increase the rate of fluid absorption from the GI tract and maintain plasma volume during exercise and recovery.

  Most physically active people do not need to replace the minerals lost in sweat immediately; a meal eaten within hours of competition replaces these minerals soon enough. Most sports drinks are relatively low in sodium, however, so those who choose to use these beverages run little risk of excessive intake.

  In strenuous, world-class competitions lasting 6 hours or more, heavy sweating coupled with consumption of large amounts of plain water dangerously dilutes blood sodium. In these few cases, intravenous fluid and electrolyte repletion is needed.[c]
- *Good taste.* Manufacturers reason that if a drink tastes good, people will drink more, thereby ensuring adequate hydration. For athletes who prefer the flavors of sports drinks over water, it may be worth paying for good taste to replace lost fluids.
- *Psychological edge.* Sports drinks provide a psychological edge for some people who associate the drinks with athletes and sports. The need to belong is valid. If the drinks boost morale and are used with care, they may do no harm.

For trained endurance athletes who exercise for an hour or more, sports drinks may provide a slight advantage over water. For most physically active people, though, water is the best fluid to replenish lost fluids. The most important thing to do is drink—even if you don't feel thirsty.

glucose polymers: compounds that supply glucose, not as single molecules, but linked in chains somewhat like starch. The objective is to attract less water from the body into the digestive tract (osmotic attraction depends on the number, not the size of particles).

[a] D. C. Nieman, *Fitness and Sports Medicine: An Introduction* (Palo Alto, Calif.: Bull Publishing, 1990), p. 239.
[b] J. M. Davis and coauthors, Fluid availability of sports drinks differing in carbohydrate type and concentration, *American Journal of Clinical Nutrition* 51 (1990): 1054–1057.
[c] N. Clark, J. Tobin, and C. Ellis, Feeding the ultraendurance athlete: Practical tips and a case study, *Journal of the American Dietetic Association* 92 (1992): 1258–1262.

Beer facts:

- *Beer is not carbohydrate-rich*. (Beer is *kcalorie*-rich, but only ⅓ of its kcalories are from carbohydrates. The other ⅔ are from alcohol.)
- *Beer is mineral-poor.* (Beer contains a few minerals, but to replace those lost in sweat, athletes need good sources such as fruit juices.)
- *Beer is vitamin-poor.* (Beer contains tiny traces of some B vitamins, but it cannot compete with rich food sources.)
- *Beer causes fluid losses*. (Beer is a fluid, but alcohol is a diuretic and causes the body to lose more fluid in urine than is provided by the beer.)

of carbohydrate—one-third the amount of carbohydrate in a glass of orange juice the same size. In addition to carbohydrate, beer also contains alcohol, of course. Energy from alcohol breakdown generates heat, but does not fuel muscle work because alcohol is metabolized in the liver.

It is hard to overstate alcohol's detrimental effects on physical activity. Alcohol's diuretic effect impairs the body's fluid balance, making dehydration likely; after exercise, a person needs to replace fluids, not lose them by drinking beer. Alcohol impairs the body's ability to regulate its temperature, making hypothermia or heat stroke much more likely.

Alcohol also alters perceptions; slows reaction time; reduces strength, power, and endurance; and hinders accuracy, balance, eye-hand coordination, and coordination in general—all opposing optimal athletic performance. In addition, it deprives people of their judgment, thereby comprising their safety in sports: many sports-related fatalities and injuries involve alcohol or other drugs.

Clearly, alcohol impairs performance, but physically active people do drink on occasion. A word of caution: do not drink alcohol before exercising and drink plenty of water after exercising before drinking alcohol.

The mixture of fuels the body uses during physical activity depends on diet, the intensity and duration of the activity, and training. During intense activity, the muscles use glucose primarily; during less intense, moderate activity fat makes a greater energy contribution and glycogen use is slower. With the possible exception of iron, well-nourished active people do not need nutrient supplements. Active people do need to drink plenty of water, especially during training or competition.

Diets for Physically Active People

No one diet supports physical performance. Active people who choose foods within the framework of the diet-planning principles presented in Chapter 2 can design many excellent diets.

CHOOSING A DIET TO SUPPORT FITNESS

First, remember that water is depleted more rapidly than any other nutrient. A diet to support fitness must provide water, energy, and all the other nutrients.

Water Even casual exercisers must attend conscientiously to their fluid needs. Physical activity blunts the thirst mechanism, especially in cold weather. During activity, thirst signals come too late, so don't wait to feel thirsty before drinking. To find out how much water is needed to replenish exercise losses, weigh yourself before and after the activity—the difference is almost all water. One pound equals roughly 2 cups (500 milliliters) fluid.

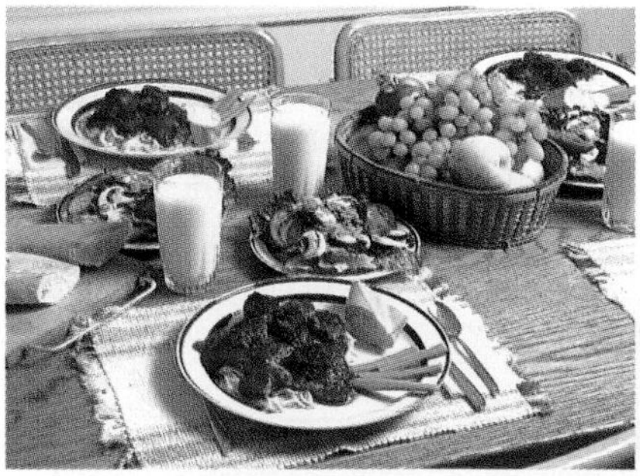

A variety of foods is the best source of nutrients for athletes.

Nutrient Density A healthful diet is based on nutrient-dense foods—foods that provide an adequate supply of vitamins and minerals for the energy they provide. Active people need to eat both for nutrient adequacy and for energy. They are not immune to heart disease and cancer and so must limit fats. A diet that is high in carbohydrate (60 percent of total kcalories or more), low in fat (25 percent or less), and adequate in protein (12 to 15 percent) ensures full glycogen and other nutrient stores.

Carbohydrate On two occasions, the active person's regular high-carbohydrate, fiber-rich diet may require temporary adjustment. Both of these exceptions involve training for competition rather than fitness. During intensive training, energy needs are high—so high that they may outstrip the person's capacity to eat enough food to meet them. At that point, added sugar and fat may be needed. The person can add concentrated carbohydrate foods such as dried fruits, sweet potatoes, nectars, and even high-fat foods such as avocados, nuts, cookies, and ice cream. Still, a nutrient-rich diet remains central for adequacy's sake. While vital, energy alone is not enough to support performance. The other special occasion is the pregame meal, when fiber-rich, bulky foods are best avoided. The pregame meal is discussed in a later section.

Carbohydrate recommendation for athletes in heavy training: 8 g/kg body weight.

Protein In addition to carbohydrate and some fat (and the energy they provide), physically active people need protein. How much of what kinds of foods supply enough protein to meet their needs? Meats and milk products are rich protein sources, but to recommend that active people emphasize these foods would be narrow advice for many reasons. For one thing, all people must protect themselves from heart disease, and even lean meats and low-fat milk products contain fat, much of it saturated fat. For another, as emphasized repeatedly, active people need diets high in carbohydrate, and of course, meats have none to offer. Legumes, grains, and vegetables provide protein with abundant carbohydrate and little fat. Table 14–4 showed some possible protein intakes for active people.

A Performance Diet Example It is likely that a person weighing 70 kilograms who engaged in vigorous physical activity on a daily basis could require more than 3000 kcalories per day. To meet this need, the person could choose a variety of nutrient-dense foods. Figure 14–5 (on p. 536) provides one example; it shows the Monday's meal selections pictured in Highlight 13 on p. 506 with enough additions to attain a 3300-kcalorie intake. These meals supply over 130 grams protein, more than even the highest recommended intake for such a person. Obviously, the more energy a person requires, the more protein that person will receive, assuming the foods chosen are nutrient dense. This relationship between energy and protein intakes breaks down only when people meet their energy needs with high-fat, high-sugar confections. The meals shown in Figure 14–5 provide almost 550 grams carbohydrate, or over 60 percent of total kcalories. Athletes who train exhaustively for endurance events may want to aim for somewhat higher carbohydrate intakes. Beyond these specific concerns of total energy, protein, and carbohydrate, the diet most beneficial to athletic performance is remarkably similar to the diet recommended for most people.

MEALS BEFORE AND AFTER COMPETITION

No single food improves speed, strength, or skill in competitive events, although some *kinds* of foods do support performance better than others as already explained. Still, a competitor may eat a particular food before or after an event

Figure 14–5

An Athlete's Meal Selections

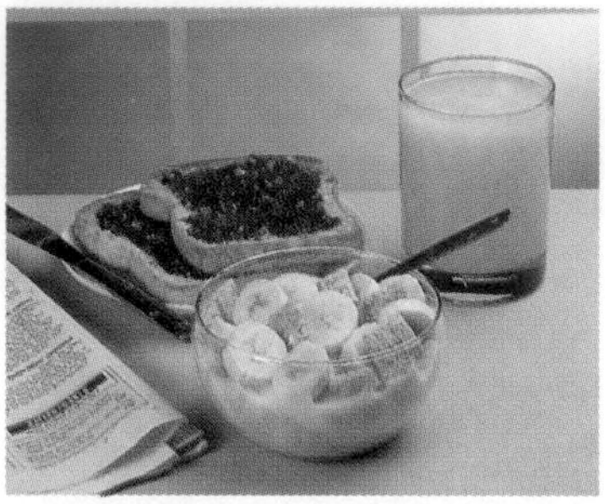

Breakfast:
1 c shredded wheat.
1 c 1% low-fat milk.
1 small banana.
2 slices whole-wheat toast.
4 tsp jelly.
1½ c orange juice.

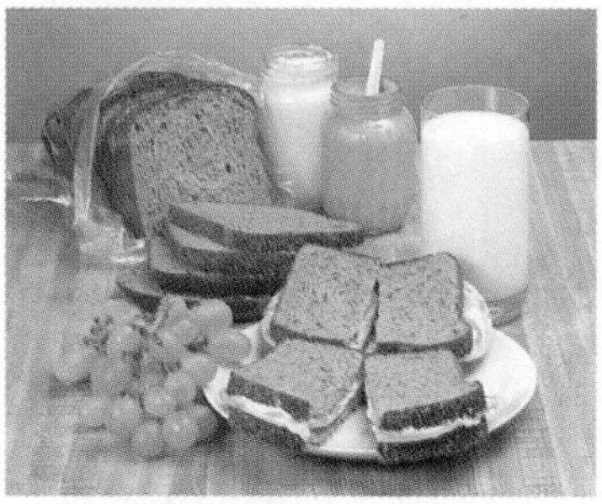

Lunch:
2 turkey sandwiches.
1½ c 1% low-fat milk.
Large bunch of grapes.

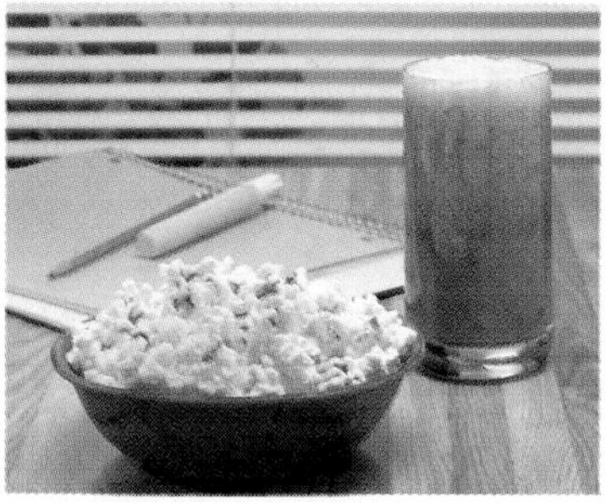

Snack:
3 c plain popcorn.
A smoothie made from:
1½ c apple juice.
1½ frozen banana.

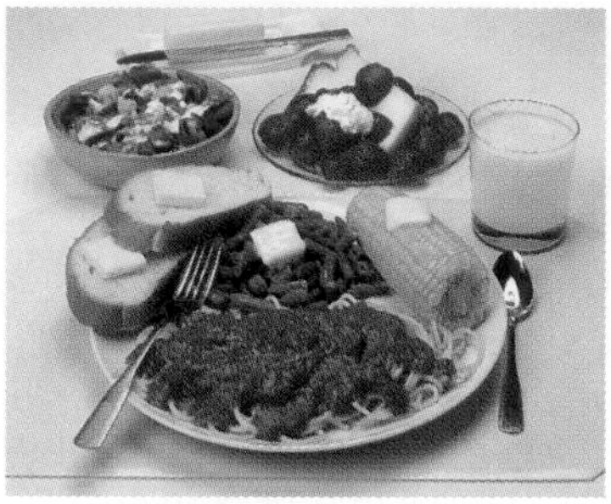

Dinner:
Salad: 1 c spinach, carrots, and mushrooms.
½ c garbanzo beans.
1 tbs sunflower seeds.
1 tbs ranch salad dressing.
1 c spaghetti with meat sauce.
1 c green beans.
1 corn on the cob.
2 slices Italian bread.
4 tsp butter.
1 piece angel food cake.
1¼ c fresh strawberries.
1 tbs whipping cream.
1 c 1% low-fat milk.

Total kcal: 3300
63% kcal from carbohydrate
22% kcal from fat
15% kcal from protein
All vitamin and mineral intakes exceed the RDA for both men and women.

for psychological reasons. One eats a steak the night before wrestling, another takes some honey five minutes after diving. As long as these practices remain harmless, they should be respected.

Pregame Meals Science indicates that the pregame meal or snack should include plenty of fluids and be light and easy to digest. It should provide between 300 and 800 kcalories, primarily from carbohydrate-rich foods that are familiar and well tolerated by the athlete. The meal should end three to five hours before competition to allow plenty of time for the stomach to empty before exertion.

Breads, potatoes, pasta, and fruit juices—that is, carbohydrate-rich foods low in fat, protein, and fiber—form the basis of the best pregame meal. Bulky, fiber-rich foods such as raw vegetables or high-bran cereals, although usually desirable, are best avoided just before competition. Fiber in the digestive tract attracts water out of the blood and can cause stomach discomfort during performance. Liquid meals are easy to digest, and many such meals are commercially available. Alternatively, athletes can mix nonfat milk or juice, frozen fruits, and flavorings in a blender.

High-carbohydrate, liquid pregame meal ideas:

- Apple juice, frozen banana, and cinnamon.
- Papaya juice, frozen strawberries, and mint.
- Nonfat milk, frozen banana, and vanilla.

Postgame Meals As mentioned earlier, eating high-carbohydrate foods *after* physical activity enhances glycogen storage. Since people are usually not hungry immediately following physical activity, carbohydrate-containing beverages such as the sports drinks discussed earlier may be preferred. If an active person does feel hungry after an event, then foods high in carbohydrate and low in protein, fat, and fiber are the ones to choose—the same ones recommended prior to competition. Foods high in protein and fat should be avoided during the first few hours after activity as these foods may suppress hunger and thus limit carbohydrate intake.[43]

To sum up, ample fluid and nutrient-dense foods best support physical activity. Carbohydrate-rich foods that are light and easy-to-digest are recommended for both the pregame and postgame meals.

The person who wants to excel physically will apply accurate nutrition knowledge along with dedication to rigorous training. A diet that provides ample fluid and consists of a variety of nutrient-dense foods in quantities to meet energy needs will enhance not only athletic performance, but overall health as well. Training and genetics being equal, who would win a competition—the athlete who habitually consumes inadequate amounts of needed nutrients or the competitor who arrives at the event with a long history of full nutrient stores and well-met metabolic needs?

Some athletes learn that nutrition can support physical performance and turn to pills and powders instead of foods. In case you need further convincing that a healthful diet surpasses such potions, the following highlight addresses this issue.

Study Questions

1. Define fitness, and list its benefits.
2. Explain the overload principle.
3. What types of activity are aerobic? Which are anaerobic?
4. What special problems do female athletes face? How do these problems relate to each other?
5. Describe the relationships among energy expenditure, type of activity, and oxygen use.
6. What factors influence the body's use of glucose during physical activity? How?
7. What factors influence the body's use of fat during physical activity? How?
8. What factors influence the body's use of protein during physical activity? How?
9. Why are some athletes likely to develop iron-deficiency anemia? Compare iron-deficiency anemia and sports anemia, explaining the differences.
10. Discuss the importance of hydration during training, and list recommendations to maintain fluid balance.
11. Describe the components of a healthy diet for athletic performance.

Notes

1. R. S. Paffenbarger and coauthors, The association of changes in physical-activity level and other lifestyle characteristics with mortality among men, *New England Journal of Medicine* 328 (1993): 538–545; L. Sandvik and coauthors, Physical fitness as a predictor of mortality among healthy, middle-aged Norwegian men, *New England Journal of Medicine* 328 (1993): 533–537.
2. U.S. Centers for Disease Control and Prevention and American College of Sports Medicine, Summary statement: Workshop on physical activity and public health, *Sports Medicine Bulletin* 28 (1993): 7.
3. American Heart Association Position Statement on Exercise: Benefits and recommendations for physical activity programs for all Americans, *Circulation* 86 (1992): 340–344; A. M. Bovens and coauthors, Physical activity, fitness, and selected risk factors for CHD in active men and women, *Medicine and Science in Sports and Exercise* 25 (1993): 572–576; R. R. Pate and coauthors, Physical activity and public health: A recommendation from the Centers for Disease Control and Prevention and the American College of Sports Medicine, *Journal of the American Medical Association* 273 (1995): 402–407.
4. W. L. Haskell, Health consequences of physical activity: Understanding and challenges regarding dose-response, *Medicine and Science in Sports and Exercise* 26 (1994): 649–660.
5. S. N. Blair and coauthors, Changes in physical fitness and all-cause mortality, *Journal of the American Medical Association* 273 (1995): 1093–1098.
6. American College of Sports Medicine, The recommended quality and quantity of exercise for developing and maintaining fitness in healthy adults, *Medicine and Science in Sports and Exercise* 22 (1990): 265–274.
7. U.S. Centers for Disease Control and Prevention and American College of Sports Medicine, 1993.
8. I. M. Lee, C. Hsieh, and R. S. Paffenbarger, Exercise intensity and longevity in men: The Harvard alumni study, *Journal of the American Medical Association* 272 (1995): 1179–1184.
9. Paffenbarger and coauthors, 1993.
10. R. R. Recker and coauthors, Bone gain in young adult women, *Journal of the American Medical Association* 268 (1992): 2403–2408; A. M. Fehily and coauthors, Factors affecting bone density in young adults, *American Journal of Clinical Nutrition* 56 (1992): 579–586; B. P. Conroy and coauthors, Bone mineral density in elite junior Olympic weightlifters, *Medicine and Science in Sports and Exercise* 25 (1993): 1103–1109; ACSM Position Stand on Osteoporosis and Exercise, *Medicine and Science in Sports and Exercise* 27 (1995): i–iv.
11. D. C. Nieman, Exercise, upper respiratory tract infection, and the immune system, *Medicine and Science in Sports and Exercise* 26 (1994): 128–139.
12. J. A. Woods and J. M. Davis, Exercise, monocyte/macrophage function, and cancer, *Medicine and Science in Sports and Exercise* 26 (1994): 147–157.
13. Paffenbarger and coauthors, 1993; A. L. Macnair, Physical activity, not diet, should be the focus of measures for the primary prevention of cardiovascular disease, *Nutrition Research Reviews* 7 (1994): 43–65.
14. S. P. Helmrich and coauthors, Physical activity and reduced occurrence of non-insulin-dependent diabetes mellitus, *New England Journal of Medicine* 325 (1991): 147–152.
15. M. A. Fiatarone and coauthors, High-intensity strength training in nonagenarians: Effects on skeletal muscle, *Journal of the American Medical Association* 263 (1990): 3029–3034; C. L. Pollock, Breaking the risk of falls: An exercise benefit for older patients, *Physician and Sportsmedicine*, November 1992, pp. 147–156; L. E. Voorrips and coauthors, The physical condition of elderly women differing in habitual physical activity, *Medicine and Science in Sports and Exercise* 25 (1993): 1152–1157.
16. American College of Sports Medicine, *Guidelines for Exercise Testing and Prescription*, 4th ed. (Philadelphia: Lea & Febiger, 1991).
17. American College of Sports Medicine, 1990.
18. J. H. Wilson, Nutrition, physical activity and bone health in women, *Nutrition Research Reviews* 7 (1994): 67–91.
19. A. A. Skolnick, "Female athlete triad" risk for women, *Journal of the American Medical Association* 270 (1993): 921–923.
20. K. K. Yeager and coauthors, The female athlete triad: Disordered eating, amenorrhea, osteoporosis, *Medicine and Science in Sports and Exercise* 25 (1993): 775–777.
21. J. Sundgot-Borgen, Risk and trigger factors for the development of eating disorders in female elite athletes, *Medicine and Science in Sports and Exercise* 26 (1994): 414–419.
22. Yeager and coauthors, 1993.
23. C. L. Otis, American College of Sports Medicine's Ad Hoc Task Force on Women's Issues in Sports Medicine, as quoted in Skolnick, 1993.
24. N. T. Frusztajer and coauthors, Nutrition and the incidence of stress fractures in ballet dancers, *American Journal of Clinical Nutrition* 51 (1990): 779–783.
25. M. Hargreaves, Carbohydrates and exercise, in *Foods, Nutrition, and Sports Performance: An International Scientific Consensus*, eds. C. Williams and J. T. Devlin (London: E & FN Spon, 1992), pp. 19–33.
26. D. C. Nieman, *Fitness and Sports Medicine: An Introduction* (Palo Alto, Calif.: Bull Publishing, 1990), p. 250.
27. P. Arnos, F. Andres, and K. Drowatzky, Fat oxidation and RPE at varied exercise intensities, *Medicine and Science in Sports and Exercise* (supplement) 25 (1993): S9; F. A. Kulling and coauthors, Identification and evaluation of the exercise intensity

which maximizes fat oxidation in young women, *Medicine and Science in Sports and Exercise* (supplement) 25 (1993): S179.
28. D. L. Ballor, J. P. McCarthy, and E. J. Wilterdink, Exercise intensity does not affect the composition of diet- and exercise-induced body mass loss, *American Journal of Clinical Nutrition* 51 (1990): 142–146.
29. A Tremblay and coauthors, Effect of intensity of physical activity on body fatness and distribution, *American Journal of Clinical Nutrition* 51 (1990): 153–157.
30. T. J. Horton and C. A. Geissler, Effect of habitual exercise on daily energy expenditures and metabolic rate during standardized activity, *American Journal of Clinical Nutrition* 59 (1994): 13–19.
31. F. Carraro and coauthors, Alanine kinetics in humans during low-intensity exercise, *Medicine and Science in Sports and Exercise* 26 (1994): 348–353.
32. M. J. Zachin, Protein requirements for athletes, *Sports Medicine Digest*, March 1990, pp. 1–2; P. W. R. Lemon, Protein and exercise: Update 1987, *Medicine and Science in Sports and Exercise* 19 (1987): S179–S188.
33. Position of The American Dietetic Association and The Canadian Dietetic Association: Nutrition for physical fitness and athletic performance for adults, *Journal of the American Dietetic Association* 93 (1993): 691–695.
34. P. W. R. Lemon, Effect of exercise on protein requirements, in *Foods, Nutrition, and Sports Performance: An International Scientific Consensus*, eds. C. Williams and J. T. Devlin (London: E & FN Spon, 1992), pp. 65–68.
35. A. Singh, F. M. Moses, and P. A. Deuster, Chronic multivitamin-mineral supplementation does not enhance physical performance, *Medicine and Science in Sports and Exercise* 24 (1992): 726–732.
36. H. M. Alessio, Exercise induced oxidative stress, *Medicine and Science in Sports and Exercise* 25 (1993): 218–224; R. R. Jenkins and A. Goldfarb, Introduction: Oxidative stress, aging, and exercise, *Medicine and Science in Sports and Exercise* 25 (1993): 210–212; E. W. Askew, Environmental and physical stress and nutrient requirements, *American Journal of Clinical Nutrition* (supplement) 61 (1995): 631–637.
37. Alessio, 1993.
38. S. K. Sumida and coauthors, Exercise-induced lipid peroxidation and leakage of enzymes before and after vitamin E supplementation, *International Journal of Biochemistry* 21 (1989): 835–838, as cited in A. H. Goldfarb, Antioxidants: Role of supplementation to prevent exercise-induced oxidative stress, *Medicine and Science in Sports and Exercise* 25 (1993): 232–236.
39. R. M. Lyle and coauthors, Iron status in exercising women: The effect of oral iron therapy vs. increased consumption of muscle foods, *American Journal of Clinical Nutrition* 56 (1992): 1049–1055.
40. J. E. Greenleaf, Problems: Thirst, drinking behavior, and involuntary dehydration, *Medicine and Science in Sports and Exercise* 24 (1992): 645–656.
41. R. J. Maughan, Fluid and electrolyte loss and replacement in exercise, in *Foods, Nutrition, and Sports Performance: An International Scientific Consensus*, eds. C. Williams and J. T. Devlin (London: E & FN Spon, 1992), pp. 147–178.
42. C. V. Gisolfi and S. M. Duchman, Guidelines for optimal replacement beverages for different athletic events, *Medicine and Science in Sports and Exercise* 24 (1992): 679–687.
43. E. F. Coyle, Timing and method of increased carbohydrate intake to cope with heavy training, competition, and recovery, in *Foods, Nutrition, and Sports Performance: An International Scientific Consensus*, eds. C. Williams and J. T. Devlin (London: E & FN Spon, 1992), pp. 37–61.

Supplements and Ergogenic Aids Athletes Use

Athletes gravitate to promises that they can enhance their performance by taking pills, powders, or potions. Unfortunately, they often hear such promises from their coaches and peers, who advise them to use nutrient supplements, take drugs, or follow procedures that claim to deliver results without effort. When such aids are harmless, they are only a waste of money; when they impair performance or harm health, they waste athletic potential and cost lives. This highlight looks at some promises of magic to improve physical performance.

Many substances or treatments claim to be *ergogenic*, meaning work enhancing (the accompanying glossary defines this and related terms). For the large majority of these so-called ergogenic aids, research findings do not support those claims. Athletes who hear that a product is ergogenic should ask who is making the claim and who will profit from the sale.

Sometimes it is difficult to distinguish valid claims from bogus ones. Fitness magazines are particularly troublesome because many of them present both valid and invalid nutrition articles alongside slick advertisements for nutrition products. Advertisements often feature colorful anatomical figures, graphs, and tables that appear scientific. Some ads even include "reviews of literature" citing such credible sources as the *American Journal of Clinical Nutrition* and the *Journal of the American Medical Association*. Such ads create the illusion of credibility to gain readers' trust. Keep in mind, however, that the ads are created not to teach, but to sell. A careful reading of the cited research might reveal that the ads have presented the research findings out of context. In one such case, ad writers cited an article to support the invalid conclusion that their supplement was "critical to maximum anabolic utilization." Researchers reporting in the cited article had reached another conclusion: regular exercise has a definite anabolic effect, and the use of supplements does not appear to enhance that effect. Scientific facts had been twisted and created to promote sales. Highlight 1 describes ways to recognize quackery.

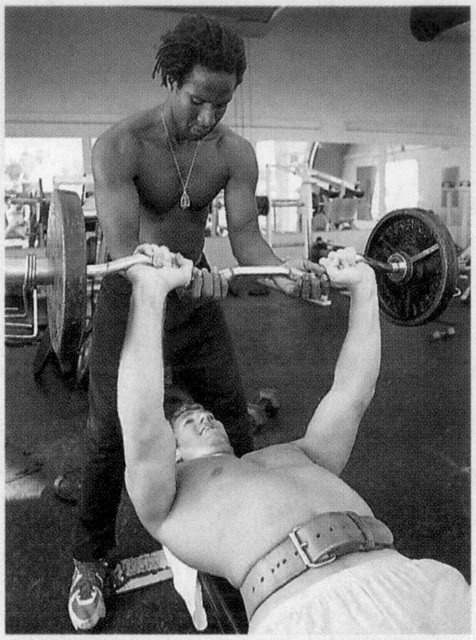

Training serves an athlete better than any pills or powders.

NUTRIENT SUPPLEMENTS

A variety of supplements make claims based on misunderstood nutrition principles. The claims may sound good, but they have no factual basis.

Protein Powders

Protein powders can supply amino acids to the body, but nature's protein sources—lean meat, milk, and legumes—supply all these amino acids and more. Because the body builds muscle protein from amino acids, many athletes take protein powders with the false hope of stimulating muscle growth. Purified protein preparations, however, contain none of the other nutrients needed to support the building of muscle, and the protein they supply is not needed by athletes who eat food. It is excess protein, and the body dismantles it and uses it for energy or stores it as body fat. The deamination of excess amino acids places an extra burden on the kidneys to excrete unused nitrogen.

Amino Acid Supplements

Most healthy athletes eating well-balanced diets do not need amino acid supplements either. Advertisers point to research that identifies the branched-chain amino acids as the main ones used as fuel by exercising muscles. What the ads leave out is that compared to glucose and fatty acids, branched-chain amino acids provide almost no fuel and that anyway, ordinary foods provide them in abundance. Any improvements in performance with amino acid supplements are apparent only in athletes competing in events lasting longer than 3 hours.[1]

Glossary

blood doping: the process of injecting red blood cells to enhance the blood's oxygen-carrying ability. Risks include dangerous blood clotting, especially in athletes who become dehydrated, infections from non-sterile equipment, transfusion reactions, and dangers of improperly transferred blood. Blood doping is banned in Olympic competitions.

caffeine: a natural stimulant found in many common foods and beverages, including coffee, tea, and chocolate, that in small amounts may produce alertness and reduced reaction time in some people, but also causes fluid losses. Overdoses cause headaches, trembling, rapid heart rate, and other undesirable side effects.

epoetin (eh-poy-EE-tin)**:** a drug derived from human erythropoietin and marketed under the trade name Epogen; illegally used to increase oxygen capacity.

ergogenic aids: the term implies "energy giving," but in fact, no products impart such a quality.
ergo = work
genic = gives rise to

hGH (human growth hormone): a hormone produced by the brain's pituitary gland that regulates normal growth and development; also called *somatotropin*. Some athletes misuse this hormone to increase their height and strength.

sodium bicarbonate: baking soda; an alkaline salt believed to neutralize blood lactic acid and thereby reduce pain and enhance possible workload. "Soda loading" may cause intestinal bloating and diarrhea.

Carnitine

Carnitine, a nonprotein amino acid, is a popular supplement among endurance athletes, who believe carnitine will help them burn more fat, thereby sparing glycogen during endurance events. Carnitine is also promoted to bodybuilders as a "fat burner."

In the body, carnitine facilitates the transfer of fatty acids across the mitochondrial membrane. The idea therefore is that with more carnitine available, fat oxidation will be enhanced. This does not seem to be the case: researchers found that carnitine supplementation for 7 to 14 days neither raised muscle carnitine concentrations nor influenced fat or carbohydrate oxidation.[2] It did, however, produce diarrhea in half of the men tested. Milk and meat products are good sources of carnitine, and supplements are not needed.

Chromium Picolinate

Chapter 13 introduced chromium as an essential trace mineral involved in carbohydrate and lipid metabolism. Advertisements in bodybuilding magazines claim that chromium picolinate, which is supposed to be more easily absorbed than chromium alone, builds muscle, enhances energy, and burns fat. Research so far does not support such claims, and use of large doses of chromium picolinate may result in iron deficiency.[3]

Complete Nutrition Supplements

Several drinks and candy bars appeal to athletes by claiming to provide "complete" nutrition. These products usually taste good and provide extra food energy, but fall short of providing "complete" nutrition. They can be useful as a pregame meal or a between-meal snack, but they should not replace regular meals.

A nutritionally "complete" drink can be of use to the nervous athlete who cannot tolerate solid food on the day of an event. A liquid meal two or three hours before competition can supply some of the fluid and carbohydrate needed in a pregame meal, but a shake of nonfat milk or juice (such as apple or papaya) and ice milk or frozen fruit (such as strawberries or bananas) can do the same thing less expensively.

SODA LOADING

Some athletes competing in short-duration, high-intensity anaerobic events, such as 400- to 800-meter races, are using baking soda (sodium bicarbonate) to help neutralize the lactic acid that accumulates in their blood. Sodium bicarbonate occurs normally in the blood, and one of its roles is to buffer lactic acid produced during anaerobic activity. Theoretically, adding an alkaline salt such as sodium bicarbonate could delay the onset of fatigue from lactic acid accumulation. Some research studies of this practice have found no benefit, others have found improved performance.[4] Any improvements, though statistically significant, are minimal, however. For competitive athletes, a savings of a second or two can be valuable, but for most people, it's not. And as is true of most performance gimmicks, there are drawbacks: severe diarrhea, dizziness, cramps, and nausea.

CAFFEINE

Although some research findings support the use of caffeine to enhance endurance, other studies suggest that caffeine has no effect on athletic performance. If caffeine does enhance endurance, it probably does so by stimulating fatty acid release, thereby slowing glycogen use. Of course, physically active people can make their work seem easier without consuming caffeine by warming up with light activity. Light activity before a workout stimulates fat release, as does caffeine, but the activity also warms the muscles and connective tissues, making them flexible and resistant to injury. Caffeine does not offer these added benefits.

Caffeine is a stimulant that elicits a number of physiological and psychological effects in the body. (The table at the start of Appendix H provides a list of common caffeine-containing items and the doses they deliver.) The possible benefits of caffeine use must be weighed against its adverse effects—stomach upset, nervousness, irritability, headaches, and diarrhea. Caffeine-containing beverages should be used in moderation, if at all, and *in addition* to other fluids, not as a substitute for them. In college, national, and international athletic competitions, the use of caffeine is forbidden in amounts greater than the equivalent of 5 or 6 cups of coffee consumed in a 2-hour period prior to competition. Urine tests that detect more caffeine than this disqualify athletes from competition.

ANABOLIC STEROIDS

Among the most dangerous and illegal ergogenic practices is the taking of anabolic steroids. These drugs are derived from the male sex hormone testosterone, which promotes the development of male characteristics and lean body mass. Athletes take steroids to stimulate muscle bulking.

To athletes struggling to excel, the promise of bigger, stronger muscles than training alone can produce has been tempting. Athletes who lack superstar genetic material and who normally would not be able to break into the elite ranks can, with the help of steroids, suddenly compete with true champions. Especially in professional circles, where monetary rewards for excellence are sky-high, steroid use is common despite its illegality and side effects.

The American Academy of Pediatrics and the American College of Sports Medicine condemn athletes' use of anabolic steroids, and the International Olympic Committee bans their use. These authorities cite the known toxic side effects and maintain that taking these drugs is a form of cheating. Other athletes are put in the difficult position of either conceding an unfair advantage to competitors who use steroids or taking them and accepting the risk of harmful side effects. Young athletes should not be forced to make such a choice.

The list of adverse reactions to steroids is long and continues to grow amid only a slight decline in use of the drugs. Table H14–1 lists the side effects of steroids.

The price for the potential competitive edge that steroids confer is high—sometimes it is life itself. The commissioner of the Food and Drug Administration (FDA) warns that steroids are not simple pills that build bigger muscles, but complex chemicals to which the body reacts in many ways, particularly when bodybuilders and other athletes take large amounts. The safest, most effective way to build muscle has always been through hard training and a sound diet, and—despite popular misconceptions—it still is.

Some manufacturers push specific herbs as legal substitutes for steroid drugs. They falsely claim that these herbs contain hormones, enhance the body's hormonal activity, or both. In some cases, an herb may contain plant sterols, such as oryzanol, but these compounds are poorly absorbed. Even if absorption occurs, the body cannot convert herbal compounds to anabolic steroids. Ironically, injections of oryzanol in rats alter metabolic pathways to favor *catabolism*.[5] None of these products has any proven anabolic steroid activity, none enhances muscles strength, and some contain natural toxins. In short, "natural" does not mean "harmless."

HUMAN GROWTH HORMONE

Some short or average-sized athletes seek human growth hormone (hGH) to build lean tissue and increase their height if they are still in their growing years. Athletes in power sports such as weight lifting and judo are most likely to experiment with hGH, believing the injectable hormone will provide the benefits of anabolic steroids without the dangerous side effects.

Abuse of hGH is not as extensive as abuse of steroids or other such drugs, in part because of the cost. A dose of hGH that will produce the effect sought might cost $2000 a week on the black market. As with other drugs sold on the black mar-

Table H14–1

Anabolic Steroids: Side Effects and Adverse Reactions

Mind

- Extreme aggression with hostility ("steroid rage"); mood swings; anxiety; dizziness; drowsiness; unpredictability; insomnia; psychotic depression; personality changes, suicidal thoughts

Face and Hair

- Swollen appearance; greasy skin; severe, scarring acne; mouth and tongue soreness; yellowing of whites of eyes (jaundice)
- In females, male-pattern hair loss and increased growth of face and body hair

Voice

- In females, irreversible deepening of voice

Chest

- In males, breathing difficulty; breathing stoppage; breast development
- In females, breast atrophy

Heart

- Heart disease; elevated or reduced heart rate; heart attack; stroke; hypertension; increased LDL; drastic reduction in HDL

Abdominal Organs

- Nausea; vomiting; bloody diarrhea; pain; edema; liver tumors (possibly cancerous); liver damage, disease, or rupture leading to fatal liver failure (peliosis hepatitis)[a]; kidney stones and damage; gallstones; frequent urination; possible rupture of aneurysm or hemorrhage

Blood

- Blood clots; high risk of blood poisoning; those who share needles risk contracting HIV (the AIDS virus) or other disease-causing organisms; septic shock (from injections)

Reproductive System

- In males, permanent shrinkage of testes; prostate enlargement with increased risk of cancer; sexual dysfunction; loss of fertility; excessive and painful erections
- In females, loss of menstruation and fertility; permanent enlargement of external genitalia; fetal damage, if pregnant

Muscles, Bones, and Connective Tissues

- Increased susceptibility to injury with delayed recovery times; cramps; tremors; seizurelike movements; injury at injection site;
- In adolescents, failure to grow to normal height

Other

- Fatigue; increased risk of cancer

[a]In peliosis hepatitis, excess buildup of bile causes destruction of liver cells. Blood pools form, and liver failure causes death.

Sources: K. L. Ropp, No-win situation for athletes, *FDA Consumer,* December 1992, pp. 8–12; National Academy of Sports Medicine policy statement and position paper: Anabolic androgenic steroids, growth hormones, stimulants, ergogenics, and drug use in sports, in B. Goldman and R. Klatz, *Death in the Locker Room II: Drugs and Sports* (Chicago: Elite Sports Medicine Publications, 1992), pp. 328–373.

ket, athletes often do not get what they think they are buying.

Taken in large quantities, hGH causes the disease acromegaly, in which the body becomes huge and the organs and bones overenlarge. Other effects include diabetes, thyroid disorder, heart disease, menstrual irregularities, diminished sexual desire, and shortened life span. The U.S. Olympic Committee bans hGH use, but tests cannot distinguish between naturally occurring hGH and hGH used as a drug. The committee maintains that use of hGH is a form of cheating that undermines the quest for physical excellence and that its use is coercive to other athletes.

BLOOD DOPING

Nutrition supplements and drugs are not the only things athletes use to improve athletic performance. Another ergogenic aid is blood doping: injecting red blood cells to enhance the blood's aerobic capacity (ability to carry oxygen). To "dope the blood," the athlete has one liter of blood drawn two to three months prior to the event and banks it in frozen storage. The body replaces these red blood cells; then, a few days before the competition, the athlete receives the stored blood, raising the total red blood cell count well above normal. This temporarily increases the oxygen-carrying capacity of the blood and improves endurance.

Some studies confirm an aerobic benefit from blood doping, but also point out that it carries negative health consequences. One possible outcome is blood clotting, especially in athletes who become dehydrated. Blood doping is considered unethical and is illegal; the International Olympic Committee forbids the

Table H14–2

Ineffective Ergogenic Aids

- **Amino acids:** the building blocks of proteins found in many foods; packaged and promoted for athletes as ergogenic aids (see *glycine*).
- **Bee pollen:** a product consisting of bee saliva, plant nectar, and pollen that supposedly aids in weight loss and boosts athletic performance; it does neither and may cause an allergic reaction in individuals sensitive to it.
- **Boron:** a nonessential mineral that is promoted as a "natural" steroid replacement.
- **Brewer's yeast:** a preparation of yeast cells, containing a concentrated amount of B vitamins and some minerals; falsely promoted as an energy booster.
- **Carnitine:** a nonprotein amino acid made in the body from glutamine and methionine that helps transport fatty acids across the mitochrondrial membrane. Carnitine supposedly "burns" fat and spares glycogen during endurance events, but in reality it does neither.
- **Cell salts:** a preparation of minerals supposedly harvested from living cells, sold as a health-promoting supplement.
- **Chaparral:** an herb that is promoted as an antioxidant and free-radical scavenger that supposedly slows aging, "cleanses" the blood, and treats skin problems; has been associated with acute, toxic hepatitis.
- **Chromium picolinate:** a trace element supplement; falsely promoted to increase lean body mass.
- **Coenzyme Q10:** a lipid found in cells (mitochondria) shown to improve exercise performance in heart disease patients, but not effective in improving performance of healthy athletes.
- **Comfrey:** a leafy plant that supposedly soothes nerves; has been associated with liver disease and at least one death.
- **Desiccated liver:** dehydrated liver powder that supposedly contains all the nutrients found in liver in concentrated form; possibly not dangerous, but it has no particular nutritional merit and is considerably more expensive than fresh liver.
- **DNA** (deoxyribonucleic acid)**:** the genetic material of cells necessary in protein synthesis; falsely promoted as an energy booster.
- **Gelatin:** a soluble form of the protein collagen, used to thicken foods; sometimes falsely promoted as a strength enhancer.
- **Germanium:** a nonessential mineral that supposedly promotes health and neutralizes heavy metal toxicity; has been associated with irreversible kidney damage and death.
- **Ginseng:** a plant whose extract supposedly boosts energy; side effects of chronic use include nervousness, confusion, and depression.
- **Glycine:** a nonessential amino acid, promoted as an ergogenic aid because it is a precursor of the high-energy compound phosphocreatine. Other amino acids commonly packaged for athletes that are equally useless include tryptophan, ornithine, arginine, lysine, and the branched-chain amino acids leucine, isoleucine, and valine, which are present in large amounts in skeletal muscle tissue.
- **Growth hormone releasers:** herbs or pills that supposedly regulate hormones; falsely promoted for enhancing athletic performance.
- **Guarana:** a reddish berry found in Brazil's Amazon valley that is used as an ingredient in carbonated sodas and taken in powder or tablet form. Guarana is marketed as an ergogenic aid to enhance speed and endurance, an aphrodisiac, a "cardiac tonic," an "intestinal disinfectant," and a smart drug that supposedly improves memory and concentration and wards off senility. Because guarana contains seven times as much caffeine as its relative the coffee bean, there are con-

cerns that high doses can stress the heart and cause panic attacks.

- **Herbal steroids:** curious mixtures of herbs, "adaptogens," and "aphrodisiacs" that supposedly enhance hormone activity. Products marketed as herbal steroids include astragalus, damiana, dong quai, fo ti teng, ginseng root, licorice root, palmetto berries, sarsaparilla, schizardra, unicorn root, yohimbe bark, and yucca.
- **Inosine:** an organic chemical that is falsely said to "activate cells, produce energy, and facilitate exercise," but has been shown actually to reduce the endurance of runners.
- **Jin bu huan:** a Chinese herbal product that supposedly relieves pain; has been associated with slowed heart rate, depressed central nervous system, and breathing difficulties.
- **Kelp:** dehydrated seaweed used by the Japanese as a foodstuff.
- **Ma huang:** an evergreen plant derivative that supposedly boosts energy and helps with weight control. Ma huang contains ephedrine, a cardiac stimulant, and has been associated with high blood pressure, rapid heart rate, nerve damage, muscle injury, psychosis, stroke, and memory loss.
- **Niacin:** a B vitamin that when taken in excess rushes blood to the skin, producing vascularity and a red tint—physical attributes bodybuilders strive to attain prior to performance. These attributes do not enhance performance and excess niacin can cause headaches and nausea.
- **Octacosanol:** an alcohol isolated from wheat germ; often falsely promoted to enhance athletic performance.
- **Oryzanol:** a plant sterol that supposedly provides the same benefits as anabolic steroids without the adverse side effects; also known as *ferulic acid, ferulate*, or *FRAC*.
- **Pangamic acid:** also called vitamin B_{15} (but not a vitamin, nor even a specific compound—it can be anything with that label); falsely claimed to speed oxygen delivery.
- **Phosphate pills:** a product demonstrated to increase the levels of a metabolically important phosphate compound (diphosphoglycerate) in red blood cells and the potential of the cells to deliver oxygen to the body's muscle cells; however, it does not extend endurance nor increase efficiency of aerobic metabolism and may cause calcium losses from the bones if taken in excess.
- **RNA** (ribonucleic acid)**:** the genetic material of cells necessary for protein synthesis; falsely promoted to enhance athletic performance.
- **Royal jelly:** the substance produced by worker bees and fed to the queen bee; falsely promoted to increase strength and enhance performance.
- **Spirulina:** a kind of alga ("blue-green manna") that supposedly contains large amounts of protein and vitamin B_{12}, suppresses appetite, and improves athletic performance; it does none of these things and is potentially toxic.
- **Succinate:** a compound synthesized in the body and involved in the TCA cycle; falsely promoted as a metabolic enhancer.
- **Superoxide dismutase (SOD):** an enzyme that protects cells from oxidation. When it is taken orally, the body digests and inactivates this protein; it is useless to athletes.
- **Wheat germ oil:** the oil from the wheat kernel; often falsely promoted as an energy aid.
- **Yohimbe:** tree bark that supposedly enhances "male performance"; has been associated with kidney failure, seizures, and death.

practice and tests for it prior to competition.

Athletes have recently discovered an alternative to blood doping in another potentially dangerous practice—taking the illegally obtained drug epoetin. Epoetin is derived from the human hormone erythropoietin, which controls the production of red blood cells. Theoretically, epoetin can amplify the oxygen-carrying capacity of the blood by as much as 10 percent. Like blood doping, taking epoetin is dangerous, especially for endurance athletes who may become dehydrated. Changes in blood chemistry and viscosity may lead to heart attack and stroke. Because epoetin must be given by injection, athletes abusing the drug face additional risks of HIV infection or hepatitis if they share nonsterile equipment.

The search for a single food, nutrient, drug, or technique that will safely and effectively enhance athletic performance will no doubt continue as long as people strive to achieve excellence in sports. Table H14–2 lists many ineffective ergogenic aids. So far, when athletic performance does improve after use of an ergogenic aid, the improvement can usually be attributed to the placebo effect, which is strongly at work in athletes. Even if a reliable source reports a performance boost from a newly tried product, give it time to fade away. Chances are excellent that the effect simply reflects the power of the mind over the body.

The overwhelming majority of potions sold for athletes are frauds. Wishful thinking will not substitute for talent, hard training, adequate diet, and mental preparedness in competition. But don't discount the power of mind over body for a

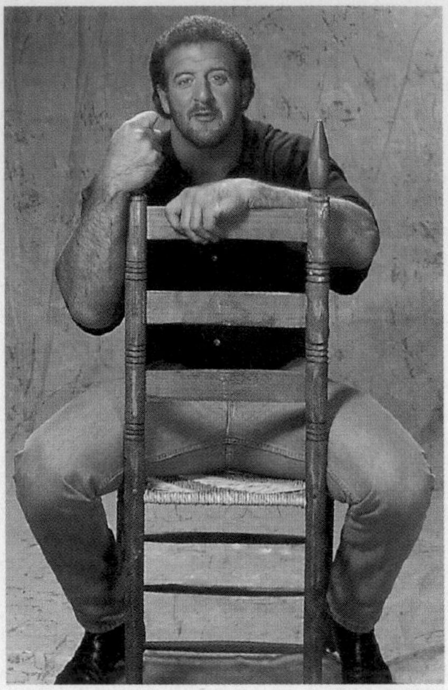

"I lied to a lot of people for a lot of years when I said I didn't use steroids. . . . If you're on steroids or human growth hormone, stop. I should have." Lyle Alzado, former NFL football player who died of cancer in May of 1992; as quoted by S. Smith, I'm sick and I'm scared, *Sports Illustrated*, July 8, 1991, pp. 21–25.

minute—it is formidable, and sports psychologists dedicate their work to harnessing it. You can use it by imagining yourself a winner and visualizing yourself excelling in your sport. You don't have to buy magic to obtain a winning edge; you already possess it—your mind.

NOTES

1. M. Mitchell and coauthors, Effects of amino acid supplementation on metabolic responses to ultraendurance triathlon performance, *Medicine and Science in Sports and Exercise* 24 (1992): S15; R. Kreider and coauthors, Effects of amino acid supplementation on substrate usage during ultraendurance triathlon performance, *Medicine and Science in Sports and Exercise* 24 (1992): S16.
2. M. Vukovich, D. L. Costill, and W. J. Fink, Carnitine supplementation: Effect on muscle carnitine and glycogen content during exercise, *Medicine and Science in Sports and Exercises* 26 (1994): 1122–1129.
3. C. Rosenbloom, M. Millard-Stafford, and J. Lathrop, Contemporary ergogenic aids used by strength/power athletes, *Journal of the American Dietetic Association* 92 (1992): 1264–1266; Chromium and athletes, *Sports Medicine Digest*, January 1994, p. 6.
4. J. Linderman and T. D. Fahey, Sodium bicarbonate ingestion and exercise performance: An update, *Sports Medicine* 11 (1991): 71–77.
5. K. B. Wheeler and K. A. Garleb, Gamma oryzanol—Plant sterol supplementation: Metabolic, endocrine, and physiologic effects, *International Journal of Sport Nutrition* 1 (1991): 170–177.

Chapter 15

Life Cycle Nutrition: Pregnancy and Lactation

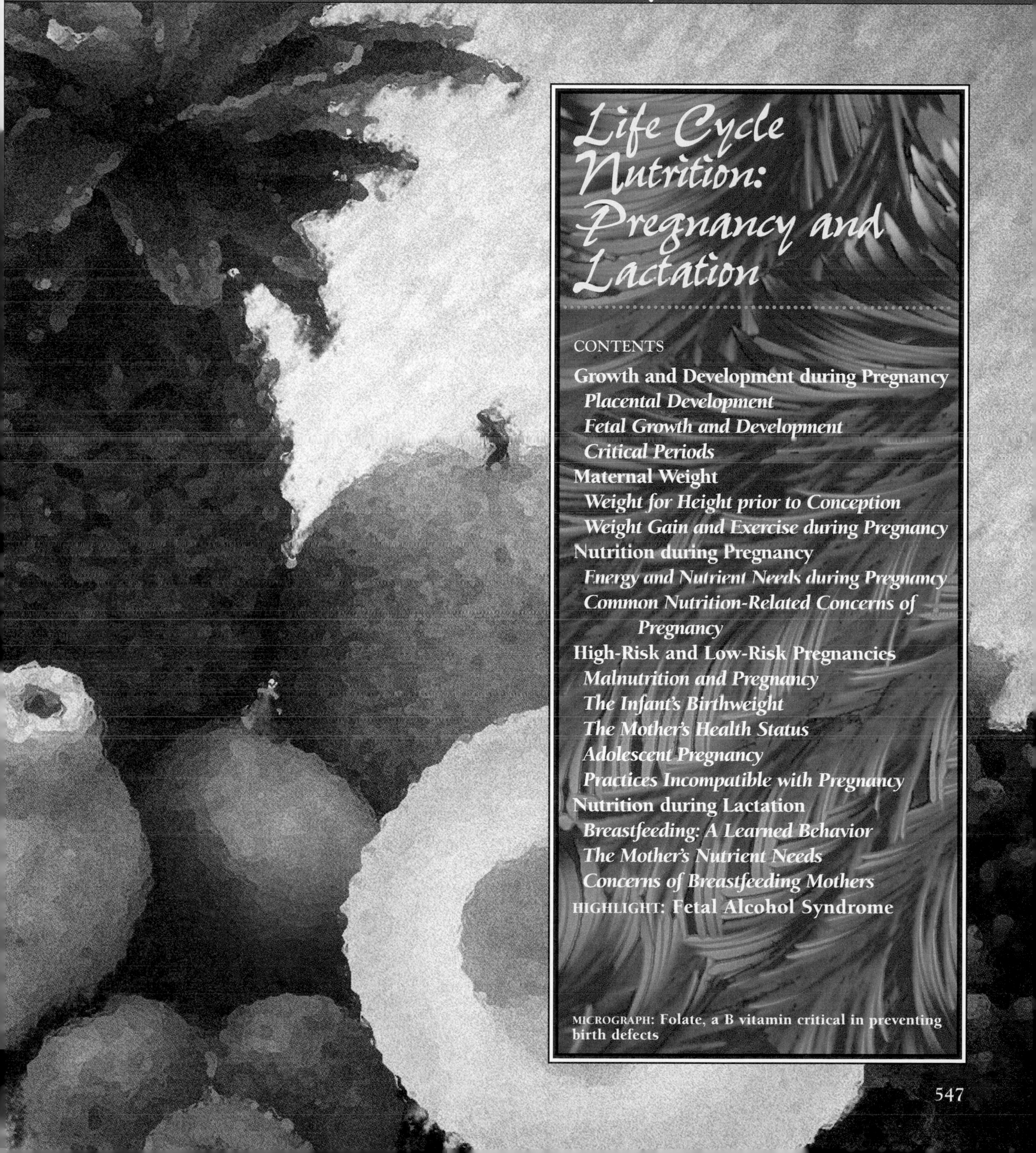

CONTENTS

MICROGRAPH: Folate, a B vitamin critical in preventing birth defects

All people need the same nutrients, but the amounts needed vary depending on the stage of life. This chapter focuses on nutrition in preparation for, and support of, pregnancy and lactation.

uterus (YOU-ter-us): the muscular organ within which the infant develops before birth; the womb.

placenta (plah-SEN-tuh): the organ that develops inside the uterus early in pregnancy, in which maternal and fetal blood circulate in close proximity so that materials can be exchanged between them. The fetus receives nutrients and oxygen across the placenta; the mother's blood picks up carbon dioxide and other waste products to be excreted.

amniotic (am-nee-OTT-ic) **sac**: the "bag of waters" in the uterus, in which the fetus floats.

umbilical (um-BILL-ih-cul) **cord**: the ropelike structure through which the fetus's veins and arteries reach the placenta; the route of nourishment and oxygen into the fetus and the route of waste disposal from the fetus. The scar in the middle of the abdomen that marks the former attachment of the umbilical cord is the **umbilicus** (um-BILL-ih-cus), commonly known as the "belly button."

ovum: the female reproductive cell, capable of developing into a new organism upon fertilization; commonly referred to as an egg.

sperm: the male reproductive cell, capable of fertilizing an ovum.

zygote (ZY-goat): the product of the union of ovum and sperm; so-called for the first two weeks after fertilization.

implantation: the stage of development in which the zygote embeds itself in the wall of the uterus and begins to develop; occurs during the first two weeks after conception.

gestation (jes-TAY-shun): the period from conception to birth; for human beings gestation lasts from 38 to 42 weeks. Pregnancy is often divided into thirds, called **trimesters**.

embryo (EM-bree-oh): the developing infant from two to eight weeks after conception.

Growth and Development during Pregnancy

A whole new life begins at conception. Organ systems develop rapidly, and nutrition plays many supportive roles. This section describes placenta and fetal development, paying close attention to times of intense activity.

PLACENTAL DEVELOPMENT

In the early days of pregnancy, a new organ develops within the uterus—the placenta, shown in Figure 15–1. Two associated structures also form. One is the amniotic sac, a fluid-filled balloonlike structure that houses the developing fetus. The other is the umbilical cord, a ropelike structure containing fetal blood vessels that extends through the fetus's "belly button" (the umbilicus) to the placenta. These three structures serve crucial roles during the pregnancy and then are expelled from the uterus following childbirth.

The placenta is composed of spongy tissue in which fetal blood and maternal blood flow side by side, each in its own vessels. The maternal blood transfers oxygen and nutrients to the fetus's blood and picks up fetal waste products. By exchanging oxygen, nutrients and waste products, the placenta performs the respiratory, absorptive, and excretory functions that the fetus's lungs, digestive system, and kidneys will provide after birth.

The placenta is a versatile, metabolically active organ. Like all body tissues, the placenta uses energy and nutrients to support its work. Like a gland, it produces an array of hormones that maintain pregnancy and prepare the mother's breasts for lactation (making milk). A healthy placenta is essential for normal fetal development.

FETAL GROWTH AND DEVELOPMENT

Fetal development begins with the fertilization of an ovum by a sperm. Three stages follow: the zygote, the embryo, and the fetus.

The Zygote The newly fertilized ovum, or zygote, begins as a single cell and divides to become many cells during the days after fertilization. Within two weeks, the zygote embeds itself in the uterine wall—a process known as implantation. Cell division continues—each set of cells divides into many other cells. Later in gestation, as development proceeds, the zygote becomes an embryo.

The Embryo The embryo accomplishes amazing developmental feats. The number of cells at first doubles approximately every 24 hours; later the rate slows, and only one doubling occurs during the final ten weeks of pregnancy. The embryo's size changes very little, but at eight weeks, the 1¼-inch embryo has a complete central nervous system, a beating heart, a digestive system, well-defined fingers and toes, and the beginnings of facial features.

Figure 15–1

The Placenta and Associated Structures

To understand how placental villi absorb nutrients without maternal and fetal blood interacting directly, think of how the intestinal villi work. The GI side of the intestinal villi is bathed in a nutrient-rich fluid (chyme). The intestinal villi absorb the nutrient molecules and release them into the body via capillaries. Similarly, the maternal side of the placental villi is bathed in nutrient-rich maternal blood. The placental villi absorb the nutrient molecules and release them to the fetus via fetal capillaries.

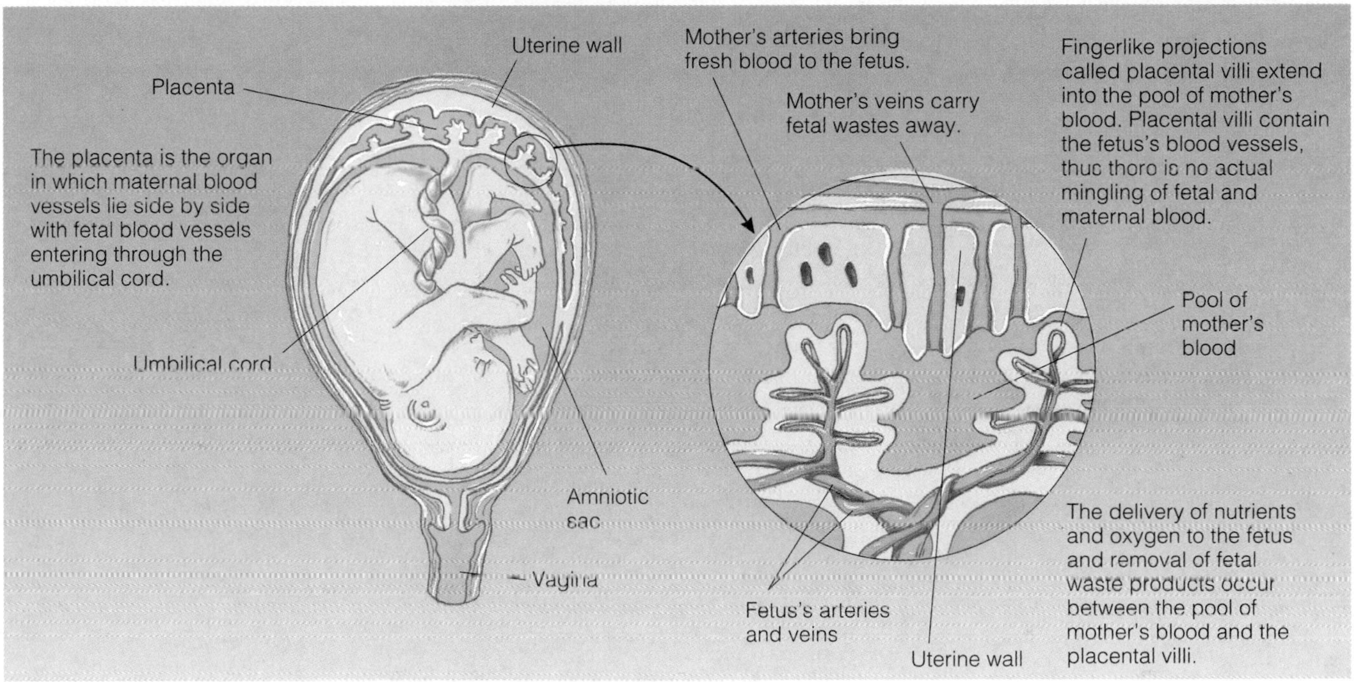

Uterine wall
Placenta
The placenta is the organ in which maternal blood vessels lie side by side with fetal blood vessels entering through the umbilical cord.
Umbilical cord
Amniotic sac
Vagina
Mother's arteries bring fresh blood to the fetus.
Mother's veins carry fetal wastes away.
Fingerlike projections called placental villi extend into the pool of mother's blood. Placental villi contain the fetus's blood vessels, thus there is no actual mingling of fetal and maternal blood.
Pool of mother's blood
The delivery of nutrients and oxygen to the fetus and removal of fetal waste products occur between the pool of mother's blood and the placental villi.
Fetus's arteries and veins
Uterine wall

The Fetus During the next seven months, each organ grows to maturity on its own schedule. As Figure 15–2 shows, fetal growth is phenomenal: weight increases from less than a gram to about 3500 grams (7½ pounds).

fetus (FEET-us): the developing infant from eight weeks after conception until term.

CRITICAL PERIODS

Times of intense development and rapid cell division are called critical periods—critical in the sense that the events scheduled for those times can occur only then, not later. If cell division and the final cell number achieved in an organ are limited during a critical period, full recovery will not occur (see Figure 15–3 on p. 551).

Each organ and tissue is most vulnerable to adverse influences during its own critical period. The critical period for neural tube development, for example, is from 17 to 30 days gestation.[1] Consequently, neural tube development is most vulnerable to nutrient deficiencies or toxins during this time—a time most women do not even realize that they are pregnant. Any abnormal development of the neural tube or its failure to close completely can produce major defects in the central nervous system, causing serious disabilities and infant death.

critical periods: finite periods during development in which certain events may occur that will have irreversible effects on later developmental stages. In a body organ, a critical period is usually a period of rapid cell division.

The neural tube forms the beginnings of the brain and spinal cord, key structures in the central nervous system.

Figure 15–2

Stages of Embryonic and Fetal Development

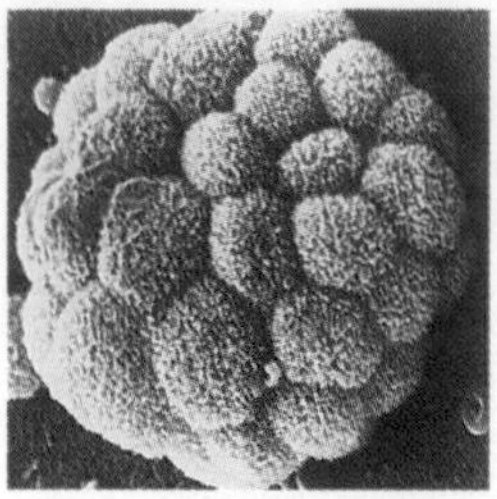

1. A newly fertilized ovum is about the size of the period at the end of this sentence. This zygote at less than one week after fertilization is not much bigger and is ready for implantation.

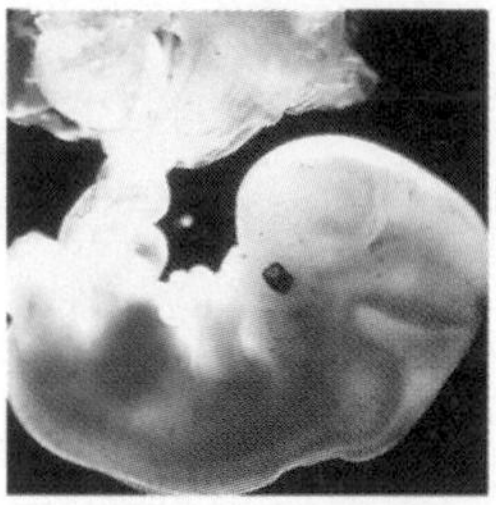

2. After implantation, the placenta develops and begins to provide nourishment to the developing embryo. An embryo five weeks after fertilization is about ½ inch long.

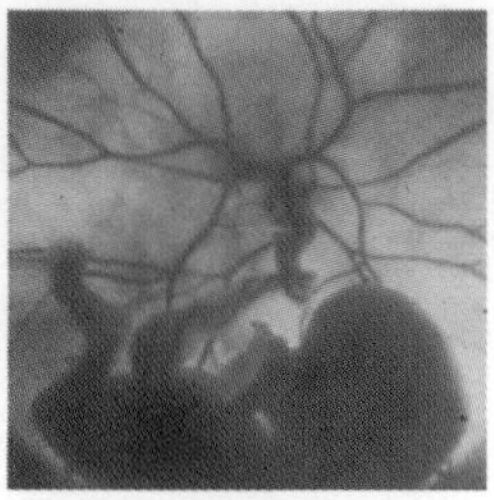

3. A fetus after 11 weeks of development is just over an inch long. Notice the umbilical cord and blood vessels connecting the fetus with the placenta.

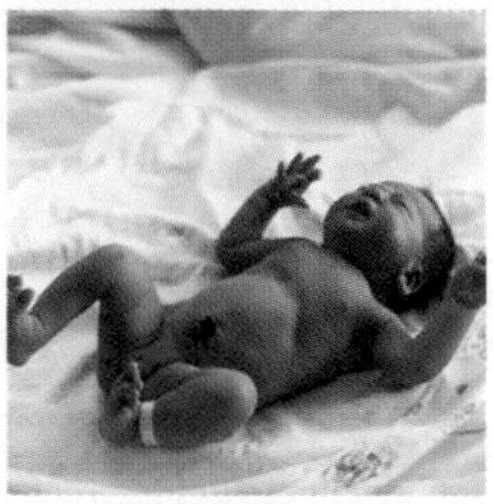

4. A newborn infant after nine months of development measures close to 20 inches in length. From eight weeks to term, this infant grew 20 times longer and 50 times heavier.

Spina Bifida, for Example One of the most common types of neural tube defects is spina bifida, a disorder characterized by incomplete closure of the spinal cord and its bony encasement. The membranes covering the spinal cord often protrude as a sac, which may rupture and lead to meningitis, a life-threatening inflammation of the membranes. Spina bifida is accompanied by varying degrees of paralysis, depending on the extent of spinal cord damage. Mild cases may not even be noticed, but severe cases lead to death. Common problems include clubfoot, dislocated hip, kidney disorders, curvature of the spine, muscle weakness, mental handicaps, and motor and sensory losses.

In the United States, approximately 1 of every 1000 newborns has a neural tube defect; some 2500 to 3000 infants are affected each year.* Many other pregnancies with neural tube defects end in abortion or stillbirths.

Folate Supplementation Chapter 10 described how folate supplements taken one month before conception and continued throughout the first trimester can prevent neural tube defects.[2] For this reason, the Public Health Service has recommended that all women of childbearing age who are capable of becoming pregnant take 0.4 milligrams of folate daily. This amount of folate is easy to obtain from a diet that includes plenty of fruits and vegetables, but supplements offer women a convenient way to ingest sufficient folate regularly and continuously enough to benefit pregnancy. Most over-the-counter multivitamin supplements contain 0.4 milligrams of folate; prenatal supplements usually contain at least 0.8 milligrams. A woman who has previously had an infant with a neural tube defect may be advised by her physician to take folate supplements in doses

Folate RDA:
- For women: 180 μg (0.18 mg)/day.
- During pregnancy: 400 μg (0.4 mg)/day.

*Worldwide, some 300,000 to 400,000 infants are born with neural tube defects each year.

ten times larger—4 milligrams daily. The risks associated with high doses of folate are not all known, but they can mask the pernicious anemia of a vitamin B_{12} deficiency. For this reason, quantities of 1 milligram or more require a prescription.

The Food and Drug Administration (FDA) is considering several approaches for delivering folate to the U.S. population, including food fortification. This decision must carefully weigh the benefits of fortification against the risks of overconsumption. On the one hand, an adequate folate intake is expected to reduce the incidence of neural tube defects by 50 percent. On the other hand, if vitamin B_{12} deficiency is masked by folate and left untreated, irreversible nerve damage may occur. The American Dietetic Association supports the FDA proposal to fortify foods with 140 micrograms of folate per 100 grams of foods, which should increase average daily intakes by 100 micrograms. Proposals suggest adding folate to pasta, flour, rolls, buns, farina, grits, cornmeal, and rice.

Figure 15–3

The Concept of Critical Periods

Critical periods occur early in development. An adverse influence felt early can have a much more severe and prolonged impact than one felt later on.

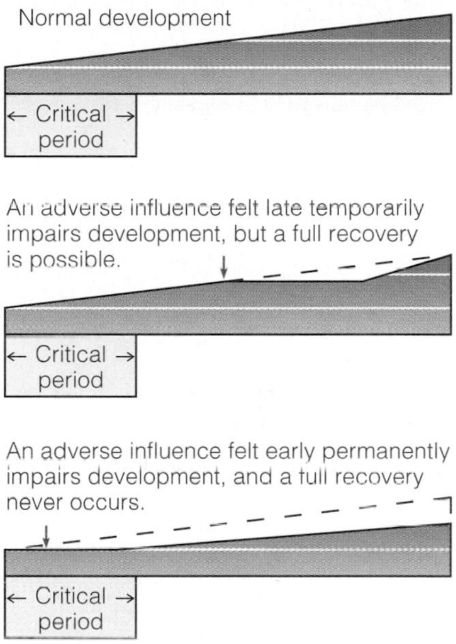
Normal development
← Critical →
period
An adverse influence felt late temporarily impairs development, but a full recovery is possible.
← Critical →
period
An adverse influence felt early permanently impairs development, and a full recovery never occurs.
← Critical →
period

Maternal nutrition before and during pregnancy affects both the mother's health and the infant's growth. As the infant develops through its three stages—the zygote, embryo, and fetus—its organs and tissues grow, each on its own schedule. Times of intense development are critical periods that depend on nutrients to proceed smoothly. Without folate, for example, the neural tube fails to develop completely during the first month of pregnancy, prompting recommendations for all women of childbearing age to take folate daily.

Because critical periods occur throughout pregnancy, a woman should continuously take good care of her health. That care should include, first, achieving and maintaining a healthy body weight and, then, gaining sufficient weight to support a healthy pregnancy.

Maternal Weight

Birthweight is the most reliable indicator of an infant's health. In general, higher birthweights present lower risks for infants. Two characteristics of the mother's weight influence an infant's birthweight: her weight for height prior to conception and her weight gain during pregnancy.

WEIGHT FOR HEIGHT PRIOR TO CONCEPTION

A woman's weight for height prior to conception influences fetal growth. Even with the same weight gain during pregnancy, underweight women tend to have smaller babies than heavier women.

Underweight An underweight woman has a high risk of having a low-birthweight infant, especially if she is unable to gain sufficient weight during pregnancy. In addition, the rates of preterm births and infant mortality are higher for underweight women. An underweight woman improves her chances of having a healthy infant by gaining sufficient weight prior to conception or by gaining extra pounds during pregnancy. To increase food energy intake, an underweight woman can follow the dietary recommendations for pregnant women (described in Table 15–3 on p. 556).

Underweight is defined as BMI <19.8.

preterm (infant)**:** an infant born prior to the 38th week of pregnancy; also called a **premature** infant. A **term** infant is born between the 38th and 42nd week of pregnancy.

Overweight is defined as BMI >26.0 to 29.0, which corresponds with 20% over the reference weight in standard weight-for-height tables. Obese is defined as BMI >29.0.

cesarean section: a surgically assisted birth involving removal of the fetus by an incision into the uterus, usually by way of the abdominal wall.

post term (infant): an infant born after the 42nd week of pregnancy.

Overweight Like underweight women, overweight women face problems related to pregnancy and childbirth. Overweight women face an especially high risk of medical complications such as hypertension, gestational diabetes, and postpartum infections. Compared with other women, overweight women are also more likely to require induced labor and cesarean section.

Infants of overweight women are likely to be born post term and to weigh more than 9 pounds. Overweight women are unlikely to have premature infants, but if they do, the infants may be large for their gestational age. Weight-loss dieting during pregnancy is never advisable, however. An overweight woman should try to achieve a healthy body weight before becoming pregnant, avoid excessive weight gain during pregnancy, and postpone weight loss until after childbirth. Weight loss is best achieved by eating moderate amounts of nutritious foods and exercising to lose body fat.

WEIGHT GAIN AND EXERCISE DURING PREGNANCY

All women must gain weight during pregnancy—fetal growth and maternal health depend on it. Maternal weight gain during pregnancy correlates closely with infant birthweight, and as mentioned earlier, infant birthweight is a strong predictor of the health and subsequent development of the infant.

Weight-gain recommendations:

- Underweight women: 28 to 40 lb (12.5 to 18 kg).
- Normal-weight women: 25 to 35 lb (11.5 to 16 kg).
- Overweight women: 15 to 25 lb (7 to 11.5 kg).
- Obese women: 13 lb minimum (6 kg minimum).

Note: Underweight is defined as BMI <19.8; normal weight, as BMI 19.8 to 26.0; overweight as BMI 26.0 to 29.0; and obese as BMI >29.0.

Recommended Weight Gains The recommended gain for a woman who begins pregnancy at a healthy weight and is carrying a single fetus is 25 to 35 pounds.[3] An underweight woman needs to gain between 28 and 40 pounds; and an overweight woman, between 15 and 25 pounds. Some women should strive for gains at the upper end of the target range, notably, adolescents who are still growing themselves. Short women (5 feet 2 inches and under) should strive for gains at the lower end of the target range. Women who are carrying twins should aim for a weight gain of 35 to 45 pounds. For the normal-weight woman, weight gain ideally follows a pattern of about 5 pounds during the first trimester, and about 1 pound per week thereafter. Health care professionals monitor weight gain using charts; Appendix E presents one example.

If a woman gains more than is recommended early in pregnancy, she should not restrict her energy intake later in order to lose weight. To be a little overweight is healthier than to be underweight. A sudden large weight gain, however, may be the first sign of preeclampsia, a serious medical complication discussed later.

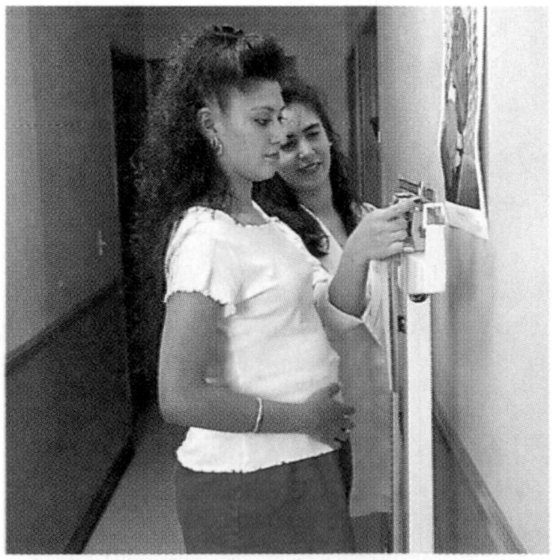

Fetal growth and maternal health depend on a sufficient weight gain during pregnancy.

Components of Weight Gain Women often express concern about the weight gain that accompanies a healthy pregnancy. They may find comfort in a reminder that most of the gain supports the growth and development of the placenta, uterus, blood, and breasts, as well as an optimally healthy 7½-pound infant. A small amount goes into maternal fat stores, and even that fat is there for a special purpose: to provide energy for labor and lactation. Table 15–1 shows the components of a typical 30-pound weight gain.

Weight Loss after Pregnancy The pregnant woman loses some of the weight at delivery. In the following weeks, she loses more as her blood volume returns to normal and she sheds accumulated fluids. The typical woman does not, however, return to her prepregnancy weight. In general, the more weight a woman gains beyond what she needs for pregnancy, the more she will retain.

Table 15–1

Components of Weight Gain during Pregnancy

Development	Weight Gain (lb)
Infant at birth	7½
Placenta	1½
Increase in mother's blood volume to supply placenta	4
Increase in mother's fluid volume	4
Increase in size of uterus and supporting muscles	2
Increase in size of mother's breasts	2
Fluid to surround infant in amniotic sac	2
Mother's fat stores	7
Total	30

Source: ACOG *Guide to Planning for Pregnancy, Birth, and Beyond* (Washington, D.C.: The American College of Obstetricians and Gynecologists, 1990), p. 109.

Even with an average weight gain, though, most women tend to retain a couple of pounds with each pregnancy.[4]

Exercise The active, physically fit woman experiencing a normal pregnancy can continue to exercise throughout pregnancy, adjusting the duration and intensity as the pregnancy progresses. Staying active can improve fitness, prevent gestational diabetes, facilitate labor, and reduce stress.[5] It also maintains the habits that help a woman lose excess weight and get back into shape after the birth. A pregnant woman should avoid sports in which she might fall or be hit by other people or objects. For example, playing tennis with one person on each side of the net is safer than a fast-moving game of racquetball in which the two competitors can collide. Swimming is ideal because it allows the body to remain cool and move freely with the water's support. Table 15–2 provides some guidelines for exercise during pregnancy. Several of the guidelines listed are aimed at

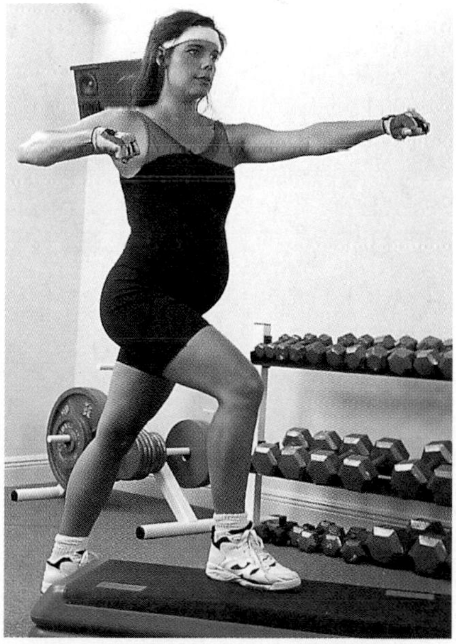

Pregnant women can enjoy the benefits of exercise.

Table 15–2

Exercise Guidelines for Pregnancy

- Limit strenuous activity to 15 minutes or less.
- Stop exercising if you feel overheated.
- Drink plenty of fluids before and after exercise.
- Avoid exercising in hot, humid weather; avoid overheating.
- Protect the abdomen from injury, especially in games like baseball or basketball in which accidents are likely.
- Discontinue any exercise that causes discomfort.
- Do not exercise while lying on your back after about the fourth month.
- Do not allow your heart rate to exceed 140 beats per minute.
- Eat enough to support the additional needs of pregnancy plus exercise.

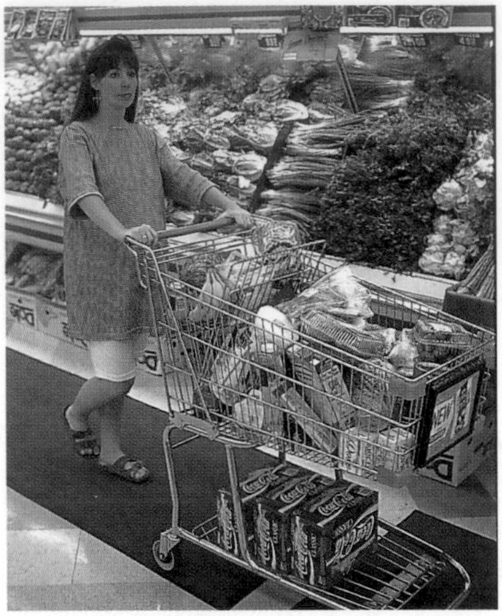

A pregnant woman's nutrition choices support both her health and her infant's growth and development.

preventing excessively high internal body temperature and dehydration, both of which can harm fetal development. To this end, pregnant women should also stay out of saunas, steam rooms, and hot whirlpools.

A healthy pregnancy depends on a sufficient weight gain. Women who begin their pregnancies at a healthy weight need to gain about 30 pounds, which covers the growth and development of the placenta, uterus, blood, breasts, and infant.

Nutrition during Pregnancy

A woman's body changes dramatically during pregnancy. Her blood volume expands; her uterus and its supporting muscles increase in size and strength; her joints become more flexible in preparation for childbirth; her feet swell in response to high concentrations of the hormone estrogen, which promotes water retention and helps to ready the uterus for delivery; and her breasts grow in preparation for lactation. The hormones that mediate all these changes may influence her mood. She can best prepare to handle these changes given a nutritious diet, regular physical activity, plenty of rest, and caring companions. This section highlights the role of nutrition.

ENERGY AND NUTRIENT NEEDS DURING PREGNANCY

From conception to birth, all parts of the infant—bones, muscles, organs, blood cells, skin, and other tissues—are made of nutrients from maternal stores and diet. For most women, nutrients needs during pregnancy and lactation are higher than at any other time (see Figure 15–4).

Energy RDA during pregnancy (2nd and 3rd trimesters):
+300 kcal/day.
Canadian RNI during pregnancy:
+100 to 300 kcal/day.*

Energy Nutrients A pregnant woman needs extra food energy, but only a little extra—300 kcalories above the allowance for nonpregnant women—and only during the second and third trimesters. A woman can easily get 300 kcalories by taking just one extra serving from each of the five food groups—a slice of bread, a serving of vegetables, an ounce of lean meat, a piece of fruit, and a cup of nonfat milk (see Table 15–3 on p. 556). Pregnant teenagers, underweight women, and exceptionally active women may require more.

For women of average size and moderate physical activity, 300 kcalories represent only 15 percent more food energy than before pregnancy. Nutrient needs expand more than this, however, so nutrient-dense foods should supply the 300 kcalories: foods such as nonfat milk; lean meats, fish, and poultry; eggs; legumes; dark green vegetables; citrus fruits; and whole-grain breads and cereals. Ample carbohydrate is needed to spare the protein for growth.

Protein RDA during pregnancy:
+10 g/day.
Canadian RNI during pregnancy:
+5 to 24/g day.†

Protein The RDA for pregnancy is 10 grams per day higher than for nonpregnant women. Because people in the United States typically exceed the RDA, most women need not add the full 10 grams to their diets. In fact, preg-

*For all Canadian RNI values during pregnancy, the lower value indicates recommendations for the first trimester, and the higher value indicates those for the second and third trimesters.

†For the first trimester, the RNI is an additional 5 grams/day; for the second trimester, it is an additional 20 grams/day; and for the third trimester, it is 24 grams/day.

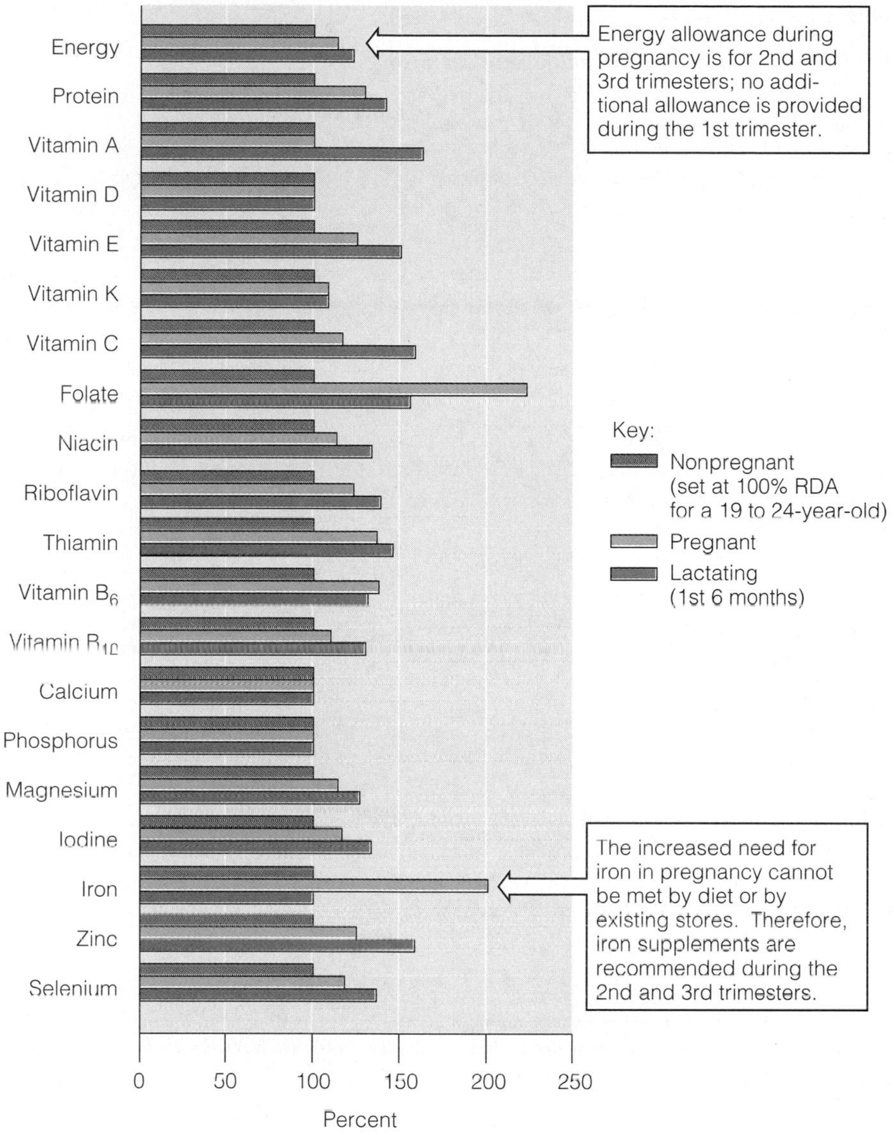

Figure 15–4

Comparison of Nutrient RDA of Nonpregnant, Pregnant, and Lactating Women

The RDA for pregnant and lactating women are not specific to age, as they are for nonpregnant women. This figure uses women aged 19 to 24 as the nonpregnant standard. For several of the nutrients, the RDA do not differ during the childbearing years of 15 to 50. For a few, however, they do, and it is important to note that:

- For protein and vitamin K, the RDA increase slightly with age, so increased needs during pregnancy are more dramatic for women in the younger age groups.
- For vitamin D, calcium, and phosphorus, the RDA decrease at 25 years, so increased needs during pregnancy are more dramatic for women over 25.

For actual values, turn to the RDA table, inside front cover, left.

nant women in the United States—even those with low incomes who are not participating in food assistance programs—generally receive between 75 and 110 grams of protein a day.[6] Pregnant vegetarian women who meet their energy needs by eating ample servings of protein-containing plant foods such as legumes, whole grains, nuts, and seeds meet their protein needs as well. Use of high-protein supplements during pregnancy can be harmful and is discouraged.

B Vitamins Associated with Energy Intake Extra B vitamins are needed in proportion to the increase in energy requirements. The Committee on Dietary Allowances recommends a slight increase above the nonpregnant woman's RDA for thiamin, riboflavin, and niacin. The usual intake of these nutrients is adequate for most pregnant women in the United States.

Thiamin RDA during pregnancy:
1.5 mg/day.
Canadian RNI during pregnancy:
+0.1 mg/day.

Riboflavin RDA during pregnancy:
1.6 mg/day.
Canadian RNI during pregnancy:
+0.1 to 0.3 mg/day

Niacin RDA during pregnancy:
17 mg NE/day.
Canadian RNI during pregnancy:
+1 to 2 NE/day.

Table 15–3

Daily Food Choices for Pregnant and Lactating Women

Food Group	Number of Servings	
	ADULT	PREGNANT OR LACTATING WOMEN
Breads/cereals	6 to 11	7 to 11
Vegetables	3 to 5	4 to 5
Fruits	2 to 4	3 to 4
Meat/meat alternatives	2 to 3	3
Milk/milk products	2	3 to 4

This sample meal plan follows the Daily Food Guide for pregnant and lactating women and provides about 2500 kcalories (50% from carbohydrate, 20% from protein, and 30% from fat).

Breakfast
2 medium bran muffins
2 tsp butter or margarine
1 c vanilla yogurt
½ c fresh strawberries
1 c orange juice

Midmorning snack
1 medium apple

Lunch
Sandwich (2 oz ham, 1 oz swiss cheese, 2 slices rye bread, 2 tsp mayonnaise, lettuce)
1¼ c salad (lettuce, tomatoes, carrots)
1 tbs salad dressing
1 c low-fat milk

Dinner
Chicken cacciatore
  4 oz chicken
  ¾ c stewed tomatoes
1 c rice
¾ c summer squash
1½ c salad (spinach, mushrooms, onions)
1 tbs salad dressing
2 slices Italian bread
2 tsp butter or margarine
1 c low-fat milk

Evening snack
1 c low-fat milk
3 oatmeal cookies

Note: Figure 2–1 in Chapter 2 provides a detailed summary of the Daily Food Guide.

Vitamin B_6 RDA during pregnancy: 2.2 mg/day.
Canadian RNI during pregnancy: 0.015 mg/g dietary protein.

Folate RDA during pregnancy: 400 μg/day.
Canadian RNI during pregnancy: +200 μg/day.

Vitamin B_{12} RDA during pregnancy: 2.2 μg/day.
Canadian RNI during pregnancy: +0.2 μg/day.

Vitamin B_6 Associated with Protein Intake Vitamin B_6 recommendations rise in parallel with protein recommendations. The RDA provides enough additional vitamin B_6 to cover the protein recommendation.

Folate and Vitamin B_{12} for Blood Production and Cell Growth New cells are laid down at a tremendous pace as the fetus grows and develops. At the same time, the mother's red blood cell mass expands, so the RDA for folate more than doubles during pregnancy. It is possible to obtain sufficient folate, without supplements, from a diet that includes fruits, juices, green vegetables, and whole-grain or fortified cereals. When dietary folate is inadequate, daily supplementation is recommended.

The pregnant woman also has a slightly greater need for the B vitamin that activates folate—vitamin B_{12}. Generally, even modest amounts of meat, fish, eggs, or milk products together with body stores easily meet the need for vitamin B_{12}. Strict vegetarians who exclude all foods of animal origin, however, may need daily supplements to prevent deficiency.

Vitamin D and Calcium for Bone Development Vitamin D and the bone-building minerals calcium, phosphorus, and magnesium are in great demand during pregnancy. Insufficient intakes may produce abnormal fetal bones and teeth.

Vitamin D plays a vital role in calcium absorption and utilization. Consequently, maternal vitamin D deficiency is associated with underdeveloped tooth enamel in the fetus and osteomalacia in the mother. Exposure to sunlight and vitamin D–fortified milk is usually sufficient to provide the recommended amount of vitamin D during pregnancy. Routine supplementation is not recommended because of the toxicity risk. Vegetarians who avoid milk, eggs, and fish may receive enough vitamin D from daily exposure to sunlight or from fortified soy milk.

Reminder: *Osteomalacia* is the vitamin D–deficiency disease characterized by softening of the bones.

Vitamin D RDA during pregnancy: 10 μg/day.
Canadian RNI during pregnancy: +2.5 μg/day.

Calcium absorption more than doubles early in pregnancy, and the mother's bones store the mineral. Calcium added to the mother's bones early in pregnancy is withdrawn to provide sufficient calcium to the fetus later in gestation.[7] During the last trimester, as the fetal bones begin to calcify, a dramatic shift of calcium across the placenta occurs. In the final weeks of pregnancy, over 300 milligrams are transferred to the fetus every day. Increasing calcium intake during pregnancy helps conserve maternal bone while meeting fetal needs.

Most pregnant women drink more milk than other women, but still their calcium intakes typically fall below the RDA. Because a woman under 25 may still be actively depositing minerals in her own bones, adequate calcium is especially important for young women. Pregnant women under age 25 who receive less than 600 milligrams of dietary calcium daily need to increase their consumption of milk, cheese, yogurt, and other calcium-rich foods. Alternatively, and less preferably, they may need a daily supplement of 600 milligrams of calcium.[8]

Calcium RDA during pregnancy: 1200 mg/day.
Canadian RNI during pregnancy: +500 mg/day.

HEALTHY PEOPLE 2000: Increase calcium intake so at least 50% of pregnant and lactating women consume three or more servings daily of foods rich in calcium.

Iron The body makes several adaptations to help meet iron needs during pregnancy. Menstruation, the major route of iron loss in women, ceases, and iron absorption nearly triples due to a rise in blood transferrin, the body's iron-absorbing and iron-carrying protein. Still, iron stores dwindle during pregnancy.

A pregnant woman needs iron to support her enlarged blood volume and to provide for placental and fetal needs. The developing fetus draws on maternal iron stores to create stores of its own to last through the first four to six months after birth when iron-poor milk will be its sole food. Also, the blood losses inevitable at birth, especially a cesarean delivery, can drain the mother's supply.*

Iron RDA during pregnancy: 30 mg/day.
Canadian RNI during pregnancy: +0 to 10 mg/day.

Few women enter pregnancy with adequate iron stores, so a daily iron supplement is recommended during the second and third trimesters for all pregnant women.[9] To enhance absorption, the supplement should be taken between meals or at bedtime on an empty stomach and with liquids other than milk, coffee, or tea, which inhibit iron absorption.[10]

*The average blood loss during a cesarean delivery is almost twice that occurring during the average vaginal delivery of a single fetus.

Zinc RDA during pregnancy: 15 mg/day.
Canadian RNI during pregnancy: +6 mg/day.

Table 15–4

Nutrient Supplements during Pregnancy[a]

Nutrient	Amount
Folate	300 µg
Vitamin B_6	2 mg
Vitamin C	50 mg
Vitamin D	5 µg
Calcium	250 mg
Copper	2 mg
Iron	30 mg
Zinc	15 mg

[a]For pregnant women at nutritional risk (see Table 15–5).

Source: Reprinted with permission from *Nutrition during Pregnancy* © by the National Academy of Sciences. Published by the National Academy Press, Washington, D.C., 1990.

To alleviate the nausea of pregnancy:
- On waking, arise slowly.
- Eat dry toast or crackers.
- Chew gum or suck hard candies.
- Eat small, frequent meals.
- Avoid foods with offensive odors.
- When nauseated, drink no citrus juice, water, milk, coffee, or tea.

To prevent or alleviate constipation:
- Eat foods high in fiber.
- Exercise daily.
- Drink at least 8 glasses of liquids a day.
- Respond promptly to the urge to defecate.
- Use laxatives only as prescribed by a physician; do not use mineral oil because it impairs fat-soluble vitamin absorption.

To prevent or relieve heartburn:
- Eat small, frequent meals.
- Drink liquids between meals.
- Avoid spicy or greasy foods.
- Sit up while eating.
- Wait an hour after eating before lying down.
- Wait 2 hours after eating before exercising.

Zinc Zinc is required for DNA and RNA synthesis and thus for protein synthesis and cell development. Low blood zinc is a significant predictor of low birthweight.[11] The zinc recommendation for pregnant women is slightly higher than for nonpregnant women. Typical zinc intakes are lower than recommendations, but routine supplementation is not advised.[12] Large doses of iron interfere with the body's absorption and use of zinc, so women taking iron supplements (more than 30 milligrams per day) may need zinc supplementation.

Nutrient Supplements A balanced diet can meet most of a pregnant woman's nutrient needs, except for iron. As mentioned, iron supplements (30 milligrams per day) are recommended during the second and third trimesters of pregnancy. Daily multivitamin-mineral supplements are recommended for women who do not eat adequately and for those in high-risk groups: women carrying multiple fetuses, cigarette smokers, and alcohol and drug abusers. Table 15–4 lists recommended amounts for supplements.

The nutrients mentioned earlier are those most intensely involved in blood production, cell growth, and bone growth. Of course, other nutrients are also needed during pregnancy. Without adequate nutrient and energy intakes, the growth and health of both fetus and mother may be compromised. Even with adequate nutrition, repeated pregnancies less than a year apart deplete nutrient reserves: fetal growth may be protected, but maternal health may decline.[13]

COMMON NUTRITION-RELATED CONCERNS OF PREGNANCY

Nausea, constipation, heartburn, and food sensitivities are common nutrition-related concerns during pregnancy. A few simple strategies can help avert them.

Nausea Many women have uneasy stomachs in the early months of pregnancy. The nausea of "morning" (actually, anytime) sickness ranges from mild queasiness to debilitating nausea and vomiting. The hormonal changes of early pregnancy seem to be responsible for a woman's sensitivities to a food's appearance, texture, or smell. Traditional strategies for quelling nausea are listed in the margin, but some women benefit most from simply eating the foods they want when they feel like eating.[14]

Constipation and Hemorrhoids As the hormones of pregnancy alter muscle tone and the growing infant crowds intestinal organs, an expectant mother may experience constipation. She may also develop hemorrhoids (swollen veins of the anus and rectum). These can be painful, and straining during bowel movements makes them worse. She can gain relief by following the strategies listed in the margin.

Heartburn Heartburn is another common complaint during pregnancy. As the growing fetus puts increasing pressure on a woman's stomach, acid may back up and create a burning sensation in the lower esophagus near the heart. Tips to help relieve heartburn are listed in the margin.

Food Cravings and Aversions Some women develop cravings for, or aversions to, some foods and beverages during pregnancy. These cravings do not seem to reflect real physiological needs. A woman who craves pickles does not necessarily need salt, nor does a woman who craves chocolate need caffeine or fat. Cravings for ice cream are common in pregnancy, but do not signify calcium deficiencies. Food cravings and aversions that arise during pregnancy are probably due to hormone-induced changes in sensitivity to taste and smell.

food craving: a deep longing for a particular food.

food aversion: a strong desire to avoid a particular food.

Reminder: The craving for a nonfood item such as clay, ice, and cornstarch is known as *pica*.

In summary, energy and nutrient needs are high during pregnancy. A balanced diet that includes an extra serving from each of the five food groups can usually meet these needs, with the exception of iron (supplements are recommended). The nausea, constipation, and heartburn that sometimes accompany pregnancy can usually be averted with a few simple strategies; food cravings do not typically reflect physiological needs.

High-Risk and Low-Risk Pregnancies

high-risk pregnancy: a pregnancy characterized by indicators that make it likely the birth will be surrounded by problems such as premature delivery, difficult birth, retarded growth, birth defects, and early infant death.

Some pregnancies are risky to the life and health of the mother and baby. Table 15–5 identifies several characteristics of "high-risk" pregnancies. A woman with

Table 15–5

High-Risk Pregnancy Factors

Factor	Condition That Raises Risk
Maternal weight	
Prior to pregnancy	Prepregnancy weight either more than 10% underweight or 20% overweight compared with standard weight-for-height tables
During pregnancy	Insufficient or excessive pregnancy weight gain
Maternal nutrition	Nutrient deficiencies or toxicities; eating disorders
Socioeconomic status	Poverty, lack of family support, low level of education, limited food available
Lifestyle habits	Smoking, alcohol or other drug use
Age[a]	Teenage, especially 15 years or younger
Previous pregnancies	
Number	Many previous pregnancies
Interval	Short intervals between pregnancies
Outcomes	Previous history of problems
Multiple births	Twins or triplets
Birthweight	Low- or high-birthweight infants
Maternal health	
High blood pressure	Development of pregnancy-related hypertension
Diabetes	Development of gestational diabetes
Chronic diseases	Diabetes; heart, respiratory, and kidney disease; certain genetic disorders; special diets and drugs

[a]Over the past several decades, many women have intentionally postponed pregnancy. First births to mothers aged 30 and older have increased, but total births to women in this age group have declined. Older women face fewer risks today than in the past, thanks to generally higher socioeconomic status and better medical care.

Food Assistance Programs for Pregnant Women, Infants, and Children

WIC (the Special Supplemental Food Program for Women, Infants, and Children) provides nutrition education and nutritious foods to low-income pregnant women and their children. WIC provides eggs, milk, cereal, juice, cheese, legumes, peanut butter, and infant formula to infants, children up to age five, and pregnant and breastfeeding women who qualify financially and are at medical or nutritional risk. The program is both remedial and preventive: services include health care referrals, nutrition education, and food packages or vouchers for specific foods to supply nutrients known to be lacking in the diets of the target population. Prenatal WIC participation can effectively reduce low birthweight and newborn medical cost.[a] For every dollar spent on WIC, an estimated three dollars are saved. In 1992, participation in WIC reduced first-year medical expenses for infants by $1.19 billion.[b]

[a] P. A. Buescher and coauthors, Prenatal WIC participation can reduce low birth weight and newborn medical costs: A cost-benefit analysis of WIC participation in North Carolina, *Journal of the American Dietetic Association* 93 (1993): 163–166.

[b] S. Avruch and A. P. Cackley, Savings achieved by giving WIC benefits to women prenatally, *Public Health Reports* 110 (1995): 27–34.

Currently, the U.S. Department of Agriculture (USDA) funds WIC, and state health departments administer the program. As congress considers various cost-cutting measures, this arrangement may be revised.

low-risk pregnancy: a pregnancy characterized by indicators that make a normal outcome likely.

none of these risk factors is said to have a low-risk pregnancy. The more factors that apply, the higher the risk. High-risk pregnancies need special management, including intervention to correct malnutrition. The accompanying box describes government efforts to provide assistance to pregnant women in the United States.

MALNUTRITION AND PREGNANCY

Good nutrition clearly supports a pregnancy. In contrast, malnutrition interferes with the ability to conceive, the likelihood of implantation, and the subsequent development of a fetus should these events occur.

fertility: the capacity of a woman to produce a normal ovum periodically and of a man to produce normal sperm; the ability to reproduce.

Malnutrition and Fertility The nutrition habits and lifestyle choices people make can influence the course of a pregnancy they are not even planning at the time. Malnutrition and food deprivation can reduce fertility: women may develop amenorrhea, and men may lose their ability to produce viable sperm. Furthermore, men and women lose their interest in sex during times of starvation. Starvation arises predictably during famines, wars, and droughts, but can also occur amidst peace and plenty. Many women who diet excessively and exercise intensely are starving and amenorrheic.

Reminder: Women who are *amenorrheic* have a temporary or permanent absence of menstrual periods. Amenorrhea is normal before puberty, after menopause, during pregnancy, and during lactation; otherwise it is abnormal.

Malnutrition and Early Pregnancy If a malnourished woman does become pregnant, she faces the challenge of supporting both the growth of a baby and her own health with inadequate nutrient stores. Malnutrition prior to and around conception prevents the placenta from developing fully.[15] A poorly developed placenta cannot deliver optimum nourishment to the fetus, and the infant will be born small and possibly with physical and cognitive abnormalities. If this small infant is a female, she may develop poorly and in turn will have an elevated risk of having a poor pregnancy outcome. Thus a woman's malnutrition during or even before her pregnancy can adversely affect not only her children but her *grandchildren*.

Malnutrition and Fetal Development Without adequate nutrition during pregnancy, fetal growth and infant health are compromised. In general, consequences of malnutrition during pregnancy include:

- Fetal growth retardation.
- Congenital malformations (birth defects).
- Spontaneous abortion and stillbirth.
- Premature birth.
- Low infant birthweight.

Of these, birthweight is most frequently used as a predictor of an infant's survival and health. Malnutrition coupled with low birthweight contributes to more than half of all deaths of children under five worldwide.

THE INFANT'S BIRTHWEIGHT

The most common outcome of a high-risk pregnancy is low birthweight. Low-birthweight infants, defined as infants who weigh 5½ pounds or less, are classified according to gestational age. Preterm, or premature, infants are born before they are fully developed; they are often underweight and have trouble breathing because their lungs are immature. Preterm infants may be small, but if their size and weight are appropriate for their age, they can catch up in growth given adequate nutrition support. In contrast, small-for-gestational-age infants have suffered growth failure in the uterus and do not catch up as well. For the most part, survival improves with increased gestational age and birthweight.[16]

Low-birthweight infants are more likely to experience complications during delivery than normal-weight babies. They also have a statistically greater chance of having physical and mental birth defects, contracting diseases, and dying early in life. Of infants who die before their first birthdays, about two-thirds are low-birthweight babies.

A strong relationship has been established between socioeconomic disadvantage and low birthweight. Low socioeconomic status impairs fetal development by causing stress and by limiting access to medical care and to nutritious foods. Low socioeconomic status often accompanies teen pregnancies, smoking, and alcohol and drug abuse—all predicators of low birthweight.

low birthweight (LBW): a birthweight of 5½ lb (2500 g) or less; indicates probable poor health in the newborn and poor nutrition status in the mother during pregnancy, before pregnancy, or both. Normal birthweight for a full-term baby is 6½ to 8¾ lb (about 3000 to 4000 g).

Some preterm infants are of a weight **appropriate for gestational age (AGA)**; others are **small for gestational age (SGA)**, often reflecting malnutrition. The latter type are also called **small-for-date** babies.

THE MOTHER'S HEALTH STATUS

Normal weight gain and adequate nutrition support the health of the mother and growth of the infant. Conversely, maternal diseases detract from growth and health. If discovered early, many diseases can be controlled—another reason early prenatal care is recommended.

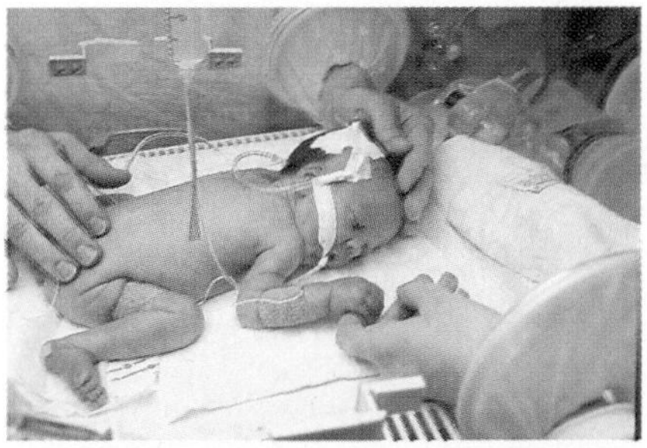

Low-birthweight babies need special care and nourishment.

Preexisting Diabetes The extent to which diabetes presents risks depends on how well it is controlled before and during pregnancy. Without proper management, women with diabetes face an exceptionally high infertility rate, and those who do conceive may experience episodes of severe hypoglycemia or hyperglycemia, spontaneous abortions, and pregnancy-related hypertension. Ideally, a woman with diabetes will have it under control before becoming pregnant and will be able to maintain glucose control throughout pregnancy.

gestational diabetes: the appearance of abnormal glucose tolerance during pregnancy, with subsequent return to normal postpartum.

Risk factors for gestational diabetes:
- Previous gestational diabetes.
- History of large infants (9 pounds or more).
- Age 30 or older.
- Obesity or excessive weight gain.
- Complications in previous pregnancies.
- Symptoms of diabetes.
- Family history of diabetes.

Gestational Diabetes Placental hormones elevate blood insulin and alter insulin resistance during pregnancy. In some women, this can precipitate a condition known as gestational diabetes. Gestational diabetes usually develops late in pregnancy, with subsequent return to normal glucose tolerance after childbirth. In about one-third of such cases, however, women develop diabetes (NIDDM) within five years. To ensure that the problems of gestational diabetes are dealt with promptly, health care professionals look for the risk factors listed in the margin.[17] Gestational diabetes requires dietary management just as other forms of diabetes do. Diet alone may control gestational diabetes, but insulin therapy may be required if blood glucose fails to normalize.

Preexisting Hypertension Hypertension complicates pregnancy. In addition to the threats hypertension always carries (such as heart attack and stroke), high blood pressure raises the risks of having a low-birthweight baby or of having the placenta detach from the wall of the uterus before the birth, resulting in stillbirth. Ideally, before a woman with hypertension becomes pregnant, her blood pressure will be normalized by diet, weight loss, and possibly medication.

Transient Hypertension of Pregnancy Some women first develop hypertension during the second half of pregnancy.* Most often, the rise in blood pressure is mild and does not affect the pregnancy adversely.[18] Blood pressure usually returns to normal during the first few weeks after childbirth. This transient hypertension of pregnancy differs from the pregnancy-induced hypertension that accompanies preeclampsia.†

pregnancy-induced hypertension (PIH): high blood pressure that develops in the second half of pregnancy.

preeclampsia: a condition characterized by hypertension, fluid retention, and protein in the urine.

The normal edema of pregnancy responds to gravity; fluid pools in the ankles. The edema of preeclampsia is a generalized edema. The differences between these two types of edema help with the diagnosis of preeclampsia.

Preeclampsia Hypertension may signal the onset of preeclampsia, a condition characterized not only by high blood pressure but by protein in the urine and fluid retention (edema). Preeclampsia usually occurs with first pregnancies after 20 weeks gestation, most often near term. Symptoms typically regress within two days of delivery. The edema of preeclampsia is a whole-body edema, distinct from the localized fluid retention women normally experience late in pregnancy. Preeclampsia effects almost all of the mother's organs—the circulatory system, liver, kidneys, and brain.

Blood flow through the vessels that supply oxygen and nutrients to the placenta diminishes. For this reason, preeclampsia often retards fetal growth. In some cases, the placenta separates from the uterus, resulting in stillbirth.

---

*Blood pressure of 140/90 millimeters mercury during the second half of pregnancy in a woman who has not previously exhibited hypertension indicates high blood pressure. So does a rise in systolic blood pressure of 30 millimeters or in diastolic blood pressure of 15 millimeters on at least two occasions more than six hours apart. By this rule, an apparently "normal" blood pressure of 120/85 would be high for a woman whose normal value was 90/70.

†The Working Group on High Blood Pressure in Pregnancy, convened by the National High Blood Pressure Education Program of the National Heart, Lung, and Blood Institute, has suggested abandoning the term "pregnancy-induced hypertension" because it fails to differentiate between the mild, transient hypertension of pregnancy and the life-threatening hypertension of preeclampsia.

Preeclampsia can progress rapidly to eclampsia—a condition characterized by convulsions and coma. Maternal mortality during pregnancy and childbirth is extremely rare in developed countries, but eclampsia is a common cause.

Preeclampsia demands prompt medical attention. Treatment focuses on regulating blood pressure and preventing convulsions. If preeclampsia develops early and is severe, induced labor or cesarean birth may be necessary. The infant will be preterm, with all of the associated problems, including poor lung development, and will need special care.

Several approaches have been proposed to prevent preeclampsia, including salt restriction, calcium supplementation, and low-dose aspirin therapy. Salt restriction does not improve the incidence or severity of preeclampsia and is not a part of treatment until and unless the kidneys prove unable to handle sodium.

Several studies have reported an inverse relationship between calcium intake and preeclampsia.[19] Furthermore, research has determined that calcium supplementation during pregnancy can lower high blood pressure.[20] In a group of over 1000 pregnant women given either a calcium supplement or a placebo during the second half of pregnancy, the women who received calcium supplements (2000 milligrams per day) had a reduced risk of hypertensive disorders.[21] Such findings are promising, but at this time evidence is insufficient to recommend routine supplementation; furthermore, calcium supplementation may create risks of its own, including the development of kidney stones.[22]

Another promising option is the use of low doses of aspirin (60 to 100 milligrams a day). Low-dose aspirin appears to reduce the incidence of preeclampsia, and some clinicians recommend its use in high-risk pregnancies (women with a history of preeclampsia, fetal death, or placental insufficiency).[23]

eclampsia: a condition characterized by convulsions and coma that develops in some women with untreated preeclampsia.

Warning signs of preeclampsia:
- Hypertension.
- Protein in the urine.
- Upper abdominal pain.
- Severe and constant headaches.
- Swelling, especially of the face.
- Dizziness.
- Blurred vision.
- Sudden weight gain (1 lb/day).

ADOLESCENT PREGNANCY

Most adolescents become sexually active before age 19, and one million adolescent girls face pregnancies each year in the United States. About half of them continue their pregnancies. Put another way, about one out of every five babies is born to a teenager, and more than a tenth of these mothers are 15 or younger. Clearly, teenage pregnancy is a major public health problem. Even when not pregnant, a teenage girl has difficulty meeting her nutrient needs. Nourishing a growing fetus adds to her burden. The competition between maternal and fetal needs places both mother and infant at risk.

Maternal illness is especially common in adolescent pregnancies. The rates of preeclampsia are 50 percent higher in teens than in older women. Other common complications of adolescent pregnancies are iron-deficiency anemia (which may reflect poor diet and inadequate prenatal care) and prolonged labor (which reflects the mother's physical immaturity).

Pregnant teenagers have higher rates of stillbirths, preterm births, and low-birthweight infants than do adult women. Many of these infants suffer physical problems, require intensive care, and die within the first year. Simply being young increases these risks independently of important socioeconomic factors.[24]

The care of infants born to teenagers costs our society an estimated $1 billion annually. Because teenagers have few financial resources, they cannot pay these costs. Furthermore, their low economic status contributes significantly to the complications surrounding their pregnancies. At a time when prenatal care is most important, it is less available.

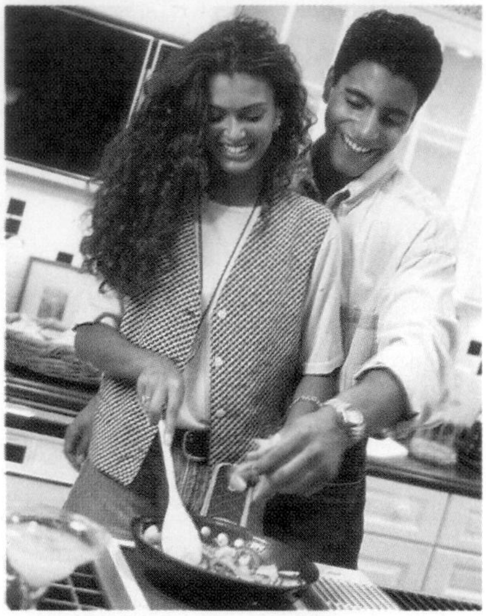

Young adults can prepare themselves for a healthy pregnancy by taking care of themselves today.

In addition to economic factors, psychosocial immaturity often hampers a teenager's ability to care for herself during her pregnancy and for her child after the birth. For those who are physically immature, the complications are even more extensive. Physically immature mothers are still growing; they have high energy and nutrient needs. Furthermore, if they are typical teenagers who depend on fast-food meals, skip meals, and pay little attention to what they eat, they will not have the nutrient stores they need for their own growth plus pregnancy.

To support the needs of both mother and fetus, young teenagers (13 to 16 years old) are encouraged to strive for the highest weight gains recommended for pregnancy. For a teen who enters pregnancy at a healthy body weight, a weight gain of approximately 35 pounds is recommended; this minimizes the risk of delivering a low-birthweight infant.[25] Gaining less may limit fetal growth.[26] Pregnant and lactating teenagers can use the Daily Food Guide presented in Table 15–3 (on p. 556), making sure to select at least 4 servings of milk or milk products daily.

Pregnant adolescents have unique economic, psychosocial, and physical vulnerabilities that jeopardize a healthy pregnancy.[27] To improve their chances for a successful pregnancy and healthy infant, they must seek prenatal care. WIC helps pregnant teenagers obtain adequate food to support a reasonable weight gain.

PRACTICES INCOMPATIBLE WITH PREGNANCY

teratogenic (ter-AT-oh-jen-ik): causing abnormal fetal development and birth defects.
terato = monster
genic = to produce

Fetal alcohol syndrome is the topic of Highlight 15.

Besides malnutrition, which presents many hazards to pregnancy, a variety of lifestyle factors can have adverse impacts; and some may be teratogenic. People who are planning to have children need to know what practices to avoid.

Alcohol Consumption Alcohol consumption during pregnancy can cause irreversible mental and physical retardation of the fetus—fetal alcohol syndrome (FAS). Of the leading causes of mental retardation, FAS is the only one that is totally *preventable*. As a consequence, the surgeon general has issued a statement that pregnant women should drink absolutely no alcohol.

Medicinal Drugs Drugs other than alcohol can also cause complications during pregnancy, problems in labor, and serious birth defects. For these reasons, pregnant women should not take any medicines without consulting their physicians. Drug labels warn: As with any drug, if you are pregnant or nursing a baby, seek the advice of a health professional before using this product. For aspirin and ibuprofen, an additional warning immediately follows: It is especially important not to use aspirin (or ibuprofen) during the last three months of pregnancy unless specifically directed to do so by a doctor because it may cause problems in the unborn child or (excessive bleeding) during delivery.

Fetal effects of abused drugs:

- Amphetamines: Suspected nervous system damage; behavioral abnormalities.
- Barbiturates: Drug withdrawal symptoms in the newborn, lasting up to six months.
- Cocaine (including "crack"): Uncontrolled jerking motions; paralysis; permanent mental and physical damage.
- Marijuana: Short-term irritability at birth.
- Opiates (including heroin): Drug withdrawal symptoms in the newborn; permanent learning disability (attention deficit disorder).

Illicit Drugs The recommendation to avoid drugs during pregnancy includes illicit drugs, of course. Unfortunately, use of illicit drugs, such as cocaine and marijuana, is common among pregnant women. One study of over 700 pregnant women found that 15 percent of them tested positive for illicit drugs—regardless of race or socioeconomic status.[28]

Drugs of abuse, such as cocaine, pass easily through the placenta and impair fetal development.[29] Furthermore, they are responsible for preterm births, low-birthweight infants, and sudden infant deaths.[30] If these newborns survive, their cries and behaviors at birth are abnormal, and their cognitive development later in life is impaired.[31] They may be hypersensitive or underaroused; those who test positive for drugs suffer the greatest effects of toxicity and withdrawal.[32]

Smoking and Chewing Tobacco Smoking and chewing tobacco at any time exerts harmful effects, and pregnancy dramatically magnifies the hazards of these practices. Smoking restricts the blood supply to the growing fetus and so limits oxygen and nutrient delivery and waste removal. Also, smokers tend to eat less nutritious foods during their pregnancies than do nonsmokers, which in turn impairs fetal nutrition.[33]

Of all preventable causes of low birthweight in the United States, smoking has the greatest impact. The more a mother smokes, the smaller her baby will be. Furthermore, smoking causes death in otherwise healthy fetuses and newborns. There is a positive relationship between sudden infant death syndrome (SIDS) and both cigarette smoking during pregnancy and postnatal exposure to passive smoke.[34] Smoking during pregnancy may even harm the intellectual and behavioral development of the child later in life.[35] Infants of mothers who chew tobacco also have lower birthweights and higher rates of fetal deaths than infants born to women who do not use tobacco.

The prevalence of smoking in pregnancy is an estimated 20 percent, with higher rates for unmarried women, teenagers, and those who lack education. A woman who smokes and is considering pregnancy or who is already pregnant should try to quit or at least cut back on the number of cigarettes smoked.

Smoking during pregnancy increases the risk of:
- Fetal growth retardation.
- Low birthweight.
- Complications at birth.
- Mislocation of the placenta.
- Premature separation of the placenta.
- Vaginal bleeding.
- Spontaneous abortion.
- Fetal death.
- SIDS.

sudden infant death syndrome (SIDS): the unexpected and unexplained death of an apparently well infant; the most common cause of death of infants between the second week and the end of the first year of life; also called *crib death*.

Environmental Contaminants Evidence of exposure to environmental contaminants such as lead and mercury has been detected in the amniotic fluid of pregnant women.[36] Infants and young children of these mothers show signs of impaired cognitive development.[37] For this reason, it is particularly important that pregnant women receive foods and beverages grown and prepared in environments free of contamination.

Highlight 19 describes how lead toxicity impairs a child's development.

Vitamin-Mineral Megadoses The pregnant woman who is trying to eat well may mistakenly assume that more is better when it comes to vitamin-mineral supplements. This is simply not true; many vitamins are toxic when taken in excess, and the minerals are even more so, some at levels not far above recommendations. A pregnant woman can obtain most of the vitamins and minerals she needs by eating whole foods and should take supplements only on the advice of a registered dietitian or physician.

Caffeine Pregnant women may wonder whether they should give up coffee, tea, and colas because of their caffeine contents. Research studies have not proven that caffeine (even in high doses) causes birth defects in human babies (as it does in animal studies), but limited evidence suggests that moderate-to-heavy use may lower infant birthweight.[38] All things considered, it might be most sensible to limit caffeine consumption to the equivalent of a cup of coffee or two 12-ounce cola beverages a day.

Weight-Loss Dieting Weight-loss dieting, even for short periods, is hazardous during pregnancy. Low-carbohydrate diets or fasts that cause ketosis deprive the fetal brain of needed glucose and may impair its development. Such diets are also likely to lack other nutrients vital to fetal growth. Regardless of prepregnancy weight, pregnant women should never intentionally lose weight.

Sugar Substitutes Artificial sweeteners have been extensively investigated and found to be safe for use during pregnancy.[39] (Women with phenylketonuria should not use aspartame, as Highlight 4 explains.) It would be prudent for pregnant women to use sweeteners in moderation and within an otherwise nutritious and well-balanced diet.

To recap, high-risk pregnancies, especially for teenagers, threaten the life and health of both mother and infant. Proper nutrition and abstinence from smoking, alcohol, and other drugs improve the outcome. In addition, prenatal care includes monitoring pregnant women for gestational diabetes and preeclampsia.

Nutrition during Lactation

For infants, breastfeeding:

- Prevents a variety of infections.
- Protects against some chronic diseases, such as NIDDM.
- Makes food allergies less likely.

For mothers, breastfeeding:

- Contracts the uterus.
- Lengthens birth intervals.
- Conserves iron stores (amenorrhea).
- Reduces risk of breast cancer.
- Protects bone density.
- Saves money and offers convenience.

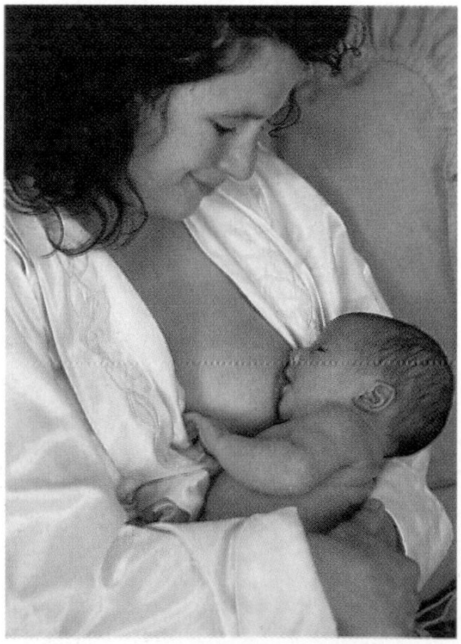

Breastfeeding is a natural extension of pregnancy—of the mother's body nourishing the infant.

Before the end of her pregnancy, a woman will need to consider whether to feed her infant breast milk, infant formula, or both. These options are the only recommended foods for an infant during the first four to six months of life.

HEALTHY PEOPLE 2000: Increase to at least 75% the proportion of mothers who breastfeed their babies in the early weeks and to at least 50% the proportion who continue breastfeeding until their babies are five to six months old.

Breastfeeding offers many benefits to both mother and infant, and every pregnant woman should seriously consider it. Still, there are valid reasons for not breastfeeding, and formula-fed infants grow and develop into healthy children. After all, the primary goal is to provide the infant with optimal nourishment in a relaxed and loving environment.

BREASTFEEDING: A LEARNED BEHAVIOR

In many countries around the world, a woman breastfeeds her newborn without considering the alternatives or consciously making a decision. In other parts of the world, a woman feeds her newborn formula simply because she knows so little about breastfeeding. She may have misconceptions or feel uncomfortable about a process she has never seen or experienced.

Although lactation is an automatic physiological process, breastfeeding is a learned behavior that is most successful in a supportive environment. Health care professionals play an important role in providing encouragement and accurate information on breastfeeding. Of women who do breastfeed, 25 to 50 percent stop within the first month, and 50 to 70 percent stop by four months; those who receive early and repeated information and support breastfeed their infants longer than other breastfeeding women.

Fathers also play an important role in encouraging breastfeeding.[40] One study reported that most of those fathers whose partners planned to breastfeed supported that decision and respected breastfeeding women. By comparison, those whose partners planned to bottle feed believed that breastfeeding would make the breasts ugly and interfere with sex. Clearly, educating fathers could change attitudes and promote breastfeeding.

In societies where few women breastfeed, appropriate breastfeeding etiquette remains undefined. A woman faces conflict, confusion, and frustration. Must she retreat to a private place to nurse? What if she cannot find such a place in a public setting? A hungry infant is impatient, and a mother must act quickly. With abundant role models, a consensus defines accepted behaviors, thus offering a nursing mother guidance and confidence. Many public buildings now provide "baby rooms" with tables for changing diapers and comfortable chairs for nursing.

Parents in today's society also have to coordinate work and family. All mothers are working women—many of them with jobs outside the home. A social system that provides extended, paid maternity leaves, breaks on the job to nurse infants or pump breasts, and job-site child care promotes breastfeeding as a feasible option.

Most healthy women who want to breastfeed can do so with a little preparation; physical obstacles to breastfeeding are rare. Successful breastfeeding requires adequate nutrition and rest. This, plus the support of all who care, will help to enhance the well-being of mother and infant.

To learn about breastfeeding, a pregnant woman can read at least one of the many books available. Appendix F provides a list of other nutrition resources.

THE MOTHER'S NUTRIENT NEEDS

By continuing to eat nutrient-dense foods throughout lactation, the mother who chooses to breastfeed her infant will be nutritionally prepared to do so. An adequate diet is needed to support the stamina, patience, and self-confidence that nursing an infant demands.

lactation: production and secretion of breast milk for the purpose of nourishing an infant.

Energy Intake and Exercise A nursing mother produces about 25 ounces of milk a day, with considerable variation from woman to woman and in the same woman from time to time, depending primarily on the infant's demand for milk.[11] To produce milk, a woman needs extra food energy–almost 650 kcalories a day above her regular need during the first six months of lactation. To meet this energy need, the woman is advised to eat an extra 500 kcalories of food each day and let the fat reserves she accumulated during pregnancy provide the rest. Some research suggests that many women need less energy for milk production; other research findings confirm current recommendations.[42] Severe energy restriction, however, hinders milk production.

Energy RDA during lactation:
+500 kcal/day (1800 kcal/day minimum).
Canadian RNI during lactation:
+450 kcal/day.

After the birth of the infant, many women are in a hurry to lose the extra body fat they accumulated during pregnancy. One study reports that the amount of weight lost does not depend on whether a woman breastfeeds her infant.[43] Another study suggests that breastfeeding enhances weight loss initially, especially fat loss from the lower body, but not thereafter.[44] Still another study indicates that weight loss is significant only if breastfeeding continues for at least six months.[45] A woman who breastfeeds her infant will gradually lose weight if she chooses nutrient-dense foods, even though her energy intake may be greater than normal. Most women lose 1 to 2 pounds a month during the first four to six months of lactation; some may lose more, and others may maintain or even gain weight.[46] Regardless of a woman's prepregnancy weight, the more weight she gains during pregnancy, the more weight she loses following delivery (when measured at six weeks and one year).[47]

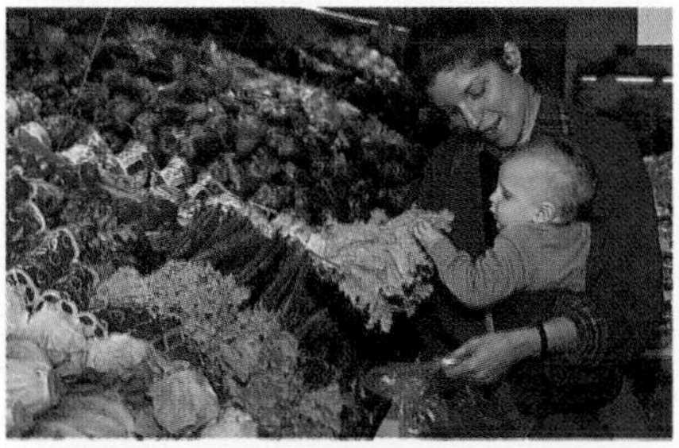

Nutritious foods support successful lactation.

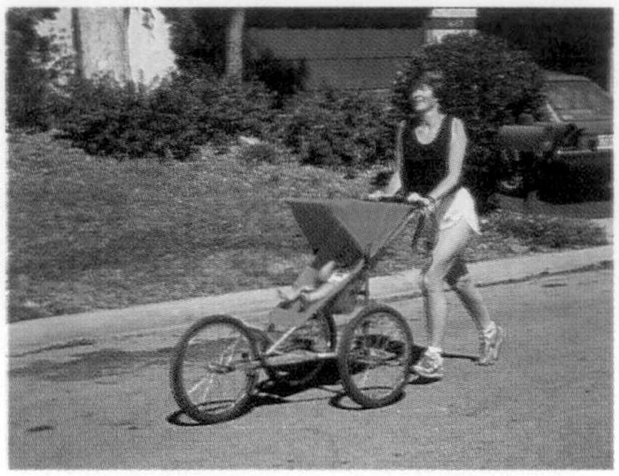

A brisk walk through the neighborhood offers a refreshing opportunity for physical activity and fresh air.

Women often exercise to reduce body fat and improve fitness, and this is compatible with breastfeeding.[48] Studies have found that lactating women who exercise compensate for their high energy expenditures by increasing their energy intakes.[49] Intense exercise can raise the lactic acid concentration of breast milk, which influences the milk's taste. Infants appear to prefer milk produced prior to exercise (which has a lower lactic acid content).[50] For this reason, mothers may want to breastfeed their infants before exercise or express their milk before exercise for use afterward.

Vitamins and Minerals In addition to providing energy, the foods consumed by the nursing mother should offer abundant nutrients and plenty of fluid. Review Figure 15–4 (on p. 555) to compare a lactating woman's nutrient needs with those of pregnant and nonpregnant women.

A question often raised is whether a mother's milk may lack a nutrient if she fails to get enough in her diet. The answer differs from one nutrient to the next, but in general, nutritional inadequacies reduce the *quantity*, not the *quality*, of breast milk. Women can produce milk with adequate protein, carbohydrate, fat, and most minerals, even when their own supplies are limited.[51] For these nutrients and for folate as well, milk quality is maintained at the expense of maternal stores. Nutrients in breast milk are most likely to decline in response to prolonged inadequate intakes of the vitamins—especially vitamins B_6, B_{12}, A, and D.[52]

Water A lactating woman needs to drink plenty of fluids to protect herself from dehydration. A sensible rule of thumb is to drink a glass of milk, juice, or water at each meal and each time the baby nurses. Despite previous misconceptions, a mother who drinks more fluid does not produce more breast milk.[53]

Supplements Most lactating women can obtain all the nutrients they need from a well-balanced diet without taking vitamin-mineral supplements; some, however, may need iron supplements. Maternal iron stores dwindle when the fetus takes iron to meet its own needs for four to six months after birth. In addition, childbirth may have incurred blood losses. A woman may therefore need iron supplements during lactation, not to augment the iron in her breast milk, but to refill her depleted iron stores.

Particular Foods Foods with strong or spicy flavors (such as garlic) may alter the flavor of breast milk.[54] A sudden change in the taste of the milk may annoy some infants. Infants who are sensitive to particular foods such as cow's milk protein may become uncomfortable when the mother's diet includes these foods. Only a few infants exhibit this sensitivity, so only a few nursing mothers need avoid cow's milk. Generally, nutrients from milk products support both the infant's and the mother's health.

In general, a nursing mother can eat whatever nutritious foods she chooses. If she suspects a particular food is causing the infant discomfort, her physician may recommend a dietary challenge: eliminate the food from the diet to see if the infant's reactions subside; then return the food to the diet, and again monitor the infant's reactions. If a food must be eliminated for an extended time, appropriate substitutions must be made to ensure nutrient adequacy.

CONCERNS OF BREASTFEEDING MOTHERS

Some substances impair milk production or enter breast milk and interfere with infant development. Some medical conditions prohibit breastfeeding. This section describes these effects.

Alcohol Alcohol easily enters breast milk. One study showed that the alcohol concentration of breast milk peaks within one hour after ingestion.[55] In this study, even small amounts of alcohol (equivalent to a can of beer) consumed by lactating women significantly reduced their infants' intakes of breast milk. The researchers suggest three possible reasons, acting separately or together. For one, the alcohol may have altered the flavor of the breast milk and thereby the infants' acceptance of it. For another, because infants metabolize alcohol inefficiently, even low doses may be potent enough to suppress their feeding behavior. Third, the alcohol may have reduced the women's milk production.

In the past, alcohol has been recommended to mothers to facilitate lactation despite a lack of scientific evidence that it does so. The research summarized here suggests that alcohol actually hinders breastfeeding. An occasional glass of wine or beer is considered within safe limits, but in general, lactating women should consume little or no alcohol.

Caffeine Caffeine taken during lactation may make a breastfed infant irritable and wakeful. As during pregnancy, caffeine consumption should be moderate—say, one to two cups of coffee a day. Larger doses of coffee may interfere with the availability of iron from the milk and impair the infant's iron status.

Smoking Cigarette smoking reduces milk volume, so smokers may produce too little milk to meet their infants' energy needs. One study of lactating women found that infants of smoking mothers gained less weight than infants of nonsmoking mothers.[56] Furthermore, infant exposure to passive smoke negates the protective effect breastfeeding offers against SIDS and increases the risks dramatically.[57]

Medical Considerations If a woman has an ordinary cold, she can go on nursing without worry. If susceptible, the infant will catch it from her anyway. (Thanks to immunological protection, a breastfed baby may be less susceptible than a formula-fed baby would be.) If a woman has a communicable disease such as tuberculosis or hepatitis that could threaten the infant's health, then mother and baby have to be separated; mothers can pump their breasts several times a day and feed breast milk by bottle.

For mothers with HIV infections, advice differs depending on context. Where safe alternatives are available, the Centers for Disease Control and the American Academy of Pediatrics recommend that HIV-positive women not breastfeed their infants. In developing countries, however, the feeding of inappropriate or contaminated formulas is the cause of 1.5 million infant deaths each year, so WHO and UNICEF urge mothers to breastfeed irrespective of HIV infection.

Women with chronic diseases such as diabetes (IDDM) may need careful monitoring and counseling to ensure successful lactation.[58] Women with IDDM need to adjust their energy intakes and insulin doses to meet the heightened needs of lactation. Maintaining good glucose control helps to initiate lactation and support milk production.[59]

Many drugs are compatible with breastfeeding, but some medicines are contraindicated, either because they suppress lactation or because they are secreted into breast milk and can harm the infant.[60] As a precaution, a nursing mother should consult with her physician prior to taking any drug. Illicit drugs, of course, are harmful to the physical and emotional health of both the mother and the nursing infant. Breast milk can deliver such high doses of illicit drugs as to cause irritability, tremors, and hallucinations in infants.

postpartum amenorrhea: the normal temporary absence of menstrual periods immediately following childbirth.

Women who breastfeed experience prolonged postpartum amenorrhea. Absent menstrual periods, however, do not protect a woman from pregnancy. To prevent pregnancy, a couple must use some form of contraception—but not oral contraceptive agents. Standard oral contraceptives contain estrogen, which reduces milk volume and the protein content of breast milk.[61]

Some women fear that breastfeeding will cause their breasts to sag. The breasts do swell and become heavy and large immediately after the birth, but even when they are producing enough milk to nourish a thriving infant, they eventually shrink back to their prepregnant size. Given proper support, diet, and exercise, breasts return to their former shape and size after weaning. Breasts change their shape as the body ages, but breastfeeding does not accelerate this process.

Environmental Contaminants Environmental contaminants, such as DDT, PCBs, and methylmercury can find their way into breast milk. Inuit mothers living in Arctic Québec who eat seal and beluga whale blubber have concentrations of DDT and PCBs in their breast milk two to ten times greater than those found in breast milk from women in southern Québec.[62] The impact of contaminated breast milk on infant development is unclear, however. Preliminary studies indicate the children of these Inuit mothers are developing normally. Researchers speculate that the abundant omega-3 fatty acids of the Inuit diet may protect against damage to the central nervous system.

In summary, the lactating woman needs extra fluid and enough energy and nutrients to produce about 25 ounces of milk a day. Alcohol, other drugs, smoking, and contaminants may impair milk production or enter breast milk and impair infant development.

This chapter has focused on the nutrition needs of the mother during pregnancy and lactation. The next chapter explores the dietary needs of infants, children, and adolescents.

Study Questions

1. Describe the placenta and its function.
2. Describe the normal events of fetal development. How does malnutrition impair fetal development?
3. Define the term *critical period*. How do adverse influences during critical periods affect later health?
4. Explain why women of childbearing age need folate in their diets. How much is recommended, and how can women ensure that these needs are met?
5. How does nutrition *prior* to conception influence a pregnancy?
6. What is the recommended pattern of weight gain

during pregnancy for a woman at a healthy weight? For an underweight woman? For an overweight woman?
7. What does a pregnant woman need to know about exercise?
8. Which nutrients are needed in the greatest amounts during pregnancy? Why are they so important? Describe wise food choices for the pregnant woman.
9. Define low-risk and high-risk pregnancies. What is the significance of infant birthweight in terms of the child's future health?
10. Describe some of the special problems of the pregnant adolescent. Which nutrients are needed in increased amounts?
11. What practices should be avoided during pregnancy? Why?
12. How do nutrient needs during lactation differ from nutrient needs during pregnancy?

Notes

1. Committee on Nutritional Status during Pregnancy and Lactation, *Nutrition during Pregnancy* (Washington, D.C.: National Academy Press, 1990), pp. 412–419.
2. American Academy of Pediatrics, Committee on Genetics, Folic acid for the prevention of neural tube defects, *Pediatrics* 92 (1993): 493–494.
3. Committee on Nutritional Status during Pregnancy and Lactation, 1990, p. 10.
4. Committee on Nutritional Status during Pregnancy and Lactation, 1990, p. 229.
5. K. G. Dewey and M. A. McCrory, Effects of dieting and physical activity on pregnancy and lactation, *American Journal of Clinical Nutrition* (supplement) 59 (1994): 446S–453S.
6. Committee on Nutritional Status during Pregnancy and Lactation, 1990, p. 384.
7. Committee on Nutritional Status during Pregnancy and Lactation, 1990, pp. 318–335.
8. Food and Nutrition Board, 1990, p. 322.
9. Committee on Nutritional Status during Pregnancy and Lactation, 1990, pp. 272–298.
10. Committee on Nutritional Status during Pregnancy and Lactation, 1990 pp. 285–293.
11. Y. H. Neggers and coauthors, A positive association between maternal serum zinc concentration and birth weight, *American Journal of Clinical Nutrition* 51 (1990): 678–684.
12. Committee on Nutritional Status during Pregnancy and Lactation, 1990, pp. 299–317.
13. K. Merchant, R. Martorell, and J. D. Haas, Consequences for maternal nutrition of reproductive stress across consecutive pregnancies, *American Journal of Clinical Nutrition* 52 (1990): 616–620.
14. M. Erick, Battling morning (noon and night) sickness: New approaches for treating an age-old problem, *Journal of the American Dietetic Association* 94 (1994): 147–148.
15. Transplacental nutrient transfer and intrauterine growth retardation, *Nutrition Reviews* 50 (1992): 56–57.
16. D. L. Phelps and coauthors, 28-day survival rates of 6676 neonates with birth weights of 1250 grams or less, *Pediatrics* 87 (1991): 7–17.
17. ACOG *Guide to Planning for Pregnancy, Birth, and Beyond* (Washington, D.C.: The American College of Obstetricians and Gynecologists, 1990), pp. 128–140.
18. F. G. Cunningham and M. D. Lindheimer, Hypertension in pregnancy, *New England Journal of Medicine* 326 (1992): 927–932.
19. Calcium supplementation prevents hypertensive disorders of pregnancy, *Nutrition Reviews* 50 (1992): 233–236.
20. K. B. Knight and R. E. Keith, Calcium supplementation on normotensive and hypertensive pregnant women, *American Journal of Clinical Nutrition* 55 (1992): 891–895; J. R. Repke and J. Villar, Pregnancy-induced hypertension and low birth weight: The role of calcium, *American Journal of Clinical Nutrition* 54 (1991): 237S–241S.
21. J. M. Belizan and coauthors, Calcium supplementation to prevent hypertensive disorders of pregnancy, *New England Journal of Medicine* 325 (1991): 1399–1405.
22. T. F. Ferris, Pregnancy, preeclampsia, and the endothelial cell, *New England Journal of Medicine* 325 (1991): 1439–1440.
23. F. G. Cummingham and N. F. Gant, Prevention of preeclampsia —A reality? *New England Journal of Medicine* 321 (1989): 606–607.
24. A. M. Fraser, J. E. Brockert, and R. H. Ward, Association of young maternal age with adverse reproductive outcomes, *New England Journal of Medicine* 332 (1995): 1113–1117.
25. M. L. Hediger and coauthors, Rate and amount of weight gain during adolescent pregnancy: Associations with maternal weight-for-height and birth weight, *American Journal of Clinical Nutrition* 52 (1990): 793–799.
26. Committee on Nutritional Status during Pregnancy and Lactation, 1990, pp. 1–23; J. M. Rees and coauthors, Weight gain in adolescents during pregnancy: Rate related to birth-weight outcome, *American Journal of Clinical Nutrition* 56 (1992): 868–873.
27. Position of The American Dietetic Association: Nutrition care for pregnant adolescents, *Journal of the American Dietetic Association* 94 (1994): 449–450.
28. I. J. Chasnoff and coauthors, The prevalence of illicit-drug or alcohol use during pregnancy and discrepancies in mandatory

reporting in Pinellas County, Florida, *New England Journal of Medicine* 322 (1990): 1202–1206.
29. D. B. Petitti and C. Coleman, Cocaine and the risk of low birth weight, *American Journal of Public Health* 80 (1990): 25–28; S. Parker and coauthors, Jitteriness in full-term neonates: Prevalence and correlates, *Pediatrics* 85 (1990): 17–23; M. van de Bor, F. J. Walther, and M. Ebrahimi, Decreased cardiac output in infants of mothers who abused cocaine, *Pediatrics* 85 (1990): 30–32; B. Zuckerman and coauthors, Effects of maternal marijuana and cocaine use on fetal growth, *New England Journal of Medicine* 320 (1989): 762–768.
30. W. T. Weathers and coauthors, Cocaine use in women from a defined population: Prevalence at delivery and effects on growth in infants, *Pediatrics* 91 (1993): 350–354.
31. S. D. Azuma and I. J. Chasnoff, Outcome of children prenatally exposed to cocaine and other drugs: A path analysis of three-year data, *Pediatrics* 92 (1993): 396–402; M. J. Corwin and coauthors, Effects of in utero cocaine exposure on newborn acoustical cry characteristics, *Pediatrics* 89 (1992): 1199–1203; L. N. Eisen and coauthors, Perinatal cocaine effects on neonatal stress behavior and performance on the Brazelton Scale, *Pediatrics* 88 (1991): 477–480; M. Mirochnick and coauthors, Circulating catecholamine concentrations in cocaine-exposed neonates: A pilot study, *Pediatrics* 88 (1991): 481–485.
32. Corwin and coauthors, 1992; L. C. Mayes and coauthors, Neurobehavioral profiles of neonates exposed to cocaine prenatally, *Pediatrics* 91 (1993): 778–783.
33. F. M. Haste and coauthors, Nutrient intakes during pregnancy: Observations on the influence of smoking and social class, *American Journal of Clinical Nutrition* 51 (1990): 29–36.
34. H. S. Klonoff-Cohen and coauthors, The effect of passive smoking and tobacco exposure through breast milk on sudden infant death syndrome, *Journal of the American Medical Association* 273 (1995): 795–798; E. A. Mitchell and coauthors, Smoking and the sudden infant death syndrome, *Pediatrics* 91 (1993): 893–896; K. C. Schoendorf and J. L. Kiely, Relationship of sudden infant death syndrome to maternal smoking during and after pregnancy, *Pediatrics* 90 (1992): 905–908; M. G. Bulterys, S. Greenland, and J. F. Kraus, Chronic fetal hypoxia and sudden infant death syndrome: Interaction between maternal smoking and low hematocrit during pregnancy, *Pediatrics* 86 (1990): 535–540; B. Haglund and S. Cnattingius, Cigarette smoking as a risk factor for sudden infant death syndrome: A population-based study, *American Journal of Public Health* 80 (1990): 29–32.
35. D. L. Olds, C. R. Henderson, Jr., and R. Tatelbaum, Intellectual impairment in children of women who smoke cigarettes during pregnancy, *Pediatrics* 93 (1994): 221–227; D. M. Fergusson, L. J. Horwood, and M. T. Lynskey, Maternal smoking before and after pregnancy: Effects on behavioral outcomes in middle childhood, *Pediatrics* 92 (1993): 815–822.
36. M. Lewis and coauthors, Prenatal exposure to heavy metals: Effect on childhood cognitive skills and health status, *Pediatrics* 89 (1992): 1010–1015.
37. Lewis, 1992; M. W. Shannon and J. W. Graef, Lead intoxication in infancy, *Pediatrics* 89 (1992): 87–90.
38. Committee on Nutritional Status during Pregnancy and Lactation, 1990, pp. 397–399.
39. Position of The American Dietetic Association: Use of nutritive and nonnutritive sweeteners, *Journal of the American Dietetic Association* 93 (1993): 816–821.
40. G. L. Freed, J. K. Fraley, and R. J. Schanler, Attitudes of expectant fathers regarding breast-feeding, *Pediatrics* 90 (1992): 224–227.
41. K. G. Dewey and coauthors, Maternal versus infant factors related to breast milk intake and residual milk volume: The DARLING Study, *Pediatrics* 87 (1991): 829–837; Committee on Nutrition Status during Pregnancy and Lactation, *Nutrition during Lactation* (Washington, D.C.: National Academy Press, 1991), pp. 1–19.
42. M. A. Guillermo-Tuazon and coauthors, Energy intake, energy expenditure, and body composition of poor rural Philippine women throughout the first 6 mo of lactation, *American Journal of Clinical Nutrition* 56 (1992): 874–880; C. Frigerio and coauthors, A new procedure to assess the energy requirements of lactation in Gambian women, *American Journal of Clinical Nutrition* 54 (1991): 526–533; J. M. A. van Raaij and coauthors, Energy cost of lactation, and energy balances of well-nourished Dutch lactating women: Reappraisal of the extra energy requirements of lactation, *American Journal of Clinical Nutrition* 53 (1991): 612–619.
43. S. Potter and coauthors, Does infant feeding method influence maternal postpartum weight loss? *Journal of the American Dietetic Association* 91 (1991): 441–446.
44. F. M. Kramer and coauthors, Breast-feeding reduces material lower-body fat, *Journal of the American Dietetic Association* 93 (1993): 429–433.
45. K. G. Dewey, M. J. Heinig, and L. A. Nommsen, Maternal weight-loss patterns during prolonged lactation, *American Journal of Clinical Nutrition* 58 (1993): 162–166.
46. Committee on Nutritional Status during Pregnancy and Lactation, 1991, pp. 1–19.
47. Potter and coauthors, 1991.
48. Dewey and McCrory, 1994; K. G. Dewey and coauthors, A randomized study of the effects of aerobic exercise by lactating women on breast-milk volume and composition, *New England Journal of Medicine* 330 (1994): 449–453.
49. Dewey and coauthors, 1994; C. A. Lovelady, B. Lonnerdal, and K. G. Dewey, Lactation performance of exercising women, *American Journal of Clinical Nutrition* 52 (1990): 103–109.
50. J. P. Wallace, G. Inbar, and K. Ernsthausen, Infant acceptance of postexercise breast milk, *Pediatrics* 89 (1992): 1245–1247.
51. Committee on Nutritional Status during Pregnancy and Lactation, 1991, p. 140.
52. Committee on Nutritional Status during Pregnancy and Lactation, 1991, p. 140.

53. L. B. Dusdieker and coauthors, Prolonged maternal fluid supplementation in breast-feeding, *Pediatrics* 86 (1990): 737–740.
54. J. A. Mennella and G. K. Beauchamp, Maternal diet alters the sensory qualities of human milk and the behavior of the nursing infant, *Pediatrics* 88 (1991): 737–747.
55. J. A. Mennella and G. K. Beauchamp, The transfer of alcohol to human milk: Effects on flavor and the infant's behavior, *New England Journal of Medicine* 325 (1991): 981–985.
56. F. Vio, G. Salazar, and C. Infante, Smoking during pregnancy and lactation and its effects on breast-milk volume, *American Journal of Clinical Nutrition* 54 (1991): 1011–1016.
57. Klonoff-Cohen, 1995.
58. A. M. Ferris and E. A. Reece, Nutritional consequences of chronic maternal conditions during pregnancy and lactation: Lupus and diabetes, *American Journal of Clinical Nutrition* (supplement) 59 (1994): 465S–473S; A. M. Ferris and coauthors, Perinatal lactation protocol and outcome in mothers with and without insulin-dependent diabetes mellitus, *American Journal of Clinical Nutrition* 58 (1993): 43–48.
59. C. M. van Beusekom and coauthors, Milk of patients with tightly controlled insulin-dependent diabetes mellitus has normal macronutrient and fatty acid composition, *American Journal of Clinical Nutrition* 57 (1993): 938–943.
60. American Academy of Pediatrics, Committee on Drugs, The transfer of drugs and other chemicals into human milk, *Pediatrics* 93 (1994): 137–150.
61. American Academy of Pediatrics, Committee on Drugs, Transfer of drugs and other chemicals into human milk, *Pediatrics* 84 (1989): 924–936.
62. E. Dewailly and coauthors, Inuit exposure to organochlorines through the aquatic food chain in Arctic Québec, *Environmental Health Perspectives* 101 (1993): 618–620.

Highlight 15

Fetal Alcohol Syndrome

As Chapter 15 mentioned, drinking alcohol during pregnancy endangers the fetus. Alcohol crosses the placenta freely and deprives the developing fetal brain of both nutrients and oxygen. The result may be fetal alcohol syndrome (FAS), a cluster of symptoms that includes:[1]

- Prenatal and postnatal growth retardation.
- Impairment of the brain and nerves, with consequent mental retardation, poor coordination, and hyperactivity.
- Abnormalities of the face and skull (see Figure H15–1).
- Increased frequency of major birth defects: cleft palate, heart defects, and defects in ears, genitals, and urinary system.

Tragically, the damage evident at birth persists: children with FAS never fully recover.[2]

Of every 10,000 children born in the United States some 6 or 7 suffer health problems because their mothers drank alcohol during pregnancy—a sixfold increase over the past 15 years.[3] In addition, many infants are born with the less serious, yet still significant, damage some clinicians describe as fetal alcohol effects (FAE; see the glossary on the next page).[4] Some children with FAE have no outward signs; others may be short or have only minor facial abnormalities. Often they go undiagnosed even when problems develop in the early school years: learning disabilities, behavioral abnormalities, motor impairments, and more.

This highlight asks two questions: How much alcohol causes FAS? When during pregnancy is the damage done? The answers are already available; researchers are now merely refining the details. To anticipate the conclusions, abstinence from alcohol is the best policy for pregnant women both because alcohol consumption during pregnancy has such severe consequences, and because FAS can only be prevented—it cannot be treated.[5] And because the most severe damage occurs around the time of conception—*before a woman*

Figure H15–1

Typical Facial Characteristics of FAS

The severe facial abnormalities shown here are just outward signs of the severe mental impairments within. The internal organs also suffer irreversible damage that, while hidden, may create major problems for a child's health.

Source: Adapted from J. O. Beattie, Alcohol exposure and the fetus, *European Journal of Clinical Nutrition* 46 (1992): S7–S17.

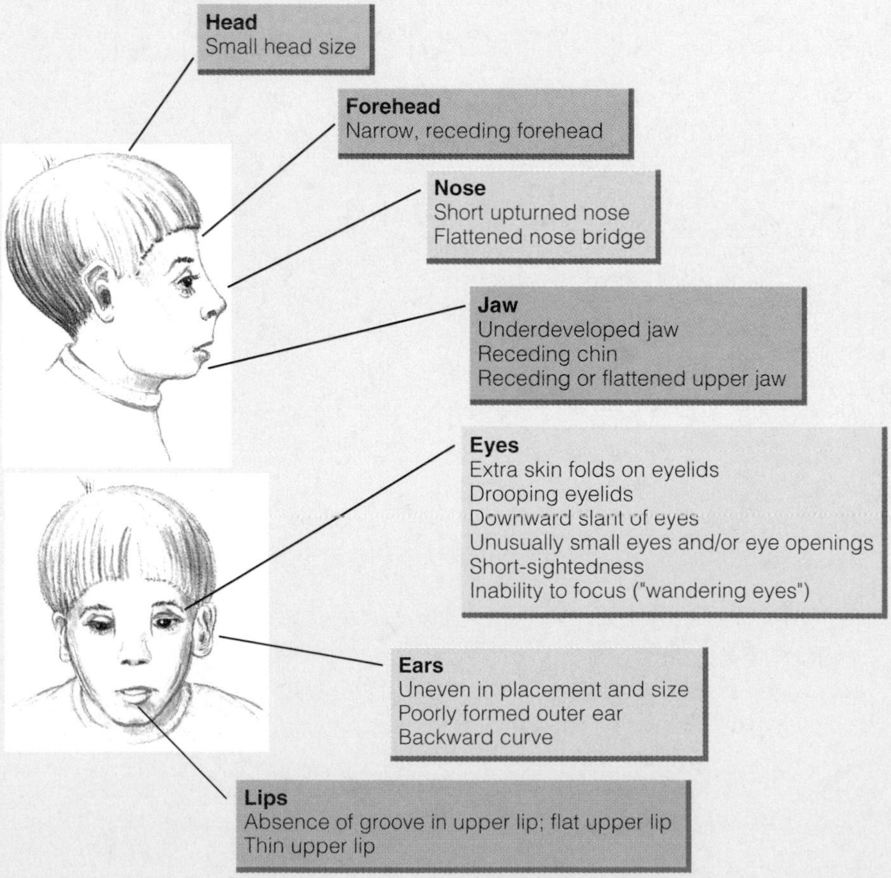

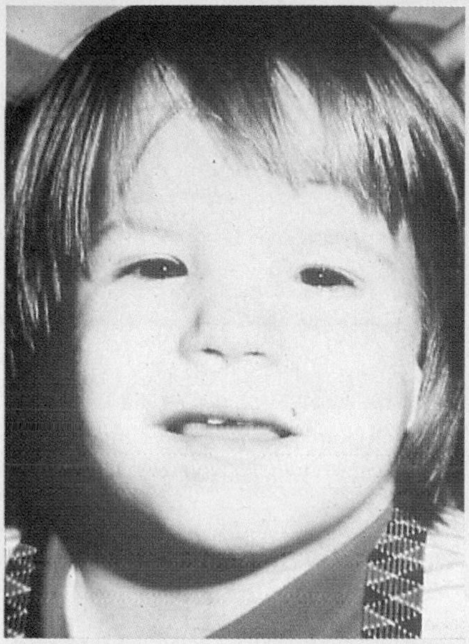

The most obvious symptoms of FAS are the abnormal facial features, but the most tragic ones are the mental disabilities.

may even realize that she is pregnant—even a woman planning to conceive should abstain.

DRINKING DURING PREGNANCY

When a woman drinks during pregnancy, she causes damage in two ways: directly, by intoxication, and indirectly, by malnutrition. Prior to the complete formation of the placenta (approximately 12 weeks), alcohol diffuses directly into the tissues of the developing embryo, causing incredible damages. When alcohol crosses the placenta, fetal blood alcohol rises until it reaches an equilibrium with maternal blood alcohol. The mother may not even appear drunk, but the fetus may be poisoned. The fetus's body is small, its detoxification system is immature, and alcohol remains in fetal blood long after it has disappeared from maternal blood. Alcohol interferes with many developmental events, reducing the number of cells produced and damaging those that are produced.[6]

Alcohol also impairs maternal nutrition status. People who abuse alcohol often are malnourished, and as Chapter 15 already described, maternal malnutrition impedes fetal development. Even if the mother eats well and maintains adequate nutrient stores, alcohol damages the placenta, and so interferes with the transport of nutrients to the fetus, causing fetal malnutrition.

HOW MUCH ALCOHOL IS TOO MUCH?

Alcohol damages the fetus to an extent that correlates directly with the quantity the mother consumes: the number of defects rises with increasing amounts of alcohol. A pregnant woman need not have an alcohol-abuse problem to give birth to a baby with FAS. She need only drink in excess of her liver's capacity to detoxify alcohol. About four drinks a day dramatically worsens the risk of having physical malformations. Even one to two drinks a day threatens to retard growth.

Does this mean that drinking, say, one drink every day or so might be safe? Probably not, for researchers have not yet defined the relationship between alcohol consumption and damage that precisely, nor do they agree on the criteria used to define safety. Although some of alcohol's effects are obvious (such as the physical malformations), others are more subtle (the neurological defects) and often become evident only after several years. Even with those ambiguities resolved, researchers could not specify an amount that would be safe for every woman because individuals respond differently to varying levels of alcohol intake.

In addition to total alcohol intake, drinking patterns play an important role. Most FAS studies report their findings in terms of average intake per day, but people usually drink more heavily on some days than on others. For example, a woman who drinks an *average* of 1 ounce of alcohol (2 drinks) a day may not drink at all during the week but then might have 14 drinks on a Saturday night, exposing the fetus to highly toxic quantities of alcohol. Whether drinking a certain number of drinks during binges or spreading them out over several days causes more damage depends on the frequency of the binges, the quantity consumed, and the stage of

Glossary

fetal alcohol effects (FAE): a subclinical version of FAS, with hidden defects including learning disabilities, behavioral abnormalities, and motor impairments; also called **alcohol-related birth defects (ARBD)**.

fetal alcohol syndrome (FAS): the cluster of symptoms seen in an infant or child whose mother consumed excess alcohol during pregnancy, including retarded growth, impaired development of the central nervous system, and facial malformations.

See Highlight 7 for other alcohol-related terms and information.

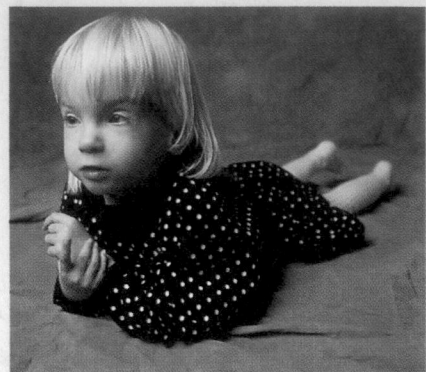

Characteristic facial features may diminish with time, but children with FAS typically continue to be short and underweight for their age.

fetal development at the time of each drinking episode.

An occasional drink may be innocuous, but researchers are unable to say how much alcohol is safe to consume during pregnancy.[7] For this reason, health care professionals urge women to stop drinking alcohol as soon as they realize they are pregnant, or better, as soon as they *plan* to become pregnant.[8] Why take any risk? Only the woman who abstains is sure of protecting her infant from FAS.

WHEN IS THE DAMAGE DONE?

The type of abnormality observed in an FAS infant depends on the developmental events occurring at the times of alcohol exposure. During the first trimester, developing organs such as the brain, heart, and kidneys may be malformed. During the second trimester, the risk of spontaneous abortion increases. During the third trimester, body and brain growth may be retarded.

In experiments on laboratory animals, the effects of alcohol on fetal development are most marked when the female takes alcohol during the earliest period—that of organ formation. Effects also appear when the female takes alcohol just *prior* to conception. Studies on human beings also find that alcohol is most potent in causing birth defects within the first eight weeks of gestation.

Male alcohol ingestion may also affect fertility and fetal development. Animal studies have found smaller litter sizes, lower birthweights, reduced survival rates, and impaired learning ability in the offspring of males consuming alcohol prior to conception.[9] One human study found an association between paternal alcohol intake one month prior to conception and low infant birthweight.[10] (Paternal alcohol intake was defined as an average of two or more drinks daily or at least five drinks on one occasion.) This relationship was independent of either parent's smoking and of the mother's use of alcohol, caffeine, or other drugs.

In view of these findings, it is important to advise women not to drink during pregnancy. Everyone should know of the potential dangers. Heavy drinkers who are sexually active urgently need effective contraception to prevent pregnancy.

All containers of beer, wine, and liquor carry the warning: "Drinking during pregnancy may cause mental retardation and other birth defects. Avoid alcohol during pregnancy." Everyone should hear the message loud and clear: Don't drink alcohol prior to conception or during pregnancy. Once present, FAS has no cure.

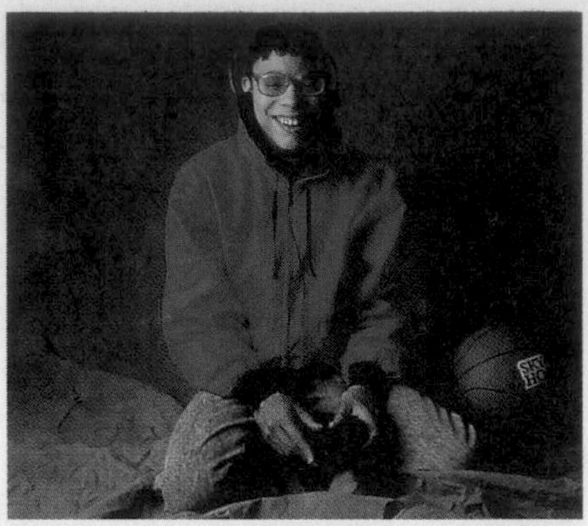

Children born with FAS must live with the long-term consequences of prenatal brain damage.

NOTES

1. Committee on Substance Abuse and Committee on Children with Disabilities, American Academy of Pediatrics, Fetal alcohol syndrome and fetal alcohol effects, *Pediatrics* 91 (1993): 1004–1006; J. O. Beattie, Alcohol exposure and the fetus, *European Journal of Clinical Nutrition* 46 (1992): S7–S17.
2. H. L. Spohr, J. Willms, and H. C. Steinhausen, Prenatal alcohol exposure and long-term developmental consequences, *Lancet* 341 (1993): 907–910.
3. Update: Trends in fetal alcohol syndrome—United States, 1979–1993, *Morbidity and Mortality Weekly Report* 44 (1995): 249–251.
4. J. M. Aase, K. L. Jones, and S. K. Clarren, Do we need the term "FAE"? *Pediatrics* 95 (1995): 428–430.
5. Committee on Nutritional Status during Pregnancy and Lactation, *Nutrition during Pregnancy* (Washington, D.C.: National Academy Press, 1990), pp. 390–411.
6. Beattie, 1992.
7. Beattie, 1992.
8. Committee on Substance Abuse and Committee on Children with Disabilities, 1993; *The Surgeon General's Report on Nutrition and Health* (Washington, D.C.: U.S. Government Printing Office, 1988), p. 72.
9. When dad drinks: Can his liquor intake impair his future offspring? *Scientific American*, February 1990, p. 23; L. F. Soyka and J. M. Joffe, Male mediated drug effects on offspring, *Progress in Clinical and Biological Research* 36 (1980): 49–66.
10. R. E. Little and C. F. Sing, Father's drinking and infant birth weight: Report of an association, *Teratology* 36 (1987): 59–65.

Chapter 16

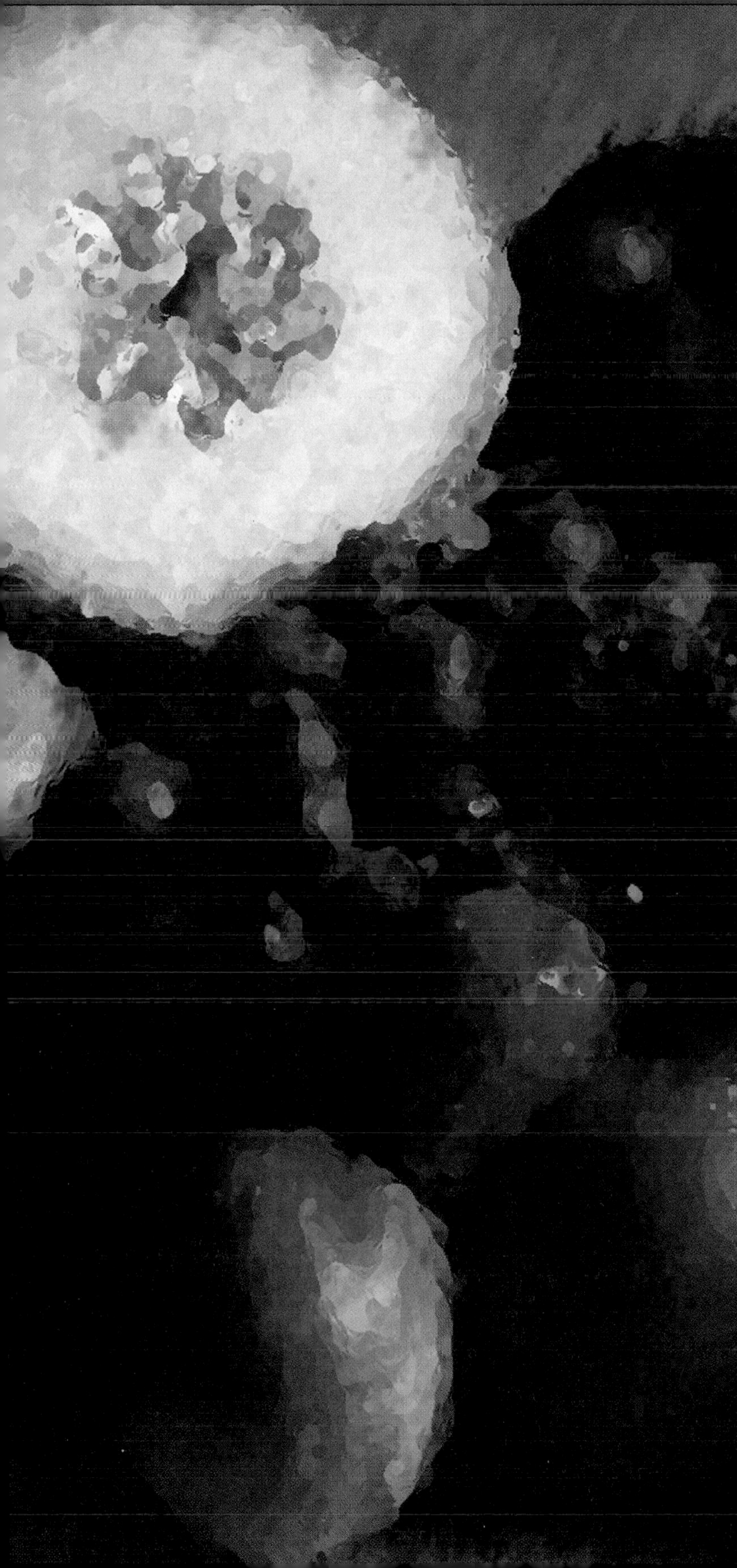

Life Cycle Nutrition: Infancy, Childhood, and Adolescence

CONTENTS

MICROGRAPH: Growth hormone, a chemical messenger active during infancy, childhood, and adolescence

The first year of life is a time of phenomenal growth and development. After the first year, a child continues to grow and change, but more slowly. Still, the cumulative effects over the next decade are remarkable. Then, as the child enters the teen years, the pace toward adulthood accelerates dramatically. This chapter examines the special nutrient needs of infants, children, and teenagers.

Figure 16–1

Weight Gain of Human Infants in Their First Five Years of Life
In the first year, an infant's birthweight may triple, but over the following several years, the rate of weight gain gradually diminishes.

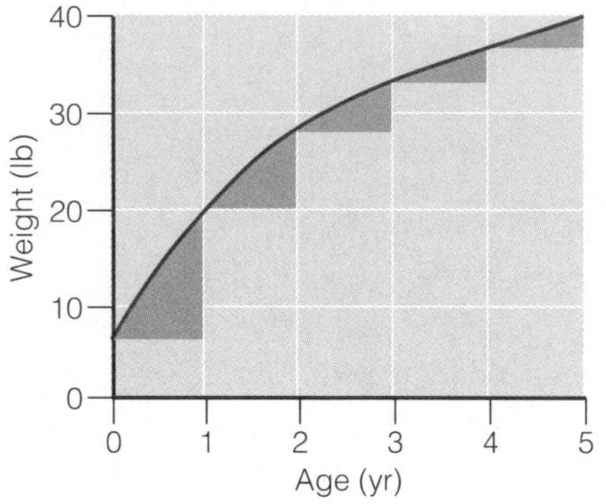

Nutrition during Infancy

For a while, the infant drinks only breast milk or formula, but later begins to eat some foods, as appropriate. Trends change and experts argue about the fine points, but properly nourishing a baby is relatively simple overall. Common sense in the selection of infant foods and a nurturing, relaxed environment go far to promote an infant's health and well-being.

ENERGY AND NUTRIENT NEEDS

An infant grows faster during the first year than ever again, as Figure 16–1 shows. Growth directly reflects nutrient intake and is an important parameter in assessing the nutrition status of infants and children. Health care professionals measure the heights and weights of infants and children at intervals and compare measures both with standard growth curves for sex and age and with previous measures of each child (see Figure 16–2).

Energy Intake and Activity A healthy infant's birthweight doubles by about four months of age and triples by the age of one year, typically reaching 20 to 25 pounds. (If an adult were to do this, a person weighing 150 pounds would increase to 450 pounds in a single year.) By the end of the first year, infant growth slows considerably; an infant gains less than 10 pounds during the second year.

Not only do infants grow rapidly, but their basal metabolic rate is remarkably high—about twice that of an adult, based on body weight.[1] Infants require about 100 kcalories per kilogram of body weight per day, whereas most adults need fewer than 40. (A 170-pound adult who tried to eat like an infant would have to ingest over 7000 kcalories a day.) After six months, metabolic needs decline as the growth rate slows down, but some of the energy saved by slower growth is spent in increased activity.

A newborn baby requires about 650 kcalories per day, whereas most adults require about 2000 kcalories per day. In comparison to body weight, the difference is remarkable.

Recommended water intake for infants:
1.5 mL/kcal energy expenditure.
For example, a six-month-old infant who expends 850 kcal a day needs:

1.5 mL/kcal × 850 kcal = 1275 mL, or about 5 c of water/day.

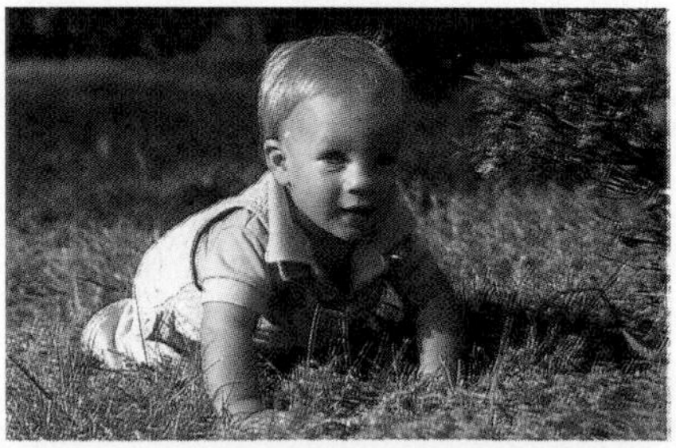

After six months, energy saved by slower growth is spent in increased activity.

Vitamins and Minerals Vitamin and mineral recommendations are based on the contents of human milk, which seems appropriate considering that neither deficiencies nor toxicities develop when infants receive these amounts.[2] Figure 16–3 (on p. 580) compares a five-month-old infant's needs per unit of body weight with those of a man and shows that some of the differences are extraordinary.

Water An important nutrient for infants, as for everyone, is the one easiest to forget: water. The younger the infant, the greater the percentage of body weight that is present as fluids between the cells and in the vascular space—fluids that are easy to lose. Breast milk or infant formula normally provides enough water to replace a healthy infant's fluid losses, but an infant who is exposed to hot weather, has diarrhea, or vomits repeatedly needs supplemental water to pre-

Figure 16–2

Examples of Growth Charts

These two charts are used for girls from birth to 36 months. The first chart gives percentiles for length and weight for age; the other, percentiles for head circumference for age and weight for length. Appendix E describes how to monitor growth and provides these and six other growth charts for both boys and girls of various ages.

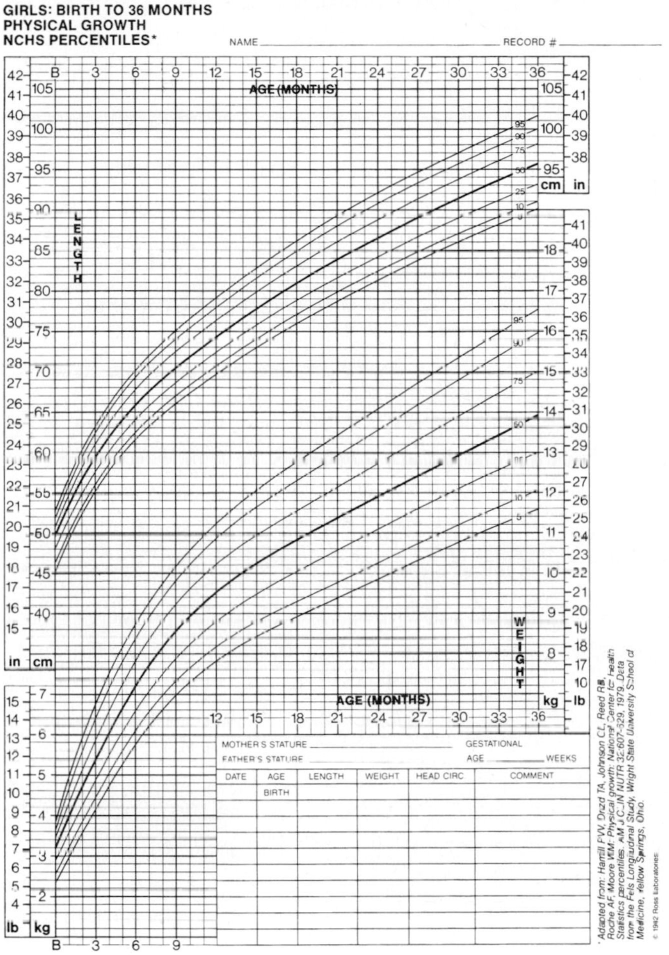

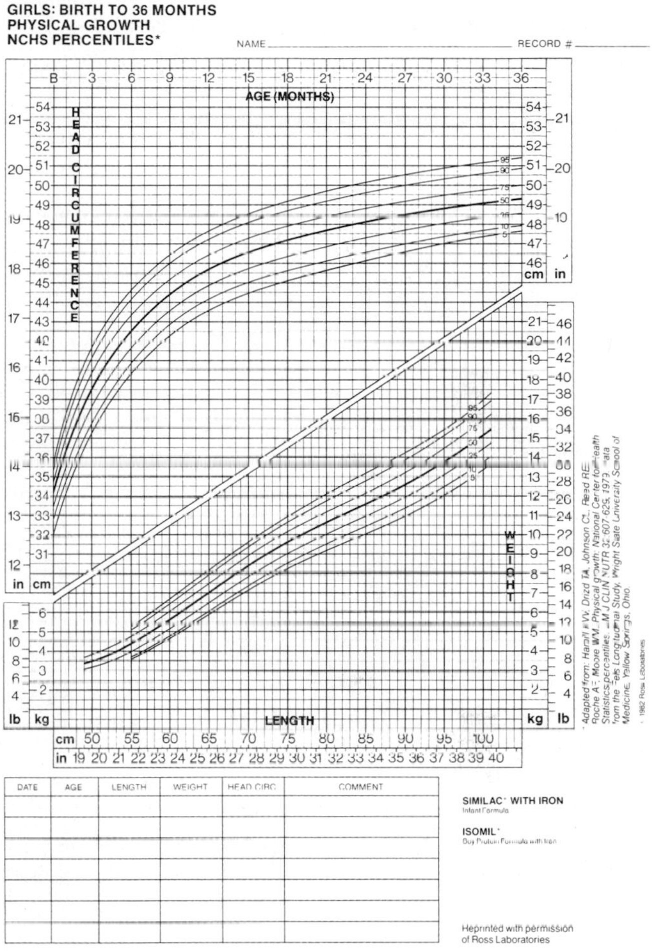

vent life-threatening dehydration.[3] Infants cannot explain why they are crying; adults must remember that an infant may need water, and then provide as much as the infant will drink.

BREAST MILK VERSUS INFANT FORMULA

The American Academy of Pediatrics recommends that infants receive breast milk for the first 6 to 12 months.[4] The American Dietetic Association also advocates breastfeeding because of its many benefits to both infant and mother.[5] Breast milk's unique nutrient composition and protective factors promote optimal infant health and development. Experts add, though, that iron-fortified for-

Figure 16–3

Nutrient RDA of a Five-Month-Old Infant and an Adult Male Compared on the Basis of Body Weight

Because infants are small, they need smaller total amounts of the nutrients than adults do, but when comparisons are based on body weight, infants need over twice as much of many nutrients. Infants use large amounts of energy and nutrients, in proportion to their body size, to keep all their metabolic processes going.

Infant's metabolism:

- Heart rate: 120 to 140 beats per minute.
- Respiration rate: 20 per minute.
- Energy needs: 45 kcalories per pound (100 kcalories per kilogram) body weight.

Adult's metabolism:

- Heart rate: 70 to 80 beats per minute.
- Respiration rate: 12 to 14 per minute.
- Energy needs: <18 kcalories per pound (<40 kcalories per kilogram) body weight.

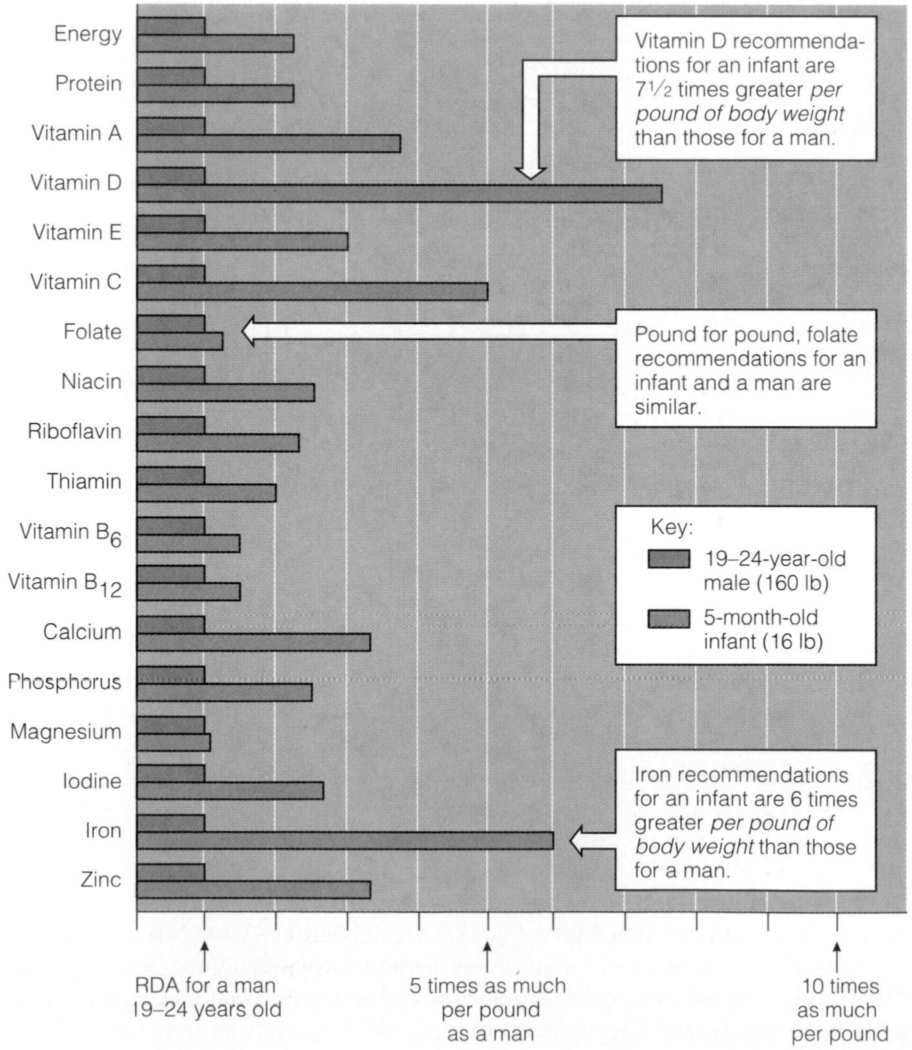

mula is an acceptable alternative to breast milk, for it imitates the composition of breast milk as closely as possible.

Even two or three months of breastfeeding give the infant immunological protection and other special advantages during the most critical period after birth—protection that persists beyond the breastfeeding period itself.[6] The mother can then shift to formula, if necessary, knowing she has given her infant those benefits.

In the United States and Canada, the two dietary practices that have the most effect on an infant's nutrition status are, first, the milk the infant receives, and second, the age at which solid foods are introduced. The next sections are devoted to feeding the infant and identifying common nutrient deficiencies.

BREAST MILK

Breast milk excels as a source of nutrients for the young infant.[7] The American Academy of Pediatrics and the Canadian Pediatric Society have issued this joint statement: "Breastfeeding is strongly recommended for full-term infants, except in the few instances where specific contraindications exist."

Breastfed infants generally gain weight at about the same rate as formula-fed infants during the first two or three months, even though they usually drink less milk and therefore have lower energy intakes.[8] For the next six months, breastfed infants tend to gain slightly less weight than formula-fed infants, but then resume gaining at a similar rate again.[9]

With the possible exception of vitamin D, breast milk provides all the nutrients a healthy infant needs for the first four to six months of life. Breast milk also confers immunological protection, described later.

Energy Nutrients The energy-nutrient composition of breast milk differs dramatically from the dietary recommendations for adults (see Figure 16–4). Yet for infants, breast milk is the most nearly perfect food, proving that people at different stages of life really do have different nutrient needs.

Breast milk's carbohydrate is lactose, which enhances calcium absorption. Breast milk's fat offers a generous proportion of the essential fatty acid linoleic acid. The total protein in breast milk is less than in cow's milk, which is good because it places less stress on the infant's immature kidneys to excrete the major end product of protein metabolism, urea. The main protein in breast milk is alpha-lactalbumin, which is easy for infants to digest.

Vitamins With the possible exception of vitamin D, the vitamins in breast milk are ample to support infant growth. Even vitamin C, for which cow's milk is a poor source, is abundant in the breast milk of a well-nourished mother. The vitamin D in breast milk is low, however, and vitamin D deficiency impairs bone mineralization in infants and children.[10] Manufacturers fortify cow's milk and infant formulas with vitamin D, and physicians routinely prescribe vitamin D supplements for breastfed infants in the United States and Canada.

Some infants can make enough vitamin D to meet their needs. The amount formed depends on skin color, exposure time, atmospheric pollution, time of year, and latitude. Vitamin D deficiency is a risk for infants who are not exposed to sunlight daily, who receive breast milk without supplementation, and who have darkly pigmented skin.

Figure 16–4

Percentages of Energy-Yielding Nutrients in Human Milk and in Recommended Adult Diets

The proportions of energy-yielding nutrients in human breast milk differ from those recommended for adults.

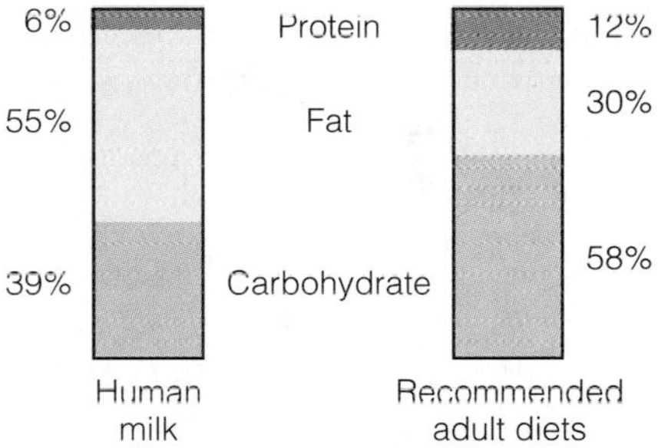

alpha-lactalbumin (lact-AL-byoo-min): the chief protein in human breast milk, as opposed to **casein** (CAY-seen), the chief protein in cow's milk.

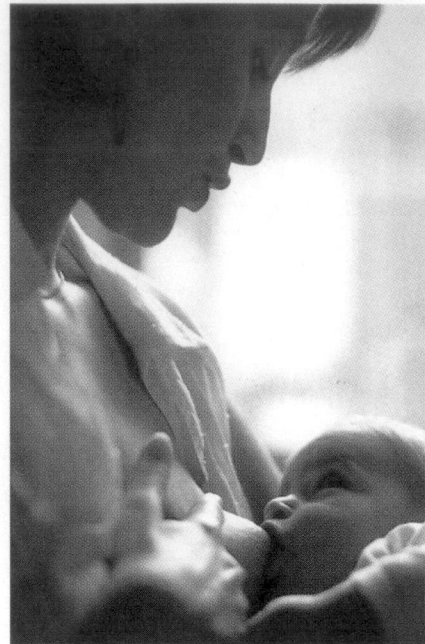

Women are encouraged to breastfeed whenever possible because breast milk offers infants many nutrients and health advantages.

colostrum (co-LAHS-trum)**:** a milklike secretion from the breast, present during the first day or so after delivery before milk appears; rich in protective factors.

Minerals The calcium-to-phosphorus ratio of breast milk is ideal for calcium absorption. The iron in breast milk is highly absorbable, as is the zinc, thanks to the presence of a zinc-binding protein. Breast milk is low in sodium, another benefit for immature kidneys.

Fluoride is not an essential nutrient, but it does help to prevent dental caries. Breast milk provides little fluoride, regardless of the mother's intake.

Supplements Breastfed newborns usually require no supplements, with the possible exception of vitamin D. At six months, depending on food and water intake, infants may require iron and fluoride supplements (see Table 16–1).

Immunological Protection Breast milk offers unsurpassed protection against infection during a time when an infant's immune system is not fully functional. It contains antiviral agents such as immunoglobulins, antibacterial agents such as lactoferrin, and other infection inhibitors.

During the first two or three days of lactation, the breasts produce colostrum, a premilk substance containing antibodies and white cells from the mother's blood. Because it contains maternal immune factors, colostrum helps protect the newborn from infections the mother has developed immunity against. These diseases are the ones in her environment and are precisely those against which the infant needs protection. The maternal antibodies swallowed with the milk inactivate disease-causing bacteria within the digestive tract before they can start infections. This explains, in part, why breastfed infants have fewer intestinal infections than formula-fed infants. Later, breast milk also delivers antibodies, although not as many as colostrum.

Table 16–1

Supplements for Full-Term Infants

	Vitamin D[a]	Iron[b]	Fluoride[c]
Breastfed infants:			
Birth to six months of age	√		
Six months to one year	√	√	√
Formula-fed infants:			
Birth to six months of age			
Six months to one year		√	√

[a]Vitamin D supplements are recommended only for as long as breast milk is the infant's major milk.

[b]Infants four to six months of age need additional iron, preferably in the form of iron-fortified cereal for both breastfed and formula-fed infants and iron-fortified infant formula for formula-fed infants.

[c]The Committee on Nutrition of the American Academy of Pediatrics recommends initiating fluoride supplements at six months of age for breastfed infants, formula-fed infants who receive ready-to-use formulas (these are prepared with water low in fluoride), and those who receive formula mixed with water that contains little or no fluoride (less than 0.3 ppm).

Source: Adapted from Committee on Nutrition, American Academy of Pediatrics, Vitamin and mineral supplement needs of normal children in the United States, in *Pediatric Nutrition Handbook,* 3rd ed., ed. L. A. Barness (Elk Grove Village, Ill.: American Academy of Pediatrics, 1993), pp. 34–42; American Academy of Pediatrics, Committee on Nutrition, Fluoride supplementation for children: Interim policy recommendations, *Pediatrics* 95 (1995): 777.

In addition to antibodies, colostrum and breast milk provide other powerful agents that help to fight against bacterial infection. Among them are bifidus factors, which favor the growth of the "friendly" bacteria *Lactobacillus bifidus* in the infant's digestive tract, so that other, harmful bacteria cannot gain a foothold there. An iron-grabbing protein in breast milk, lactoferrin, keeps bacteria from getting the iron they need to grow, helps absorb iron into the infant's bloodstream, and kills some bacteria directly. Also present is a growth factor that stimulates the development and maintenance of the infant's digestive tract and its protective factors. Several breast milk enzymes, hormones, and lipids also help protect the infant against infection. Much remains to be learned about the composition and characteristics of human milk, but clearly it is a very special substance.

bifidus (BIFF-id-us, by-FEED-us) **factors:** factors in colostrum and breast milk that favor the growth of the "friendly" bacteria *Lactobacillus* (lack-toh-ba-SILL-us) *bifidus* in the infant's intestinal tract, so that other, less desirable intestinal inhabitants will not flourish.

lactoferrin (lak-toh-FERR-in)**:** a factor in breast milk that binds iron and keeps it from supporting the growth of the infant's intestinal bacteria.

INFANT FORMULA

Breastfeeding offers many benefits to both mother and infant, and every woman should seriously consider it. Still, there are valid reasons for not breastfeeding, and formula-fed infants grow and develop into healthy children. The mother who chooses to feed formula to her infant can offer the same closeness, warmth, and stimulation during feedings as the breastfeeding mother can. Other family members can help with feedings, thus allowing the mother additional time to rest.

Formula preparation:

- Liquid concentrate (inexpensive, relatively easy)—mix with equal part water.
- Powdered formula (cheapest, lightest for travel)—read label directions.
- Ready-to-feed (easiest, most expensive)—pour directly into clean bottles.
- Whole milk—do not use during first year.

Appropriate Uses of Formula A woman who breastfeeds for a year can wean her infant to cow's milk, bypassing the need for infant formula. Many breastfeeding women use some infant formula, however. Some substitute formula for breastfeeding on occasion. Some wean from breast milk to formulas within the first year. And some women, of course, feed formula to their infants from birth. Whatever the case, a woman who uses formula must select an appropriate formula and learn to prepare it.

wean: to gradually replace breast milk with infant formula or other foods appropriate to an infant's diet.

Infant Formula Composition Formulas made from cow's milk closely resemble human milk in nutrient content. Figure 16–5 illustrates the energy-nutrient balance of both, and Table 16–2 compares breast milk, cow's milk, and a standard infant formula.

The American Academy of Pediatrics recommends iron-fortified infant formula for all formula-fed infants. The increasing use of iron-fortified formulas during the past few decades is a major reason for the decline in iron-deficiency anemia among U.S. infants.

Infant formulas contain no protective antibodies for infants, but in general, vaccinations, clean water, and clean environments in the developed countries make this deficit less important than in the past. Formulas can be prepared safely by following the rules of proper food handling and using water that is sanitary and free of contamination. Lead-contaminated water is a major source of lead poisoning in infants (see Highlight 19).[11]

Figure 16–5

Percentages of Energy-Yielding Nutrients in Human Milk and in Infant Formula

The proportions of energy-yielding nutrients in human breast milk and formula differ slightly.

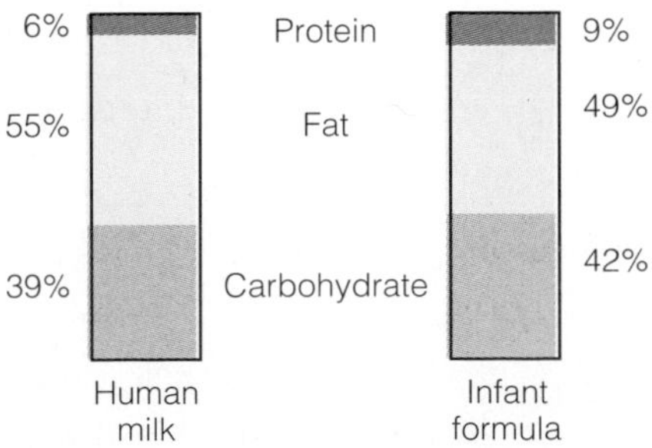

Risks of Formula Feeding In developing countries and in poor areas of this country, formula may be unavailable or may be prepared with contaminated water or overdiluted in an attempt to save money. More than 1.2 billion people in developing countries have no safe drinking water. Contaminated formulas often cause infections, leading to diarrhea, dehydration, and failure to absorb

Table 16–2

Comparison of Human Milk, Cow's Milk, and Infant Formula

Nutrient (per 100 mL)	Human Milk	Cow's Milk	Infant Formula[a]
ENERGY-YIELDING NUTRIENTS			
Energy (kcal)	64	66	67
Protein (g)	0.9	3.4	1.5
Fat (g)	3.4	3.7	3.7
Carbohydrate (g)	6.6	4.9	7.1
MINERALS			
Sodium (mg)	17	58	20
Potassium (mg)	55	138	68
Chloride (mg)	43	103	43
Calcium (mg)	26	125	47
Phosphorus (mg)	14	96	35
Magnesium (mg)	4	12	5
Iron (mg)	0.5	0.5	1.2[b]
Zinc (mg)	0.2	0.4	0.5
Copper (mg)	0.04	0.01	0.06
VITAMINS			
Vitamin A (IU)	190	103	255
Thiamin (μg)	16	44	63
Riboflavin (μg)	36	175	110
Vitamin B_6 (μg)	10	64	41
Niacin (μg)	159	93	700
Pantothenic acid (μg)	198	352	277
Biotin (μg)	1	4	1.4
Folate (μg)	5	5	9
Vitamin B_{12} (μg)	0.04	0.04	0.14
Vitamin C (mg)	4.6	1.2	5.6
Vitamin D (IU)	2.2	3.4	41
Vitamin E (IU)	0.2	0.04	1.7
Vitamin K (μg)	1.5	6.0	5.7
Inositol (μg)	37	17	3
Choline (μg)	6	20	10

[a]Values represent the average for three major commercial products: (1) Similac, Ross Laboratories, (2) Enfamil, Mead-Johnson Laboratories, and (3) SMA, Wyeth Laboratories.

[b]The value represents formulas with iron fortification. The value for unfortified formula is 0.1 milligram.

Source: Adapted with permission from K. J. Motil, Breast-feeding: Public health and clinical overview, in *Pediatric Nutrition*, eds. R. J. Grand, J. L. Sutphen, and W. H. Dietz, Jr. (Stoneham, Mass.: Butterworths, 1987), pp. 251–263.

nutrients. Without sterilization and refrigeration, bottles of formula are an ideal breeding ground for bacteria. Whenever such risks are present, breastfeeding can be a lifesaving option. Wherever sanitation is poor, breastfeeding is preferred: breast milk is sterile, and its antibodies enhance an infant's resistance to disease. An infant who lives in a house without indoor plumbing and is not breastfed is twice as likely to die early in life as a breastfed infant who lives in a house with good sanitation.

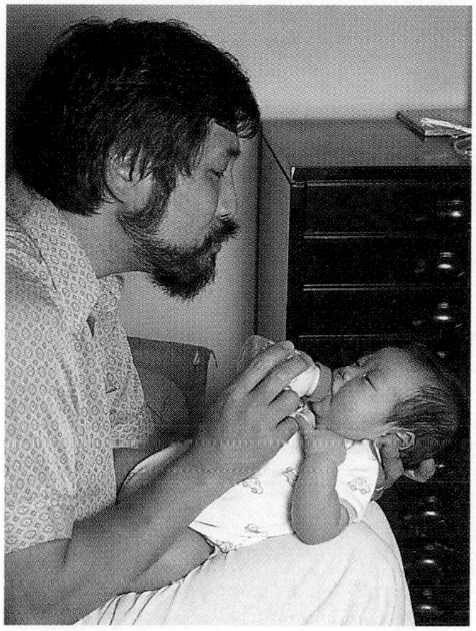

The infant thrives on infant formula offered with affection.

Infant Formula Standards National and international standards have been set for the nutrient contents of infant formulas. U.S. standards are based on American Academy of Pediatrics recommendations, and the Food and Drug Administration (FDA) mandates quality control procedures to ensure that they are met. All formulas that meet the standards are nutritionally similar; small differences are sometimes confusing, but usually not important unless infants have special needs.

Special Formulas Standard formulas are inappropriate for some infants. For example, infants with inherited diseases may need special formulas. Special formulas based on soy protein are available for infants allergic to milk protein. Soy formulas are usually lactose-free, and so can be used for infants with lactose intolerance as well. Other variations have been formulated for infants with other special needs.

Inappropriate Formulas Caretakers must use only products designed for infants; soy *beverages*, for example, are nutritionally incomplete and inappropriate for infants.[12] Goat's milk is also inappropriate for infants because of its low folate content. An infant receiving goat's milk is likely to develop "goat's milk anemia," an anemia characteristic of folate deficiency.

nursing bottle tooth decay: extensive tooth decay due to prolonged tooth contact with formula, milk, fruit juice, or other carbohydrate-rich liquid offered to an infant in a bottle.

Nursing Bottle Tooth Decay Dentists advise against putting a baby to bed with a bottle. Salivary flow, which normally cleanses the mouth, diminishes as the baby falls asleep. Sucking for long times pushes the jawline out of shape and causes a bucktoothed profile, with protruding upper and receding lower teeth. Furthermore, prolonged sucking on a bottle of formula, milk, or juice bathes the upper teeth in a carbohydrate-rich fluid that nourishes decay-producing bacteria. (The tongue covers and protects most of the lower teeth, but they, too, may be affected.) The result is extensive and rapid tooth decay. To prevent it, no child should be put to bed with a bottle of nourishing fluid. If a bottle is given, it should contain water. In fact, caregivers are wise to offer infants water after each feeding to rinse the mouth.

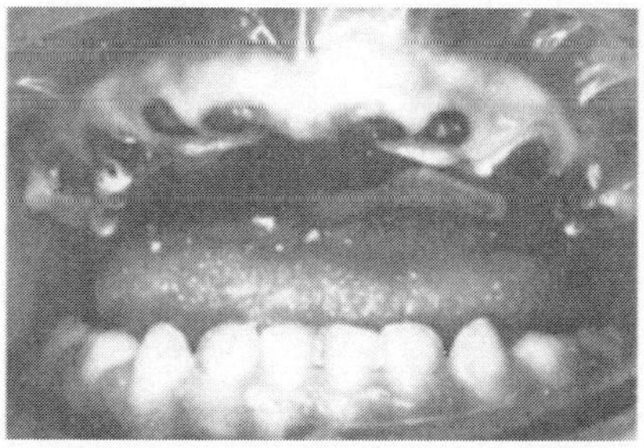

An extreme example of nursing bottle tooth decay. This child was frequently put to bed sucking on a bottle filled with apple juice, so that the teeth were bathed in carbohydrate for long periods of time—a perfect medium for bacterial growth. The upper teeth have decayed all the way to the gum line.

HEALTHY PEOPLE 2000: Increase to at least 75% the proportion of parents and caregivers who use feeding practices that prevent nursing bottle tooth decay.

SPECIAL NEEDS OF PRETERM INFANTS

The terms *preterm* and *premature* imply incomplete fetal development, or immaturity, of many body systems. The preterm infant faces physical independence before some of the organs and tissues are ready. The fastest fetal weight gain occurs during the last trimester of gestation, so a preterm infant is most often a low-birthweight infant. With a premature birth, the infant is forced to endure the time of maximal growth without the continued nutritional support of the placenta.

The last trimester of gestation is also a time when nutrients are stored for later use. Having limited nutrient stores intensifies the precarious situation for premature infants, and their metabolic immaturity further compromises their nutrition status. Their absorption of nutrients, especially of fat and calcium, is also limited. Preterm, low-birthweight infants are likely candidates for nutrient deficiencies.

Infants who are born eight to ten weeks prior to term have acquired only about 30 percent as much calcium as full-term infants, so their calcium requirements are high. They miss out on the normal mineralization of bone that takes place during the last trimester of gestation. As a result, they often develop the metabolic bone disease osteopenia, the rickets of prematurity. Susceptibility to osteopenia varies directly with the infant's weight: the smaller the infant, the greater the risk.

osteopenia: a metabolic bone disease common in preterm infants; also called **rickets of prematurity**.

Preterm infants often receive both breast milk and formula. Breast milk provides protection against infection, and its composition is excellent for the immature intestine, kidneys, and liver. Breast milk cannot, however, fully meet the calcium and phosphorus needs of the preterm infant. Formulas for preterm infants contain more highly concentrated calcium and phosphorus than standard formulas, and breastfed preterm infants receive human milk supplemented with these minerals.[13] Special formulas designed for preterm infants offer the advantages of known composition and precise measurement of intake.

INTRODUCING FIRST FOODS

Changes in body organs during the first year affect the baby's readiness to accept solid foods. For example, the stomach and intestines can easily digest the milk sugar lactose at birth, but they cannot digest starch for several months. One reason why breast milk or formula is the ideal first food is that its easily digested carbohydrate can best supply energy for the baby's intense growth and activity. Breast milk or infant formula should therefore be the baby's major food, at first. Cow's milk is inappropriate during the first year because it provides insufficient vitamin C and iron and excessive sodium and protein. If introduced too soon, cow's milk displaces iron-fortified formula or breast milk and causes GI blood loss in many infants.

Supplemental, or weaning, foods are sometimes called **beikost** (BYE-cost).

When to Introduce Solid Food In addition to formula or breast milk, an infant needs to begin eating other foods around four to six months. Infants who do not receive solid foods before the end of the first year may suffer delayed growth.

Physical readiness for solid foods develops in small steps. Teeth begin to erupt, and the infant develops the ability to swallow solid foods at around four to six months. Offering food by spoon and liquids by cup helps an infant learn to swallow. At nine months to a year, a baby can sit up and handle objects; at that time, hard crackers and other finger foods can help the infant develop manual dexterity and control of the jaw muscles.

Table 16–3

First Foods for the Infant

Breast milk or iron-fortified formula is the only source of nourishment for the first 4 to 6 months. Throughout the first year, the infant's intake of breast milk or iron-fortified formula will gradually decline as solid food intake increases.

Age (mo)	Addition
4 to 6	Iron-fortified rice cereal, followed by other single-grain cereals, mixed with breast milk, formula, or water
	Pureed vegetables and fruits, one by one (perhaps vegetables before fruits, so the baby will learn to like their less sweet flavors)
6 to 8	Infant breads and crackers
	Mashed vegetables and fruits, and their juices[a]
8 to 10	Breads and cereals from the table
	Soft, cooked vegetables and fruit from the table
	Finely cut meats, fish, chicken, casseroles, cheeses, yogurts, tofu, eggs, and legumes
10 to 12	Continue to introduce a variety of nutritious foods

[a]All baby juices are fortified with vitamin C. Orange juice may cause allergies; apple juice may be a better juice to feed first. Dilute juices with water and offer in a cup to prevent nursing bottle tooth decay.

Source: Adapted in part from Committee on Nutrition, American Academy of Pediatrics, *Pediatric Nutrition Handbook,* 3rd ed., ed. L. A. Barness (Elk Grove Village, Ill.: American Academy of Pediatrics, 1993), pp. 23–33.

Infants differ, and each program of adding foods should depend on the infant, not on a rigid schedule. Indications of readiness for solid foods include:

- The infant's birthweight has doubled.
- The infant can sit with support and can control head movements.
- The infant is four to six months old.

Table 16–3 presents a suggested sequence for adding foods to the infant's diet.

Some parents want to feed solids at an earlier age on the mistaken belief that "stuffing the baby" at bedtime promotes sleeping through the night. On the average, babies start to sleep through the night at about three to four months, regardless of when solid foods are introduced.

The Need for Water An infant's kidneys are unable to concentrate waste efficiently, so the infant must excrete relatively more water than an adult to carry off a comparable amount of waste. When solid foods are introduced, the risk of dehydration becomes greater, and infants may require supplemental water.

Allergy-Causing Foods New foods should be introduced singly and at intervals spaced to permit detection of allergies. For example, when cereals are introduced, rice cereal is offered first for several days because it is least likely to cause an allergy. When it is clear that rice cereal is not causing an allergy, another grain is introduced. Wheat cereal is offered last because it is the most common

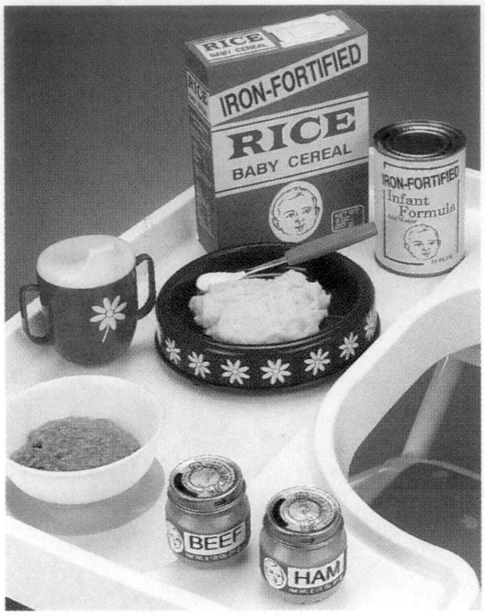

Foods such as iron-fortified cereals and formulas, mashed legumes, and strained meats provide iron.

offender. If a cereal causes an allergic reaction such as skin rash, digestive upset, or respiratory discomfort, its use should be discontinued before introducing the next food. A later section in this chapter offers more on food allergies.

Choice of Infant Foods Commercial baby foods in the United States and Canada are generally safe, nutritious, and of high quality. They contain little or no salt, less sugar than in the past, and few or no additives. Except for mixed dinners and heavily sweetened desserts, commercial baby foods typically have high nutrient density. Alternatively, parents who want to feed the baby family foods can follow safe food handling practices, cook foods without salt, and "blenderize" small portions at each meal. The foods offered should include good sources of iron and vitamin C.

Foods to Provide Iron Iron deficiency is common in children throughout the world, especially between six months and three years when they are growing fast and milk, which is a poor source of iron, has a large place in their diets. The iron an infant stored during gestation typically runs out after the birthweight doubles, long before the end of the first year.

In addition to breast milk or formula with iron, infants can receive iron from iron-fortified cereals and, later, from meat or meat alternates such as legumes. Iron-fortified cereals contribute a significant amount of iron to an infant's diet, but the iron's bioavailability is poor. Consequently, cereal alone, or in combination with cow's milk, is insufficient to meet iron needs.[14] During the first year, cereals should be mixed with iron-fortified formula, breast milk, or water rather than cow's milk. Parents or caretakers can enhance iron absorption from iron-fortified cereals by selecting vitamin C–rich foods to go with meals.

Foods to Provide Vitamin C The best sources of vitamin C are fruits and vegetables. Some authorities suggest that an infant who is introduced to fruits before vegetables may develop a preference for sweets and find the vegetables less palatable. To prevent this, introduce vegetables first, fruits later.

Fruit juices should be diluted and served in a cup, not a bottle. They should also be served in reasonable quantities as part of a balanced selection of foods. Cases have been reported of children failing to grow and thrive because they were drinking such large amounts of juice daily that other more energy- and nutrient-dense foods were displaced from their diets.[15] Such findings prove that any one food—even a healthful and nutritious one—can create nutrient imbalances and impair growth when consumed in excess.

Foods to Omit Sweets of any other kind, including baby food "desserts," have no place in an infant's diet. They convey no nutrients to support growth, and the extra food energy can promote obesity. Canned vegetables are also inappropriate for infants, as they often contain too much sodium. Honey and corn syrup should never be fed to infants because of the risk of botulism.* Babies and even young children cannot safely chew and swallow popcorn, whole grapes,

botulism (BOT-chew-lism)**:** an often fatal food-borne illness caused by the ingestion of foods containing a toxin produced by bacteria that grow in improperly canned acidic foods (see Chapter 19 for details).

*In infants, but not in older individuals, ingestion of *Clostridium botulinum* spores can cause illness when the spores germinate in the intestine and produce toxin, which is absorbed. Symptoms include poor feeding, constipation, loss of tension in the arteries and muscles, weakness, and respiratory compromise. Infant botulism has been implicated in 5 percent of cases of sudden infant death syndrome (SIDS).

Table 16–4

Meal Plan for a One-Year-Old

Breakfast	**Afternoon snack**
½ c whole milk	½ c whole milk
3 tbs cereal	Teething crackers
1 to 2 tbs fruit[a]	1 tbs peanut butter
Teething crackers	**Dinner**
Morning snack	1 c whole milk
½ c whole milk	1 egg
1 to 2 tbs fruit[a]	2 tbs cereal or potato
Teething crackers	2 to 3 tbs vegetables[b]
Lunch	2 to 3 tbs fruit[a]
1 c whole milk	
2 to 3 tbs vegetables[b]	
2 tbs chopped meat or well-cooked, mashed legumes	

[a]Include citrus fruits, melons, and berries.
[b]Include dark green, leafy and deep yellow vegetables.

whole beans, hot dog slices, hard candies, and nuts; they can easily choke on these foods, a risk not worth taking.

Foods at One Year At one year of age, whole cow's milk becomes the primary source of most of the nutrients an infant needs; 2 to 3½ cups a day meets those needs sufficiently. More milk than this displaces foods necessary to provide iron and can lead to milk anemia. Children one to two years old should drink whole milk, not low-fat or nonfat milk. If they use powdered milk, it should be one of the fat-containing varieties. Other foods—meats, iron-fortified cereals, enriched or whole-grain breads, fruits, and vegetables—should be supplied in variety and in amounts sufficient to round out total energy needs. Ideally, a one-year-old will sit at the table, eat many of the same foods everyone else eats, and drink liquids from a cup, not a bottle. Table 16–4 shows a meal plan that meets a one-year-old's requirements.

milk anemia: iron-deficiency anemia that develops when an excessive milk intake displaces iron-rich foods from the diet.

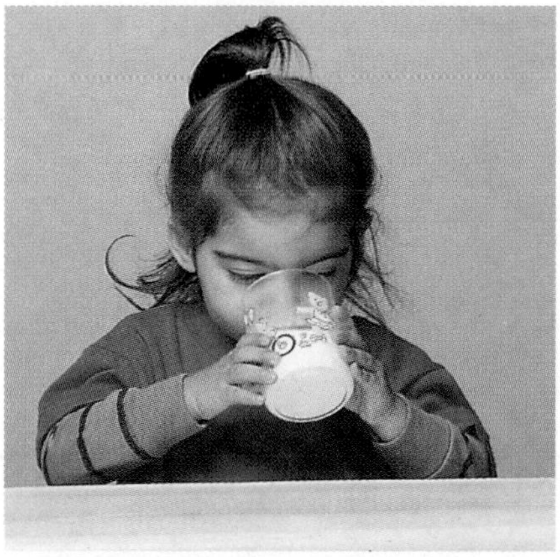

Toddlers need vitamin A– and vitamin D–fortified whole milk.

MEALTIMES WITH INFANTS

The wise parent of a one-year-old offers nutrition and love together. "Feeding with love" produces better growth and brain development than feeding the same food without love.

The person feeding a one-year-old has to be aware that exploring and experimenting are normal and desirable behaviors at this time in a child's life. The child is developing a sense of autonomy that, if fostered, will provide the foundation for later confidence and effectiveness as an individual. The child's impulses, if consistently denied, can turn to shame and self-doubt. In light of the developmental needs of one-year-olds and their often willful behavior, a few

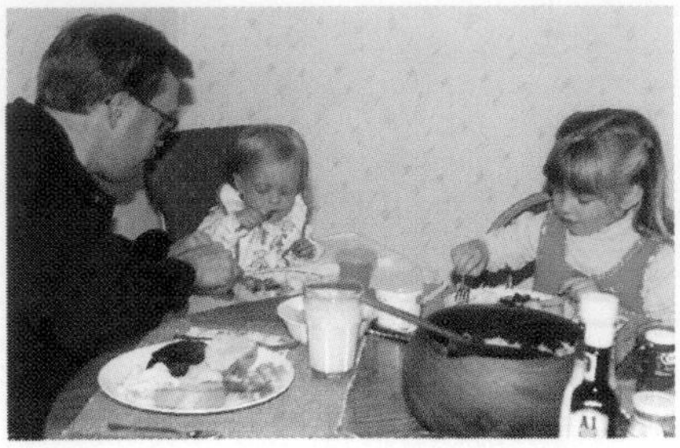

Ideally, a one-year-old eats many of the same foods as the rest of the family.

feeding guidelines may be helpful:

- Discourage unacceptable behavior, such as standing at the table or throwing food, by removing the child from the table to wait until later to eat. Be consistent and firm, not punitive. The child will soon learn to sit and eat.
- Let the child explore and enjoy food, even if this means eating with fingers for a while. Use of the spoon will come in time.
- Don't force food on children. Rejecting new foods is normal; acceptance is more likely as infants and children become familiar with new foods through repeated opportunities to taste them.[16]
- Provide children with nutritious foods, and let them choose which ones and how much they will eat. Gradually, they will acquire a taste for different foods.
- Limit sweets. Infants have little room in their daily energy allowance for empty-kcalorie foods. Do not use sweets as a reward for eating meals.
- Don't turn the dining table into a battleground. Make mealtimes enjoyable. Teach children healthy food choices and eating habits in a pleasant environment.

These recommendations reflect the spirit of tolerance that best serves the emotional and physical interests of the young child.

To recap, the primary food for infants during the first 6 to 12 months is either breast milk or iron-fortified formulas. In addition to nutrients, breast milk also offers immunological protection. At about 4 to 6 months, infants should gradually begin eating solid foods so that by 1 year, they are drinking from a cup and eating many of the same foods as the rest of the family.

Nutrition during Childhood

Each year from age one to adolescence, a child typically grows taller by 2 to 3 inches and heavier by 5 or so pounds. Growth charts provide valuable clues to a child's health. Weight gains out of proportion to height gains may reflect overeating and inactivity, whereas measures significantly below the standard suggest malnutrition.

Increases in height and weight are only two of the many developmental changes occurring during childhood. At age one, children can stand alone and are learning to toddle; by two, they can walk and are learning to run; by three, they can jump and are climbing with confidence. Bones and muscles increase in mass and density to make these accomplishments possible. Thereafter, further lengthening of the long bones and increases in musculature proceed, unevenly and more slowly, until adolescence.

ENERGY AND NUTRIENT NEEDS

Children's appetites begin to diminish around one year, consistent with the slowing of growth. Thereafter, children spontaneously vary their food intakes to coincide with their growth patterns; they demand more food during periods of rapid growth than during slow periods. At times they seem to be insatiable, and at other times they seem to live on air and water.

Although children's energy intakes may vary widely from meal to meal, their total daily intakes are remarkably constant.[17] If children eat less at one meal, they typically eat more at the next, and vice versa. Overweight children are an exception: they do not always adjust their energy intakes appropriately and may eat in response to external cues, disregarding appetite-regulation signals.

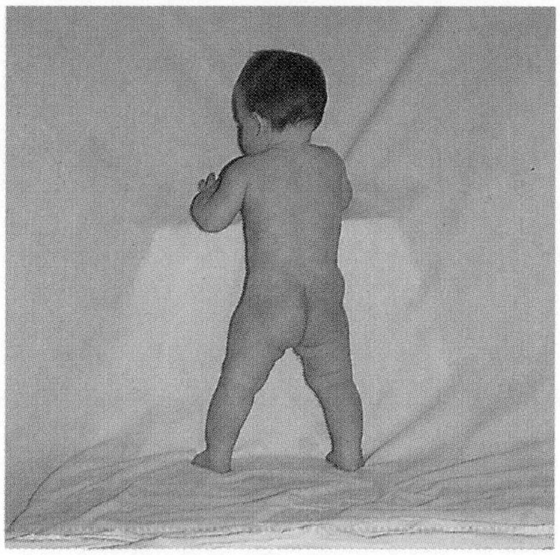

The body shape of a one-year-old (above) changes dramatically by age two (below). The two-year-old has lost much of the baby fat; the muscles (especially in the back, buttocks, and legs) have firmed and strengthened; and the leg bones have lengthened.

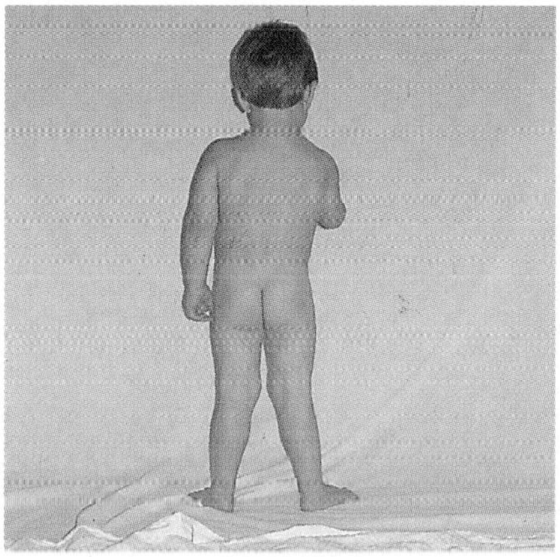

Energy Intake and Activity A one-year-old child needs perhaps 1000 kcalories a day; a three-year-old needs only 300 kcalories more. By age ten, a child needs about 2000 kcalories a day. Total energy needs increase slightly with age, but energy needs per kilogram body weight actually decline gradually.

Individual children's energy needs vary widely, depending on their physical activity. Inactive children can become obese even when they eat less food than the average. They would do well to learn to enjoy physical play and exercise.

Vitamins and Minerals Steady growth during childhood implies gradually increasing needs of all nutrients. The RDA table and the RNI for Canadians list incremental additions to the recommended intakes for each span of three years.

Before adolescence, children accumulate stores of nutrients. Then, when they take off on the adolescent growth spurt and their nutrient intakes cannot meet the demands of rapid growth, they draw on those stores. This is especially true of calcium; the denser the bones grow in childhood, the better they can support teen growth and still withstand the inevitable bone losses of later life. The way preteen children eat, then, influences their nutritional health during childhood, during their teen years—and in their old age.

Planning Children's Meals To provide all the needed nutrients, children's meals should include a variety of foods from each food group—in amounts suited to their appetites and needs. Serving sizes increase with age. A portion of meat, grains, fruits, or vegetables for children is loosely defined as 1 tablespoon per year. Thus, at four years of age, a portion is about 4 tablespoons, or ¼ cup. This rule of thumb applies until they reach the teen years. Table 16–5 offers a daily food pattern for children.

To ensure that children have healthy appetites and plenty of room for nutritious foods when they are hungry, parents and teachers must limit access to candy, cola, and other concentrated sweets. If such foods are permitted in large quantities, the only possible outcomes are nutrient deficiencies, obesity, or both. The preference for sweets is innate; most children do not naturally select nutritious foods on the basis of taste. In one study, when children were allowed to create meals freely from a variety of foods, they selected foods that provided 25 percent of the kcalories from sugar.[18] When their parents were watching, or even when they thought their parents were watching, the children improved their selections. Overweight children, especially, need help in sticking to nutrient-dense foods that will meet their nutrient needs within their energy allowances.

Sweets need not be banned altogether. Children who are exceptionally active can enjoy high-kcalorie foods such as ice cream or pudding from the milk group or pancakes or cookies from the bread group. These foods carry valuable nutrients and bring pleasure. As for sedentary children, they need to become more active, and then they, too, can enjoy some of these foods without unhealthy weight gain.

Table 16–5

Children's Daily Food Patterns for Good Nutrition

Food Group	Servings per Day	Average Size of Serving		
		1 TO 3 YEARS	4 TO 6 YEARS	7 TO 12 YEARS
Bread and cereals (whole grain or enriched)[a]	6 or more	½ slice	1 slice	1 to 2 slices
Vegetables[b]	3 or more	2–4 tbs or ½ c juice	¼–½ c or ½ c juice	½–¾ c or ½ c juice
Fruits[b]	2 or more	2–4 tbs or ½ c juice	¼–½ c or ½ c juice	½–¾ c or ½ c juice
Meat and meat alternates[c]	2 or more	1–2 oz	1–2 oz	2–3 oz
Milk and milk products[d]	3 to 4	½–¾ c	¾ c	¾–1 c

[a]1 slice bread = ¾ c dry cereal, ½ c cooked cereal, ½ c potato, rice, or noodles.

[b]Vitamin C source (citrus fruits, berries, tomatoes, broccoli, cabbage, cantaloupe) daily; vitamin A source (spinach, carrots, squash, tomato, cantaloupe) 3 to 4 times weekly.

[c]1 oz meat, fish, poultry = 1 egg, 1 frankfurter, 2 tbs peanut butter, ½ c cooked legumes.

[d]½ c milk = ½ c cottage cheese, pudding, yogurt; ¾ oz cheese; 2 tbs dried milk.

Source: Adapted from P. M. Queen and R. R. Henry, Growth and nutrient requirements of children, in *Pediatric Nutrition,* eds. R. J. Grand, J. L. Sutphen, and W. H. Dietz, Jr. (Boston: Butterworths, 1987), p. 347.

HUNGER AND MALNUTRITION IN CHILDREN

Most U.S. and Canadian children are well nourished. Their average energy intakes are sufficient to support normal growth, and their average nutrient intakes, except for iron, meet or exceed recommendations. Some low-income children, however, are malnourished and have suffered growth retardation. An estimated 11 million U.S. children under age 12 are hungry and living in poverty.

Chapter 20 examines the causes and consequences of hunger in the United States and around the world.

HEALTHY PEOPLE 2000: Reduce growth retardation among low-income children aged five years and younger to less than 10%.

Malnutrition and Health When hunger is chronic, children become malnourished. Worldwide, malnutrition takes a devastating toll on children, contributing to nearly half of the deaths of children under four years old. Vitamin A deficiency afflicts more than 5 million children worldwide, inducing blindness, stunted growth, and infections. Zinc deficiency also retards growth and typically accompanies protein-energy malnutrition and vitamin A deficiency.

Hunger and Behavior Even when hunger is temporary, as when a child misses one meal, behavior and academic performance are affected. Children who eat nutritious breakfasts function better than their peers who do not. Young children who participate in the federally funded School Breakfast Program improve their scores on achievement tests and are tardy or absent significantly less often than children who qualify for the program, but do not participate. Without breakfast, children perform poorly in tasks requiring concentration, their attention spans are shorter, and they even show lower IQs on testing than their well-fed peers; malnourished children are particularly vulnerable. Common sense dictates that it is unreasonable to expect anyone to learn and perform work when no fuel has been provided. By late morning, discomfort from hunger may become distracting even if a child has eaten breakfast.

The problem children face when attempting morning schoolwork on an empty stomach appears to be at least partly due to low blood glucose. The average child up to age ten or so needs to eat every four to six hours to maintain a blood glucose concentration high enough to support the activity of the brain and nervous system. A child's brain is as big as an adult's, and the brain is the body's chief glucose consumer. A child's liver is much smaller than an adult's, however, and the liver is the organ responsible for storing glucose as glycogen and releasing it into the blood as needed. A child's liver can store only about four hours' worth of glycogen—hence the need to eat fairly often. Teachers aware of the late-morning slump in their classrooms wisely request that midmorning snacks be provided; snacks improve classroom performance all the way to lunchtime. For the child who hasn't had breakfast, the morning's lessons may be lost altogether.

Eating breakfast also helps children to meet their nutrient needs each day. Children who skip breakfast typically do not make up the deficits at later meals—they simply have lower intakes of energy, vitamins, and minerals than those who eat breakfast.[19]

The brain uses about three times as much glucose per day as the rest of the body.

Iron Deficiency Iron deficiency anemia is a major problem worldwide, as well as being the most prevalent nutrient deficiency among U.S. and Canadian children. The high iron needs of growth combined with typically low iron intakes leave many children with marginal iron status. Reducing iron deficiency among young children is one of the foremost health priorities in the United States.[20] Internationally, the World Health Organization is collaborating with a United Nations subcommittee on nutrition to develop a ten-year plan to eliminate iron deficiency.[21]

HEALTHY PEOPLE 2000: Reduce iron deficiency to less than 3% among children aged one through four years.

To prevent iron deficiency, children's foods must deliver approximately 10 milligrams of iron per day. To achieve this goal, snacks and meals should include the iron-rich foods listed in Table 16–6, and milk should be limited to 3 or 4 cups a day, so that it will not displace lean meats, fish, poultry, eggs, legumes, and whole-grain or enriched products.

Iron Deficiency and Behavior Iron deficiency has well-known and widespread effects on children's behavior. In addition to carrying oxygen in the blood, iron transports oxygen within cells, which use it to help produce energy. Iron is also used to make neurotransmitters—most notably, those that regulate the ability to pay attention, which is crucial to learning. An iron deficiency not only causes an energy crisis but also directly affects mood, attention span, and learning ability.

Iron deficiency is usually diagnosed by a deficit of iron in the *blood,* after the deficiency has progressed all the way to anemia. A child's *brain*, however, is sensitive to low iron concentrations long before the blood effects appear. Research has shown that iron deficiency lowers the "motivation to persist in intellectually

Table 16–6

Iron-Rich Foods Children Like[a]

Breads, cereals, and grains
- Canned macaroni (½ c)
- Canned spaghetti (½ c)
- Cream of wheat (¼ c)
- Fortified dry cereals (1 oz)[b]
- Noodles, rice, or barley (½ c)
- Tortillas (1 flour, 2 corn)
- Whole-wheat, enriched, or fortified bread (1 slice)
- Bran muffins

Vegetables
- Baked flavored potato skins (½ skin)
- Cooked mushrooms (½ c)
- Cooked mung bean sprouts or snow peas (½ c)
- Green peas (½ c)
- Mixed vegetable juice (1 c)

Fruits
- Apple juice (1 c)
- Canned plums (3 plums)
- Cooked dried apricots (½ c)
- Dried peaches (4 halves)
- Raisins (1 tbs)

Meats and legumes
- Bean dip (¼ c)
- Canned pork and beans (⅓ c)
- Mild chili or other bean/meat dishes (¼ c) such as burritos
- Liverwurst (½ oz)
- Meat casseroles (½ c)
- Peanut butter and jelly sandwich (½ sandwich)
- Lean roast beef or cooked ground beef (1 oz)
- Sloppy joes (½ sandwich)

[a]Each serving provides at least 1 milligram iron, or one-tenth of a child's RDA for iron. Vitamin C–rich foods included with these snacks increase iron absorption.

[b]Some fortified breakfast cereals contain more than 10 milligrams iron per half-cup serving (read the labels).

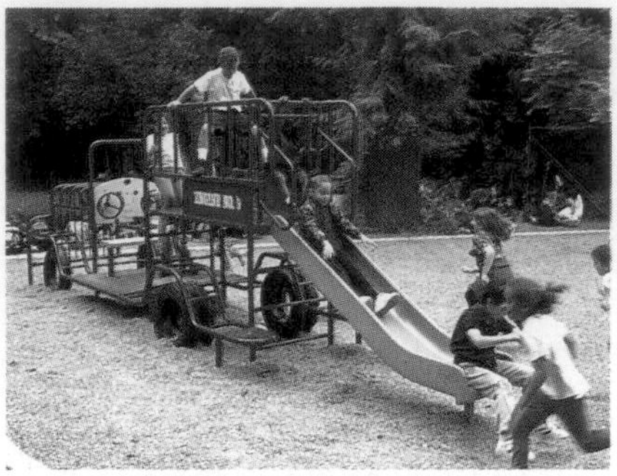

Healthy, well-nourished children are alert in the classroom and energetic at play.

challenging tasks," shortens the attention span, and impairs overall intellectual performance. Anemic children perform less well on tests and are more disruptive than their nonanemic classmates. At least one study found that children who had had iron-deficiency anemia *as infants* still continued to perform poorly at age five compared with their peers, even though they had regained excellent iron status.[22] The long-term damaging effects on mental development make prevention of iron deficiency during infancy and early childhood a high priority.[23]

Other Nutrient Deficiencies and Behavior Iron is not the only nutrient that can be displaced from a diet by nutrient-poor foods. Several dozen other nutrients may be lacking as well, causing both physical and behavioral symptoms.

A child with nutrient deficiencies may be irritable, aggressive, disagreeable, or sad and withdrawn. Such a child may be labeled "hyperactive," "depressed," or "unlikable," when in fact these traits may arise from simple, even marginal, malnutrition. In any such case, inspection of the child's diet by a qualified health care professional is clearly in order. Should suspicion of dietary inadequacies be raised, no matter what causes may be implicated, the people responsible for feeding the child should take steps to correct those inadequacies promptly.

Lead Toxicity and Malnutrition Malnutrition is quite often a complex condition involving multiple nutrients and other environmental factors. An example of a possible complicating factor is lead poisoning. Lead toxicity can cause iron deficiency, and iron deficiency can impair the body's defenses against lead absorption. Highlight 19 describes the mental, behavioral, and other health problems associated with lead toxicity. Such problems are important to investigate, but even before they have been identified, the child should be fed properly.

Parents and medical practitioners often overlook the possibility that malnutrition may account for abnormalities of appearances and behavior. Any departure from normal healthy appearance and behavior is a sign of possible poor nutrition (see Table 16–7).

NUTRITION, HYPERACTIVITY, AND "HYPER" BEHAVIOR

Because malnutrition can impair children's functioning in many ways, people tend to look to food habits for explanations of hyperactivity. Hyperactivity is not caused by a poor diet, but a poor diet may be part of a cluster of factors seen in a hyperactive child's life.

Tension-Fatigue Syndrome Children can become excitable, rambunctious, and unruly out of a desire for attention, lack of sleep, overstimulation, too much television, or a lack of physical activity. Together, these factors produce the tension-fatigue syndrome, which suggests that more consistent care, and not just better food, is needed. It helps most to insist on regular hours of sleep, regular mealtimes, and regular outdoor activity.

Hyperactivity Disorder Hyperactivity is a disorder that affects behavior and learning in about 5 percent of young school-age children. Left untreated, hyperactivity can interfere with a child's social development and ability to learn. Treatment focuses on relieving the symptoms and controlling the associated problems; there is no cure.

tension-fatigue syndrome: apparent hyperactivity produced in a child by the combination of lack of sleep, overstimulation, and anxiety.

hyperactivity: a disorder characterized by chronic behavior and learning problems. Behavior problems include impulsiveness and restlessness that are inappropriate for a child's age. Learning problems reflect a short attention span. Professionals call this syndrome **attention deficit hyperactivity disorder (ADHD)**.

Table 16–7

Physical Signs of Health and Malnutrition in Children

	Healthy	Malnourished
Hair:	Shiny, firm in the scalp	Dull, brittle, dry, loose; falls out
Eyes:	Bright, clear pink membranes; adjust easily to darkness	Pale membranes; spots; redness; adjust slowly to darkness
Teeth and gums:	No pain or cavities, gums firm, teeth bright	Missing, discolored, decayed teeth; gums bleed easily and are swollen and spongy
Face:	Good complexion	Off-color, scaly, flaky, cracked skin
Glands:	No lumps	Swollen at front of neck and cheeks
Tongue:	Red, bumpy, rough	Sore, smooth, purplish, swollen
Skin:	Smooth, firm, good color	Dry, rough, spotty; "sandpaper" feel or sores; lack of fat under skin
Nails:	Firm, pink	Spoon-shaped brittle, ridged
Behavior:	Alert, attentive, cheerful	Irritable, apathetic, inattentive, hyperactive
Internal systems:	Heart rate, heart rhythm, and blood pressure normal; normal digestive function; reflexes and psychological development normal	Heart rate, heart rhythm, or blood pressure abnormal; liver and spleen enlarged; abnormal digestion; mental irritability, confusion; burning, tingling of hands and feet; loss of balance and coordination
Muscles and bones:	Good muscle tone and posture; long bones straight	"Wasted" appearance of muscles; swollen bumps on skull or ends of bones; small bumps on ribs; bowed legs or knock-knees

Note: The physical signs shown here are consistent with malnutrition but not diagnostic of it.

Physicians often manage hyperactivity through behavior modification, special educational techniques, psychological counseling, and drug therapy. The drugs most commonly prescribed are stimulants. Normally, stimulants speed up people's activity, but they have a paradoxical effect on hyperactivity: they normalize it by stimulating control centers in the brain. If a child calms down when given stimulant drugs, the response indicates that the drugs may be correcting a biochemical imbalance in the nervous system and can help control the behavior.

Many parents mistakenly believe a solution may lie in manipulating the diet—most commonly, by eliminating sugar or food additives. Diet is one area of a child's life in which parents feel they can exert some control. If problems can be solved by adding carrots or eliminating candy, then parents are eager to give diet advice a try. While nutrition should be considered whenever a person's health is less than optimal, it is unwise to jump at appealing solutions that are unfounded. Several studies have found no convincing evidence that sugar causes hyperactivity or worsens behavior.[24] Recommendations to restrict sugar in children's diets to prevent or treat behavior problems are groundless. Sugar can influence children's behavior only by displacing nutritious foods and contributing to nutrient deficiencies.

Caffeine and Behavior Caffeine is often overlooked as a source of "hyper" behavior in children, but it is a matter of some concern to pediatricians. A 12-

ounce cola beverage may contain as much as 50 milligrams caffeine; in the body of a 60-pound child, two or more such beverages are equivalent to the caffeine in 8 cups of coffee for a 175-pound adult. Children who are troubled by sleeplessness, restlessness, and irregular heartbeats may need to limit their caffeine consumption. Children not accustomed to caffeine who are given doses equivalent to about two cola beverages a day become noticeably inattentive and restless. As long as children are surrounded by attractive temptations such as cola beverages, adults must prevent abuse until the children learn to control consumption themselves. (Appendix H presents a table that lists the caffeine contents of foods, beverages, and medicines.)

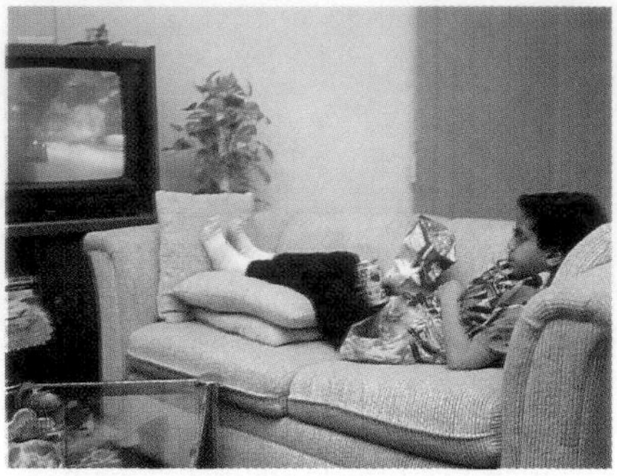

Television watching influences children's eating habits and activity patterns.

TELEVISION AND CHILDREN'S NUTRITION

The average child watches 5000 hours of television before the end of preschool and has seen 19,000 hours by the end of high school.[25] Watching television is second only to sleeping among children's uses of time.

Besides contributing to tension-fatigue syndrome, watching television adversely affects children's nutritional health in several ways. As Chapter 9 reported, studies have found that the prevalence of obesity increases with each hour of television viewed; even daydreaming appears to use more energy than watching television.[26] Children who watch more than two hours of television per day also have higher serum cholesterol than do more active children.

TV fosters obesity because it:

- Requires no energy beyond basal metabolism.
- Replaces vigorous activities.
- Encourages snacking.
- Promotes a sedentary lifestyle.

The average child sees an estimated 10,000 commercials a year—almost all luring viewers to purchase sugar-coated breakfast cereals, candy bars, chips, fast foods, and carbonated beverages. These foods add sugar, fat, and salt to the diet and displace foods that provide needed nutrients. Many parents and pediatricians believe that food ads aimed at children should be banned because they support corporate profits rather than children's health. Alternatively, parents can teach their children how to evaluate food ads and make healthful choices.

ADVERSE REACTIONS TO FOODS

adverse reactions: unusual responses to food (including intolerances and allergies).

Adverse reactions to foods can threaten nutritional health to varying extents, depending on the severity and duration of the reactions and the foods they involve. Temporary reactions may lead to permanent avoidance of foods; permanent reactions, if not detected and treated, can cause chronic illness.

food intolerances: adverse reactions to foods that do not involve the immune system.

Food Intolerances Not all adverse reactions to foods are food allergies, although even physicians may describe them as such. Signs of adverse reactions to foods include stomachaches, headaches, pain, rapid pulse rate, nausea, wheezing, hives, bronchial irritation, coughs, and other such discomforts. Among the causes may be reactions to chemicals in foods, such as the flavor enhancer monosodium glutamate (MSG), the natural laxative in prunes, or the mineral sulfur; digestive diseases, such as obstructions or injuries; enzyme deficiencies, such as lactose intolerance; and even psychological aversions. These reactions involve symptoms but no antibody production. Therefore, they are food intolerances, not allergies.[27]

food allergies: adverse reactions to foods that involve an immune response; also called *food-hypersensitivity reactions*.

Food Allergies A true food allergy occurs when a whole food protein or other large molecule enters the body and elicits an immunologic response.

(Recall that large molecules of food are normally dismantled in the digestive tract to smaller ones that are absorbed without such a reaction.) The body's immune system reacts to a large food molecule as it does to other antigens—by producing antibodies, histamines, or other defensive agents.

Allergies may have one or two components. They always involve antibodies; they may or may not involve symptoms. This means that allergies can be diagnosed only by testing for antibodies. Even symptoms exactly like those of an allergy may not be caused by one.

Allergic reactions to food may be immediate or delayed. In both cases, the antigen interacts immediately with the immune system, but the timing of symptoms varies from minutes to 24 hours. Identifying the food that causes an immediate allergic reaction is easy because the symptoms may not appear until a day later. By this time, many other foods have been eaten, complicating the picture.

Almost 75 percent of adverse reactions are caused by three major foods—eggs, peanuts, or milk.[28] Allergic reactions to single foods are common. Reactions to multiple foods are the exception, not the rule.

Identifying a true food allergy requires a thorough health history, physical examination, and diagnostic tests to eliminate other diseases.[29] Skin pricks with food extracts are one of the most common tests for food allergies, even though the high incidence of false positive results can complicate diagnosis. Physicians also conduct dietary trials that first eliminate the offending food and then reintroduce it in small quantities to substantiate that reactions occur only when that particular food is eaten.[30] Once a food allergy has been diagnosed, therapy requires strict elimination of the offending food.

Food allergies are most common during the first few years of life, but then children typically outgrow (become tolerant to) their hypersensitivity. Between 2 and 8 percent of young children are allergic to certain foods, whereas only 2 percent of adults have food allergies.[31] Tolerance is most likely if the offending food can be identified and eliminated from the diet for at least a year or two.[32]

When parents stop serving a suspected food to their child, they risk the child's suffering nutrient deficiencies. They should be sure to include other foods that offer the same nutrients as the omitted food. Children with allergies, like all children, need all their nutrients.

histamine (HISS-tah-mean, or HISS-tah-men)**:** a substance produced by cells of the immune system as part of a local immune reaction to an antigen; participates in causing inflammation.

A person who produces antibodies *without* having any symptoms has an **asymptomatic allergy**; a person who produces antibodies *and* has symptoms has a **symptomatic allergy**.

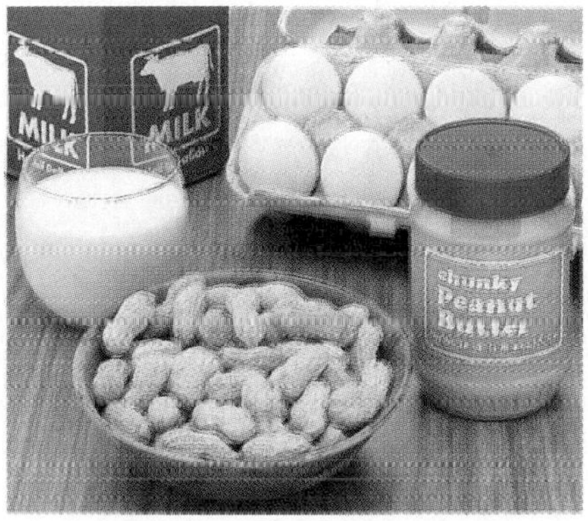

Eggs, peanuts, and milk are most likely to induce symptoms in people with food allergy

Healthful food choices and regular physical activity both promote growth and help prevent the degenerative diseases of later life—cardiovascular disease, cancer, diabetes, and osteoporosis. In contrast, poor food choices and lack of exercise can lead to obesity, elevated cholesterol levels, and hypertension—major risk factors for degenerative diseases. The highlight that follows this chapter describes how behaviors during the childhood and teen years influence disease in adulthood. The next two sections examine how children's eating behaviors are shaped both at home and at school.

MEALTIMES AT HOME

The childhood years represent a parent's best, and maybe last, chance to influence food choices. Parents are gatekeepers; they determine what foods and activities will be available in their children's environments. Then the children make their own selections. One survey reports that 65 percent of fourth through eighth graders choose their own breakfasts, 46 percent select their lunches, and 74 per-

gatekeepers: with respect to nutrition, key people who control other people's access to foods and thereby exert profound impacts on their nutrition. Examples are the spouse who buys and cooks the food, the parent who feeds the children, and the caretaker in a day-care center.

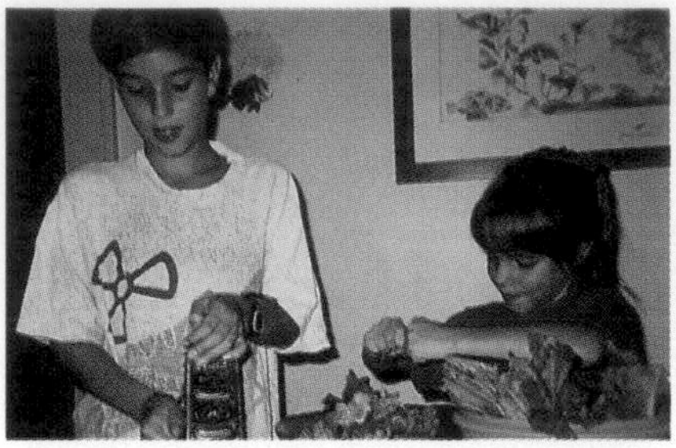

Children enjoy eating the foods they help to prepare.

cent select their snacks.[33] Gatekeepers who want to promote nutritious choices and healthful habits provide access to nutrient-dense, delicious foods and opportunities for active play at home.

- Child feeding pointer: Provide child-sized portions and utensils.
- Child feeding pointer: Serve vegetables raw or slightly undercooked and crunchy.
- Child feeding pointer: Encourage children to help plan and prepare meals.

Honoring Children's Preferences Little children like to eat at little tables and to be served little portions of food. They also like to eat with other children, and they tend to eat more in the company of their peers. Children also more easily overcome their prejudices against foods when they see their peers eating them.

Children usually like raw vegetables better than cooked ones, so it is wise to offer vegetables that are raw or slightly undercooked and crunchy, served separately, and easy to eat. Foods should be warm, not hot, because a child's mouth is much more sensitive than an adult's. The flavor should be mild because a child has more taste buds, and smooth foods such as mashed potatoes or pea soup should contain no lumps (a child wonders, with some disgust, what the lumps might be). Children prefer foods that are familiar, so offer various foods regularly.

Learning through Participation Helping to plan and prepare family meals can be an enjoyable learning experience. Children are also more likely to eat the foods they have prepared. Vegetables are pretty, especially when fresh, and provide opportunities for children to learn about color, about growing things and their seeds, and about shapes and textures—all of which are fascinating to young children. Measuring, stirring, washing, and arranging vegetables are skills that even a young child can practice with enjoyment and pride.

- Child feeding pointer: Offer children nutritious foods, but don't insist that they eat.

Avoiding Power Struggles When introducing new foods at the table, parents are advised to offer them one at a time and only in small amounts at first. The more often a food is presented to a young child, the more likely the child will like that food. Whenever possible, offer the new food at the beginning of the meal, when the child is hungry, and allow the child to make the decision to accept or reject it. Never make an issue of food acceptance, not even to reward acceptance. Children who are pushed to try new foods are less likely to try those foods again than children who are left to decide for themselves. The parent is responsible for *what* the child is offered to eat, but the child is responsible for *how much* and even *whether* to eat.

A bright, unhurried atmosphere free of conflict is conducive to good appetite. Parents who serve meals in a relaxed and casual manner, without anxiety, provide a climate that minimizes a child's negative emotions. Unaware parents can promote conflicts, despite their good intentions. Parents who beg, cajole, and demand that their children eat deny opportunities to develop self-control. Instead, the children engage in battles that take on more importance than their own hunger. A power struggle almost invariably results in a confirmed pattern of resistance and a permanently closed mind on the child's part.

- Child feeding pointer: To prevent choking, watch children eat and enforce a "sit-down" rule.

Young children can easily choke on:

- Popcorn
- Whole grapes
- Whole beans
- Hot dog slices
- Hard candies
- Nuts

Choking Prevention Parents must always be alert to the dangers of choking. A choking child is a silent child, and an adult should be present whenever a child is eating. Serve foods cut into small bite-size pieces and encourage children to sit when eating; choking is more likely when a child is running or falling. (Highlight 3 describes the Heimlich maneuver for children.)

- Child feeding pointer: Play first, then eat.

Play First Ideally, each meal is preceded, not followed, by fun activities. A number of schools have discovered that children eat a much better lunch if recess occurs before, rather than after, the meal—otherwise children "hurry up and eat" so that they can go play.

Snacks Parents may find that their children snack so much that they aren't hungry at mealtimes. Instead of teaching children *not* to snack, parents might be wise to teach them *how* to snack. Provide snacks that are as nutritious as the foods served at mealtime. Snacks can even be mealtime foods served individually over time, instead of all at once on one plate. When providing snacks to children, a smart parent thinks of the food groups and offers such snacks as pieces of cheese, tangerine slices, carrot sticks, and peanut butter on whole-wheat crackers. Snacks need to be easy to prepare, especially for children who arrive home from school before parents.

- Child feeding pointer: Provide healthful snacks.

Preventing Dental Caries Children frequently snack on sticky, sugary foods that stay on the teeth and provide an ideal environment for the growth of bacteria that cause dental caries. Teach children to eat sweets at mealtimes, to brush and floss after meals, to brush or rinse after eating snacks, to avoid sticky foods, and to select crisp or fibrous foods instead. Table 16–8 lists food suggestions for controlling dental caries.

Serving as Role Models In an effort to practice these many tips, parents may overlook perhaps the single most important influence on their children's food habits—themselves. Parents who don't eat carrots shouldn't be surprised when their children refuse to eat carrots. Likewise, parents who dislike the smell

- Child feeding pointer: Set a good example—enjoy nutritious foods.

Table 16–8

Food Suggestions for Controlling Dental Caries

Food Group	Frequent Use Recommended	Infrequent Use Suggested[a]
Milk/ milk products	Milk, cheese, plain yogurt	Chocolate milk, ice cream, ice milk, milk shakes, fruited yogurt
Meat/meat alternates	Lean meat, fish, poultry; eggs; legumes	Peanut butter with added sugar, lunch meats with added sugar, meats with sugared glazes
Fruits	Fresh or packed in water	Dried, packed in syrup or juice, jams, jellies, preserves, fruit juices or drinks
Vegetables	Salad greens, cauliflower, cucumbers, radishes, carrots, celery	Candied sweet potatoes, glazed carrots
Bread/cereal	Popcorn, soda crackers, toast, hard rolls, pretzels, corn chips, pizza	Cookies, sweet rolls, pies, cakes, potato chips, ready-to-eat sweetened cereals as between-meal snacks
Other	Sugarless gum	Sugared soft drinks, candy, fudge, caramels, honey, sugars, syrups

[a]It is particularly important to brush, floss, and rinse after eating these foods.

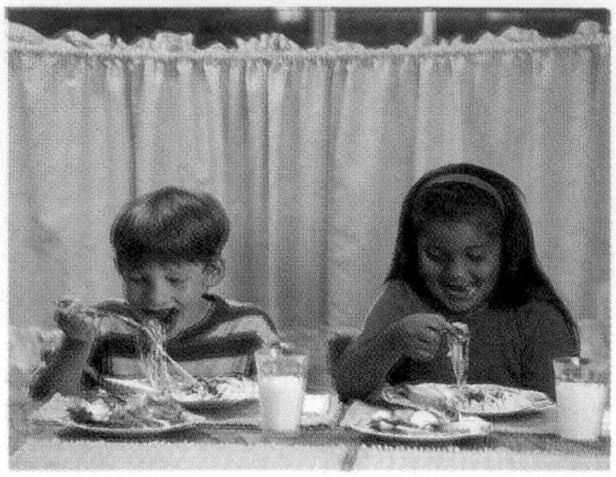

Eating is more fun when your friends are there.

of brussels sprouts may not be able to persuade children to try them. Children learn much through imitation. Parents and older siblings set an irresistible example by enjoying nutritious foods.

While serving and enjoying food, caretakers can promote both physical and emotional growth at every stage of a child's life. They can help their children to develop both a positive self-concept and a positive attitude toward food. If the beginnings are right, children will grow without the conflicts and confusions over food that can lead to nutrition and health problems.

NUTRITION AT SCHOOL

While parents are doing what they can to establish good eating habits in their children at home, child-care centers and schools are introducing foods prepared and served by others. In addition, children begin to learn about food and nutrition in the classroom. Meeting the nutrition and education needs of children is critical to supporting their healthy growth and development.[34]

School Meals The U.S. government funds several programs to provide nutritious meals for children at school. Both the School Breakfast Program and the National School Lunch Program provide meals at a reasonable cost to children from families with the financial means to pay. Meals are available free or at reduced cost to children from low-income families. (School lunches in Canada are administered locally and therefore vary from area to area.) Several studies have reported that children who participate in school food programs show improvements in learning. The accompanying box describes food programs for children, and Table 16–9 shows school lunch patterns for children of different ages.

HEALTHY PEOPLE 2000: Increase to at least 90% the proportion of school lunch and breakfast services and increase to at least 50% the proportion of child-care foodservices with menus that are consistent with the nutrition principles in the *Dietary Guidelines for Americans*.

Table 16–9

School Lunch Patterns for Different Ages

Food Group	Preschool (Age)		Grade School through High School (Grade)		
	1 TO 2	3 TO 4	K TO 3	4 TO 6	7 TO 12
Meat or meat alternate					
1 serving:					
Lean meat, poultry, or fish	1 oz	1½ oz	1½ oz	2 oz	3 oz
Cheese	1 oz	1½ oz	1½ oz	2 oz	3 oz
Large egg(s)	1	1½	1½	2	3
Cooked dry beans or peas	½ c	¾ c	¾ c	1 c	1½ c
Peanut butter	2 tbs	3 tbs	3 tbs	4 tbs	6 tbs
Vegetable and/or fruit					
2 or more servings, both to total	½ c	½ c	½ c	¾ c	¾ c
Bread or bread alternate					
Servings	5 per week	8 per week	8 per week	8 per week	10 per week
Milk					
1 serving of fluid milk	¾ c	¾ c	1 c	1 c	1 c

Food Assistance Programs for Children

The federal School Lunch and School Breakfast Programs assist schools financially so that every student can receive a nutritious lunch, breakfast, or both. These programs enable schools to provide low-income students with meals at no cost while charging other students somewhat less than the full costs of their meals. In addition, schools that participate in the programs can obtain food commodities. Nationally, the U.S. Department of Agriculture (USDA) administers the programs; on the state level, state departments of education operate them (although congress may change this arrangement in its efforts to cut federal spending). The programs usually cost school districts little.

Nearly 25 million children receive lunches through the National School Lunch Program—half of them at a free or reduced price. School lunches are designed to provide at least a third of the RDA for each of many nutrients and must include specified numbers of servings of milk, protein-rich foods (meat, poultry, fish, cheese, eggs, legumes, or peanut butter), vegetables, fruits, and breads or other grain foods.

The School Breakfast Program is available in slightly more than half of the nation's schools, and about 5 million children participate in it. The school breakfast must provide at least a fourth of the RDA for each of many nutrients and contain at least one serving of milk; one serving of fruit, juice, or vegetable; and either two servings of bread (or bread alternates), two servings of meat (or meat alternates), or one serving of each.

Another federal program, the Child Care Food Program, operates similarly and provides funds to organized child-care programs. All eligible children, centers, and family day-care homes have the right to participate. Meal reimbursements cover most of the meal and administration costs. Sponsors may also receive USDA commodity foods.

School lunches offer a variety of food choices and are available to most children. To their credit, these lunches help our nation's children meet at least one-third of their daily RDA. These lunches are supposed to meet the Dietary Guidelines, but unfortunately, almost all of the participating schools exceed recommendations for fat, saturated fat, and sodium and fall short on recommendations for carbohydrate.[35] Yet given the choice, many children will select low-fat meals.[36] Schools that have made special efforts to lower fat in school lunches typically have trouble providing enough energy and nutrients, especially iron, to meet the RDA specifications. The American Dietetic Association (ADA) advocates the development of dietary guidelines specifically for children to ensure that school lunches will both provide adequate energy and nutrients and support health.[37] According to the ADA, the guidelines currently used may be appropriate for adults, but may not be adequate to meet children's unique needs.

Nutrition Education at School Coincident with the school breakfast and lunch programs is a program of nutrition education and training (NET) in all the public schools. This program is minimally funded, but program administrators are ingenious and creative in accomplishing its highest-priority objectives. Children need to be fed well *and* learn enough about nutrition to make healthful food choices when the choices become theirs to make.

HEALTHY PEOPLE 2000: Increase to at least 75% the proportion of the nation's schools that provide nutrition education from preschool through grade 12, preferably as part of quality school health education.

In summary, children's appetites and nutrient needs reflect their stage of growth. Those who are chronically hungry and malnourished suffer growth retardation; when hunger is temporary and nutrient deficiencies are mild, the problems are usually more subtle—such as poor academic performance. Iron deficiency is widespread and has many physical and behavioral consquences. "Hyper" behavior is not caused by poor nutrition, but may reflect too much caffeine and inconsistent care, including too much television watching, which can contribute to obesity by promoting inactivity and an overconsumption of snack foods. Adults at home and at school need to provide children with nutrient dense foods and teach them how to make healthful choices.

Nutrition during Adolescence

adolescence: the period from the beginning of puberty until maturity.

Nutrient needs are greater during adolescence than at any other time of life, except for pregnancy and lactation. In general, nutrient needs rise throughout childhood and then level off or even diminish slightly as the adolescent passes into adulthood.

Teenagers make many more choices for themselves than they did as children. They are not fed, they eat; they are not sent out to play, they choose to go. At the same time, social pressures thrust choices at them: whether to drink alcoholic beverages and whether to develop their bodies to meet extreme ideals of slimness or athletic prowess.

Adolescents learn about nutrition—both valid information and misinformation—from personal, immediate experiences. They are concerned with how diet can improve their lives now—they engage in crash dieting in order to buy a new bathing suit, avoid greasy foods in an effort to clear acne, or eat a pile of spaghetti to prepare for a big sporting event. The person concerned with the nutrition and health of adolescents, then, must learn about these subjects of interest and show the relationships with nutrition.

GROWTH AND DEVELOPMENT

The steady growth of childhood speeds up abruptly and dramatically with the onset of adolescence, and female and male growth patterns become distinct. A female's adolescent growth spurt beings at age 10 or 11 and reaches its peak at 12. A male's growth spurt begins at 12 or 13 and peaks at 14.

Gender differences become apparent in the skeletal system, lean body mass, and fat stores. In females, fat becomes a larger percentage of the total body weight, and in males, the lean body mass—muscle and bone—becomes much greater. On the average, males grow 8 inches taller during the growth spurt;

females, 6 inches. Males add approximately 45 pounds to their weight; females, about 35 pounds. Hormonal changes profoundly affect every organ of the body, including the brain, and within two or three years, physically mature adults emerge.

Teenagers' rates and patterns of growth exhibit such wide variations that growth charts used for children must be abandoned when the signs of puberty begin to appear. Age in years indicates little about development; one way to be sure a teenager is growing normally is to compare his or her height and weight with previous measures. To record developmental changes during puberty, health care professionals use standard rating scales based on stages of adolescent development.[38]

puberty: the period in life in which a person becomes physically capable of reproduction.

ENERGY AND NUTRIENT NEEDS

As children become adults, they change in many ways. Their physical changes make their nutrient needs high, and their emotional, intellectual, and social changes make meeting those needs a challenge.

Energy Intake and Activity The energy needs of adolescents vary to a great extent, depending on the current rate of growth, body size, and physical activity. Boys' energy needs may be especially high; they grow faster and, as mentioned, develop more lean body mass. An active boy of 15 may need 4000 kcalories or more a day just to maintain his weight. Girls start growing earlier than boys and attain lower body weights, so their energy needs peak sooner and decline more quickly than those of their male peers. An inactive girl of 15 whose growth is nearly at a standstill may need fewer than 2000 kcalories a day if she is to avoid excessive weight gain. Thus adolescent girls need to pay special attention to being physically active and selecting foods of high nutrient density in order to meet their nutrient needs without exceeding their energy needs.

The insidious problem of obesity becomes apparent in adolescence and often continues into adulthood; it occurs mostly in females, especially in African-American females.[39] Young women who become interested in nutrition may make choices that will benefit their fitness, or they may become unhealthily obsessed with weight control (see Highlight 9).

Iron Iron remains a nutrient of special concern. Iron needs increase in females as they start to menstruate and in males as their lean body mass develops. Adolescent iron intakes often fail to keep pace with increasing needs, especially for females, who typically consume less iron-rich meat and fewer total kcalories than males.[40]

Calcium Adolescence is a crucial time for bone development, and the requirement for calcium reaches its peak during these years.[41] Unfortunately, many adolescents have calcium intakes below current recommendations.[42] Low calcium intakes during the adolescent growth spurt, especially if paired with physical inactivity, may compromise the development of peak bone mass. As emphasized earlier, the attainment of maximal bone mass is considered the best protection against age-related bone loss and fractures.[43] Once again, teenage girls are at greatest risk, for their milk—and therefore calcium—intakes begin to decline at the time when their calcium needs are greatest.

HEALTHY PEOPLE 2000: Increase calcium intake, so that at least 50% of youth aged 12 through 24 years consume three or more servings of calcium-rich foods daily.

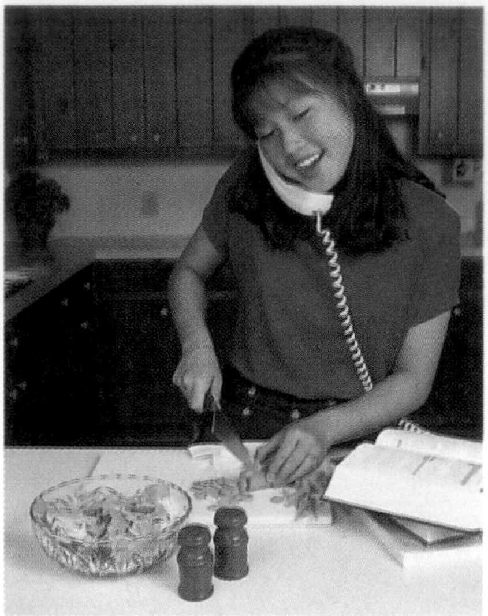

Nutritious snacks play an important role in an active teen's diet.

FOOD CHOICES AND HEALTH HABITS

Teenagers come and go as they choose and eat what they want when they have time. With a multitude of after-school, social, and job activities, they almost inevitably fall into irregular eating habits. The teenage snacker who finds only nutritious foods around the house is well provided for.

Snacks Snacks typically provide at least a fourth of the average teenager's daily food energy intake. Snacks often fail to provide enough calcium, iron, vitamin A, and folate. (Wherever vitamin A is lacking, folate generally is, too, because both are found in green vegetables.) Many adolescents need to eat a greater variety of foods to obtain these nutrients. Table 16–10 shows how to combine foods from different food groups to create healthy snacks. Most vending machines offer few nutrient-dense options, and nutrition information alone does not convince people to make healthy choices.[44]

The nutritive values of selected fast foods are presented in Appendix H.

Eating Away from Home Inevitably, adolescents do a lot of eating away from home, and their nutritional welfare is enhanced or hindered by the choices they make. A lunch of a hamburger, a chocolate shake, and french fries supplies substantial quantities of many nutrients, as shown in Table 16–11, at a kcalorie cost of 800, an energy cost many adolescents can afford. When they eat this sort of lunch, teens can balance their diets by adjusting their breakfast and dinner choices. They need to select fruits and vegetables for vitamins A, C, folate, and fiber, and lean meats for iron and zinc at their other meals.

Table 16–11

Selected Nutrients in a Hamburger, Chocolate Shake, and Small Serving of French Fries

Nutrient	Male[a] % RDA	Female[a] % RDA
Energy	30	35
Protein	47	64
Fat[b]	26	31
Calcium	38	38
Iron	30	24
Zinc	16	20
Vitamin A	9	11
Thiamin	41	48
Riboflavin	42	49
Niacin	35	41
Folate	18	20
Vitamin C	7	7
Sodium[b]	34	34

[a]RDA for a 15- to 18-year-old, moderately active, person of average height and weight.
[b]Daily Values used for fat and sodium.

Peer Influence Many of the food and health choices adolescents make reflect the opinions and actions of their peers. When others perceive milk as "babyish," a teen will choose soft drinks instead; when others skip lunch and hang out in the parking lot, a teen may join in for the camaraderie, regardless of hunger. Adults need to remember that teenagers have the right to make their own decisions—even if they are contrary to the adults' views. Gatekeepers can set up the environment so that nutritious foods are available and can stand by with reliable nutrition information and advice, but the rest is up to the adolescents. Ultimately, they make the choices.

PROBLEMS ADOLESCENTS FACE

Physical maturity and growing independence present adolescents with new choices to make. The consequences of those choices will influence their nutritional health both today and throughout life. Some teenagers begin using drugs, alcohol, and tobacco; others wisely refrain. Information about the use of these substances is presented here because most people are first exposed to them during adolescence, but it actually applies to people of all ages.

The dangers of steroid use are presented in Highlight 14.

Marijuana Three of every five high school seniors report that they have at least tried an illicit drug, most commonly marijuana. The body processes all sub-

Table 16–10

Healthful Snack Ideas—Think Food Groups, Alone and in Combination

Selecting two or more foods from different food groups adds variety and nutrient balance to snacks. The combinations are endless, so be creative.

Grain Products

Grain products are filling snacks, especially when combined with other foods:
- Cereal with fruit and milk.
- Crackers and cheese.
- Wheat toast with peanut butter.
- Popcorn with grated cheese.
- Oatmeal raisin cookies with milk.

Vegetables

Cut-up fresh, raw vegetables make great snacks alone or in combination with foods from other food groups:
- Celery with peanut butter.
- Broccoli, cauliflower, and carrot sticks with a flavored cottage cheese dip.

Fruits

Fruits are delicious snacks and can be eaten alone—fresh, dried, or juiced—or combined with other foods:
- Apples and cheese.
- Bananas and peanut butter.
- Peaches with yogurt.
- Raisins mixed with sunflower seeds or nuts.

Meats and Meat Alternates

Meat and meat alternates add protein to snacks:
- Refried beans with nachos and cheese.
- Tuna on crackers.
- Luncheon meat on wheat bread.

Milk and Milk Products

Milk can be used as a beverage with any snack, and many other milk products, such as yogurt and cheese, can be eaten alone or with other foods as listed above.

stances, and marijuana is no exception. The active ingredients are rapidly and almost completely absorbed from the lungs.* Then, being fat soluble, these substances are packaged in lipoproteins before traveling in the blood to the various body tissues. The liver and other tissues metabolize these substances, and their remnants linger in the body for several days, being gradually excreted for a week or more after the smoking of a single marijuana cigarette. With repeated exposure, these substances accumulate in body fat, the lungs, the liver, the reproductive organs, and the brain.

---

*The active ingredient of marijuana, which is primarily responsible for its intoxicating effects, is delta-9-tetrahydrocannabinol, or THC.

Smoking a marijuana cigarette seems to enhance the enjoyment of eating, especially of sweets, a phenomenon commonly known as "the munchies." Why or how this effect occurs is not known; it may be a social effect induced by suggestibility, or it may be that the drug stimulates appetite. Prolonged use of the drug does not seem to bring about a weight gain.

Marijuana users may think that because they usually smoke fewer marijuana cigarettes in a day than they would tobacco cigarettes, their lungs will incur fewer harmful, long-term effects. This is a myth. One marijuana cigarette is as bad for the body as four or five tobacco cigarettes, because people who smoke marijuana inhale more smoke and hold it in their lungs longer. People who regularly smoke several marijuana cigarettes a day face the same risk of lung cancer as people who smoke a pack of tobacco cigarettes a day.[45]

Reminder: *Euphoria* is an inflated sense of well-being and pleasure brought on by some drugs; popularly called a *high*.

Cocaine One in 20 high school seniors reports having used cocaine at least once.[46] Cocaine elicits diverse effects: intense euphoria, restlessness, heightened self-confidence, irritability, insomnia, and loss of appetite. Weight loss is common, and cocaine abusers often develop eating disorders. Notably, the craving for cocaine replaces hunger; rats given unlimited cocaine will choose it over food until they starve to death. Thus, unlike marijuana use, cocaine use has major nutritional consequences.

Cocaine can cause rapid and irregular heartbeats, heart attacks, and even death. Its use continues to escalate as cheaper and more addictive forms become available. In its smokable form, crack cocaine is more addicting than any other drug. One former crack addict tells of holding a gun to his brother's head to steal money for his next drug purchase.

Nutrition problems of drug abusers:

- They spend money for drugs that could be spent on food.
- They lose interest in food during "highs."
- Some drugs depress appetite.
- Their lifestyle fails to promote good eating habits.
- If they use intravenous (IV) drugs, they may contract AIDS, hepatitis, or other infectious diseases, which increase their nutrient needs. Hepatitis also causes taste changes and loss of appetite.
- Medicines used to treat drug abusers may alter their nutrition status.

Drug Abuse, in General The effects of other addictive drugs vary in degree but are similar in kind to those caused by cocaine. Drug abusers face the multiple nutrition problems listed in the margin. During withdrawal from drugs, an important part of treatment is to identify and correct these nutrition problems.

Alcohol Abuse Sooner or later all teenagers face the decision whether to drink alcohol. The law forbids the sale of alcohol to people under a specific age, but most adolescents who seek alcohol find it easy to obtain.

Many adolescents find that alcohol and marijuana serve similar purposes, and the pattern of substance use indicates parallel consumption, not a displacement of one by the other. Some adolescents use alcohol as an escape or for support—an ineffective way to cope with problems that leads to greater problems. Dependency on any drug severely impairs development and deserves attention, but is beyond the scope of this text.

Highlight 7 describes how alcohol affects nutrition status. To sum it up, alcohol is an empty-kcalorie beverage that can displace nutritious foods from the diet. It alters nutrient absorption and metabolism, so that imbalances develop. People who cannot keep their alcohol use moderate must abstain to maintain their health.

Tobacco Cigarette smoking is a pervasive health problem causing thousands of people to suffer from cancer and diseases of the cardiovascular, digestive, and respiratory systems. These effects are beyond the scope of nutrition, but smoking cigarettes does influence hunger, body weight, and nutrient status. Links between nutrients and lung cancer are also known.

Smoking a cigarette eases feelings of hunger. When smokers receive a hunger signal, they can quiet it with cigarettes instead of food. Such behavior ignores body signals and postpones energy and nutrient intake. Studies on rats confirm that nicotine reduces food intake, causing weight loss.[47]

Indeed, smokers tend to weigh less than nonsmokers and to gain weight when they stop smoking.[48] Weight gain is often a concern for people contemplating giving up cigarettes. They should know that the average person who quits smoking gains less than 10 pounds. Smokers wanting to quit need to prepare for this possibility and adjust their diet and activity habits so as to maintain weight during and after quitting. Smoking cessation programs need to include strategies for weight management.

Nutrient intakes of smokers and nonsmokers differ. Smokers tend to have lower intakes of dietary fiber, vitamin A, beta-carotene, folate, and vitamin C.[49] The association between smoking and low vitamin intake may be noteworthy, considering the altered metabolism of vitamin C in smokers and the protective effect of vitamin A and beta-carotene against lung cancer.

Research shows that compared to nonsmokers, smokers require almost twice as much vitamin C to maintain steady body pools. Oxidants in cigarette smoke accelerate vitamin C metabolism and deplete smokers' body stores of this antioxidant; this depletion is even evident to some degree in nonsmokers who are exposed to passive smoke.[50]

The vitamin C RDA for people who regularly smoke cigarettes is 100 mg/day. The Canadian RNI suggests smokers should add 50% to the vitamin C recommendation.

Beta-carotene enhances the immune response and protects against some cancer activity.[51] Specifically, the risk of lung cancer is greatest for smokers who have the lowest intakes of carotene. Of course, such evidence should not be misinterpreted. It does not mean that as long as people eat their carrots, they can safely use tobacco. Smokers are ten times more likely to get lung cancer than nonsmokers. Both smokers and nonsmokers can, however, reduce their cancer risks by eating fruits and vegetables rich in carotene (see Highlight 11 for details on antioxidant nutrients and disease prevention).

To review, nutrient needs rise dramatically as children enter the rapid growth phase of the teen years. The busy lifestyles of teenagers add to the challenge of meeting their nutrient needs—especially for iron and calcium. In addition to making wise foods choices, teenagers need to refrain from using substances that will impair their health including illicit drugs, tobacco, and alcohol.

The nutrition and lifestyle choices people make as children and teenagers have long-term, as well as immediate, effects of their health. Highlight 16 describes how sound choices and good habits during childhood can help prevent disease later in life.

Study Questions

1. Describe some of the nutrient and immunological attributes of breast milk.
2. What are the appropriate uses of formula feeding? What criteria would you use in selecting an infant formula?
3. Why are solid foods not recommended for an infant during the first few months of life? When is an infant ready to start eating solid food?
4. Name foods that are inappropriate for infants and explain why they are inappropriate.

(continued on the next page)

5. What nutrition problems are most common in children? What strategies can help prevent them?
6. Describe the relationships between nutrition and behavior. How does television influence nutrition?
7. Describe a true food allergy. Which foods most often cause allergic reactions? How do food allergies influence nutrition status?
8. List strategies for introducing nutritious foods to children.
9. What impact do school meal programs have on the nutrition status of children?
10. Describe the changes in nutrient needs from childhood to adolescence. Why is a teenaged girl more likely to develop an iron deficiency than is a boy?
11. How do teen eating habits influence their nutrient intakes?
12. How does the use of illicit drugs influence nutrition status?
13. How do the nutrient intakes of smokers differ from those of nonsmokers? What impacts can those differences exert on health?

Notes

1. P. S. W. Davies, Energy requirements and energy expenditure in infancy, *European Journal of Clinical Nutrition* (supplement 4) 46 (1992): S29–S35.
2. H. L. Greene and coauthors, Vitamins for newborn infant formulas: A review of recommendations with emphasis on data from low birth-weight infants, *European Journal of Clinical Nutrition* 46 (1992): S1–S8.
3. Committee on Nutrition, American Academy of Pediatrics, *Pediatric Nutrition Handbook*, 3rd ed., ed. L. A. Barness (Elk Grove Village, Ill.: American Academy of Pediatrics, 1993), pp. 23–33.
4. American Academy of Pediatrics, Committee on Nutrition, The use of whole cow's milk in infancy, *Pediatrics* 89 (1992): 1105–1109.
5. Position of The American Dietetic Association: Promotion and support of breast feeding, *Journal of the American Dietetic Association* 93 (1993): 467–469.
6. J. S. Forsyth, Is it worthwhile breast-feeding? *European Journal of Clinical Nutrition* (supplement 1) 46 (1993): 519–525.
7. A. C. Goedhart and J. G. Bindels, The composition of human milk as a model for the design of infant formulas: Recent findings and possible applications, *Nutrition Research Reviews* 7 (1994): 1–23.
8. N. F. Butte, E. O. Smith, and C. Garza, Energy utilization of breast-fed and formula-fed infants, *American Journal of Clinical Nutrition* 51 (1990): 350–358.
9. M. J. Heinig and coauthors, Energy and protein intakes of breast-fed and formula-fed infants during the first year of life and their association with growth velocity: The DARLING Study, *American Journal of Clinical Nutrition* 58 (1993): 152–161.
10. Committee on Nutritional Status during Pregnancy and Lactation, *Nutrition during Lactation* (Washington, D.C.: National Academy Press, 1991), pp. 155–156.
11. M. W. Shannon and J. W. Graef, Lead intoxication in infancy, *Pediatrics* 89 (1992): 87–90.
12. D. Stehlin, Soy beverages not complete formulas, *FDA Consumer*, September 1990, p. 29.
13. S. Ryan, Bone mineralization and growth, *European Journal of Clinical Nutrition* 46 (1992): S41–S44.
14. T. Walter and coauthors, Effectiveness of iron-fortified infant cereal in prevention of iron deficiency anemia, *Pediatrics* 91 (1993): 976–982; G. J. Fuchs and coauthors, Iron status and intake of older infants fed formula vs cow milk with cereal, *American Journal of Clinical Nutrition* 58 (1993): 343–348.
15. M. M. Smith and F. Lifshitz, Excess fruit juice consumption as a contributing factor in nonorganic failure to thrive, *Pediatrics* 93 (1994): 438–443.
16. S. A. Sullivan and L. L. Birch, Infant dietary experience and acceptance of solid foods, *Pediatrics* 93 (1994): 271–277.
17. L. L. Birch and coauthors, Effects of a nonenergy fat substitute on children's energy and macronutrient intake, *American Journal of Clinical Nutrition* 58 (1993): 326–333; S. Shea and coauthors, Variability and self-regulation of energy intake in young children in their everyday environment, *Pediatrics* 90 (1992): 542–546; L. L. Birch and coauthors, The variability of young children's energy intake, *New England Journal of Medicine* 324 (1991): 232–235.
18. R. E. Klesges and coauthors, Parental influence on food selection in young children and its relationships to childhood obesity, *American Journal of Clinical Nutrition* 53 (1991): 859–864.
19. T. A. Nicklas and coauthors, Breakfast consumption affects adequacy of total daily intake in children, *Journal of the American Dietetic Association* 93 (1993): 886–891.
20. P. L. Splett and M. Story, Child nutrition: Objectives for the decade, *Journal of the American Dietetic Association* 91 (1991): 665–668.
21. N. S. Scrimshaw, Iron deficiency, *Scientific American*, October 1991, pp. 46–52.
22. B. Lozoff, E. Jimenez, and A. W. Wolf, Long-term developmental outcome of infants with iron deficiency, *New England Journal of Medicine* 325 (1991): 687–694.

23. F. A. Oski, Iron deficiency in infancy and childhood, *Pediatrics* 329 (1993): 190–193; S. J. Fairweather-Tait, Iron deficiency in infancy: Easy to prevent—or is it? *European Journal of Clinical Nutrition* (supplement 4) 46 (1992): S9–S14.
24. D. A. Gans, Sucrose and unusual childhood behavior, *Nutrition Today*, May/June 1991, pp. 8–14; E. H. Wender and M. V. Solanto, Effects of sugar on aggressive and inattentive behavior in children with attention deficit disorder with hyperactivity and normal children, *Pediatrics* 88 (1991): 960–966; J. A. Bachorowshi and coauthors, Sucrose and delinquency: Behavioral assessment, *Pediatrics* 86 (1990): 244–253.
25. R. Zoglin, Is TV ruining our children? *Time*, October 15, 1990, p. 75.
26. R. C. Klesges, M. L. Shelton, and L. M. Klesges, Effects of television on metabolic rate: Potential implications for childhood obesity, *Pediatrics* 91 (1993): 281–286.
27. H. A. Sampson and D. D. Metcalfe, Food allergies, *Journal of the American Medical Association* 268 (1992): 2840–2844.
28. S. A. Bock and F. M. Atkins, Patterns of food hypersensitivity during sixteen years of double-blind, placebo-controlled food challenges, *Journal of Pediatrics* 117 (1990): 561–567.
29. Sampson and Metcalfe, 1992.
30. V. L. Olejer, Food hypersensitivities, *Handbook of Pediatric Nutrition* (Gaithersburg, Md.: Aspen Publishers, 1993), pp. 206–231.
31. A. T. Hingley, Food allergies: When eating is risky, *FDA Consumer*, December 1993, pp. 27–31.
32. Sampson and Metcalfe, 1992.
33. National Center for Nutrition and Dietetics, International Food Information Council, Kids at the table: Who's placing the orders? (Chicago: American Dietetic Association, 1991).
34. Position of The American Dietetic Association: Nutrition standards for child care programs, *Journal of the American Dietetic Association* 94 (1994): 323.
35. K. Schuster, Feds put schools on a lowfat diet, *Food Management* 29 (1994): 78–84; J. Burghardt and B. Devaney, The School Nutrition Dietary Assessment Study: Summary of findings, Food and Nutrition Service, U.S. Department of Agriculture, October 1993.
36. R. C. Whitaker and coauthors, An environmental intervention to reduce dietary fat in school lunches, *Pediatrics* 91 (1993): 1107–1111.
37. Timely statement of The American Dietetic Association: Dietary guidance for healthy children, *Journal of the American Dietetic Association* 95 (1995): 370.
38. L. E. Underwood, Normal adolescent growth and development, *Nutrition Today*, March/April 1991, pp. 11–16.
39. T. A. Wadden and coauthors, Obesity in black adolescent girls: A controlled clinical trial of treatment by diet, behavior modification, and parental support, *Pediatrics* 85 (1990): 345–352.
40. J. B. Anderson, The status of adolescent nutrition, *Nutrition Today*, March/April 1991, pp. 7–10.
41. S. M. Ott, Bone density in adolescents, *New England Journal of Medicine* 325 (1991): 1646–1647.
42. S. I. Barr, Associations of social and demographic variables with calcium intakes of high school students, *Journal of the American Dietetic Association* 94 (1994): 260–266, 269.
43. V. Matkovic, Diet, genetics, and peak bone mass of adolescent girls, *Nutrition Today*, March/April 1991, pp. 21–24.
44. S. M. Hoerr and V. A. Louden, Can nutrition information increase sales of healthful vended snacks? *Journal of School Health* 63 (1993): 386–390.
45. T. C. Wu and coauthors, Pulmonary hazards of smoking marijuana as compared with tobacco, *New England Journal of Medicine* 318 (1988): 347–351.
46. American Council on Science and Health, *Cocaine: Facts and Dangers* (New York: American Council on Science and Health, 1990).
47. S. R. Schwid, M. D. Hirvonen, and R. E. Keesey, Nicotine effects on body weight: A regulatory perspective, *American Journal of Clinical Nutrition* 55 (1992): 878–884.
48. D. F. Williamson and coauthors, Smoking cessation and severity of weight gain in a national cohort, *New England Journal of Medicine* 324 (1991): 739–745.
49. T. A. B. Sanders and coauthors, Essential fatty acids, plasma cholesterol and fat-soluble vitamins in subjects with age-related maculopathy and matched control subjects, *American Journal of Clinical Nutrition* 57 (1993): 428–433; A. F. Subar, L. C. Harlan, and M. E. Mattson, Food and nutrient intake differences between smokers and non-smokers in the US, *American Journal of Public Health* 80 (1990): 1323–1329.
50. D. L. Tribble, L. J. Giuliano, and S. P. Fortmann, Reduced plasma ascorbic acid concentrations in nonsmokers regularly exposed to environmental tobacco smoke, *American Journal of Clinical Nutrition* 58 (1993): 886–890.
51. G. van Poppel, S. Spanhaak, and T. Ockhuizen, Effect of β-carotene on immunological indexes in healthy male smokers, *American Journal of Clinical Nutrition* 57 (1993): 402–407; T. V. Ringer and coauthors, Beta-carotene's effects on serum lipoproteins and immunologic indices in humans, *American Journal of Clinical Nutrition* 53 (1991): 688–694.

Childhood Obesity and the Early Development of Chronic Diseases

When people think of the health problems of children and adolescents, they typically think of measles and acne, not cardiovascular disease (CVD). They think of CVD as the number-one killer of adults in the United States and Canada, but CVD begins in childhood.[1]

Much of our knowledge about the early development of CVD comes from the Bogalusa Heart Study, a long-term epidemiological study of some 14,000 young people. For nearly three decades, researchers have been observing how changes in body weight, blood lipids, blood pressure, and individual behaviors correlate with the development of CVD over time—from infancy to childhood through adolescence and into young adulthood. Some major findings have emerged from the research:

- Changes inside the arteries—changes predictive of CVD—are evident in childhood.
- Obesity in children affects these changes.
- Behaviors that influence the development of obesity and of CVD are learned and begin early in life. These behaviors include overeating, eating high-fat foods, physical inactivity, and cigarette smoking.

This highlight focuses on efforts to prevent childhood obesity and CVD, but the benefits extend to cancer, diabetes, and other chronic diseases as well. The years of childhood are emphasized here, for the earlier in life health-promoting habits become established, the better they will stick. Chapter 18 fills in the rest of the story of nutrition's role in reducing chronic disease risk.

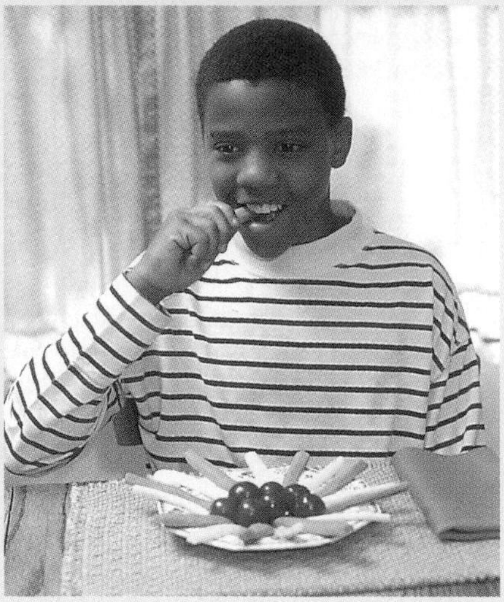

Take care of your body and your body will take care of you.

Invariably, questions arise as to what extent genetics is involved in CVD development. Children who are obese and who have high blood lipids and high blood pressure are often from families with a history of CVD. Genetics does not appear to play a *determining* role in CVD; that is, a person is not simply destined at birth to develop CVD.[2] Instead, genetics appears to play a *permissive* role—the potential is inherited and then will develop, if given a push by poor health choices such as excessive weight gain, poor diet, sedentary lifestyle, and cigarette smoking.

EARLY DEVELOPMENT OF CVD

Most people consider CVD to be an adult disease: its incidence rises with advancing age, and symptoms rarely appear before age 30. The disease process begins much earlier, though.

Atherosclerosis

Most CVD involves atherosclerosis—the accumulation of cholesterol and other blood lipids along the walls of the arteries. Atherosclerosis eventually blocks the flow of blood to the heart and causes a heart attack, or cuts off blood flow to the brain and causes a stroke. Infants are born with healthy, smooth, clear arteries, but within the first decade of life, fatty streaks may begin to appear (see Figure H16–1). During adolescence, these fatty streaks may begin to turn to fibrous plaques. By early adulthood, the fibrous plaques may begin to calcify and become raised lesions, especially in boys and young men.[3] As the lesions grow more numerous and enlarge, the heart disease rate begins to rise, and the rise becomes dramatic at about age 45 in men and 55 in women.[4] From this point on, arterial damage and blockage progress rapidly, and heart attacks and strokes threaten life. In short, the consequences of atherosclerosis, which become apparent only in adulthood, have their beginnings in the first decades of life.[5]

Atherosclerosis is not inevitable; people can grow old with relatively clear arteries. Early lesions may either progress or regress, depending on several factors, many of which reflect lifestyle behaviors. Smoking, for example, is strongly associated

Figure H16–1

The Formation of Plaques in Atherosclerosis
When plaques have covered 60 percent of the coronary artery walls, the critical phase of heart disease begins.

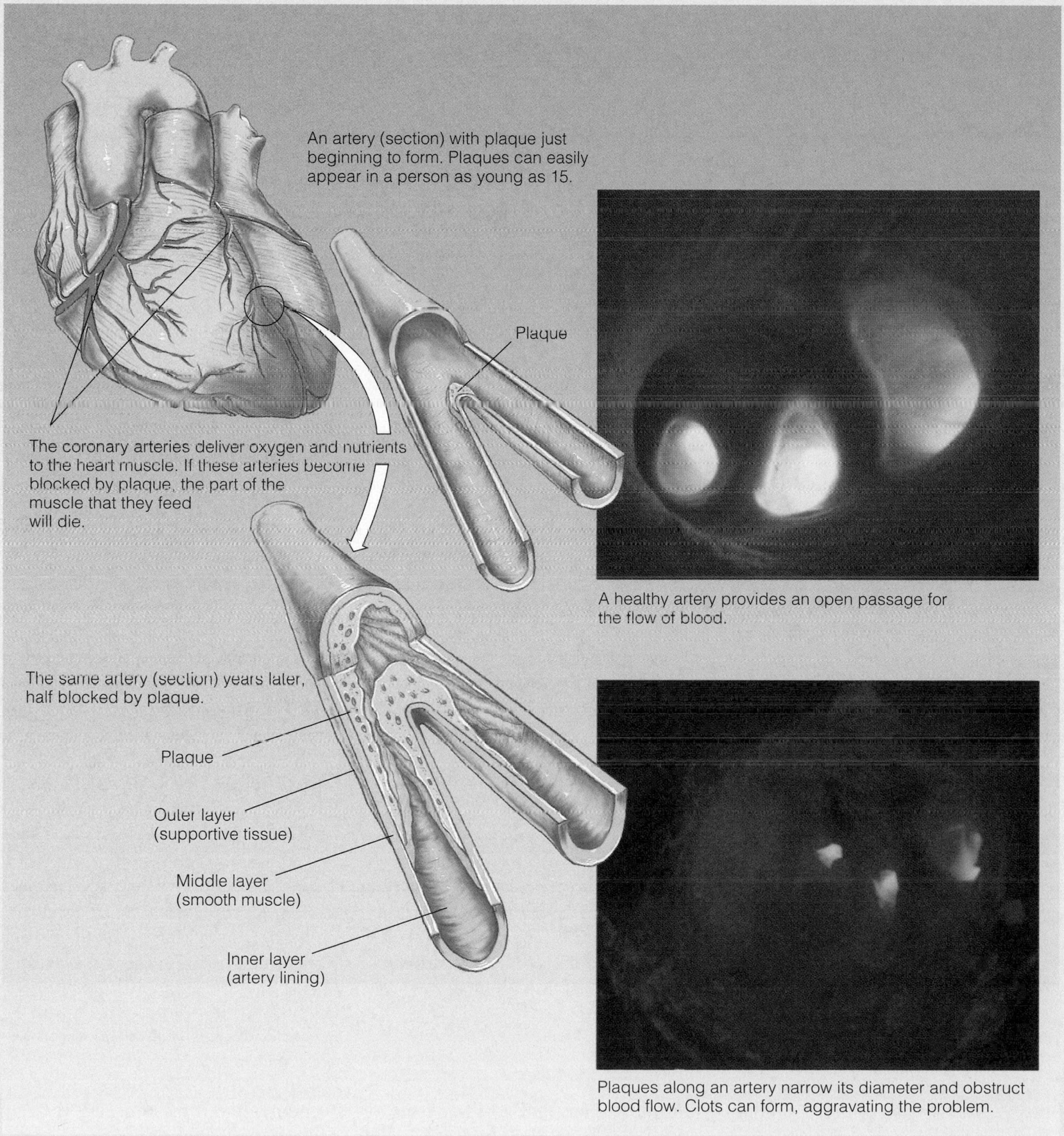
An artery (section) with plaque just beginning to form. Plaques can easily appear in a person as young as 15.
Plaque
The coronary arteries deliver oxygen and nutrients to the heart muscle. If these arteries become blocked by plaque, the part of the muscle that they feed will die.
The same artery (section) years later, half blocked by plaque.
Plaque
Outer layer (supportive tissue)
Middle layer (smooth muscle)
Inner layer (artery lining)

A healthy artery provides an open passage for the flow of blood.

Plaques along an artery narrow its diameter and obstruct blood flow. Clots can form, aggravating the problem.

with the prevalence of raised lesions, even in young adults.[6]

Blood Cholesterol

Atherosclerotic lesions reflect blood cholesterol: as blood cholesterol increases, lesion coverage increases.[7] Cholesterol values at birth are similar in all populations; differences emerge in early childhood. In countries where the adults have high blood cholesterol and high rates of CVD, the children also tend to have high blood cholesterol. Conversely, in countries where the adults have low blood cholesterol and low rates of CVD, the children tend to have low blood cholesterol, suggesting that adult heart disease tracks early trends and that early preventive efforts might reduce the incidence of later CVD.[8]

The studies just described examined population trends; but individual cholesterol status also becomes established in early childhood. At one year, cholesterol values predict the values that will be seen later in childhood, especially for those with high blood cholesterol.[9] Studies examining children for more than a decade have found that the best predictor of their blood cholesterol is earlier baseline values: childhood values correlate with values in young adulthood.[10] Quite simply, if you want to know a child's future cholesterol, measure it now.

Blood cholesterol also correlates with obesity, especially central obesity. LDL cholesterol correlates positively, and HDL negatively.[11] These relationships are apparent throughout childhood and their magnitude increases with age.

Research has also confirmed an association between blood lipids and physical activity in children similar to that seen in adults.[12] Inactive children have higher total cholesterol and LDL and lower HDL than physically active children.

Blood Pressure

An elevated blood pressure accelerates the development of CVD. On the average, children's blood pressure is lower than adults', but blood pressure increases as children grow, rising sharply at puberty and then leveling off. Like blood cholesterol, blood pressure correlates with obesity, especially central obesity.[13] Blood pressure tends to increase at a slower rate in children who participate in regular aerobic activity or who have either lost weight or maintained their weight as they grew taller.[14]

DEVELOPMENT OF OBESITY IN CHILDREN

Many experts agree that preventing or treating obesity in childhood will reduce the rate of CVD in adulthood. Without intervention, overweight children become overweight adolescents who become overweight adults, and being overweight exacerbates every chronic disease that adults face.[15]

Growing Fatter

Children are heavier today than they were 10 to 20 years ago. On the average, they have gained more than 5 pounds over the past two decades. This pattern is a secular trend—that is, one that cannot be explained by genetics. Diet and physical activity must be responsible.

Not Eating More

Reports from the Bogalusa Heart Study indicate that children's energy intakes have remained relatively stable over the past 15 years. There has even been a slight decline in fat intake, from 38 to 36 percent of kcalories from fat daily.[16] This slight decline in dietary fat is not enough, however, to have influenced body weight, nor is it enough to meet current dietary recommendations.

Children's dietary fat intakes vary, of course, and some children do eat high-fat diets. Children who prefer high-fat foods tend to consume a relatively large percentage of their energy intake from fat.[17] They also tend to be more overweight than their peers. Particularly noteworthy is the finding that the children's fat preferences and consumption correlate with their parents' obesity as well. Such findings confirm the significant roles parents play—teaching children about healthy food choices, providing children with low-fat selections, and serving as role models.

Growing Less Active

Most likely, children have grown more overweight because of their lack of physical activity.[18] An inactive child can become obese even while eating less food than an active child. Today's children are more sedentary and less physically fit than children were 20 years ago.

Watching television accounts for some 24 hours a week of sedentary behavior. Beyond these 24 hours, children spend more sedentary time working at computers and playing video games. As mentioned in earlier chapters, studies have found that both obesity and blood cholesterol correlate with hours of television viewed.[19] TV uses no more energy than it takes to rest, displaces participation in more vigorous activities, and fosters snacking on high-fat foods.

Just as blood cholesterol and obesity track over the years, so does a person's level of physical activity. A study of almost 1000 teenagers reported that over half of those who were initially described as inactive remained inactive six years later.[20] Similarly, almost half of those who were physically active remained so. Compared with inactive teens, those who were physically active weighed less, smoked less, ate a diet lower in saturated fats, and had a better blood lipid profile. The message is clear: physical activity offers numerous health benefits and children who are active today are most likely to be active for years to come.

PREVENTING CHILDHOOD OBESITY

In light of all these findings, parents and teachers of children are encouraged to make major efforts to prevent child obesity. Among directives are the following: encourage children to eat slowly, to pause and enjoy their table companions, and to stop eating when they are full. Teach them how to select low-fat snacks and to serve themselves appropriate portions. Never force children to clean their plates. Encourage physical activity daily to promote strong skeletal, muscular, and cardiovascular development and to instill in children the desire to be physically active throughout life. Physical activity is a natural and lifelong behavior of healthy living.[21] It can be as simple as riding a bike, playing tag, jumping rope, or doing chores. It need not be an organized sport; it just needs to be some activity on a regular basis.

It is important to use sensitivity in teaching children nutrition principles that can help to prevent obesity. Children can easily get the idea that their worth is tied to their body weight. Some parents fail to realize that society's ideal of slimness can be perilously close to starvation, and that a child encouraged to "diet" cannot obtain the energy and nutrients required for normal growth and development. Even healthy children without diagnosable eating disorders have been observed to limit their growth through "dieting."[22] Weight gain in truly overweight children can be controlled safely without compromising growth, but should be overseen by a health care professional.

DEALING WITH CHILDHOOD OBESITY

The child who is already obese needs careful management. Weight loss is not ordinarily recommended because restrictive diets can easily impair growth in children. Instead, aim to maintain a constant weight while the child grows taller. The object is to support normal lean body development, while letting children "grow out" of their obesity.

CHOLESTEROL SCREENING FOR CHILDREN

Many children in the United States are not only overweight but also have high blood cholesterol.[23] The question of whether to screen children for high blood cholesterol is controversial.[24] Currently, selective screening for children and adolescents whose parents or grandparents have CVD is recommended.[25] Since blood cholesterol in children is a good predictor of adult values, however, some experts recommend universal screening to identify all children with high blood cholesterol.[26] They note that many children who have high blood cholesterol do not have family histories of CVD and would be missed under current screening criteria.[27] Opponents argue that some children with high blood cholesterol may reach adulthood with normal blood cholesterol and that treating adults who have high blood cholesterol should be sufficient. They believe screening will create unnecessary anxiety and lead to an overuse of drug therapy and overly restrictive dieting during childhood and adolescence.[28] Furthermore, studies have found that few children follow up with additional testing or dietary changes anyway.[29] Standard values for cholesterol screening in children and adolescents are listed in Table H16–1.

In some cases, parents are too young to have a CVD history. In many other cases, children, or their parents, may not know their family histories. For these reasons, it may be most effective for physicians of adult heart patients to refer the children and grandchildren of these patients for cholesterol screening.[30]

Some research shows that overweight children should also be con-

Table H16–1

Cholesterol Values for Children and Adolescents

Disease Risk	Total Cholesterol (mg/dL)	LDL Cholesterol (mg/dL)
Acceptable	<170	<110
Borderline	170–199	110–129
High	≥200	≥130

Note: Adult values appear in Table 18–2 on p. 650.

sidered for cholesterol screening, even if they do not satisfy the current criteria.[31] The incidence of high blood cholesterol in obese children with no other criteria is similar to that of nonobese children with family histories of CVD.

Considering the many lifestyle factors that accompany the development of CVD, questions regarding a child's health behaviors might also be informative. Health care professionals should determine whether children smoke, and how physically active they are, especially when family history is unknown.[32]

Early—but not advanced—atherosclerotic lesions are reversible, making screening and education a high priority. Both those with family histories of CVD and those with multiple risk factors need intervention. Children with the highest risks of developing CVD are sedentary and obese, with high blood pressure and high blood cholesterol. In contrast, children with the lowest risks of heart disease are physically active and of normal weight, with low blood pressure and favorable lipid profiles. Routine pediatric care should identify these known risk factors and provide education when needed (see Table H16–2).

Table H16–2

Health Professional's Schedule of Cardiovascular Disease Assessment in Children

Birth	• Family history for early heart disease, high blood lipids (if positive, discuss risk factors and refer parents to health care). • Start growth chart. • Parental smoking history (if positive, refer to smoking cessation program).
0–2 years	• Update family history, growth chart. • With introduction of solids, begin teaching about healthy diet (nutritionally adequate, low in salt, low in saturated fats). • Recommend healthy snacks as finger foods. • Change to whole milk from formula or breastfeeding at approximately 1 year of age.
2–6 years	• Update family history, growth chart (review growth chart[a] with family and discuss concept of weight for height). • Introduce moderately low-fat diet. • Change to low-fat milk. • Start blood pressure chart at approximately 3 years of age[b]; review for concept of lower salt intake. • Encourage active parent-child play. • Lipid determination in children with positive family history or with parental cholesterol >240 mg/dl (if abnormal, initiate nutrition counseling).
6–10 years	• Update family history, blood pressure, and growth charts. • Complete cardiovascular health profile with child; determine family history, smoking history, blood pressure percentile, weight for height, fingerstick cholesterol, and level of activity and fitness. • Reinforce low-fat diet. • Begin active antismoking counseling. • Introduce fitness for health and encourage lifelong sport activities for child and family. • Discuss role of watching television in sedentary lifestyle and obesity.
>10 years	• Update family history, blood pressure, and growth charts annually. • Review low-fat diet, risks of smoking, fitness benefits whenever possible. • Consider lipid profile in all patients. • Final review of personal cardiovascular health status.

[a]If weight is >120% of normal for height, diagnosis of obesity should be considered and the subject addressed with the child and family.
[b]If three consecutive interval blood pressure measurements exceed the 90th percentile and blood pressure is not explained by height or weight, diagnosis of hypertension should be made and appropriate evaluation considered.

Source: Adapted with permission from W. B. Strong and coauthors, Integrated cardiovascular health promotion in childhood: A statement for health professionals from the Subcommittee on Atherosclerosis and Hypertension in Childhood of the Council on Cardiovascular Disease in the Young, American Heart Association, *Circulation* 85 (1992): 1638–1650. Copyright 1992 American Heart Association.

DIETARY RECOMMENDATIONS FOR CHILDREN

An expert panel on blood cholesterol in children and adolescents recommends that, regardless of family history, all children over age two should eat a variety of foods and maintain desirable weight.[33] Children should receive less than 30 percent of total energy from fat, less than 10 percent from saturated fat, and less than 300 milligrams of cholesterol per day. The American

Academy of Pediatrics agrees, but cautions against fat intakes of less than 30 percent of total kcalories for growing children.

Not before Two

Recommendations limiting fat and cholesterol are not intended for infants or children under two years old. Infants and toddlers need a higher percentage of fat to support their rapid growth.

Moderation, Not Deprivation

Healthy children over age two can begin the transition to eating according to recommendations. Even then, meals can include moderate amounts of a child's favorite foods, even if they are high-fat selections such as french fries and ice cream.[34] Without such additions, diets might be too low in fat, not to mention unappetizing and boring.

Balanced meals need to provide lean meat, poultry, fish, and vegetable sources of protein; fruits and vegetables; whole grains; and low-fat milk products. Such meals can provide enough food energy and nutrients to support growth and maintain blood cholesterol within a healthy range.[35] Pediatricians warn parents to avoid extremes; they caution that while intentions may be good, excessive food restriction may create nutrient deficiencies and impair growth. Furthermore, parental control over eating may instigate battles and foster attitudes about foods that can lead to inappropriate eating behaviors.

Diet First, Drugs Later

Experts agree that children at high risk should first be treated with diet. If, in children ten years and older, blood cholesterol remains high after 6 to 12 months of dietary intervention, then drugs may be used to lower blood cholesterol.[36] Pharmacological doses of niacin effectively lower LDL cholesterol in children, but adverse effects are common; such treatment should be reserved only for severe cases.[37]

SMOKING

Another risk factor for CVD that starts in childhood and carries over into adulthood is cigarette smoking. Each day 3000 children begin to use tobacco, 40 percent of them in grade school. Among high school students, two out of three have tried smoking, and one in eight smokes regularly. Over half of all adult smokers began smoking before the age of 18.

Efforts to teach children about the dangers of smoking need to be aggressive to compete with the tobacco industry's promotional campaigns. The tobacco industry spends millions of dollars on advertising aimed at young people and makes over $200 million a year on sales to children under 18. Cigarette companies use cartoon characters, advertise in youth-oriented publications, and sponsor sporting events. Children and teenagers are not likely to consider the long-term health consequences of tobacco use. They are more likely to be struck by the immediate health consequences, such as shortness of breath when playing sports, or social consequences, such as having bad breath. Whatever the context, the message to all children and teens should be clear: don't start smoking. If you've already started, quit.

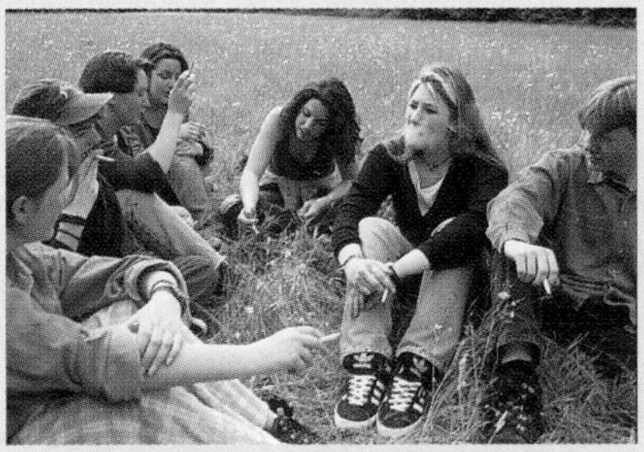

Cigarette smoking is the number-one cause of premature deaths.

In conclusion, *adult* CVD is a major *pediatric* problem. Without intervention, some 60 million children are destined to suffer its consequences within the next 30 years. Optimal prevention efforts focus on children, especially on those who are overweight.

Just as young children receive vaccinations against infectious diseases, they need screening for, and education about, CVD. Many health education programs have been implemented in schools around the country.[38] These programs are most effective when they include education in the classroom, heart-healthy meals in the lunchroom, fitness activities on the playground, and parental involvement at home.

NOTES

1. G. S. Berenson and coauthors, Review: Atherosclerosis and its evolution in childhood, *American Journal of the Medical Sciences* 30 (1987): 429–440; W. B. Strong and coauthors, Integrated cardiovascular health promotion in childhood: A statement for health professionals from the Subcommittee on Atherosclerosis and Hypertension in Childhood of the Council on Cardiovascular Disease in the Young, American Heart Association, *Circulation* 85 (1992): 1638–1650.

2. W. B. Kannel, R. B. D'Agostino, and A. Belanger, Concept of bridging the gap from

youth to adulthood—The Framingham Study, an address presented at the Recognition and Prevention of Heart Disease: State of the Art conference, New Orleans, Louisiana, April 27 and 28, 1994.

3. G. S. Berenson and coauthors, Atherosclerosis of the aorta and coronary arteries and cardiovascular risk factors in persons aged 6 to 30 years and studied at necropsy (the Bogalusa Heart Study), *American Journal of Cardiology* 70 (1992): 851–858.

4. Kannel, D'Agostino, and Belanger, 1994.

5. Committee on Nutrition, Statement on cholesterol, *Pediatrics* 90 (1992): 469–473; National Cholesterol Education Program, Report of the Expert Panel on Blood Cholesterol Levels in Children and Adolescents, Overview and summary, *Pediatrics* (supplement) 89 (1992): 525–527.

6. Pathobiological Determinants of Atherosclerosis in Youth (PDAY) Research Group, Relationship of atherosclerosis in young men to serum lipoprotein cholesterol concentrations and smoking: A preliminary report from the Pathobiological Determinants of Atherosclerosis in Youth (PDAY) Research Group, *Journal of the American Medical Association* 264 (1990): 3018–3024.

7. Pathobiological Determinants of Atherosclerosis in Youth (PDAY) Research Group, 1990.

8. L. Snetselaar and R. M. Lauer, Childhood, diet and the atherosclerotic process, *Nutrition Today*, January/February 1992, pp. 22–28.

9. M. J. T. Kallio and coauthors, Tracking of serum cholesterol and lipoprotein levels from the first year of life, *Pediatrics* 91 (1993): 949–954.

10. S. Guo and coauthors, Serial analysis of plasma lipids and lipoproteins from individuals 9–21 years of age, *American Journal of Clinical Nutrition* 58 (1993): 61–67.

11. W. A. Wattigney and coauthors, Increasing impact of obesity on serum lipids and lipoproteins in young adults: The Bogalusa Heart Study, *Archives of Internal Medicine* 151 (1991): 2017–2022.

12. E. Suter and M. R. Hawes, Relationship of physical activity, body fat, diet, and blood lipid profile in youths 10–15 yr, *Medicine and Science in Sports and Exercise* 25 (1993): 748–754.

13. C. L. Shear and coauthors, Body fat patterning and blood pressure in children and young adults: The Bogalusa Heart Study, *Hypertension* 9 (1987): 236–244.

14. S. Shea and coauthors, The rate of increase in blood pressure in children 5 years of age is related to changes in aerobic fitness and body mass index, *Pediatrics* 94 (1994): 465–470.

15. S. S. Guo and coauthors, The predictive value of childhood body mass index values for overweight at age 35 y, *American Journal of Clinical Nutrition* 59 (1994): 810–819.

16. T. A. Nicklas and coauthors, Secular trends in dietary intakes and cardiovascular risk factors of 10-year-old children: The Bogalusa Heart Study (1973–1988), *American Journal of Clinical Nutrition* 58 (1993): 930–937.

17. J. O. Fisher and L. L. Birch, Fat preferences and fat consumption of 3- to 5-year-old children are related to parental obesity, *Journal of the American Dietetic Association*95 (1995): 759–764.

18. S. A. Schlicker, S. T. Borra, and C. Regan, The weight and fitness status of United States children, *Nutrition Reviews* 52 (1994): 11–17.

19. E. Obarzanek and coauthors, Energy intake and physical activity in relation to indexes of body fat: The National Heart, Lung, and Blood Institute Growth and Health Study, *American Journal of Clinical Nutrition* 60 (1994): 15–22.

20. O. T. Raitakari and coauthors, Effects of persistent physical activity on coronary risk factors in children and young adults: The Cardiovascular Risk in Young Finns Study, *American Journal of Epidemiology* 140 (1994): 195–205.

21. Committee on Sports Medicine and Fitness, Fitness, activity, and sports participation in the preschool child, *Pediatrics* 90 (1992): 1002–1004.

22. F. Lifshitz and N. Moses, Nutritional dwarfing: Growth, dieting, and fear of obesity, *Journal of the American College of Nutrition* 7 (1988): 367–376.

23. G. S. Berenson, S. R. Srinivasan, and L. S. Webber, Cardiovascular risk prevention in children: A challenge or a poor idea? *Nutrition, Metabolism and Cardiovascular Diseases* 4 (1994): 46–52.

24. S. S. Gidding, The rationale for lowering serum cholesterol levels in American children, *American Journal of Diseases of Children* 147 (1993): 386–392; P. T. Einhorn and B. M. Rifkind, Cholesterol measurement in children, *American Journal of Diseases of Children* 147 (1993): 373–375; G. S. Berenson, Cholesterol: Myth vs reality in pediatric practice, *American Journal of Diseases of Children* 147 (1993): 371–373.

25. Report of the Expert Panel on Blood Cholesterol Levels in Children and Adolescents, *Pediatrics* 89 (1992): entire supplement.

26. Berenson, Srinivasan, and Webber, 1994.

27. S. J. Wadowski and coauthors, Family history of coronary artery disease and cholesterol: Screening children in disadvantaged inner-city population, *Pediatrics* 93 (1994): 109–113; K. Resnicow and D. Cross, Are parents' self-reported total cholesterol levels useful in identifying children with hyperlipidemia? An examination of current guidelines, *Pediatrics* 92 (1993): 347–354.

28. National Cholesterol Education Program, Overview and summary, 1992.

29. C. M. Lannon and J. Earp, Parents' behavior and attitudes toward screening children for high serum cholesterol levels, *Pediatrics* 89 (1992): 1159–1163.

30. L. E. Muhonen and coauthors, Coronary risk factors in adolescents related to their knowledge of familial coronary heart disease and hypercholesterolemia: The Muscatine Study, *Pediatrics* 93 (1994): 444–451.

31. M. S. Glassman and S. M. Schwarz, Cholesterol screening in children: Should obesity be a risk factor? *Journal of the American College of Nutrition* 12 (1993): 270–273.

32. Committee on Nutrition, 1992.

33. NCEP Expert Panel on Blood Cholesterol Levels in Children and Adolescents, National Cholesterol Education Program (NCEP): Highlight of the report of the Expert Panel on Blood Cholesterol Levels in Children and Adolescents, *Pediatrics* 89 (1992): 495–501.

34. N. Sigman–Grant, S. Zimmerman, and P. M. Kris–Etherton, Dietary approaches for reducing fat intake of preschool-age children, *Pediatrics* 91 (1993): 955–960.

35. Timely statement on NCEP report on children and adolescents, *Journal of the American Dietetic Association* 91 (1991): 983; Is there a relationship between dietary fat and stature or growth in children three to five years of age? *Pediatrics* 92 (1993): 579–586.

36. Committee on Nutrition, 1992.

37. R. B. Colletti and coauthors, Niacin treatment of hypercholesterolemia in children, *Pediatrics* 92 (1993): 78–82.

38. A. M. Downey, J. L. Cresanta, and G. S. Berenson, Cardiovascular health promotion in children: "Heart Smart" and the changing role of physicians, *American Journal of Preventive Medicine* 5 (1989): 279–295.

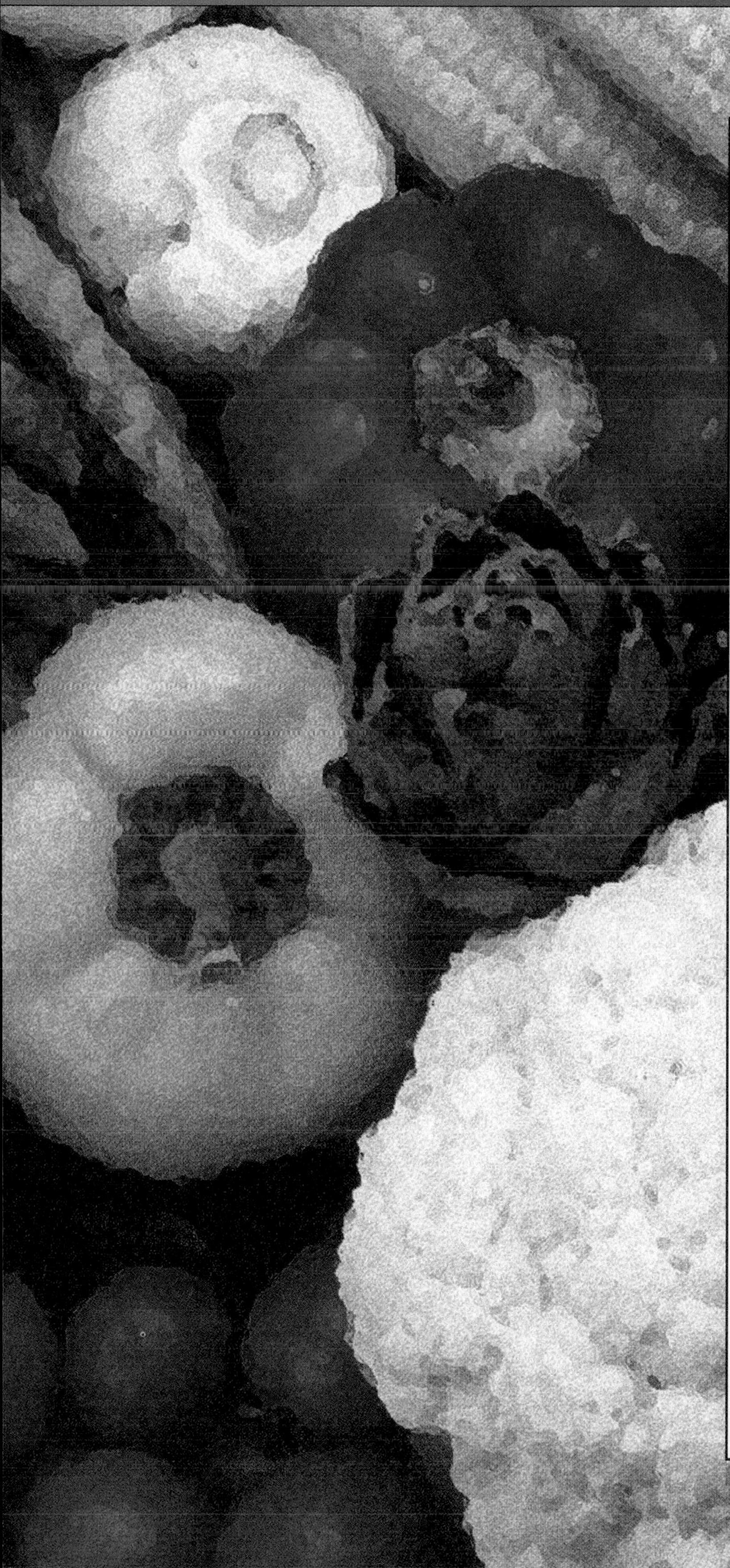

## Chapter 17

Life Cycle Nutrition: Adulthood and the Later Years

CONTENTS

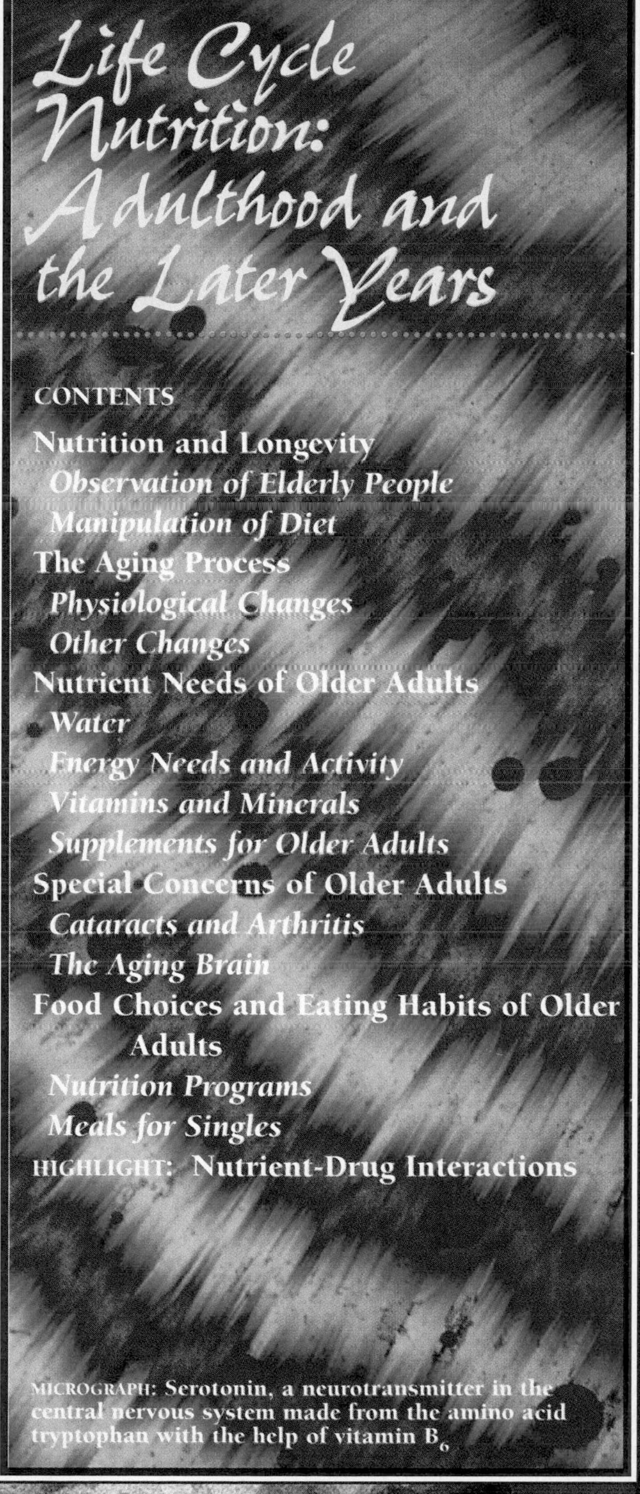

MICROGRAPH: Serotonin, a neurotransmitter in the central nervous system made from the amino acid tryptophan with the help of vitamin B_6

Wise food choices, made throughout adulthood, can support a person's ability to meet physical, emotional, and mental challenges and to achieve freedom from disease. Three goals inspire adults to take responsibility for their nutritional health: promotion of overall wellness, prevention of disease, and slowing of aging. Much of this text has focused on nutrition to support wellness during adulthood; Chapter 18 discusses prevention of disease; and this chapter presents information on aging and the nutrition needs of older adults.

The U.S. population is "graying." The majority is now middle-aged, and the ratio of old people to young is becoming greater, as Figure 17–1 shows. Our society uses the arbitrary age of 65 years to define the transition point between middle age and old age, but growing "old" happens day by day, with change occurring gradually over time. Since 1950 the population of those over 65 has more than doubled. Remarkably, the fastest-growing age group is people over 85 years (see Figure 17–2).[1]

life expectancy: the average number of years lived by people in a given society.

longevity: long duration of life.

life span: the maximum number of years of life attainable by a member of a species.

The life expectancy for U.S. women is 79 years and for men, 72 years—up from about 47 years in 1900. Advances in medical science—antibiotics and other treatments—are largely responsible for almost doubling the life expectancy in this century. Improved nutrition and an abundant supply of food have also contributed to lengthening life expectancy.[2] Still, there appears to be an upper limit on human longevity that even nutrition cannot extend. The human life span is about 115 years and has not changed much over the years.

Figure 17–1

The Aging of the U.S. Population (= 65 years or older)

In 1940, 6.8 percent of the population was 65 or older. In 1990, 12.7 percent of us had reached age 65, with 1.2 percent of the population 85 years or older; by 2040, 21.7 percent will have reached age 65; and a century from now, nearly one of four Americans will be 65 and older. An estimated 25,000 Americans now living are 100 years old or older.

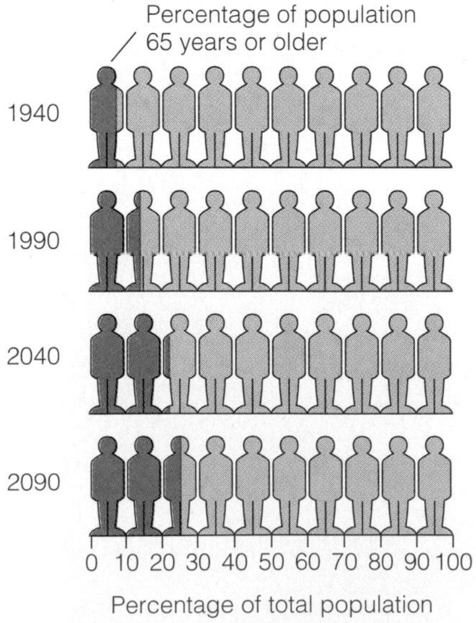

Nutrition and Longevity

Only in this century have human beings achieved a life expectancy that permits science to study aging. Research in the field now is active—and difficult. Researchers are challenged by the diversity of older adults. When older adults experience health problems, it is hard to know whether to attribute them to normal, age-related processes or to other reasons and relationships. If some of the health problems of later life are preventable, then research that focuses on how nutrition and other factors affect aging and disease processes is of great value. The findings will be vital to ensuring that more and more people can look forward to long, healthy lives.

The idea that nutrition can influence the aging process is particularly appealing, because people can control and change their eating habits. Among the questions researchers are asking are:

- To what extent is aging inevitable, and can it be slowed through changes in lifestyle and environment?
- What role does nutrition play in the aging process, and what role can it play in retarding aging?

With respect to the first question, it seems that aging is an inevitable, natural process, programmed into the genes at conception. People can, however, slow the process within the natural limits set by heredity. They need to adopt healthy lifestyle habits such as engaging in physical activity.

With respect to the second question, good nutrition helps to maintain a healthy body and can therefore ease the aging process in many significant ways. Clearly, nutrition can improve the quality of the later years.

OBSERVATION OF ELDERLY PEOPLE

One approach researchers use to search out the secret of long life has been to study older people. No doubt, you have noticed that some people are young for their ages, others old for their ages. What makes the difference?

Healthy Habits Six healthy habits seem to have a profound influence on physiological age:[3]

- Abstinence from, or moderation in, alcohol use.
- Regularity of meals.
- Weight control.
- Regular, adequate sleep.
- Abstinence from smoking.
- Regular physical activity.

The effects of all these factors are cumulative—that is, those who follow all of the practices are in better health, even if older in chronological age, than people who fail to do so. In fact, the physical health of people who report all positive health practices is comparable to that of people *30 years younger* who follow few or none. Other studies have confirmed that these health habits both extend longevity and support independence in later life.[4] The findings suggest that even though people cannot alter the years of their births, they can alter the probable lengths and quality of their lives.

Especially Physical Activity Vigorous physical activity and long life seem to go together.[5] Even a moderate amount of physical activity—for example, a brisk 30-minute walk each day—is protective against early mortality. An extensive study of more than 16,000 men demonstrates this clearly.[6] The men were between 35 and 74 years of age and were studied for 12 to 16 years. The group whose members expended 2000 or more kcalories in exercise per week (equal to walking or running about 20 miles per week) had a death rate 25 to 33 percent lower than the less active group's rate. Exercise seemed to affect the risk of death even more than did heredity, smoking, hypertension, or extremes in body weight. Physical activity slows cardiovascular aging and reduces heart disease risks. The numerous benefits derived from regular physical activity emphasize the importance of making it a priority in everyone's life.

MANIPULATION OF DIET

Another approach researchers use to learn about longevity has been to manipulate animals' diets. This research has given rise to some interesting and suggestive findings.

physiological age: a person's age as estimated from her or his body's health and probable life expectancy.

chronological age: a person's age in years from his or her date of birth.

Figure 17–2

U.S. Population Growth, 1960 to 1990

The "oldest old"—those 85 years and older—are the fastest-growing age group in the United States. Between 1960 and 1990, the U.S. population grew 39 percent, but the population of those over 85 more than doubled.

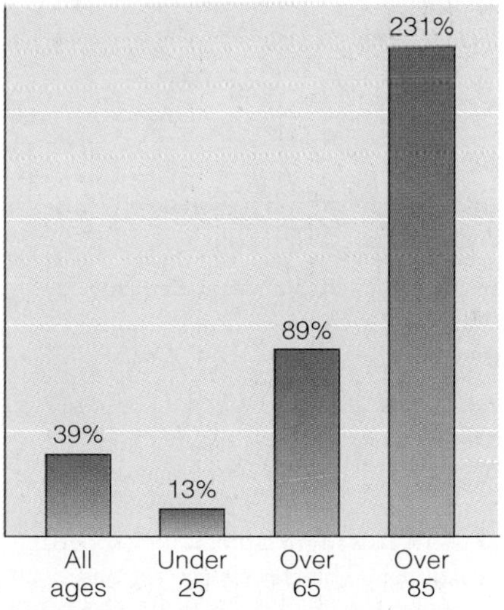

Energy Restriction in Rats Rats live longer when their food intakes are restricted in the early weeks of their lives or even after they are mature. Extensive research shows that it is the restriction of food energy rather than restriction of a specific nutrient that exerts the antiaging effect.[7]

Several mechanisms to explain how energy restriction prolongs life in rats have been proposed but not proven. Food restriction may extend the life span by delaying age-related diseases, retarding growth and development, reducing body fat, slowing the metabolic rate, controlling blood glucose, and preventing lipid oxidation.[8]

While restricting energy intake is the most effective way to lengthen rats' lives, no evidence suggests that these findings apply to human beings. To apply the results of animal studies to human beings is often unrealistic and, in this case, would even be dangerous. The animals given restricted feedings suffered distinct disadvantages: half of them died *very* early (before 300 days); the surviving animals were retarded and malformed in a number of ways. Extreme starvation to extend life, like any extreme, is probably never worth the price.

Energy Restriction in Human Beings One group of researchers studied the relationship between *moderate* energy restriction and the retardation of aging in human beings.[9] Sixteen middle-aged, nonobese men were studied during 10 weeks of energy restriction (80 percent of their usual weight-maintaining intake). They lost weight, mostly due to loss of fat. Their blood pressures dropped significantly, and their HDL cholesterol concentrations rose significantly. Energy restriction had no adverse effects on their mental and physical performances. For these men, moderate energy restriction favorably changed disease risk factors such as obesity, blood pressure, and blood cholesterol.

In summary, life expectancy in the United States has increased dramatically in the last century. Factors that enhance longevity include limited or no alcohol use, regular balanced meals, weight control, adequate sleep, abstinence from smoking, and regular physical activity. Nutrition alone, even if ideal, cannot guarantee a long and robust life. At the very least, however, nutrition can influence aging and longevity in human beings by helping to prevent disease. The next chapter is dedicated to the relationships between diet and disease prevention; the focus here is on changes that commonly accompany the aging process.

The Aging Process

As people get older, each person becomes less and less like anyone else. Everyday stresses and habits have had more time to affect the body's health. Both physical stressors, such as alcohol abuse, other drug abuse, smoking, pain, heat, and illness, and psychological stressors, such as exams, divorce, moving, and death of a loved one, elicit the body's stress response. The body responds to such stressors with an elaborate series of physiological steps, using the nervous and hormonal systems to bring about defensive readiness in every body part. The effects all favor physical action—the classic fight-or-flight response. Stress that is prolonged or severe can drain the body of its reserves and leave it weakened, aged, and vulnerable to illness, especially if physical action is not taken. As people age, they lose their ability to adapt to both external and internal disturbances. When

stress: any threat to a person's well-being; a demand placed on the body to adapt.

stressor: an environmental element, physical or psychological, that causes stress.

stress response: the body's response to stress, mediated by both nerves and hormones initially; begins with an *alarm reaction*, proceeds through a stage of *resistance*, and then leads to *recovery* or, if prolonged, to *exhaustion*. This three-stage response has also been termed the **general adaptation syndrome**.

disease strikes, the reduced ability to adapt makes the aging individual more vulnerable to death than a younger person.

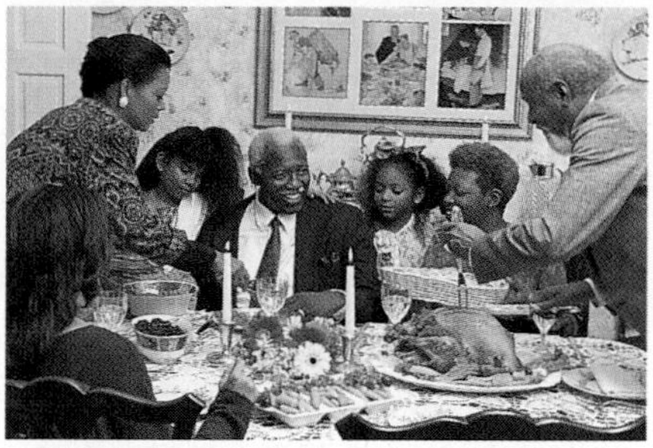

Growing old is enjoyable for people who take care of their health and live each day fully.

PHYSIOLOGICAL CHANGES

As aging progresses, inevitable changes in each of the body's organs contribute to the body's declining function. These physiological changes influence nutrition status, just as growth and development do in the earlier stages of the life cycle.

Body Composition Optimal nutrition and physical activity can minimize the body composition changes associated with aging. In general, though, older people tend to lose bone and lean body mass and gain body fat.[10] Many of these changes in body composition occur because some hormones that regulate metabolism become less active with age while others become more active. The action of insulin, for example, diminishes with age as the pancreas begins to secrete less of the hormone and the cells lose their ability to respond efficiently.*

Immune System Changes in the immune system also bring declining function with age.[11] The immune system is also compromised by nutrient deficiencies, and so the combination of age and malnutrition makes older people vulnerable to infectious diseases.[12] Adding insult to injury, antibiotics often are not effective against infections in people with compromised immune systems.[13] Consequently, infectious diseases are a major cause of death in older adults.

GI Tract In the GI tract, the intestinal wall loses strength and elasticity with age, and this slows motility. Constipation is four to eight times more common in the elderly than in the young.[14] Atrophic gastritis, a condition that affects almost one-third of those over 60, is characterized by an inflamed stomach, abundant bacteria, and a lack of hydrochloric acid—all of which can impair the digestion and absorption of nutrients, most notably, vitamin B_{12}, biotin, calcium, and iron.

Reminder: *Atrophic gastritis* is a condition characterized by chronic inflammation of the stomach accompanied by a diminished size and functioning of the mucosa and glands.

Tooth Loss Tooth loss and gum disease are common in old age, making chewing difficult or painful. Dentures, even when they fit properly, are less effective than natural teeth, and inefficient chewing can cause choking. People with tooth loss, gum disease, and ill-fitting dentures tend to limit their selections to soft foods. If foods such as corn on the cob, apples, and hard rolls are replaced by creamed corn, applesauce, and rice, then nutrition status may not be greatly affected, but when food groups are eliminated and variety is limited, nutrient deficiencies follow.

Other Physical Problems A multitude of other physical problems can also interfere with an older person's ability to obtain adequate nourishment. Failing eyesight, for example, can make driving to the grocery store impossible and shopping for food a frustrating experience. It may become so difficult to read food

*Other examples of hormones that change with age include the growth hormone and androgens, which decline with advancing age, thus contributing to the decrease in lean body mass, and the hormone prolactin, which increases with age, helping to maintain body fat.

labels and count money that the person doesn't buy the needed foods. Carrying bags of groceries may be an unmanageable task. Similarly, a person with limited mobility may find cooking and cleaning up too hard to do.

Sensory losses can interfere with a person's ability or willingness to eat. Taste and smell sensitivities tend to diminish with age and may make eating less enjoyable.[15] Loss of vision and hearing may contribute to social isolation.[16]

OTHER CHANGES

In addition to the physiological changes that accompany aging, adults are changing in many other ways that influence their nutrition status. Psychological, economic, and social factors play big roles in a person's ability and willingness to eat.

Psychological Changes Though not an inevitable component of aging, depression is common among older adults. It is frequently accompanied by loss of appetite and of the motivation to cook. These feelings are especially apparent when a person has recently lost a loved one. When a person is suffering the heartache and loneliness of bereavement, cooking meals may not seem worthwhile. The support and companionship of family and friends, especially at mealtimes, can help overcome depression and enhance appetite. In addition to depression, older adults are often troubled by insomnia, worry, anxiety, apathy, and forgetfulness.

Economic Changes Overall, the older population today has a higher income than their cohorts of previous generations. Still, poverty, is a major problem for about 20 percent of the people over age 65. Factors such as living arrangements and income make significant differences in the food choices, eating habits, and nutrition status of older adults, especially those over age 80.[17] People of low socioeconomic status are likely to have inadequate food and nutrient intakes. For example, studies report a consistent relationship between low income and low intakes of vitamin B_6.[18]

Social Changes Malnutrition among older adults is most likely to occur among those with the least education, those living alone in federally funded housing (an indicator of low income), and those who have recently experienced a change in lifestyle. The risk of nutrient deficiencies is high among people living alone, especially men.[19] One study on home-delivered meals confirmed that men living alone eat less than men living with others; interestingly, women living alone eat more than women living with others.[20] Adults who live alone do not necessarily make poor food choices, but they often consume too little food: loneliness is directly related to inadequacies, especially of energy intake.[21]

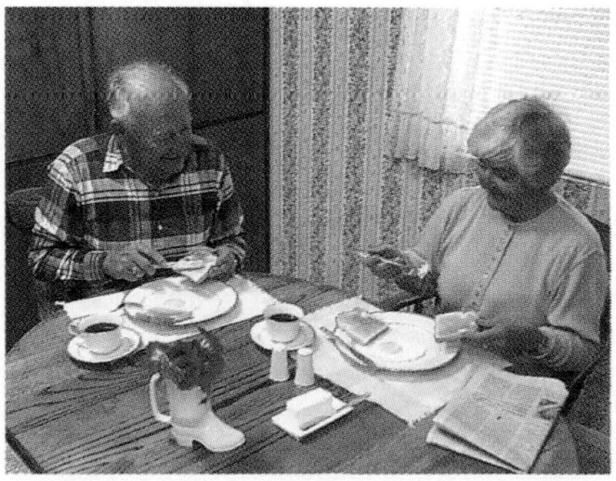

Shared meals can brighten the day and enhance the appetite.

To quickly review, many changes that accompany aging can impair nutrition status. Among physiological changes, hormone activity alters body composition, immune system changes raise the risk of infections, atrophic gastritis interferes with nutrient digestion and absorption, and tooth loss limits food choices. Psychological changes such as depression, economic changes such as loss of income, and social changes such as loneliness contribute to poor food intake.

Nutrient Needs of Older Adults

Knowledge about the nutrient needs and nutrition status of older adults has grown considerably in the last decade or so. The current RDA, however, still combine all people over 50 into one group. Future editions are likely to split this group into at least two age categories—perhaps one group of 50 to 70 years old and one of over 70.*[22] After all, the needs of people 50 to 60 years old may be very different from those of people over 80. The need for more age-specific RDA is becoming more and more urgent as the population ages.

Setting standards for older people, is difficult, though, because individual differences become more pronounced as people grow older. One person may tend to omit vegetables from his diet, and by the time he is old, he will have an associated set of nutrition problems. Another may have omitted milk and milk products all her life—her nutrition problems will be different. Also, as people age, they suffer different chronic diseases and take different drugs—both having impacts on nutrient needs. Even before all this, people start out with different genetic predispositions and ways of handling nutrients, and the effects of these became magnified with the years. Researchers have difficulty even defining "healthy aging," a prerequisite to developing RDA that are designed to meet the "needs of practically all healthy persons."[23] Still some generalizations are valid, and although new RDA may be needed, the present RDA for adults are of some use. The next sections give special attention to a few nutrients of concern.

WATER

Dehydration is a risk for older adults, who may not notice or pay attention to their thirst, or who find it difficult and bothersome to get a drink or to get to a bathroom. Older adults who have lost bladder control may be afraid to drink too much water. Despite real fluid needs, older people do not seem to feel thirsty or notice mouth dryness.[24] Many nursing home employees say it is hard to persuade their elderly clients to drink enough water and fruit juices.

Total body water also decreases as people age, so that even mild stresses such as fever or hot weather can precipitate rapid dehydration in older adults.[25] Chapter 12 described the importance of water and recommended an intake of 6 to 8 glasses of water a day. Milk and juices may replace some of this water, but beverages containing alcohol or caffeine cannot because of their diuretic effect.

Water recommendation for adults: 1 to 1½ oz/kg actual body weight.

- Older adult feeding pointer: Drink plenty of water.

ENERGY NEEDS AND ACTIVITY

Energy needs decline with advancing age. As a rule of thumb, adult energy needs decline an estimated 5 percent per decade. For one thing, as people age, they usually reduce their physical activity, although they need not do so. For another, lean body mass diminishes, slowing the basal metabolic rate. The lower energy expenditures require that older adults eat less food energy to maintain their weights. Accordingly, the energy RDA for adults decreases slightly, beginning at age 51. Energy intakes typically decline in parallel with needs. Still, many older

*The Canadian RNI divide older people into two age groups—50 to 74, and 75 and older.

adults are overweight, indicating that their food intakes do not decline enough to compensate for their reduced energy expenditure.[26]

• Older adult feeding pointer: Select nutrient-dense foods low in fats, sugars, and alcohol.

On limited energy allowances, people must select mostly nutrient-dense foods. There is little leeway for sugars, fats, oils, or alcohol. Because overweight creates many health problems and shortens the life span, these seem to be life-sustaining recommendations. The Daily Food Guide (on pp. 44–45) offers a dietary framework for adults of all ages. Those who need additional food energy should choose extra servings from each of the groups listed.[27]

Regular Physical Activity The many and remarkable benefits of regular physical activity are not limited to the young: older adults who are active weigh less and have greater flexibility, more endurance, and better balance than those who are inactive.[28] They reap additional benefits as well; for example, evening exercise helps to eliminate late night trips to the bathroom, and strength training significantly improves mobility and resistance to injury.*[29] In fact, regular physical activity is the most powerful predictor of a person's mobility in the later years.[30]

• Older adult pointer: Exercise to maintain muscle and bone mass.

Activities of all kinds are recommended to maintain and promote health: strength training can build muscles, and aerobic exercise can improve cardiorespiratory endurance and lower blood lipid concentrations.[31] While aging affects both speed and endurance to some degree, older adults can still train and achieve exceptional performances.

Ideally, physical activity should be part of each day's schedule and should be intense enough to prevent muscle atrophy and to speed up the heartbeat and respiration rate. Healthy older adults who have not been active can ease into a suitable routine. They can start by walking short distances until they can walk at least a mile three times a week; then they can gradually increase their pace to achieve a 20-to-25 minute mile.[32]

Muscle mass and muscle strength tend to decline with aging, making older people vulnerable to falls and immobility. Falls are a major cause of fear, injury, disability, dependence, and even death among older adults. Regular exercise tones, firms, and strengthens muscles, helping to improve confidence, reduce the risk of falling, and minimize the risk of injury should a fall occur. Strength training, even in frail, elderly people over 85 years of age, has been shown to not only improve muscle strength and mobility but to increase energy expenditure and energy intake, thereby enhancing nutrient intakes.[33] This finding highlights another reason to exercise: a person spending energy on physical activity can afford to eat more food and with it, more nutrients. People who are committed to an ongoing fitness program have higher energy and nutrient intakes than more sedentary people.[34]

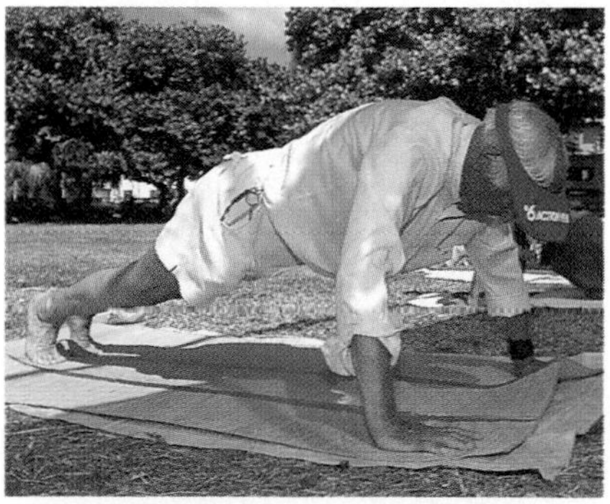

Strength training promotes strong muscles and bones and healthy appetites.

One expert suggests the following physical activity program to maintain good health and function in older adults:[35]

• *Every day.* 60 minutes of some physical activity: gardening, walking, climbing stairs, or simply moving about. This can be for 5 minutes at a time, 12 times a

*Exercising keeps body fluids circulating; when sedentary people lie down, the excess fluid that has pooled in their lower extremities begins to circulate again, creating the need to urinate. Interview with W. E. Wooldridge, MD, professor emeritus of clinical medicine at the University of Missouri in Columbia as reported in *The Physician and Sportsmedicine* 19 (1991): 49.

day; 12 minutes at a time, 5 times a day; or any combination of activity to total 60 minutes.

- *Three days a week.* 30 to 45 minutes of vigorous and continuous physical activity, such as swimming, dancing, rowing, or brisk walking.

With persistence, people can achieve great improvements at any age. Training not only tones, firms, and strengthens muscles but also increases the blood flow to the brain, thereby improving mental ability.

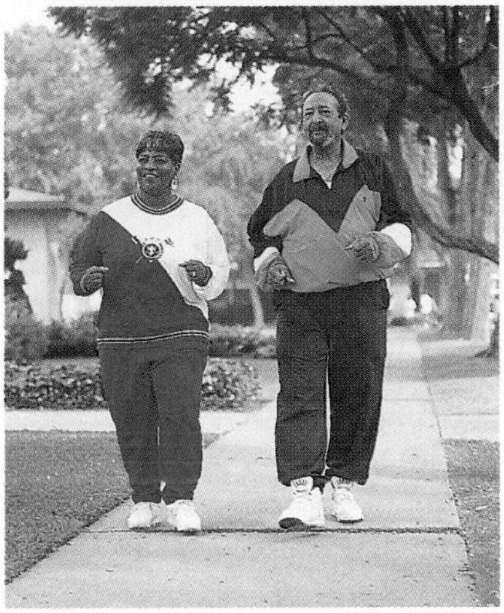

A walk in the neighborhood provides many physical benefits and a time to visit with others.

Protein The protein needs of older adults appear to be about the same as, or even greater than, those of younger people. Since energy needs decrease, however, the protein has to be obtained from low-kcalorie sources of high-quality protein, such as lean meats, poultry, fish, and eggs; nonfat and low-fat milk products; and legumes and grains.

Carbohydrate Abundant carbohydrate is needed to protect protein from being used as an energy source. Complex carbohydrate foods such as vegetables, whole grains, and fruits are also rich in fiber and essential vitamins and minerals.

The combination of ample water and high-fiber foods can alleviate constipation—a condition common among older adults, and especially among nursing home residents. Physical inactivity and medications probably contribute to the high incidence of constipation, but lack of water and fiber does, too, in many cases. In fact, average fiber intakes are lower than current recommendations.

Fat As is true for people of all ages, fat needs to be limited in the diet of most older adults. Cutting fat may help retard the development of cancer, atherosclerosis, and other degenerative diseases. Restricting fat intakes to less than 30 percent of total energy presents a challenge for many older adults, given their limited energy allowances and food intakes. For some older adults, limiting fat intake too severely may lead to nutrient deficiencies and weight loss—two problems that carry greater health risks in the elderly than overweight.[36]

VITAMINS AND MINERALS

Most people can achieve adequate vitamin and mineral intakes simply by including foods from all food groups in their diets, but studies show that older adults often omit fruits and vegetables.[37] About 18 percent of people 60 years and older are reported to eat no vegetables at all, and up to one of every three older adults reports never eating fruit. When almost 500 participants in a meal program were asked about their food likes and dislikes, nine of the ten most-disliked foods were vegetables. Similarly, few older adults consume the recommended amounts of milk products.[38]

Vitamin A Vitamin A stands alone in that it is absorbed and stored more efficiently by the aging GI tract and liver, although its processing within the body slows slightly.[39] Several studies have reported that healthy older adults have normal levels of plasma vitamin A even when their dietary intakes fall below the RDA, suggesting that the current RDA may be too high.[40] The Committee on Dietary Allowances must balance the research for preventing vitamin

A deficiency against findings that the vitamin A precursor beta-carotene might prevent or delay the onset of some age-related diseases.

Vitamin D Older adults face a greater risk of vitamin D deficiency than younger people do. Only vitamin D–fortified milk provides significant vitamin D, and many older adults drink little or no milk. Consequently, many older adults have vitamin D intakes of less than half of the RDA. Further compromising the vitamin D status of many older people, especially those in nursing homes, is their limited exposure to sunlight. Finally, aging reduces the skin's capacity to make vitamin D and the kidneys' ability to convert it to its active form. Not only are older adults not getting enough vitamin D, but they may actually need more than the RDA to maintain bone health.[41] Some research indicates that a vitamin D intake greater than the RDA may be necessary to prevent bone loss and to maintain vitamin D status in older people, especially in those who engage in minimal outdoor activity.[42]

Vitamin B_6 Studies on vitamin B_6 reveal that its metabolism is altered with age, resulting in a higher requirement. The current RDA for people over 50 may need to be raised.[43]

Vitamin B_{12} People with atrophic gastritis are particularly vulnerable to vitamin B_{12} deficiency for two reasons. First, digestion in the inflamed stomach is inefficient. Second, the abundant bacteria that accompany this condition use the vitamin. Given the devastating effects of a vitamin B_{12} deficiency, an RDA higher than the current one may be appropriate.[44]

Iron Among the minerals, iron deserves first mention. Iron-deficiency anemia is less common in older adults than in younger people, but it still occurs in some, especially in those with low food energy intakes. Aside from diet, other factors in many older people's lives make iron deficiency likely: chronic blood loss from disease conditions and medicines, and poor iron absorption due to reduced stomach acid secretion and antacid use. Anyone concerned with older people's nutrition should keep these possibilities in mind.

Zinc Zinc intake is commonly low in older people. As many as 95 percent of older adults may not get the zinc they need, and many receive less than half of the recommended amount.[45] In addition, older adults may absorb zinc less efficiently than younger people do. A number of different factors, including medications that older adults commonly use, can impair zinc absorption or enhance its excretion and thus lead to deficiency.[46] Older adults who do not make special efforts to eat zinc-rich foods such as meats, fish, and poultry will no doubt fail to meet the zinc RDA. Some of the symptoms of zinc deficiency resemble symptoms associated with aging—for example, decline in taste acuity and dermatitis. Whether these symptoms are attributable to zinc deficiency remains unclear.

Reminder: The calcium RDA for adults 25 years and older is 800 mg/day.

Calcium The appropriate calcium intake for older adults remains controversial. A National Institutes of Health panel has concluded that women over 50 who are not on estrogen replacement therapy and all adults over 65 should receive 1500 milligrams of calcium daily.[47] The Committee on Dietary

Allowances contends that evidence is insufficient to warrant raising the calcium RDA for older women.[48]

While researchers attempt to reach agreement about the calcium requirements of older adults, especially those of women, one thing is clear: the calcium intakes of many people, especially women, in the United States are well below the RDA. If fresh milk causes stomach discomfort, as some older people report, then special efforts should be made to eat other calcium-rich foods. One simple solution is to incorporate dry nonfat milk into recipes; Chapter 12 offers many other strategies.

The importance of abundant dietary calcium throughout life, and especially for women after menopause, to protect against osteoporosis was discussed in Chapter and Highlight 12.

HEALTHY PEOPLE 2000: Increase calcium intake so that at least 50% of people aged 25 years and older consume two or more servings of calcium-rich foods daily.

Malnutrition It has been estimated that as many as 50 percent of nursing home residents may be malnourished and underweight.[49] For these people, a diet that emphasizes fiber-rich foods such as whole grains, fruits, and vegetables may be too low in concentrated protein and energy. Protein- and energy-dense snacks such as hard-boiled eggs, tuna fish and crackers, peanut butter on graham crackers, and homemade soups are valuable additions to the diets of underweight or malnourished older adults. Table 17–1 lists risk factors for malnutrition in elderly people.

Table 17–1

Risk Factors for Malnutrition in Older Adults

Difficulties in chewing or swallowing
Difficulties in procuring or preparing food
Recent loss of spouse
Oral health problems
Poverty
Multiple drug use
Confusion or depression
Neurologic disorders
Chronic lung disease
Eating fewer than three meals per day
Anorexia
Institutionalization
Inability to self-feed
Alcoholism
Altered taste or smell
Recent surgery
Diabetes
Loneliness

Source: Adapted from R. Chernoff, Meeting the nutritional needs of the elderly in the institutional setting, *Nutrition Reviews* 52 (1994): 132–136.

SUPPLEMENTS FOR OLDER ADULTS

Advertisers target older people with appeals to take supplements and eat "health" foods, claiming that these products prevent disease and promote longevity. About half of all women over 65 years of age take some type of nutrient supplement, while about one-fifth of older men do. Quite often those who take supplements are not deficient in the nutrients being supplemented.[50] Certain diseases or health problems may necessitate the taking of supplements, but quite often, supplements have not been prescribed by health care professionals and are inappropriate.

When recommended by a physician, vitamin D and calcium supplements for osteoporosis or iron for iron-deficiency anemia may be beneficial. In most cases, though, the money spent on supplements would be better spent on nutritious foods. Older adults with food energy intakes less than about 1500 kcalories should probably take supplements—not megavitamins, but just the once-daily type of vitamin-mineral supplements.

People with small energy allowances would do well to become more active and earn the right to eat more food. Food is the best source of nutrients for everybody. Supplements are just that—supplements to foods, not substitutes for them. For anyone who is motivated to obtain the best possible health, it is never too late to learn to eat well, exercise regularly, and adopt other lifestyle changes such as quitting smoking, moderating alcohol use, and the like.

Table 17–2 summarizes the nutrient concerns of aging. While some nutrients need special attention in the diet, supplements are not routinely recommended.

Table 17–2

Summary of Nutrient Concerns in Aging

Nutrient	Effect of Aging	Comments
Energy	Need decreases.	Physical activity moderates the decline.
Fiber	Likelihood of constipation increases with low intakes and changes in the GI tract.	Inadequate water intakes and lack of physical activity, along with some medications, compound the problem.
Protein	Needs stay the same.	Low-fat, high-fiber legumes and grains meet both protein and other nutrient needs.
Vitamin A	Absorption increases.	RDA may be high.
Vitamin D	Increased likelihood of inadequate intake; skin synthesis declines.	Daily limited sunlight exposure may be of benefit.
Water	Lack of thirst and decreased total body water make dehydration likely.	Mild dehydration is a common cause of confusion. Difficulty obtaining water or getting to the bathroom may compound the problem.
Iron	In women, status improves after menopause; deficiencies are linked to chronic blood losses and low stomach acid output.	Adequate stomach acid is required for absorption; antacid or other medicine use may aggravate iron deficiency; vitamin C and meat increase absorption.
Zinc	Often inadequate intakes and reduced absorption; but needs may also decrease.	Medications interfere with absorption; deficiency may depress appetite and sense of taste.
Calcium	Intakes may be low; osteoporosis common.	Stomach discomfort commonly limits milk intake; calcium substitutes are needed.

The ever-growing number of older people in the world presents an urgent need to know more about how their nutrient requirements differ from those of younger people and how such knowledge can enhance their health.

Special Concerns of Older Adults

Nutrition through the prime years may play a greater role than has been realized in preventing many changes once thought to be inevitable consquences of growing older. The following discussions of cataracts, arthritis, and the aging brain show that nutrition may provide at least some protection against some of the conditions associated with aging.

CATARACTS AND ARTHRITIS

Two common causes of distress among older people are cataracts and arthritis. Both of these conditions have nutrition links.

cataracts: thickenings of the eye lenses that impair vision and can lead to blindness.

Cataracts Cataracts are age-related thickenings in the lenses of the eye that impair vision. If not surgically removed, they ultimately lead to blindness. Cataracts occur even in well-nourished individuals due to ultraviolet light exposure, free-radical damage, injury, viral infections, toxic substances, and genetic disorders. Many cataracts, however, are vaguely called senile cataracts—meaning "caused by aging." In the United States, some 46 percent of people between the ages of 75 and 85 have cataracts, compared to only 5 percent of those between the ages of 52 and 64.[51]

Oxidative stress appears to play a significant role in the development of cataracts, and the antioxidant nutrients may help minimize the damage.[52] Studies have reported an inverse relationship between cataracts and dietary intakes of vitamin C, vitamin E, and carotenoids.[53] One study found that people who had no cataracts took significantly more supplements of vitamins C and E than those who had cataracts.[54]

Reminder: *Free radicals* are highly reactive molecules that arise during oxidative reactions and readily attack other molecules; see Highlight 11 for more details.

Arthritis Another condition that disables older people is arthritis, a painful swelling of the joints. During movement, the ends of bones are normally protected from wear by cartilage and by small sacs of fluid that act as a lubricant; but with age, bones sometimes disintegrate, and the joints become malformed and painful to move. Arthritis afflicts millions of people around the world, especially the elderly. Nutrition quackery to treat arthritis is abundant, but no known diet prevents, relieves, or cures.

One possibly valid link between arthritis and diet is through the immune system. Researchers believe that in rheumatoid arthritis, the immune system mistakenly attacks the bone coverings as if they were made of foreign tissue.[55] The integrity of the immune system depends on adequate nutrition, and a poor diet may worsen arthritis. It is also possible that in some individuals, certain foods may stimulate the immune system to attack. For example, milk and milk products seem to aggravate arthritis in some people.[56]

Another nutrient linked to arthritis is the omega-3 fatty acid found in fish oil, EPA. Research shows that the same diet recommended for heart health—one low in saturated fat from meats and milk products and high in oils from fish—helps prevent or reduce the inflammation in the joints that makes arthritis so painful.[57] Researchers theorize that EPA probably interferes with the action of prostaglandins, chemicals involved in inflammation.

Another possible link between nutrition and arthritis involves the lipid peroxidation reaction described in Highlight 11—which vitamin E helps to prevent. Lipid peroxidation of the membranes within joints causes inflammation and swelling.[58] Vitamin E has not improved active cases of arthritis, but this is not surprising since the vitamin's role in lipid peroxidation is preventive, not restorative.

A known connection between arthritis and nutrition is overweight. Weight loss is important for overweight persons with arthritis, partly because the joints affected are often weight-bearing joints that are stressed and irritated by having to carry excess poundage. Interestingly, though, weight loss often relieves the worst of the pain of arthritis in the hands as well, even though they are not weight-bearing joints. Jogging and other weight-bearing exercises do not worsen arthritis, even in marathon runners.

Drugs used to relieve arthritis can impose nutrition risks.[59] Many drugs affect appetite and alter the body's use of nutrients, as Highlight 17 explains.

arthritis: a usually painful inflammation of a joint caused by many conditions, including infections, metabolic disturbances, or injury; joint structure is usually altered, with loss of function.

Not effective against arthritis:

- Alfalfa tea.
- Amino acid supplements.
- Blackstrap molasses.
- Burdock root.
- Calcium.
- Celery juice.
- Cod liver oil.
- Copper supplements.
- Dimethyl sulfoxide (DMSO).
- Fasting.
- Fresh fruit.
- Garlic.
- Honey.
- Inositol.
- Kelp.
- Lecithin.
- Para-amino benzoic acid (PABA).
- Raw liver.
- *Aloe vera* liquid.
- Superoxide dismutase (SOD).
- Vitamin D.
- Vitamin megadoses.
- Watercress.
- Yeast.
- 100 other substances.

These brief discussions of cataracts and arthritis show that nutrition may provide at least some protection against certain conditions associated with aging. In fact, it is beginning to look as though nutrition through the prime years may play a greater role than has been realized in preventing many changes once thought to be inevitable consequences of growing older.

THE AGING BRAIN

The brain, like all of the body's organs, responds to both inherited and environmental factors that can enhance or diminish its amazing capacities. One of the challenges researchers face when studying aging of the brain in human beings is to distinguish among normal age-related physiological changes, changes caused by diseases, and changes that result from cumulative, extrinsic factors such as diet.

neuron: a nerve cell; the structural and functional unit of the nervous system. Neurons initiate and conduct nerve transmissions.

cerebral cortex: the outer surface of the cerebrum.

The brain normally changes in some characteristic ways as it ages. For one thing, its blood supply decreases. For another, the number of neurons, the brain cells that specialize in transmitting information, diminishes as people age. When the number of nerve cells in one part of the cerebral cortex diminishes, hearing and speech are affected. Losses of neurons in other parts of the cortex can impair memory and cognitive function. When the number of neurons in the hindbrain diminishes, balance and posture are affected. Losses of neurons in other parts of the brain affect still other functions.

Clinicians now recognize that much of the cognitive loss and forgetfulness generally attributed to aging is due in part to extrinsic, and therefore controllable, factors such as nutrient deficiencies. In some instances, the degree of cognitive loss is extensive and attributable to a specific disorder such as a brain tumor. In cases such as Alzheimer's disease, deterioration may be genetically determined and will not yet yield to external approaches.

senile dementia: the loss of brain function beyond the normal loss of physical adeptness and memory that occurs with aging.

senile dementia of the Alzheimer's type (SDAT): a degenerative disease of the brain involving memory loss and major structural changes in neuron networks; also known as primary degenerative dementia of senile onset or chronic brain syndrome, but often simply called Alzheimer's disease.

Alzheimer's Disease Much attention has focused on the *abnormal* deterioration of the brain called senile dementia of the Alzheimer's type (SDAT), which affects 5 percent of U.S. adults by age 65 and 20 percent of those over 80.[60] Diagnosis of SDAT depends on its characteristic symptoms: the victim gradually loses memory and reasoning, the ability to communicate, physical capabilities, and eventually life itself. Nerve cells in the brain die and communication between the cells breaks down.

To date, the causes of SDAT continue to elude researchers, although genetic factors are apparently involved. Consequently, researchers have yet to find a cure for this devastating degenerative disease. Treatment involves providing care to clients and support to their families. One drug (trade-named Tacrine) seems to slow the advance of the disease in about 20 percent of those who use it, but it does not reverse the damage already done. Meanwhile, some drugs seem to favorably influence the ability to remember and so hold promise for improving the lives of those with Alzheimer's disease. Other drugs may be used to control depression or behavior problems.

Nutrition may be somehow linked to SDAT. For example, as blood flow to the brain diminishes with age, the brain normally compensates by absorbing more glucose and oxygen. In SDAT, no such compensation occurs, the glucose and oxygen uptake declines. Whether the brain's diminished capacity to take up glucose and oxygen causes or results from SDAT remains unclear.

Reminder: A *neurotransmitter* is a chemical that is released by one nerve cell that acts upon a second nerve cell, altering its electrical state or activity.

Another abnormality of interest involves the extremely low concentrations of the enzyme that makes the neurotransmitter acetylcholine from choline and acetyl CoA. Acetylcholine is essential to memory. To date, supplements of choline (or of lecithin, which contains choline) have had no effect on memory or on the progression of the disease. Trials of lecithin in combination with drugs show some improvement in limited areas of cognitive deficiencies.

Most people have heard of an association between aluminum and the development of SDAT, although a causal connection seems unlikely. Brain concentrations of aluminum in SDAT people exceed normal brain concentrations by some 10 to 30 times, but blood and hair aluminum remains normal, indicating that the accumulation is caused by something in the brain itself, not by an overload of aluminum in the body. Thus the high brain aluminum must be at least partly a result, rather than a cause, of SDAT. Researchers are still investigating the relationship between dietary aluminum and SDAT in individuals, and the question is still open whether aluminum cookware, which slightly increases the aluminum content of foods, significantly affects the progress of SDAT.

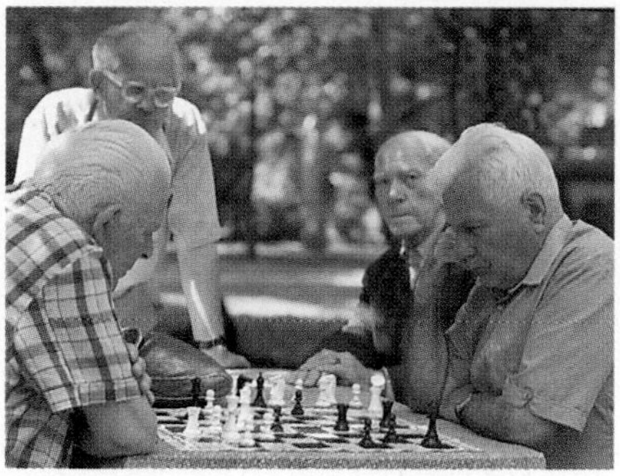

The brain is nourished by both foods and mental challenges.

Maintaining appropriate body weight may be the most important nutrition concern for the person with SDAT. Depression and forgetfulness can lead to poor food intake, and restlessness may increase energy needs. Perhaps the best that a caretaker can do nutritionally for an SDAT client is to supervise food planning and mealtimes. Providing well-liked and well-balanced meals and snacks in a cheerful atmosphere encourages food consumption. To minimize confusion, offer a few ready-to-eat foods, in bite-size pieces, with seasonings and sauces. To avoid mealtime disruptions, control distractions such as television, children, and the telephone.

SDAT is an identifiable disease, the course of which is probably not influenced by nutrition. But poor nutrition in general does affect the brain in other ways.

Nutrient Deficiencies and Brain Function Moderate, long-term nutrient deficiencies may contribute to the loss of memory and cognition that some older adults experience. For example, the ability of neurons to synthesize specific neurotransmitters depends in part on the availability of precursor nutrients that are obtained from the diet. The neurotransmitter serotonin derives from the amino acid tryptophan. To function properly, the enzymes involved in neurotransmitter synthesis require vitamins and minerals. Severe dietary deficiencies of thiamin, vitamin B_6, vitamin B_{12}, folate, and vitamin C impair mental ability, including memory. Trace elements such as iron and zinc also support normal brain function. Table 17–3 summarizes some of the better known connections between impaired brain function and severe nutrient deficiencies. If long-term,

Table 17–3

Summary of Nutrient-Brain Relationships

Brain Function	Inadequate Intake or Deficiency of:
Short-term memory loss	Vitamin B_{12}, vitamin C
Poor performance in problem-solving tests	Riboflavin, folate, vitamin B_{12}, vitamin C
Dementia	Thiamin, zinc
Cognition	Folate, vitamin B_6, vitamin B_{12}, iron
Degeneration of brain tissue	Vitamin B_6

moderate nutrient deficiencies influence the loss of cognitive function that accompanies aging, then the loss may be preventable or at least diminished or delayed through diet.

Senile dementia and other losses of brain function afflict millions of older adults. As the number of people over age 65 continues to grow, the need for solutions to the problems that this major portion of the population faces is becoming urgent. Some problems may be inevitable, but others are preventable.

We can now state with certainty that a person's nutrition status affects the health and functioning of the whole body. Eating a nutritious, balanced diet throughout life seems a small effort in light of the rewards of continued health and enjoyment in later life.

In addition, there is much people can do, besides obtaining adequate nutrition, to support a high quality of life into old age. By practicing stress-management skills, maintaining physical fitness, participating in activities of interest, and cultivating spiritual health, a person can grow old gracefully (see Table 17–4 for some strategies).

Table 17–4

Strategies for Growing Old Gracefully

- Choose nutrient-dense foods.
- Maintain appropriate body weight.
- Reduce stress.
- For women, see a physician about estrogen replacement.
- For people who smoke, quit.
- Expect to enjoy sex, and learn new ways of enhancing it.
- Use alcohol only moderately, if at all; use drugs only as prescribed.
- Take care to prevent accidents.
- Expect good vision and hearing throughout life; obtain glasses and hearing aids if necessary.
- Be alert to confusion as a disease symptom, and seek diagnosis.
- Control depression through activities and friendships.
- Drink 8 glasses of water every day.
- Practice mental skills. Keep on solving math problems and crossword puzzles, playing cards or other games, reading, writing, imagining, and creating.
- Make financial plans early to ensure security.
- Accept change. Work at recovering from losses; make new friends.
- Cultivate spiritual health. Cherish personal values. Make life meaningful.
- Go outside for sunshine and fresh air as often as possible.
- Be physically active. Walk, run, dance, swim, bike, row, or climb for aerobic activity. Lift weights, do calisthenics, or pursue some other activity to tone, firm, and strengthen muscles. Change activities to suit changing abilities and tastes.
- Be socially active—play bridge, join an exercise group, take a class, teach a class, eat with friends, volunteer time to help others.
- Stay interested in life—pursue a hobby, spend time with grandchildren, take a trip, read, grow a garden, or go to the movies.
- Enjoy life.

Food Choices and Eating Habits of Older Adults

Older people are an incredibly diverse group, and for the most part they are independent, socially sophisticated, mentally lucid, fully participating members of society who report themselves to be happy and healthy. Most people over 65 live in their own or relatives' homes; only 5 percent of those 65 to 85, and 20 percent of those over 85, live in facilities such as nursing homes.

Older people spend more money per person on foods to eat at home than other age groups and less money on foods away from home. Manufacturers would be wise to cater to the preferences of older adults by providing good-tasting, nutritious foods in easy-to-open, single-serving packages with labels that are easy to read. Such services enable older adults to maintain their independence; most of them want to take care of themselves and need to feel a sense of control and involvement in their own lives.

- Older adult feeding pointer: Try to maintain independence.

Familiarity, taste, and health beliefs are most influential on older people's food choices. Eating foods that are familiar, especially those that recall family meals and pleasant times, can be comforting. The importance of diet and health beliefs in food selection is evidenced by surveys indicating that older adults are choosing low-fat poultry and fish, low-fat milk and milk products, and high-fiber breads and grains.[61] People 65 and over are less likely to diet to lose weight than younger people are, but are more likely to diet in pursuit of medical goals such as controlling blood glucose, cholesterol, and sodium.

- Older adult feeding pointer: Select familiar foods, especially ethnic favorites.

NUTRITION PROGRAMS

Nutrition services are an integral part of health care, and different subgroups of the aging population need different programs designed to meet their specific needs.[62] People living alone can benefit from congregate meal programs; people confined to their homes need meals delivered. The Nutrition Screening Initiative is part of a national effort to identify and treat nutrition problems in older persons; it uses a screening checklist (see Table 17–5 on p. 634). To *determine* the risk of malnutrition in older clients, health care providers can keep in mind the characteristics listed in the margin.[63]

Risk factors for malnutrition in older adults:

- Disease.
- Eating poorly.
- Tooth loss or oral pain.
- Economic hardship.
- Reduced social contact.
- Multiple medications.
- Involuntary weight loss or gain.
- Needs assistance with self-care.
- Elderly person older than 80 years.

HEALTHY PEOPLE 2000: Increase to at least 80% the receipt of home foodservices by people aged 65 and older who have difficulty in preparing their own meals or are otherwise in need of home-delivered meals.

The U.S. government funds programs to provide nutritious meals to older adults at congregate meal sites. These meals are a valuable source of nutrients for many older adults. Like the school lunches, though, congregate meals do not typically meet current dietary recommendations to limit sodium, fat, and cholesterol.[64] The box on p. 635 describes food assistance programs for older adults.

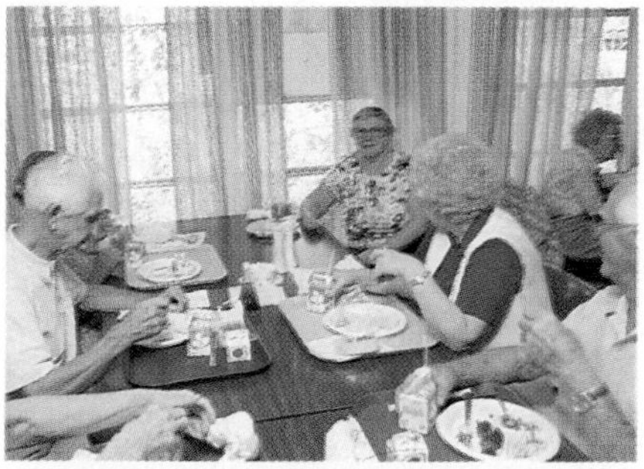

Social interactions at a congregate meal site can be as nourishing as the foods served.

MEALS FOR SINGLES

Singles of all ages face difficulties in purchasing, storing, and preparing food. Large packages of meat and vegetables are often intended for families of four or more, and even a head of lettuce can spoil before one person can use it all. Many

Table 17–5

Nutrition Screening Initiative Checklist

Circle the number to the right if the statement applies to you.

Statement	Yes
I have an illness or condition that made me change the kind and/or amount of food I eat.	2
I eat fewer than 2 meals per day.	3
I eat few fruits or vegetables or milk products.	2
I have 3 or more drinks of beer, liquor, or wine almost every day.	2
I have tooth or mouth problems that make it hard for me to eat.	2
I don't always have enough money to buy the food I need.	4
I eat alone most of the time.	1
I take 3 or more different prescribed or over-the-counter drugs a day.	1
Without wanting to, I have lost or gained 10 pounds in the last 6 months.	2
I am not always physically able to shop, cook, and/or feed myself.	2
Total	

SCORE:

0–2: Good. Recheck your score in 6 months.

3–5: Moderate nutritional risk. Visit your local office on aging, senior nutrition program, senior citizens center, or health department for tips on improving eating habits.

6 or more: High nutritional risk. See your doctor, dietitian, or other health care professional for help in improving your nutrition status.

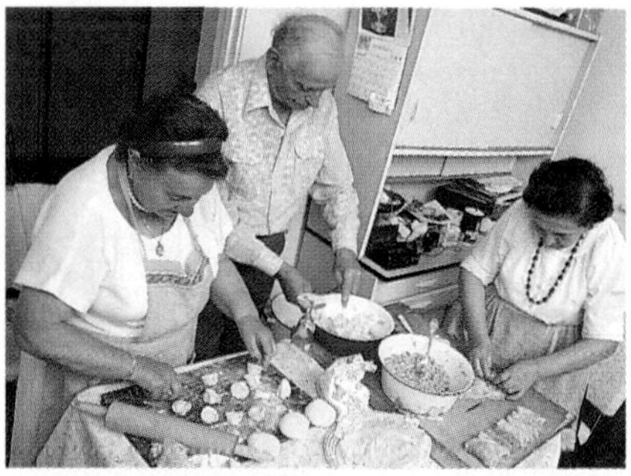

Taking time to nourish your body well is a gift you give yourself.

singles live in small dwellings and have little storage space for foods. A limited income presents additional obstacles. This section presents ideas that can help to solve some of these problems.

Spend Wisely People who have the means to shop and cook for themselves can cut their food bills just by being wise shoppers. The first decision a person with a tight grocery budget must make is where to shop. Large supermarkets are usually less expensive than convenience stores, but the cost of transportation to the market is a consideration. A grocery list helps reduce impulse buying, and specials and coupons can save money when the items featured are those that the shopper needs and uses.

Buy Bulk Many foods that offer a variety of nutrients for practically pennies have a long shelf life and can be purchased in bulk. Staples such as rice, pastas, nonfat dry powdered milk, and dried beans and peas can be stored on a shelf for months at room temperature. Other foods that are usually a good buy include whole pieces of cheese rather than sliced or shredded cheese; fresh produce in season; variety meats such as chicken livers; and cereals that require cooking instead of ready-to-serve cereals.

A person who has ample freezing space can buy large packages of meat, such as pork chops, ground beef, or chicken, when they are on sale. Then, the pack-

Food Assistance Programs for Older Adults

The federal Nutrition Program for Older Americans (Title III) is intended to improve older people's nutrition status and enable them to avoid medical problems, continue living in communities of their own choice, and stay out of institutions. Its specific goals are to provide low-cost, nutritious meals; opportunities for social interaction; homemaker education and shopping assistance; counseling and referral to social services; and transportation.

Title III provides for congregate meal programs. Administrators try to select sites for congregate meals so as to feed as many eligible people as possible. Volunteers may also deliver meals to those who are homebound either permanently or temporarily; these efforts are known as Meals on Wheels. The home-delivery program ensures nutrition, but its recipients miss out on the social benefit of the congregate meal sites; every effort is made to persuade older people to come to the shared meals, if they can. All persons aged 60 years and older are eligible to receive meals from these programs, regardless of their income. Priority is given to those who are economically and socially needy. These programs provide at least one meal a day that meets a third of the RDA for this age group; they must operate five or more days a week. Many programs voluntarily offer additional services: provisions for therapeutic diets, food pantries, ethnic meals, and delivery of meals to the homeless.

Older adults can learn about the available programs in their communities by looking in the yellow pages of the telephone book under "Social Services" or "Senior Citizens' Organizations." In addition, the local senior center and hospital can usually direct people to programs providing nutrition and other health related services.

age can be immediately divided into individual servings and wrapped in aluminum foil, not freezer paper: the foil can become the liner for the pan in which to bake or broil the meat, thus saving work over the sink. All the individual servings can be put in a bag marked "hamburger" or "chicken thighs" or whatever, along with the date. The bag will be easy to locate in the freezer, and a person can easily see when the supply is running low.

Frozen vegetables are more economical in large bags than in small boxes. The amount needed can be taken out, and the bag closed tightly with a rubber band. If the package is returned quickly to the freezer each time, the vegetables will stay fresh for a long time.

Finally, breads and cereals usually must be purchased in larger quantities. Again the amount needed for a few days can be taken out and the rest stored in the freezer.

Buy Small Buying the right amount in order not to waste any food is a challenge for people eating alone. They can buy fresh milk in the size best suited for personal needs. Pint-size and even cup-size boxes of milk are also available and can be stored unopened on a shelf for up to three months without refrigeration.

Boxes of milk kept at room temperature on the shelves of grocery stores have been treated with a process called **ultrahigh temperature (UHT)**; the milk is exposed to temperatures above those of pasteurization just long enough to sterilize it.

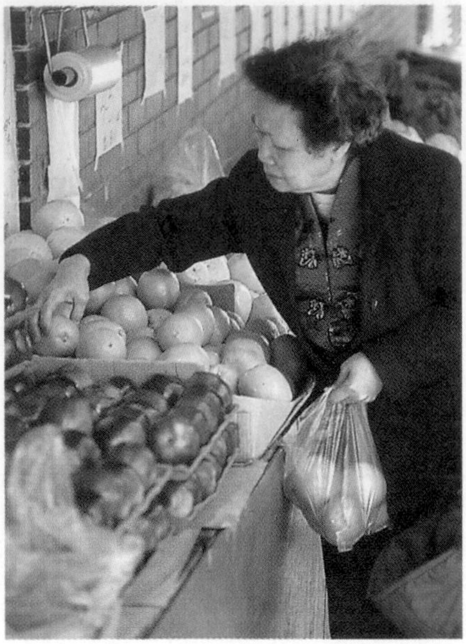

Buy only what you will use.

Grocers will break open a package of wrapped meat and rewrap the portion needed. Similarly, eggs can be purchased by the half-dozen. Eggs do keep for long periods, though, if stored properly in the refrigerator.

Fresh fruits and vegetables can be purchased individually. A person can buy three pieces of each kind of fresh fruit: a ripe one to eat right away, a semiripe one to eat soon after, and a green one to ripen on the windowsill. If vegetables are packaged in large quantities, the grocer can break open the package so that a smaller amount can be purchased. Small cans of fruits and vegetables, even though they are more expensive per unit, are a reasonable alternative, considering that it is expensive to buy a regular-size can and let the unused portion spoil.

Be Creative For times when a person has to buy more food than one person can use, here are a few hints. Mixtures of leftovers can be prepared and served again. A thick stew made from leftover green beans, carrots, cauliflower, broccoli, and any meat with added onion, pepper, celery, and potatoes makes a complete and balanced meal—except for milk, but then powdered milk can be added to the stew.

Glass jars are ideal for storing shelf staple items—rice, tapioca, lentils or other dry beans, flour, cornmeal, nonfat dry milk, macaroni, cereal, and the like. Freezing each filled jar for one night first kills any insect eggs that might be present. The jars will then keep bugs out of the food indefinitely. They make an attractive display and serve to remind the cook of different choices to vary menus. The directions-for-use labels from the packages can be stored in the jars.

Creative chefs think of various ways to use a vegetable when only large amounts are available. For example, a head of cauliflower can be divided into thirds. Then one-third is cooked and eaten hot. Another third is put into a vinegar and oil marinade for use in a salad. And the last third can be used in a casserole or stew.

Also, single people shouldn't hesitate to invite someone to share meals with them whenever there is a lot of food. It's likely that that person will return the invitation, and both parties will get to enjoy companionship and a meal prepared by others.

An occasional frozen TV dinner can also be useful—although expensive—if it makes the difference between a person's eating and not eating. Many such dinners that are now available are low in fat and nutritious. Adding a fresh salad, a whole-wheat roll, and a glass of milk can make a nice meal. Another option for those who can afford it is to eat meals from restaurants. Most restaurants offer take-out meals and many provide delivery services.

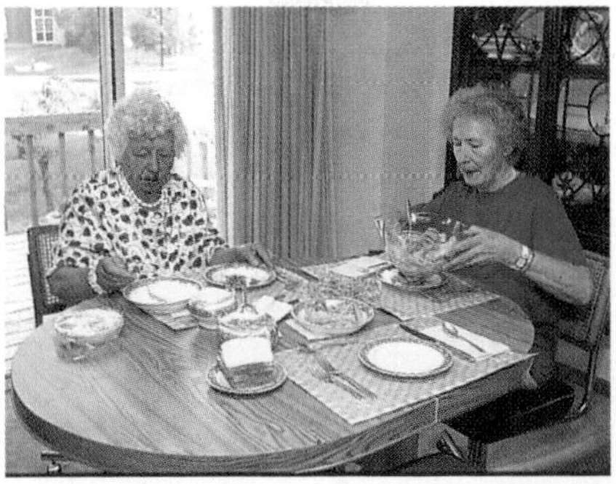

Invite guests to share a meal.

One more suggestion for those who are alone at mealtime is this: make it a special occasion. One way to do this is to set the table with a tablecloth, a napkin, a full set of utensils, and fresh flowers. Set a pot of stew or homemade soup with vegetables and fresh herbs on low heat to cook, and make a salad. Get comfortable in a stuffed chair, and enjoy a book or some soothing music until the rich aroma of a simmering dinner beckons. After serving your plate, light a candle, dim the lights, savor the food, and relish some of the best company you will have—your own.

Study Questions

1. What are some of the physiological changes that occur in the body's systems with aging? To what extent can aging be prevented?
2. What roles does nutrition play in aging, and what roles can it play in retarding aging?
3. Why does the risk of dehydration increase as people age?
4. Why do energy needs usually decline with advancing age?
5. Which vitamins and minerals need special consideration for the elderly? Explain why. Name some factors that complicate the task of setting nutrient standards for older adults.
6. What characteristics contribute to malnutrition in older people?

Notes

1. R. Chernoff, Demographics of aging, in *Geriatric Nutrition: The Health Professional's Handbook*, ed. R. Chernoff (Gaithersburg, Md.: Aspen Publishers, 1991), pp. 1–9.
2. K. G. Kinsella, Changes in life expectancy 1900–1990, *American Journal of Clinical Nutrition* 55 (1992): 1196S–1202S; S. Kobayashi, A scientific basis for the longevity of Japanese in relation to diet and nutrition, *Nutrition Reviews* 50 (1992): 353–359.
3. L. Breslow and N. Breslow, Health practices and disability: Some evidence from Almeda County, *Preventive Medicine* 22 (1993): 86–95.
4. A. Z. LaCroix and coauthors, Maintaining mobility in late life: Smoking, alcohol consumption, physical activity, and body mass index, *American Journal of Epidemiology* 137 (1993): 858–869.
5. R. S. Paffenbarger and coauthors, The association of changes in physical-activity level and other lifestyle characteristics with mortality among men, *New England Journal of Medicine* 328 (1993): 538–545; S. N. Blair and coauthors, Physical fitness and all-cause mortality, *Journal of the American Medical Association* 262 (1989): 2395–2401.
6. R. S. Paffenbarger and coauthors, Physical activity, all-cause mortality, and longevity of college alumni, *New England Journal of Medicine* 314 (1986): 605–611.
7. E. J. Masoro, Retardation of aging processes by food restriction: An experimental tool, *American Journal of Clinical Nutrition* (supplement) 55 (1992): 1250–1252.
8. E. J. Masoro, Assessment of nutritional components in prolongation of life and health by diet, *Proceedings of the Society for Experimental Biology and Medicine* 193 (1990): 31–34; Energy intake restriction and oxidant defense, *Nutrition Reviews* 49 (1991): 278–280.
9. E. J. M. Velthuis-te Wierik and coauthors, Energy restriction, a useful intervention to retard human ageing? Results of a feasibility study, *European Journal of Clinical Nutrition* 48 (1994): 138–148.
10. R. Roubenoff and L. C. Rall, Humoral mediation of changing body composition during aging and chronic inflammation, *Nutrition Reviews* 51 (1993): 1–11.
11. T. Tada, Nutrition and the immune system in aging: An overview, *Nutrition Reviews* 50 (1992): 360.
12. R. K. Chandra, Nutrition and immunity in the elderly, *Nutrition Reviews* 50 (1992): 367–371.
13. K. Hirokawa, Understanding the mechanism of the age-related decline in immune function, *Nutrition Reviews* 50 (1992): 361–366.
14. S. Hosoda and coauthors, Age-related changes in the gastrointestinal tract, *Nutrition Reviews* 50 (1992): 374–377.
15. C. Murphy, Age-associated changes in taste and odor sensation, perception, and preference, in *Nutrition of the Elderly*, eds. H. Munro and G. Schlierf (New York: Raven Press, 1992), pp. 79–87.
16. C. O. Mitchell and R. Chernoff, Nutritional assessment of the elderly, in *Geriatric Nutrition: The Health Professional's Handbook*, ed. R. Chernoff (Gaithersburg, Md.: Aspen Publishers, 1991), pp. 363–395.
17. J. V. White and coauthors, Consensus of the Nutrition Screening Initiative: Risk factors and indicators of poor nutritional status in older Americans, *Journal of the American Dietetic Association* 91 (1991): 783–787.
18. A. K. Kant and G. Block, Dietary vitamin B-6 intake and food sources in the US population: NHANES II, 1976–1980, *American Journal of Clinical Nutrition* 52 (1990): 707–716.
19. M. A. Davis and coauthors, Living arrangements and dietary quality of older U.S. adults, *Journal of the American Dietetic Association* 90 (1990): 1667–1672; I. Darnton-Hill, Psychosocial aspects of nutrition and aging, *Nutrition Reviews* 50 (1992): 476–479.
20. E. Fogler-Levitt and coauthors, Utilization of home-delivered meals by recipients 75 years of age or older, *Journal of the American Dietetic Association* 95 (1995): 552–557.
21. D. Walker and R. E. Beauchene, The relationship of loneliness, social isolation, and physical health to dietary adequacy of independently living elderly, *Journal of the American Dietetic Association* 91 (1991): 300–304.
22. R. M. Russell and P. M. Suter, Vitamin requirements of elderly

people: An update, *American Journal of Clinical Nutrition* 58 (1993): 4–14; J. Blumberg, Nutrient requirements of the elderly—Should there be specific RDAs? *Nutrition Reviews* 52 (1994): S15–S18.

23. A. Bendich, Criteria for determining recommended dietary allowances for healthy older adults, *Nutrition Reviews* 53 (1995): S105–S110.
24. B. J. Rolls and P. A. Phillips, Aging and disturbances of thirst and fluid balance, *Nutrition Reviews* 48 (1990): 137–144.
25. R. Chernoff, Physiologic aging and nutritional status, *Nutrition in Clinical Practice*, February 1990, pp. 5–8.
26. E. T. Poehlman and E. S. Horton, Regulation of energy expenditure in aging humans, *Annual Review of Nutrition* 10 (1990): 255–275.
27. A. Greeley, Nutrition and the elderly, *FDA Consumer*, October 1990, pp. 25–28.
28. L. E. Voorrips and coauthors, The physical condition of elderly women differing in habitual physical activity, *Medicine and Science in Sports and Exercise* 25 (1993): 1152–1157.
29. M. A. Fiatarone and coauthors, High-intensity strength training in nonagenarians: Effects on skeletal muscle, *Journal of the American Medical Association* 263 (1990): 3029–3034; W. E. Wooldridge as cited by *The Physician and Sportsmedicine* 19 (1991): 49.
30. A. Z. LaCroix and coauthors, Maintaining mobility in late life: Smoking, alcohol consumption, physical activity, and body mass index, *American Journal of Epidemiology* 137 (1993): 858–869; Breslow and Breslow, 1993.
31. Fiatarone and coauthors, 1990; D. E. Danforth and coauthors, Report on the fourth conference for federally supported human nutrition research units and centers, *American Journal of Clinical Nutrition* 54 (1991): 164–168; M. Whitehurst and E. Menendez, Endurance training in older women, *The Physician and Sportsmedicine* 19 (1991): 95–102.
32. J. Posner, M. D., professor of medicine and chief of the divisions of Geriatric Medicine at the Medical College of Pennsylvania in Philadelphia, as cited in C. L. Pollock, Breaking the risk of falls, *The Physician and Sports Medicine* 20 (1992): 146–156.
33. M. A. Fiatarone and coauthors, Exercise training and nutritional supplementation for physical frailty in very elderly people, *New England Journal of Medicine* 330 (1994): 1769–1775; W. W. Campbell and coauthors, Increased energy requirements and changes in body composition with resistance training in older adults, *American Journal of Clinical Nutrition* 60 (1994): 167–175.
34. D. E. Butterworth and coauthors, Exercise training and nutrient intake in elderly women, *Journal of the American Dietetic Association* 93 (1993): 653–657.
35. P. Astrand, Physical activity and fitness, *American Journal of Clinical Nutrition* (supplement) 55 (1992): 1231–1236.
36. P. J. Nestel, Dietary fat for the elderly: What are the issues? in *Nutrition of the Elderly*, eds. H. Munro and G. Schlierf (New York: Raven Press, 1992), pp. 119–127.
37. V. Holt, J. Nordstrom, and M. B. Kohrs, Food preferences of older adults, *Journal of Nutrition for the Elderly* 6 (1987): 47.
38. J. G. Fischer and coauthors, Dairy product intake of the oldest old, *Journal of the American Dietetic Association* 95 (1995): 918–921.
39. Processing of dietary retinoids is slowed in the elderly, *Nutrition Reviews* 49 (1991): 116–119.
40. Russell and Suter, 1993.
41. Russell and Suter, 1993.
42. A. R. Webb and coauthors, An evaluation of the relative contributions of exposure to sunlight and of diet to the circulating concentrations of 25-hydroxyvitamin D in an elderly nursing home population in Boston, *American Journal of Clinical Nutrition* 51 (1990): 1075–1081.
43. Russell and Suter, 1993.
44. Russell and Suter, 1993.
45. C. A. Swanson and coauthors, Zinc status of elderly adults: Response to supplement, *American Journal of Clinical Nutrition* 48 (1988): 343–349.
46. G. J. Fosmire, Trace mineral requirements, in *Geriatric Nutrition: The Health Professional's Handbook*, ed. R. Chernoff (Gaithersburg, Md.: Aspen Publishers, 1991), pp. 77–105.
47. D. V. Porter, Washington update: NIH consensus development conference statement optimal calcium intake, *Nutrition Today*, September/October 1994, pp. 37–40.
48. Committee on Dietary Allowances, *Recommended Dietary Allowances*, 10th ed.(Washington, D.C.: National Academy Press, 1989), pp. 174–184.
49. A. A. Abbase and D. Rudman, Undernutrition in the nursing home: Prevalence, consequences, causes and prevention, *Nutrition Reviews* 52 (1994): 113–122.
50. W. A. McIntosh and coauthors, The relationship between beliefs about nutrition and dietary practices of the elderly, *Journal of the American Dietetic Association* 90 (1990): 671–675; H. Payette and K. Gray-Donald, Do vitamin and mineral supplements improve the dietary intake of elderly Canadians? *Canadian Journal of Public Health* 82 (1993): 58–60.
51. G. E. Bunce, J. Kinoshita, and J. Horwitz, Nutritional factors in cataract, *Annual Review of Nutrition* 10 (1990): 233–254.
52. Bunce, Kinoshita, and Horwitz, 1990; S. D. Varma, Scientific basis for medical therapy of cataracts by antioxidants, *American Journal of Clinical Nutrition* 53 (1991): 335S–345S.
53. P. F. Jacques and L. T. Chylack, Epidemiologic evidence of a role for the antioxidant vitamins and carotenoids in cataract prevention, *American Journal of Clinical Nutrition* 53 (1991): 352S–355S; G. E. Bunce, Antioxidant nutrition and cataract in women: A prospective study, *Nutrition Reviews* 51 (1993): 84–86.
54. J. M. Robertson, A. P. Donner, and J. R. Trevithick, A possible role for vitamins C and E in cataract prevention, *American Journal of Clinical Nutrition* 53 (1991): 346S–351S.
55. E. D. Harris, Rheumatoid arthritis: Pathophysiology and implications for therapy, *New England Journal of Medicine* 322

(1990): 1277–1289.

56. R. S. Panush, Nutritional therapy for rheumatic diseases, *Annals of Internal Medicine* 106 (1987): 619–621.
57. J. M. Kremer and coauthors, Fish-oil fatty acid supplementation in active rheumatoid arthritis: A double-blind, controlled crossover study, *Annals of Internal Medicine* 106 (1987): 497–503.
58. P. Merry and coauthors, Oxidative damage to lipids within the inflamed human joint provides evidence of radical-mediated hypoxic-reperfusion injury, *American Journal of Clinical Nutrition* 53 (1991): 362S–369S.
59. R. Roubenoff and coauthors, Catabolic effects of high-dose corticosteroids persist despite therapeutic benefit in rheumatoid arthritis, *American Journal of Clinical Nutrition* 52 (1990): 1113–1117.
60. R. N. Butler, Senile dementia of the Alzheimer type (SDAT), in *The Merck Manual of Geriatrics* (Rahway, NJ: Merck & Co., Inc., 1990), pp. 933–938.
61. Are older Americans making better food choices to meet diet and health recommendations? *Nutrition Reviews* 51 (1993): 20–22.
62. Position of The American Dietetic Association: Nutrition, aging, and the continuum of health care, *Journal of the American Dietetic Association* 93 (1993): 80–82.
63. J. Dwyer and coauthors, Screening older Americans' nutritional health: Future possibilities, *Nutrition Today*, September/October 1991, pp. 21–24.
64. M. B. Moran and E. Reed, Are congregate meals meeting clients' needs for "heart healthy" menus? *Journal of Nutrition for the Elderly* 13 (1993): 3–10.

Nutrient-Drug Interactions

People over the age of 65 take about 25 percent of all the over-the-counter and prescription drugs sold in the United States. They often go to different doctors for different conditions and receive different prescriptions from each. The drugs prescribed enable many older adults to enjoy long, healthy lives, but they also bring side effects and risks.

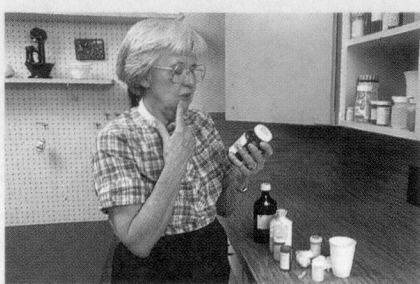

Taking several drugs over long periods intensifies the risk of nutrient-drug interactions.

THE ACTIONS OF DRUGS

Most people think of drugs either as medicines that help them recover from illnesses or as illegal substances that lead to bodily harm and addiction. Actually, both uses of the term *drug* are correct because any substance that modifies one or more of the body's functions is, technically, a drug. Even when people use medical drugs, the drugs set in motion not only desirable, but also undesirable, events within the body.

Consider aspirin. One action of aspirin is to retard the production of certain prostaglandins. Some prostaglandins help to produce fevers, some sensitize pain receptors, some cause contractions of the uterus, some stimulate digestive tract motility, some control nerve impulses, some regulate blood pressure, some promote blood clotting, and some cause inflammation. By interfering with prostaglandin actions, aspirin reduces fever and inflammation, relieves pain, and slows blood clotting, among other things.

A person cannot use aspirin to produce one of its effects without producing all of its other effects. Someone who is prone to strokes and heart attacks might take aspirin to prevent blood clotting, but it would also dull that person's sense of pain. In another person who took aspirin only for pain, it would also slow blood clotting. For the second person, the anticlotting effect might be dangerous because it might cause abnormal bleeding. A single two-tablet dose of aspirin doubles the bleeding time of wounds, an effect that lasts from four to seven hours. For this reason, physicians caution clients to refrain from taking aspirin before surgery.

This discussion focuses on some of the nutrition-related consequences of medical drugs, both prescription drugs and nonprescription, or over-the-counter, drugs. (Highlight 7 described the relationships between nutrition and the drug alcohol.)

THE INTERACTIONS BETWEEN DRUGS AND NUTRIENTS

Hundreds of medical drugs interact with nutrients. The possibility of nutrient imbalances arises whenever a person takes drugs. Drugs can profoundly affect nutrition status, and conversely, nutrition status and nutrients can profoundly affect the body's responses to drugs. When the intestinal cells of a malnourished person atrophy, for instance, drug absorption diminishes. If the liver produces too few protein carriers for substances in the blood, then some drugs may not reach their sites of action or may not be transported back to the liver and kidneys for detoxification and excretion. In the latter case, the drugs may remain active too long, intensifying side effects.

Drug-nutrient interactions sometimes pose no significant problems. Adverse interactions are most likely in elderly people, especially those with serious illnesses that raise nutrient needs, for these people are most likely to be in poor nutrition status, to suffer chronic disorders, to use many drugs, and to take them over long periods.

Nutrients and drugs may interact in many ways:

- Drugs can alter food intake and the absorption, metabolism, and excretion of nutrients.
- Foods and nutrients can alter the absorption, metabolism, and excretion of drugs.

Table H17–1 summarizes the mechanisms by which these interactions occur and provides specific examples. The following sections describe these interactions in more detail.

DRUGS AND FOOD INTAKE

Many drugs can lead to malnutrition by interfering with food intake. Drugs can influence appetite, alter

Table H17–1

Mechanisms and Examples of Food-Drug Interactions

Drugs Can Alter Food Intake by:	
• Altering the appetite (amphetamines suppress the appetite). • Interfering with taste or smell (methotrexate changes taste sensations). • Inducing nausea or vomiting (digitalis can do both). • Changing the oral environment (phenobarbital can cause dry mouth). • Irritating the GI tract (cyclophosphamide induces mucosal ulcers). • Causing sores or inflammation of the mouth (methotrexate can cause painful mouth ulcers to form).	
Drugs Can Alter Nutrition Absorption by:	**Foods Can Alter Drug Absorption by:**
• Changing the acidity of the digestive tract (antacids can interfere with iron absorption). • Altering digestive juices (cimetidine can improve fat absorption). • Altering motility of the digestive tract (laxatives speed motility, causing the malabsorption of many nutrients). • Inactivating enzyme systems (neomycin may reduce lipase activity). • Damaging mucosal cells (chemotherapy can damage mucosal cells). • Binding to nutrients (antacids bind phosphorus).	• Changing the acidity of the digestive tract (candy can change the acidity, thus dissolving slow-acting asthma medication too quickly). • Stimulating secretion of digestive juices (griseofulvin is absorbed better when taken with foods that stimulate the release of digestive enzymes). • Delaying digestive processes (aspirin is absorbed more slowly when taken with food). • Binding to drugs (tetracycline binds to calcium in dairy foods, limiting drug absorption). • Competing for absorption sites in the intestines (dietary amino acids interfere with levodopa absorption this way).
Drugs Can Alter Nutrient Metabolism by:	**Foods Can Alter Drug Metabolism by:**
• Acting as structural analogs (as anticoagulants and vitamin K do). • Interfering with metabolic enzyme systems (phenobarbital competes for folate coenzymes).	• Interfering with a drug's action (phenobarbital action is limited by large amounts of folate in the diet). • Contributing pharmacologically active substances (tyramine from cheese remains active with monoamine oxidase inhibitors).
Drugs Can Alter Nutrient Excretion by:	**Foods Can Alter Drug Excretion by:**
• Altering reabsorption in the kidneys (some diuretics increase the excretion of sodium and potassium). • Displacing nutrients from their plasma protein carriers (aspirin displaces folate).	• Changing the acidity of the urine (vitamin C can alter urinary pH and limit the excretion of aspirin).

taste or smell, cause sores or irritation in the mouth, reduce the flow of saliva, or induce nausea or vomiting. Amphetamines used to treat hyperactivity in children provide an example of how drug side effects can interfere with food intake. Amphetamines may effectively improve behavior, but they also diminish appetite, alter taste perceptions, dry the mouth, and cause nausea.

Conversely, some drugs enhance food intake and lead to undesirable weight gain. An example is astemizole (Hismanal), an antihistamine used by some people to relieve allergy symptoms.

ABSORPTION AND DRUG-NUTRIENT INTERACTIONS

Foods can enhance, delay, or reduce drug absorption, and drugs can do the same thing to nutrient absorption. The interactions between the antibiotic tetracycline and the minerals calcium and iron are a classic example. People are advised not to take tetracycline with milk, milk products, or calcium-containing antacids, such as Tums. When calcium and tetracycline are taken at the same time, they bind to each other, thus reducing the absorption of both. Iron has a similar effect. Therefore, iron supplements should be taken two hours apart from tetracycline doses.

Another example of how foods can interfere with the absorption of a drug is the interaction between acidic foods and the nicotine gum that is sometimes prescribed to help people quit smoking cigarettes. The acidity from certain foods and beverages changes the chemical balance in the mouth, thus limiting nicotine absorption through the lining of the mouth into the blood.[1] This interference may help to explain why nicotine gum is successful in helping only about one-fourth of the people who use it to quit smoking. For maximum effectiveness, people should refrain from ingesting foods and beverages during or immediately after chewing nicotine gum, especially those listed in Table H17–2. This food-drug interaction has other side effects as well: a person may develop nausea and hiccups when the unabsorbed nicotine arrives in the stomach. Thus the combination of acidic foods and nicotine gum both interferes with the drug's effectiveness and creates uncomfortable side effects.

Conversely, foods can enhance the absorption of some drugs. For this reason, the antifungal drug griseofulvin is always given with meals. Similarly, some drugs can enhance the absorption of nutrients. Enzyme replacements, designed specifically to improve the absorption of proteins, carbohydrates, and fats, are an example.

Table H17–2

Foods and Beverages That Limit the Effectiveness of Nicotine Gum

- Apple juice.
- Beer.
- Catsup.
- Coffee.
- Colas.
- Grape juice.
- Lemon-lime soda.
- Mustard.
- Orange juice.
- Pineapple juice.
- Soy sauce.
- Tomato juice.

The ways foods and drugs influence absorption determine how drugs are administered. Drugs are absorbed rapidly when they are taken on an empty stomach; foods delay the rate at which the stomach empties. An aspirin given on an empty stomach, for example, works faster than when it is given with food. But aspirin can irritate the stomach to such an extent that repeated over time it can cause iron-deficiency anemia by inducing bleeding in the GI tract. The presence of food can minimize this irritation. As a guideline, then, if rapid action is not essential, take food with aspirin or other drugs that irritate the GI tract to help reduce nausea and protect the GI lining.

METABOLISM AND DRUG-NUTRIENT INTERACTIONS

Foods can affect drug metabolism in two basic ways: first, nutrients can change the way the body uses a drug, and second, substances in foods can alter the drug's action. To appreciate the way that nutrients can change the body's use of a drug, consider the interactions between vitamin K and the anticlotting medication warfarin (Coumadin). Warfarin works by interfering with vitamin K's clot-promoting action. The drug's effectiveness depends on maintaining a balance between the dosage and a consistent vitamin K intake. If a person's vitamin K intake increases, the warfarin's effectiveness diminishes. If the person wishes to continue eating many foods high in vitamin K, then the physician has to increase the drug dose.

An example of a substance in foods that alters a drug's action is tyramine, which interacts with monoamine oxidase (MAO) inhibitors, drugs that physicians sometimes prescribe to treat some forms of severe depression. MAO inhibitors block the action of the enzyme monoamine oxidase. Normally, monoamine oxidase converts tyramine, a substance found in some foods (see Table H17–3), into an inactive form. When people take the inhibitors, tyramine remains active and stimulates the release of norepinephrine. This action can lead to severe hypertension and headaches. If blood pressure rises high enough, it can be fatal. For this reason, people taking MAO inhibitors must restrict their intakes of foods rich in tyramine.

Drugs that are similar in structure to vitamins can displace vitamins from enzymes or other cell constituents and interfere with normal metabolism. Many drugs used to treat cancer are of this type. Cancer cells, like normal cells, need real vitamins to multiply. When the vitamins are not available, cancer cells die. Unfortunately, other grow-

Table H17–3

Foods Restricted in a Tyramine-Controlled Diet

Beverages	Chianti, sherry, sauterne, champagne, imported beer, nonalcoholic beer, ale[a]
Cheeses	Aged cheeses, American, camembert, cheddar, gouda, gruyère, mozzarella, parmesan, provolone, romano, roquefort, stilton;[b] cheese-filled breads, crackers, and desserts
Meats	Liver; dried, salted, smoked, or pickled fish; meat processed with tenderizers; sausage, pepperoni; dried meats; meat extracts
Vegetables	Fava beans; Italian broad beans; sauerkraut; fermented pickles and olives
Other	Brewer's yeast; monosodium glutamate; all aged and fermented products; caffeine and chocolate in large amounts

Note: The tyramine contents of foods vary from product to product depending on the methods used to prepare, process, and store the food. The amount of tyramine a person consumes depends on the quantity of the food eaten. In some cases, as little as 1 ounce of cheese can cause a severe hypertensive reaction in people taking monoamine oxidase inhibitors. The items listed in this table contain significant enough quantities of tyramine that they are not allowed. In general, the following foods contain small enough amounts of tyramine that they can be consumed in small quantities: ripe avocado, banana, yogurt, sour cream, acidophilus milk, buttermilk, raspberries, and peanuts.

[a]Most wine and domestic beer can be consumed in small quantities.

[b]Unfermented cheeses, such as ricotta, cottage cheese, and cream cheese, are allowed.

ing cells in the body also need vitamins, and so vitamin deficiencies develop. Both methotrexate, used to treat cancer and psoriasis, and pyrimethamine, used to prevent malaria, are structurally similar to the B vitamin folate and can cause severe folate deficiency (see Figure H17–1 on p. 644).

Aspirin can also alter vitamin metabolism. Aspirin competes with folate for its protein carrier, thus interfering with the body's use of the vitamin.

EXCRETION AND DRUG-NUTRIENT INTERACTIONS

The acidity of the urine affects the relative extents to which some drugs are excreted by the kidneys or retained in the body. For example, a low urinary pH limits the excretion of acidic drugs like aspirin. Some nutrients, such as vitamin C, can lower the pH of urine, making it more acidic. Therefore, when large doses of vitamin C are given with aspirin, aspirin remains in the blood longer.

Drugs can also alter the excretion of nutrients. For example, some diuretics and laxatives speed up the excretion of calcium, potassium, magnesium, and zinc. Drugs can also interfere with nutrient excretion by displacing nutrients from their blood protein carriers. As mentioned, aspirin displaces folate from its carrier protein and so accelerates the vitamin's excretion. When folate is bound to the larger protein, it is not filtered by the kidneys; in contrast, the smaller unbound vitamin is readily excreted.

THE HEALTH PROFESSIONAL AND DRUG-NUTRIENT INTERACTIONS

Hundreds of drug-nutrient interactions have been identified, and information continues to accumulate. It would be difficult, if not impossible, to remember and apply all of this information.

Instead, health care professionals would serve their clients well to:[2]

- Keep in mind that drug-nutrient interactions can and do occur, especially when drug use is long term.
- Review drug and diet histories with potential interactions in mind.
- Be aware of groups of people who are likely to develop nutrient deficiencies and assess their nutrition status frequently.
- Provide appropriate foods or supplements to prevent or correct nutrient problems.
- Become familiar with the nutrient interactions of drugs commonly used to treat the disorders of their clients.
- Be prepared to look up the nutrition effects of drugs that clients are taking.

Health care professionals can play a significant role in limiting potentially harmful drug-nutrient interactions. One study, in a hospital with an established drug-nutrient interaction policy, found clinically significant drug-nutrient interactions in only 2 of 493 cases that were reviewed.[3] The researchers attributed the low incidence of interactions to the policy, which guided health care professionals to prevent, recognize, and treat the most common and clinically significant interactions before problems developed.

Nutrient interactions and risks

Figure H17–1

Two Antivitamins

Methotrexate (an antineoplastic drug) and pyrimethamine (an antimalaria drug) are structurally similar to the vitamin folate. When these drugs are used, they compete for the enzyme that normally activates folate, creating a secondary deficiency of folate. Interestingly, folate deficiency protects against malaria by limiting the parasites' ability to double their DNA and divide.

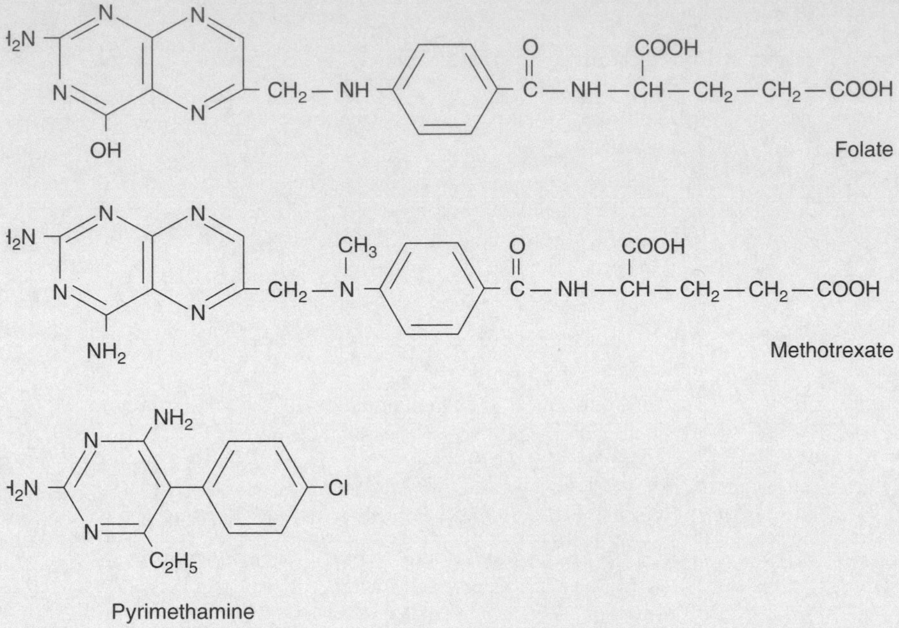

are not unique to prescription drugs. People who buy over-the-counter drugs also need to protect themselves. About 300,000 nonprescription drug products are marketed in the United States; more than 400 of these were available only by prescription 15 years ago.[4] The increasing availability of over-the-counter drugs allows people to treat themselves for many ailments from arthritis to yeast infections. Many older adults take over-the-counter laxatives and antacids regularly. Excessive use of either of these drugs may impair nutrition status by interfering with absorption, increasing excretion, or both. Consumers need to ask their physicians about potential interactions and check with their pharmacists for instructions on taking drugs with foods. Should problems arise, they should seek professional care without delay.

NOTES

1. J. E. Henningfield and coauthors, Drinking coffee and carbonated beverages blocks absorption of nicotine from nicotine polacrilex gum, *Journal of the American Medical Association* 264 (1990): 1560–1564.
2. R. N. Varma, Risk for drug-induced malnutrition is unchecked in elderly patients in nursing homes, *Journal of the American Dietetic Association* 94 (1994): 192–194.
3. V. L. Franse, N. Stark, and T. Powers, Drug-nutrient interactions in a Veterans Administration medical center teaching hospital, *Nutrition in Clinical Practice* 3 (1988): 145–147.
4. Nonprescription Drug Manufacturers Association, *Facts and Figures* (Washington, D.C.: Nonprescription Drug Manufacturers Association, 1993).

Chapter 18

Diet and Health

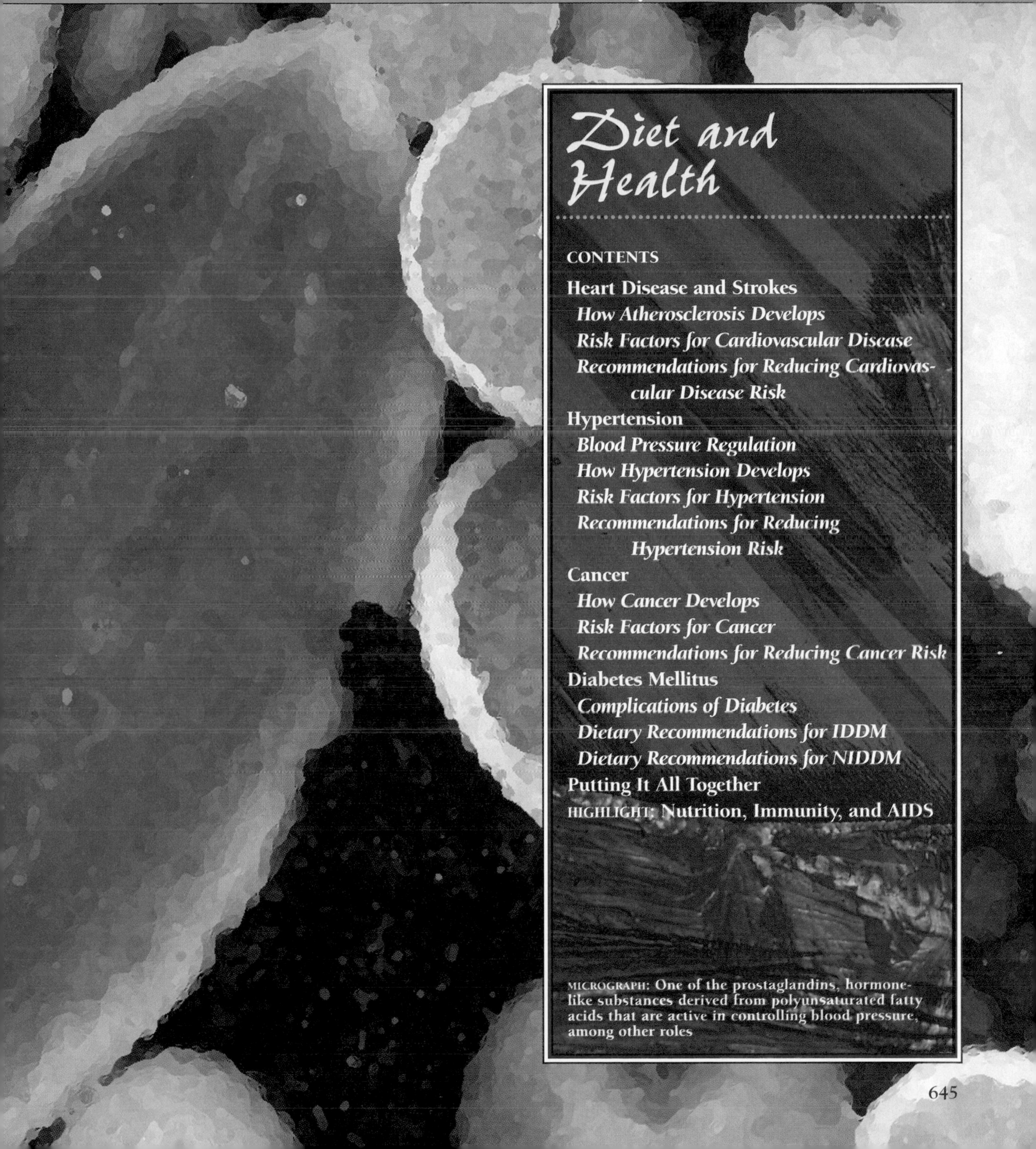

CONTENTS

MICROGRAPH: One of the prostaglandins, hormone-like substances derived from polyunsaturated fatty acids that are active in controlling blood pressure, among other roles

A century ago our ancestors feared infectious and communicable diseases such as smallpox—diseases that claimed many children's lives and limited the average life expectancy of adults. Today far fewer infectious diseases threaten us, thanks to medical science's ability to identify disease-causing microorganisms and develop vaccines. In developed nations, purification of water prevents the spread of infection, and immunizations protect individuals. Most people live well into their later years, and today's average life expectancy far exceeds that of our ancestors.

Still, some infectious diseases threaten many lives despite public health measures and medical treatments. Perhaps the most infamous is AIDS (acquired immune deficiency syndrome). AIDS develops from infection by the human immunodeficiency virus (HIV), which attacks the immune system and disables the body's defenses against other diseases. Then these diseases, which would produce only mild, if any, illness in people with healthy immune systems, destroy health and life. The highlight that follows this chapter describes the immune system and the nutrition-related problems of people with HIV infections.

Although some infectious diseases remain serious threats in developed countries, most of the diseases that threaten life develop as a result of metabolic abnormalities induced by such factors as genetics, age, sex, lifestyle, and environment. Diet is among the many lifestyle factors that influence the risks of developing chronic diseases, and dietary factors that advance or prevent the progression of chronic diseases are the primary focus of this chapter.

Table 18–1 lists the ten leading causes of death in the United States.[1] Four of these causes, including the top three, have some relationship with diet. Taken together, these four conditions account for two-thirds of the nation's 2 million deaths each year.

Table 18–1

Ten Leading Causes of Death in the United States

1. **Heart disease.**
2. **Cancers.**
3. **Strokes.**
4. Chronic obstructive lung disease.
5. Unintentional injuries.
6. Pneumonia and influenza.
7. **Diabetes mellitus.**
8. HIV infection.
9. Suicide.
10. Homicide.

Note: The diseases in bold type have relationships with diet.

This chapter explains how each of these four chronic diseases develops and summarizes their major links with nutrition. Earlier chapters described individual nutrients' connections with diseases and may have left the mistaken impression of "one disease–one nutrient" relationships.[2] Indeed, valid links do exist between fiber and diabetes, fat and heart disease, calcium and osteoporosis, and antioxidant vitamins and cancer, but to focus just on these links oversimplifies the story. In reality, each nutrient may have connections with several diseases because its role in the body is not specific to a disease, but to a body function. Fiber—because it binds substances in the GI tract—helps prevent both diabetes and cancer. Vitamin C—because it acts as an antioxidant—helps prevent both cancer and heart disease. Furthermore, each of the chronic diseases develops in response to multiple factors—including many nondietary factors such as genetics, physical activity, and smoking. An integrated and balanced approach to disease prevention therefore includes attention to all of the many factors involved. Figure 18–1 illustrates some of the relationships between risk factors and degenerative diseases.

Reminder: Factors that are associated with a high incidence of a disease are *risk factors*. Some risk factors, such as diet and physical activity, are *modifiable*, meaning that they can be changed; others, such as genetics, age, and sex, cannot be changed.

synergistic: multiple factors operating together in such a way that their combined effects are greater than the sum of their individual effects.

Notice how many of the diseases have a genetic component. A family history of a certain disease is a powerful indicator of a person's tendency to contract that disease. Still, environmental factors are often pivotal in determining whether that tendency will be expressed. Genetics and environmental factors often work synergistically; for instance, cigarette smoking is especially likely to bring on heart disease in people who are predisposed to develop it.

Degenerative Diseases	Diet Risk Factors: High fat diet	Excessive alcohol intake	Low complex carbohydrate/fiber intake	Low vitamin and/or mineral intake	High sugar intake	High intake of salty or pickled foods	Other Risk Factors: Genetics	Age	Sedentary lifestyle	Smoking and tobacco use	Stress	Environmental contaminants
Cancers	✔	✔	✔	✔		✔	✔	✔	✔	✔		✔
Hypertension	✔	✔		✔		✔	✔	✔	✔	✔	✔	
Diabetes (NIDDM)	✔		✔				✔	✔	✔			
Osteoporosis		✔		✔			✔	✔	✔	✔		
Atherosclerosis	✔	✔	✔	✔			✔	✔	✔	✔	✔	
Obesity	✔	✔	✔		✔		✔		✔			
Stroke	✔	✔	✔				✔	✔		✔	✔	
Diverticulosis	✔		✔	✔				✔	✔			
Dental and oral disease				✔	✔		✔			✔		

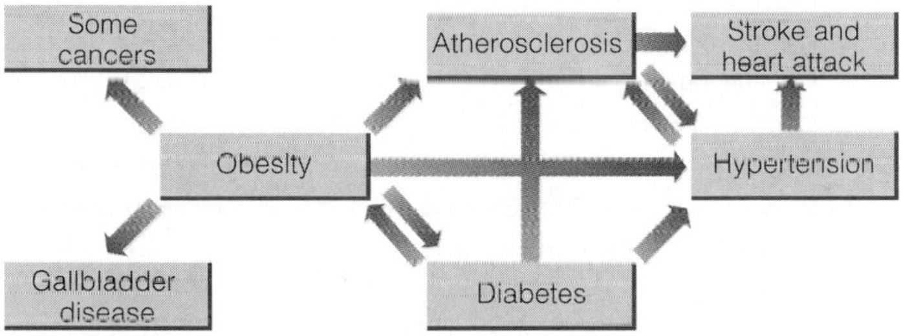

Figure 18–1

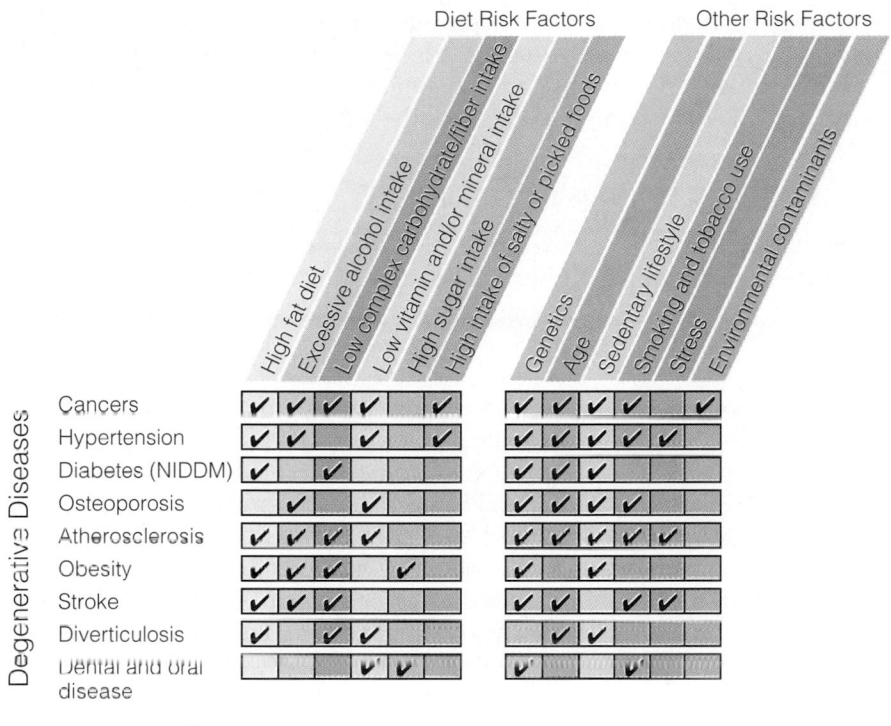

Diet/Lifestyle Risk Factors and Degenerative Diseases

The chart at the top shows that the same risk factor can affect many chronic diseases. Notice, for example, how many diseases have been linked to a high-fat diet. The chart also shows that a particular disease, such as atherosclerosis, may have several risk factors.

The flow chart at the bottom shows that many of these conditions are themselves risk factors for other chronic diseases. For example, a person with diabetes is likely to develop atherosclerosis and hypertension. These two conditions, in turn, worsen each other. Notice how all of these diseases are linked to obesity.

Heart Disease and Strokes

Diseases of the heart and blood vessels, collectively known as cardiovascular diseases, are the leading single cause of death around the world today.[3] In the United States, death rates from cardiovascular diseases in young men (35 to 40 years old) are three times greater than in young women, but in later years (65 to 74), the incidence is similar. The consequences of cardiovascular disease are usually heart disease and strokes, the first and third leading causes of death for adults, respectively.[4]

Reminder: *Cardiovascular disease (CVD)* is a general term for all diseases of the heart and blood vessels.

HEALTHY PEOPLE 2000: Reduce coronary heart disease deaths to no more than 100 per 100,000 people.

Reminder: *Coronary heart disease (CHD)* describes the damage that occurs when the blood vessels carrying blood to the heart become narrow and occluded. The narrowing is usually caused by *atherosclerosis*, a condition characterized by plaques along the inner walls of the arteries. *Hypertension* is high blood pressure.

plaques (PLACKS): mounds of lipid material, mixed with smooth muscle cells and calcium, which develop in the artery walls in atherosclerosis. This type of plaque is known as **atheromatous plaque**.
placken = patch or plate

Coronary heart disease (CHD) is the most common form of cardiovascular disease and usually involves both atherosclerosis and hypertension. Atherosclerosis is the accumulation of lipids and other materials in the arteries, and hypertension is high blood pressure. Each makes the other worse.

HOW ATHEROSCLEROSIS DEVELOPS

As Highlight 16 pointed out, no one is free of the fatty streaks that may one day become the fibrous plaques of atherosclerosis. For most adults, the question is not whether you have them, but how far advanced they are and what you can do to retard or reverse their progression.

Plaques Develop Atherosclerosis usually begins with the accumulation of soft fatty streaks along the inner arterial walls, especially at branch points (see Figure H16–1 on p. 611). These fatty streaks gradually enlarge and become hardened with minerals, forming plaques. Plaques stiffen the arteries and narrow the passages through them. Most people have well-developed plaques by the age of 30. The progression of atherosclerosis in the coronary arteries may restrict blood flow to the heart muscle and limit the delivery of oxygen. As Chapter 5 pointed out, a diet high in saturated fat is a major contributor to the development of atherosclerosis.[5]

Blood Pressure Rises Normally, the arteries expand with each heartbeat to accommodate the pulses of blood that flow through them. Arteries stiffened and narrowed by plaques cannot expand, and so each pulse raises the blood pressure instead. This damages the artery walls further, and plaques are especially likely to form at damage points; thus the development of atherosclerosis is a self-accelerating process. As the arteries harden, blood flows less freely through the kidneys; then the kidneys respond by raising the blood pressure further, and the high blood pressure strains the heart.

platelets: tiny, disc-shaped bodies in the blood, important in blood clot formation.

Blood Clots Form Small, cell-like bodies in the blood, known as platelets, cause clots to form whenever they encounter injuries in blood vessels. Clots normally form and dissolve in the blood all the time. When the clot-forming and clot-dissolving processes are balanced, the clots do not harm, but in atherosclerosis, platelets respond to plaques as they normally do to injuries: they form clots, and the clots form faster than they dissolve.

Reminder: *Eicosanoids* are hormonelike compounds that help regulate many of the body's functions including blood pressure, clot formation, lipid concentrations, and the immune response.

prostaglandins (PROS-tah-GLAND-ins): eicosanoid compounds with a multitude of diverse effects on the body, including contraction of blood vessels, transmission of nerve impulses, immune assistance, and hormone responses.

thromboxanes: eicosanoid compounds with effects on the blood-clotting system.

The action of platelets is under the control of certain eicosanoids, known as prostaglandins and thromboxanes. Various eicosanoids can be made from the omega-6 and omega-3 fatty acids. Platelets are less likely to form clots when omega-3 fatty acids are abundant in the diet because the same enzymes are needed to convert both omega-3 and omega-6 fatty acids to eicosanoids. With omega-3 fatty acids abundant, the omega-6 fatty acids have less access to the needed enzymes, fewer omega-6 eicosanoids are made, and fewer clots are formed.

Abnormal blood clotting can trigger life-threatening events. A clot, once formed, may stick to a plaque in an artery and gradually enlarge until it shuts off the blood supply to the portion of the tissue supplied by that artery. The tissue may die slowly and give way to scar tissue. The blood clot, called a thrombus, may grow large enough to close off a blood vessel. Coronary thrombosis is the blockage of a vessel that feeds the heart muscle. Cerebral thrombosis is the blockage of a vessel that feeds the brain.

A clot can also break loose, becoming an embolus, and travel along the system until it reaches an artery too small to allow its passage. Then the tissues fed by this artery will be robbed of oxygen and nutrients and will die suddenly. Such a clot lodged in an artery of the heart causes sudden death of part of the heart muscle—a heart attack. When the clot lodges in an artery of the brain, it kills a portion of the brain tissue—a stroke.

thrombus: a blood clot that may obstruct a blood vessel or the heart cavity. The formation or development of a thrombus is called a **thrombosis.**
thrombo = clot

embolus (EM-boh-luss): a thrombus or other material that breaks loose from accumulated matter in the circulatory system and travels through the system. The obstruction of a blood vessel by an embolus is called an **embolism.**
embol = to insert, plug

RISK FACTORS FOR CARDIOVASCULAR DISEASE

The margin lists the major risk factors for heart disease.[6] Organizations such as the American Heart Association name other risk factors as well—notably, obesity and physical inactivity. The expert panel that prepared the list presented here does not consider obesity and lack of physical activity to be *independent* risk factors, but rather factors that significantly modify the major risk factors. Both obesity and physical inactivity contribute to high LDL cholesterol, low HDL cholesterol, hypertension, and diabetes.[7] The criteria for defining blood lipids, blood pressure, and obesity in relation to CHD risk are shown in Table 18–2 (on p. 650).

Most middle-aged and older adults have at least one risk factor, and many have more than one.[8] Such findings have prompted campaigns in both the United States and Canada to screen adults for risk factors. These programs identify individuals at high risk and use a population approach to prevention. Such public health programs are proving successful: since 1960, both blood cholesterol levels and deaths from cardiovascular disease among U.S. adults have shown a continuous and substantial downward trend.[9] These trends reflect behavior changes in individuals. As adults grow older, many of them stop smoking and drinking alcohol and start following a low-fat diet or taking medication in an effort to improve their cardiovascular health.[10]

Major risk factors for CHD:
- **High LDL cholesterol.**
- Male, 45 years or older.
- Female, 55 years or older, or with premature menopause and not on estrogen replacement therapy.
- **Low HDL cholesterol.** (Subtract 1 risk factor if HDL cholesterol ≥60 mg/dL.)
- **Hypertension.**
- Smoking.
- **Diabetes mellitus.**
- Family history of heart attacks or sudden death prior to age 55 in a male parent or sibling or prior to age 65 in a female parent or sibling.

Note: Risk factors in bold type have relationships with diet.

Reminder: The *population approach* to diet advice aims to lower disease risks among all people through population-wide changes in eating patterns. The *individual approach* aims to identify and treat only people who are at the greatest risk of disease development. Chapter 1 provides more explanation.

It befits a nutrition book to focus on dietary strategies to prevent heart disease, but it should be noted that diet is not itself a major risk factor. Four of the eight major risk factors, however, can be modified by diet or weight loss: high LDL cholesterol, low HDL cholesterol, hypertension, and diabetes. Three cannot be modified by diet or otherwise: sex, age, and family history. The other major risk factor—smoking—is, of course, modifiable, and may indeed be the most influential. As appealing as the solution may sound, diet may not reduce the risk of heart disease and stroke as successfully as other interventions do. Quitting smoking and taking prescribed medicines to lower blood lipids or blood pressure, for example, may be far more effective than dietary changes alone. Dietary changes can be effective, however, especially when combined with other strategies, such as quitting smoking and being physically active. These three strategies—dietary changes, quitting smoking, and physical activity—are always recommended before drug therapy.

High LDL Cholesterol, Low HDL Cholesterol The blood cholesterol linked to atherosclerosis risk is LDL cholesterol. HDL also carry cholesterol, but raised HDL represent cholesterol returning from the arteries to the liver and thus indicate a reduced risk of atherosclerosis and heart attack (see Figure 18–2).

Reminder: Cholesterol is carried in several lipoproteins, chief among them LDL and HDL (see Chapter 5 for details). Remember them this way:
- LDL = Low-density lipoproteins = Less healthy.
- HDL = High-density lipoproteins = Healthy.

Figure 18–2

HDL and LDL Compared

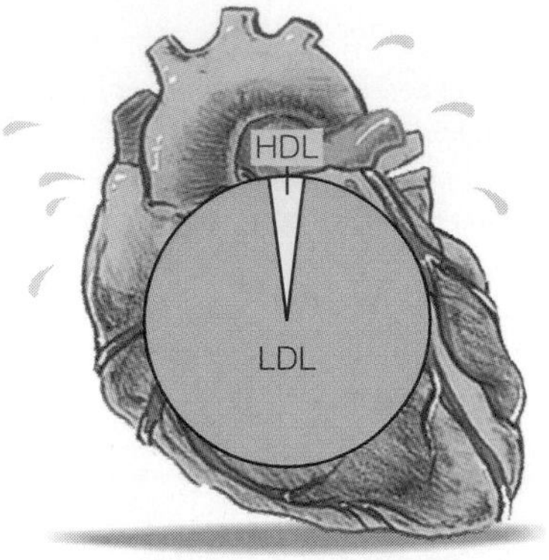

Low HDL relative to **LDL**
Increased risk of heart attack

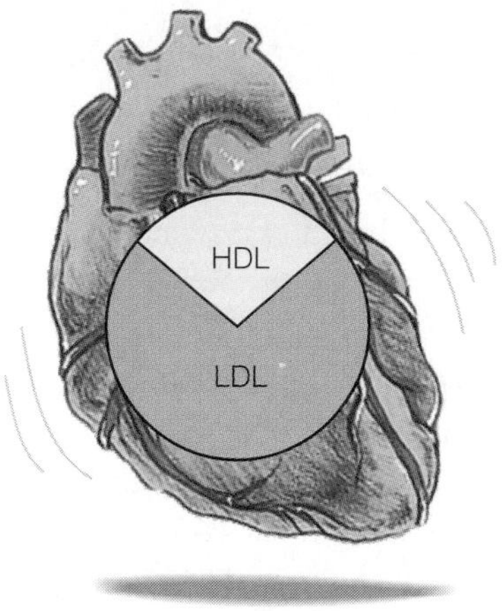

High HDL relative to **LDL**
Decreased risk of heart attack

Table 18–2

Standards for CHD Risk Factors

LDL Cholesterol	Total Cholesterol[b]
<130 mg/dL = desirable.[a] 130–159 mg/dL = borderline high. ≥160 mg/dL = high.	<200 mg/dL = desirable. 200–239 mg/dL = borderline high. ≥240 mg/dL = high.
HDL Cholesterol	**Triglycerides (Fasting)[d]**
HDL: ≤35 mg/dL indicates risk.[c] LDL-to-HDL ratio:[f] Men: >5.0 indicates risk. Women: >4.5 indicates risk.	<200 mg/dL = desirable. 200–400 mg/dL = borderline high. 400–1000 mg/dL = high. >1000 mg/dL = very high.
Hypertension	**Obesity**
Diastolic pressure:[e] <85 = normal. 80–89 = high-normal. 90–99 = mild. 100–109 = moderate. 110–119 = severe. >120 = very severe.	Body mass index: Men: >27.8. Women: >27.3.

[a] For people with existing CHD, desirable LDL cholesterol values are lower (≤100 mg/dL).

[b] To convert cholesterol (mg/dL) to standard international units (mmol/L), multiply by 0.02586.

[c] This HDL value may be too low for women; no alternative value has yet been proposed. NIH Consensus Development Panel on Triglyceride, High-Density Lipoprotein, and Coronary Heart Disease, Triglyceride, high-density lipoprotein, and coronary heart disease, *Journal of the American Medical Association* 269 (1993): 505–510.

[d] High triglycerides alone normally do not indicate *direct* risk, but may reflect lipoprotein abnormalities associated with CHD. The risk of CHD increases as triglyceride levels increase in people with other risk factors. High triglycerides also occur in conditions such as kidney disease and diabetes, which suggest a high CHD risk.

[e] Diastolic pressure is the lower of the numbers in the blood pressure reading—for example, the 70 in 105/70.

[f] The LDL-to-HDL ratio compares the concentration of LDL to that of HDL. A ratio of 5.0 really means "5 to 1," or that the first value (in this case LDL) is 5 times greater than the second (HDL). Similarly, a ratio of 4.5 means that LDL is 4.5 times greater than HDL.

Source: Blood lipid standards adapted from The Expert Panel, Summary of the second report of the National Cholesterol Education Program (NCEP), Expert Panel on Detection, Evaluation, and Treatment of High Blood Cholesterol in Adults (Adult Treatment Panel), *Journal of the American Medical Association* 269 (1993): 3015–3023; hypertension standards adapted from the Fifth Report of the Joint National Committee on Detection, Evaluation, and Treatment of High Blood Pressure, National High Blood Pressure Education Program, National Heart, Lung, and Blood Institute, National Institutes of Health, October 30, 1992, p. 5.

Research confirms that high LDL correlate *directly* with heart disease, whereas high HDL correlate *inversely* with risk.[11] In general, the higher the LDL cholesterol the greater the risk of CHD (review Table 18–2 on p. 650).

To a lesser extent, other blood lipids have also been linked to CHD. Triglycerides, mostly concentrated in VLDL, are elevated in some people with CHD, especially in those with diabetes and those who are overweight. Yet other people with high triglycerides and VLDL do not appear to have a high risk of heart disease. Elevated triglycerides are also associated with a high fasting blood glucose and low HDL.[12] Further studies are needed to determine whether triglycerides directly increase heart disease risk.[13]

Male, 45 Years or Older In general, men have higher blood cholesterol and a greater risk of CHD at an earlier age than women. Their blood cholesterol early in adulthood strongly correlates with their risk of developing heart disease later in life.[14] Almost half of all deaths from CHD occur among men with blood cholesterol in the borderline-high range.

Female, 55 Years or Older Cardiovascular disease seems to occur about 10 to 12 years later in women than in men.[15] Women younger than 45 tend to have lower LDL cholesterol than men of the same age, but a woman's blood cholesterol typically begins to rise between ages 45 and 55. Independently of age, a lack of estrogen influences blood cholesterol: at menopause, LDL tend to rise and HDL to decline, so that women's LDL cholesterol becomes greater than men's for the first time. About one-third of the women in the United States have LDL cholesterol high enough to pose a serious risk of heart disease.[16] Estrogen replacement therapy after menopause and regular physical activity reduce CHD risks in older women by lowering LDL and raising HDL. Estrogen replacement therapy increases the risk of some cancers, however, so a woman must carefully consider her health history when balancing the apparent benefits against the potential risks of such treatment.[17]

Estrogen replacement therapy:
- Alleviates menopausal symptoms.
- Reduces CHD risks.
- Reduces osteoporosis risks.
- Increases cancer risks.

Hypertension Chronic high blood pressure frequently accompanies cardiovascular disease: the higher the blood pressure above normal, the greater the risk. A stiffened artery, already strained by each pulse of blood surging through it, is more greatly stressed if the internal pressure is high. Lesions (injured places) develop more frequently, and plaques grow faster.

As mentioned, atherosclerosis makes hypertension worse. As the arteries harden, they are unable to expand with each beat of the heart, so the pressure rises instead. This increased pressure leads to further hardening of the arteries, as already explained. Hardened arteries also inhibit blood from flowing freely through the body's blood pressure–sensing organs, the kidneys. The kidneys respond as if the blood pressure were too low, and raise it further. (Hypertension receives more attention later in this chapter.)

Smoking Low HDL cholesterol is among the many health problems associated with cigarette smoking.[18] Smoking also damages the heart directly by increasing blood pressure and the heart's workload. It deprives the heart of oxygen and damages platelets, making blood clot formation likely. Toxins in cigarette smoke damage blood vessels, setting the stage for atherosclerosis.

Diabetes In diabetes, blood vessels often become blocked and circulation diminishes. Atherosclerosis progresses rapidly. More than 80 percent of people with diabetes die of some type of cardiovascular disease, often a heart attack. Women with diabetes have a higher risk of death from cardiovascular disease than do men with diabetes.[19] In fact, diabetes doubles the risk of death from heart disease in women. Diabetes, like CHD, is associated with high LDL, high triglycerides, low HDL, hypertension, and obesity, particularly central obesity.

RECOMMENDATIONS FOR REDUCING CARDIOVASCULAR DISEASE RISK

Recommendations to reduce cardiovascular disease risk include both screening and intervention. Once a person's risks have been identified, treatment options focus first on dietary measures and then on drug therapy for those who cannot adequately normalize blood lipids using diet alone. The accompanying box presents a scorecard to assist you in assessing your heart disease risk.

Cholesterol Screening To determine an individual's risk of CHD, health care professionals measure several blood lipids including total cholesterol, LDL cholesterol, HDL cholesterol, and triglycerides. Ideally, at least two measurements are taken at least one week apart and then compared to standards (shown in Table 18–2). Single measurements may fail to identify those at risk or may misclassify them because blood cholesterol and other lipid concentrations vary significantly from day to day.[20] One study reported variability ranging from 5 to 20 percent.[21] On retesting, a person in the "desirable" category could move to the "high-risk" category, or vice versa.[22]

Two-Step Diet Plan Dietary recommendations to reduce the risk of CHD focus on reducing LDL cholesterol. To that end, people are advised to control their body weights and their intakes of saturated fat, total fat, and dietary cholesterol.[23] A panel of experts recommends a two-step plan, shown in Table 18–3.[24] Step 1 reflects recommendations for reducing chronic disease risk (introduced in Chapter 1).[25] The Step 1 diet was originally designed for people with borderline-high or high LDL cholesterol, but because atherosclerotic disease is so common, many experts advocate its use for everyone. If blood lipids improve, good; if not, the therapy goes on to Step 2. People with existing CHD are immediately placed on the Step 2 diet.

Table 18–3

Characteristics of Diets to Reduce High LDL Cholesterol

	Step 1	Step 2
Energy	Adequate to achieve or maintain desirable weight	Adequate to achieve or maintain desirable weight
Total fat[a]	<30%	<30%
Saturated fat[a]	8–10%	<7%
Polyunsaturated fat[a]	Up to 10%	Up to 10%
Monounsaturated fat[a]	10–15%	10–15%
Cholesterol	<300 mg/day	<200 mg/day

[a] Expressed as percentages of total food energy when energy intake is adequate to achieve and maintain desirable weight.

Source: Adapted from The Expert Panel, Summary of the second report of the National Cholesterol Education Program (NCEP) Expert Panel on Detection, Evaluation, and Treatment of High Blood Cholesterol in Adults (Adult Treatment Panel II), *Journal of the American Medical Association* 269 (1993): 3015–3023.

How to Assess Your Heart Disease Risk

Do you know your heart disease risk score? Respond to the statements below, and score yourself as directed. Be aware that a high risk score does not mean you *will* develop heart disease, but it should warn you of the possibility. Consult your physician if you have questions about your score results.

Heart Disease Risk Scorecard

Age	If you are 56 or over:	1	______
	If you are 55 or under:	0	______
Sex	If you are male:	1	______
	If you are female:	0	______
Family history	If you have blood relatives who have had a heart attack or stroke before age 60:	12	______
	If you have blood relatives who have had a history of heart disease at or before age 60:	10	______
	If you have blood relatives who have had a heart attack or stroke after age 60:	6	______
	If you have no history of heart disease:	0	______
Personal history	If you are 50 or under and have had a heart attack, stroke, or cardiovascular surgery:	20	______
	If you are 51 or over and have had any of the above:	10	______
	If you have had none of the above:	0	______
Diabetes	If onset of diabetes appeared before age 40 and you take insulin:	10	______
	If onset of diabetes appeared at or after 40 and you take insulin or pills:	5	______
	If onset of diabetes appeared after age 55 and you control it with diet:	3	______
	If you have not had diabetes:	0	______
Smoking	If you smoke 2 packs/day:	10	______
	If you smoke 1 to 2 packs/day or quit within past year:	6	______
	If you smoke 6 or more cigars/day or use a pipe regularly:	6	______
	If you smoke less than 1 pack/day or quit over a year ago:	3	______
	If you never smoked:	0	______
Cholesterol[a]	If your cholesterol level is 240 or higher:	10	______
	If your cholesterol level is 200 to 239:	5	______
	If your cholesterol level is 199 or lower:	0	______
Diet[a]	If you normally eat:		
	Red meat daily; more than 7 eggs weekly; and butter, whole milk, and cheese daily:	8	______
	Red meat 4 to 6 times weekly; margarine, low-fat dairy products, and some cheese:	4	______
	Poultry, fish, little or no red meat; 3 or fewer eggs weekly; some margarine, nonfat milk and milk products:	0	______
Blood pressure	If either number is 160 over 100 or higher:	10	______
	If either number is 140 over 90 but less than 160 or over 100:	5	______
	If both numbers are less than 140 over 90:	0	______
Weight[b]	If you are 25 lb overweight:	4	______
	If you are 10 to 24 lb overweight:	2	______
	If you are less than 10 lb overweight:	0	______
Exercise	If you engage in aerobic exercise more than 20 minutes less than once a week:	4	______
	If you engage in aerobic exercise more than 20 minutes 1 to 2 times a week:	2	______
	If you engage in aerobic exercise more than 20 minutes 3 or more times a week:	0	______
Stress	When waiting, if you are frustrated and easily angered:	4	______
	When waiting, if you are impatient and occasionally moody:	2	______
	When waiting, if you are comfortable and easygoing:	0	______
		TOTAL POINTS	______

[a]Answer the diet question only if you do not know your cholesterol level.

[b]Use the formula 106 lb + 6 lb per inch over 5 feet for men, or 100 lb + 5 lb per inch over 5 feet for women.

If you answered the blood pressure question:

High risk . . . . .36 and above
Medium risk . . . . .19 to 35
Low risk . . . . .18 and below

If you did not answer the blood pressure question:

High risk . . . . .40 and above
Medium risk . . . . .20 to 30
Low risk . . . . .19 and below

Source: Adapted from Arizona Heart Institute, Cardiovascular Risk Factor Analysis.

Control Weight Dietary plans to reduce LDL cholesterol include attention to weight reduction or weight maintenance (see Chapter 9). Both steps recommend energy intake to achieve and maintain desirable weight. With weight loss, heart disease risk factors improve: blood pressure, blood cholesterol, and blood triglycerides decline.[26]

Reduce Fat, Especially Saturated Fat In addition to limiting total energy intake, the Step 1 diet recommends a total fat intake of less than 30 percent of daily kcalories, with saturated fat no more than one-third of that and dietary cholesterol less than 300 milligrams a day. Chapter 5 (pp. 180–183) provides practical suggestions for reducing fat and saturated fats in the diet.

The Step 1 diet eliminates obvious sources of saturated fat and cholesterol from meals. These changes can be made without radically modifying the diet. Step 2 reduces saturated fat and cholesterol further, as shown. For persons undertaking the Step 2 diet, the help of a registered dietitian can ensure that saturated fat and cholesterol are cut as needed without sacrificing nutritional quality.

Interestingly, men may benefit more from such a dietary regimen than women do.[27] Even though total blood cholesterol levels decrease similarly, the decline in LDL is greater and the decline in HDL is smaller in men than in women.

Sources of soluble fiber:
- Legumes.
- Oats.
- Apples and other fruits.

Other Dietary Interventions Other dietary strategies may also reduce blood cholesterol. For example, soluble fiber lowers blood cholesterol, especially in those with high blood cholesterol.[28] Foods rich in the antioxidant vitamins C and E may help limit the oxidation of LDL and protect against heart disease (see Highlight 11 for details).[29]

Some research suggests that *moderate* alcohol consumption (one or two drinks a day) reduces the risk of heart disease by raising HDL cholesterol and preventing blood clot formation.[30] These benefits are most apparent in people over age 50 and in those with one or more risk factors.[31] Studies also report that heavy alcohol consumption (three or more drinks a day) increases the risk of death from other causes.[32] As Highlight 7 described, alcohol has many negative effects on body systems, and a later section in this chapter describes its link with cancer. Any benefits that alcohol may confer on cardiovascular health must be weighed against the risks of incurring these negative effects, as well as the possibility of alcohol abuse.[33] An individual's age and health history are critical to the decision of whether to drink alcohol. The number of deaths attributed to alcohol is greatest for people between the ages of 15 and 44—and their risk of heart disease is relatively minor. Clearly, for these people, the benefits do not outweigh the risks.

In addition to alcohol, wine contains phenols and other phytochemicals that may protect against cardiovascular disease.[34] These substances may act as antioxidants, reducing LDL oxidation, and may alter prostaglandin metabolism, reducing blood clot formation. These protective effects may explain the so-called French paradox: that the wine-drinking population of France enjoys a lower incidence of CHD even though they have many of the same risk factors as people in the United States. In general, though, most experts hesitate to recommend the taking of alcohol to benefit health.[35]

Dietary interventions alone may not be enough to reduce CHD risk. Physical activity combined with a low-fat diet offers many advantages. If this approach fails to normalize blood lipids, drugs may be used.

Physical Activity Physical activity deserves attention in any program to reduce CHD risk. Some evidence suggests that weight training can raise HDL somewhat if undertaken regularly, but frequent and sustained *aerobic* activity may be most effective in lowering LDL and raising HDL. Furthermore, aerobic, endurance-type activities, such as brisk walking, undertaken faithfully as a daily or every-other-day routine can strengthen the heart and blood vessels; alter body composition in favor of lean over fat tissue; expand the volume of oxygen the heart can deliver to the tissues at each beat and so reduce the heart's workload; change the hormonal climate in which the body does its work in such a way as to lower blood pressure; and bring about a redistribution of body water that eases the transit of blood through the peripheral arteries. These changes are so beneficial that some experts believe that physical activity, not diet, should be the primary focus of cardiovascular disease prevention efforts.[36]

Chapter 14 describes exercise for cardiovascular endurance.

If heart and artery disease has already set in, a monitored program of physical activity may actually help to reverse it.[37] Activity may stimulate development of new arteries to feed the heart muscle. This may help account for the excellent recovery seen in some heart attack victims who exercise.

Some researchers wonder if physical activity itself raises HDL or if the weight loss that often accompanies exercise is the real factor. For women, diet alone appears to *lower* HDL, but when diet is combined with moderate aerobic activity, HDL do not decline.[38] In men, diet raises HDL, and the combination of activity and diet results in a significantly greater rise in HDL than diet alone.

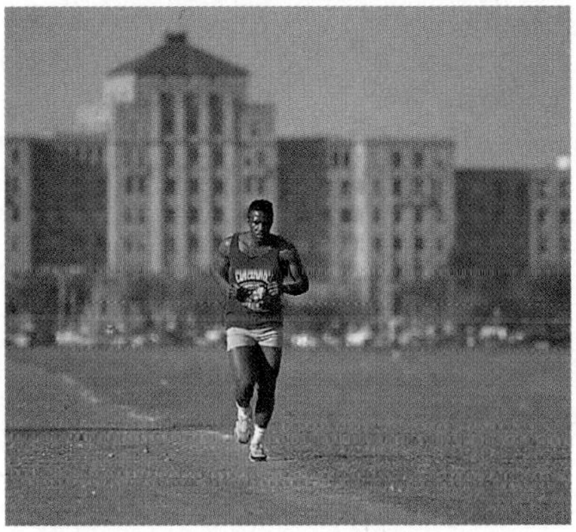

Regular aerobic exercise can help to defend against heart disease by strengthening the heart muscle, promoting weight loss, and improving blood lipid and blood glucose levels.

Diet helps a little, physical activity helps a little, and the combination is better still. People with CHD have been able to reduce plaque buildup in their arteries by following a comprehensive plan combining a low-fat vegetarian diet, no cigarette smoking, stress management training, and moderate exercise.[39] Without such a program, atherosclerosis would most likely have progressed; instead, it regressed and did so without lipid-lowering drugs.

Drug Therapy The potential risks and costs of drug therapy to lower blood lipids make it a second choice to diet and physical activity programs. Although data are inconsistent, some research suggests that lipid-lowering drugs may reduce the risk of CHD, but may be associated with higher mortality from other causes.[40] These drugs are associated with many side effects. The risk of side effects is heightened in the case of CHD, because once drug therapy begins, it usually continues for many years or even for life.

As Chapter 10 explained, large doses of niacin can effectively lower blood cholesterol, but they have adverse side effects as well. Self-medication is never advisable.

To sum up, plaques in atherosclerosis raise blood pressure and trigger abnormal blood clotting, which can cause heart attacks and strokes. Dietary recommendations to lower the risks of these cardiovascular diseases focus on reducing saturated fat and cholesterol intake. Quitting smoking and engaging in regular physical activity are also important. Anyone concerned with atherosclerosis and the risk it presents must also be concerned about hypertension. As described earlier, the two together are a life-threatening combination.

Hypertension

Chronic elevated blood pressure, or hypertension, is a major CHD risk factor; it is believed to affect some 60 million people in the United States, more than a third of the entire adult population.[41] It contributes to half a million strokes and

hypertension: higher-than-normal blood pressure. Hypertension that develops without an identifiable cause is known as **essential** or **primary hypertension**; hypertension that is caused by a specific disorder such as kidney disease is known as **secondary hypertension**.

over a million heart attacks each year. The higher the blood pressure is above normal, the greater the risk of heart disease. (Low blood pressure, on the other hand, is generally a sign of long life expectancy and low heart disease risk.) People cannot feel the physical affects of high blood pressure, but it can impair life's quality and end life prematurely.

BLOOD PRESSURE REGULATION

Blood pressure is vital to life. It is the blood pressure that pushes the blood through the major arteries into the smaller arteries and finally into the tiny capillaries, whose thin, porous walls permit fluid exchange between the blood and the tissues (see Figure 18–3). When the pressure is right, the cells receive a constant supply of nutrients and oxygen and give up their wastes.

Figure 18–3

How Normal Blood Pressure Supports Fluid Exchange

At the same time the heart pushes blood into an artery, the small-diameter arteries and capillaries at its other end resist the blood's flow (peripheral resistance). Both actions contribute to the pressure inside the artery. Another determining factor is the volume of fluid in the circulatory system, which depends in turn on the number of dissolved particles in that fluid.

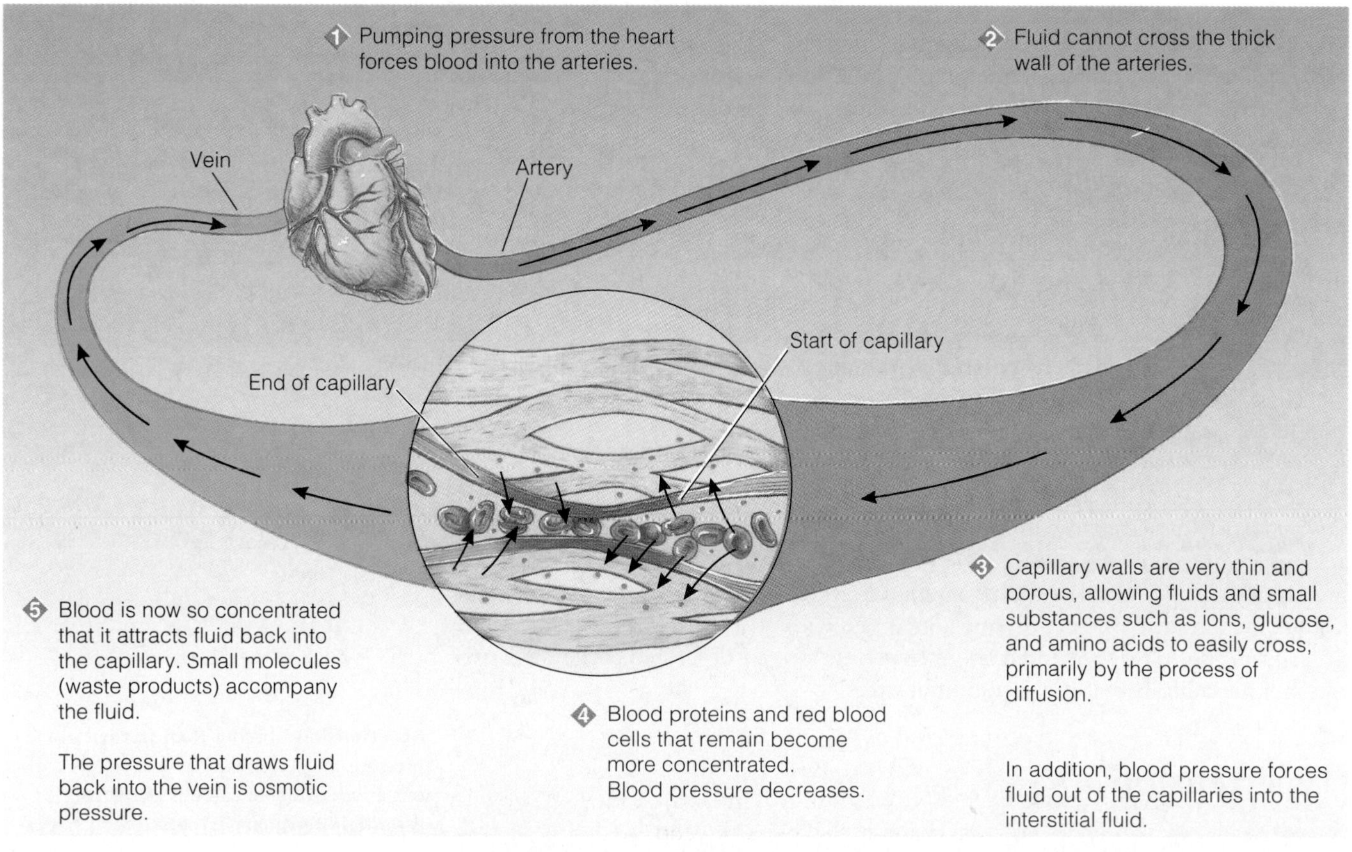
1 Pumping pressure from the heart forces blood into the arteries.
2 Fluid cannot cross the thick wall of the arteries.
Vein
Artery
Start of capillary
End of capillary
3 Capillary walls are very thin and porous, allowing fluids and small substances such as ions, glucose, and amino acids to easily cross, primarily by the process of diffusion.
In addition, blood pressure forces fluid out of the capillaries into the interstitial fluid.
4 Blood proteins and red blood cells that remain become more concentrated. Blood pressure decreases.
5 Blood is now so concentrated that it attracts fluid back into the capillary. Small molecules (waste products) accompany the fluid.
The pressure that draws fluid back into the vein is osmotic pressure.

The Arteries The pressure the blood exerts on the inner arterial walls results from two actions occurring together: at the body's center, the heart is pushing the blood into the arteries, and at the periphery, the smallest arteries and capillaries are resisting its flow. The heart's push ensures that the blood circulates through the whole system; the peripheral resistance and resulting pressure force oxygen and nutrients across the capillary walls to feed the tissues.

peripheral resistance: resistance to the flow of blood caused by the reduced diameter of the vessels at the periphery of the body—the smallest arteries and capillaries.

The Blood Volume The volume of fluid in the vascular system also contributes to blood pressure. That volume, in turn, depends on the number of dissolved particles the fluid contains. By the rule of osmosis, the more dissolved particles in the blood, the more water there will be.

The Kidneys The kidneys depend on the blood pressure to help them filter waste materials out of the blood into the urine (you may want to review Figure 3–8 on p. 98). The pressure has to be high enough to force the blood's fluid out of the capillaries into the kidneys' filtering networks. If the blood pressure is too low, the kidneys set in motion actions to raise it (as shown in Figure 12–1 on p. 433). One action is to retain sodium and water, expanding blood volume. Another is to constrict the peripheral blood vessels. Both raise blood pressure.

Normally, dehydration sets these actions in motion. This is beneficial, because in dehydration the blood volume falls, and higher blood pressure is needed to deliver substances to the tissues. The kidneys maintain normal blood pressure by constricting the blood vessels and conserving water and sodium until the dehydrated person can drink water and replenish the blood volume.

HOW HYPERTENSION DEVELOPS

What triggers chronic hypertension remains for the most part unknown, although some of the mechanisms have been defined. Sometimes the kidneys take action to raise the blood pressure as if trying to remedy dehydration when dehydration is not present. This occurs in atherosclerosis. Atherosclerosis obstructs blood vessels, limiting the flow of blood to the kidneys. In response to this deficiency, the kidneys create enough pressure to acquire the fluid they need to filter the blood properly. Unfortunately, however, the pressure increases not only in the kidneys, but all over the body. High blood pressure stresses the heart, which has to pump extra hard to push the blood against resistant arteries. Hypertension worsens atherosclerosis, as described earlier, by mechanically injuring the artery linings and accelerating plaque formation. Then the plaques induce a further rise in blood pressure, intensifying the problem.

Effect of Obesity Obesity makes hypertension still worse. Added adipose tissue means miles of extra capillaries through which the blood must be pumped. The combination of hypertension, atherosclerosis, and obesity puts a severe strain on the heart and arteries, leading to cardiovascular disease and death.

Another relationship between obesity and hypertension involves insulin's effect on sodium. In obesity, even though insulin is abundant, it is ineffective in moving glucose into the cells. High blood insulin signals the kidneys to retain sodium and may precipitate the development of hypertension.[42]

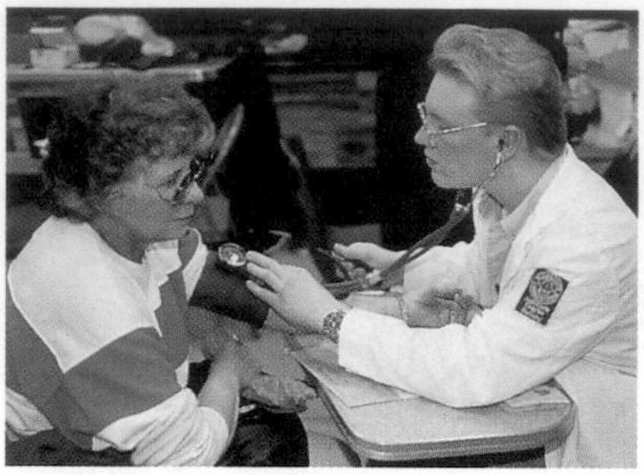

Screening people for high blood pressure is a first step in reducing CHD risk from hypertension.

Complications Strain on the heart's pump, the left ventricle, can enlarge and weaken it, until finally it fails (heart failure). Pressure in the aorta may cause it to balloon out and burst (aneurysm), which can lead to massive bleeding and death. Pressure in the small arteries of the brain may make them burst and bleed (stroke). The kidneys can be damaged when the heart is unable to adequately pump blood through them (kidney disease).

RISK FACTORS FOR HYPERTENSION

Epidemiological studies have identified several risk factors to predict the development of hypertension, including:

- *Age*. Arteries lose their elasticity and blood pressure increases with age; most people who develop hypertension do so in their 50s and 60s.
- *Heredity*. A family history of hypertension and heart disease raises the risk of developing hypertension two to five times.
- *Obesity*. Obese people are more likely to develop hypertension.
- *Race*. Hypertension is twice as common among African Americans as among whites; it tends to develop earlier and become more severe.

Of these risk factors, obesity is the only one that might be modified by diet. Notice that salt intake is not a risk factor for the development of hypertension, although it may aggravate existing hypertension in some people, as a later section explains.

RECOMMENDATIONS FOR REDUCING HYPERTENSION RISK

The most effective single step people can take against hypertension is to find out whether they have it. At checkup time, a health care professional can provide an accurate resting blood pressure reading. Under normal conditions, blood pressure fluctuates continuously in response to a variety of factors including such things as talking or shifting position. Some people react emotionally to the procedure, which raises the blood pressure reading. For these reasons, if the resting blood pressure is above normal, the reading should be repeated before confirming the diagnosis of hypertension. Thereafter, it should be checked regularly.

Blood pressure is measured in millimeters of mercury (mm Hg), a standard unit for the measurement of pressure.

The normal resting blood pressure for adults averages about 120 over 70. At readings of 140 over 90 or higher, the risks of heart attacks and strokes increase in direct proportion to increasing blood pressure, especially diastolic pressure (see Table 18 2).

A major national effort to identify and treat hypertension is currently under way. Even mild hypertension can be serious.[43] Individuals who have hypertension benefit from treatment, enjoying better health and longer lives.

Weight Control Efforts to reduce high blood pressure focus on weight control because excess body fat, especially abdominal fat, can precipitate hypertension, thus increasing the risks of heart attack and stroke. Weight loss alone is one of the most effective nondrug treatments for hypertension.[44] Those who are using drugs to control their blood pressure can often reduce or discontinue the drugs if they lose weight. Even a modest weight loss of 10 pounds may significantly lower blood pressure.[45] Many professionals recommend a fat-controlled diet, such as the Step 1 diet shown in Table 18–3 on p. 652, both for weight loss and to control blood lipids and blood pressure.

Increase Physical Activity The higher the blood pressure and the less active a person is to begin with, the greater the likelihood that physical activity will be effective in reducing blood pressure.[46] Physical activity helps with weight control, of course, but moderate aerobic activity also helps to lower blood pressure directly. Those who engage in regular, aerobic activity may not need medication for mild hypertension.[47]

Reduce Sodium/Salt Intake Salt may aggravate hypertension in some people who are genetically sensitive, but most studies clearly show that weight loss lowers blood pressure more effectively than sodium or salt restriction.[48] For most people, blood pressure responses to sodium or salt are modest at best.

Still, many health care professionals advocate moderate salt restriction for everyone, reasoning that at best it may help and at worst it will do no harm. Salt-sensitive people should certainly limit their salt intakes to 5 to 6 grams per day following the suggestions in the box on p. 442. People taking certain antihypertensive drugs may need a low-sodium, high-potassium diet.

Reminder:
- 1 tsp salt = 5 g salt.
- 5 g salt = 2 g sodium.

Reduce Alcohol Intake Alcohol, especially if taken in high doses (an average of two or more drinks per day), is associated with hypertension. Furthermore, alcohol is associated with strokes independently of hypertension. The surgeon general's advice on alcohol use is: if you drink, do so in moderation—no more than one to two drinks a day. Such amounts seem safe from a blood pressure point of view.[49]

Count as one drink:
- 12 oz of beer.
- 4 to 5 oz of wine.
- 1 oz of hard liquor.

For more on alcohol, see Highlight 7.

Other Dietary Interventions Other dietary factors may play a role in the prevention of hypertension, even though evidence is insufficient to warrant specific recommendations. Potassium, calcium, and magnesium, for example, appear to help prevent and treat hypertension in certain populations. Similarly, vitamin C status and blood pressure appear to have an inverse relationship.[50]

As mentioned earlier, a low-fat, high-fiber diet rich in omega-3 fatty acids can improve atherosclerosis, and the same diet may lower blood pressure, especially in people with hypertension and atherosclerosis. Also, because hypertension may be an insulin-resistant state, measures preventive against diabetes may also protect against hypertension.

Chapter 12 reviewed the relationships between hypertension and the minerals potassium, calcium, and magnesium.

Drug Therapy When diet and physical activity fail to reduce blood pressure, diuretics and antihypertensive agents may be prescribed. Diuretics lower blood pressure by increasing fluid loss. Some diuretics can lead to a potassium deficiency. People taking these diuretics must be particularly careful to include good sources of potassium in their daily diets; their physicians may even advise them to use potassium supplements. Blood potassium should be monitored regularly to prevent hypokalemia, and clients should watch for its signs, such as weakness (particularly of the legs), unexplained numbness or tingling sensation, cramps, irregular heartbeats, and excessive thirst and urination.

hypokalemia (HIGH-po-ka-LEE-me-ah): low levels of potassium in the blood.

Although some diuretics can lead to a potassium deficiency, others spare potassium. A combination of these two types of diuretics may be prescribed to prevent potassium deficiency. In such cases, excessive potassium intakes and potassium supplements should be avoided; hyperkalemia can be life-threatening.

hyperkalemia (HIGH-per-ka-LEE-me-ah): high levels of potassium in the blood.

Of the risk factors that contribute to hypertension, obesity is the only one with a dietary relationship; weight control is the most effective treatment. When atherosclerosis and hypertension run their courses without treatment, they may lead to heart attacks and strokes. The other leading cause of death, cancer, develops in significantly different ways, yet many of the preventive measures are the same.

Cancer

cancer: a disease in which abnormal cells multiply out of control and disrupt the normal functioning of the body's cells or organs.

A carcinoma (KAR-see-NO-mah) is a cancer that develops from epithelial tissue. A sarcoma (sar-KO-mah) is a cancer that arises from muscle, bone, or other connective tissue. A hematopoietic (HEE-ma-toe-poy-ET-ik) neoplasm is a cancer of the blood and immune system. A cancer that spreads from one part of the body to another is said to metastasize (me-TAS-tah-size).

The thought of cancer often strikes fear in people. This fear arises in part from personal experiences with cancer and in part from knowledge that some cancers are incurable. The prognosis for most people today, however, is far brighter than in the past. Some cancers are preventable, and many are curable, especially when they are detected early. People can turn their fears into positive action by learning about cancer prevention and early detection. They can take comfort in knowing they are not alone in the battle against cancer; medical science refuses to give up the fight. New techniques for detecting cancers early and innovative therapies to wipe out cancers offer hope and encouragement.

HEALTHY PEOPLE 2000: Reverse the rise in cancer deaths to achieve a rate of no more than 130 per 100,000 people.

Cancer is not a single disorder. The word *cancer* refers to any uncontrolled growth of abnormal cells, resulting in many different kinds of malignancies. They have different characteristics, occur in different locations in the body, take different courses, and require different treatments.

A growing tumor, or neoplasm, interferes with the normal functioning of an organ or tissue. The growth seemingly has no built-in brakes and is supported by nutrients from the diet or body reserves.

tumor: an unchecked new growth of tissue forming an abnormal mass with no function; also called a neoplasm (NEE-oh-plazm). Tumors that pose no problem are called benign (bee-NINE); those that resist treatment and are harmful are malignant.
benign = mild
mal = bad

HOW CANCER DEVELOPS

Cancer is believed to develop in steps:

1. Exposure to a carcinogen.
2. Entry of the carcinogen into a cell.
3. Initiation, probably by the carcinogen's altering the cellular DNA.
4. Enhancement of cancer development by promoters, probably involving several more steps before the cell begins to multiply out of control.
5. Formation of a tumor or other malignancy.

Because cancer development is a process rather than a single event, it takes time, and the time allows opportunities for intervention.

Researchers think that the first three steps, which culminate with initiation, are the key ones. The initiating event may be either chemical or physical. The chemical event may occur when a carcinogen intrudes into the cell and alters the genetic material. The physical event may occur when radiation—either the

carcinogen (car-SIN-oh-jen): a cancer-initiating substance. A carcinogen is one kind of initiator; radiation is another.
carcin = cancer
gen = gives rise to

initiation: an event caused by radiation or chemical reaction that can give rise to cancer.

promoters: factors that favor the development of cancer once the initiating event has taken place. Other factors, antipromoters, oppose the development of cancer.

Figure 18–4

Tumor Formation

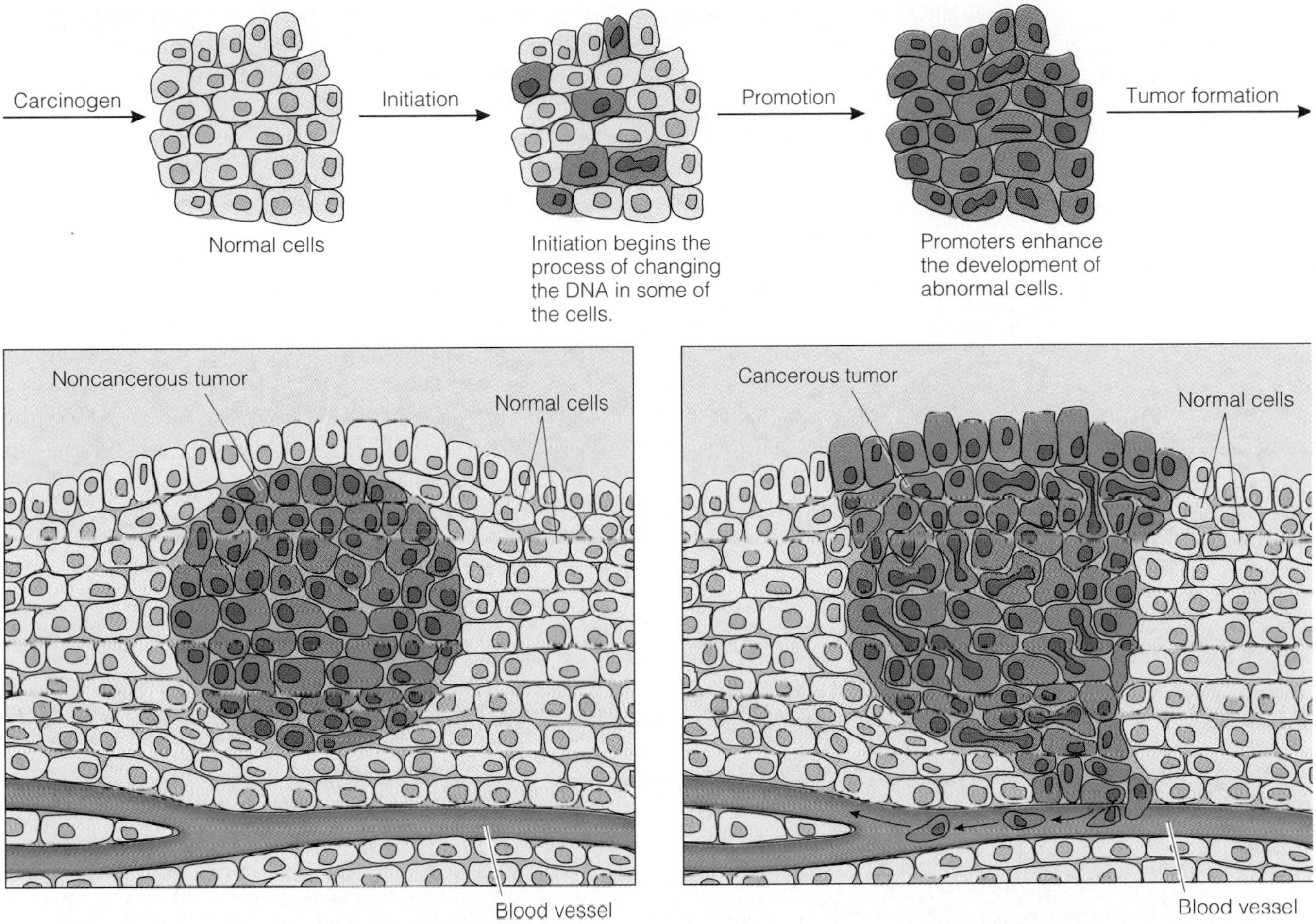

A noncancerous (benign) tumor usually grows within a self-contained capsule. It does not invade nearby tissue, nor does it spread.

A cancerous (malignant) tumor usually grows out of control and may spread to other parts of the body through the blood or lymph systems.

general radiation that is always present, or medical or industrial radiation—bombards the cell and alters the genetic material. In either case, the protein-making machinery of the cell changes so that the DNA produces an odd structural protein or an enzyme that produces abnormal products. The end result is a cell that is unable to halt its own multiplication; the neoplasm grows uncontrollably. Figure 18–4 illustrates tumor formation.

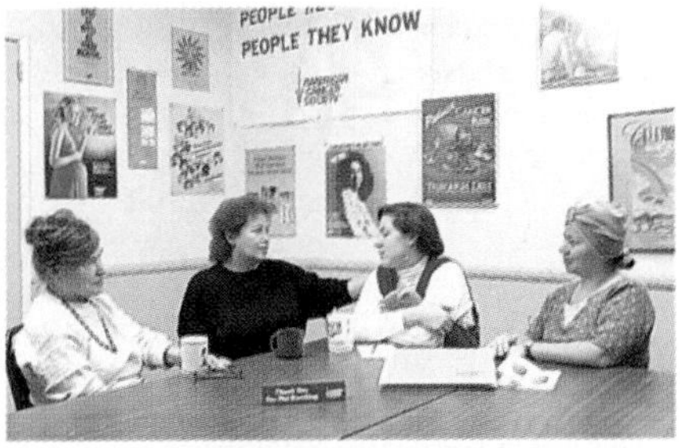

Until medical science wins the battle against cancer, people with cancer take comfort from the support of others.

RISK FACTORS FOR CANCER

Genetic, environmental, and dietary factors can play roles in cancer development. Cancer risk increases with repeated exposure to carcinogens. People who wish to reduce their cancer risks can reduce their exposure to environmental and

Table 18–4

Factors Associated with Cancer at Specific Sites

Cancer Sites	High Incidence Associated with:	Protective Effect Associated with:
Esophageal cancer	High alcohol use, tobacco use, and especially combined use; use of preserved foods (such as pickles); low intakes of vitamins and minerals; high intakes of vitamin A supplements	
Stomach cancer	High intakes of salt-preserved foods (such as dried, salted fish); low intakes of fresh fruits and vegetables	Fresh fruits and vegetables
Colorectal cancer	High intakes of fat (particularly saturated fat), meat, and alcohol (especially beer); low intakes of fiber, folate, and vegetables; inactivity	High intake of vegetables
Liver cancer	Infection with hepatitis B or aflatoxins; high intakes of alcohol; iron overload	
Pancreatic and lung cancer	No dietary risk factors have been established; correlated primarily with cigarette smoking	Fruits and vegetables, especially green and yellow ones
Breast cancer	High intakes of food energy and alcohol; little or no association with dietary fat specifically	Fruits and vegetables, especially green and yellow ones
Ovarian cancer	No dietary risk factors have been established; inversely correlated with oral contraceptive use	Fruits and vegetables, especially green and yellow ones
Cervical cancer	Folate deficiency	
Endometrial cancer	No dietary risk factors have been established; associated with estrogen therapy, obesity, hypertension, and diabetes (NIDDM)	
Bladder cancer	*Possible* associations with coffee, artificial sweeteners, and alcohol; associated with cigarette smoking	Fruits and vegetables, especially green and yellow ones
Prostate cancer	High fat intake, especially saturated fats from meats	Fruits and vegetables, especially green and yellow ones

Note: Findings based on epidemiological studies.

Source: Diet and Health: Implications for Reducing Chronic Disease Risk (Washington, D.C.: National Academy Press, 1989), pp. 594–600; J. H. Weisburger, Nutritional approach to cancer prevention with emphasis on vitamins, antioxidants, and carotenoids, *American Journal of Clinical Nutrition* (supplement) 53 (1991): 226–237; R. G. Ziegler, Vegetables, fruits, and carotenoids and the risk of cancer, *American Journal of Clinical Nutrition* (supplement) 53 (1991): 251–259; Potential mechanisms for food-related carcinogens and anticarcinogens: A scientific status summary by the Institute of Food Technologists' Expert Panel on Food Safety and Nutrition, *Food Technology* 47 (1993): 105–118.

dietary factors that have been linked to cancer. This section focuses primarily on diet and cancer in general; Table 18–4 lists various types of cancers and their specific carcinogens and protective factors.

Genetic Factors Some cancers are programmed by genes to develop. A person with a family history of a specific cancer, such as breast cancer, has a greater risk of developing that cancer than a person without such a genetic predisposition. This does not mean, however, that the person *will* develop cancer, only that the risk is greater.

Environmental Factors Among environmental factors, smoking, water and air pollution, and sun exposure are known to cause cancer. Dietary constituents can also be carcinogens, and the emphasis here is on these factors.

Dietary Factors—Cancer Initiators We do not know to what extent diet contributes to cancer development, although some experts estimate that diet may be linked to a third or more of all cases. Consequently, many people think that certain foods are carcinogenic, most likely those that contain additives or pesticides. As Chapter 19 will explain, our food supply is one of the safest in the world. Additives that have been approved for use in foods are not carcinogenic. Some pesticides are carcinogenic at high doses, but not at the concentrations allowed on fruits and vegetables.[51]

Additives and pesticides receive full attention in Chapter 19.

The incidence of cancers, especially stomach cancers, is high in parts of the world where people eat a lot of heavily smoked, pickled, or salt-cured foods that produce carcinogenic nitrosamines. Most commercial manufacturers in the United States use different preservative methods, and all are carefully controlled to minimize carcinogen contamination.

Chapter 19 describes nitrosamine formation.

Alcohol has also been associated with a high incidence of some cancers, especially cancers of the mouth and throat. Beverages such as beer and scotch may contain damaging nitrosamines as well as alcohol.[52] Other beverages, such as wine and brandy, may contain the carcinogen urethane, which is produced during fermentation.[53] The amounts of these compounds found in alcoholic beverages currently on the market are not considered harmful—assuming consumption in moderate amounts. These findings illustrate clearly why any potential benefit of moderate alcohol consumption on cardiovascular disease must be weighed against the potential dangers.

Dietary Factors—Cancer Promoters Unlike carcinogens, which initiate cancers, some dietary components promote cancers. That is, once the initiating step has taken place, these components may accelerate tumor development. Studies suggest that dietary fats eaten in excess may promote cancer, in part by contributing to obesity. (Energy restriction is the single most effective dietary strategy for reducing cancer risk in rats.)[54] More specifically, linoleic acid, the omega-6 fatty acid of vegetable oils, has been implicated in enhancing cancer development in rats.[55] (In contrast, omega-3 fatty acids appear to delay cancer development.)

Dietary Factors—Antipromoters It seems apparent that, besides promoters, foods may contain antipromoters. Almost without exception, epidemiological studies find a link between eating plenty of fruits and vegetables and a low incidence of cancers.[56] The fiber in fruits and vegetables helps to protect against some cancers by speeding up the transit time of all materials through the colon so that the colon walls are not exposed to cancer-causing substances for long. In addition to fiber, fruits and vegetables contain both nutrients and nonnutrients that protect against cancer. By acting as scavengers of oxygen-derived free radicals, the antioxidant nutrients beta-carotene, vitamin C, and vitamin E may help to prevent cell and tissue damage that can give rise to cancer.[57] Phytochemicals common to many vegetables, especially those of the cabbage family, can activate enzymes that are capable of destroying carcinogens (see Highlight 11 for more details).[58]

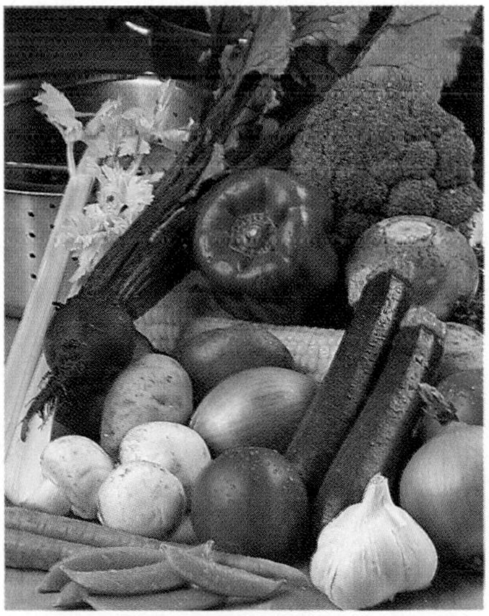

Vegetables rich in fiber and the antioxidant nutrients (beta-carotene, vitamin C, and vitamin E) help to protect against cancer.

RECOMMENDATIONS FOR REDUCING CANCER RISK

On the basis of current knowledge and available evidence, the following guidelines are recommended for cancer prevention:

- Control weight and prevent obesity.
- Reduce consumption of total fat to 30 percent or less of total energy intake.
- Increase fiber intake to 20–30 grams per day.
- Include a variety of vegetables and fruits in the daily diet.
- Minimize consumption of salt-cured, salt-pickled, and smoked foods.
- Consume alcoholic beverages in moderation, if at all.

One additional recommendation is in order: vary food choices. This last suggestion is based on an important concept that applies specifically to the prevention of cancer initiation—dilution. Switching from food to food dilutes whatever is in one food with what is in the others. For example, it is safe to eat *some* salt-cured or smoked meats, but not all the time. Combine such foods with a variety of others so that any carcinogens that may be present will be diluted in the total diet.

To review, some dietary factors, such as alcohol and heavily smoked or salted foods, may initiate cancer development; others, such as dietary fat, may promote cancer once it has gotten started; and still others, such as fiber and antioxidant nutrients and nonnutrients, may serve as antipromoters that protect against the development of cancer. Eating many green, yellow, and orange vegetables, including high-fiber foods, and reducing fat intake offer the best possible nutrition at the lowest possible risk.

Diabetes Mellitus

diabetes (DYE-uh-BEET-eez) mellitus (MELL-ih-tus or mell-EYE-tus)**:** a metabolic disorder characterized by altered glucose regulation and utilization, usually caused by insufficient or relatively ineffective insulin.

mellitus = honey-sweet (sugar in urine)

Reminder: *Insulin* is the hormone that, among other things, enables cells to take up glucose from the blood.

Diabetes mellitus ranks seventh among the leading causes of death. In addition, diabetes underlies, or contributes to, a variety of other major diseases, including heart disease and stroke. In fact, people with diabetes are twice as likely to develop these cardiovascular problems as those without diabetes.

Several disorders have been called diabetes, but by far the most common ones are the two forms of *diabetes mellitus* described here. They are metabolic disorders characterized by high blood glucose and either insufficient or ineffective insulin.

To appreciate the problems presented by an absolute or relative lack of insulin, consider insulin's normal action. After a meal, insulin enhances cellular uptake of the energy nutrients—amino acids, glucose, and fatty acids. It helps to maintain blood glucose within normal limits and stimulates protein synthesis, glycogen synthesis in liver and muscle, and fat synthesis. Without insulin, glucose regulation falters, and metabolism of energy-yielding nutrients changes.

insulin-dependent diabetes mellitus (IDDM)**:** the less common type of diabetes in which the person produces no insulin at all; also known as type I diabetes or juvenile-onset diabetes, although some cases arise in adulthood.

Insulin-Dependent Diabetes Mellitus In insulin-dependent diabetes, which is the less common type (about 5 to 10 percent of all cases), the pancreas loses its ability to synthesize the hormone insulin. Without insulin, when a person eats carbohydrate and absorbs the glucose from it, the glucose remains in the blood, even though the body's cells may be starved for glucose. The person must inject insulin regularly to assist the cells in taking up the needed glucose from the blood; hence the name insulin-dependent diabetes mellitus (IDDM). The insulin must be injected; it cannot be taken orally because insulin is a protein and the GI enzymes would digest it.

Noninsulin-Dependent Diabetes Mellitus The predominant type of diabetes mellitus (90 to 95 percent of all cases) is called noninsulin-dependent diabetes mellitus (NIDDM); it develops most often in people over 40 years old. Although the exact cause of NIDDM remains unknown, high blood glucose and insulin resistance are the hallmarks of the disorder. In the initial stages, the pancreas produces insulin. In fact, the person may actually have higher-than-average insulin levels, but the cells become resistant to it and respond less sensitively. Cell receptors for insulin, the sites at which insulin signals the cell, are often reduced in number or function. As in IDDM, blood glucose rises too high. The high blood glucose stimulates the pancreatic cells to make insulin, exhausting these cells and reducing their ability to make insulin. Thus, NIDDM appears to be a self-aggravating condition.

noninsulin-dependent diabetes mellitus (NIDDM): the more common type of diabetes in which the cells resist insulin; also called type II diabetes or adult-onset diabetes.

insulin resistance: the condition of having a normal amount of insulin producing a subnormal effect; a metabolic consequence of obesity.

NIDDM usually develops later in life, for in all people, pancreatic insulin-producing cells progressively lose their function with age. NIDDM is also associated with obesity; about 90 percent of U.S. adults with NIDDM are obese. Compared with normal-weight people, obese people require much more insulin to maintain normal blood glucose. This state of insulin resistance is one of many metabolic consequences of obesity. As body fat increases, insulin receptors are reduced in number or function, insulin resistance increases, and adipose and muscle tissues become less and less able to take up glucose. At some point, individuals cannot produce enough insulin to keep up and they develop NIDDM. Age and obesity alone do not predict the onset of NIDDM; genetics also plays a role.[59]

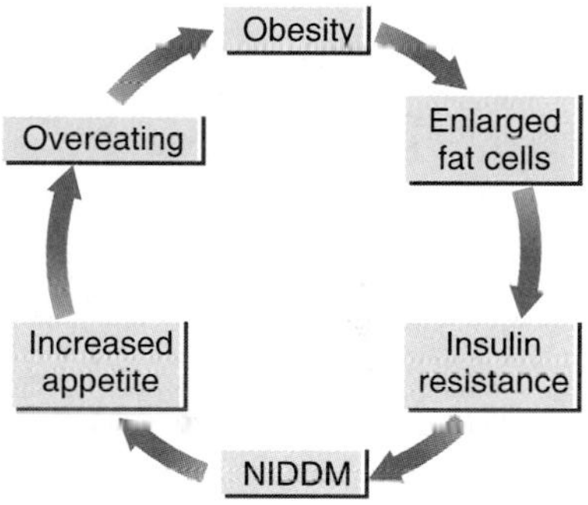

COMPLICATIONS OF DIABETES

In both types of diabetes, glucose fails to gain entry into the cells and accumulates in the blood. These two problems lead to both acute and chronic complications. Figure 18–5 (on p. 666) summarizes the metabolic complications and physical symptoms that can arise. Notice that when some glucose enters the cells, as in NIDDM, many of the symptoms of IDDM do not occur.

Over the long term, the person with diabetes suffers not only from the acute complications shown in Figure 18–5, but also from its chronic effects.[60] Infections are likely, especially in the urinary tract, because bacteria thrive on glucose-rich blood and urine. Chronically elevated blood glucose also affects the structures of the blood vessels and nerves, leading to loss of circulation and nerve function. Blood vessel disorders involve both the large blood vessels and the smaller ones.

Diseases of the Large Blood Vessels Atherosclerosis in the large blood vessels is the same as that found in the general population, except that it tends to develop early, progress rapidly, and be more severe in people with diabetes. To complicate the picture, people with NIDDM are often obese, and they may also have hypertension. If blood glucose is poorly controlled, triglycerides rise and HDL decline. All of these factors increase the risk of cardiovascular disease and help explain why atherosclerosis is a major cause of death for people with NIDDM.

In diabetes, large blood vessels serving the legs and feet often become blocked. The loss of circulation and nerve function causes pain and the sensation of coldness; the affected limbs also tire easily. Reduced circulation can lead to tissue death and ulcers. In severe cases, an affected limb must be amputated.

The death of tissue, usually due to deficient blood supply, is gangrene (GANG-green).

Figure 18–5

Metabolic Consequences of Untreated IDDM and NIDDM

The metabolic consequences of IDDM are more immediate and severe than those of NIDDM, because in IDDM no insulin is available to allow any glucose to enter the cells. As you can see, when glucose cannot enter the cells, a cascade of metabolic changes follows. In NIDDM, some glucose enters the cells. Because the cells are not "starved" for glucose, the body does not shift into the metabolism of fasting (losing weight and producing ketones).

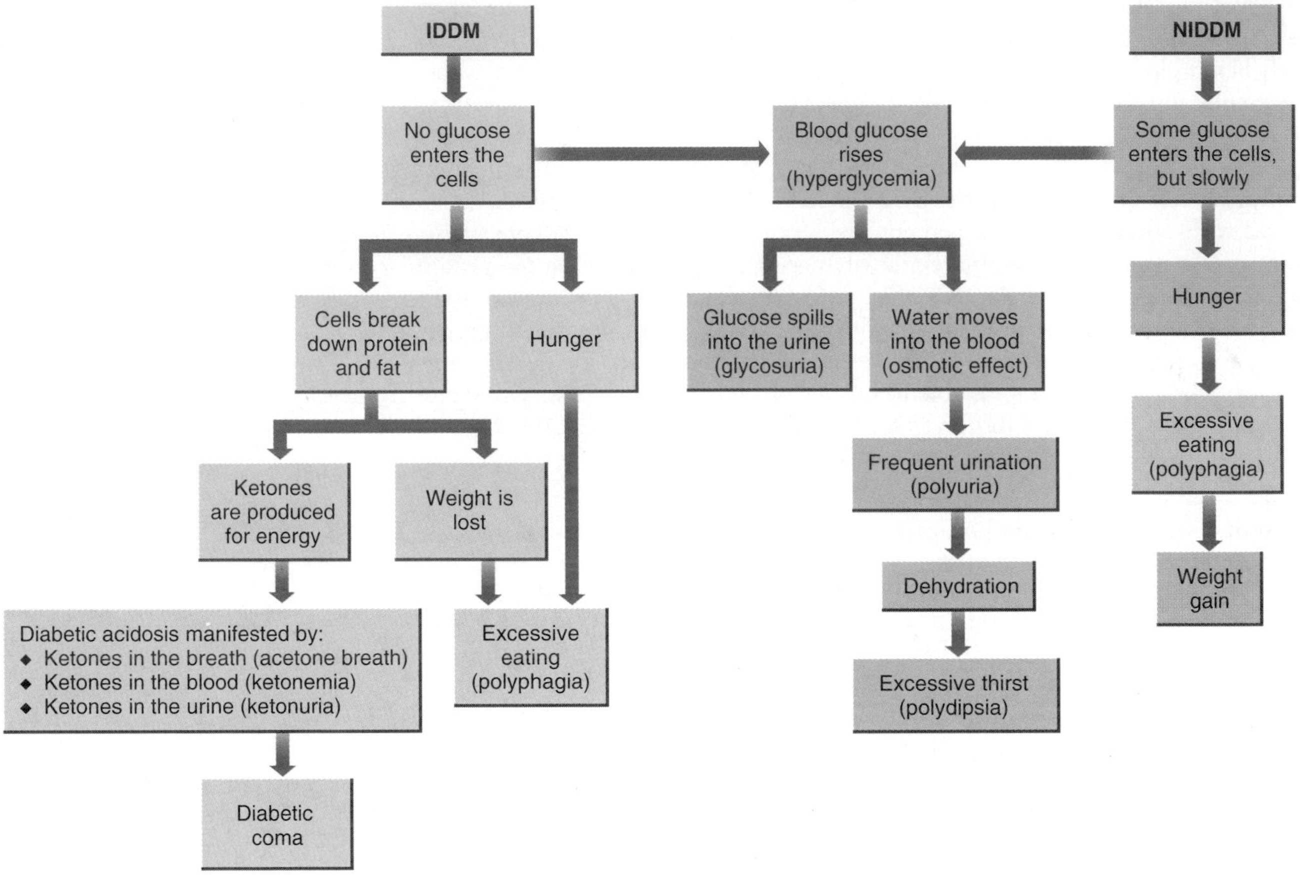

Diseases of the Small Blood Vessels Disorders of the small blood vessels (capillaries) may also develop and are far more common in people with diabetes than in the general population. In these disorders, which are caused by poor blood circulation through the capillaries, blood stagnates and the membranes surrounding the capillaries thicken, impairing circulation and increasing the risk of infection. The results are retinal degeneration, leading to loss of vision, and impaired kidney function, sometimes requiring hospital care or kidney transplant. Diabetes is a leading cause of both blindness and kidney failure.

Diseases of the Nerves Nerve tissue deterioration expresses itself as a painful prickling sensation, often in the arms and legs. Later, the individual loses sensation in the hands and feet. Thereafter, injuries to these areas may go unnoticed, and infections can progress rapidly. The combination of loss of circulation and nerve function, undetected injury, and infection often necessitates amputation of the limbs (usually the legs and feet).

DIETARY RECOMMENDATIONS FOR IDDM

Diet is an important component of IDDM treatment. To maintain blood glucose within a fairly normal range requires a lifelong commitment to a carefully coordinated diet, physical activity, and insulin program.

Nutrition therapy focuses on maintaining optimal nutrition status, controlling blood glucose at near-normal levels, achieving a desirable blood lipid profile, and preventing and treating the complications of diabetes.[61] In addition to meeting basic nutrient requirements, the diet must provide for carbohydrate intake to be fairly consistent from day to day and at each meal and snack to help minimize fluctuations in blood glucose. Further alterations in diet may be necessary for the person with chronic complications such as cardiovascular or kidney disease. Diet planners often use the exchange system described in Chapter 2 and Appendixes G and I for planning diabetic diets.

Recent research suggests that pharmacological doses of the vitamin niacin may prevent IDDM by protecting pancreatic cells from damage by free radicals.[62] A large international study involving over 30,000 people is currently underway to determine whether niacin treatment reduces the incidence of IDDM in high-risk individuals.

DIETARY RECOMMENDATIONS FOR NIDDM

Obesity, especially central obesity, triples the likelihood of a person's developing NIDDM. Consequently, prevention efforts focus on weight control, and in treatment, too, weight loss is often prescribed. Physical activity helps to control weight, and both weight loss and physical activity can improve blood glucose, blood lipids, and blood pressure. In fact, vigorous physical activity may delay or prevent the onset of NIDDM.[63] Those who must take insulin or insulin-eliciting drugs sometimes find that they can reduce their daily drug doses if they exercise regularly because physical activity enhances insulin's effect. Weight loss also improves insulin resistance in people with NIDDM. A diet low in fat helps with both weight loss and lowering blood lipids. In addition to weight loss and physical activity, people with elevated blood lipids may benefit from a moderate increase in monounsaturated fatty acids (up to 20 percent).[64] These strategies will in turn help forestall cardiovascular disease.

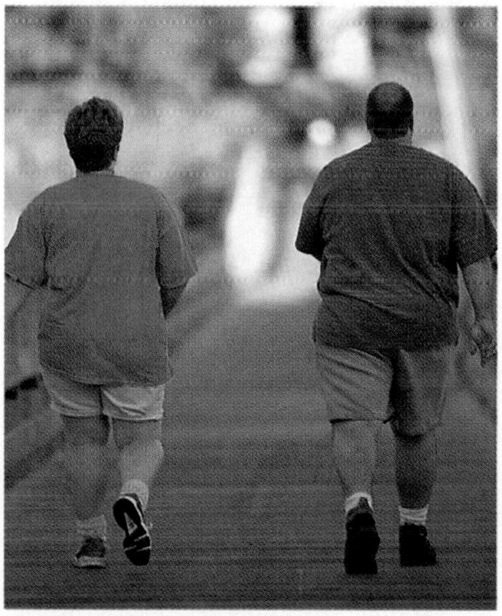

Even a moderate weight loss of, say, 10 to 20 pounds can help improve blood glucose, blood lipids, and blood pressure.

In summary, diabetes is characterized by high blood glucose and either insufficient insulin (IDDM) or ineffective insulin (NIDDM). People with IDDM coordinate diet, insulin injections, and physical activity to help control their blood glucose. Those with NIDDM benefit most from a low-fat diet and physical activity to help control their weight.

Putting It All Together

This chapter began with the major cardiovascular diseases, went on to cancer, and concluded with the metabolic disorder, diabetes—three different conditions with distinct sets of causes. Yet all are responsive to diet, and in some ways, the responses are similar. Dietary excesses, particularly excess food energy and fat intakes, increase the likelihood of all three diseases. Not all recommendations apply equally to all of the diseases, but fortunately for the consumer, dietary recommendations do not contradict one another. In fact, they support each other. A person designing a low-fat diet would need to select plenty of vegetables, fruits, and grain products—foods that supply fiber, vitamins, and minerals in abundance. Especially when combined with physical activity, such a diet would help a person to maintain a healthy weight—and weight control is central to the prevention of each of the diseases described in this chapter. Clearly, a nutritious diet plays a key role in keeping people healthy. Every recommendation mentioned since the start of Chapter 1 was established to promote optimal health. A person can do no better than to incorporate those suggestions into his or her daily life.

Study Questions

1. How do the major diseases of today as a group differ from those of several decades ago as a group? Why is nutrition considered so important in connection with today's major diseases?
2. Explain what a risk factor is and how it differs from a cause (such as a microbial cause) of a disease.
3. Identify the major diet-related risk factors for atherosclerosis, hypertension, cancer, and diabetes.
4. Describe some ways in which people can alter their diets to lower their blood cholesterol levels.
5. Describe some steps that people with hypertension can take to lower their blood pressure.
6. Differentiate between cancer initiators, promoters, and antipromoters. Which nutrients or foods fit into each of these categories?
7. Describe the characteristics of a diet that might offer the best protection against the onset of cancer.
8. Name the two major types of diabetes and describe some differences between them. How do dietary recommendations for each type of diabetes compare with the healthy diet recommended for all people?

Notes

1. Centers for Disease Control, Mortality patterns—United States, 1989, *Morbidity and Mortality Weekly Report* 41 (1992): 121–125.
2. W. Mertz, A balanced approach to nutrition for health: The need for biologically essential minerals and vitamins, *Journal of the American Dietetic Association* 94 (1994): 1259–1262.
3. A. Leaf and H. A. Hallaq, The role of nutrition in the functioning of the cardiovascular system, *Nutrition Reviews* 50 (1992): 402–406.
4. National Institutes of Health, National Heart, Lung, and Blood Institute, *The Healthy Heart Handbook for Women*, NIH Publication No. 92–2720, 1992.
5. G. S. Tell and coauthors, Dietary fat intake and carotid artery wall thickness: The Atherosclerosis Risk in Communities (ARIC) Study, *American Journal of Epidemiology* 139 (1994): 979–989.
6. The Expert Panel, Summary of the second report of the National Cholesterol Education Program (NCEP) Expert Panel on Detection, Evaluation, and Treatment of High Blood Cholesterol in Adults (Adult Treatment Panel II), *Journal of the American Medical Association* 269 (1993): 3015–3023.
7. R. J. Garrison, The role of adiposity in the prevention of cardiovascular disease, in *Obesity: New Directions in Assessment and Management*, eds. T. B. VanItallie and A. P. Simopoulos (Philadelphia: The Charles Press, 1995), pp. 22–23.
8. L. Kuller and coauthors, Prevalence of subclinical atherosclerosis and cardiovascular disease and association with risk fac-

tors in the Cardiovascular Health Study, *American Journal of Epidemiology* 139 (1994): 1164–1179.
9. C. L. Johnson and coauthors, Declining serum total cholesterol levels among US adults—The National Health and Nutrition Examination Surveys, *Journal of the American Medical Association* 269 (1993): 3002–3008.
10. R. Benfante and coauthors, To what extent do cardiovascular risk factor values measured in elderly men represent their midlife values measured 25 years earlier? A preliminary report and commentary from the Honolulu Heart Study, *American Journal of Epidemiology* 140 (1994): 206–216.
11. M. J. Stampfer and coauthors, A prospective study in cholesterol, apolipoproteins, and the risk of mycardial infarction, *New England Journal of Medicine* 325 (1991): 373–381.
12. M. H. Criqui and coauthors, Plasma triglyceride lèvel and mortality from coronary heart disease, *New England Journal of Medicine* 328 (1993): 1220–1225.
13. NIH Consensus Development Panel on Triglyceride, High-Density Lipoprotein, and Coronary Heart Disease, Triglyceride, high-density lipoprotein, and coronary heart disease, *Journal of the American Medical Association* 269 (1993): 505–510; Criqui and coauthors, 1993.
14. M. J. Klag and coauthors, Serum cholesterol in young men and subsequent cardiovascular disease, *New England Journal of Medicine* 328 (1993): 313–318.
15. P. M. Kris-Etherton and D. Krummel, Role of nutrition in the prevention and treatment of coronary heart disease in women, *Journal of the American Dietetic Association* 93 (1993): 987–993.
16. National Institutes of Health, 1992.
17. N. E. Davidson, Hormone-replacement therapy—Breast versus heart versus bone, *New England Journal of Medicine* 332 (1995): 1638–1639.
18. The Bezafibrate Infarction Prevention (BIP) Study Group, Israel, Lipids and lipoproteins in symptomatic coronary heart disease: Distribution, intercorrelations, and significance for risk classification in 6,700 men and 1,500 women, *Circulation* 86 (1992): 839–848.
19. Y. Liao and coauthors, Sex differences in the impact of coexistent diabetes on survival in patients with coronary heart disease, *Diabetes Care* 16 (1993): 708–713.
20. D. Kritchevsky, Variation in plasma cholesterol levels, *Nutrition Today*, September/October 1992, pp. 21–23.
21. L. Bookstein and coauthors, Day-to-day variability of serum cholesterol, triglyceride, and high-density lipoprotein cholesterol levels: Impact on the assessment of risk according to the National Cholesterol Education Program Guidelines, *Archives of Internal Medicine* 150 (1990): 1653–1657.
22. M. Mogadam and coauthors, Within-person fluctuations of serum cholesterol and lipoproteins, *Archives of Internal Medicine* 150 (1990): 1645–1648.
23. R. A. Carleton and coauthors, Report of the Expert Panel on Population Strategies for Blood Cholesterol Reduction, *Circulation* 83 (1991): 2154–2161.
24. Expert Panel on Detection, Evaluation, and Treatment of High Blood Cholesterol in Adults, 1993.
25. *Diet and Health: Implications for Reducing Chronic Disease Risk* (Washington, D.C.: National Academy Press, 1989).
26. R. E. Andersen and coauthors, Relation of weight loss to changes in serum lipids and lipoproteins in obese women, *American Journal of Clinical Nutrition* 62 (1995): 350–357; A. M. Dattilo and P. M. Kris-Etherton, Effects of weight reduction on blood lipids and lipoproteins: A meta-analysis, *American Journal of Clinical Nutrition* 56 (1992): 320–328; R. R. Wing and coauthors, Change in waist-hip ratio with weight loss and its association with change in cardiovascular risk factors, *American Journal of Clinical Nutrition* 55 (1992): 1086–1092.
27. P. M. Clifton and P. J. Nestel, Influence of gender, body mass index, and age on response of plasma lipids to dietary fat plus cholesterol, *Arteriosclerosis and Thrombosis* 12 (1992): 955–962.
28. C. Dubois and coauthors, Chronic oat bran intake alters postprandial lipemia and lipoproteins in healthy adults. *American Journal of Clinical Nutrition* 61 (1995): 325–333; S. R. Glore and coauthors, Soluble fiber and serum lipids: A literature review, *Journal of the American Dietetic Association* 94 (1994): 425–436; C. M. Ripsin and coauthors, Oat products and lipid lowering, *Journal of the American Medical Association* 267 (1992): 3317–3325.
29. P. Knekt and coauthors, Antioxidant vitamin intake and coronary mortality in a longitudinal population study, *American Journal of Epidemiology* 139 (1994): 1180–1189.
30. J. M. Gaziano and coauthors, Moderate alcohol intake, increased levels of high-density lipoprotein and its subfractions, and decreased risk of myocardial infarction, *New England Journal of Medicine* 329 (1993): 1829–1834; P. R. Ridker and coauthors, Association of moderate alcohol consumption and plasma concentration of endogenous tissue-type plasminogen activator, *Journal of the American Medical Association* 272 (1994): 929–933.
31. C. S. Fuchs and coauthors, Alcohol consumption and mortality among women, *New England Journal of Medicine* 332 (1995): 1245–1250.
32. T. A. Pearson and P. Terry, What to advise patients about drinking alcohol—The clinician's conundrum, *Journal of the American Medical Association* 272 (1994): 967–968.
33. G. D. Friedman and A. L. Klatsky, Is alcohol good for your health? *New England Journal of Medicine* 329 (1993): 1882–1883.
34. Inhibition of LDL oxidation by phenolic substances in red wine: A clue to the French paradox? *Nutrition Reviews* 51 (1993): 185–187.
35. R. N. Amarasuriya and coauthors, Ethanol stimulates apolipoprotein A-1 secretion by human hepatocytes: Implications for a mechanism for atherosclerosis prevention, *Metabolism* 41 (1992): 827–832; NIH Consensus Development Panel on Triglyceride, High-Density Lipoprotein, and Coronary

Heart Disease, 1993; Gaziano and coauthors, 1993; Ethanol stimulates apo A-1 secretion in human hepatocytes: A possible mechanism underlying the cardioprotective effect of ethanol, *Nutrition Reviews* 51 (1993): 151–152.

36. A. L. Macnair, Physical activity, not diet, should be the focus of measures for the primary prevention of cardiovascular disease, *Nutrition Research Reviews* 7 (1994): 43–65.
37. P. D. Wood and coauthors, The effects on plasma lipoproteins of a prudent weight-reducing diet, with or without exercise in overweight men and women, *New England Journal of Medicine* 325 (1991): 461–466.
38. Wood and coauthors, 1991.
39. D. Ornish and coauthors, Can lifestyle changes reverse coronary heart disease? The Lifestyle Heart Trial, *Lancet* 336 (1990): 129–133.
40. Expert Panel on Detection, Evaluation, and Treatment of High Blood Cholesterol in Adults, 1993.
41. D. Farley, High blood pressure: Controlling the silent killer, *FDA Consumer*, December 1991, pp. 28–33.
42. K. M. Finta and coauthors, Urine sodium excretion in response to an oral glucose tolerance test in obese and nonobese adolescents, *Pediatrics* 90 (1992): 442–446.
43. P. R. Liebson and coauthors, Echocardiographic correlates of left ventricular structure among 844 mildly hypertensive men and women in the Treatment of Mild Hypertension Study (TOMHS), *Circulation* 87 (1993): 476.
44. Hypertension Prevention Collaborative Research Group, The effects of nonpharmacologic interventions on blood pressure of persons with high normal levels, *Journal of the American Medical Association* 267 (1992): 1213–1220.
45. S. A. Corrigan and coauthors, Weight reduction in the prevention and treatment of hypertension: A review of representative clinical trials, *American Journal of Health Promotion* 5 (1991): 208–214.
46. B. M. Massie, To combat hypertension, increase activity, *The Physician and Sportsmedicine*, May 1992, pp. 89–111.
47. M. H. Keleman and coauthors, Exercise training combined with antihypertensive drug therapy: Effects on blood lipids, blood pressure, and left ventricular mass, *Journal of the American Medical Association* 263 (1990): 2766–2771.
48. Hypertension Prevention Collaborative Research Group, 1992; J. Wylie-Rosett and coauthors, Trial of Antihypertensive Intervention and Management: Greater efficacy with weight reduction than with a sodium-potassium intervention, *Journal of the American Dietetic Association* 93 (1993): 408–415.
49. R. G. Victor and J. Hansen, Alcohol and blood pressure—A drink a day . . . *New England Journal of Medicine* 332 (1995): 1782–1783.
50. J. P. Moran and coauthors, Plasma ascorbic acid concentrations relate inversely to blood pressure in human subjects, *American Journal of Clinical Nutrition* 57 (1993): 213–217; D. L. Trout, Vitamin C and cardiovascular risk factors, *American Journal of Clinical Nutrition* 53 (1991): 322S–325S.
51. Council on Scientific Affairs, American Medical Association, Report of the Council on Scientific Affairs, Diet and cancer: Where do matters stand? *Archives of Internal Medicine* 153 (1993): 50–56.
52. H. Hwang, J. Dwyer, and R. M. Russel, Diet *Heliobacter pylori* infection, food preservation and gastric cancer risk: Are there new roles for preventative factors? *Nutrition Reviews* 52 (1994): 75–83.
53. J. E. Foulke, Urethane in alcoholic beverages under investigation, *FDA Consumer*, January/February 1993, pp. 19–23.
54. G. A. Boissonneault, Calories and carcinogenesis: Modulation by growth factors, in *Nutrition, Toxicity, and Cancer*, ed. I. R. Rowland (Boca Raton, Fla.: CRC Press, 1991), pp. 413–437.
55. R. A. Karmali, Fatty acid metabolism and biochemical mechanisms in cancer, in *Health Effects of Dietary Fatty Acids*, ed. G. J. Nelson (Champaign, Ill.: American Oil Chemists Society, 1991), pp. 150–156.
56. J. H. Weisburger, Nutritional approach to cancer prevention with emphasis on vitamins, antioxidants, and carotenoids, *American Journal of Clinical Nutrition* (supplement) 53 (1991): 226–237.
57. A. T. Diplock, Antioxidant nutrients and disease prevention: An overview, *American Journal of Clinical Nutrition* (supplement) 53 (1991): 189–193.
58. I. T. Johnson, G. Williamson, and S. R. R. Musk, Anticarcinogenic factors in plant foods: A new class of nutrients? *Nutrition Research Reviews* 7 (1994): 175–204.
59. J. Walston and coauthors, Time of onset of non-insulin-dependent diabetes mellitus and genetic variation in the β_3-adrenergic-receptor gene, *New England Journal of Medicine* 333 (1995): 343–347; L. C. Groop and coauthors, Association between polymorphism of the glycogen synthase gene and non-insulin-dependent diabetes mellitus, *New England Journal of Medicine* 328 (1993): 10–14; J. L. Leahy and A. E. Boyd III, Diabetes genes in non-insulin-dependent diabetes mellitus, *New England Journal of Medicine* 328 (1993): 56–57.
60. D. M. Nathan, Long-term complications of diabetes mellitus, *New England Journal of Medicine* 328 (1993): 1676–1685.
61. American Diabetes Association, Nutrition recommendations and principles for people with diabetes mellitus, *Journal of the American Dietetic Association* 94 (1994): 504–506.
62. M. T. Behme, Nicotinamide and diabetes prevention, *Nutrition Reviews* 53 (1995): 137–139.
63. J. Manson and coauthors, A prospective study of exercise and incidence of diabetes among U.S. male physicians, *Journal of the American Medical Association* 268 (1992): 63–67; S. P. Helmrich and coauthors, Physical activity and reduced occurrence of non-insulin-dependent diabetes mellitus, *New England Journal of Medicine* 325 (1991): 147–152.
64. American Diabetes Association Position Statement: Nutrition recommendations and principles for people with diabetes mellitus, *Diabetes Care* 5 (1994): 519–522.

Nutrition, Immunity, and AIDS

Chapter 18 focused on the degenerative diseases that are prevalent in later life, for they are the ones most people have to face today. The present is not like earlier times when *infectious* diseases most often threatened life. Some infectious diseases still threaten people today, however, and nutrition supports defenses against them.

The immune system defends the body so alertly and silently that people are normally not even aware of the thousands of enemy attacks mounted against them every day. If the immune system fails, though, the body suddenly becomes vulnerable to every wayward disease-causing agent that comes its way; infectious disease invariably follows.

Of all the body's systems, the immune system responds most sensitively to subtle changes in nutrition status. When people become ill and are unable to eat well, malnutrition often sets in, compromising immunity. Impaired immunity then opens the way for disease, disease raises nutrient needs and reduces food intake, and nutrition status suffers further. Thus disease and malnutrition create a synergistic downward spiral that must be broken for recovery to occur (see Figure H18–1).

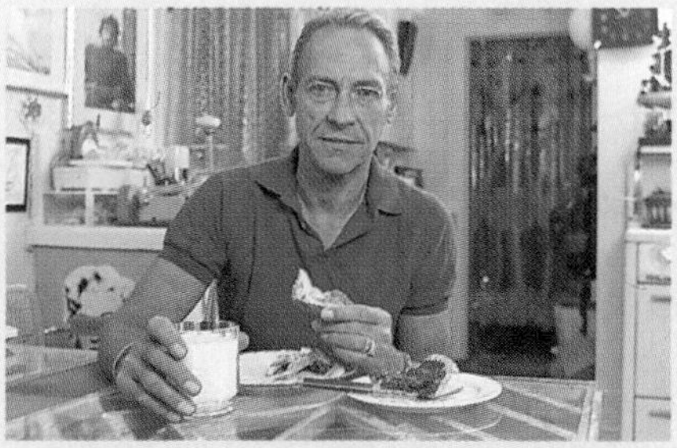

For people with AIDS, nutrition provides an edge in maintaining quality of life and encouraging independence.

This highlight begins with a description of the roles the immune system and nutrition play in the body's defenses against infectious diseases. It then describes the special connections between nutrition and AIDS (acquired immune deficiency syndrome). In contrast to Chapter 18, which described nutrition's role in preventing disease, the discussion on AIDS describes how nutrition can improve the quality of life after people have become ill.

IMMUNITY

The immune system resides in no single organ, but depends on the interactions and secretions of various organs and white blood cells. (The glossary on p. 672 defines related terms.) The body's first lines of defense against foreign substances—the skin, the mucous membranes, and the GI tract—normally deter invaders.

The Skin

The skin is thick and is coated with protective waxes. Furthermore, it is constantly shedding its outermost layers while its associated glands secrete sweat and oily secretions that are toxic to some types of bacteria.

The Mucous Membranes

Mucous membranes line all of the body's openings—eyes, nose, mouth, lungs, GI tract, and genitourinary tract—and secrete a protective coating of mucus. The sticky mucus catches foreign materials and expels them as it continuously flows out of the body. Moreover, it contains antimicrobial chemicals and enzymes that are lethal to invading organisms.

Figure H18–1

Nutrition and Immunity

Malnutrition and infections worsen each other.

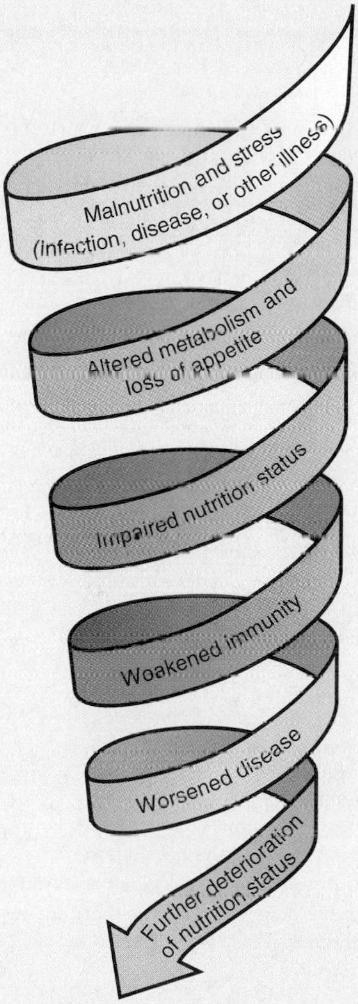

Glossary

acquired immune deficiency syndrome (AIDS): the end stage of HIV infection, in which severe complications are manifested. In the early, symptomless stages, the person is said to have an HIV infection.

AIDS-related complex (ARC): a condition of mild AIDS symptoms that sometimes occurs early in the course of the disease AIDS.

B-cells: lymphocytes that produce antibodies.

cell-mediated immunity: immunity conferred by the reaction of T-cells to an invading organism.

cytokines (SIGH-toe-kines)**:** proteins secreted by phagocytes that activate metabolic and immune responses to infections.

herpes virus: a virus that can lead to mouth lesions and may also affect the lower GI tract, causing diarrhea.

human immunodeficiency virus (HIV): the virus that causes AIDS. The infection progresses to become an immune system disorder that leaves its victims defenseless against numerous infections.

humoral immunity: immunity conferred by antibodies secreted by B-cells and carried to the invaded area by way of the body fluids.
humor = fluid

immune system: the body's natural defense system against foreign materials that have penetrated the skin or mucous membranes.

immunoglobulin: a protein capable of acting as an antibody.

Kaposi's (cap-OH-seez) **sarcoma:** a type of cancer rare in the general population but common in people with HIV infections.

lymphocytes: white blood cells that participate in acquired immunity; *B-cells* and *T-cells*.

nonspecific immunity: immunity directed at many kinds of organisms (also called **general** or **innate immunity**). Phagocytes, the skin, and mucous membranes confer this type of immunity.

opportunistic infections: infections from microorganisms that normally do not cause disease in the general population but can infect people once their immune systems are compromised (as in HIV infection).

phagocytes: white blood cells that have the ability to ingest and destroy foreign substances.
phagein = to eat
kytos = cell

phagocytosis (FAG-oh-sigh-TOE-sis)**:** the process by which phagocytes engulf and destroy foreign materials.
osis = intensive

specific immunity: immunity directed at specific organisms (also called **acquired immunity**). The lymphocytes mediate this type of immunity, which depends on prior exposure, recognition, and reaction to invading organisms. Two types of specific immunity are **cell-mediated immunity** and **humoral immunity**.

T-cells: lymphocytes that attack antigens.

thrush: a fungal infection of the mouth caused by *Candida albicans;* the technical term for this infection is *candidiasis*.

Reminders: *Immunity* is the body's ability to recognize and eliminate foreign invaders. An *antibody* is an immunoglobulin produced by the B-cells in response to invasion of an antigen. An *antigen* is a foreign substance that induces the formation of antibodies. A *synergistic* effect occurs when multiple factors have a greater influence than their combined individual effects.

The GI Tract

The remarkably efficient cells of the GI tract rarely allow microorganisms to pass into the body, even though over 500 species of bacteria normally reside in the intestines.[1] Healthy intestinal cells are crowded so close together that they form a physical barrier. In addition some bacteria in the intestines prevent other more harmful bacteria from multiplying in the body. The action of intestinal bacteria and GI secretions such as saliva, gastric acid, bile, and mucus also prevent harmful substances from entering the body.[2] If an invader penetrates all these barriers and gains entry into the body, then the organs and cells of the immune system race into action.

CELLS OF THE IMMUNE SYSTEM

The immune system depends primarily on the white blood cells. Two types of white blood cells, the phagocytes and lymphocytes, travel over the entire body, but their primary residence is the lymph tissue—the thymus, lymph nodes, spleen, bone marrow, and areas lining the GI tract. Of the 100 trillion cells that make up the human body, one in every hundred is a white blood cell.

Nonspecific Immunity

Phagocytes, the scavengers of the immune system, are the first to arrive at the scene if an invader gains entry. When a phagocyte spots a substance it recognizes as foreign, if engulfs and digests that substance, if it can, in a process called phagocytosis (see Figure H18–2). Phagocytes also secrete proteins that activate

Figure H18–2

Phagocytosis

During phagocytosis, a white blood cell engulfs a foreign substance and eventually surrounds and digests it.

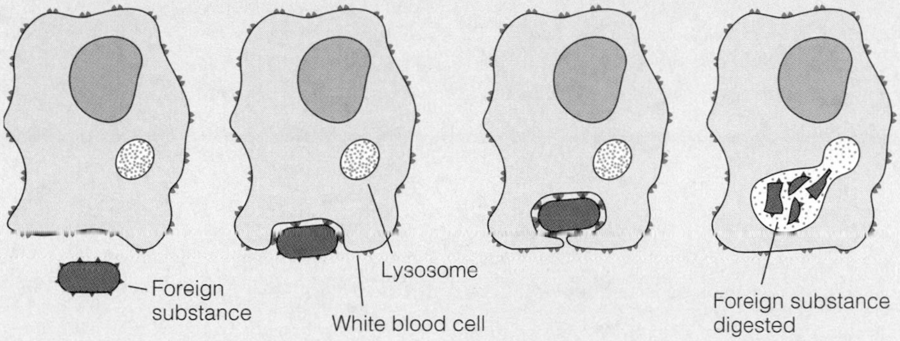

the metabolic and immune responses to infection.*

Some phagocytes perform the special task of facilitating recognition, the hallmark of immunity. Immunity depends on these phagocytes being able to recognize foreign materials and destroy or otherwise neutralize them. As a phagocyte engulfs an invading organism, it detaches a portion of the invading antigen and displays that portion on its own cell surface. The presence of the antigen on the cell's surface activates a special group of lymphocytes. This way, if the phagocytes cannot work fast enough to rid the body of the invader, lymphocytes will be ready to aid in the body's defense.

Specific Immunity

The lymphocytes are of two distinct types: T-cells and B-cells. *T* stands for the thymus gland, where the T-cells are stored for a while; *B* stands for bursa, an organ in the chicken associated with the first identification of the B-cells. The T-cells participate in cell-mediated immunity, so named because the T-cells travel directly to the invasion site to battle the foreign organisms. T-cells recognize the antigens displayed on the surfaces of their partner phagocyte cells and multiply in response. Then they release powerful chemicals to destroy all the foreign particles that have this antigen on their surfaces. As the T-cells begin to win the battle against infection, they release signals to slow down the immune response.

Unlike the phagocytes, which are capable of inactivating many different types of invaders, T-cells are highly specific. Each T-cell can attack only one type of antigen. This specificity is remarkable, for nature creates millions of antigens. After making enough T-cells to destroy a particular antigen, some lymphocytes retain the necessary information to serve as memory cells so that the immune system can rapidly produce the same type of T-cells again should the identical infection recur.

T-cells actively defend the body against fungi, viruses, parasites, and a few types of bacteria; they can also destroy cancer cells. T-cells participate in the rejection of newly transplanted tissues, which is why physicians prescribe immunosuppressive drugs following such surgery. The T-cells are also inactivated by the human immunodeficiency virus that causes AIDS, as explained later.

The B-cells are important in a different type of immunity—humoral immunity, so named because the cells' secretions, not the cells themselves, mount the defensive effort. B-cells respond to infection by rapidly dividing and then producing the large proteins known as antibodies. Antibodies then travel in the bloodstream to the site of the infection. There they stick to the surfaces of the foreign particles and kill or otherwise inactive them, making the foreign particles easy for the phagocytes to ingest.

The antibodies are members of a class of proteins known as immunoglobulins—literally, large globular proteins that produce immunity. Antibodies react selectively to a specific foreign organism just as T-cells do, and the B-cells retain a memory of how to make them. The next time the same foreign organism is encountered, the immune system can respond with greater speed than it did the first time. B-cells play a big-

* The proteins secreted by phagocytes are called *cytokines*. The cytokine *interleukin-1* (in-ter-LOO-kin) activates lymphocytes and is also responsible for the fever-induced anorexia that commonly accompanies an infection. The cytokine *cachectin* (ka-KEK-tin) also induces anorexia. The cytokine *gamma-interferon* (in-ter-FEAR-on) induces the fever and malaise that frequently occur during an infection.

ger role in resistance to infection than do T-cells.

In summary, the body's first line of defense against foreign materials is provided by the skin, the mucous membranes, the GI tract, and various body secretions. Should a microorganism pass these barriers, the immune system calls phagocytes into play. Phagocytes produce chemicals that activate T-cells and display antigens from the unwelcome cells on their surfaces so that the T-cells can recognize and destroy the invader. At the same time, the B-cells secrete specific antibodies that can kill invading organisms directly and also make them easier targets for attack by phagocytes. These changes enable the immune system to respond quickly and forcefully to future exposures. Table H18–1 summarizes the functions of the immune system cells.

THE ROLES OF NUTRIENTS IN IMMUNITY

To function at its best, the immune system must have nutrients available. For this reason, people who suffer from malnutrition develop more infections than well-nourished people. Table H18–2 shows how general malnutrition affects immune system components.

Listed first on the table are the initial barriers a foreign invader encounters when trying to enter the body—the skin and the mucous membranes. During malnutrition the skin becomes thinner with less connective tissue, and the absorptive microvilli of the mucous membranes become flattened. They lose their integrity and permit antigens that would normally be barred to invade the bloodstream. Once antigens are inside, defenses against them are weak.

Malnutrition seems to affect T-cell function more than B-cell function. Cell-mediated immunity, a function of the T-cells, appears to be markedly depressed. People with severe malnutrition consistently are found to have low levels of circulating lymphocytes, and their thymus, spleen, lymph nodes, and lymph-associated areas of the intestinal tract are reduced in size. The areas of the lymph tissues that house the T-cells are depleted of lymphocytes.

Our understanding of the immune system has grown dramatically during the last decade or so as researchers have tried to discover the cause and possible cures for AIDS. This knowledge has unraveled a few of the mysteries surrounding this fatal infection and other immune system disorders as well.

Table H18–1

Functions of Cells of the Immune System

Phagocytes	Lymphocytes	
	T-CELLS (CELL-MEDIATED IMMUNITY)	B-CELLS (HUMORAL IMMUNITY)
Engulf foreign organisms. Activate lymphocytes. Suppress appetite. Induce fever and malaise. Display antigens.	Recognize antigens and send chemical signals. Stimulate T-cell development. Release killer chemicals. Suppress immune response when battle against infection has been won.	Produce antibodies. Kill invaders directly or make them easy targets for phagocytosis.

Table H18–2

Effects of Malnutrition on the Body's Immune System

Immune System Component	Effects of Malnutrition
Skin	Thinned, with less connective tissue
Mucous membranes	Microvilli flattened; antibody secretions reduced
GI tract	Atrophy of intestinal cells
Lymph tissues	Thymus gland, lymph nodes, and spleen reduced in size; T-cell areas depleted of lymphocytes
Phagocytosis	Kill time delayed
Cell-mediated immunity	Circulating T-cells reduced
Humoral immunity	Circulating immunoglobulin levels normal; antibody response possibly impaired

HIV INFECTION AND AIDS

Infection by the human immunodeficiency virus (HIV) eventually causes AIDS, the devastating disorder that affects young and old, rich and poor, urban and rural dwellers, men and women. The only saving grace is that in most cases, HIV infection can be prevented (see Table H18–3). Transmission of the virus requires sexual activity, direct blood contact, or passage of the infection from a mother to her infant during pregnancy, birth, or breastfeeding.

By the year 2000, an estimated 30 to 110 million adults and more than 10 million children worldwide will be infected with HIV. Approximately 25 million adults and several million children will have developed AIDS.[3] As this incidence rises to affect one in every 20 persons worldwide, prevention and treatment of HIV infection will become more and more critical concerns of health care professionals around the world.

Table H18–3

Strategies to Prevent HIV Transmission

HIV is transmitted from one person to another by direct contact with contaminated body fluids, most often through sexual intercourse, through contaminated needles or blood products, or from mother to infant during pregnancy or lactation. To prevent the transmission of HIV infection:

- Avoid sexual contact with anyone with HIV infection.
- Use a latex condom and a spermicidal agent if you have sexual contact with anyone whose sexual history you do not know.
- Do not share toothbrushes, razors, or other implements that could be contaminated with blood.
- Exercise caution when undergoing procedures such as acupuncture, tattooing, or ear piercing, in which needles might be contaminated.
- If you are an IV drug user, seek help for your addiction. Meanwhile, use only sterile, unused needles and dispose of them so that others will not use them. Avoid unprotected sexual contact with others.

Consequences of HIV Infection

HIV infection attacks the immune system and leaves its victims defenseless against opportunistic infections and disorders from which most people are protected. The disorder begins with infection by the virus and progresses in stages. At first, the HIV-infected individual is symptom-free. Later, as the infection progresses, symptoms may include fatigue, skin rashes, fever, diarrhea, muscle pain, night sweats, weight loss, oral lesions, and opportunistic infections. In the final stages, frequent and often fatal complications arise, such as severe weight loss; tuberculosis; recurrent bacterial pneumonia; serious infections of the central nervous system, GI tract, and skin; cancers; and severe diarrhea.

Treatment for HIV Infection

AIDS is a fatal disease. HIV infection has no cure, so prevention is imperative. Currently, treatment can only focus on slowing its course and controlling its symptoms to improve the individual's comfort and quality of life.

THE HIV WASTING SYNDROME

People with HIV infection frequently experience severe protein-energy malnutrition (PEM) and wasting. The wasting often begins early in the disease and becomes progressively worse. People with AIDS lose a lot of weight in the four to five months before death—an amount similar to that seen in people who die from starvation.[4] Some clinicians speculate that the severe wasting itself can cause death in some individuals with AIDS.[5] Even when other complications ultimately cause death, malnutrition contributes either directly or through its adverse effects on the immune system. The combined effects on the immune system of both PEM and HIV infection may hasten the course of the disease. For people with AIDS, malnutrition and weight loss correlate strongly with a diminished survival time.[6]

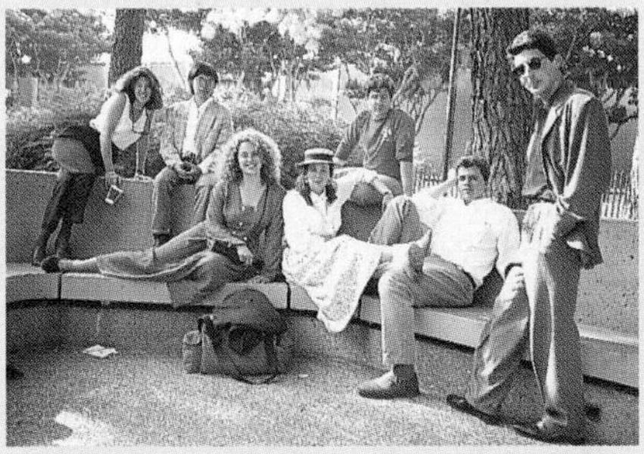

AIDS is the number 1 killer of men, and the number 4 killer of women, ages 25 to 44 years old, in the United States. One out of every five deaths in this age group is caused by AIDS.

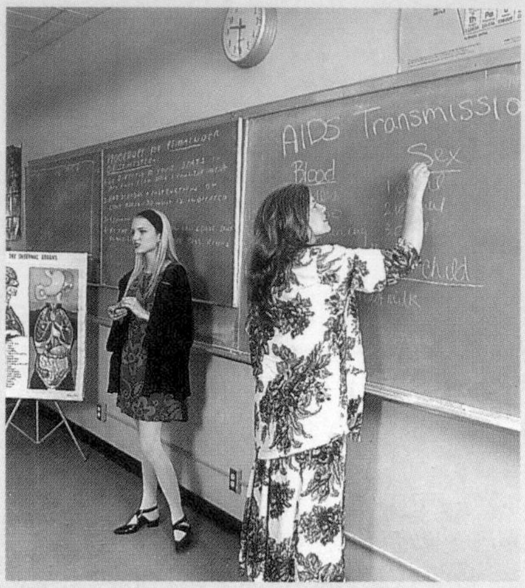

The incidence of AIDS among women has increased dramatically in the United States—through heterosexual relations.

Table H18–4

Causes of Malnutrition in HIV Infections

Reduced Food Intake	Accelerated Nutrient Losses
• Drug therapy causes anorexia, nausea, and vomiting; food aversions arise • Lethargy and exhaustion drain the energy to eat • Fever, pain, and infection cause anorexia • Psychological stresses such as fear and depression make eating seem unimportant • Oral infections (thrush) alter taste sensations, cause pain, and reduce saliva flow • Oral infections (herpes virus) cause painful mouth ulcers and problems with chewing and swallowing • Esophageal infections and lesions make swallowing painful • Respiratory infections and use of oxygen masks make eating difficult • Kaposi's sarcoma (a cancer associated with AIDS) causes esophageal lesions and obstructions	• Cancers of the GI tract and cancer therapy lead to malabsorption • Chronic or recurrent diarrhea interferes with nutrient absorption • Malabsorption limits nutrient absorption • Low serum albumin levels provide too few nutrient carriers • PEM leads to diarrhea and malabsorption • Drug therapy causes diarrhea and malabsorption • High gastric pH limits absorption and promotes bacterial growth, leading to infections **Altered Metabolism** • Infections and fever accelerate metabolism (high BMR) • Cancer accelerates metabolism • Drug therapy interferes with nutrient use

Preventing and treating malnutrition and wasting should be a high priority in the care of HIV-infected people.[7]

Inadequate nutrient intake is the prime determinant of the wasting and malnutrition associated with HIV.[8] Other factors also contribute: excessive nutrient losses, accelerated metabolism, and drug-nutrient interactions. The exact causes of wasting depend on the particular complications each individual develops. Repeated infections and cancer accelerate wasting dramatically. Table H18–4 lists the many factors that lead to malnutrition and progressive wasting in HIV infections.

NUTRIENT SUPPORT FOR HIV INFECTION

Attention to nutrition cannot change the ultimate outcome of HIV infection, but it may slow its progression and improve the quality of life. At a minimum, meeting nutrient needs eliminates the additional stresses posed by malnutrition. Good nutrition status may also improve people's responses to drug therapy, reduce duration of hospital stays, and promote physical independence.[9] Furthermore, it may help people with AIDS to maintain or regain their weight; weight loss need not be inevitable.[10]

Benefits of Early Nutrition Support

A positive test for HIV infection in an individual alerts the health care professional to the need for immediate and aggressive attention to nutrition. Early intervention may detect and correct subclinical deficiencies in preparation for the stresses ahead; it also establishes baseline assessment parameters to assist in monitoring changes in nutrition status. Clinicians can begin to encourage gradual changes in eating habits before such a task becomes monumental for a debilitated person.

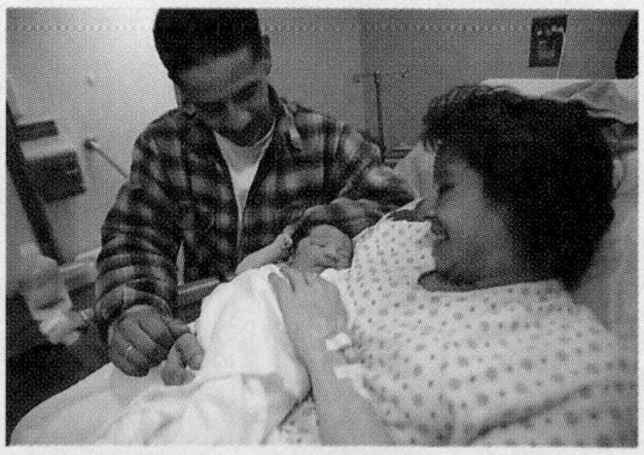
AIDS will leave 72,000 to 125,000 U.S. children orphaned by the year 2000.

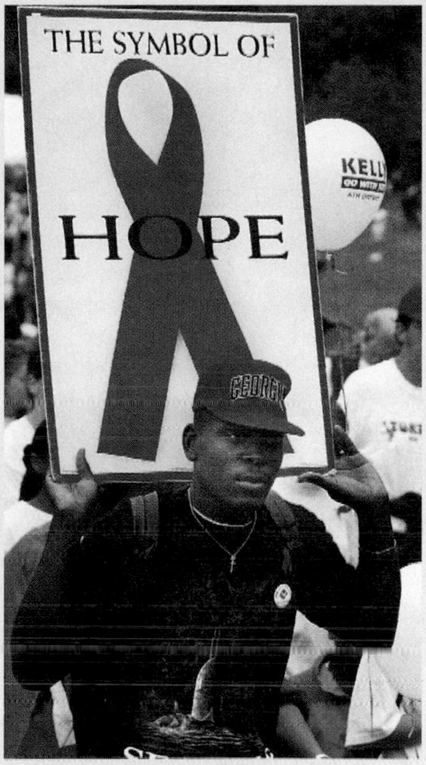

The fight against AIDS, like the fight against cancer, is bolstered by both medical science and people who refuse to give up hope.

Weight loss, reduced percent body fat, and reduced body mass index are early signs of deterioration in people with HIV infections.[11]

Dietary Interventions

A dietary strategy for the treatment of AIDS has not been devised. Instead, practitioners rely on clinical experience to make nutrient recommendations, basing their judgments on the complications that arise in each case. Efforts are aimed primarily at controlling weight loss.[12]

Although the exact vitamin and mineral needs of people with AIDS have not been determined, at least 100 percent of the RDA for these nutrients should be provided daily. People who are unable to eat enough food to provide an adequate intake might benefit from a multivitamin-mineral supplement.[13] Many physicians prescribe a daily prenatal vitamin supplement for people with HIV infections.[14] Individuals who are unable to eat enough food to prevent nutrition complications and unintentional weight loss may need aggressive nutrition support.

Susceptibility to food-borne illnesses requires that the individual with HIV be given written and oral instructions on the safe handling of foods. Chapter 19 describes such precautions. In addition, the Food and Drug Administration (FDA) advises people with HIV infections to avoid eating raw or undercooked seafood.[15]

AIDS is frightening, but in most cases, it can be prevented. It is urgent that every person not yet infected with HIV adopt an effective personal strategy to prevent it from occurring. Review Table H18–3 on p. 675 and call the AIDS hotline for the information you need.*

NOTES

1. J. W. Alexander, Nutrition and translocation, *Journal of Parenteral and Enteral Nutrition* (supplement) 14 (1990): 170–174.
2. B. Langkamp-Henken, J. A. Glezer, and K. A. Kudsk, Immunologic structure and function of the gastrointestinal tract, *Nutrition in Clinical Practice* 7 (1992): 100–108.
3. As cited in an interview with Jonathan Mann, director of the International AIDS Center at Harvard University and one of the authors of a report by the Global AIDS policy coalition, June 1992.
4. D. P. Kotler and coauthors, Magnitude of body-cell-mass depletion and the timing of death from wasting in AIDS, *American Journal of Clinical Nutrition* 50 (1989): 444–447.
5. D. O. Jacobs, Bioelectrical impedance analysis: A way to assess changes in body cell mass in patients with acquired immunodeficiency syndrome? *Journal of Parenteral and Enteral Nutrition* 17 (1993): 401–402.
6. R. T. Chlebowski and coauthors, Nutritional status, gastrointestinal dysfunction and survival in patients with AIDS, *American Journal of Gastroenterology* 84 (1989): 1288–1293.
7. Position of The American Dietetic Association and The Canadian Dietetic Association: Nutrition intervention in the care of persons with human immunodeficiency virus infection, *Journal of the American Dietetic Association* 94 (1994): 1042–1045.
8. D. C. Macallan and coauthors, Energy expenditure and wasting in human immunodeficiency virus infection, *New England Journal of Medicine* 333 (1995): 83–88.
9. Federation of American Societies for Experimental Biology, Nutrition and HIV infection: A review and evaluation of the extant knowledge of the relationship between nutrition and HIV infection, *Nutrition in Clinical Practice* (supplement) 6 (1991): 16–18.
10. D. C. Macallan and coauthors, Prospective analysis of patterns of weight change in stage IV human immunodeficiency virus infection, *American Journal of Clinical Nutrition* 58 (1993): 417–424; C. Parisien, M. D. Gélinas and M. Cossette, Comparison of anthropometric measures of men with HIV: Asymptomatic, symptomatic, and AIDS, *Journal of the American Dietetic Association* 93 (1993): 1404–1408.
11. C. McCorkindale and coauthors, Nutritional status of HIV-infected patients during the early disease stages, *Journal of the American Dietetic Association* 90 (1990): 1236–1241.
12. S. L. Gorbach, T. A. Knox, and R. Roubenoff, Interactions between nutrition and infection with human immunodeficiency virus, *Nutrition Reviews* 51 (1993): 226–234.
13. Task Force on Nutrition Support in AIDS, Guidelines for nutrition support in AIDS, *Nutrition* 5 (1989): 39–46.
14. Department of Continuing Education in Health Sciences, UCLA Extension, *Nutritional Aspects of the AIDS Patient* (Los Angeles, 1989).
15. P. Kurtzweil, Warding off HIV wasting syndrome, *FDA Consumer*, April 1995, pp. 16–20.

* AIDS hotline: (800) 342–AIDS.

Chapter 19

Consumer Concerns About Foods and Water

CONTENTS

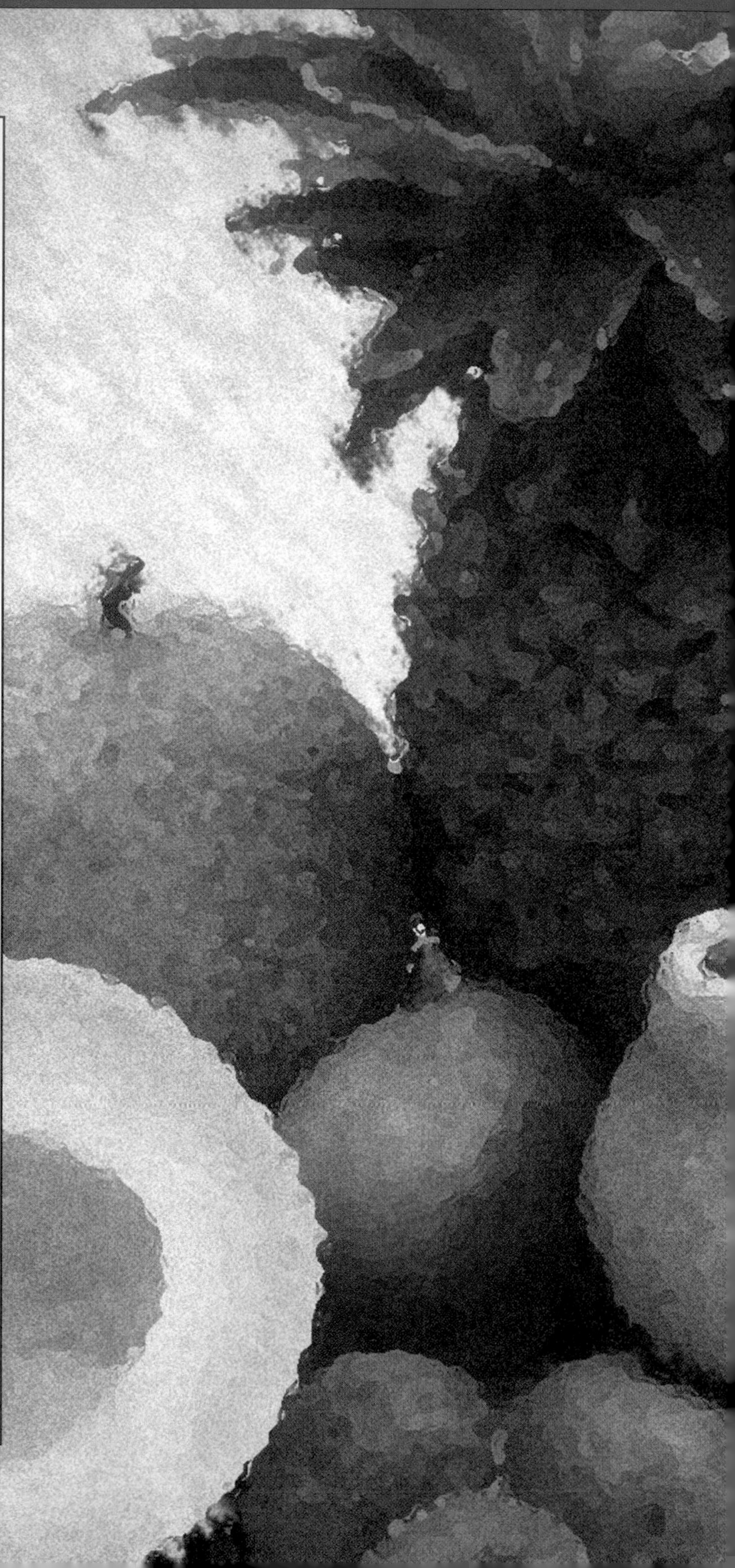

MICROGRAPH: **Capsaicin, the nonnutrient that makes hot peppers hot**

Much of this book has focused on the nutrients in foods and in the body, but no chapter has focused on what is in foods besides nutrients. What causes food poisoning? Are the amounts of contaminants and pesticides found in foods harmful? Are food additives safe? What does public water contain, and is it safe to drink?

This chapter takes up these concerns in the order listed in the margin. This is the order in which the Food and Drug Administration (FDA) has ranked them according to the risks they pose. The rank order of these food hazards is remarkably similar for nations around the world.[1] The chapter closes with a look at public drinking water.

FDA's food safety concerns:

1. Food-borne illnesses.
2. Nutritional adequacy of foods.
3. Environmental contaminants.
4. Naturally occurring toxicants.
5. Pesticide residues.
6. Food additives.

risk: a measure of the probability and severity of harm.

By way of introduction, take a moment to consider the vastness of the task at hand—supplying food to over 250 million people in the United States. To feed this nation requires farmers to grow and harvest crops; dairy producers to supply milk products; ranchers to raise livestock; shippers to deliver foods to manufacturers by land, sea, and air; manufacturers to prepare, process, preserve, and package products for refrigerated food cases and grocery-store shelves; and grocers to store the food and supply it to consumers. After much time, much labor, and extensive transport, an abundant supply of a large variety of safe foods finally reaches consumers at reasonable market prices.

Government and international agencies monitor this huge system using a nationwide network of people and sophisticated equipment. The accompanying glossary identifies the various food regulatory agencies by their acronyms. These agencies focus on the potential hazard of foods, which differs from the toxicity of a substance—a distinction worth understanding. Anything can be toxic. Toxicity simply means that a substance *can* cause harm *if* enough is consumed. We eat lots of things that are toxic, without risk, because the amounts consumed are so

hazard: source of danger; used to refer to circumstances in which toxicity is possible under normal conditions of use.

toxicity: the ability of a substance to harm living organisms. All substances are toxic if high enough concentrations are used.

Glossary of Agencies That Monitor the Food Supply

CDC (Centers for Disease Control): a branch of the Department of Health and Human Services that is responsible for, among other things, monitoring food-borne diseases.

EPA (Environmental Protection Agency): a federal agency that is responsible for, among other things, regulating pesticides and establishing water quality standards.

FAO (Food and Agriculture Organization): an international agency (part of the United Nations) that has adopted standards to regulate pesticide use among other responsibilities.

FDA (Food and Drug Administration): a part of the Department of Health and Human Services' Public Health Service that is responsible for ensuring the safety and wholesomeness of all foods sold in interstate commerce except meat, poultry, and eggs (which are under the jurisdiction of the USDA); inspecting food plants and imported foods; and setting standards for food composition.

USDA (U.S. Department of Agriculture): the federal agency responsible for enforcing standards for the wholesomeness and quality of meat, poultry, and eggs produced in the United States; conducting nutrition research; and educating the public about nutrition.

WHO (World Health Organization): an international agency that has adopted standards to regulate pesticide use among other responsibilities.

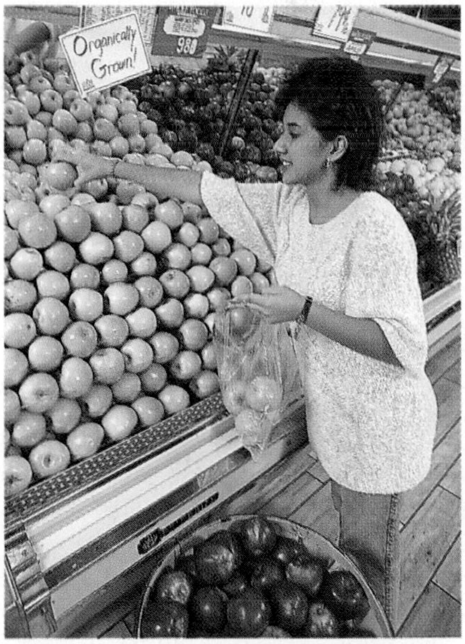

With the benefits of a safe and abundant food supply comes the responsibility to select, prepare, and store foods safely.

small. The term *hazard,* on the other hand, is more relevant to our daily lives because it refers to the harm that is *likely* under real-life conditions. Consumers rely on these monitoring agencies to set sound standards and can learn to protect themselves from food hazards by taking a few preventive steps.

Food-Borne Illnesses

food-borne illnesses: illnesses transmitted to human beings through food, caused by either an infectious agent *(food-borne infection)* or a poisonous substance *(food intoxication)*; commonly known as **food poisoning.**

The FDA lists food-borne illness as the leading food safety concern because episodes of food poisoning far outnumber episodes of any other kind of food contamination. Just about everyone experiences a food-borne illness (whether they realize it or not) at least once a year. Some 6.5 million cases of food-borne illness

Table 19–1

Food-Borne Illnesses

Disease and Organism That Causes It	Most Frequent Food Source	Onset and General Symptoms	Prevention Methods[a]
FOOD-BORNE INFECTIONS			
Campylobacteriosis *Campylobacter jejuni* bacteria	Raw poultry, beef, lamb, unpasteurized milk (foods of animal origin eaten raw or undercooked or recontaminated after cooking).	Onset: 2 to 5 days. Diarrhea, nausea, vomiting, abdominal cramps, fever; sometimes bloody stools; lasts 7 to 10 days.	Cook foods thoroughly; use pasteurized milk; use sanitary food-handling methods.
Giardiasis *Giardia lamblia* protozoa	Contaminated water; uncooked foods.	Onset: 5 to 25 days. Diarrhea (but occasionally constipation), abdominal pain, gas, abdominal distention, digestive disturbances, anorexia, nausea, and vomiting.	Use sanitary food-handling methods; avoid raw fruits and vegetables where protozoa are endemic; dispose of sewage properly.
Hepatitis Hepatitis A virus	Undercooked or raw shellfish.	Onset: 15 to 50 days (28 to 30 days average). Inflammation of the liver with tiredness; nausea, vomiting, or indigestion; jaundice (yellowed skin and eyes from buildup of wastes); muscle pain.	Cook foods thoroughly.
Listeriosis *Listeria monocytogenes* bacteria	Raw meat and seafood, raw milk, and soft cheeses.	Onset: 7 to 30 days. Mimics flu; blood poisoning, complications in pregnancy, and meningitis (stiff neck, severe headache, and fever).	Use sanitary food-handling methods; cook foods thoroughly; use pasteurized milk.
Perfringens food poisoning *Clostridium perfringens* bacteria	Meats and meat products stored at between 120 and 130°F.	Onset: 8 to 12 hr (usually 12). Abdominal pain, diarrhea, nausea, and vomiting; symptoms last a day or less and are usually mild; can be serious in old or weak people.	Use sanitary food-handling methods; cook foods thoroughly; refrigerate foods promptly and properly.
Salmonellosis *Salmonella* bacteria	Raw or undercooked eggs, meats, poultry, milk and other dairy products, shrimp, frog legs, yeast, coconut, pasta, and chocolate.	Onset: 6 to 48 hr. Nausea, fever, chills, vomiting, abdominal cramps, diarrhea, and headache; can be fatal.	Use sanitary food-handling methods; use pasteurized milk; cook foods thoroughly; refrigerate foods promptly and properly.

are reported in the United States each year; millions more go unreported. For some 9000 people each year, the symptoms can be so severe as to cause death.[2] Most vulnerable are the very young, the very old, the sick, and the malnourished. By taking the proper precautions, however, people can minimize their chances of contracting food-borne illnesses.

FOOD-BORNE INFECTIONS AND FOOD INTOXICATIONS

The term *food-borne illness* refers to both infections and intoxications. Table 19–1 summarizes some of the more common food-borne illnesses, their most frequent food sources, general symptoms, and prevention methods.

Disease and Organism That Causes It	Most Frequent Food Source	Onset and General Symptoms	Prevention Methods[a]
FOOD-BORNE INFECTIONS (*continued*)			
Traveler's diarrhea *Escherichia coli* (usually)	Contaminated water, undercooked ground beef, raw foods, imported soft cheeses	Onset: 12 to 18 hr. Loose and watery stools, nausea, bloating, and abdominal cramps	Cook foods thoroughly; use safe, treated water and pasteurized milk; wash fruits and vegetables.
Trichinosis *Trichinella spiralis* parasite	Raw or undercooked pork or wild game (bear). Worms burrow through the body tissues to reach muscle tissue where they remain alive.	Onset: 24 hr. Abdominal pain, nausea, vomiting, diarrhea, and fever. One to two weeks later, muscle pain, low-grade fever, pain on breathing, edema (swelling), skin eruptions, loss of appetite, and weight loss. Drug therapy kills the worms and deaths are rare.	Cook foods thoroughly.
FOOD INTOXICATIONS			
Botulism Botulinum toxin (produced by *Clostridium botulinum* bacteria)	Anaerobic environment of low acidity (canned corn, peppers, green beans, soups, beets, asparagus, mushrooms, ripe olives, spinach, tuna, chicken, chicken liver, liver pâte, luncheon meats, ham, sausage, stuffed eggplant, lobster, and smoked and salted fish).	Onset: 4 to 36 hr. Nervous system symptoms, including double vision, inability to swallow, speech difficulty, and progressive paralysis of the respiratory system; often fatal; leaves prolonged symptoms in survivors.	Use proper canning methods for low-acid foods; avoid commercially prepared foods with leaky seals or with bent, bulging, or broken cans.
Staphylococcal food poisoning Staphylococcal toxin (produced by *Staphylococcus aureus* bacteria)	Toxin produced in meats, poultry, egg products, tuna, potato and macaroni salads, and cream-filled pastries.	Onset: ½ to 8 hr. Diarrhea, nausea, vomiting, abdominal cramps, and fatigue; mimics flu; lasts 24 to 48 hr; rarely fatal.	Use sanitary food-handling methods; cook food thoroughly; refrigerate foods promptly and properly.

[a]The box on pp. 684–685 provides more details on the proper handling, cooking, and refrigeration of foods.

Food-Borne Infections Food-borne infections are caused by eating foods contaminated by infectious microbes. Two of the most common infectious microbes are *Campylobacter jejuni* and *Salmonella*, which enter the GI tract in contaminated foods such as undercooked poultry and unpasteurized milk. Symptoms generally include abdominal cramps, fever, and diarrhea. If a person experiences these symptoms as the major or only symptoms of a bout of "flu," chances are excellent that what the person really has is a food-borne illness.*

Food Intoxications Food intoxications are caused by eating foods containing natural toxins or, more likely, microbes that produce toxins. The most infamous, but not common, example is *Clostridium botulinum*, the organism that produces a deadly toxin in improperly canned foods. Botulism requires immediate medical attention, and even then, survivors may suffer the effects for months or years. An amount of toxin as tiny as a single crystal of salt can kill several people within an hour.

Reminder: *Botulism* is an often-fatal food-borne illness caused by the ingestion of foods containing a toxin produced by bacteria that grow without oxygen in improperly canned nonacidic foods. The **botulinum** (BOT-chew-line-um) **toxin** responsible for botulism is called **botulin** (BOT-chew-lin).

Botulism danger signs:
- Double vision.
- Slurred speech.
- Weakening muscles.
- Difficulty swallowing.
- Difficulty breathing.

pasteurization: a process of heating milk sufficiently to kill many disease-causing microbes commonly transmitted through milk; not a sterilization process. Pasteurized milk retains bacteria that cause milk spoilage. Unpasteurized ("certified" raw) milk transmits many food-borne diseases to people each year and should be avoided.

FOOD HAZARDS IN THE MARKETPLACE

Commercially prepared food is usually safe, but infected food from one major supplier can make thousands of people sick. Milk producers, for example, rely on pasteurization to make milk safe for consumption. When a major dairy in Chicago experienced a flaw in its pasteurization system, over 16,000 confirmed, and as many as 200,000 suspected, cases of food-borne illness resulted. Similarly, some 1000 residents of St. Paul became sick after eating *Samonella*-contaminated ice cream made by a local manufacturer. In another episode, over 100 people in California got sick and 50 of them died of listeriosis from eating contaminated cheese. In still another, a fast-food restaurant in Seattle served burgers tainted with the infectious organism *Escherichia coli*, causing illness in some 500 patrons and at least one child's death. The meat had been improperly handled at the slaughterhouse and undercooked at the restaurant.

Fortunately, such large-scale incidents, though dramatic, make up only a small fraction of total food poisoning cases each year. Most arise from one person's error in a small setting and affect just a few victims. Some people have come to accept a yearly bout or two of intestinal illness as inevitable, but in truth, most of these illnesses can be prevented.

Canned and packaged foods sold in grocery stores are controlled more easily than raw foods, but still, rare accidents do happen. Batch numbering makes it possible for suppliers to recall contaminated foods through public announcements via newspapers, television, and radio. In the grocery store, consumers can carefully inspect the seals, safety "buttons," and wrappers of packages. A broken seal or mangled package fails to protect the product against microbes, insects, spoilage, or even vandalism.

Raw foods from the grocery store, especially meats and poultry, contain microbes. Whether microbes multiply and cause illness depends, in part, on what consumers do or fail to do in their kitchens.

---

*Some viruses do cause intestinal distress, and those that do are usually transmitted via food; true influenza viruses cause symptoms primarily in the upper respiratory tract.

FOOD SAFETY IN THE KITCHEN

Almost one-third of all food-borne illnesses arise from mistakes made in home kitchens.[3] For the most part, these illnesses can be prevented by doing three simple things: keeping hot foods hot; keeping cold foods cold; and keeping hands, utensils, and the kitchen clean.

Keeping hot foods hot includes cooking foods long enough to reach internal temperatures that will kill microbes, keeping them hot enough to prevent bacterial growth until served, and refrigerating them immediately after serving a meal. Keeping cold foods cold entails going directly home upon leaving the grocery store and immediately unpacking foods into the refrigerator or freezer upon arrival. Keeping a clean, safe kitchen requires that cooks wash the countertops, their hands, and utensils in hot, soapy water before and after each step of food preparation. See the box on pp. 684–685 for specific food safety tips.

The "2–40–140" rule will help you to remember the time and temperature danger zone for foods—allow them to stay for no more than 2 hr between 40°F and 140°F.

Meat Meat requires special handling. It contains bacteria, and its moist, nutrient-rich environment favors microbial growth. Ground meat is especially susceptible because it receives more handling than other kinds of meat and has more surface exposed to bacterial contamination. Consumers have no way to detect the harmful bacteria in or on meat. A USDA seal indicates that the product has been inspected for quality. It does not guarantee that the meat is free of potentially harmful bacteria, although the USDA has recently strengthened its inspection system to include microbial testing and prohibit fecal contamination.

When buying meat, consumers take on the responsibility of handling it in such a way that the bacteria present won't cause a food-borne illness (see Figure 19–1). Wash any utensils and surfaces (such as cutting boards or platters) that have been in contact with raw meat with hot, soapy water before using them again for the cooked meat or raw produce. Bacteria inevitably left on the surfaces from the raw meat can recontaminate the cooked meat or start to grow in the other foods—a problem known as *cross-contamination*. Cook meat thoroughly, using a thermometer to test the internal temperature (see Figure 19–2).

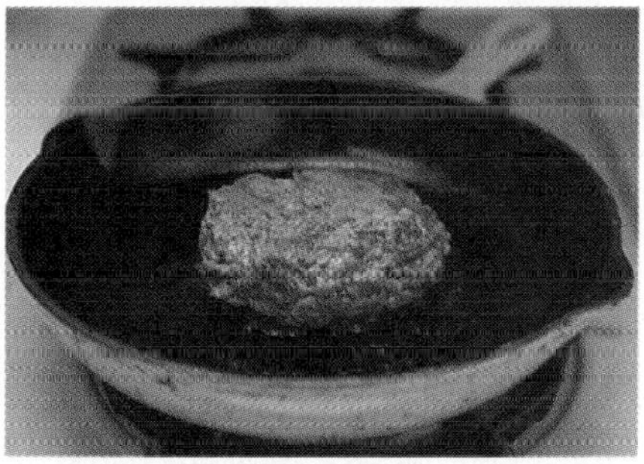

Cook hamburgers until they are brown (not pink) throughout, the juices run clear, and the inside is steaming hot.

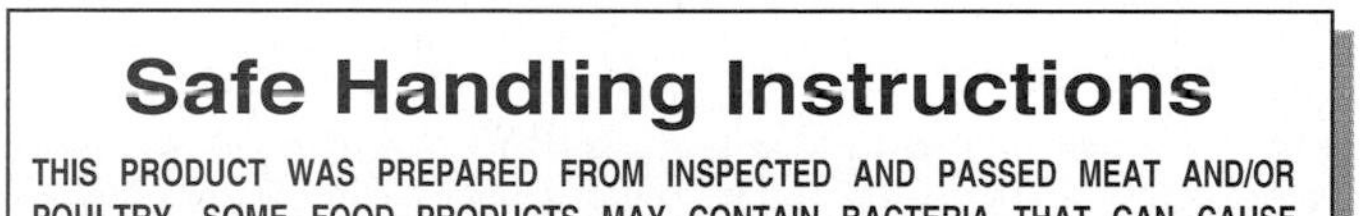
Safe Handling Instructions
THIS PRODUCT WAS PREPARED FROM INSPECTED AND PASSED MEAT AND/OR POULTRY. SOME FOOD PRODUCTS MAY CONTAIN BACTERIA THAT CAN CAUSE ILLNESS IF THE PRODUCT IS MISHANDLED OR COOKED IMPROPERLY. FOR YOUR PROTECTION, FOLLOW THESE SAFE HANDLING INSTRUCTIONS.
KEEP REFRIGERATED OR FROZEN. THAW IN REFRIGERATOR OR MICROWAVE.
KEEP RAW MEAT AND POULTRY SEPARATE FROM OTHER FOODS. WASH WORKING SURFACES (INCLUDING CUTTING BOARDS), UTENSILS, AND HANDS AFTER TOUCHING RAW MEAT OR POULTRY.
COOK THOROUGHLY.
KEEP HOT FOODS HOT. REFRIGERATE LEFTOVERS IMMEDIATELY OR DISCARD.

Figure 19–1

Safe Handling Instructions for Meat and Poultry

Figure 19–2

Safe Internal Temperatures for Cooking Meats and Poultry (Fahrenheit)

Source: USDA, 1993.

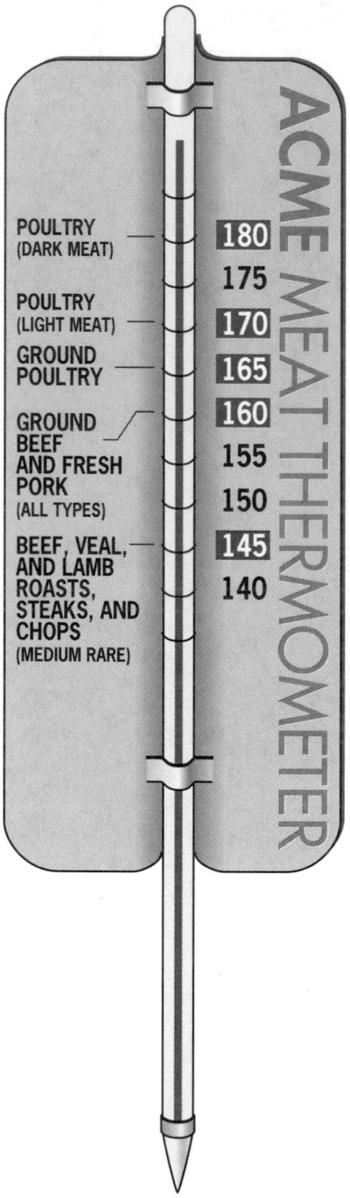

How to Prevent Food-Borne Illnesses

Most food-borne illnesses can be prevented by following three simple rules: keep hot foods hot, keep cold foods cold, and keep a clean kitchen.

Keep Hot Foods Hot

- When cooking meats or poultry, use a thermometer to test the internal temperature. Insert the thermometer between the thigh and the body of a turkey or into the thickest part of other meats, making sure the tip of the thermometer is not in contact with bone or the pan. Cook to the temperature indicated for that particular meat; cook hamburgers to at least medium well-done. If you have safety questions, call the USDA Meat and Poultry Hotline: (800) 535–4555.
- Cook stuffing separately, or stuff poultry just prior to cooking.
- Do not cook large cuts of meats or turkeys in a microwave oven; they leave some parts undercooked while overcooking others.
- Marinate meats in the refrigerator, not on the counter. Don't use marinade that was in contact with raw meat for basting or sauces.
- Cook eggs before eating them (soft-boiled for at least 3½ min; scrambled until set, not runny; fried for at least 3 min on one side and 1 min on the other).
- Cook seafood thoroughly. If you have safety questions call the FDA Seafood Hotline: (800) FDA–4010.
- When serving foods maintain temperatures at 140°F or higher.
- Heat leftovers thoroughly to at least 165°F.

Keep Cold Foods Cold

- When running errands, stop at the grocery store last. When you get home, refrigerate the perishable groceries (such as meats and dairy products) immediately. Do not leave perishables in the car any longer than it takes for ice cream to melt.
- Buy only those foods that are solidly frozen and stored below the frost line in store freezers.
- Keep cold foods at 40°F or less; keep frozen foods at 0°F or less (keep a thermometer in the refrigerator).
- Refrigerate leftovers promptly; use shallow containers to cool foods faster.
- Thaw meats or poultry in the refrigerator, not at room temperature. If you must hasten thawing, use cool running water or a microwave oven.

Keep a Clean and Safe Kitchen

- Wash fruits and vegetables with a scrub brush.
- Use hot, soapy water to wash hands, utensils, dishes, nonporous cutting boards, and countertops. Use a bleach solution on wooden cutting boards.
- Cover cuts with clean bandages before food preparation; dirty bandages carry harmful microorganisms.
- Avoid cross-contamination by washing all surfaces that have been in contact with raw meats, poultry, or eggs before reusing.

- Mix foods with utensils, not hands; keep hands and utensils away from mouth, nose, and hair.
- Anyone may be a carrier of bacteria and should avoid coughing or sneezing over food. A person with a skin infection or infectious disease should not prepare food.
- Wash or replace sponges and towels regularly.
- Clean up food spills and crumb-filled crevices.

In General

- Do not taste food that is suspect. "If in doubt, throw it out."
- Throw out foods with danger-signaling odors. Be aware, though, that most food poisoning bacteria are odorless, colorless, and tasteless.
- Do not buy or use items that appear to have been opened; check safety seals, buttons, and expiration dates.
- Follow label instructions for storing and preparing packaged and frozen foods.
- Discard foods that have decayed or been contaminated by insects or rodents.

For Specific Food Items

- *Canned goods*. Discard food from cans that leak or bulge in a manner that will protect other people and animals from accidentally ingesting it; before canning, seek professional advice from the USDA Extension Service (check your phone book under U.S. government listings, or ask directory assistance).
- *Milk and cheeses*. Use only pasteurized milk and milk products. Aged cheeses, such as cheddar and swiss, do well for an hour or two without refrigeration, but should be refrigerated or stored in an ice chest for longer periods.
- *Eggs*. Use clean eggs with intact shells. Do not eat eggs raw.
- *Honey*. Honey may contain dormant bacterial spores, which can awaken in the human body to produce botulism. In adults, this poses little hazard, but infants under one year of age should never be fed honey. Honey can accumulate enough toxin to kill an infant; it has been implicated in several cases of sudden infant death. (Honey can also be contaminated with environmental pollutants picked up by the bees.)
- *Mayonnaise*. Commercial mayonnaise may actually help a food to resist spoilage because of the acid content. Still, keep it cold after opening.
- *Mixed salads*. Mixed salads of chopped ingredients spoil easily because they have extensive surface area for bacteria to invade, and they have been in contact with cutting boards, hands, and kitchen utensils that easily transmit bacteria to food (regardless of their mayonnaise content). Chill them well before, during, and after serving.
- *Picnic foods*. Choose foods that last without refrigeration such as fresh fruits and vegetables, breads and crackers, and canned spreads and cheeses that can be opened and used immediately. Pack foods cold, layer ice between foods, and keep foods out of water.

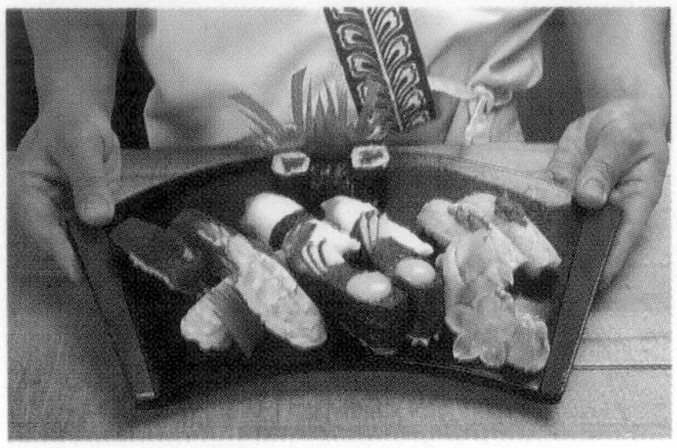

Eating raw seafood is a risky proposition even if it is prepared in sushi by a master chef.

sushi: vinegar-flavored rice and seafood, typically wrapped in seaweed and stuffed with colorful vegetables. Some sushi is stuffed with raw fish; other varieties contain only cooked ingredients.

Seafood Most seafoods available in the United States and Canada are safe, but eating undercooked seafood or raw seafood can cause severe illnesses—hepatitis, worms, parasites, viral intestinal disorders, and other diseases. The microorganisms in raw seafood are undetectable, even to an expert. Rumor has it that freezing fish will make it safe to eat raw, but this is only partly true. Freezing fish will kill mature parasitic worms, but only cooking can kill all worm eggs and other microorganisms that can cause illness. For safety's sake, all seafood should be cooked. Even sushi can be enjoyed this way: many sushi chefs combine cooked seafood, vegetables, avocado, and other ingredients into delicacies that are perfectly safe to enjoy.

At least 10 species of bacteria found in raw oysters cause illness in people. Raw oysters may also carry the hepatitis A virus, which can cause liver disease. Some hot sauces can kill many of these bacteria, but not the virus; alcohol may also protect against oyster-borne illnesses, but not completely. One study reported that among people who had eaten contaminated oysters, those who consumed an alcoholic beverage were less likely to have gotten sick, or their symptoms were less severe, than those who had not consumed alcoholic beverages.[4] Of course, this is not sufficient evidence to guarantee protection or to recommend drinking alcohol.

Frequently unsafe:
- Raw milk.
- Raw or undercooked seafood, meat, or eggs.

Occasionally unsafe:
- Soft cheeses (Mexican style, feta, brie, camembert, blue-veined).
- Salad bar items.
- Unwashed berries and grapes.
- Sandwiches.
- Hamburgers.
- Airline food.

Rarely unsafe:
- Peeled fruit.
- High-sugar foods.
- Steaming-hot foods.

As population density increases along the shores of seafood-harvesting waters, pollution inevitably invades the seafood living there. Watchdog agencies monitor commercial fishing waters to keep harvesters out of contaminated areas, but some unwholesome foods taken illegally from closed harvesting areas do reach the market.[5] Preventing seafood-borne illness is in large part a task of controlling water pollution.

Chemical pollution and microbial contamination lurk not only in the water, but in the boats and warehouses where seafood is cleaned, prepared, and refrigerated. Seafood is one of the most perishable foods: time and temperature are critical to its freshness and flavor. To keep seafood as fresh as possible, people in the industry "keep it cold, keep it clean, and keep it moving."[6] Wise consumers eat it cooked.

Precautions and Procedures Fresh food generally smells fresh. Not all types of food poisoning are detectable by odor, but some bacterial wastes produce "off" odors. If an abnormal odor exists, the food is spoiled. Throw it out or, if it was recently purchased, return it to the grocery store. Do not taste it. Table 19–2 lists safe storage times for selected foods.

Local health departments and the USDA Extension Service can provide further information about food safety. Should precautions fail and mild food-borne illness develop, drink clear liquids to replace fluids lost through vomiting and diarrhea. If serious food-borne illness is suspected, first call a physician. Then wrap the remainder of the suspected food and label its container so that it cannot be mistakenly eaten, place it in the refrigerator, and hold it for possible inspection by health authorities.

Call a doctor if you develop these potentially dangerous conditions:
- Bloody diarrhea.
- A stiff neck, severe headache, and fever (signs of meningitis).
- Excessive diarrhea or vomiting.
- Any food poisoning symptoms that last longer than 3 days.

biosensor: a genetically altered microbe that provides a rapid, low-cost, and accurate test for the products of spoilage in foods.

New advances in biotechnology offer promise for the future purity of foods, and especially of seafoods. Geneticists can couple a strand of synthetic DNA with one from bacteria to create a combined version that possesses a new talent—the hybrid is a biosensor that can detect chemicals that disease-causing microorganisms produce in foods.[7] These biosensors surpass today's methods in their sensitivity, simplicity, and reliability in detecting harmful organisms.[8]

How to Achieve Food Safety while Traveling

Food-borne illnesses contracted while traveling are colloquially known as traveler's diarrhea. A bout of this ailment can ruin the most enthusiastic tourist's trip. To avoid food-borne illness while traveling:

- Wash your hands often with soap and water, especially before handling food or eating.
- Eat only cooked or canned foods. Eat raw fruits or vegetables only if you have washed them in boiled water and peeled them yourself. Skip salads and raw fish and shellfish.
- Be aware that water, and ice made from it, may be unsafe. Take along disinfecting tablets or a device to boil water. Do not use the local water supply, even to brush your teeth, unless you boil or disinfect it first. Do not use ice.
- Drink no beverages made with tap water. Drink only treated, boiled, canned, or bottled beverages, and drink them without ice, even if they are not chilled to your liking. Refuse dairy products unless they have been properly pasteurized and refrigerated.
- Before you leave on the trip, ask your physician to recommend medicines to take with you in case your efforts to avoid illness fail.

One journalist succinctly sums up these recommendations, "Boil it, cook it, peel it, or forget it."[a] Chances are excellent that if you follow these rules, you will remain well.

[a]R. D. Williams, Boil it, cook it, peel it or forget it, *FDA Consumer*, September 1991, p. 17.

Table 19–2

Safe Refrigerator Storage Times (40°F)

1 to 2 days	Raw ground meats, breakfast or other raw sausages, raw fish or poultry; gravies
3 to 5 days	Raw steaks, roasts, or chops; cooked meats, vegetables, and mixed dishes; ham slices; mayonnaise salads (chicken, egg, pasta, tuna)
1 week	Hard-cooked eggs, bacon or hot dogs (opened packages); smoked sausages
2 to 4 weeks	Raw eggs (in shells); bacon or hot dogs (packages unopened); dry sausages (pepperoni, hard salami); most aged and processed cheeses (swiss, brick)
2 months	Mayonnaise (opened jar); most dry cheeses (parmesan, romano)

Sources: A. Hecht, Preventing food-borne illnesses, *FDA Consumer,* January/February 1991, p. 21; Refrigerator storage times for selected foods, *Consumer Reports on Health,* December 1991, p. 93.

Someday their use may dramatically improve the safety of fish and other foods for sale on the market.

FOOD SAFETY WHILE TRAVELING

People who travel to other countries have a 50–50 chance of contracting traveler's diarrhea. Like many other food-borne illnesses, traveler's diarrhea is a sometimes serious, always annoying bacterial infection of the digestive tract. The risk is high because, for one thing, some countries' cleanliness standards for food and water may be lower than those in the United States and Canada. For another, every region's microbes are different, and while people are immune to those in their own neighborhoods, they have had no chance to develop immunity to the pathogens in places they are visiting for the first time. The accompanying box offers tips to travelers on avoiding food-borne infections.

pathogens (PATH-oh-jens): microorganisms or substances capable of producing disease.

In summary, millions of people suffer from mild to life-threatening symptoms caused by food-borne illnesses. As the box on pp. 684–685 describes, most of these illnesses can be prevented by storing and cooking foods at their proper temperatures and by preparing them in sanitary conditions.

Nutritional Adequacy of Foods and Diets

Among the FDA's priority concerns, the nutritional adequacy of foods and diets ranks second only to food-borne illness. In years past, when most foods were whole and farm fresh, the task of meeting nutrient needs primarily involved balancing servings from the various food groups. Today, however, foods have changed. Many "new" foods are available to appeal to people's tastes and health needs, but not necessarily to deliver a balanced assortment of needed nutrients.

To assist consumers in finding their way among these foods, the FDA has developed extensive nutrition labeling regulations intended to help consumers combine foods into healthful diets, as Chapter 2 described. In addition, the USDA's dietary guidelines help consumers "eat to stay healthy," and the Food Guide Pyramid helps them to put those recommendations into practice (see Chapter 2).

Environmental Contaminants

The third concern, environmental contamination of foods, is growing in importance as the world becomes more populated and more industrialized. A food contaminant is anything that does not belong there.

contaminant: a substance that does not normally occur in a food.

HARMFULNESS OF ENVIRONMENTAL CONTAMINANTS

The potential harmfulness of a contaminant depends in part on its persistence—the extent to which it lingers in the environment or in the body. Some contaminants in the environment are short-lived because microorganisms or agents such as sunlight or oxygen can break them down. Some contaminants in the body may linger for only a short time because the body rapidly excretes them or metabolizes them to harmless compounds. These contaminants present little cause for concern. Some contaminants, however, resist breakdown and can accumulate. Each level of the food chain, then, has a greater concentration than the one below (bioaccumulation). Figure 19–3 shows how bioaccumulation leads to high concentrations of toxins in people at the top of the food chain, and Figure 19–4 (on p. 690) shows how contaminants find their way into food.

How much of a threat do environmental contaminants pose to the food supply? For the most part, the hazards appear to be small because the FDA regulates the presence of contaminants in foods and requires foods with unsafe amounts to be removed from the market. In the event of an accidental spill, however, the hazards can suddenly become great.

persistence: stubborn or enduring continuance; with respect to food contaminants, the quality of persisting, rather than breaking down, in the bodies of animals and human beings.

food chain: the sequence in which living things depend on other living things for food.

bioaccumulation: the accumulation of contaminants in the flesh of animals high on the food chain.

EXAMPLES OF ENVIRONMENTAL CONTAMINANTS

The following paragraphs describe how two different types of contaminants have found their way into the food supply in the past. One is a heavy metal that was released into waterways by industry and ingested by fish that people ate. The other is an organic halogen that was accidentally spilled into livestock feed and ingested by animals that people ate.

heavy metal: any of a number of mineral ions such as mercury and lead, so called because they are of relatively high atomic weight. Many heavy metals are poisonous.

organic halogen: an organic compound containing one or more atoms of a **halogen**—fluorine, chlorine, iodine, or bromine.

Figure 19–3

Bioaccumulation of Toxins in the Food Chain

If none of the chemicals are lost along the way, one person ultimately receives all of the toxic chemicals that were present in the original several tons of producer organisms.

4 A person whose principal animal-protein source is fish may consume about 100 pounds of fish in a year.

3 These fish consume a few tons of plankton-eating fish in the course of their lifetimes and the toxic chemicals become more concentrated.

2 The toxic chemicals become more concentrated in the plankton-eating fish that consume several tons of producer organisms in their lifetimes.

1 Producer organisms may become contaminated with toxic chemicals.

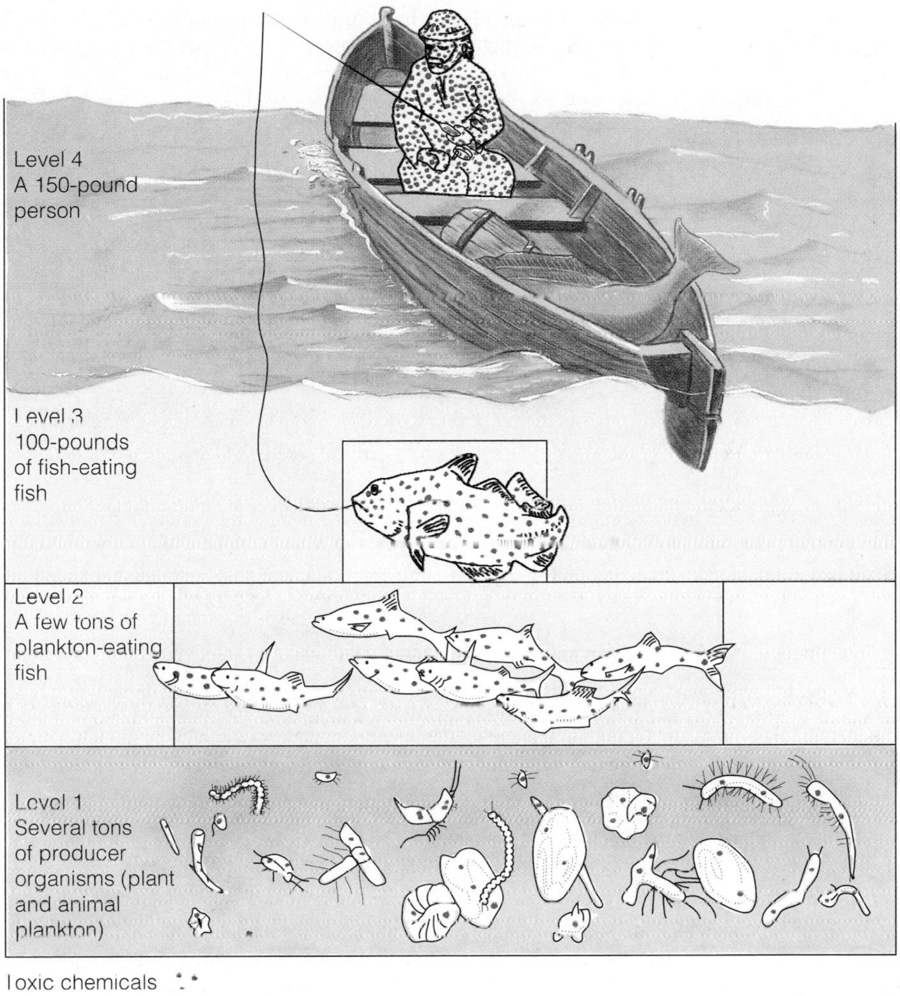

Methylmercury A classic example of acute contamination occurred in 1953 when a number of people in Minamata, Japan, became ill with a disease no one had seen before. By 1960, 121 cases had been reported, including 23 in infants. Mortality was high; 46 died, and the survivors suffered blindness, deafness, incoordination, and intellectual deterioration. The cause was ultimately revealed to be methylmercury contamination of fish from the bay where these people lived. The infants who contracted the disease had not eaten any fish, but their mothers had, and even though the mothers exhibited no symptoms during their pregnancies, the poison had been affecting their unborn babies. Manufacturing plants in the region were discharging mercury into the waters of the bay, the mercury was turning to methylmercury on leaving the factories, and the fish in the

Figure 19–4

Contaminants Find Their Way into Foods

Heavy metals and other contaminants entering the air in smokestack emissions return to the soil in rainfall. Contaminants in the soil are absorbed by plants. People either eat the plants (fruits and vegetables) or the meat from livestock that have eaten the plants. Sewage sludge and pesticides leave residues in the soil; runoff pollutes ground and surface water and contaminates the seafood that people eat.

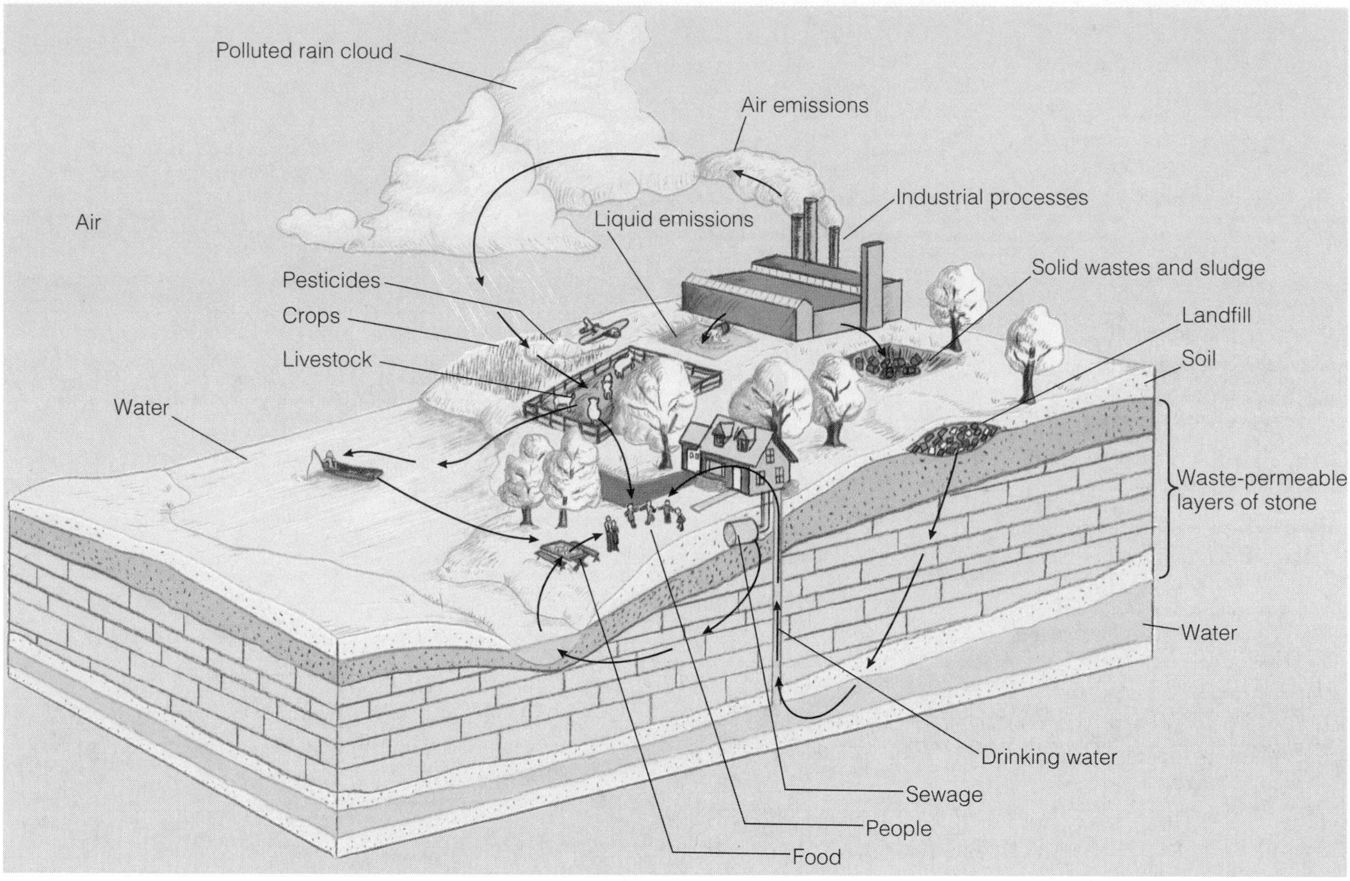

bay were accumulating this poison in their bodies. Some of the affected families had been eating fish from the bay every day.

PBB In 1973, in Michigan, half a ton of polybrominated biphenyl (PBB), a toxic organic compound, was accidentally mixed into some livestock feed that was distributed throughout the state. The chemical found its way into millions of animals and then into people who ate the meat. The seriousness of the accident began to come to light when dairy farmers reported their cows were going dry, aborting their calves, and developing abnormal growths on their hooves. Although more than 30,000 cattle, sheep, and swine and more than a million chickens were destroyed, an estimated 97 percent of Michigan's residents had been exposed to PBB. Some of the exposed farm residents suffered nervous system aberrations and liver disorders.

Methylmercury and PCB (polychlorinated biphenyl, a compound similar to PBB) are still found in our food supply today. Fish harvested from contaminated waters have relatively high amounts of these two pollutants. Thousands of other contaminants exist as well; Highlight 19 focuses on the heavy metal lead and its toxic effects.

To briefly sum up, environmental contamination of foods is a growing concern, but so far, the hazards appear small. In all cases, two principles apply: First, remain alert to the possibility of contamination of foods, and keep an ear open for public health announcements and advice. Second, do not eat any one food too often; vary your choices. Switching from food to food is an effective defensive strategy against the accumulation of toxins in your body. This is the principle of dilution: each food eaten dilutes contaminants that may be present in other components of the diet.

Natural Toxicants in Foods

Consumers concerned about food contamination may naively think that they can eliminate all poisons from their diets by eating only "natural" foods. On the contrary, nature has provided plants with an abundant array of toxicants. A few examples will show how even "natural" foods may contain potentially harmful substances. They also show that while the *potential* for harm exists, actual harm rarely occurs.

Poisonous mushrooms are a familiar example of plants that everyone knows can be harmful when eaten. Few people know, though, that other foods they commonly eat contain substances that can cause illnesses. Cabbage, turnips, mustard greens, and radishes contain small quantities of goitrogens—compounds that can enlarge the thyroid gland. Eating exceptionally large amounts of goitrogen-containing vegetables can aggravate a preexisting thyroid problem, but usually does not initiate one.

Reminder: *Goitrogens* are thyroid antagonists found in such foods as cabbage, kale, brussels sprouts, cauliflower, broccoli, and kohlrabi.

Lima beans and fruit seeds such as apricot pits contain cyanogens—inactive compounds that produce the deadly poison cyanide upon activation by a specific plant enzyme. For this reason, many countries restrict commercially grown lima beans to those varieties with the lowest cyanogen contents. As for fruit seeds, they are seldom deliberately eaten. An occasional swallowed seed or two presents no danger, but a couple of dozen seeds can be fatal to a small child. Perhaps the most infamous cyanogen in seeds is laetrile—a compound erroneously represented as a cancer cure. True, laetrile kills cancer, but only at doses that kill the person, too. Research over the past 100 years has never proven laetrile to be an effective cancer treatment. In fact, laetrile is more dangerous than no treatment at all. The combination of cyanide poisoning and lack of medical attention is life threatening.

Potatoes contain many natural poisons including solanine—a powerful narcotic-like substance. The small amounts of solanine normally found in potatoes are harmless, but solanine is toxic and presents a hazard when consumed in large quantities. Solanine production increases when potatoes are improperly stored in the light and in either very cold or fairly warm places. Cooking does not destroy solanine, but because most of a potato's solanine is in the green layer that develops just beneath the skin, it can be peeled off, making the potato safe to eat.

solanine (SO-lah-neen)**:** a poisonous narcotic-like substance present in potato peels and sprouts. Physical symptoms of solanine poisoning include headache, vomiting, abdominal pain, diarrhea, and fever; neurological symptoms include apathy, restlessness, drowsiness, confusion, stupor, hallucinations, and visual disturbances.

To review, natural toxicants include the goitrogens in cabbage, cyanogens in lima beans, and solanine in potatoes. These examples of naturally occurring toxicants illustrate two familiar principles. First, any substance can be toxic when consumed in excess. Second, poisons are poisons, whether made by people or by nature. Remember: it is not the source of a chemical that makes it hazardous, but its chemical structure and the quantity consumed.

Pesticides

pesticides: chemicals used to control insects, diseases, weeds, fungi, and other pests on plants, vegetables, fruits, and animals. Used broadly, the term includes herbicides (to kill weeds), insecticides (to kill insects), and fungicides (to kill fungi).

residues: whatever remains. In the case of pesticides, those amounts that remain on or in foods when people buy and use them.

Efforts to manage pests using a combination of natural pesticides and biological controls are presented in Highlight 20.

The use of pesticides is controversial. They do help to ensure the survival of some crops, but they leave residues in the environment and on some of the foods we eat.

Ideally, a pesticide would destroy the pest, not accumulate in the food chain, and quickly degenerate to nontoxic products. Then by the time consumers ate the food, no harmful residues would remain. Unfortunately, no such perfect pesticide exists. Developing new pesticides and monitoring their use are ongoing activities that require continued vigilance on the part of government agencies.

Hazards of Pesticides Many pesticides are broad-spectrum poisons that damage all living cells, not just those of pests. Their use, therefore, is hazardous to those who work with them: manufacturers, field workers, truck drivers, and anyone else who is exposed to them. The danger of misuses or accidental spills is ever present, despite safety regulations and precautions.

Consumers have reason to be concerned, too, because pesticides may linger in the foods to which they were applied in the field.[9] Health risks from pesticide exposure are probably small for healthy adults, but children may be vulnerable to some types of pesticide poisoning.[10] The FDA, EPA, and USDA are considering proposals to revise food safety and pesticide laws to protect infants and children from pesticide risks.[11] When setting tolerance levels, the agencies will first identify foods that children commonly eat in large amounts and then consider the effects of pesticide exposure during developmental stages.[12]

tolerance level: the maximum amount of a residue permitted in a food when a pesticide is used according to label directions.

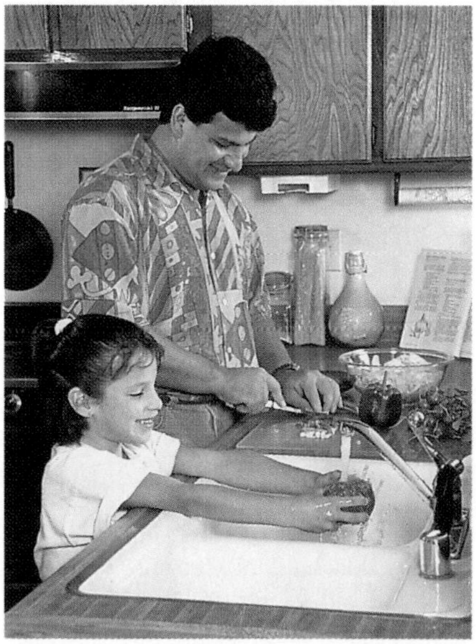

Washing fresh fruits and vegetables removes most, if not all, of the pesticide residues that might have been present.

Whether consumers are ingesting pesticide residues depends on a number of factors. How much of a given food is the consumer eating? What pesticide was used in it? How much was used? How long ago was the food last sprayed? Did environmental conditions promote pest growth or pesticide breakdown? How well was the produce washed? Was it peeled or cooked? With so many factors, consumers cannot know for sure whether any pesticide residues remain on foods.

Regulation of Pesticides Consumers depend on the EPA and the FDA to keep pesticide use within safe limits. These two agencies have joint responsibility for registering pesticides and regulating their use. To register a pesticide, the manufacturer submits results of studies on its biological effects, persistence in crops, and environmental fate to the EPA. The EPA then evaluates the risks and benefits of the pesticide's use by asking such questions as, How dangerous is it? How much residue is left in the crop? How much harm does the pesticide do to the environment? How necessary is it? What are the alternatives to its use?

If the pesticide is approved, the EPA registers the chemical and establishes a tolerance level for its presence in foods, well below that at which it could cause any conceivable harm. Tolerance levels are generally 1/100 to 1/1000 the amount that caused "no effect" in laboratory animals; actual residues may be much lower than that. Tolerance regulations also state the specific crops for which each pesticide can be used. If a pesticide is misused, growers risk fines, lawsuits, and destruction of their crops.

Once tolerances are set, the FDA enforces them by monitoring foods and livestock feeds for the presence of pesticides. In 25 years of testing, the FDA has seldom found residues above tolerance levels, so it appears that pesticides are generally used according to regulations. Minimal pesticide use means lower costs for growers. In addition to costs, many farmers are concerned about the environment, the quality of their farmland, and a safe food supply. Where violations are found, they are usually due to unusual weather conditions, use of unapproved pesticides, or misuse—for example, use of a particular pesticide on a crop for which it has not been approved.

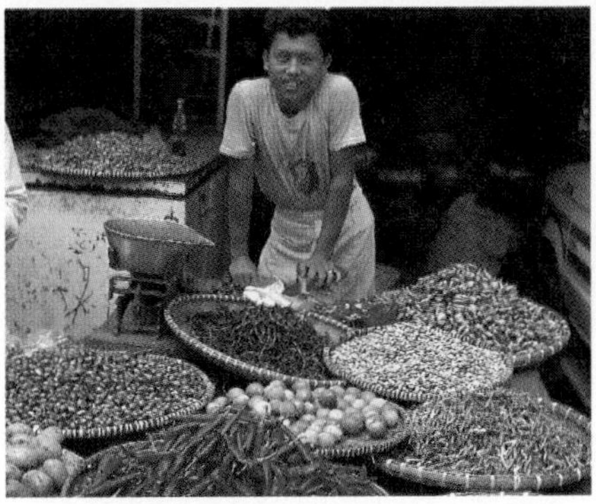

Foods imported from other countries may contain residues of pesticides that are banned from use here.

Pesticides from Other Countries Regulations in foreign countries differ from those in the United States. Imported foods may contain both pesticides that have been banned in this country and permitted pesticides at concentrations higher than are allowed in domestic foods. A loophole in federal regulations allows U.S. companies to manufacture and sell, to other countries, pesticides that are banned in this country. The banned pesticides then return to the United States on imported foods—a circuitous route that concerned consumers have called the "circle of poison." Federal inspectors do monitor imported foods and refuse entry if they are found to contain illegal residues.

Monitoring Pesticides: Food in the Fields The FDA collects and analyzes samples of both domestic and imported foods. If the agency finds samples in violation of regulations, it can seize the products or order them destroyed. The FDA may also invoke a certification requirement that forces manufacturers, at their own expense, to have their foods periodically inspected and certified safe by an independent testing agency. Individual states can also scan for pesticides (as well as for industrial chemicals) and share information with the FDA.

certification: the process in which a private laboratory inspects shipments of a product for selected chemicals and then, if the product is free of violative levels of those chemicals, issues a guarantee to that effect.

In addition to its ongoing surveillance, the FDA also conducts selective surveys to determine the presence of particular pesticides in specific crops. For example, selective surveys for one year included a search for aldicarb in potatoes, captan in cherries, and diaminozide (the chemical name for Alar) in apples, among others. Actions taken that year required several certifications. Thus one shipper in Australia had to certify apples, one in Canada, peppers; one in Costa Rica, chayotes; eight in the Dominican Republic, eggplant; 11 in Spain, lemons; and there were other similar actions. All grapes from Mexico had to be certified and so did all mangoes from anywhere. This shows, incidentally, how many foods come from abroad—not only those already named, but also bitter melons, long beans, okra, snow peas, squash, broccoli, coriander, cucumbers, grapes, strawberries, and currants—and that the FDA monitors them as carefully as it does the domestic food supply.

Monitoring Pesticides: Food on the Plate In addition to monitoring foods in the field for pesticides, the FDA also monitors people's actual intakes. The agency conducts the Total Diet Study (sometimes called the "Market Basket Survey") to estimate the dietary intakes of pesticide residues by eight age and sex groups from infants to senior citizens. Four times a year, FDA surveyors buy over 200 foods from U.S. grocery stores, each time in several cities, prepare the foods table ready, and then analyze them not only for pesticides, but for essential minerals, industrial chemicals, heavy metals, and radioactive materials. In all, the survey reports on over 10,000 samples a year, and recently more than half have been imported foods. Most heavily sampled are fresh vegetables, then fruits, and then dairy foods.

The Total Diet Study provides a direct estimate of the amounts of pesticide residues that remain in foods as they are usually eaten—after they have been washed, peeled, and cooked. The FDA finds the intake of almost all pesticides to be less than 1 percent of the amount considered acceptable. The amount considered acceptable is "the daily intake of a chemical which, if ingested over a lifetime, appears to be without appreciable risk"; it is established by the United Nations Food and Agriculture Organization and the World Health Organization. All in all, these findings corroborate "the continuing safety of the U.S. food supply relative to pesticide residues."[13]

safety: a judgment that considers the risks acceptable.

Consumer Concerns Despite these reassuring reports, consumers still worry that the monitoring of foods may not be adequate. For one thing, new pesticides keep appearing before the EPA can evaluate and register them. For another, as described, other countries use pesticides that are illegal for use here. For still another, although the regulations described here may protect U.S. foods adequately, they do not necessarily protect the environment or the people who work with them nearly as well. Concerns over poisoning of soil, waterways, wildlife, and workers may well be valid.

The FDA does not sample *all* food shipments and test for *all* pesticides in each sample. Budget constraints limit the FDA to fewer than 700 inspectors and scientists nationwide to test food samples from a multitude of farms, groves, docks, airports, warehouses, and processing plants. The FDA is a *monitoring* agency, and as such, it cannot, nor can it be expected to, guarantee 100 percent safety in the food supply. Instead, it sets conditions so that substances do not become a hazard, checks enough samples to adequately assess average food safety, and acts promptly when problems or suspicions arise.

Minimizing Risks Consumers must assume some responsibility for their own health and safety with respect to pesticides. They can learn about the potential benefits and possible dangers of pesticide use, discuss regulations and alternatives with others, advise their government representatives of their findings, and apply pressure wherever it will help change procedures. Meanwhile, people can minimize their risks by following the guidelines offered in the accompanying box.

In addition to the suggestions in the box, consumers can buy fresh foods grown locally, especially when they can confirm that produce has been grown using responsible methods. Consumers who want pesticide-free produce shouldn't look for "perfect" fruits and vegetables; pesticide-free produce may have a few blemishes, but minor blemishes are not a hazard. It is also important to buy a variety of foods and not to rely too heavily on any one. The food supply is protected well enough that consumers who take these precautions can feel secure that the foods they eat are safe.

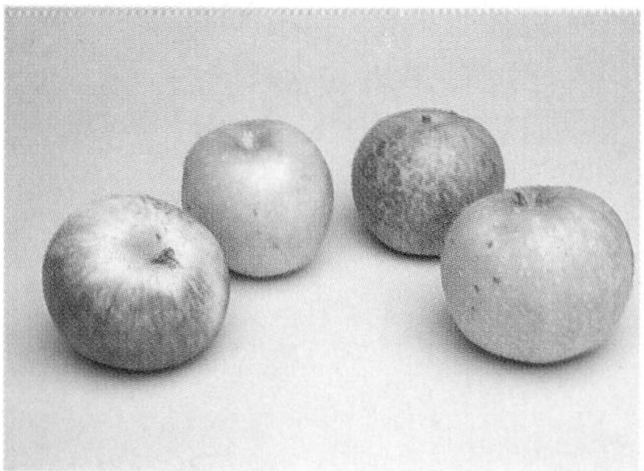

Pesticide-free produce may not be perfectly free of blemishes, but may be a healthy choice.

Alternatives to Pesticides To feed a nation while employing fewer pesticides requires creative farming methods. Highlight 20 describes such methods,

How to Prepare Foods to Minimize Pesticide Residues

To remove or reduce any pesticide residues from foods:

- Trim the fat from meat, and remove the skin from poultry and fish; discard fats and oils in broths and pan drippings. (Pesticide residues concentrate in the animals' fat.)
- Wash fresh produce in water. Use a scrub brush, and rinse thoroughly.
- Use a knife to peel an orange or grapefruit; do not bite into the peel.
- Discard the outer leaves of leafy vegetables such as cabbage and lettuce.
- Peel waxed fruits and vegetables; waxes don't wash off and can seal in pesticide residues.
- Peel vegetables such as carrots and fruits such as apples when appropriate. (Peeling removes pesticides that remain in or on the peel, but also removes fibers, vitamins, and minerals.)

recommended by the National Academy of Sciences as part of a system known as alternative, or sustainable, agriculture. This system depends on crop rotation and the use of plants that produce natural pesticides rather than on synthetic, toxic pesticides. Among natural pesticides are the nicotine in tobacco and psoralens in celery. Natural pesticides are less damaging to other living things and less persistent in the environment than most human-made ones.

Other alternatives to heavy pesticide use include releasing organisms into fields to destroy pests and planting nonfood crops nearby to kill pests or attract them away from the food crops. For example, sterile male fruit flies have been released into orchards, thus helping to curb the population growth of these pests; some flowers, such as marigolds, release natural insecticides and are often planted near crops such as tomatoes. In addition, farmers can plow compost into the soil, which enriches the nutrient content of the soil, increases moisture retention, and reduces erosion. Such alternative farming methods are more labor-intensive and may produce smaller yields than conventional methods, at least initially. Given a fair chance to compete with present methods, however, these alternatives may actually cut costs more than they cut yields, by eliminating expensive pesticides, fertilizers, and fuels.

Consumers with questions about pesticides can call the pesticide hotline.* Meanwhile, the most important thing consumers can do to protect their *food* supply is to defend the *environment*, as Chapter 20 and Highlight 20 explain.

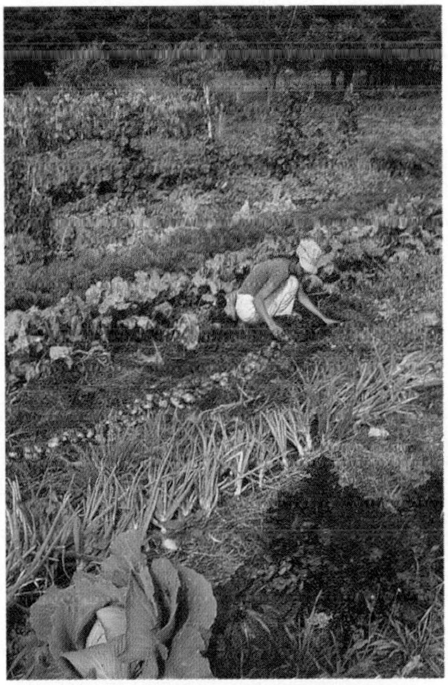

People can avoid the use of pesticides and fertilizers when their gardens or farms are relatively small.

In short, pesticides can safely improve crop yields when used according to regulations, but can also be hazardous when used inappropriately. The FDA tests both domestic and imported foods for pesticide residues in the fields and in market basket surveys of foods prepared table ready. Consumers can minimize their ingestion of pesticide residues on foods by following the suggestions in the box above.

*The National Pesticide Hotline, funded by the EPA, is 1–800–858–PEST. Call anytime day or night, 365 days a year. The Canadian Pesticide Information Line is 1–800–267–6315.

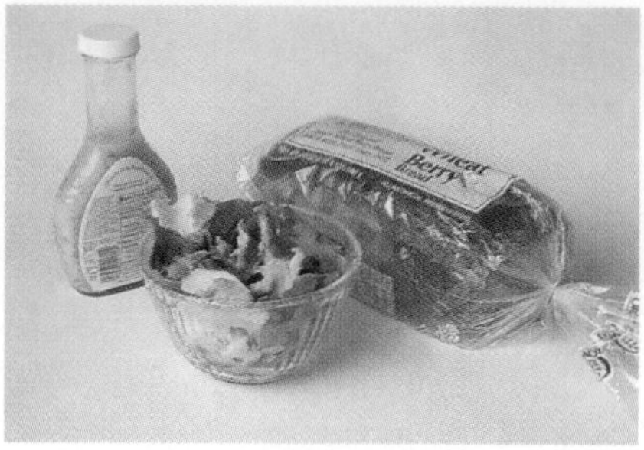

Without additives, bread would quickly get moldy and salad dressing would go rancid.

Food Additives

Additives confer many benefits on foods. Some reduce the risk of food-borne illness (for example, nitrites used in curing meat prevent poisoning from the botulinum toxin). Others enhance nutrient quality (as in vitamin D–fortified milk). Most additives help prevent spoilage during the time it takes to deliver foods long distances to grocery stores and then to kitchens. Some additives simply make foods look and taste good.

Intentional additives are put into foods on purpose, while indirect additives may get in unintentionally before or during processing. This discussion begins with the regulations that govern additives, then presents intentional additives class by class, and finally goes on to say a word about the indirect additives.

additives: substances not normally consumed as foods but added to food either intentionally or by accident.

intentional additives: additives intentionally added to foods, such as nutrients, colors, and preservatives.

indirect additives: substances that can get into food as a result of contact with foods during growing, processing, packaging, storing, cooking, or some other stage before the foods are consumed; also called incidental or accidental additives.

REGULATIONS GOVERNING ADDITIVES

The FDA's concern with additives hinges primarily on their safety. To receive permission to use a new additive in food products, a manufacturer must satisfy the FDA that the additive is:

- Effective (it does what it is supposed to do).
- Detectable and measurable in the final food product.
- Safe (when fed in large doses to animals under strictly controlled conditions, it causes no cancer, birth defects, or other injury).

On approving an additive's use, the FDA writes a regulation stating in what amounts and in what foods the additive may be used. No additive receives permanent approval; all must undergo periodic review.

GRAS (generally recognized as safe) list: a list, established by the FDA in 1958, of food additives that had long been in use and were believed safe. The list is subject to revision as new facts become known.

The GRAS List Many familiar substances are exempted from complying with this procedure because they are generally recognized as safe (GRAS), based either on their extensive, long-term use in foods or on current scientific evidence. Several hundred substances are on the GRAS list, including such items as salt, sugar, caffeine, and herbs. Whenever substantial scientific evidence or public outcry has questioned the safety of any substance on the GRAS list, it has been reevaluated. All substances about which any legitimate question has been raised have been removed or reclassified. Meanwhile, the entire GRAS list is subjected to ongoing review.

The Delaney Clause One risk that the U.S. law on additives refuses to tolerate at any level is the risk of cancer. To remain on the GRAS list, an additive must not have been found to be a carcinogen in any test on animals or human beings. The Delaney Clause (the part of the law that states this criterion) is uncompromising in addressing carcinogens in foods and drugs; in fact, it has been under fire for many years for being too strict and inflexible.

Delaney Clause: a clause in the Food Additive Amendment to the Food, Drug, and Cosmetic Act that states that no substance that is known to cause cancer in animals or human beings at any dose level shall be added to foods.

Reminder: A *carcinogen* is a substance that initiates cancer development.

The Delaney Clause states that "no additive shall be deemed to be safe if it is found to induce cancer when ingested [at any level] by man or animal." That sounds clear enough, yet some products that fail to meet that standard still remain on the market. The artificial sweetener saccharin was the first exception to the rule. In the 1970s, when the FDA tried to ban saccharin because tests had revealed that it caused cancer in animals, consumers raised an outcry asking that it still be allowed in foods. In response, Congress created a special exception that allowed saccharin to remain on the market as long as products containing it carried a warning. This was an attempt to balance the Delaney Clause with current food safety and cancer knowledge.

The Delaney Clause is best understood as a product of a different historical era. It was adopted more than 35 years ago at a time when scientists knew little about carcinogens and cancer development and most substances were detectable in foods only in relatively large amounts, such as parts per thousand. Today, scientific understanding of cancer has progressed, and technology has advanced so that carcinogens in foods can be detected even when they are present only in parts per billion or even per trillion. Earlier, "zero risk" may have seemed attainable, but today we know it is not: all substances, no matter how pure, can be shown to be contaminated at some level with one carcinogen or another. For these reasons, the FDA prefers to deem additives (and pesticides and other contaminants) safe if lifetime use presents no more than a one-in-a-million risk of cancer to human beings. Thus, instead of the "zero-risk" policy of the Delaney Clause, the FDA uses a "negligible-risk" standard, sometimes referred to as a *de minimis* rule. This policy has been challenged and overruled in court.[14] Experts continue to debate the controversial Delaney Clause. One congressional report called the Delaney Clause "scientifically unmanageable" and noted that it does not allow food safety to keep up with science.[15]

For perspective, one part per trillion is equivalent to about one grain of sugar in an Olympic-sized swimming pool; or 1 second in 32,000 years; or one hair on 10 million heads, assuming none are bald.

The *de minimis* rule defines risk as a cancer rate of less than one cancer per million people exposed to a contaminant over a 70-year lifetime.

Margin of Safety Whatever risk level is permitted, actual risks must be determined by experiments. Experiments to determine risks posed by an additive involve feeding test animals the additive at several concentrations throughout their lives. The additive is then permitted in foods 100 times below the lowest level that is found to cause any harmful effect, that is, at a 1/100 margin of safety. In many foods, *naturally* occurring substances occur with narrower margins of safety, such as 1/10. Even nutrients pose risks at dose levels above those normally consumed: the margin of safety for vitamins A and D is 1/25 to 1/40 for adults and may be less than 1/10 for infants. For some trace elements, the margin of safety is about 1/5. People consume common table salt daily in amounts only three to five times less than those that pose a hazard.

margin of safety: when speaking of food additives, a zone between the concentration normally used and that at which a hazard exists. For common table salt, for example, the margin of safety is 1/5 (five times the amount normally used would be hazardous).

Risks versus Benefits Of course, additives would not be added to foods if they only presented risks. Additives are in foods because they offer benefits that outweigh the risks they present, or make the risks worth taking. In the case of color additives that only enhance the appearance of foods but do not improve their health value or safety, no amount of risk may be deemed worth taking. In contrast, the FDA finds that it is worth taking the small risks associated with the use of nitrites on meat products, for example, because nitrites inhibit the formation of the deadly botulinum toxin. The choice involves a compromise between the risks of using additives and the risks of doing without them.

It is the manufacturers' responsibility to use only the amounts of additives that are necessary to get the needed effect, and no more. The FDA also requires that additives *not* be used:

- To disguise faulty or inferior products.
- To deceive the consumer.

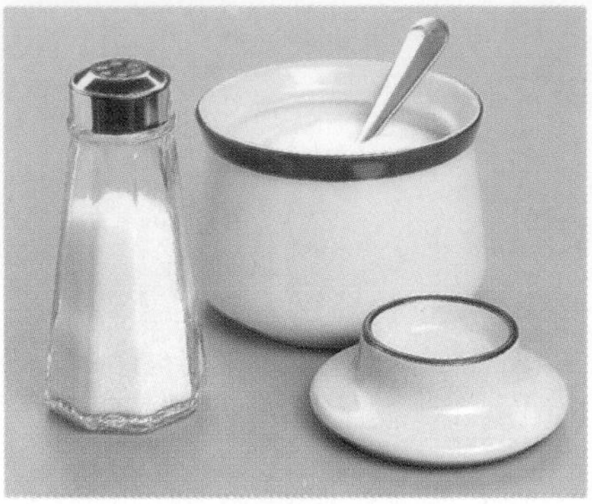

Both salt and sugar act as preservatives by withdrawing water from food; microbes cannot grow without water.

Common examples of antimicrobial additives:
- Salt.
- Sugar.
- Nitrites and nitrates (such as sodium nitrate).

nitrites: salts added to food to prevent botulism; one example is sodium nitrite, which is used to preserve meats.

nitrates: salts that are converted to nitrites by bacteria.

nitrosamines (nigh-TROHS-uh-meens)**:** derivatives of nitrites that may be formed in the stomach when nitrites combine with amines; nitrosamines are carcinogenic in animals.

- Where they significantly destroy nutrients.
- Where their effects can be achieved by economical, sound manufacturing processes.

INTENTIONAL FOOD ADDITIVES

Intentional food additives are added to foods to give them some desirable characteristic: resistance to spoilage, color, flavor, texture, stability, or nutritional value. The accompanying glossary defines the categories of additives, and the next sections describe additives people most often ask about.

Antimicrobial Agents Foods can go bad in two ways. One way is relatively harmless: by losing their flavor and attractiveness. (Additives to prevent this kind of spoilage include antioxidants, discussed later.) The other way is by becoming contaminated with microbes that cause food-borne illnesses, a hazard that justifies the use of antimicrobial agents.

The most widely used antimicrobial agents are ordinary salt and sugar. Salt has been used throughout history to preserve meat and fish; sugar serves the same purpose in canned and frozen fruits and in jams and jellies. Both exert their protective effect primarily by capturing water and making it unavailable to microbes. Other additives, such as potassium sorbate and sodium propionate, are used to extend the shelf life of baked goods, cheeses, beverages, mayonnaise, margarine, and other products.

Other antimicrobial agents, the nitrites and nitrates, are added to foods for three main purposes: to preserve color, especially the pink color of hot dogs and other cured meats; to enhance flavor by inhibiting rancidity, especially in cured meats; and to protect against bacterial growth. In amounts smaller than those needed to confer color, nitrites prevent the growth of the bacteria that produce the deadly botulinum toxin.

Nitrites clearly serve a useful purpose, but their use has been controversial. In the human body, nitrites can be converted to nitrosamines. At nitrite levels higher than those used in food products, nitrosamine formation causes cancer in

Glossary of Intentional Food Additives

antimicrobial agents: preservatives that prevent microorganisms from growing.

artificial colors: certified food colors added to enhance appearance. (*Certified* means approved by the FDA.)

artificial flavors, flavor enhancers: chemicals that mimic natural flavors and those that enhance flavor.

nutrient additives: vitamins and minerals added to improve nutritive value.

preservatives: antimicrobial agents, antioxidants, and other additives that retard spoilage or maintain desired qualities, such as softness in baked goods.

radiation: ionizing rays used to sterilize and protect food.

Reminder: An *antioxidant* is a compound that protects others from oxidation; with respect to food additives, chemicals that prevent rancidity of fats and other damage to food caused by oxygen.

animals. The food industry uses the minimal amount of nitrites necessary to achieve results, and nitrosamine formation has not been shown to cause cancer in human beings.

Detectable amounts of nitrosamine-related compounds are found in malt beverages (beer) and cured meats (primarily, bacon). Yet even the quantities found in beer and bacon hardly make a difference in a person's overall exposure to nitrosamine-related compounds. An average cigarette smoker inhales 100 times the nitrosamines that the average bacon eater ingests. A beer drinker ingests twice as much as the bacon eater, but even so, exposure from new car interiors and cosmetics is higher than this.

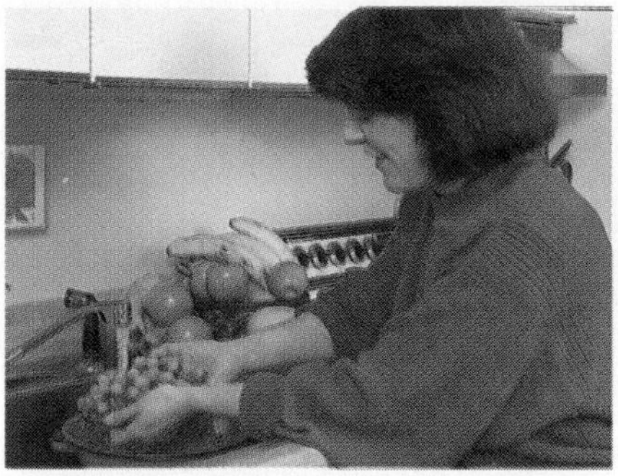

Raw grapes may legally be treated with sulfites, so wash them thoroughly before eating them.

Antioxidants Another way food can go bad is by undergoing changes in color and flavor caused by exposure to oxygen (oxidation). Oftentimes, these changes involve no hazard to health, but they damage the food's appearance, flavor, and nutritional quality. Oxidation is easy to see when sliced apples or potatoes turn brown or when oil goes rancid. Antioxidants prevent these reactions. Among the antioxidants approved for use in foods are vitamin C (ascorbate) and vitamin E (tocopherol).

Common examples of antioxidant additives:

- Vitamin C (ascorbate).
- Vitamin E (tocopherol).
- Sulfites.
- BHA and BHT.

Another group of antioxidants, the sulfites, cost less than the vitamins. Sulfites prevent oxidation in many processed foods, alcoholic beverages (especially wine), and drugs. Restaurant owners used to use sulfites to keep raw fruits and vegetables on salad bars looking fresh, but this practice was banned after some people experienced adverse reactions. The FDA now prohibits sulfite use on foods intended to be consumed raw, with the exception of grapes, and requires foods and drugs that contain sulfite additives to declare it on their labels. For most people, sulfites pose no hazard in the amounts used in products, but there is one more consideration: sulfites destroy thiamin. For this reason, the FDA prohibits their use on foods that are important sources of the vitamin, such as enriched grain products.

sulfites: salts containing sulfur that are added to foods to prevent spoilage.

Sulfites appear on food labels as:

- Sulfur dioxide.
- Sodium sulfite.
- Sodium bisulfite.
- Potassium bisulfite.
- Sodium metabisulfite.
- Potassium metabisulfite.

Two other antioxidants in wide use are BHA and BHT, which prevent rancidity in baked goods and snack foods.* Several tests have shown that animals fed large amounts of BHT developed *less* cancer when exposed to carcinogens and lived *longer* than controls. BHT apparently protects against cancer through its antioxidant effect, which is similar to that of the antioxidant vitamins. The amount of BHT ingested daily from the U.S. diet, however, contributes little to the body's antioxidant defense system. A caution: at intake levels higher than those that protect against cancer, the substance has experimentally *produced* cancer. Vitamin E and vitamin C remain the most important dietary antioxidants to strengthen defenses against cancer.

BHA and BHT: preservatives commonly used to slow the development of off-flavors, odors, and color changes caused by oxidation.

Artificial Colors Only a few artificial colors remain on the FDA's list of color additives approved for use in foods—a highly select group that has survived considerable testing. Artificial colors are among the most intensively investigated of all additives. In fact, coloring agents are much better known than the natural pigments of plants, and the safety of their use can be stated with greater certainty. Examples of natural pigments commonly used by the food industry are the caramel that tints cola beverages and the carotenoids that color margarine, cheeses, and pastas.

Common examples of color additives:

- Carotenoids.
- Blue (brilliant blue and indigotine).
- Green (fast green).
- Red (allura red and erythrosine).
- Yellow (tartrazine and sunset yellow).

*BHA is butylated hydroxyanisole; BHT is butylated hydroxytoluene.

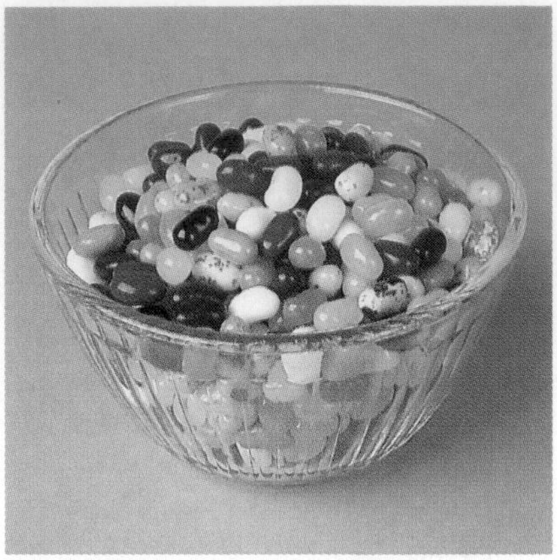

Color additives not only make foods attractive, but identify flavors as well. Everyone agrees that yellow jellybeans should taste lemony and black ones like licorice.

Artificial Flavors and Flavor Enhancers Flavoring agents are the largest single group of food additives. One of the best-known members of this group is monosodium glutamate, or MSG—a sodium salt of the amino acid glutamic acid. MSG is used widely in a number of foods, and especially in Asian foods, as a flavor enhancer. Besides enhancing the well-known sweet, salty, bitter, and sour tastes, MSG may, itself, possess a pleasant flavor.

MSG has received publicity because it may produce an adverse reaction in some individuals—the so-called Chinese restaurant syndrome—involving burning sensations, chest and facial flushing or pain, and throbbing headaches. MSG has been investigated extensively enough to be deemed safe for all adults except the 1 to 2 percent of the population who are sensitive to it. Food labels require ingredient lists to itemize all additives, including MSG.

Chinese restaurant syndrome: an intolerance reaction that may occur in 1 to 2 percent of the population 20 minutes after the ingestion of the additive MSG (monosodium glutamate). Symptoms include burning sensations, chest and facial flushing and pain, and throbbing headaches.

Nutrient Additives As mentioned earlier, manufacturers sometimes add nutrients to improve or maintain the nutritional quality of foods. Included among nutrient additives are the four nutrients added to refined grains to enrich them; the iodine added to salt; the vitamins A and D added to milk products; and the nutrients added to fortified breakfast cereals. A nutrient-poor food with nutrients added may appear to be nutrient-rich, but it is rich only in those nutrients chosen for addition, and the absorption of these nutrients may be poor. Appropriate uses of nutrient additives are to:

- Correct dietary deficiencies known to result in deficiency diseases.
- Restore nutrients to levels found in the food before storage, handling, and processing.
- Balance the vitamin, mineral, and protein contents of a food in proportion to the energy content.
- Correct nutritional inferiority in a food that replaces a more nutritious traditional food.

Common examples of nutrient additives:

- Thiamin, niacin, riboflavin, and iron in grain products.
- Iodine in salt.
- Vitamins A and D in milk.
- Vitamin C in fruit drinks.

Nutrients are sometimes also added for other purposes. Vitamins C and E were already mentioned for their antioxidant properties; beta-carotene (a vitamin A precursor) is sometimes used for its color.

On the whole, the benefits of food additives seem to justify the risks associated with their use. The FDA closely regulates and monitors all intentional additives.

INDIRECT FOOD ADDITIVES

Indirect or incidental additives are substances that find their way into foods during harvesting, production, processing, storage, or packaging. For example, incidental additives include tiny bits of plastic, glass, paper, tin, and other substances from packages as well as chemicals from processing, such as the solvent used to decaffeinate some types of coffee. The following paragraphs discuss three different types of indirect additives that sometimes make headline news.

Microwave Packaging When the FDA regulations were established in the 1950s, the writers did not foresee the use of microwave ovens. Consequently, they did not specify temperatures at which packages should be tested to determine if incidental additives migrated to foods at high temperatures. Some microwave products are sold in "active packaging" that helps to cook the food; for example, pizzas are often heated on a metalized film laminated to paperboard. This film absorbs the microwave energy in the oven and reaches temperatures as high as 500°F. In testing such products, the FDA found that packaging components migrate into the food.[16]

Most microwave products are sold in "passive packaging" that is transparent to microwaves and simply holds the food as it cooks. These containers don't get much hotter than the foods, but materials still migrate at high temperatures. Migration from packages may turn out to be harmless, but until more is known, consumers are advised to use only glass or ceramic containers designed for use in microwave ovens and to avoid reusing disposable containers such as margarine tubs.

Quick test for using glass containers in a microwave:
Microwave the empty container for 1 min.
- If it's warm, it's unsafe for the microwave.
- If it's lukewarm, it's safe for short-term reheating in the microwave.
- If it's cool, it's safe for long-term cooking in the microwave.

Dioxins Coffee filters, milk cartons, paper plates, and frozen food packages, if made from bleached paper, can contaminate foods with minute quantities of dioxins—compounds formed during chlorine treatment of wood pulp during paper manufacture. Dioxin contamination of foods from such products appears only in trace quantities—in the parts per trillion range (recall, for perspective, that one part per trillion is equal to 1 second in 32,000 years). Such levels appear to present no health risks to people, but scientists recognize that dioxins are extremely toxic, and they are known to cause cancer in animals. Accordingly, the paper industry has reduced its use of chlorine to cut dioxin exposure; in the meantime, the FDA has concluded that drinking milk from bleached-paper cartons presents no health hazard.[17]

dioxins: any of 75 structurally related compounds that contain both nitrogen and chlorine. See Chapter 20 for more on dioxins.

Decaffeinated Coffee Many consumers have tried to eliminate caffeine from their diets by selecting decaffeinated coffee. Is decaffeinated coffee a safe alternative? To answer that question, one first has to learn the facts about the decaffeination process.[18] What substances do manufacturers use? How much remains in the final cup of coffee? And are those residues harmful to health?

To remove caffeine from coffee beans, manufacturers often use methylene chloride in a process that leaves traces of the chemical in the final product. The FDA estimates that the average cup of coffee treated this way contains about 0.1 part per million of methylene chloride, which seems to pose no significant threat. A person drinking 2½ cups of decaffeinated coffee containing 100 times as much methylene chloride every day for a lifetime has a one in a million chance of developing cancer from it. People are exposed to much more methylene chloride from other sources such as hair sprays and paint stripping solutions. Still, some consumers prefer either to return to caffeine or to select coffee decaffeinated in another way. Unfortunately, manufacturers are not required to state on their labels the type of decaffeination process used in their products. Many labels provide consumer-information telephone numbers for those who have such questions.

Incidental additives sometimes find their way into foods, but adverse effects are rare. All food packagers are required to perform specific tests to discover whether materials are migrating into foods; if they are, their safety must be confirmed by strict procedures similar to those governing intentional additives.

HORMONES

Hormones are a unique type of incidental additive in that their use is intentional, but their presence in the final food product is not. The FDA has approved about a dozen hormones for use in food-producing animals, and the USDA has established limits for residues allowed in meat products.

bovine growth hormone (BGH): a hormone produced naturally in the pituitary gland of a cow that promotes growth and milk production; now produced for agricultural use by transgenic bacteria (described in the text).
bovine = of cattle

BGH Some ranchers in the United States treat young calves with bovine growth hormone (BGH). Hormone-treated meat animals produce leaner meats, and dairy cows produce more milk.[19] All cows make BGH naturally: the pituitary gland produces it and releases it into the bloodstream. Now scientists can stimulate bacteria to produce BGH, which allows laboratories to harvest huge quantities of the hormone and sell it to farmers as a drug.[20] This practice has some consumers concerned that an "artificial" drug is being given to cows that will be used for meat and milk.

Indeed, traces of BGH do remain in the meat and milk of both hormone-treated and untreated cows. BGH residues have not been tested for safety in human beings because residues of the natural hormone have always been present in milk and meat and the amount found in treated cows is within the range that can occur naturally.[21] Furthermore, BGH, being a peptide hormone, is denatured by the heat used in processing milk and cooking meat, and is also digested by enzymes in the GI tract. If any BGH were to enter the bloodstream, it would have no effect because the chemical structures of animal growth hormones differ from those in human beings; BGH does not stimulate receptors for *human* growth hormone. In a report from its Technology Assessment Conference, the National Institutes of Health concludes, "As currently used in the United States, meat and milk from [hormone] treated cows are as safe as those from untreated cows."[22]

Opponents of BGH Whether treating animals with hormones is wise is debated. Opponents say that a vast surplus of milk will flood the market, driving milk prices down. Huge farms that can weather price fluctuations will not be affected, but small farms may be forced to close, further reducing an already dwindling agricultural landscape across the United States.

Another concern is that BGH-treated cows suffer more udder infections (mastitis) and so are given more antibiotics—then, these drugs show up in the cows' milk and meat.[23] Furthermore, increased agricultural use of antibiotics helps to spread antibiotic-resistant microorganisms. These microorganisms can cause life-threatening food-borne illnesses that do not respond to antibiotic therapy.

Proponents of BGH Supporters of BGH say that we need and use all the milk that can be produced. A greater output of milk per cow will simply mean fewer cows to feed, smaller feed bills, and larger profits for farmers. Similarly, beef cattle will reach their market weights earlier and require less food and care. The environment will suffer less damage. Smaller herds can live on smaller plots of cleared land and eat less food, which means less production, transportation, and overall environmental degradation.

Despite reassurances, some U.S. consumers still have concerns. The outcry against BGH has prompted farmers and grocers in several milk-producing states to pledge not to produce or sell milk from hormone-like cows. The beef industry has responded by providing beef "certified as untreated." Several European countries refuse to import meat from animals treated with hormones. Consumers will have the final word on BGH by deciding whether to accept milk and meat from hormone-treated animals.

RADIATION

The FDA has approved the use of ionizing radiation on certain foods and treats irradiation as an additive. Radiation kills microorganisms and insects in postharvest wheat, spices, and teas (postharvest pesticide fumigation); kills *Trichinella*, the parasitic worms that sometimes contaminate pork; kills *Salmonella*, the bacteria that contaminate poultry; inhibits the growth of sprouts on potatoes and onions; and delays ripening in some fruits such as strawberries and mangoes.[24] Milk products change flavor when irradiated and so are not candidates for the treatment. (Incidentally, the milk in those boxes kept at room temperature on grocery-store shelves is not irradiated, but processed with an ultrahigh temperature treatment for just long enough to sterilize it.)

ultrahigh temperature (UHT) treatment: short-time exposure of a food to temperatures above those normally used in order to sterilize it.

In many cases, the flavor, texture, and color of foods treated with radiation do not change. Vitamin loss is minimal and comparable to amounts lost from foods processed by other commercial processing methods.

Consumer Concerns Irradiation does not make foods radioactive and therefore does not expose people to radiation. Radiation sterilizes foods and, as a side effect, slightly alters their chemistry. When radiation strikes the atoms in the molecules of the food, they lose electrons and form ions or free radicals. How these particles react with one another and with other food constituents is the focus of much research.

Compounds produced as a result of the irradiation process are called radiolytic products. A few radiolytic products are unique to irradiated foods. The higher the radiation dose, the more unique radiolytic products are formed. Most radiolytic products (approximately 90 percent), however, are also found in foods that have not been irradiated, leading to the conclusion that radiolytic products are probably not hazardous.[25] Research on irradiation safety continues.

radiolytic (RAY-dee-oh-LIT-ic) products: chemicals formed during the irradiation of food.

Many customers, associating radiation with cancer, birth defects, and mutations, have strong negative emotions about the use of radiation on foods. Some confuse it with food contamination by radioactive particles, such as occurs in the aftermath of a nuclear accident. Many food producers are eager to use irradiation, but hesitate to do so until consumers are ready to accept it. Proponents believe that once consumers understand the benefits of irradiation and are no longer afraid of it, they will demand to have foods sterilized by this process. Some proponents suggest renaming irradiation *pico wave*, because consumers readily accepted microwaves.

Speaking of microwaves, like irradiation, microwaves can sterilize foods under certain conditions of time and temperature.* Unlike irradiation, though, microwaves cook food, and they do not create unique radiolytic products.

---

*Gamma waves (pico waves) used in the irradiation of foods have a wavelength of 10^{-12} meters; microwaves have a wavelength of 10^{-2} meters. As a point of reference, lightbulbs emit wavelengths in the range of 10^{-7} meters.

This international symbol identifies retail foods that have been irradiated. The words "Treated by irradiation" or "Treated with irradiation" must accompany the symbol. The irradiation label is not required on commercially prepared foods that contain irradiated ingredients, such as spices.

Irradiation cuts down on food wastage and can replace some costly pesticides, thus reducing those residues in food. Alternatively, the same goals could be achieved by less expensive methods—such as higher cleanliness standards for food-animal facilities to prevent microbial contamination and selective breeding of produce to achieve longer storage times. These methods pose none of the hazards associated with transport and handling of radioactive materials, and they are proven safe for the human food supply. Whether irradiation will become widely used for food processing may depend on the ability of its backers to prove its safety beyond doubt.

Where irradiation technology is available, its use must be carefully scrutinized. There is no possibility of a meltdown or nuclear disaster because food irradiation plants are not nuclear reactors. However, strict controls on the transport of radioactive materials, adequate safety operations at facilities, and proper disposal of the wastes generated are indispensable to prevent hazards to workers and the environment.

Regulation of Radiation The FDA has established regulations governing the specific uses of irradiation and allowed doses. Each food that has been treated with radiation must say so on its label. Labels can be misleading however, if consumers interpret the *absence* of the irradiation symbol to mean that the food was produced without any kind of treatment. This is not true; it is just that the FDA does not require label statements for other treatments used for the same purpose, such as postharvest fumigation with pesticides. If all treatment methods were declared, consumers could make fully informed choices.

FOOD BIOTECHNOLOGY

For centuries farmers have manipulated the genetics of plants and animals to shape the characteristics of their crops and livestock. Consider corn, for example. Wild, native corn bears only two or three kernels on a cob, but many years of patient selective breeding have produced the large, full, sweet ears people enjoy today, and many types of wild corn are now all but extinct. Half of the increases in U.S. crop yields this century are due to such genetic improvements; the use of irrigation, fertilizers, and pesticides have also contributed.[26] Farmers are still using selective breeding to provide consumers with low-fat meats, high-yield grains, and a seemingly endless variety of fruits and vegetables.

biotechnology: the use of biological systems or organisms to create or modify products; also called **biogenetic engineering.**

Recently, scientists have discovered a way of speeding up the process of genetic change through biotechnology. Farmers need no longer wait patiently for breeding to yield improved crops and animals, nor must they even respect natural lines of reproduction among species. Laboratory scientists can now select desirable traits from any of a number of species and insert those traits into the genetic material of crops and animals.

So far, most of the traits that have been selected for transfer help to produce foods more efficiently. For example, the enzyme rennin, which is essential for making cheese, was previously harvested from the stomachs of calves, a costly process. Now scientists can convey into bacteria the genetic material to mass-produce rennin.

rennin: an enzyme that coagulates milk; found in the gastric juice of cows, but not human beings.

Among the new products of biotechnology are tomatoes that stay fresh much longer than others and so promise less waste and higher profits. Soybeans may soon be implanted with a gene that will upgrade soy protein to a quality approaching that of milk. Corn may be modified to contain lysine and tryptophan, its two limiting amino acids.[27] Fats and oils with a predetermined fatty acid composition may be possible within the decade.[28] Crops that produce their own insecticides upon receiving genes from bacteria may render pesticides unnecessary. Shrimp may soon fight diseases with genetic ammunition borrowed from sea urchins. Livestock may receive growth-promoting hormones from bacteria as mentioned earlier. Overall, biotechnology offers solutions to enhance the quality, nutritional value, and variety of foods.[29] The possibilities seem unlimited, and though they sound fantastic, many are waiting on laboratory shelves for the time when they will be fully employed in agriculture.

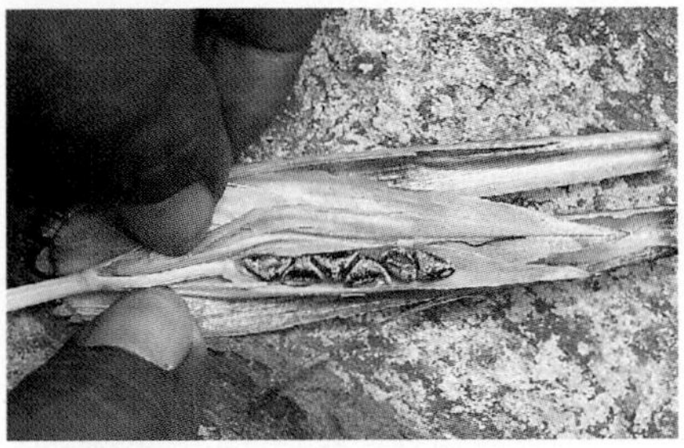

Today's large, full, sweet ears bear little resemblance to the original wild, native corn with its sparse two or three kernels to a cob.

While food industrialists hail biotechnology as a miracle, some other people fear that tampering with genetics may change organisms in ways not yet fully understood, even by the scientists who developed the techniques. They wonder what unknown changes take place when the genes of living things are manipulated, and what the long-term consequences might be.

DNA Technology To understand the issues, it is necessary to understand the basic process of recombinant DNA technology.[30] To transfer genes, scientists first employ enzymes to snip from an organism's genetic material the bit of DNA responsible for a desirable trait. Then, they "recombine" the snipped bit with the DNA from viruses, yeasts, bacteria, or other sources to yield a complete DNA molecule. They then insert this "recombinant DNA" into the target plant, animal, or bacterial cell where it produces the proteins responsible for the desired trait. When the receiving cell happens to be an embryonic, stem, or germ cell, it gives rise to a whole new transgenic organism.

recombinant DNA technology: methods of joining (recombining) pieces of the genetic material DNA in order to change the proteins produced by the altered DNA.

The transgenic organism carries the desired DNA code in every one of its cells. For example, when scientists implant a piece of DNA from a virus that attacks potato plants into a stem cell, that cell develops into a new potato plant that replicates a piece of the viral protein coat in each of its cells. That transgenic potato plant can then effectively repel the virus when it attacks.

transgenic organism: an organism that grows from an embryonic, stem, or germ cell into which a gene is inserted; the organism then carries the new gene in all of its cells.

The technique just described allows an organism to make proteins native to another living thing. Another way that biotechnology can change the internal chemistry of an organism is by blocking, or suppressing, production of a protein the organism normally makes. One example is the long-lasting tomato, mentioned earlier. Normally, tomatoes produce a protein that softens them after they have been picked. Scientists introduce into a tomato plant an antisense gene, that is, a gene that is a mirror image of the one that codes for the "softening" enzyme. The antisense gene fastens itself to the RNA of the native gene and blocks its action. A vine-ripe tomato with the antisense gene rots much more slowly than a normal tomato. This means growers can harvest tomatoes at their most flavorful and nutritious red stage, and the tomatoes will still last much longer during shipping and marketing than regular, green-harvested tomatoes.

antisense gene: the chemical opposite of a native gene that adheres to the native working gene and blocks its production of proteins.

Safety and Regulation The case for regulating technology's products is strong.[31] New substances, additives in a sense, are present in genetically engineered foods. The source of the new materials may be unique—never before seen in foods in exactly the same way. If a disease-producing microorganism donates genetic material to make recombinant DNA, scientists must prove that no dangerous characteristic from the microorganism exists in the food. If the new genetic material creates proteins never before encountered by the human body, their effects should be understood and their presence regulated to ensure their safety for human consumption.[32]

So far, FDA safety and labeling regulations apply only if the technology creates new ingredients in the food. The FDA has taken the position that foods produced through biotechnology that are not substantially different from others require no special safety testing or labeling.[33] A product with an antisense gene, such as the tomato described earlier, need not be tested since antisense genes *prevent* synthesis of a protein and add nothing but a tiny fragment of genetic material. On the other hand, any substances introduced into a food by way of bioengineering must meet the same safety standards applied to all additives.[34] A tomato plant with a gene that, for example, produces an insecticide cannot be marketed until it proves safe for consumption. Foods produced via biotechnology are not required to be labeled as such unless they pose known problems, such as allergy, to some people.

Some people object to genetic tampering and want labels to help them identify "old-fashioned" tomatoes. They may not realize that most foods available today have already been altered genetically by selective breeding. The new vegetable broccoflower, a product of sophisticated cross-breeding of broccoli with cauliflower, met no testing or approval barriers on its way to the dinner plate. Only after the vegetables became popular with consumers did scientists study its nutrient contents (see Appendix H for their findings).

Scientists are continuing to study the effects not only of biotechnology but of all sorts of new food-processing techniques. Their efforts to enhance food production will help meet the challenge of feeding an ever-increasing world population.[35] Chapter 20 explores other possible solutions and the issues of world hunger.

To summarize food additives, FDA regulates the use of the following intentional additives: antimicrobial agents (such as nitrites) to prevent microbial spoilage; antioxidants (such as vitamins C and E, sulfites, and BHA and BHT) to prevent oxidative changes; colors (such as tartrazine) and flavor enhancers (such as MSG) to appeal to senses; and nutrients (such as iodine in salt) to enrich or fortify foods. Incidental additives sometimes get into foods during processing, but rarely present a hazard. Other processes such as treating livestock with hormones, irradiating fruits and vegetables, and using biotechnology enhance crop yields and make some foods safer to eat, but raise consumer concerns.

The Public Water Supply

Water may contain the same impurities that foods do: microorganisms, environmental contaminants, pesticides, and additives such as chlorine used to kill pathogenic microorganisms and fluoride used to protect against dental caries. A glass of "water" is more than just H_2O.

SOURCES OF DRINKING WATER

Drinking water comes from two sources—surface water and groundwater. Each source supplies water for about half of the population.

Surface Water Surface water comes from lakes, rivers, and reservoirs and supplies drinking water for most major cities. Surface water is readily contaminated because it is directly exposed to acid rain, runoff from highways and urban areas, pesticide runoff from agricultural areas, and industrial wastes that are dumped directly into it. Surface water contamination is reversible, however, because the water is constantly replaced by fresh rain. It is also cleansed to some degree by aeration, sunlight, and the plants and microorganisms that live in it.

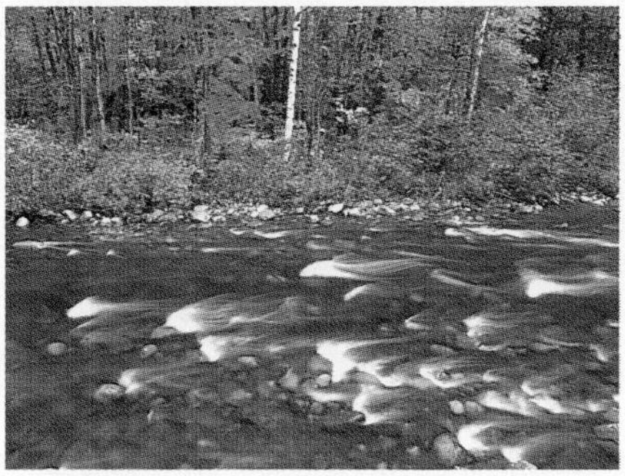
Clean rivers represent irreplaceable water resources.

Groundwater Groundwater comes from underground aquifers—rock formations that are saturated with and yield usable water. People who live in rural areas rely mostly on groundwater pumped up from private wells.

Groundwater is contaminated more slowly than surface water, but also more permanently. Contaminants deposited on the ground migrate slowly through the soil before reaching groundwater. Slow replacement combined with lack of aeration, sunlight, and aerobic microorganisms means that contaminants break down more slowly in groundwater than in surface water. Groundwater is especially susceptible to contamination from hazardous waste sites, dumps and landfills, underground tanks storing gasoline and other chemicals, and improperly discarded household chemicals and solvents.

Contaminants via Plumbing Contamination can also occur as water travels from the main water supply to homes. Lead or asbestos from corroded pipes can contaminate drinking water, as can bacteria and dirt from leaking pipes. People who suspect contamination of their water should have it tested where it flows out, at the tap.

The Cleansing Process In the wilderness, water is purified each time it cycles through living systems. The soil filters out animal waste excreted onto the earth, preventing it from reaching the groundwater; plants use the waste as fertilizer instead. Soil holds pollutants, too—not beneficial to the soil, of course, but protective of the water. Surface waters also leave behind their pollutants as rivers flow along. But neither the soil nor the rivers can completely purify the heavily polluted water expelled as city sewage or industrial waste. Water leaving a factory may contain higher and higher concentrations of toxic metals as time passes, especially if the same water cycles repeatedly through a factory. Human technology is responsible for purifying water contaminated by human technology.

Public water systems treat water to remove contaminants that have been detected above acceptable levels. During treatment, a disinfectant (usually, chlorine) is added to kill bacteria. The addition of chlorine to public water is an important public health measure that appears to offer both great benefits and small risks.[36] On the one hand, chlorinated water has eliminated such waterborne diseases as typhoid fever, which once ravaged vast areas, killing thousands of people. On the other hand, it has been associated with a slight increase in bladder and rectal cancers and with contamination of the environment with the toxic by-product dioxin. Private well water is usually not chlorinated or cleansed, so the 40 million Americans who consume water from private wells are most at risk of drinking contaminated water.

DRINKING WATER CONTAMINANTS

Hundreds of contaminants, including heavy metals, pathogenic microorganisms, and organic compounds, have been detected in public drinking water. The health implications of these contaminants are just becoming known.

Heavy Metals The metals of greatest concern are mercury, cadmium, and lead. These metals may be absorbed into the body, where they damage cell structures and impair enzyme or coenzyme functions. When combined with organic compounds, these metals may be absorbed especially rapidly and may damage body tissues even more. Heavy metals can alter the genetic material DNA, causing mutations that can produce cancer or birth defects. If the mutations occur in the DNA of the germ cells (eggs or sperm), the changes are hereditary.

Pathogenic Microorganisms While the water supply naturally contains few, if any, heavy metals, it does naturally contain bacteria from the soil and from contamination with sewage. Before a sewage treatment plant releases water into the public supply, it must cut the bacterial count.

Water that is suitable for drinking is potable (POTE-ah-bul).

High standards for sewage treatment in the developed countries ensure that most people have safe drinking water. For the rest of the world, however, microbial contamination remains the primary cause of human diseases and epidemics. Two of the most basic public health needs of the world's people are safe drinking water and an acceptable standard of waste disposal.

Organic Compounds Organic compounds from sewage, pesticides, petroleum-based industries, highway runoff, and other sources may also appear in water. Researchers have found that some of these compounds cause birth defects, some cause cancer, and some cause genetic mutations. Many of these organic compounds contain chlorine, and some may be formed during the chlorination of water. The risks they present remain unknown; standards are being established, and if public water exceeds them, new treatment systems may be needed.

WATER SYSTEMS AND REGULATIONS

The EPA is responsible for ensuring that public water systems meet minimum standards for protecting the public health. The agency's tasks include developing maximum permitted levels for all regulated contaminants, monitoring for contaminants in drinking water, identifying the appropriate technology for removing excess contaminants, and providing protection for groundwater sources. Critics have charged that existing laws are inadequate to protect drinking water supplies and are not enforced. Some consumers have adopted alternatives to the public water system.

Home Water Treatments To ease concerns about drinking water quality, some people purchase home water-treatment systems. Manufacturers offer a variety of units for removing contaminants from drinking water. None of them removes all contaminants, and each has its own advantages and disadvantages. Choosing the right treatment unit depends on the kinds of contaminants in the water. Therefore, before purchasing a home water-treatment unit, a consumer must first determine the quality of the water. In some cases, a state or county health department will test water samples or can refer the consumer to a certified laboratory.

Rather than purchasing a home treatment unit, some people boil their water. This kills microorganisms and removes some organic chemicals, but may concentrate inorganic chemicals such as lead.

Bottled Water Many people turn to bottled water as an alternative to tap water. Bottled water is classified as a food, so it is regulated nationwide by the FDA and locally by state health and environmental agencies. The FDA has established quality and safety standards for bottled drinking waters compatible with those set by the EPA for public water systems. In addition, all bottled waters must be processed, packaged, and labeled in accordance with FDA regulations.

Approximately 75 percent of bottled waters derive from protected groundwater (from springs or wells) that has been disinfected with ozone rather than chlorine. Ozone kills microorganisms, then disintegrates spontaneously into water and oxygen, leaving behind no toxic by-products. Other bottled waters derive from municipal tap water that has been treated by carbon filtration to remove chlorine and inorganic compounds. Bottled waters may also be treated by reverse osmosis or ion exchange to remove inorganic compounds. Alternatively, the water may be distilled or deionized to remove dissolved solids. Some bottled waters may also have minerals or carbonation added. "Carbonated," "seltzer," "soda," and "tonic" waters are not considered waters, however, but soft drinks.

The FDA has proposed regulations for labels to disclose the sources of bottled waters and to use legally defined descriptive terms.[37] Some of the terms used to describe water are listed in the glossary.

Glossary of Water Terms

artesian water: water that is drawn from a well that taps a confined aquifer in which the water level stands above the natural water table.

distilled water: water that has been vaporized and recondensed, leaving it free of dissolved minerals.

fluoridated water: water that has been treated so as to contain at least 0.8 mg fluoride per liter.

hard water: water with a high calcium and magnesium concentration.

mineral water: water from a spring or well that typically contains 250 to 500 ppm of minerals. Minerals give water a distinctive flavor. Many mineral waters are high in sodium.

natural water: water obtained from a spring or well that is certified to be safe and sanitary. The mineral content may not be changed, but the water may be treated in other ways such as by filtration or ozonization.

public water: water from a municipal or county water system that has been treated and disinfected.

purified water: water that has been processed through distillation, deionization, or reverse osmosis and meets U.S. Pharmacopoeia standards for medical and research purposes.

soft water: water with a high sodium concentration.

spring water: water originating from an underground spring or well. It may be carbonated or not ("flat" or "still"). Brand names such as "Spring Pure" do not necessarily mean that the water comes from a spring.

well water: water drawn from groundwater by tapping into an aquifer.

Despite government regulations, some contamination has been detected in some bottled waters.[38] While the amounts of most contaminants found in bottled waters are probably insignificant, consumers should be aware that bottled water is not always purer than the water from their taps.

Protection of drinking water is, and will continue to be, the subject of an ongoing battle between environmentalists and industry. Many consumers and industries are unwilling to pay the financial costs of a clean, safe environment. Long-term solutions are most likely to emerge when consumers demand safe environmental practices and stringent environmental legislation and, especially, enforcement. Better handling of industrial wastes in some areas is an obvious need. Alternative farming techniques are also needed to reduce large-scale use of pesticides. Consumer education for proper disposal of solvents and household wastes is also important. A lack of attention to the problem of water contamination will only ensure that it gets worse. To learn about the water supply in your area, call the local public health agency.

As this chapter said at the start, supplying food safely to over 250 million people is an incredible challenge—one that gets met, for the most part, with remarkable efficiency. The next chapter describes a contrasting situation—that of the food supply not reaching the people.

Study Questions

1. To what extent does food poisoning present a real hazard to U.S. consumers eating U.S. foods? How often does it occur?
2. Distinguish between the two types of food-borne illnesses and provide an example of each. Describe measures that help prevent food-borne illnesses at home and while traveling.
3. What special precautions apply to meats? To seafood?
4. What is meant by a "persistent" contaminant of foods? Describe how contaminants get into foods and build up in the food chain.
5. What dangers do natural toxicants present?
6. How do pesticides become a hazard to the food supply, and how are they monitored? In what ways can people reduce the concentrations of pesticides in and on foods that they prepare?
7. What is the difference between a GRAS substance and a regulated food additive? Give examples of each. Name and describe the different classes of additives.
8. Explain the differences between surface water and groundwater. Which is more easily contaminated and why?
9. Describe some of the health implications of water contamination. What steps has the government taken to ensure a safe water supply?

Notes

1. R. L. Hall, Food safety and biotechnology, *Nutrition Today*, May/June 1991, pp. 15–20.
2. M. P. Doyle, Reducing foodborne diseases—What are the priorities? *Nutrition Reviews* 51 (1993): 346–347.
3. A. Hecht, The unwelcome dinner guest: Preventing food-borne illness, *FDA Consumer*, January/February 1991, pp. 19–25.
4. J. A. Desenclos and coauthors, The protective effect of alcohol on the occurrence of epidemic oyster-borne hepatitis A, *Epidemiology* 3 (1992): 371–374.
5. M. Segal, Operation pearl, *FDA Consumer*, January/February 1991, pp. 35–36.
6. P. M. Schantz, The dangers of eating raw fish, *New England Journal of Medicine* 320 (1989): 1143–1145.
7. J. H. T. Luong, C. A. Groom, and K. B. Male, The potential role of biosensors in the food and drink industries, *Biosensors and Bioelectronics* 6 (1991): 547–554.

8. P. I. Peterkin, E. S. Idziak, and A. N. Sharpe, Detection of *Listeria monocytogenes* by direct colony hybridization on hydrophobic grid-membrane filters by using a chromogen-labeled DNA probe, *Applied and Environmental Microbiology* 57 (1991): 586–591; M. Hoshi, Y. Sasamoto, and M. Nonaka, Microbial sensor system for nondestructive evaluation of fish meat quality, *Biosensors and Bioelectronics* 6 (1991): 15–20.
9. C. F. Chaisson, B. Petersen, and J. S. Douglass, *Pesticides in Foods: A Guide for Professionals* (Chicago: American Dietetic Association, 1991), pp. 2–3.
10. National Academy of Sciences Committee, as quoted by J. Raloff and D. Pendick, Pesticides in produce may threaten kids, *Science News* 144 (1993): 4–5.
11. Three agencies propose pesticide reforms, *FDA Consumer*, January/February 1994, p. 3.
12. C. Marwick, Pesticides pose concern about children's diet, *Journal of the American Medical Association* 270 (1993): 802, 805.
13. Food and Drug Administration Pesticide Program, 1991.
14. C. K. Winter, Pesticide residues and the Delaney Clause, *Food Technology* 47 (1993): 81–86; Government regulation of food safety: Interaction of scientific and societal forces, *Food Technology* 46 (1992): 73–80.
15. Federal update: Delaney Clause called "scientifically unmanageable," *Journal of the American Dietetic Association* 93 (1993): 268.
16. D. Farley, Keeping up with the microwave revolution, *FDA Consumer*, March 1990, pp. 17–21.
17. D. Blumenthal, Deciding about dioxins, *FDA Consumer*, February 1990, pp. 11–13.
18. Much of the discussion on decaffeinated coffee came from P. L. Cerrato, Is decaffeinated coffee dangerous to your health? *Issues in Nutrition*, ed. A Heinz (New York: American Council on Science and Health, 1991), pp. 107–108.
19. T. D. Etherton and coauthors, Mechanisms by which somatotropin decreases adipose tissue growth, *American Journal of Clinical Nutrition* (supplement) 58 (1993): 287S–295S; Bovine somatotropin and the safety of cow's milk: National Institutes of Health Technology Assessment Conference Statement, *Nutrition Reviews* 49 (1991): 227–232.
20. T. D. Etherton, P. M. Kris-Etherton, and E. W. Mills, Recombinant bovine and porcine somatotropin: Safety and benefits of these biotechnologies, *Journal of the American Dietetic Association* 93 (1993): 177–180.
21. J. C. Juskevich and C. G. Guyer, Bovine growth hormone: Human food safety evaluation, *Science* 249 (1990): 875–884; R. W. Rhein, BST = A Safe, More Plentiful Milk Supply (1990), a booklet available from the American Council on Science and Health at 1995 Broadway, 16th floor, New York, NY 10023–5860.
22. Bovine somatotropin and the safety of cow's milk, 1991.
23. Bovine somatotropin and the safety of cow's milk, 1991.
24. D. Blumenthal, Food irradiation: Toxic to bacteria, safe for humans, *FDA Consumer*, November 1990, pp. 11–15.
25. Blumenthal, 1990.
26. R. L. Phillips, Plant genetics: Out with the old, in with the new? *American Journal of Clinical Nutrition* (supplement) 58 (1993): 259S–263S.
27. B. A. Larkins, C. R. Lending, and J. C. Wallace, Modification of maize-seed-protein quality, *American Journal of Clinical Nutrition* (supplement) 58 (1993): 264S–269S.
28. C. R. Somerville, Future prospects for genetic modification of the composition of edible oils from higher plants, *American Journal of Clinical Nutrition* (supplement) 58 (1993): 270S–275S.
29. Position of The American Dietetic Association: Biotechnology and the future of food, *Journal of the American Dietetic Association* 93 (1993): 189–192.
30. W. L. Carroll, Introduction to recombinant-DNA technology, *American Journal of Clinical Nutrition* (supplement) 58 (1993): 249S–258S.
31. R. J. Goldburg, Why the U.S. should regulate gene-altered foods, 1991; American Medical Association Council on Scientific Affairs, Biotechnology and the American agricultural industry, *Journal of the American Medical Association* 265 (1991): 1429–1436.
32. Goldburg, 1991.
33. Statement of policy: Foods derived from new plant varieties, *Federal Register*, May 29, 1992, pp. 22983–23005.
34. Biotechnology of food: Background information from the FDA, *Nutrition Today*, July/August 1994, pp. 19–20.
35. T. D. Etherton, The impact of biotechnology on animal agriculture and the consumer, *Nutrition Today*, July/August 1994, pp. 12–18.
36. K. Napier, Chlorinated water: Risks and benefits, *Priorities*, Fall 1992, p. 23.
37. V. Lambert, Bottled water: New trends, new rules, *FDA Consumer*, June 1993, pp. 8–11.
38. D. Farley and coauthors, Contaminated bottled water dumped, *FDA Consumer*, January/February 1991, pp. 39–40.

Our Children's Daily Lead*

At nine months, Joey crawled about exploring the world around him—touching and tasting everything, as all babies do. He chewed on table legs, toys, and spindles of flaky paint railings—whatever was in his reach. He eagerly drank his morning bottle of formula, which his mother prepared with the first water drawn from the tap. Not until he was two did he begin to toddle about while his parents watched proudly. At four, he amused his parents when he'd chase after balls tossed his way, but he couldn't catch them. By age five, he was a cautious, quiet preschooler who clung tightly to stair railings with both hands as he slowly climbed up or down.

Joey was late in walking, small for his age, seldom played as vigorously as other children, and was prone to small health disturbances such as diarrhea, irritability, and lethargy. His kindergarten teacher reported that Joey had some difficulty hearing and that his progress was slower than expected. While his health quietly deteriorated, his parents thought these subtle symptoms were within the range of normal variations seen in children. Finally, a pediatrician detected lead toxicity and started treating Joey with lead-scavenging drugs.[1] Joey is now growing normally and playing vigorously, although he still has minor learning disabilities. His physician expects the deficits in brain function to persist into adulthood.[2]

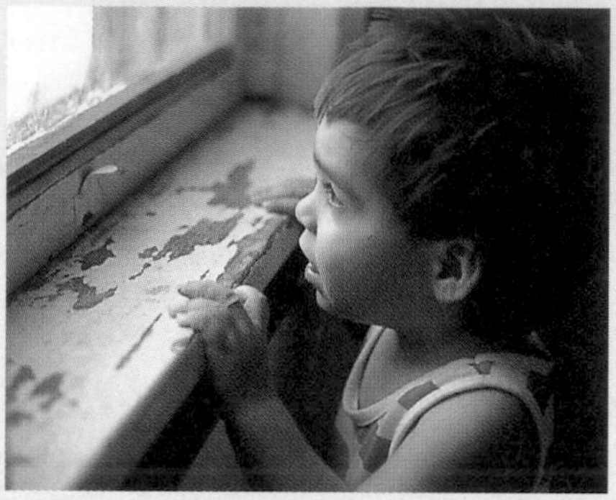
Old, lead-based paint threatens the health of an exploring child.

For children like Joey, the diagnosis often comes too late. Even one year of lead exposure can permanently injure the brain, nervous system, and psychological functioning. Furthermore, the effects occur with even low exposure.[3] The lead poisoning threshold—the amount of lead in the blood recognized to cause harm —is now known to be 10 micrograms per 100 milliliters of blood; earlier it was thought to be 25.[4] Health agencies point to lead poisoning as the most serious environmental threat to young children.[5] The FDA has proposed reducing the acceptable level of lead in foods tenfold—from its 1958 limit of 10 parts per million to 0.5 to 1.0 parts per million.[6]

This highlight describes how lead disrupts the body processes and impairs nutrition status then points out sources of lead in the environment. Perhaps, with awareness, we can make changes that will safeguard the health of our children.

LEAD IN THE BODY

Chapters 12 and 13 told of the many ways minerals serve the body—maintaining fluid and electrolyte balance, providing structural support to the bones, transporting oxygen, and assisting enzymes. In contrast to those minerals that the body requires, the mineral lead impairs the body's growth, work, and general heath.

Like other minerals, lead is indestructible; the body cannot change its chemistry. Chemically similar to nutrient minerals like iron, calcium, and zinc, lead displaces them from some of the slots they normally occupy, but is then unable to perform their roles. For example, lead interferes with the enzymes that facilitate heme formation (see Figure H19–1). Lead damages many body systems, particularly the vulnerable nervous system, kidneys, and bone marrow. It impairs such normal activities as growth by interfering with hormone activity.[7] Table H19–1 lists symptoms of lead toxicity. The greater the exposure, the more damaging the effects.

LEAD AND GROWING CHILDREN

The body absorbs lead greedily, especially during times of rapid growth. Thereafter, it hoards lead possessively. During pregnancy, lead readily moves across the placenta, inflicting severe damage on the developing fetal nervous system. Infants and young children absorb five to ten times as much lead as adults do. One out of every six children from six months to five years old and one out of every nine fetuses are exposed to harmful doses of lead. Lead toxicity is most prevalent among children under six—as many

*Title borrowed form M. A. Wessel and A. Dominski, Our children's daily lead, *American Scientist* 65 (1977): 294–298.

Figure H19–1

Lead Displaces Iron

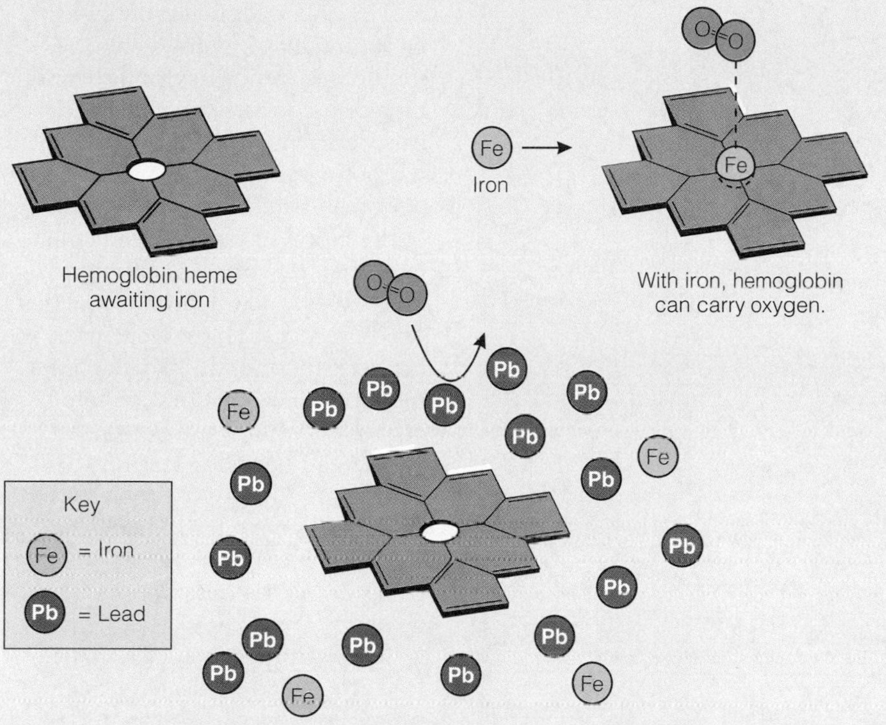

With high levels of lead, the placement of iron in the heme structure is blocked, and so hemoglobin cannot carry oxygen.

as 3 to 4 million children (10 to 15 percent of all preschoolers) may have blood lead concentrations high enough to cause mental, behavioral, and other health problems.[8]

Lead poisoning in infants most often comes from infant formula made with contaminated water.[9] The water, in turn, receives its lead burden from lead-soldered plumbing. The first water drawn from the tap each day is highest in lead—therefore, a person living in a house with old, lead-soldered plumbing should let the water run a few minutes before drinking or using it to prepare formula or food.

Lead intoxication in young children comes from their own behaviors and activities—putting their hands in their mouths, playing in dirt, and eating nonfood items (see Figure H19–2 on p. 714). The toddler years see a marked rise in blood lead. Tragically, a child's neuromuscular system is maturing at precisely the same time. No wonder children with high blood lead experience impairment of balance, motor development, and the relaying of nerve messages to and from the brain. Children two and three years old with the highest blood lead suffer the greatest developmental delays at age four. Researchers studying young children's development must now consider the possible effects of lead poisoning.

Excess lead in the blood also deranges the structure of red blood cell membranes, making them leaky and fragile. Lead interacts with white blood cells, too, impairing their ability to fight infection, and it binds to antibodies, thereby impairing the body's resistance to disease.

THE MALNUTRITION-LEAD CONNECTION

Among children, those who are malnourished are most vulnerable to lead poisoning. Children absorb more lead if their stomachs are empty, if they have low calcium or zinc intakes, and, of greatest concern because it is so common, if they have iron deficiencies.

As Chapter 13 mentioned, lead poisoning can cause iron deficiency, and iron deficiency weakens the body's defenses against lead absorption. In fact, the interactions

Table H19–1

Symptoms of Lead Toxicity

In children:
- Learning disabilities
- Low IQ
- Behavior problems
- Slow growth
- Iron-deficiency anemia
- Nervous system disorders
- Impaired concentration
- Reduced short-term memory
- Slow reaction time
- Seizures
- Impaired hearing
- Poor coordination

In adults:
- Hypertension
- Reproductive complications

Figure H19–2

Sources of Lead Exposure

Lead finds its way into the bodies of children when they ingest lead-containing foods, water, dust, or paint chips, or when they breathe lead-laden air.

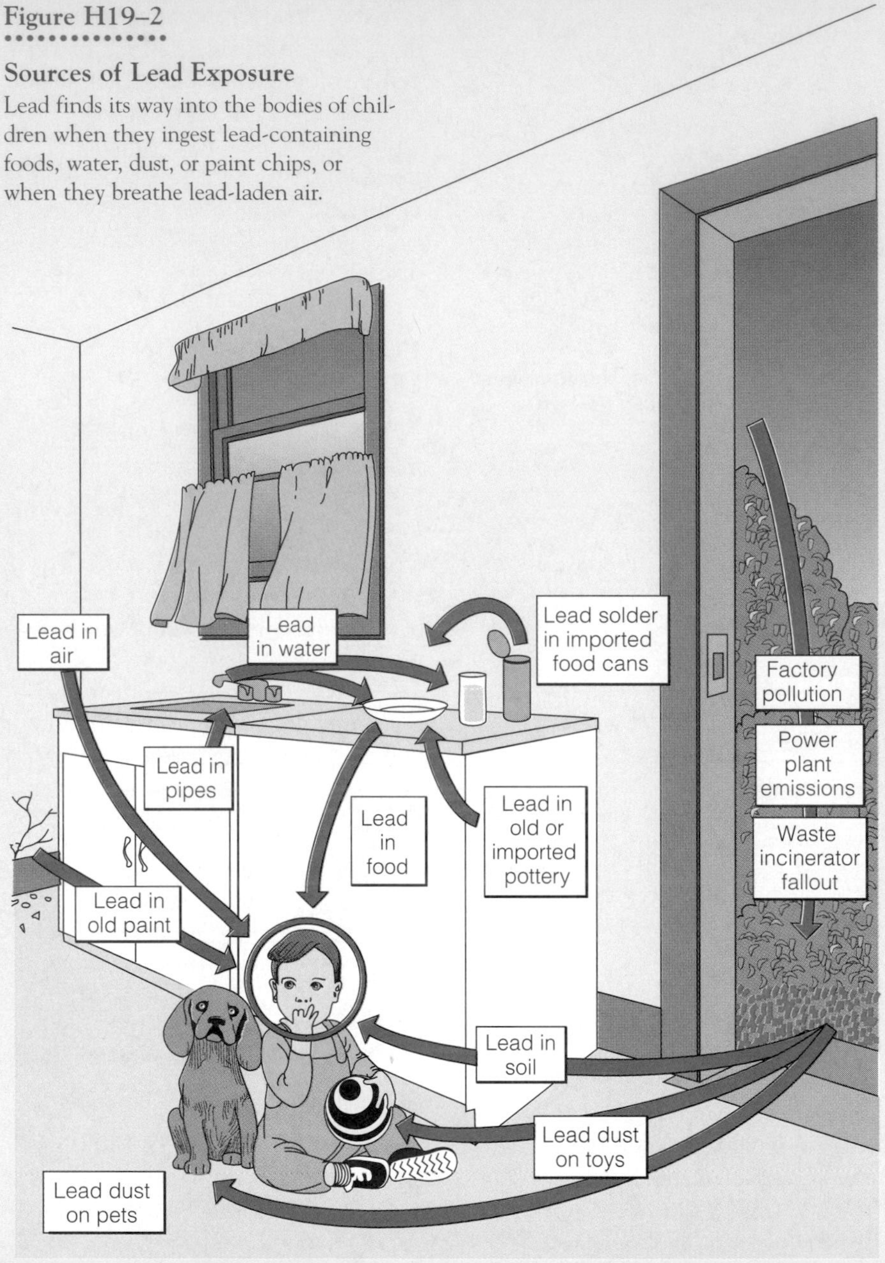

between lead poisoning and iron deficiency are so strong that lead poisoning is considered an adverse consequence of iron deficiency. A child with adequate iron stores is not immune, but a child with iron-deficiency anemia is three times as likely to have high blood lead. Common to both iron deficiency and lead poisoning is a low socioeconomic background. Another common factor is pica—a craving for nonfood items. Many children with lead poisoning eat dirt or newspapers, two common sources of lead.

The anemia brought on by lead poisoning may be mistaken for a simple iron deficiency, and therefore may be incorrectly treated. Like iron deficiency, mild lead toxicity has nonspecific symptoms, including diarrhea, irritability, reduced ability of the blood to carry oxygen, and fatigue. The symptoms are not reversible by adding iron to the diet; exposure to lead must stop. With further exposure, the signs become more pronounced: children lose cognitive, verbal, and perceptual abilities and develop learning disabilities and behavior problems. Still more severe lead toxicity can cause irreversible nerve damage, paralysis, mental retardation, and death.

Just as iron deficiency enhances lead uptake, an inadequate calcium intake enhances lead absorption and retention. Zinc deficiency also enhances both tissue accumulation of lead and sensitivity to its effects; serum zinc is frequently low in children with high blood lead. Prevention of lead toxicity rests primarily on reduced exposure, but parents can protect their children, at least to some degree, by making sure that they eat adequate foods rich in iron, calcium, zinc, and other nutrients.

LEAD IN THE ENVIRONMENT

All foods contain some lead. Most, perhaps all, of it derives from industrial pollution. People are exposed to lead in some types of gasoline, paint, newspaper ink, batteries, shotgun ammunition, and pesticides as well as in the air and water that carry lead from industrial processes and landfills. Lead works its way through rainfall and soil into plants and animals that people use for food. Lead also enters food from containers such as tin cans sealed with lead solder. (Manufacturers in the United States no longer use lead solder in canning, but many in foreign countries still do.) Old, handmade, or imported pottery decorated with lead glazes can also leach lead into foods.

Pipelines soldered with lead or coupled with brass fixtures also release lead into drinking water, making lead the nation's most significant water contaminant. A recent sampling by the EPA found unsafe levels of lead in the public water systems that serve 30 million people. Exposures are highest in older communities along the nation's east coast; in urban and industrial areas; near highways; and in slums where old leaded paint peels from the buildings. People suffering the effects of lead exposure are most often black, male, and from low-income families, but it is also seen in upper-middle-class families as they move into inner-city areas and renovate older homes.

Federal law has mandated reductions in the use of leaded gasolines, lead-based solder, and other products in recent years. These efforts have helped to reduce the amounts of lead in the environment—and in children's blood. The decline in blood lead in children during the late 1970s paralleled exactly the decline in the nation's use of leaded gasolines, leaded house paints, and lead-soldered food cans. Even so, lead still contaminates the blood of some 4 percent of our nation's children. Paint remains the primary source;[10] 70 percent of homes built before 1960 are covered with lead paint and are likely to cause lead poisoning, especially during times of renovation. A routine question asked when screening children for lead poisoning is whether they have ever lived in a house built before 1960.[11] If leaded surfaces in these homes are peeling and deteriorating, the children are either already poisoned or at immediate risk of lead poisoning.

STRATEGIES FOR PROTECTION

Three major discoveries about lead toxicity occurred simultaneously: lead poisoning has *subtle* effects; the effects are *permanent*; and they occur at *low levels of exposure*. Consumers would be wise to take ultraconservative measures to protect themselves, and especially their infants and young children, from lead poisoning.

Defensive strategies include:

- Test children for lead poisoning; lead screening is essential to preventing its devastating effects.[12]
- In contaminated environments, keep small children from putting dirty or old painted objects in their mouths, and make sure children wash their hands before eating.
- Be aware that other countries do not have the same regulations protecting consumers against lead. Children have been poisoned by eating crayons made in China and drinking fruit juice canned in Mexico.
- Make baby formula from lead-free ingredients. Do not use milk from lead-soldered cans and do not use lead-contaminated water.
- Once you have opened canned food, immediately move it to a lead-free storage container to prevent lead migration into the food.
- Do not store acidic foods or beverages (such as orange juice) in ceramic dishware.
- Many manufacturers are now making lead-safe products.* Old, handmade, or imported ceramic cups and bowls may contain lead and should not be used to heat coffee or tea, or acidic foods such as tomato soup.
- Do not store alcoholic beverages in pewter or crystal decanters.
- Some wineries still use lead in their foil seals; to be safe, wipe the foil-sealed rim of the wine bottle with water or lemon juice before removing the cork.
- Feed children nutritious meals regularly (see Chapter 16 for more details).
- Confirm with the publisher that your newspaper uses no lead in its ink before using the paper to wrap food, mulch garden plants, or add to your compost.

The EPA also publishes a booklet, *Lead and Your Drinking Water,* in which the following cautions appear:

- Have the water in your home tested by a competent laboratory.
- Use only cold water for drinking, cooking, and making formula (cold water absorbs less lead).
- When water has been standing in pipes for more than two hours, flush the cold-water pipes by running water through them for at least a minute before using it for drinking, cooking, or mixing formulas.

*Shopper's Guide to Low-Lead China is available from the Environmental Defense Fund, 257 Park Avenue South, New York, NY 10010; telephone (212) 505–2100.

- If lead contamination of your water supply seems probable, obtain additional information and advice from the EPA and your local public health agency.[13]

By taking these steps, parents can protect themselves and their children from this preventable danger.*

This highlight may appear to have been just about lead, but its actions typify the ways all heavy metals behave in the body: they interfere with nutrients that are trying to do their jobs. The "good guy" nutrients are shoved aside by the "bad guy" contaminants. Then the contaminants—whether lead, mercury, cadmium, or some other—cannot perform the roles of the nutrients, and health declines. To safeguard our health, we must defend ourselves against contamination by eating nutrient-rich foods and preserving a clean environment.

*The National Lead Information Center provides two hotlines; call (800) LEAD–FYI (532–3394) for general information or (800) 424–LEAD (424–5323) with specific questions.

NOTES

1. The majority of children with high blood lead levels (45 µg/dL) are treated using a process called chelation—using drugs (most often succimer or calcium-disodium EDTA) that bind to lead in the blood and carry it out in the urine. American Adademy of Pediatrics Committee on Drugs, Treatment guidelines for lead exposure in children, *Pediatrics* 96 (1995): 155–160.
2. P. A. Baghurst and coauthors, Environmental exposure to lead and children's intelligence at the age of seven years, *New England Journal of Medicine* 327 (1992): 1279–1284; D. C. Bellinger, K. M. Stiles, and H. L. Needleman, Low-level lead exposure, intelligence and academic achievement: A long-term follow-up study, *Pediatrics* 90 (1992): 855–961; H. L. Needleman and coauthors, The long-term effects of exposure to low doses of lead in childhood: An 11-year follow-up report, *New England Journal of Medicine* 322 (1990): 83–88.
3. K. N. Dietrich, O. G. Berger, and P. A. Succop, Lead exposure and the motor developmental status of urban six-year-old children in the Cincinnati Prospective Study, *Pediatrics* 97 (1993): 301–307.
4. J. Murphy, Federal agencies gearing up for new efforts against lead, *Nation's Health*, May/June 1991, pp. 1, 23.
5. A. Greeley, Getting the lead out of just about everything, *FDA Consumer*, July/August 1991, pp. 27–36.
6. FDA seeks lower lead levels in food additives and GRAS ingredients, *Journal of the American Dietetic Association* 94 (1994): 495.
7. C. A. Huseman, M. M. Varma, and C. R. Angle, Neuroendocrine effects of toxic and low blood lead levels in children, *Pediatrics* 90 (1992): 186–189.
8. Murphy, 1991.
9. M. W. Shannon and J. W. Graef, Lead intoxication in infancy, *Pediatrics* 89 (1992): 87–90.
10. Childhood lead poisoning: A disease for the history texts (editorial), *American Journal of Public Health* 81 (1991): 685.
11. H. J. Binns, Is there lead in the suburbs? Risk assessment in Chicago suburban pediatric practices, *Pediatrics* 93 (1994): 164–171.
12. Committee on Environmental Health, Lead poisoning: From screening to primary prevention, *Pediatrics* 92 (1993): 176–183; S. J. Schaffer, P. G. Szilagyi, and M. Weitzman, Lead poisoning risk determination in an urban population through the use of a standardized questionnaire, *Pediatrics* 93 (1994): 159–163.
13. U.S. Environmental Protection Agency, Office of Water, *Lead and Your Drinking Water*, publication no. OPA 87–006 (Washington, D.C.: U.S. Government Printing Office, April 1987).

Chapter 20

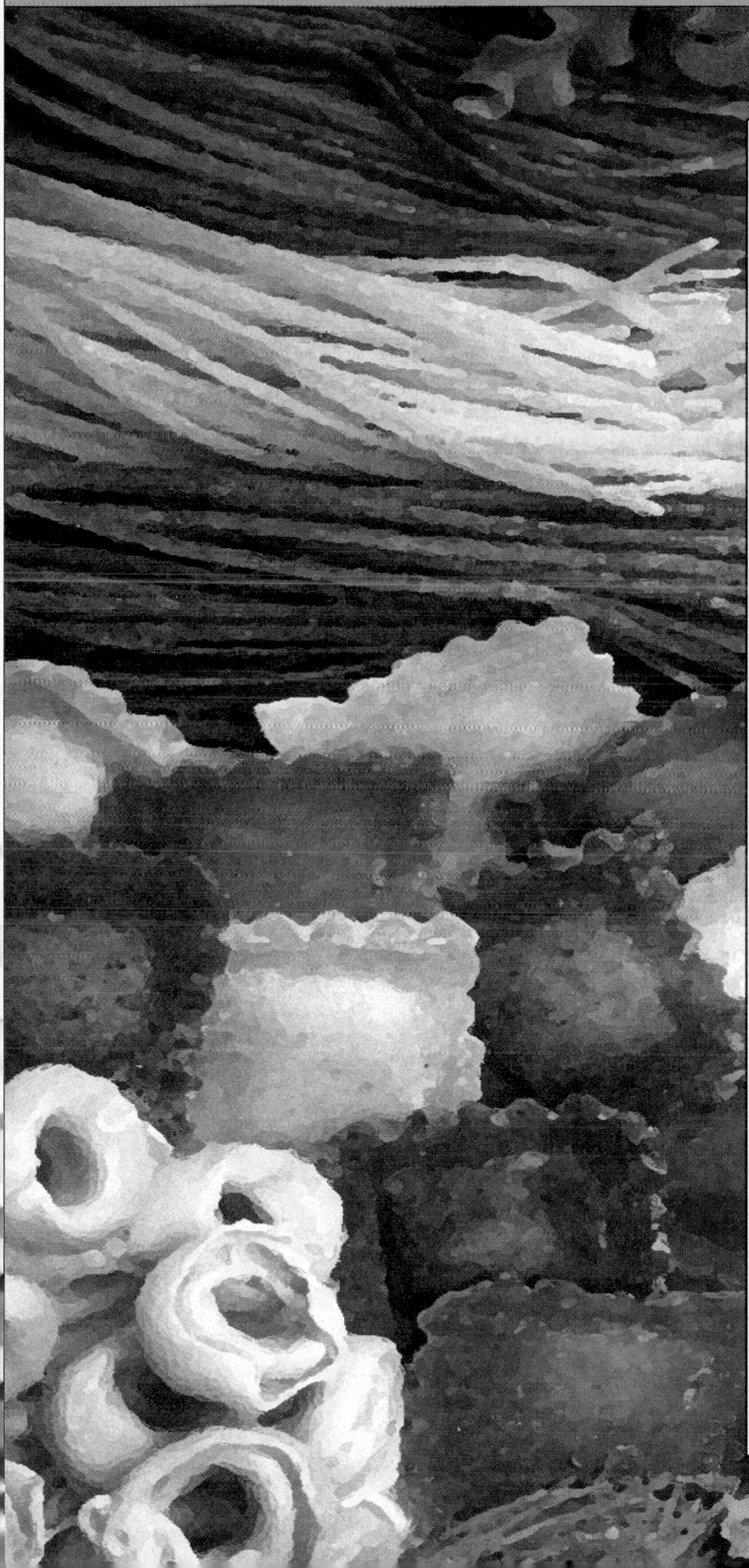

Hunger and Global Environmental Problems

CONTENTS

MICROGRAPH: Vitamin A, the most common vitamin deficiency among the hungry people of the world

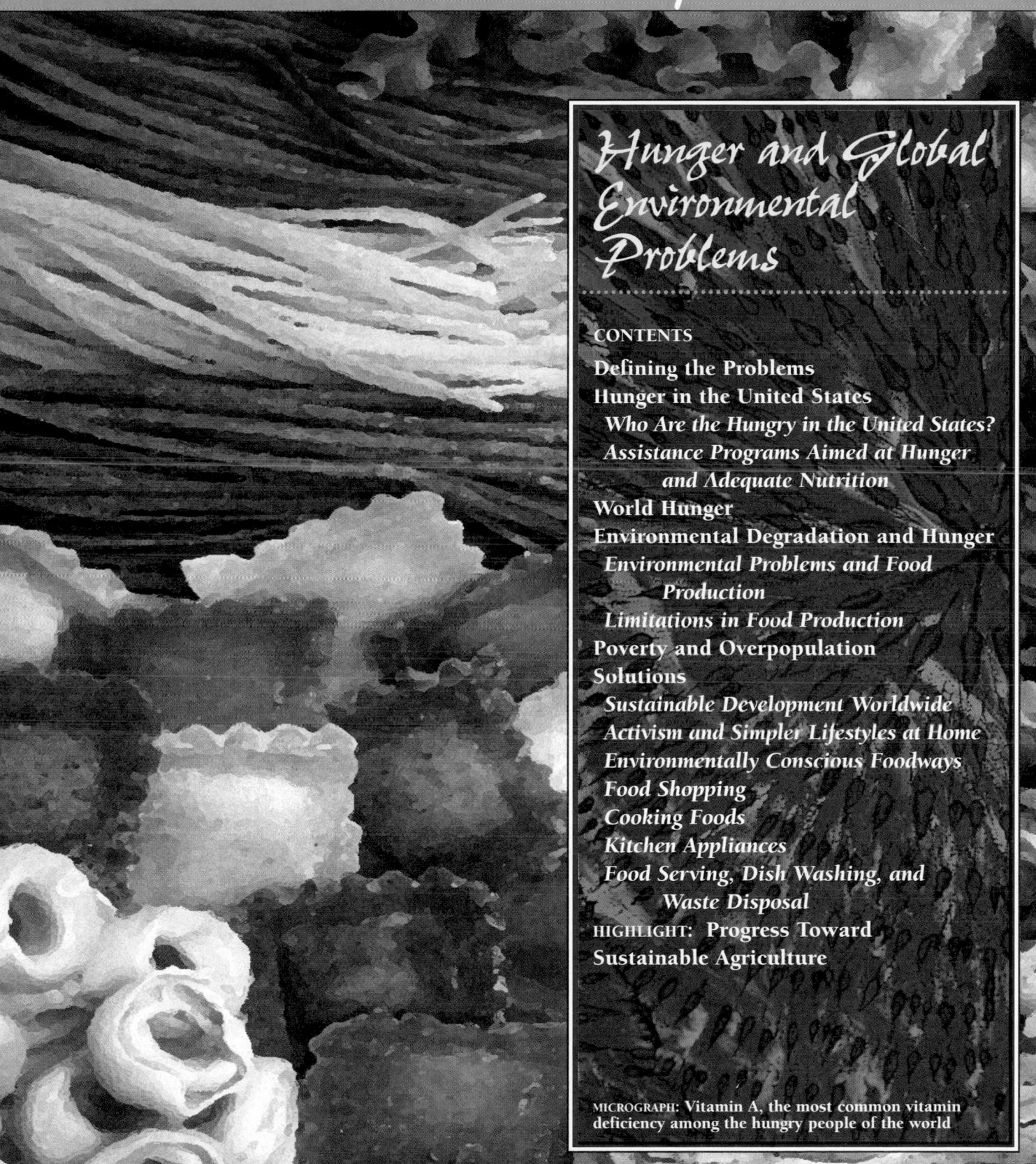

Defining the Problems

In the early 1990s, one person in every ten worldwide was experiencing hunger—not the healthy hunger we all feel, which leads us to sit down and eat a hearty meal, but the chronic, painful hunger people feel when no food is available. Today, hundreds of millions of people are suffering from chronic hunger, both in the developing world and at home in the United States. Many are dying of starvation: tens of thousands each day, one every two seconds.[1] Many are children. Tragic scenes of people starving in drought- and flood-stricken areas are a familiar sight on television. Some of the causes (such as war) are obvious, but the environmental factors that often underlie these situations are less apparent.

During the 1990s, all of the following trends are taking place at once:

- *Hunger, poverty, and population growth.* Millions of people are starving. Fifteen children die of malnutrition every 30 seconds, but more than 75 children are born in that same 30 seconds.[2]
- *Losses of food-producing land.* Food-producing land is eroding, becoming more salty, and being paved over. Each year, the world's farmers try to feed over 90 million more people with 24 billion fewer tons of topsoil.[3]
- *Accelerating fossil fuel use.* Fossil fuel use is accelerating, with attendant pollution of air, soil, and water; ozone depletion; and global warming.
- *Increasing air pollution.* Air quality is diminishing all over the globe, despite increased awareness of this problem and successful measures to control certain pollutants, such as lead and chlorofluorocarbons (CFCs).
- *Global warming, droughts, and floods.* Atmospheric concentrations of heat-trapping carbon dioxide are now 26 percent higher than the preindustrial level and are continuing to climb. As a result, a massive warming trend seems to be taking place.[4] It is changing the climate, causing both droughts and floods, and threatening to destroy crops and people's homelands.
- *Ozone loss from the outer atmosphere.* The outer atmosphere's protective ozone layer is growing thinner, permitting harmful radiation from the sun to damage crops and ecosystems and to cause cancers and cataracts in people and animals.[5]
- *Water shortages.* The world's supplies of fresh water are dwindling and becoming polluted.
- *Deforestation and desertification.* Forests are being destroyed, and with the loss of trees, natural water cycles are disrupted. Desert areas are increasing and cultivable land is decreasing.
- *Ocean pollution.* Ocean pollution is killing fish; overfishing is depleting the numbers of those that remain. Marine scientists report that all 17 of the world's major fishing grounds are currently harvested at or beyond their capacity and 9 are in a state of decline.[6] Per capita fish supplies are down by 8 percent from the 1989 historic high seafood harvest.[7]
- *Extinctions of species.* Many animals and plants are becoming extinct, a minimum of 140 species a day. An additional 20 percent of all species are expected to die out in the next ten years.[8] Many kinds of whales, birds, giant mammals, colorful butterflies, and thousands of other animals and plants will never again be seen on this planet.

fossil fuel: coal, oil, and natural gas; these are nonrenewable fuels that pollute. (Renewable or alternative fuels, such as solar and wind energy, pollute less or not at all.)

These global problems are all related: their causes overlap, and so do their solutions. Any initiative a person takes to help solve one problem will help solve many others. Figure 20–1 (pp. 720–721) shows a few of the many interconnections among today's global environmental problems, and Figure 20–2 (p. 722) shows ways in which U.S. consumers may unknowingly contribute to these problems.

This chapter examines hunger in the United States and around the world and discusses how environmental problems contribute to world hunger. Aside from the constant struggle to overcome the devastation wrought by civil unrest and wars, the ultimate solutions to the problem of world hunger involve both large- and small-scale choices made with an awareness of environmental consequences. The objective is to identify sustainable ways of doing things. Sustainable development permits economic growth without environmental destruction. Sustainable use consumes resources at a rate that nature, forestry, or agriculture can replace. Numerous examples of environmentally conscious choices related to food consumption are presented in this chapter.

sustainable: able to continue indefinitely. Here, the term means the use of resources at such a rate that the earth can keep on replacing them—for example, cutting trees no faster than new ones grow and producing pollutants at a rate with which the environment and human cleanup efforts can keep pace, so that no net accumulation of pollution occurs.

Readers may be concerned such lifestyle changes could result in lost jobs and harm the U.S. economy. Fortunately, however, to a large extent new jobs can take the place of the old. Renewable energy facilities employ more workers than coal or oil facilities; the recycling industry employs more workers than do landfill operations; and railroads employ more workers than the automobile industry.[9] In some cases new kinds of jobs can be created, such as in environmental cleanup work and pollution control. If people learn to place more reliance on goods produced sustainably from renewable resources and less on goods produced with intense negative environmental impacts, jobs and the economy may expand, not decline.

Overwhelming evidence shows that the widely held belief that we can take care of the environment *or* the economy, but not both, is a fallacy.[10] Careful planning will be needed, but given the state of the environment today, jobs are most likely to sustain people in the future if they also sustain the environment. Meanwhile, all individuals can begin the process of shifting to a sustainable economy by making environmentally conscious choices such as the ones described in this chapter.

In short, the global environment, which supports all life, is deteriorating rapidly, largely because of our irresponsible use of resources and energy. Environmentally conscious choices may help solve the hunger problem, improve the quality of life, and generate jobs.

Hunger in the United States

Much as it should surprise us, even in the United States, hunger is a problem. It is estimated that 30 million Americans, including 12 million children, cannot afford to buy enough food to maintain good health.[11] Soup kitchens are numerous and are needed as badly in some regions of the country as were the bread lines of the Great Depression in the 1930s. The prevalence of malnutrition and other health problems associated with chronic hunger—stunted growth, failure to thrive, low-birthweight babies, infant mortality, and anemia—is declining more slowly than in earlier decades; some problems are growing worse. Some studies

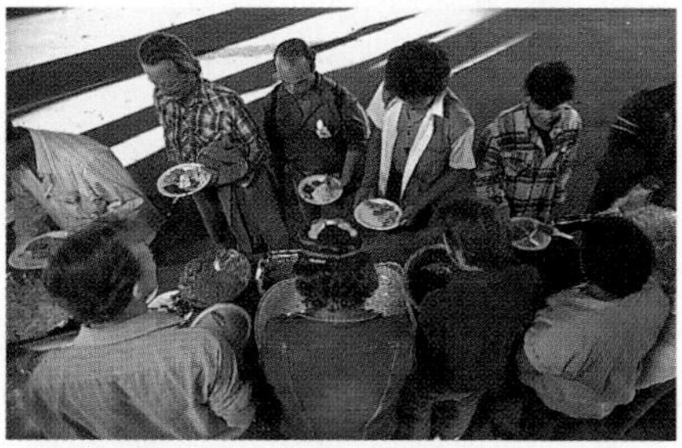

Feeding the hungry—in the United States.

Figure 20–1 The Giant Web of Global Problems

Follow the arrows to see how each problem intensifies others. Read the key opposite to understand the relationships.

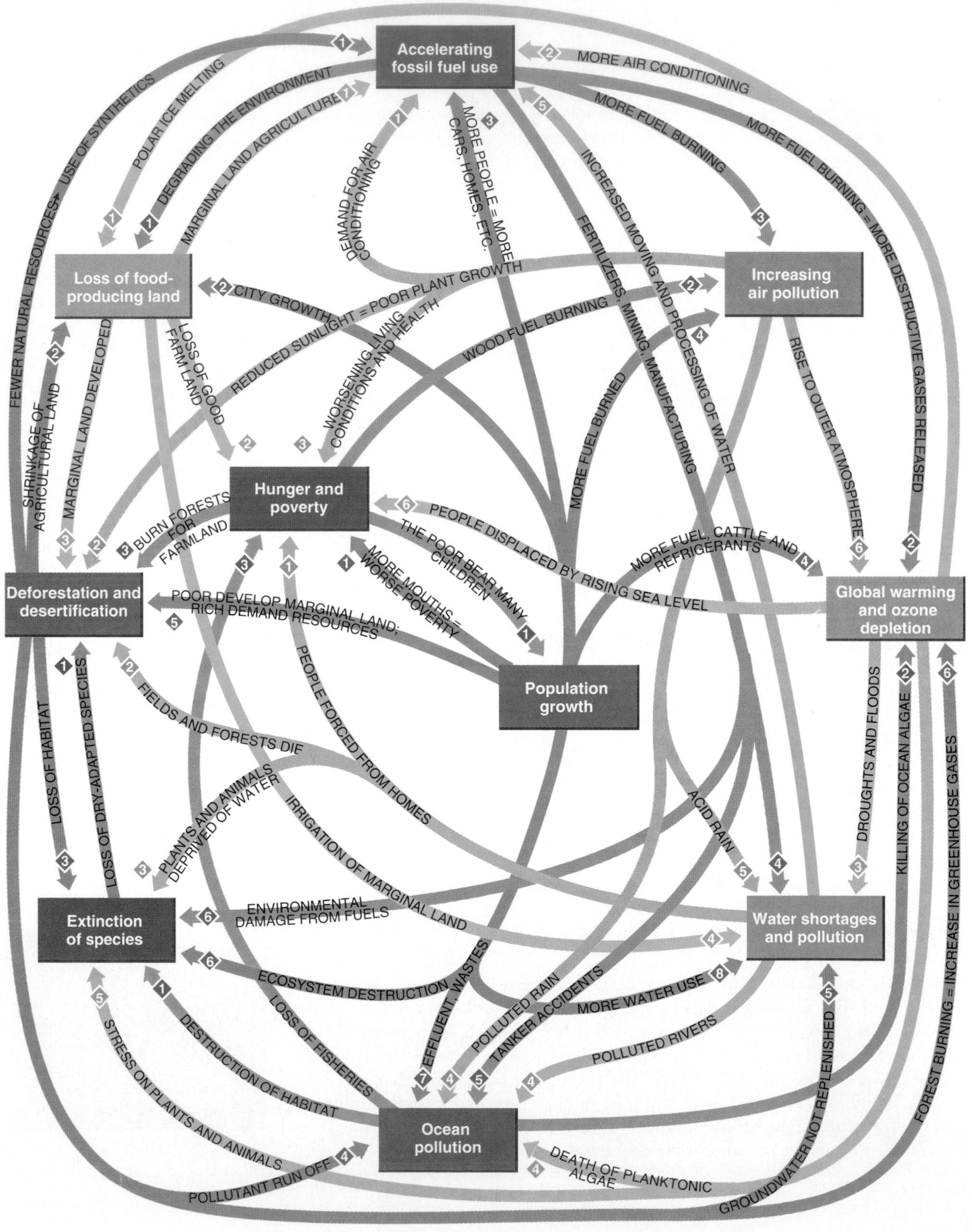

Each colored number explains an arrow on the diagram opposite and shows how one problem intensifies another.

Hunger and poverty

1. People living in hunger and poverty are not sure their children will survive, so they bear as many children as they can.
2. Poor people burn wood for fuel.
3. Poor people, being landless, venture into wilderness areas and cut and burn trees to establish plots where they can grow food. Deforested lands tend to dry out and turn to deserts.

Population growth

1. The more mouths there are to feed, the worse the poverty.
2. Growing cities expand into former farmlands.
3. Growing populations and growing use of consumer goods, appliances, and cars intensifies use of gas, coal, and oil for homes, cars, and factories.
4. The more people, the more fuels burned, and the greater the release of global-warming and ozone-destroying gases. Also, more people mean more cattle, which release methane that hastens global warming and ozone loss. More people mean more home and car air conditioners, refrigerators, and freezers and more ozone-destroying refrigerants.
5. Growing populations of poor spread onto marginal lands and destroy the balance of nature that supports plant life.
6. The growing human population, by devouring land and polluting air and water, destroys ecosystems and uses up resources that are required to support other forms of life.
7. Growing populations of poor, living near the ocean, pollute it with their sewage and their garbage. Growing wealthy populations overuse fertilizers and pesticides near coastlines.
8. The more poor, the more water they need to drink and grow their food, and the more human waste they produce. Added wealthy people also use water to support mining and manufacturing and produce consumer goods. The wealthy also produce agricultural and industrial pollution.

Loss of food-producing land

1. As good farmland is paved over, marginal land is recruited for agriculture. Marginal land requires more intensive cultivation and more fertilizer, both using fossil fuels.
2. As good farmland diminishes, food shortages intensify.
3. Some marginal land being recruited for agriculture formerly supported forests; some cannot withstand the pressures of agriculture and become deserts.
4. Marginal land used to grow food crops demands more irrigation, which devours water, salts the land, pollutes waterways.

Accelerating fossil fuel use

1. Air and water pollution from increasing fossil fuel use renders more and more land unsuitable for agriculture.
2. Oil, coal, and gas release carbon dioxide and other gases which accumulate in the atmosphere, trap heat, warm the climate, and destroy outer-atmosphere ozone.
3. Oil, coal, and gas release air pollutants.
4. Fuels and fertilizers made from them pollute rivers. Mining, manufacturing, and other industries deplete and pollute water supplies.
5. Tankers carrying fuels have accidents and oil spills.
6. Fossil fuel pollutants are damaging the environment and upsetting the natural conditions on which all life depends.

Increasing air pollution

1. Polluted air leads people to use more fuel to run air conditioners and purifiers.
2. Air pollution deprives plants of needed sunlight and harms animal and plant life, including food crops.
3. Air pollution destroys health and worsens poverty.
4. Polluted air, scrubbed by rain, drops pollutants in the ocean.
5. Polluted rain contaminates surface water and groundwater.
6. Air pollutants rise, trap heat, and destroy ozone.

Global warming and ozone depletion

1. As the earth warms, the polar ice caps are melting, causing sea level to rise and landmasses to shrink.
2. Warmer climate leads to use of more air conditioning and refrigeration.
3. Global warming causes both droughts and floods, which alternately deplete and pollute water supplies.
4. In a warmer climate, the ocean's planktonic algae, a major global consumer of carbon dioxide and producer of oxygen, may sicken and die. Since these algae also cleanse the ocean, their death may destroy the cleansing mechanism.
5. Warmer climate stresses plants and animals and leads to extinctions. Loss of earth's protective ozone layer lets harmful ultraviolet radiation and heat from the sun reach earth's surface, stressing plants and animals more.
6. Rising seas and shrinking landmasses displace people from their homes.

Water shortages and pollution

1. Water shortages render areas unsuitable for human habitation, forcing people from their homes.
2. Water shortages cause fields and forests to dry up and die.
3. Water shortages often wipe out the few remaining members of endangered plant and animal species.
4. Polluted rivers pollute the ocean.
5. More transportation of water over land, desalting of ocean water, and purification of polluted water for reuse mean more energy use.

Deforestation and desertification

1. Without wood, people use fossil fuels both for energy and to make wood substitutes such as plastics.
2. As deserts grow, land areas useful for agriculture shrink.
3. Losses of forested or fertile lands rob species of needed habitat.
4. Deforested lands and dried-up wetlands cannot absorb and detain pollutants. Instead, they run off.
5. Forests capture and return water to the earth. Trees also transpire water to the air, contributing to rainfall. Without this cycle, water runs off into rivers and the ocean, for a net loss of fresh water. Forests also purify water; without them, there is more water pollution.
6. Burning of tropical forests releases carbon dioxide that traps planetary heat and leaves fewer trees to remove carbon dioxide from the air.

Ocean pollution

1. Severe ocean pollution may destroy the conditions necessary for life.
2. Ocean pollution is beginning to kill ocean algae, which help moderate the planet's temperature.
3. Ocean pollution kills ocean life, leading to losses of fisheries.

Extinction of species

1. Extinction reduces the number of trees and plants that can grow in marginal areas.

Figure 20–2 U.S. Consumption Patterns Contributing to Global Problems

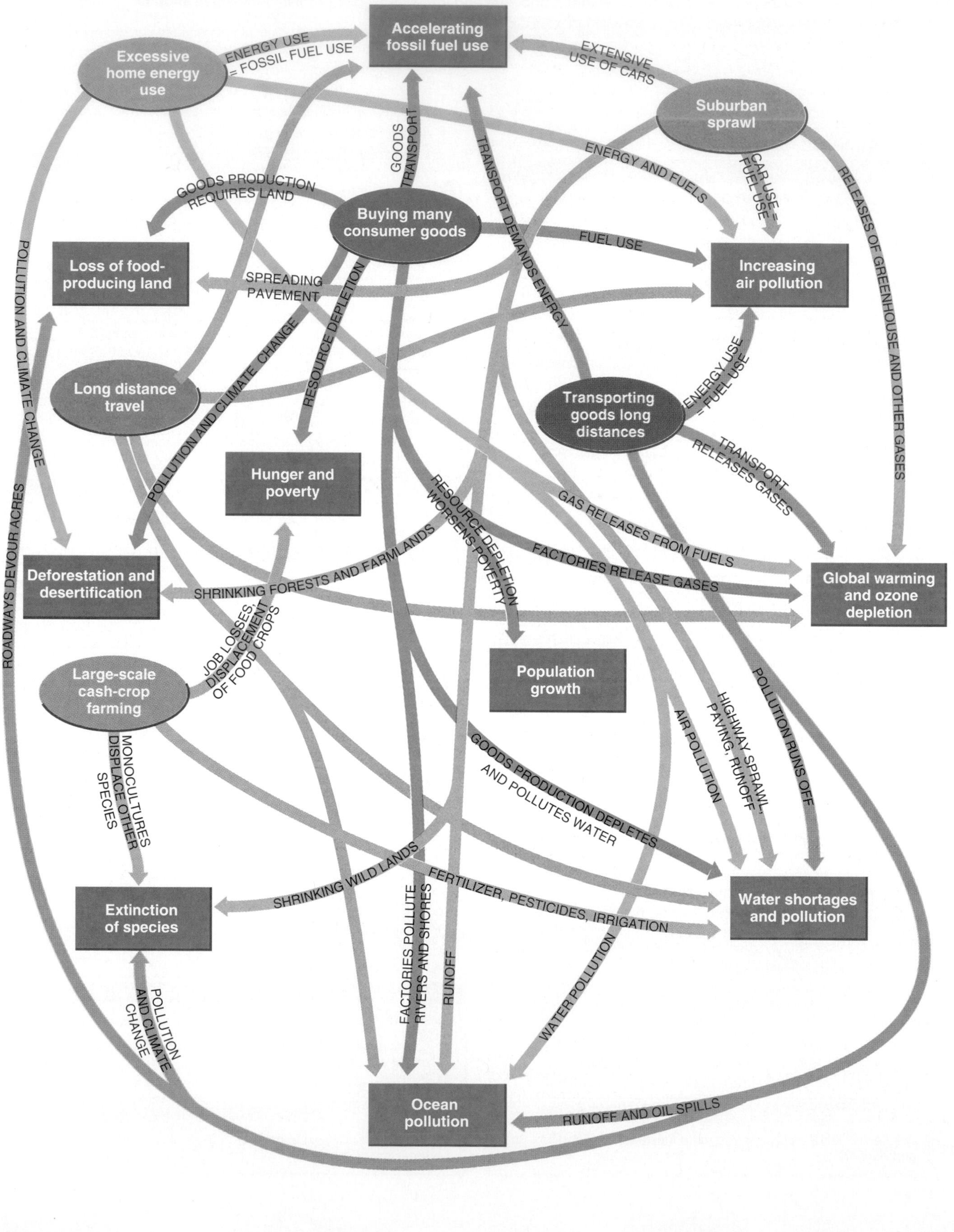

show that one of every five children in the United States is chronically hungry; these children live in families that do not know where their next meal is coming from or when it will come.[12] Their hunger stems, not from the lack of available food, but from the lack of money with which to buy it.[13]

WHO ARE THE HUNGRY IN THE UNITED STATES?

Hunger is not always easy to recognize. The accompanying box shows how national surveys identify "food insecurity" and hunger in the United States. Questions like these provide crude, but necessary, data to estimate the degree of hunger in this country.

food insecurity: intermittent hunger caused by lack of money or lack of control over other resources needed to assure a reliable food supply; the predominant form of hunger in the United States today.

Hunger has many causes, but a major one is poverty. Other causes that contribute to hunger are abuse of alcohol and other drugs; physical and mental illness; lack of awareness of available food assistance programs; and the reluctance of people, particularly the elderly, to accept what they perceive as "welfare" or

How to Identify Food Insecurity in a U.S. Household

Questions like these are asked on surveys to determine the extent of food insecurity in a household. The more questions that receive a "Yes" answer, the more intense the hunger the household is experiencing.

- Do you usually have enough food to eat? If you don't have enough food to eat, is it because:
  a. you sometimes run out of money to buy food?
  b. you do not have transportation?
  c. you do not have working appliances (stove, refrigerator)?
- Do you ever rely on nutritionally inferior foods to feed yourself or your children because you lack any of these resources?
- Do you ever eat less than you feel you should because you lack any of these resources?
- Do you ever skip meals or cut the size of meals because you lack any of these resources?
- Do you ever rely on neighbors, friends, relatives, or schools to feed any of your children because there is not enough food in the house?
- Do your children ever say they are hungry because there is not enough food in the house?
- Do you or any of your children ever go to bed hungry because there is not enough food in the house?

Sources: Adapted from C. A. Wehler, R. I. Scott, and J. J. Anderson, The Community Childhood Hunger Identification Project: A model of domestic hunger—demonstration project in Seattle, Washington, Journal of Nutrition Education (1 supplement) 24 (1992): 29S–35S; and R. R. Briefel and C. E. Woteki, Development of food sufficiency questions for the Third National Health and Nutrition Examination Survey, Journal of Nutrition Education (1 supplement) 24 (1992): 24S–28S.

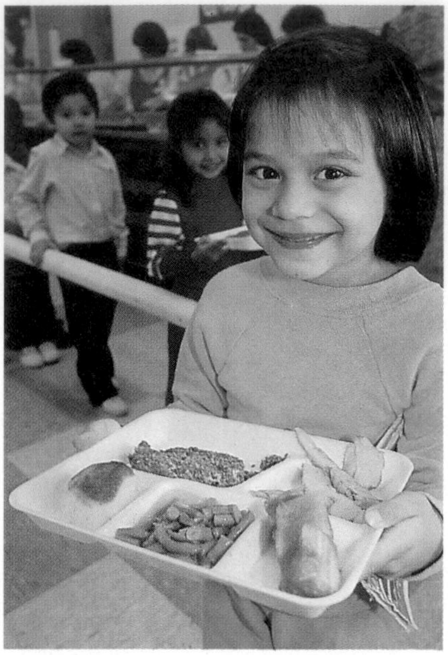

School lunches provide children with nourishment at little or no charge.

"charity."[14] Still, poverty remains the major cause of hunger, and solving the poverty problem would do a lot to solve the hunger problem.

In the United States, poverty and hunger reach into all segments of society, affecting not only the chronic poor (migrant workers, the unskilled and unemployed, the homeless, and some elderly) but also the so-called new poor. Some are displaced farm families. Some are former blue-collar and white-collar workers forced out of their trades and professions into minimum-wage jobs. These people outnumber the chronic poor, and they are not on welfare; they have jobs, but the pay is low. Families with incomes below a certain level are simply unable to buy sufficient amounts of nourishing foods, even if they are wise food shoppers.

ASSISTANCE PROGRAMS AIMED AT HUNGER AND ADEQUATE NUTRITION

At present, many U.S. programs aimed at preventing or remediating domestic malnutrition and hunger are in effect. In addition, local programs provide food to those in need.

Federal Programs Several food assistance programs have been described in earlier chapters: the school lunch, breakfast, and child care food programs for children; the WIC program for low-income pregnant women, mothers, and their young children; and food assistance programs for older adults such as congregate meals and Meals on Wheels. Another program aimed directly at the poor is the Food Stamp Program, administered by the U.S. Department of Agriculture (USDA). The Food Stamp Program is the largest of the federal food assistance programs, both in amount of money spent and in number of people participating. Over 27 million people in the United States receive food stamps at a budget cost of over $22 billion per year.[15] Over 80 percent of food stamp recipients are families with children.[16]

Food Stamp Program: a federal food assistance program. The USDA issues food stamp coupons through state social services or welfare agencies to households—people who buy and prepare food together. The number of stamps a household receives depends on the household's size and income. Recipients may use the coupons like cash to purchase food and seeds, but not to buy tobacco, cleaning items, alcohol, or other nonfood items.

To what extent these federal programs will continue to feed those who are hungry is unknown, given the current political climate; many federal programs are being targeted in cost-saving measures.

These federal programs support both health and well-being. For example, children in Project Head Start, an educational program that includes breakfast, are twice as likely to graduate from high school and to become employed as their peers in the same circumstances who do not participate.[17]

Although these programs reach millions of people daily with life-sustaining foods, hunger continues to plague the United States. Of the estimated 2 million homeless people in the United States who are eligible for food assistance, only 15 percent of single adults and 50 percent of families receive food stamps.

Local Programs To supplement federal programs and reach those who are still hungry, private efforts have sprung up in many communities, where concerned citizens work through local agencies and churches to feed the hungry. Community-based soup kitchens and shelters generally provide good-quality meals. The meals often average 1000 kcalories each, but most homeless people receive fewer than 1½ meals a day, so many are inadequately nourished.[18] Table 20–1 shows how individuals can assist in local hunger relief efforts; it presents a 14-step program for developing a hunger-free community.

Table 20–1

Fourteen Ways Communities Can Address Their Hunger Problems

1. Establish a community-based emergency food delivery network.
2. Assess community hunger problems and evaluate community services. Create strategies for responding to unmet needs.
3. Establish a group of individuals, including low-income participants, to develop and implement policies and programs to combat hunger and the threat of hunger; monitor responsiveness of existing services; and address underlying causes of hunger.
4. Participate in federally assisted nutrition programs that are easily accessible to targeted populations.
5. Integrate public and private resources, including local businesses, to relieve hunger.
6. Establish an education program that addresses the food needs of the community and the need for increased local citizen participation in activities to alleviate hunger.
7. Provide information and referral services for accessing both public and private programs and services.
8. Support programs to provide transportation and assistance in food shopping, where needed.
9. Identify high-risk populations and target services to meet their needs.
10. Provide adequate transportation and distribution of food from all resources.
11. Coordinate food services with parks and recreation programs and other community-based outlets to which residents of the area have easy access.
12. Improve public transportation to human service agencies and food resources.
13. Establish nutrition education programs for low-income citizens to enhance their food purchasing and preparation skills and make them aware of the connections between diet and health.
14. Establish a program for collecting and distributing nutritious foods—either agricultural commodities in farmers' fields or prepared foods that would have been wasted.

Source: House Select Committee on Hunger, legislation introduced by Tony P. Hall, excerpted in *Seeds,* Sprouts edition, January 1992, p. 3 with permission, © SEEDS Magazine, P.O. Box 6170; Waco, TX 76706. For more guidance on developing a hunger-free community, write: Hunger Free, House Select Committee on Hunger, 505 Ford House Office Building, Washington, DC 20515.

To summarize, poverty and hunger are widespread in the United States both among the unemployed and the underemployed. Government assistance programs help to relieve poverty and hunger, but they fall short.

World Hunger

In developing countries, which face more extreme hunger problems than the United States, the causes of hunger are more diverse. Again, the primary cause of hunger is poverty, but the poverty is more extreme. Most people would find it almost impossible to comprehend the severity of poverty in the developing world. One-fifth of the world's 5 billion people have no land and no possessions *at all.* They survive on less than one dollar a day each, they lack water that is safe to drink, and they cannot read or write.[19] The average U.S. housecat eats twice as much protein every day as one of these people, and the cost of keeping that cat is greater than such a person's annual income.[20]

Causes of Famine When we think of world hunger, most frequently we visualize the victims of famine. However, the natural causes of famine—drought, flood, and pests—have become less important in recent years than the social

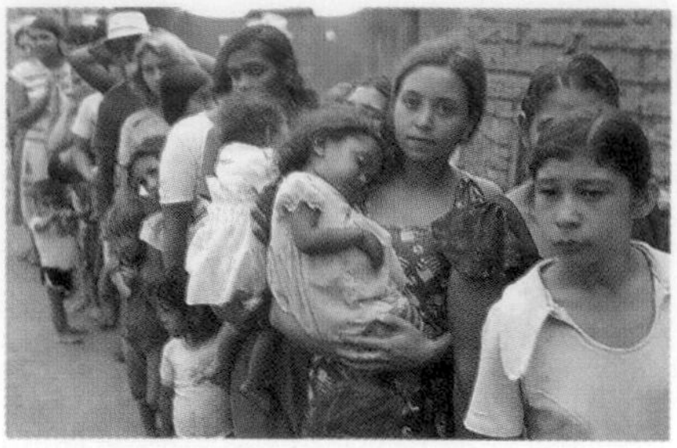

Feeding the hungry—in Nicaragua.

causes. Widespread hunger and starvation can occur even when food is available, if people have lost their ability to obtain that food. Thus a sudden increase in food prices, a drop in workers' incomes, or a change in government policy can create hunger for millions even in the absence of the more familiar obstacles of drought, flood, disease, or even war and civil unrest. Between 15 and 30 million people died during the Chinese famine of 1959 through 1961, the worst famine of this century; it was primarily a result of government policies associated with the "great leap forward," which devastated the Chinese agricultural system.[21]

In the 1990s, armed conflict has become the dominant cause of famine worldwide. In all of the countries that have reported famine so far in the 1990s—Angola, Ethiopia, Liberia, Mozambique, Somalia, and Sudan—armed conflict has been a major cause. Not only do armed conflicts create famines, but they often are the key obstacle preventing famine relief by destroying or blocking food supplies from getting to those in need. The world continues to struggle to find a middle ground between respecting the sovereignty of nations and refusing to allow any nation to prevent humanitarian assistance from reaching its people.

International Food Assistance Since the 1950s, food aid has provided a backup for countries threatened with harvest failures. But the program has shifted in more recent years from just offsetting poor harvests to providing food relief to countries, such as Ethiopia, that are chronically short of food and without resources to buy it. Some people are concerned that as many countries decrease their funding for foreign aid, this food aid backup may become insufficient.

Chronic Malnutrition While famine is the image we usually associate with world hunger, the numbers affected by famine are relatively small compared with those suffering less acute forms of hunger. Nearly 800 million people in developing countries suffer from chronic malnutrition.[22] In addition, one child in six in the world is born underweight, and almost two in five children are underweight by the age of five. Around 2 billion people, mostly women and children, are deficient in one or more of these micronutrients: iron, iodine, and vitamin A.[23]

Tens of thousands die each day as a result of malnutrition. Many are children afflicted by the diseases of poverty: parasitic and infectious diseases such as dysentery, whooping cough, measles, tuberculosis, cholera, and malaria. These diseases interact with poor nutrition in a vicious cycle that leads to death—at the rate of one every two seconds. Because of poverty, infection, and malnutrition, the life expectancy in some African countries averages 50 years; in Uganda it is only 38 years, half of the U.S. life expectancy.[24]

Overpopulation versus Food Production Until 1988, the world celebrated an increase nearly every year in its reserves of stored grain, an index of the sufficiency of the world food supply. The often-repeated statement that "We have enough food to feed everyone" was true. Efforts at relieving hunger focused on transporting food to where it was needed and on improving storage. Also, because in many developing countries most of the men were involved in producing cash crops for export, hunger-relief efforts focused on educating and empowering women to grow and use nutritious food to feed their families. These efforts were addressing the causes of the world's hunger problem and were expected to solve it.

cash crops: crops grown for cash, as opposed to crops grown for food; examples include cotton and tobacco.

Since 1988, however, the situation has changed. The world's population is growing at the rate of about 90 million persons each year, and food production is no longer keeping pace. In recent years, grain reserves have fallen to dangerously low levels (see Figure 20–3). Current grain reserves are estimated to be sufficient to feed the world for only 50 to 60 days.[25] Further growth in the world's food output is being slowed by environmental degradation.

Figure 20–3

World Grain Carryover Stocks, 1961–1995

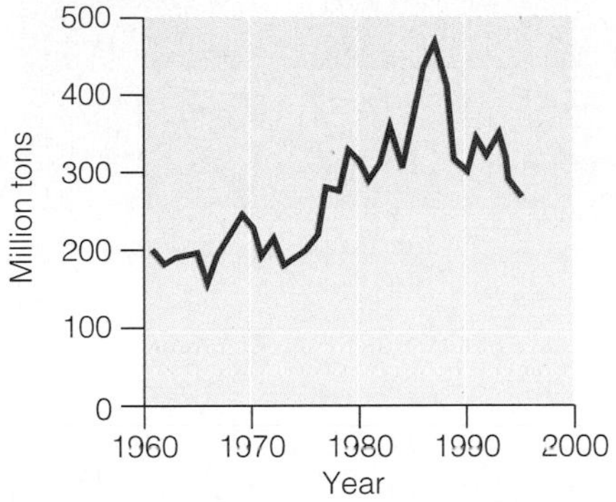

Natural causes such as drought, flood, and pests and social causes such as armed conflicts and overpopulation all contribute to the extreme hunger and poverty seen in the developing countries. International food assistance programs are insufficient to resolve the problems.

Environmental Degradation and Hunger

Today, environmental degradation is beginning to threaten the world's ability to produce enough food to feed its people. Not only are we losing our resources, but we are losing our ability to compensate for the losses.

ENVIRONMENTAL PROBLEMS AND FOOD PRODUCTION

One element of environmental degradation is soil erosion, which is occurring in every nation and is resulting in crop losses estimated at 6 percent per year.[26] Other environmental problems slowing food outputs are deforestation, air pollution, climate change, water scarcity, deterioration of rangelands, and declining fisheries.

Deforestation Deforestation along the watersheds of the Blue Nile led to erosion and during just nine years laid down so much silt behind the Roseires Reservoir dam in Sudan, which supplies irrigation water for the dry season, that one-third of its capacity was lost.[27] In Sierra Leone, where 60 percent of the land was primarily rainforest in 1961, only 6 percent is now.[28] For the world as a whole, if present rates continue, by 2010 per capita forested area will have dropped 30 percent.[29]

Air Pollution Damage to crops from air pollution is now measurable in the car-centered societies of Western Europe, the United States, and Canada and in societies that burn coal to generate electricity—notably, Eastern Europe and China. In the United States, according to a seven-year study by two government agencies, the most damaging air pollutants are ozone, sulfur dioxide, and nitrous oxide, which come from the burning of fossil fuels. Crops are especially sensitive to ground-level ozone concentrations, which increasingly are detected and measured in rural as well as urban areas in ranges that reduce crop yields. An estimate puts the increase in annual crop losses ascribable to ozone pollution at 1 percent per year.

Not only is ground-level ozone pollution reducing agricultural outputs, but outer-atmosphere ozone depletion is doing so, too—especially to radiation-sensitive crops such as soybeans. For each 1 percent loss of outer-atmosphere

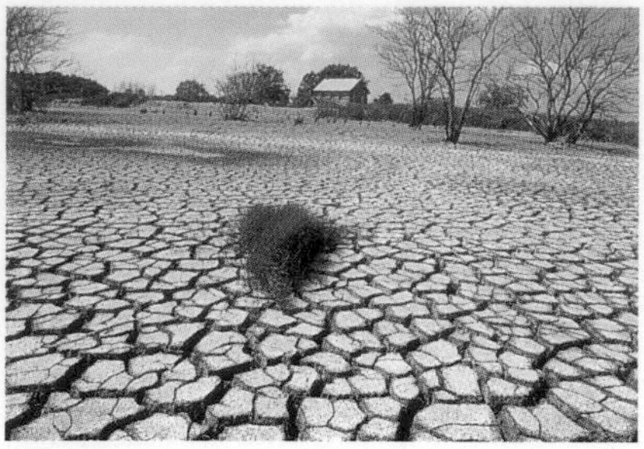

As ground water is used up, deserts spread.

ozone, the amount of damaging ultraviolet radiation reaching the earth increases by 2 percent. Based on studies of experimental plots, soybean yields fall 1 percent for each 1 percent rise in radiation. Soybeans are the world's leading protein crop, and at last report, no one was monitoring radiation-induced losses.

Climate Change Climate change may also affect crop yields. At whatever rate climate change is occurring, it is potentially disruptive. If summers become hotter, droughts during the growing season may become more common. An unusually hot and dry summer in 1988 pushed the U.S. grain harvest below consumption for the first time in history. In 1994, new heat records were set throughout the western United States, northern Europe, the Baltic, and Japan.[30] A rise of only a degree or so in average global temperature may reduce soil moisture, impair pollination of major food crops such as rice and corn, slow growth, weaken disease resistance, and disrupt many other factors affecting crop yields.

Water Scarcity Water supplies, too, are becoming limited. Decreases in available water result in reduced crop yields, most obviously on irrigated cropland. Two-thirds of all water taken from rivers and underground aquifers is used for irrigation.[31] Agricultural lands that require irrigation water play a disproportionate role in meeting the world's food needs. Although they account for only one-sixth of total cropland, irrigated croplands yield more than one-third of the total global harvest. The amount of irrigated land per capita, however, peaked in 1978 and has fallen almost 6 percent since then.[32]

Deteriorating Rangelands Grazing land is decreasing along with agricultural cropland. Grasslands for raising beef are already being fully used or misused on every continent. One-fifth of the world's land area is rangeland, twice as much area as is farmed. This land supports most of the world's 3.2 billion cattle, sheep, and goats.[33] Although world beef and mutton production per capita increased 37 percent between 1950 and 1972, more recent yields have dropped.[34] These decreases reflect deterioration in the condition of the rangelands due to environmental problems and extensive overgrazing. The feed needs of livestock in nearly all developing countries now exceed the capacity of their rangelands. In Africa, where this problem is most visible, the annual loss of rangeland productivity is estimated at $7 billion, more than the gross national product of Ethiopia and Uganda combined.[35]

Diminishing Fisheries The yield of fish from the oceans is also declining, for the first time in history, due to overfishing and pollution. Big fish, such as tuna, swordfish, and shark, are becoming threatened because they are being overfished. Atlantic stocks of the heavily fished bluefin tuna have dropped by 94 percent.[36] Cod are rapidly disappearing off the New England coast and are almost gone farther north.

Inland fisheries have also suffered tremendous drops in yield as a result of environmental damage. The Aral Sea, located between Kazakhstan and Uzbekistan, yielded 40,000 tons of fish per year in 1960 and today is biologically dead. As water was diverted for irrigation over the last 30 years, the sea became increasingly salty until finally fish could no longer live in it.[37] Acidification has also taken a toll on inland fisheries. In Canada, 14,000 lakes are considered biologically dead as a result of acid rain.[38]

LIMITATIONS IN FOOD PRODUCTION

All in all, then, environmental problems are reducing the world's ability to feed its people. With fish yields and rangelands decreasing, can advances in agriculture compensate for the losses caused by environmental degradation? Historically, agriculture has improved yields by making greater investments in irrigation, fertilizer, and improved genetic strains. Today, however, the contributions these measures can make are reaching limits for the first time in history: the improvements are leveling off. Irrigation can no longer compensate by improving crop yields because almost all the land that can benefit from irrigation is already receiving it. In fact, rising concentrations of salt in the soil—a by-product of irrigation—are *lowering* yields on close to a quarter of the world's irrigated cropland. Nor can fertilizer use enhance agricultural production much. Much of the fertilizing that can be done is being done—and with great effect; fertilizer use supports some 40 percent of the world's total crop yields. Adding more fertilizer, however, brings no further rise in yield. As for the development of high-yielding strains of crops, some advances have been dramatic, but they show little potential to change the overall trends described here. Furthermore, the raw materials necessary for developing new crops are becoming less and less available as genetic variety is lost due to the extinction of many plant species. Of the 5000 food plants used throughout the world a few centuries ago, only 150 are grown in modern agriculture today. Most of the world's population relies on only five cereals, three legumes, and three root crops to meet their energy needs. Even among these, valuable strains are vanishing.[39]

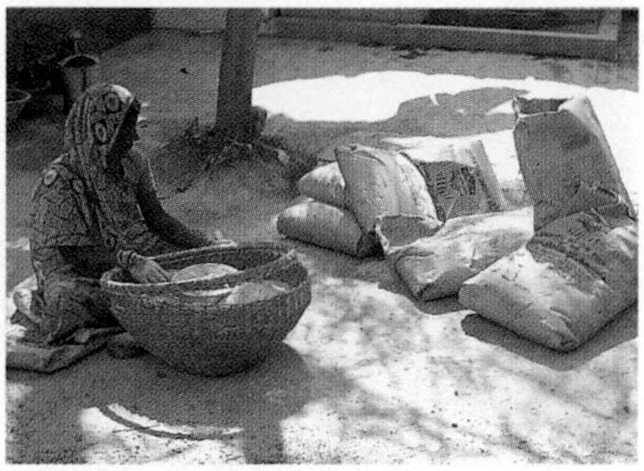

International efforts help to relieve hunger and poverty around the world.

Estimates are that the world grain harvest can be increased by no more than 1 percent a year. The increase might be higher, but for the many forms of environmental degradation described earlier. Meanwhile, the world's population is rising at the rate of at least 2 percent per year.[40] Many authorities in many fields—and more every year—are calling for a reduction in the growth rate of the world's population as the only way to enable the world's food output to keep pace with people's growing numbers.

The world still produces enough food to feed all its people, and the problem of hunger today remains a problem of unequal distribution of resources. If present trends continue, however, the time is approaching when there will be an absolute deficit of food. This conclusion seems inescapable. The world's increasing population threatens the world's capacity to produce adequate food. Population control has become one of the most pressing needs of this time in history. Until the nations of the world resolve the population problem, they can neither support the lives of people already born nor remedy global trends toward environmental deterioration. And to resolve the population problem, a necessary first step is to remedy the poverty problems, for reasons discussed next. Of the 90 million people being added to the population each year, the vast majority are in the most poverty-stricken areas of the world.

To review, increasing environmental degradation reduces our ability to produce enough food to feed the world's people. Exacerbating the situation is the rapid increase in the world population.

Poverty and Overpopulation

The giant web of global problems shown in Figure 20–1 presented population growth as one of the many factors contributing to poverty and hunger. The fig-

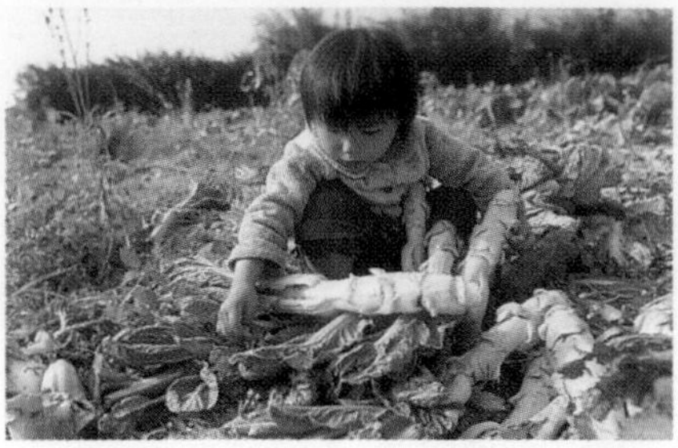
Families in developing countries depend on their children to help provide for daily needs.

ure also showed the reverse: poverty and hunger contribute to population growth.

Population Growth Leads to Hunger and Poverty The first of these cause-effect relationships is easy to understand. Population growth contributes to poverty and hunger, for the more mouths there are to feed, the worse poverty and hunger become. The sheer magnitude of our annual population increase of 90 million people is difficult to comprehend. Each month the world adds the equivalent of another New York City.[41] During six months of the terrible 1992 famine in Somalia, an estimated 300,000 people starved to death. Yet it took the world only 29 *hours* to replace their numbers! Ninety million people a year, spread over 365 days, comes to a quarter-million people a day—or just over 10,000 people born every hour.[42]

Population growth also contributes to hunger indirectly by preempting good agricultural land for growing cities and industry and forcing people onto marginal land, where they cannot produce sufficient food for themselves. The world's poorest people live in the world's most damaged and inhospitable environments. There they experience, daily, tens of thousands of early deaths from malnutrition and disease.

Hunger and Poverty Lead to Population Growth Overpopulation, then, together with the environmental degradation that it causes, worsens poverty. How, though, does poverty lead to overpopulation? Poverty and hunger are believed to exert an ironic effect on people, making them bear more children. Poverty and hunger typically go hand in hand with ignorance, including ignorance of how to control family size. Also, a family depends on its children to farm the land, haul water, and care for adults in their old age. If a family faces ongoing poverty with its associated high rates of childhood disease and mortality, the parents will choose to have many children to ensure that some will survive to adulthood. People are willing to risk having fewer children only if they are sure that their children will live.

Relieving poverty and hunger, then, may be a necessary first step in curbing population growth. When people attain better access to health care, education, and family planning, the death rate falls. At first there is a "bulge" in the population, because births outnumber deaths, but as the standard of living continues to improve, families become willing to risk having smaller numbers of children. Then the birth rate falls. Thus, after a short but necessary lag time, improvements in economic status help stabilize the population.

The link between improved economic status and slowed population growth has been demonstrated in country after country.[43] Sustainable development is central to this success and must include not only economic growth, but a sharing of resources among all groups. In parts of Sri Lanka, Taiwan, Malaysia, and Costa Rica, where this has happened, population growth has slowed the most. Where economic growth has occurred but only the rich have grown richer, population growth has remained high. Examples include Brazil, Mexico, the Philippines, and Thailand, where large families continue to be a major economic asset for the poor.

In brief, more people means more mouths to feed, which worsens the poverty and hunger problems. Poverty and hunger, on the other hand, encourage parents to have more children. Breaking this cycle requires improving the economic status of the people and providing them with health care, education, and family planning.

Solutions

Both the poor and the rich nations must contribute to solving the world's hunger, environmental, and poverty problems, but in different ways. The poor nations need to gain control of their rampaging population growth and to slow and reverse the destruction of their environmental resources: forests, waterways, and soil. To do this, they must, among other things, find ways to relieve their people's poverty. The rich nations need to stem their wasteful and polluting uses of resources and energy, which are contributing to global environmental degradation. They also must become willing to help relieve the debtor nations of their poverty in ways that effectively reach the poor.

SUSTAINABLE DEVELOPMENT WORLDWIDE

Many nations now recognize that improving all nations' economies is a prerequisite to meeting the world's other urgent needs: relief of hunger, population stabilization, arrest of environmental degradation, and sustainable treatment of resources. An important step was taken when a United Nations convention on the Rights of the Child was ratified by over 100 nations. Significantly, for the first time in world history, the convention cited *nutrition* as an internationally recognized human right.[11]

Another important step was taken in 1992, when more than 100 nations met for the Earth Summit in Rio de Janeiro, Brazil, and discussed the relationship of the environment to poverty and hunger.* At this meeting, many nations agreed for the first time to 27 principles of sustainable development, which the conferees defined as development that would equitably meet both the economic and the environmental needs of present and future generations.

Participants discussed climate change and the possibility of setting legally binding targets and timetables for every nation to cut its emissions of global-warming gases. They began to approach agreement on this issue. They also signed agreements to protect the earth's remaining species of plants and animals and to preserve the world's forests.

The Earth Summit's discussions opened vistas of hope. Much remains to be done, and all nations have major parts to play. For our part, in the United States, the challenges are many. Can we reduce our consumption of fossil fuel and thereby our disproportionate contribution to global environmental degradation? The willingness of U.S. consumers to take responsibility for their individual shares in solving global problems could make a substantial contribution to the quality of life for future generations. Our decision to use fewer goods, devour fewer resources, create less pollution, and consume less energy would go a long way toward remedying global environmental problems and conditions that contribute to world hunger. In addition, the United States can help directly by sup-

---

*The formal name of the summit was the United Nations Conference on Environment and Development: UNCED, for short.

porting international moves to relieve poverty and environmental degradation worldwide. The following steps have been recommended.

Relieve Debt First, the developing countries need to be relieved of the gigantic interest payments they have been making to U.S. and international banks. Ten years ago those countries received $50 billion more a year from the developed world than they paid out, and they were able to make some progress toward solving their internal poverty and environmental problems. Today, however, they pay out $50 billion more than they take in, so they are becoming poorer every year.[45] The developing countries supply the developed world with a variety of cash crops, such as cotton, tobacco, coffee, sugar, and palm oil, but they cannot put the proceeds back into their economies. They have to use all the money they make to pay the interest on their loans and even have to borrow more. It has been called "one of the great ironies of the world" that some of the world's richest farmland is being used to produce nonnutritious crops for U.S. dollars, only to pour the money down the interest-payment drain while the producing nations' people starve. The debtor nations could use that same land to grow food crops to feed their own people.

Land Reform Second, the debt relief needs to reach those within the countries who need it, and not just the wealthy. In some poor countries, astronomically wealthy upper classes control all the good agricultural land and use it to produce luxury cash crops for export while the landless poor starve and multiply. Relieving hunger requires land reform—returning sufficient land to the dispossessed so that they can live and grow food on it. Simultaneous community development is needed to ensure that the people become able to support themselves permanently.

Labor-Intensive Systems Third, rather than emphasizing *technology*-intensive methods of *harvesting* their resources, developing countries might shift toward *labor*-intensive means of *maintaining* their resources. That way, succeeding generations can benefit from those resources. Labor-intensive agricultural practices are often perceived as inefficient, because yields per farmer are low compared to more technology-intensive mechanized systems. However, the actual efficiency in terms of number of people fed per unit of fossil energy used is extremely high.

Account for Resources Fourth, to account for the great value of environmental resources such as soil, water, and trees, a new system of economic accounting must come into use. Soil, water, and trees should be counted in economic balance sheets. Systems of national accounting must recognize that the depletion of these natural assets is a backward economic step and subtract lost resources from the gross national product. Such accounting would force decision makers to weigh future environmental costs and benefits more accurately and would promote the use of investment criteria that would stem the loss of natural capital.

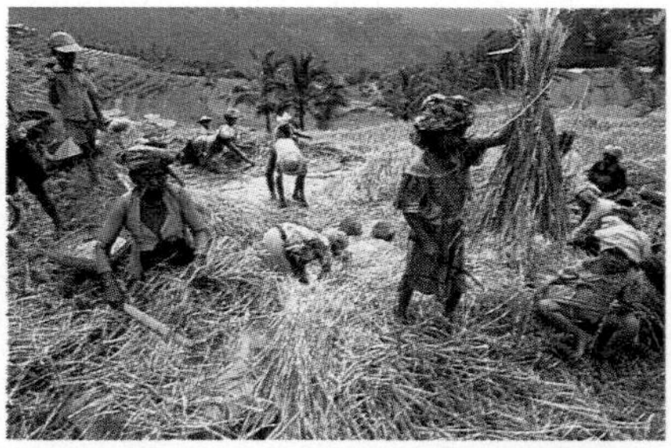

Labor-intensive technology is most often the appropriate technology in developing countries.

The United States can exert international leadership by adopting these strategies and encouraging other developed nations to support similar measures. The idea behind all these measures is that relieving poverty will help relieve environmental degradation and hunger. To rephrase a well-known adage: If you give a man a fish, he will eat for a day. If you teach him to fish and enable him to buy and maintain his own gear and bait, he will eat for a lifetime and help to feed others. Unlike food giveaways and money doles, which are only stop-gap measures, social programs that will permanently better the lot of the poor can permanently solve the hunger problem.

ACTIVISM AND SIMPLER LIFESTYLES AT HOME

Every segment of our society can have a place in the fight against hunger, poverty, and environmental degradation. The federal government, the states, local communities, big business and small companies, educators, and all individuals, including dietitians and foodservice managers, have many opportunities to forward the effort.

Government Action Government policies can change to promote sustainability. For example, the government can stop using tax money to pay for the wasteful use of fossil fuels and of fertilizers and pesticides made from them. Instead, it can pay for energy-conservation services and crop protection. Tax laws could be revised to reward energy conservation efforts, which would have a major impact on the research and development of conservation industries and sustainable agriculture. All of these actions are possible, but they depend on the support of elected officials. Keep in mind that you can affect the direction of such government actions by voting and writing letters that express your views on hunger, poverty, and environmental degradation.

Business Involvement Businesses can take initiative to help; some already have. Several large corporations are currently major supporters of anti-hunger programs. Many grocery stores and restaurants give their out-of-date and leftover food to hunger organizations such as Third Harvest, which then distribute the food where needed in the community.

Education Educators, including nutrition educators, have a crucial role to play. They can teach others about the underlying social and political causes of poverty, the root cause of hunger. At the college level, they can teach the relationship between hunger and population, hunger and environmental degradation, hunger and the status of women, and hunger and the global debt crisis. They can advocate legislation to address these problems. They can teach the poor to develop and run nutrition programs in their own communities and to fight on their own behalf for antipoverty, antihunger legislation.

Foodservice Efforts Dietitians and foodservice managers have a special role to play. Their professional organization, the American Dietetic Association (ADA), is urging them to promote the saving of resources by reuse, recycling (including composting), energy conservation, and water conservation, in both their professional and their personal lives. In addition, the ADA urges its members to work for policy changes in private and government food assistance programs, to intensify education about hunger, and to be advocates on the local, state, and national levels to help end hunger in the United States.[46]

Other Opportunities Individuals can support organizations that lobby for the needed economic policy changes toward developing countries. They can join and work for international hunger relief organizations. Appendix F includes some of the major ones.

Most importantly, at every level, individuals can try to make lifestyle choices that consider the environmental consequences. Several possible choices relating to typical U.S. foodways are presented next.

ENVIRONMENTALLY CONSCIOUS FOODWAYS

Most people eat familiar foods out of habit. They often notice food prices, but seldom do they think to ask what price the global environment pays for food. Yet food production does tax environmental resources and cause pollution, and some aspects of the food industry are more destructive than others. If we realized the impact of our foodways, we might choose differently, yet still eat as well and enjoy our foods as much as we do now.

Among the global resources involved in producing food are irrigation water, fertilizers, pesticides, fuel, land, and fisheries. Tons of packaging materials and a massive transportation network convey foods to consumers, using immense quantities of fossil fuel. This is especially true of foods for U.S. consumers, who demand many products in many kinds of packages. Each truckload of food produced in this country travels, on the average, 1300 miles to reach the market.[47] It costs 800 kcalories in fuel to make a can of diet soda that provides only 1 kcalorie of food energy, and more water is used to make the can than to make the soda.[48]

Choices that are more environmentally benign are available. In place of vegetables shipped in from far away, people might choose to eat local produce. In place of several sodas in aluminum cans, the consumer might use one large recyclable bottle. An individual can make environmentally conscious choices such as these at every step from food shopping to cooking and use of kitchen appliances to serving, cleanup, and waste disposal.

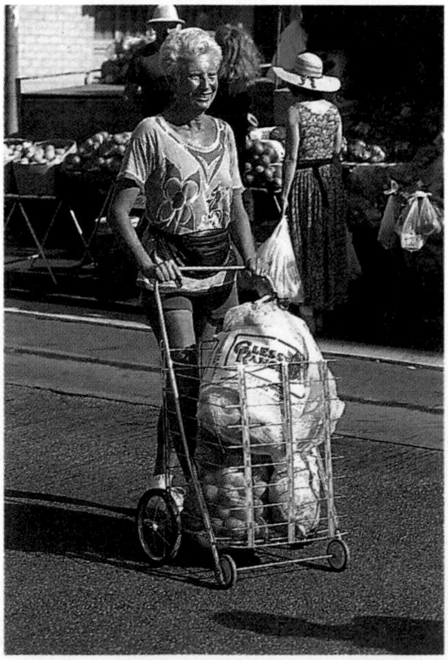
Shopping without a car can be a pleasure.

FOOD SHOPPING

Food shopping in the United States typically involves going to the store, selecting foods, choosing among the packages in which products are sold, and choosing bags in which to carry the groceries home. All of these actions exert impacts on the environment, and consumers can choose to minimize those impacts. Consider the shopping trips first.

Transportation In late 1990, 400 million cars were in use around the world and 19 million more cars were being added every year. Even without that increase, motor vehicles were the world's single largest source of air pollution.[49] Air pollution in many regions harms children, the elderly, and people with lung problems; reduces crop yields; causes acid rain; and damages forests.

Alternatives to the use of private cars include car pools, mass transit, walking, and bicycling. These can be made feasible by rearranging cities to bring residences, workplaces, and shopping centers closer together and creating safe pathways for walking and cycling. While pushing for such changes in city design, food shoppers can make the following choices: shop only once a week, share trips, or take turns shopping for each other. When selecting homes, people can choose to live close enough to walk or bicycle to and from the store. When buying a car, a buyer can choose the most fuel-efficient model available of the size needed. By the early 1990s, the U.S. market was offering several cars with fuel efficiency rated at 40 to 50 miles to the gallon or better. The impacts of these choices can become globally significant, if more and more families use less and less fuel.

Tips for making once-a-week shopping feasible were presented in Chapter 17 on pp. 633–636.

Food Choices Once in the store, the consumer faces many food choices. For good health, the Daily Food Guide recommends that adults eat 11 or more servings of plant foods daily (especially grains and vegetables) and only 4 or 5 servings of milk products and meats combined. Environmentally, too, it is beneficial to eat low on the food chain, that is, to eat plants, rather than to eat the animals that eat plants (see Figure 20–4 on p. 736; and also Figure H20–1 on p. 755 in the highlight that follows this chapter).

Reminder: The *food chain* is the sequence in which living things depend on other living things for food.

Thirty-eight percent of total global grain production is fed to cattle, pigs, and chickens.[50] It is much more efficient to consume the world's grain resources directly, rather than indirectly by eating meat and dairy products. Feedlot cattle take roughly 7 kilograms of grain to make 1 kilogram of meat. Pigs need roughly 4 kilograms of grain to add a kilogram. Eggs and cheese require about 2.5 to 3 kilograms of grain for each kilogram increase in output.[51] Poultry and fish are more efficient, requiring about 2 kilograms for each kilogram of live weight gain.

Raising animals for their meat and dairy products by feeding them grain also uses more land than growing grain for direct use by people. In addition, raising livestock uses more water, adds more pollution to waterways, and, in general, causes destruction of more native vegetarian and wildlife than growing plants. More fossil fuels are required just to grow the feed for animals: to run tractors, harvest feed grain, and transport it. Growing the feed pollutes the environment with fertilizers and pesticides, and the animals' waste pollutes it further.[52]

Some 70% of the grain we raise in the United States—and almost half the energy we produce—goes to feed livestock; the water used to supply each person with meat, milk, and eggs each day almost matches a typical citizen's water use at home, about 380 liters.

Meat and dairy producers can change the ways they raise animals so as to do less harm. Some have already done so. Guidelines for environmentally sound ways to raise animals for meat and dairy products are available; some are described in the highlight that follows this chapter.

It also makes sense, as far as possible, to avoid buying canned beef products of any kind, including soups, stews, chili, corned beef, and even pet food. Some of these foods come at the expense of cleared rainforest land in Central and South America: 200 square feet of rainforest are lost *permanently* for each *pound* of beef produced from cattle raised on the cleared land.[53] Rainforest soil wears out within only a few years when used to raise cattle; the practice is not sustainable. To keep raising cattle, ranchers have to clear more land, and the forest cannot grow back on the ruined soil.

Consumers cannot tell which products contain rainforest beef because labeling laws require no such disclosures. Once inspected at the ports of entry, beef coming into the country is simply labeled "USDA inspected"; it is not labeled as to country of origin. Even bulk buyers, such as canners and fast-food chains, cannot know whether the beef they buy is domestic or imported, unless they make special efforts to find out. The only way consumers can be sure they are not buying rainforest beef is to buy no canned beef at all.

For those who do eat meat, choose to eat it less often and in smaller portions, and select range-fed beef, buffalo, poultry, and fish more often than feedlot beef or pork. Range-fed beef and buffalo meat are preferable environmentally to feed-

Figure 20–4

Eating Low on the Food Chain Saves Resources

It takes ten times as much land and fuel to feed people meat as to feed them plants.

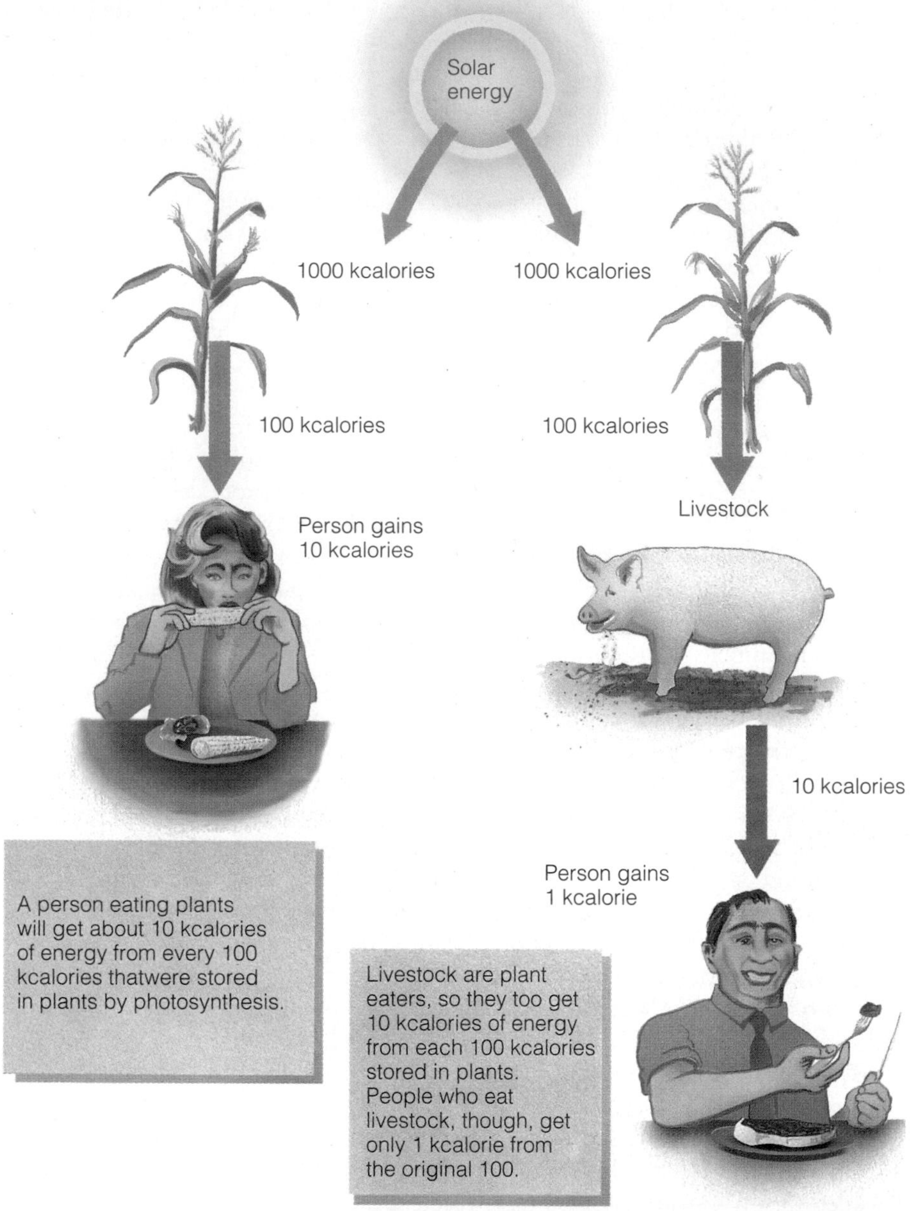

Solar energy
1000 kcalories
1000 kcalories
100 kcalories
100 kcalories
Person gains 10 kcalories
Livestock
10 kcalories
Person gains 1 kcalorie
A person eating plants will get about 10 kcalories of energy from every 100 kcalories thatwere stored in plants by photosynthesis.
Livestock are plant eaters, so they too get 10 kcalories of energy from each 100 kcalories stored in plants. People who eat livestock, though, get only 1 kcalorie from the original 100.

lot beef because cattle on the range eat grass, which people cannot eat, and because the cattle's manure and urine fertilize the range vegetation. In contrast, cattle in a feedlot eat grain that could serve as food for people, and their manure and urine run off to pollute waterways. Chickens are raised in most local regions at a lower cost in grain, land, and pollution than other meats.

Among fish, choose small and medium-sized fish, which are lower on the food chain than the large predators that eat them. Along the southeastern coast, this means fish such as mullet, snapper, and flounder; along the west coast, it means salmon and ocean fish like cod; and inland, it means river and lake fish such as walleyed pike and bass. These choices also make sense for health reasons. The fat of buffalo meat, poultry, and fish is less saturated than beef fat, and fatty acids from fish are valued for their purported blood pressure-lowering, cancer-opposing effects.

In selecting foods, local foods should be emphasized because they are transported shorter distances and less fuel is required to pack them, label them, and keep them cold if fresh. Figure 20–5 shows the energy required to produce canned and frozen corn, compared with the energy in the corn itself. Clearly, from this point of view, local farmers' markets are an excellent place to shop, if they are not too far from home. For nutrition's sake, frozen and canned foods are often nutritionally equal or even superior to fresh foods, but for the environment's sake, fresh foods grown nearby may be preferable.

Food Packages Foods come in a multitude of packages, including cans, shrink-wrap, foam trays, waxed cardboard, clay-coated cardboard, plastic bottles, glass jars, and dozens of others. It costs energy and resources to make these packages, and it may cost land pollution to dispose of them. In general, what is best for the environment is *no* packages; next best are minimal, reusable, or recyclable ones.

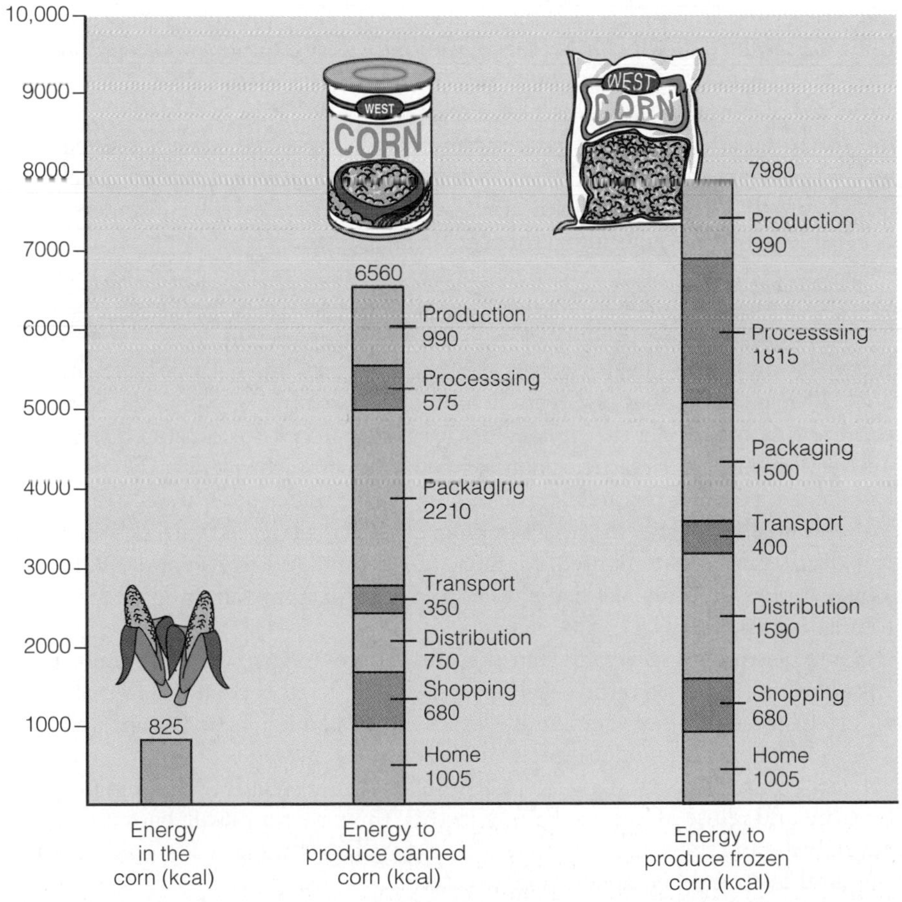

Figure 20–5

Energy Costs of Canned and Frozen Corn

The corn contains only 825 kcalories per kilogram, but look how much energy goes to produce it.

Source: D. Pimentel, *Food, Energy and the Future of Society* (Boulder, Colo.: Associated University Press, 1980).

Fresh produce can often be bought with minimal or no packaging. Most large stores package meats in foam trays, but shoppers can ask that they be wrapped in butcher paper and can always get fish that way. As for processed foods, shoppers can buy juices in large glass or recyclable plastic bottles (not small individual cartons); grain products in bulk (not in separate little packages); and eggs in compostable pressed fiber cartons (not foam, unless it is recycled locally). Shoppers can look for labels that boast of environmentally sound products and packaging. Although such labels may sometimes be misleading, they do show that the company is aware of the need.

Grocery Bags As for grocery bags, they represent a huge drain on energy and resources, and many consumers are demanding alternatives to throwaway bags. In response, some stores offer incentives to encourage reuse and recycling. Some offer a few cents back on used bags. Others accept bags for recycling. Some sell permanent shopping bags.

Every 700 paper bags not used represent one 15- to 20-year-old tree that need not be cut down.[54] Trees are a renewable resource, but trees are being cut in this country faster than they are being grown.[55] Furthermore, in making paper, pulp mills employ chemicals, such as chlorine bleach, and then dump them into waterways in quantities so large and so destructive that they can destroy whole bays and fisheries.[56] Discharges from paper mills may kill all life along long stretches of rivers, bays, or coastlines where the plants are located. Chlorine combines with ammonia, a chemical always naturally present in the environment, to produce dioxins. In waterways, dioxins cause tumors and reproductive abnormalities in aquatic life, including fish. Arriving in the ocean, dioxins are suspected of contributing to diseases and deaths of dolphins, sea turtles, seabirds, and other wildlife. Groundwater contaminated with dioxins may cause cancers and birth defects in people; when such contamination is discovered, the wells are closed, and the people must obtain their water elsewhere. Many consumers avoid disposable paper products altogether for these reasons.

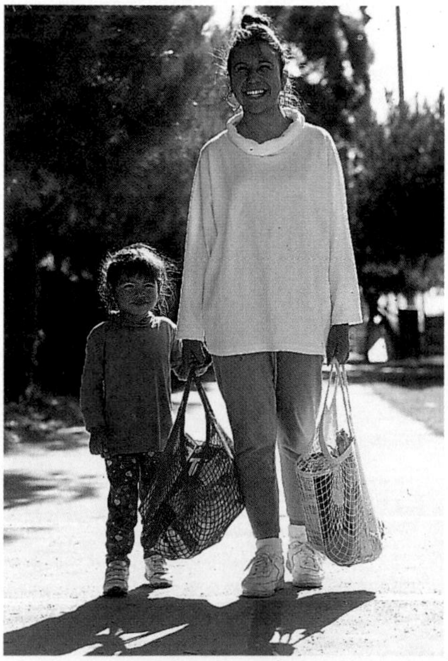
Reusable bags require the fewest resources.

Plastic bags, like most plastics, are petroleum products. Except for the recycled ones, these bags are made from oil, nearly all of which has to be transported from far away at a great cost in fuel, oil spills, and military preparedness. Then, when thrown away, many plastics persist for years or decades in landfills. Some are labeled "degradable," but few degrade fully to pure, simple compounds. Some are made of tiny bits of plastic interlaced with cornstarch; the cornstarch degrades, but the tiny pieces of plastic remain with unknown consequences. Some would degrade if exposed to sun and air, but end up buried under other trash. Some plastics contain the toxic heavy metal mercury, which is released into the air when they disintegrate or are burned. Mercury bioaccumulates in fish and wildlife; its concentration in some lake fish has led to advisories that warn people to refrain from eating the fish.

Some plastics are recyclable, but the process is cumbersome. Consumers must learn and remember to return each type of plastic to its special bin free of other materials. If a consumer accidentally drops a degradable plastic bag into a batch of recyclable ones, it renders the entire batch nonrecyclable.

For all these reasons, many shoppers prefer to carry reusable shopping bags to the store and refuse all others. Failing in this, they ask for plastic bags if they are recyclable—and then take care to recycle them. The third choice would be paper bags, and last would be nonrecyclable plastic.

COOKING FOOD

Fast cooking saves fuel and so pollutes less. Asian meals exemplify this principle: they are made of precut, bite-sized pieces of food, stir-fried fast in small amounts of oil. This cooking style both saves energy and preserves nutrients.

Pressure Cookers and Microwaves The pressure cooker or the microwave can also cook foods quickly. The pressure cooker can greatly speed preparation of dried beans and grains or the occasional big piece of meat the cook wants to serve whole; the microwave can cook vegetables, casseroles, or leftovers. Both may save using several burners on the stove, and both preserve nutrients better than most stove-top methods.

Ovens The oven, in contrast, can be a fuel waster. Efficient oven use is possible if the cook bakes or roasts a lot of food at one time and keeps the oven door closed. To keep the stove top from being an energy waster, a cook can use flat-bottomed pots with close-fitting lids that completely cover the burners. That way, each burner will donate all its heat to cooking something, not just heating the kitchen (and the planet). One can also turn electric burners and ovens off before the food is fully cooked and let the cooking finish as the stove cools.

Cooking Utensils A cook rightly refuses throwaway utensils and instead prizes pots and pans that heat well and evenly, prove durable over repeated uses, and clean up easily. Even when first equipping a kitchen, a person need not buy all-new pots, pans, and utensils. Thrift shops have pre-owned ones that may be of higher quality than new ones. If well cared for, pots and pans can be kept in condition so that foods will not stick to them. To prevent foods from sticking, the user can apply a little oil or shortening by hand or with the corner of a clean washable cloth.

Cooking Aids to Avoid Spray products other than pump sprays have several environmental disadvantages. Many of the propellants used in them pollute the air and even rise to destroy outer-atmosphere ozone. The most damaging of the propellants used in spray products, chlorofluorocarbons (or CFCs), have been banned from such use, but their replacements are not innocuous. Furthermore, once empty, spray cans are hard to recycle, for they are made of so many different materials. They are, in fact, a classic example of the use-once, throwaway mentality that keeps our society from developing a sustainable lifestyle.

Aluminum foil, used to line pans, is another throwaway product. Aluminum mining is one of the world's most environmentally destructive industries: it consumes large amounts of fuel and water, utilizes land-destroying strip-mining, and pollutes the soil, water, and groundwater with toxic materials. Aluminum use approaches sustainability only if the aluminum is recycled.[57] (Remember, even recycling costs energy.) Cans are recyclable, but in most places foil is not.

Other cooking aids that people thoughtlessly use and throw away include paper towels, plastic wrap, plastic storage bags, sponges, and more. For each of these, a permanent substitute is available: cloth towels, reusable storage containers with lids, and dishcloths.

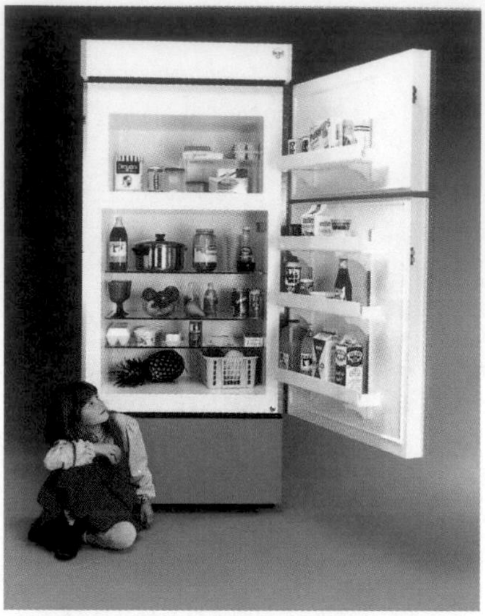

This DC refrigerator requires less than 1/20 the energy of a regular AC refrigerator, but chills and freezes food as well. The motor is small, releases little heat, and is on top. In contrast, a "regular" refrigerator's large motor, which is below the unit, heats the very unit it is trying to cool—an inefficient design.

KITCHEN APPLIANCES

All appliances use energy, which is almost invariably generated from fossil fuels. A naive consumer might say, "I don't use fossil fuels to cook with; my kitchen is all electric." But electricity, of course, is most often generated by burning fossil fuels—at the power plant rather than at the point of use. Therefore, the fewer the appliances, and the shorter the times they are used, the better for the air, water, soil, and atmosphere. Realizing this, many consumers today are returning to "old-fashioned" ways of doing things, such as beating eggs with whisks and cutting vegetables with knives rather than using electric mixers and food processors.

Doing without small electrical appliances saves more than just the small bits of energy the appliances would consume during use. It also saves the energy it would have cost to manufacture, package, transport, advertise, and market the appliances themselves. In addition, it saves the landfill space they take up when discarded.

What is true of small appliances is more true of large ones, but with exceptions. The appliances that use the most energy per minute are not necessarily the biggest energy guzzlers. Many people believe, for example, that the range uses more energy than the refrigerator, but this is not true. While in use, the range uses more, but most ranges are in use for only an hour or so a day at most, whereas most refrigerators run almost continuously. Therefore refrigerators are by far the greater energy consumers. Refrigerators are, in fact, the appliances that use the most energy in most people's homes. Figure 20–6 shows their estimated impacts on global warming, as well as the impacts of some other large energy users.

Refrigerators Consumers can take several steps to minimize the energy a refrigerator uses, within the limits of food safety requirements. If operated at 37° to 40°F (3° to 4°C), with the freezer at 0°F (-18°C), the refrigerator will keep foods fresh and gain in energy savings. A refrigerator kept 10 F degrees (5.5 C degrees) too cold may use up to 25 percent more energy than necessary.[58] Other energy-conserving steps include putting a reminder on the calendar to clean the coils at least once a year; keeping the insulating gaskets around the door clean and in good repair; and keeping the freezer and refrigerator compartments full—if not with food, then with closed containers of ice or air. That way, when opened, the doors will not let in a lot of room-temperature air. Most of the work the refrigerator and freezer do is to recool air admitted when the doors have been opened. When buying a new refrigerator, read the energy label. Choose a model based on its energy use, not on bells and whistles such as ice makers and picnic compartments.

Solar Energy About 20,000 U.S. families are now using solar energy to meet most of their homes' electricity needs and can refrigerate their foods this way. In an active solar home, the sun's light strikes photovoltaic (PV) panels on the roof, and these convert the light energy to electrical energy, which is stored in a large battery. Having a battery permits the option of purchasing DC (direct current) appliances. *No* fossil fuel is used to run a DC refrigerator operated this way.* Sun-

active solar: use of photovoltaic panels to generate electricity from sunlight. (A *passive solar* home is built to minimize heating and cooling costs by taking advantage of the available sun and shade.)

photovoltaic (PV) panels: panels that convert light (photons) into electricity (volts).

*This book was written in an office that the authors converted to run on solar PV panels. They keep their lunches in a DC refrigerator there.

Figure 20–6

Estimated Contributions to Global Warming by Cars and Home Appliances

Each year the United States increases the carbon dioxide (CO_2) content of the atmosphere by almost five trillion pounds, mostly as a result of using fossil fuels for energy. Emissions of chlorofluorocarbons (CFCs), methane, and other gases have a heat-trapping effect equivalent to another four trillion pounds of CO_2. Although the United States has less than $\frac{1}{20}$ of the world's population, it is responsible for more than $\frac{1}{5}$ of global-warming emissions.

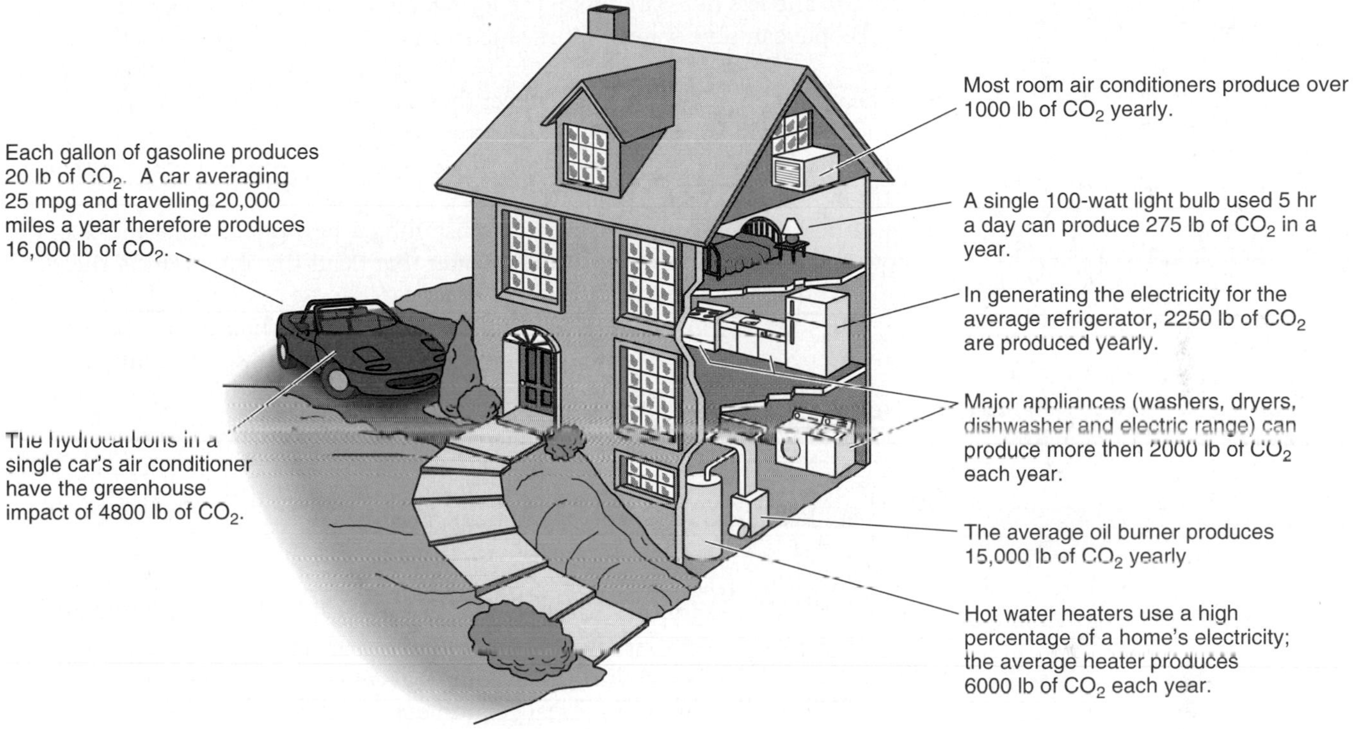
Each gallon of gasoline produces 20 lb of CO_2. A car averaging 25 mpg and travelling 20,000 miles a year therefore produces 16,000 lb of CO_2.
The hydrocarbons in a single car's air conditioner have the greenhouse impact of 4800 lb of CO_2.
Most room air conditioners produce over 1000 lb of CO_2 yearly.
A single 100-watt light bulb used 5 hr a day can produce 275 lb of CO_2 in a year.
In generating the electricity for the average refrigerator, 2250 lb of CO_2 are produced yearly.
Major appliances (washers, dryers, dishwasher and electric range) can produce more then 2000 lb of CO_2 each year.
The average oil burner produces 15,000 lb of CO_2 yearly
Hot water heaters use a high percentage of a home's electricity; the average heater produces 6000 lb of CO_2 each year.

Source: Adapted from a figure, "Household Sources of Greenhouse Gases," *Nucleus*, Summer 1990, p. 5. Permission granted by the Union of Concerned Scientists.

light is free, reliable, and pollution-free. PV panels do not work equally efficiently in all parts of the world, but they do make electricity even in cloudy weather and at temperate latitudes.

The high initial costs of PV panels, battery, and DC refrigerator prohibit most people from taking this option readily, but those who can afford to get started can meet most of their homes' electrical needs with solar energy, reduce electric bills, and recoup their initial investments within 5 to 15 years. Thereafter, their electricity is virtually free, compliments of the sun. (Most electrical appliances such as television sets, microwave ovens, and the like run on alternating current, or AC. Direct current from a battery can be converted to AC by running it through a device called an inverter; it can then be used to operate all but the largest energy guzzlers in a home.)

If this discussion of solar energy seems to have strayed far from the subject of food and nutrition, remember that energy is the major raw "material" in food production. When energy costs rise, food costs rise, too. Also, the energy use associated with U.S. food production, transport, preparation, and storage is contributing to air pollution, ozone depletion, and global warming. According to the Worldwatch Institute's *State of the World, 1992*, converting to solar energy and reducing use of automobiles are among the highest priorities in the race to save the planet.[59]

Water Heaters Other than kitchen appliances, a big energy user associated with food preparation and cleanup is the water heater (again, look at Figure 20–6). The less hot water used, the less fuel must be burned to heat that water.

People can save water-heating energy in many ways. They can set the water heater at 130°F (54°C), not hotter. They can put it on a timer, so that each day it heats just enough hot water to meet that day's needs. They can wrap it in insulation to keep it from losing heat to the surroundings. They can wrap the hot-water pipes all the way to the points of use. They can install water-saving faucets and shower heads.

When replacing a water heater or installing a new one, a consumer can opt for a small instantaneous-type water heater that heats the water only at the point of use, and only when needed. A consumer can choose a gas water heater, rather than an electric one. Natural gas is a cleaner fossil fuel than the coal or oil usually burned to make electricity. Solar water heaters work well in sunny regions; unlike PV panels, though, thermal water panels do require direct sun to heat the water. Perhaps rebates or loans to make these conversions are available from the utility company or from the local, state, or federal government. The utility company may offer an energy audit or survey in which an expert will visit the customer's home and make energy-saving suggestions.

FOOD SERVING, DISH WASHING, AND WASTE DISPOSAL

Having rendered the kitchen as nonpolluting and energy-efficient as possible, people can do the same thing in the dining room, at the kitchen counter, or on the TV tray. People can use "real" plates, cups, and glasses. They can use cloth napkins, which demand no extra energy to wash and dry because they can fit into existing washloads. School cafeterias can take similar steps and will do so if students support them in making the change.

Dish Washing As for cleanup, someone who washes many dishes at a time should consider using a dishwasher, if it is affordable. People may think that the cost of the water, heat, and soap would be higher than the cost of washing by hand, but this is not the case. One school found that a normal machine cycle used on full loads consumed less than two-thirds the water used in hand washing.[60] Using less hot water also means using less electricity to heat it. The savings are greatest if the dishes are not prerinsed and are allowed to air-dry.

Waste Disposal Once the meal is over and the dishes are washed, the trash and garbage remain to be disposed of. An average American household of four people produce about 100 pounds of trash a week, much of it from the kitchen.[61] National concern has focused on this issue because the nation is running out of landfill space in which to dispose of all the trash. Landfill space is, however, only one of many problems associated with trash. Every item thrown away is a resource lost; an aluminum can could be used to make a new aluminum can; a cereal box, but for its clay coating, could become recycled paper; a plastic bottle could become part of a beautiful carpet.* Trash need not become an undesirable mess; recycled trash could be viewed as a usable resource. Yet, as it is now, about 70 percent of all metal mined in the United States is used only once and then discarded. The aluminum thrown away every three months could rebuild the entire U.S. air fleet.[62]

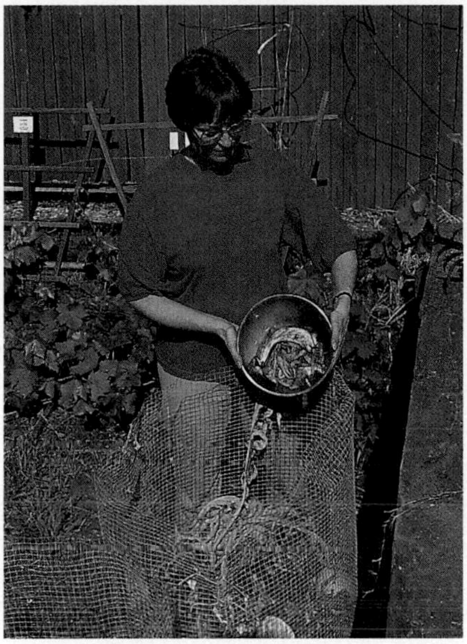

Compost nourishes plants as food nourishes people.

Recycling In many college settings, students have successfully mobilized to demand recycling on campus. Once all the recyclable materials have been collected, students can study their own trash to identify what remains to be thrown away. They can then demand recycling of those items or stop buying them. As an example, suppose you recycle glass, plastic, and cans, but cannot recycle foam. On the next trip to the store, choose only vegetables, meats, and eggs that are packaged in compostable fiber cartons. (Write to the stores and manufacturers to make sure your action is felt where it counts.) Some people pride themselves on generating only one small bag of trash a week. Some even find ways to generate no trash at all.

Composting Garbage is a special case of a resource generated in the kitchen. Vegetable scraps, fruit peelings, and leftover plant foods are organic and biodegradable, like the leaves and grass cuttings people rake up in their yards. All of these materials can be piled up together with some soil and allowed to decompose naturally, forming compost, a rich, crumbly material that can be used to fertilize growing things. Natural, organic fertilizers such as compost and manure are environmentally preferable to synthetic fertilizers on both a large and a small scale. Some schools and communities, recognizing this, conduct composting programs to recycle people's organic debris; some homeowners maintain their own composting piles. Composting can even be done indoors in small odor-free bins, and the resulting material used to pot plants.

Eating Away from Home Having adopted foodways that respect the environment at home, people can apply the same principles elsewhere. When they buy take-out food, they can bring their own reusable cups and containers to put it in. When eating out at school, at work, or on trips, they can continue to recycle throwaways. Even when ordering from fast-food places, customers can patronize only those that use no plastic packaging and no rainforest beef. They can refuse the tiny packages of catsup, salt, and sauces that amount to many tons of trash every year. At work, people can institute recycling programs, insist on using their own china mugs for coffee, and adopt many other resource-saving, energy-saving practices.

In summary, governments, businesses, and all individuals have many opportunities to promote sustainability worldwide and wise resource use at home. Personal choices, made by many people, can have a great impact.

The suggested lifestyles changes in this chapter have focused largely on our foodways, although it is easy to generalize from food to other areas. All aspects of our lifestyles relate to global problems. Recommendations include personal actions:

*The authors' office floor is covered with a luxurious wall-to-wall carpet made of recycled plastic soda and catsup bottles—45 bottles per square yard.

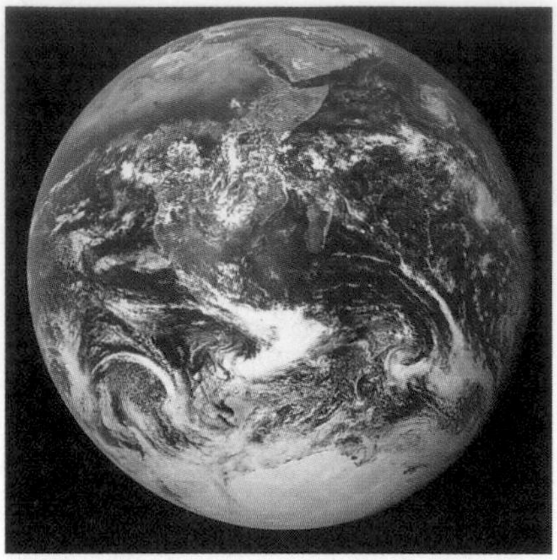

Good planets are hard to find.

Never doubt that a small group of thoughtful, committed people can change the world. Indeed, it is the only thing that ever has. —Margaret Mead

reduce, reuse, recycle, and cut energy use. Admittedly, these approaches to solving today's global problems seem simplistic, but because we number 5 billion plus, individual actions can add up to exert an immense impact. The problems are complex, they are not fully understood, and high-level scientific research is needed to solve them. But even as that research is being done and the world's best minds are translating the results into recommended actions, individuals can be doing what they already know how to do.

Emphasis on personal lifestyle choices is important because it raises awareness and paves the way for larger actions. Individual choices are, however, only part of the solution to today's problems. Institutional changes are the other part—changes in the way agriculture, industry, and governments do their business domestically and internationally. Students can become involved in promoting both kinds of change: make personal lifestyle changes and then vote for government changes.

Students everywhere are helping change governments, human predicaments, and environmental problems for the better. Student movements persuaded 127 universities and many institutions, corporations, and government agencies to withdraw investments of funds in South Africa, aiding the successful effort to end apartheid. Student pressure led to the installation of the first deaf president at a university for the deaf. Students offer major services to communities in soup kitchens, home repair, and child education. Student movements have hastened the coming of cultural and political autonomy in the former Soviet Union and other countries, encouraged the reform of universities, and advanced peace and human rights causes. Students have launched significant protests against totalitarianism in China and mounted successful environmental cleanups and defense efforts.[63]

Simple approaches sometimes are the most effective, for everyone can understand and act on them. If each of the world's 5 billion people takes one–five-billionth share of the responsibility for improving things, the job can get done. Just to be sure, though, those who can do more are encouraged to do so to compensate for those who are, as yet, too poor, ignorant, powerless, or inflexible to join in.

Finally, it makes sense for everyone in this world, rich or poor, in the United States or in any other country, to plan on bearing no more than one or two children. For those who want large families, there are plenty of children to adopt. And for those who love children and want to help them in other ways, there are numerous opportunities to play with, teach, and nurture the world's children, from the community center downtown to the remotest primitive village on earth.

"Be part of the solution, not part of the problem," an adage says. In other words, don't waste time or energy moaning and groaning about how tough things are; do something to improve them. This adage is as applicable to today's global environmental problems as it is to an unwashed dish in the kitchen sink. They are our problems: human beings created them, and human beings must solve them.

Study Questions

1. Identify several of the global environmental trends of today.
2. Choose one of the global environmental trends depicted in Figure 20–1 and, from the figure, explain (a) how other trends intensify the one you have chosen, and (b) how this trend intensifies others.
3. Identify some reasons why hunger is present in a country as wealthy as the United States.
4. Explain why relieving environmental problems will also help to alleviate hunger and poverty.
5. Discuss the different paths by which rich and poor countries can attack the problems of world hunger and the environment.
6. Describe some steps that food shoppers can take to minimize negative environmental impacts.
7. Identify some ways of cooking foods that have minimal environmental impacts.
8. Explain what domestic use of electricity has to do with air pollution and global climate change.
9. Identify the home appliances that are usually the largest users of electricity, and for each, describe ways of reducing its energy use.
10. Recall the changes identified as most urgent if we are to save the planet (see p. 732).
11. Describe some environmentally benign ways of disposing of trash and garbage.
12. Design a simple action plan for one day for a family of four to introduce changes in their lifestyles to benefit the environment.

Notes

1. L. N. Burby, *World Hunger* (San Diego, Calif. Lucent Books, 1995), pp. 13–16; P. L. Kutzner, *World Hunger: A Reference Handbook* (Santa Barbara, Calif.: ABC–CL10, 1991) pp. 158–159.
2. Burby, 1995; Kutzner, 1991; G. Arnold, *The Third World Handbook* (Chicago: Fitzroy Dearborn Publishers, 1994), p. 157.
3. Arnold, 1994; V. A. Kovda, Loss of productive land due to salinization, *Ambio* 12 (1983), as cited in S. Postel, *Water for Agriculture: Facing the Limits*, Worldwatch Paper 93 (Washington, D.C.: World Watch Institute, December 1989), p. 16; T. Peterson, Hunger and the environment, *Seeds*, October 1987, pp. 6–13; L. R. Brown, Feeding six billion, *World Watch*, September/October 1989, pp. 32–40.
4. R. A. Kerr, Greenhouse science survives skeptics, *Science* 256 (1992): 1138–1140; W. R. Cline, Scientific basis for the greenhouse effect, *The Economic Journal* 101 (1991): 904–919; J. T. Houghton, G. T. Jenkins, and J. J. Ephraums, eds., *Climate Change: The IPCC Scientific Assessment* (Cambridge: Cambridge University Press, 1990); B. Hileman, Web of interactions makes it difficult to untangle global warming data: Despite the complexities, experts have made progress, *Chemical and Engineering News*, April 27, 1992, pp. 7–19; D. L. Wheeler, Scientists studying "the greenhouse effect" challenge fears of global warming [but consensus is, it's occurring], *Journal of Forestry*, July 1990, pp. 34–36.
5. S. Postel, Denial in the decisive decade, in L. R. Brown and coauthors, *State of the World 1992* (New York: W. W. Norton, 1992).
6. United Nations Food and Agriculture Organization (FAO), *The State of Food and Agriculture, 1993* (Rome: 1993), as cited in L. R. Brown and H. Kane, *Full House* (New York: W. W. Norton, 1994), pp. 75–88.
7. FAO, *Yearbook of Fishery Statistics: Catches and Landings* (Rome: various years), FAO, Rome, private communications, December 20, 1993, as cited in L. R. Brown and H. Kane, *Full House* (New York: W. W. Norton, 1994), pp. 75–88.
8. Postel, 1992.
9. M. Renner, *Jobs in a Sustainable Economy*, Worldwatch Paper 104 (Washington, D.C.: Worldwatch Institute, September 1991), pp. 31–33.
10. Renner, 1991.
11. *Tallahassee Democrat*, October 14, 1994; P. Univ, The state of world hunger, *Nutrition Reviews* 52 (1994): 151–161.
12. *Fact Sheet on Childhood Hunger and Poverty*, (c. 1992), available from Bread for the World, 802 Rhode Island Avenue NE, Washington, DC 20018.
13. S. Lewis, Food security, environment, poverty, and the world's children, *Journal of Nutrition Education* (1 supplement) 24 (1992): 3S–5S.
14. L. D. McBean, ed., with D. Derelian, R. J. Fersh, and L. Parker, Hunger and undernutrition in America, *Dairy Council Digest*, March/April 1992.
15. U.S. Department of Commerce, *Statistical Abstract of the United States, 1994* (Washington, D.C.: Bureau of the Census, 1994), p. 386.
16. Food Research and Action Center, *Community Childhood*

Hunger Identification Project: A Survey of Childhood Hunger in the United States, Executive Summary (Washington, D.C.: Food Research and Action Center, March 1991), as cited in McBean, 1992.

17. *Fact Sheet on Childhood Hunger and Poverty*, c. 1992.
18. J. Ç. Wolgemuth and coauthors, Wasting malnutrition and inadequate nutrient intakes identified in a multiethnic homeless population, *Journal of the American Dietetic Association* 92 (1992): 834–839; M. A. Drake, The nutritional status and dietary adequacy of single homeless women and their children in shelters, *Public Health Reports* 107 (1992): 312–319; B. E. Cohen, N. Chapman, and M. R. Burt, Food sources and intake of homeless persons, *Journal of Nutrition Education* (1 supplement) 24 (1992): 45S–51S.
19. World Bank, *World Development Report 1991* (New York: Oxford University Press, 1991); Postel, 1992, pp. 3–8.
20. L. Timberlake, *Only One Earth*, cited in Food for thought, *Seeds*, Sprouts edition, 1988.
21. R. W. Kates, Ending deaths from famine: The opportunity in Somalia, *New England Journal of Medicine* 328 (1993): 1055–1057.
22. *Tallahassee Democrat*, October 14, 1994.
23. Kates, 1993.
24. U.S. Department of Commerce, 1994, pp. 854–855.
25. L. R. Brown and coauthors, *State of the World 1995* (New York: W. W. Norton, 1995), p. 11; *Tallahassee Democrat*, June 10, 1995.
26. L. R. Brown and J. E. Young, Feeding the world in the nineties, in L. R. Brown, *State of the World 1990* (New York: W. W. Norton, 1990).
27. J. W. Clay and coauthors, *The Spoils of Famine: Ethiopian Famine Policy and Peasant Agriculture* (Cambridge, Mass.: Cultural Survival, 1988), as cited in L. R. Brown and H. Kane, *Full House* (New York: W. W. Norton, 1994), pp. 146–157.
28. R. D. Kaplan, The coming anarchy, *Atlantic Monthly*, February 1994, pp. 44–76.
29. L. R. Brown and coauthors, *State of the World, 1994* (New York: W. W. Norton, 1994), p. 202.
30. Brown and coauthors, 1995, p. 191.
31. Brown and coauthors, 1995, p. 192.
32. Brown and coauthors, 1994, p. 201.
33. FAO, *FAO Production Yearbook 1992* (Rome: 1993); FAO, *FAO Production Yearbook 1991* (Rome: 1992); FAO, *1948–1985 World Crop and Livestock Statistics* (Rome: 1987), as cited in L. R. Brown and H. Kane, *Full House* (New York: W. W. Norton, 1994), pp. 89–95.
34. U.S. Department of Agriculture (USDA), *Dairy, Livestock, and Poultry: World Livestock Situation* (Washington, D.C., October 1993), as cited in L. R. Brown and H. Kane, *Full House* (New York: W. W. Norton, 1994), pp. 89–95.
35. H. Dregne and coauthors, A new assessment of the world status of desertification, *Desertification Control Bulletin* 20 (1991), as cited in L. R. Brown and H. Kane, *Full House* (New York: W. W. Norton, 1994), pp. 89–95.
36. FAO, cited in World Resources Institute (WRI), *World Resources 1992–93* (New York: Oxford University Press, 1992); bluefin tuna figure from D. Meadows and coauthors, *Beyond the Limits* (Post Mills, Vt.: Chelsea Green Publishing Company, 1992), as cited in L. R. Brown and H. Kane, *Full House* (New York: W. W. Norton, 1994), pp. 75–88.
37. L. Brown, The Aral Sea: going, going . . ., *World Watch*, January/February 1991.
38. Government of Canada, *The State of Canada's Environment* (Ottawa: 1991).
39. K. Dixit, The shrinking pool, *New Internationalist*, March 1991, p. 20.
40. Brown and Young, 1990, pp. 64–65.
41. Population Reference Bureau (PRB), *1993 World Population Data Sheet* (Washington, D.C.: 1993), as cited in L. R. Brown and H. Kane, *Full House* (New York: W. W. Norton, 1994), pp. 49–61.
42. Centers for Disease Control, Population based mortality assessment: Baidoa and Afgoi, Somalia, 1992, *Journal of the American Medical Association* (1993), as cited in L. R. Brown and H. Kane, *Full House* (New York: W. W. Norton, 1994), pp. 49–61.
43. P. S. Dasgupta, Population, poverty and the local environment, *Scientific American*, February 1995, pp. 40–45.
44. Lewis, 1992.
45. Lewis, 1992.
46. Position of The American Dietetic Association: Environmental issues, *Journal of the American Dietetic Association* 93 (1993): 589–591; Position of The American Dietetic Association: Domestic hunger and inadequate access to food, *Journal of the American Dietetic Association* 90 (1990): 1437–1441.
47. A. D. Basiago, The house where the future lives, *Calypso Log*, September 1986, p. 11.
48. J. E. Young, Aluminum's real tab, *World Watch*, March/April 1992, pp. 26–33; Earth Works Group, *50 Simple Things That You Can Do to Save the Earth* (Berkeley, Calif.: Earthworks Press, 1989), p. 64–65.
49. M. D. Lowe, *Alternatives to the Automobile: Transport for Livable Cities, Worldwatch Paper 98*, October 1990, p. 5.
50. A. T. Durning and H. B. Brough, Reforming the livestock economy, in L. R. Brown and coauthors, *State of the World 1992* (New York, W. W. Norton, 1992), as cited in J. D. Gussow, Ecology and vegetarian considerations: Does environmental responsibility demand the elimination of livestock? *American Journal of Clinical Nutrition* (supplement) 59 (1994): 1110S–1116S.
51. Grain-to-beef conversion ratio based on Allen Baker, Feed Situation and Outlook Staff, Economic Research Service (ERS), USDA, Washington, D.C., private communications, April 27, 1992; pork conversion data from Leland Southard, Livestock and Poultry Situation and Outlook Staff, ERS, USDA, Washington, D.C., private communication, April 27, 1992; feed-to-poultry conversion ratio derived from data in R. V. Bishop and coauthors, *The World Poultry Market—Government Intervention*

and Multilateral Policy Reform (Washington, D.C.: USDA, 1990); fish conversion ratio from Ross Garnaut and Guonan Ma, East Asian Analytical Unit, Department of Foreign Affairs and Trade, *Grain in China* (Canberra: Australian Government Publishing Service, 1992); cheese and egg conversion ratios from A. B. Durning and H. B. Brough, *Taking Stock: Animal Farming and the Environment*, Worldwatch Paper 103 (Washington, D.C.: Worldwatch Institute, July 1991), citing USDA, Foreign Agricultural Service, *World Livestock Situation* (Washington, D.C.: April 1991), and Linda Bailey, agricultural economist, USDA, Washington, D.C., private communication, September 11, 1990, as cited in L. R. Brown and H. Kane, *Full House* (New York: W. W. Norton, 1994), pp. 62–72.

52. Durning and Brough, 1991.
53. J. D. Nations and D. I. Komer, Rainforests and the hamburger society, *Environment*, April 1983, pp. 12–20.
54. Earth Works Group, 1989, p. 39.
55. J. C. Ryan, Timber's last stand, *World Watch*, July/August 1990, pp. 27–34; Ecological economics: Its implications for forest management and research (a workshop summary), *Conservation Biology*, September 1990, pp. 221–226; A. Leopold, Standards of conservation, *Conservative Biology*, September 1990, pp. 227–228; R. K. Anderberg, Wall Street and the great north woods, *The Amicus Journal*, Winter 1989, pp. 40–43; C. Wille, Ancient forest heritage going fast, *Audubon*, March 1989, pp. 130–131; Forest Service: Admissions and additions, *Wilderness*, Spring 1989, pp. v–vi; J. Stiak, Old growth! Battle cry of the Northwest, *The Amicus Journal*, Winter 1990, pp. 35–41; E. A. Norse, What good are ancient forests? Global resources, global concern, *The Amicus Journal*, Winter 1990, pp. 42–45; D. Doak, Spotted owls and old growth logging in the Pacific Northwest, *Conservation Biology*, December 1989, pp. 389–396; M. Lipske, Who runs America's forests? *National Wildlife*, October/November 1990, pp. 24–28.
56. P. Von Stackelberg, Whitewash: The dioxin coverup, *Greenpeace*, March/April 1989, pp. 7–11; National Wildlife Federation calls for ban on chlorine use, *International Wildlife*, January/February 1991, p. 26.
57. Young, 1992.
58. Earth Works Group, 1989, p. 31.
59. Postel, 1992.
60. At home, *Executive Fitness*, April 1989, p. 8.
61. Earth Works Group, 1989, p. 9; *Tallahassee Democrat*, April 24, 1995, p. 11a, Sue Ellyn Scaletta, Good earthkeeping begins in your home and garden.
62. Earth Works Group, 1989, p. 9.
63. Examples: M. Countryman, Lessons of the divestment drive, *The Nation*, March 26, 1988, pp. 406–409; H. Orlans, The revolution at Gallaudet: Students provoke break with the past, *Change, The Magazine of Higher Learning*, January/February 1989, pp. 8–18; S. Conn, Thoughts on national service: An open letter to William F. Buckley, Jr., *Change, The Magazine of Higher Learning*, May/June 1991, pp. 6–7, 52; R. G. Braungart and M. M. Braungart, Young movements in the 1980s: A global perspective, *International Sociology*, June 1990, pp. 157–181; E. Larsen, Youth environmental movement, *Utne Reader*, March/April 1991, pp. 30–31; J. Smith, The 1989 Chinese student movement: Lessons for nonviolent activists, *Peace and Change, A Journal of Peace Research*, January 1992, pp. 82–101; Windmill at Hamilton College generates heat, light, and a conservation campaign, *Chronicles of Higher Education*, April 1, 1992; A dollars-and-cents moral crusade in recycling, *Chronicles of Higher Education*, April 15, 1992, p. A5. The Rainforest Action network (450 Sansome, Suite 700, San Francisco, CA 94111), which now puts effective pressure on governments and corporations all over the world to stop destroying rainforests, originated and is maintained largely as a student effort.

Progress Toward Sustainable Agriculture

While some individuals are attempting to make their own personal lifestyles more environmentally benign, as suggested in the chapter, others are seeking ways to improve whole sectors of human enterprise, among them, agriculture. Large agricultural enterprises have, to date, been among the world's biggest polluters and resource users. Is it possible for agriculture to become sustainable? And if so, can the change be made without hurting farmers?

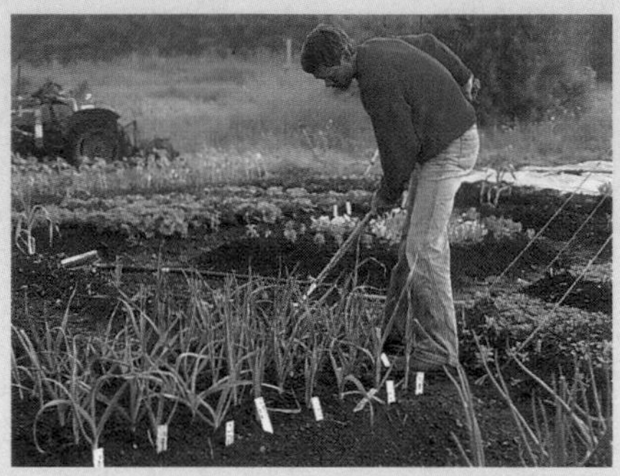

The small farm managed for variety, and the farmer, are valuable resources.

COST OF PRODUCING FOOD UNSUSTAINABLY

The environmental and social costs of current unsustainable agricultural practices take many forms. Among them are resource waste and pollution, energy overuse, and disruption of farm communities.

Resources and Pollution

Producing food costs the earth dearly. First of all, to grow food, we clear land—prairie, wetland, or forest. This always incurs losses of native ecosystems and wildlife.

Then we plant crops or graze animals on the land. Negative impacts on soil and water follow. The soil loses nutrients as each crop is taken from it, so fertilizer is applied. The fertilizer that runs off pollutes the waterways; so does the plowed soil, which clouds the water and interferes with the growth of aquatic plants and animals.

Then, to protect crops against weeds and pests, we apply herbicides and pesticides. These chemicals also pollute the water and, wherever the wind carries them, the air. Most herbicides and pesticides are nonspecific; they kill not only weeds and pests, but also native plants, native insects, and animals that eat those plants and insects.

Finally, to add insult to injury, we irrigate. Unlike rain, irrigation water contains salts and other compounds. The water evaporates, but its salts do not, so the soil becomes more and more salty. These salts combine with organic materials and impede the flow of water, make the land soggy, and hinder plant growth. Also, irrigation depletes the water supply over time, because irrigation water is pulled from surface waters or pumped up from underground; then, it evaporates or runs off, leaving the area. This process dries up rivers and lakes and lowers the water table, making whole regions drier and setting a vicious cycle in motion: the drier the region becomes, the more the farmers need irrigation water, and the more water they use, the drier the region becomes.

Many national and world agencies are concerned about the environmental damage agriculture can do. In 1989, the nation's most prestigious national scientific research body, the National Research Council of the National Academy of Sciences, produced a report that said, in part, that agriculture is the largest single source of nonpoint water pollution of surface water in the nation (the accompanying glossary defines "nonpoint pollution" and related terms). (Pollution from "point sources," such as sewage plants or factories, is relatively easy to control, but runoff from fields and pastures enters waterways from all over broad regions and is nearly impossible to control.)

Ironically, widespread use of pesticides and herbicides promote the survival of the very pests and weeds they are intended to wipe out. Consider a pesticide aimed at some insects that are attacking a crop. The pesticide may kill *almost* 100 percent of them, but thanks to the genetic variability of large populations, some insects are likely to survive exposure. The resistant insects can then multiply free of competition and produce many offspring that are resistant to the pesticide and can attack the crop with new vigor. To control these resistant insects, a new and more powerful pesticide must be applied, and this leads to the appearance of a population of still more resistant insects. Consequently, still more pesticides and herbicides must be used.

Some farmers rely so heavily on pesticides, herbicides, fertilizers, and soil boosters that the expense is becoming prohibitive. For people who eat foods produced this way, pesticide residues are becoming a

Glossary

agribusiness: agriculture practiced on a massive scale by large corporations owning vast acreages and employing intensive technological, fuel, and chemical inputs.

alternative agriculture: agriculture practiced on a small scale using individualized approaches that vary with local conditions so as to minimize technological, fuel, and chemical inputs.

externalities: hidden costs that are not reflected in the prices of things, such as the costs of environmental deterioration or subsidies that permit agribusiness foods to be sold at artificially low prices.

integrated pest management (IPM): management of pests using a combination of natural and biological controls rather than indiscriminate application of pesticides.

nonpoint water pollution: water pollution caused by runoff from all over an area rather than from discrete "point" sources. An example is the pollution caused by runoff from agricultural fields.

subsidies: government money, derived from taxes, used to support (subsidize) practices that otherwise would force recipients to price their products too high to compete successfully.

---

safety concern. In short, our way of producing foods is, for the most part, not sustainable.[1]

In 1992, the World Resources Institute presented the results of a massive study that came to the same conclusion: agriculture is destroying its own foundation. In just the past 40 years, human agricultural activities have ruined more than 10 percent of the earth's most fertile land, an area the size of China and India combined. Over 20 million acres have been so damaged by overgrazing, deforestation, and other unsustainable agricultural practices that they will be impossible to reclaim. Soil erosion, if unchecked, is predicted to result in a 20 percent loss in global food production by the end of this century, and by the year 2025 food-producing land per person may shrink by nearly 40 percent.[2]

Agriculture is also cutting out its own underpinnings by failing to conserve species diversity. By the year 2050, the number of plant species remaining on earth may be reduced by some 40,000 from the number that existed in 1990. The United Nations' Food and Agriculture Organization attributes many of the losses, which are already occurring daily, to modern farming practices, as well as to population growth. The increasing uniformity of global eating habits is also having an effect. As people everywhere eat the same limited array of foods, demand for local regions' native, genetically diverse plants declines, and the plants no longer seem worth preserving. Yet, in the future, as the climate warms and the earth changes, those may be "the very plants that can serve as important sources of food for large numbers of people."[3] A wild species of corn that grows in a hot climate, for example, might contain the genetic information necessary to help make domestic corn resistant to drought.

These culprits that attend the growing of crops—land clearing, irrigation, fertilizer overuse, pesticide and herbicide overuse, and loss of biogenetic diversity—have always taken a toll on the earth. Today, the damage is accelerating as the population grows faster and uses more technology every year. Agriculture has already destroyed many of the world's once-fertile regions, where high civilizations once flourished. All of North Africa, now desert, was once wheat fields—the breadbasket of the Roman Empire. Mistreatment of soil and water is now causing destruction on a scale never known before.[4]

Like growing crops, raising livestock also takes a toll on the environment. Like plant crops, herds of livestock occupy land that once maintained itself in a natural state. The land pays a price in losses of native plants and animals, soil erosion, water depletion, and desert formation. Raising animals in concentrated areas (such as feedlots) is not a solution. Not only do their wastes pollute the soil and water, but animals in feedlots still have to be fed; grain is grown for them on other land that requires fertilizers, herbicides, pesticides, and irrigation. One-fifth of all cropland in the United States is used to produce feed grains for livestock, more land than is used to produce grain for people.[5]

When people turn to fishing, still other prices are paid. Fishing easily becomes overfishing and depletes stocks of the very food fish that people need to eat. Some fishing methods (such as nets and filament line) kill aquatic animals other than the ones sought and deplete large populations of nonfood animals, such as dolphins.

Energy

The entire food industry, whether based on growing crops, raising livestock, or fishing, requires energy, which entails burning fossil fuel. As

Chapter 20 discussed, massive fossil fuel use causes air and water pollution, global warming, ozone depletion, and other environmental ills.

In the United States, the food industry's energy consumption is huge, about 20 percent of all the energy the nation uses. Each year, we spend 1500 liters of oil (over 350 gallons) *per person* to produce, process, distribute, and prepare our food.[6] Most of this energy is used to run farm machinery and to produce fertilizers and pesticides. Energy is also used to prepare, package, transport, refrigerate, store, cook, and wash our foods. As an example of how much goes into nonfood items associated with the foods we eat, consider this: consumers paid $29 million in 1985 just for the packages on their foods. In the same year, farmers received less than $29 million for the food itself.[7]

The amount of energy used in agricultural production differs sharply between the developed and developing countries. Developed countries consume five times as much energy as the developing world. North America alone uses 28 percent of total worldwide agricultural energy. Because the developing countries account for the majority of the world's population, differences in per capita annual energy use are even greater. Developed countries use 16 times more energy per capita than the developing world, and the United States uses nearly twice as much per capita as the other industrialized nations.[8]

Losses of Family Farms

During the early and mid-1980s, U.S. agriculture encountered serious economic hardships. Exports of farm produce fell worldwide. Recession occurred. Federal loans became expensive. Other countries increased their agricultural production and exports. Many U.S. farmers, particularly those who specialized in export crops, suffered heavy financial losses. Some became unable to pay their debts and had to leave farming. Between 1980 and 1993, more than 350,000 farms, representing 15 percent of the farms in the United States, disappeared.[9] Tens of thousands of farms were still struggling at the start of the 1990s, especially mid-sized family farms.

U.S. farmers today lack significant control over what products they produce, the costs of their supplies, and the prices they receive for their goods. Just prior to 1980, the USDA urged farmers to increase corn and soybean production for export. To expand their production capabilities, the farmers borrowed heavily. Since that time, the costs of seed, fertilizer, equipment, and loans have risen, and the crop prices have dropped. Thousands of U.S. farmers are frustrated and in debt.

Farmers and ranchers can theoretically obtain financial support from the government in the form of subsidies and tax write-offs. Subsidies use taxpayer money to support practices such as the use of irrigation, pesticides, fertilizers, and fuels that farmers could not otherwise afford. Farmers and ranchers who receive subsidies can charge lower prices for their crops and meats, which helps them compete for buyers. Tax write-offs permit farmers and ranchers to pay fewer taxes than other citizens, in effect making their enterprises more profitable.

Unfortunately, huge corporation-owned farms find it much easier to obtain and use subsidies than do small family farms. Subsidies usually

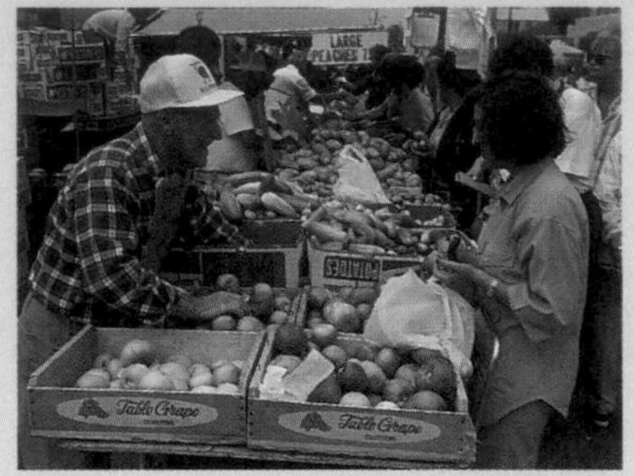

Locally grown foods offer benefits to both the local economy and the global environment.

support technology-intensive practices that employ large machinery and large land areas. Huge farms and ranches, collectively part of the massive food-producing enterprise called agribusiness, tend to use little local labor, and the profits they make tend not to stay in local communities. In fact, subsidies to agribusiness may actually be helping to drive families out of farming.

Farm subsidies also tend to promote unsustainable practices. Subsidies make it a higher priority to produce abundant food than to protect the resource base—that is, the soil, the water, and local biodiversity. Subsidies make it easy to overuse fertilizers and pesticides, to overuse land at the cost of soil erosion, and to use irrigation water wastefully.[10] Evidence suggests that both economically and environmentally, subsidies are unsound. If, for example, price supports for pesticides were eliminated, farmers would use them perhaps a third more sparingly and to better effect.[11]

It has been suggested that farm subsidies could be altered to support desirable agriculture methods rather than paying for environmentally harmful practices. The Rocky Mountain Institute of Snowmass, Colorado, which studies the environmental impacts of agriculture, has published a book called *Farm Subsidies: Consequences and Alternatives*, showing how farm subsidies often support unsustainable practices, and what some alternatives may be.[12]

Another problem is that subsidies permit sellers to set the prices of their products lower than other producers. As a result, people buy products from agribusiness, rather than from smaller, local farms. Family farms can't compete, and the environment continues to pay with its own losses. People buy the foods that are priced the lowest and think they are getting bargains. The pocket that holds their food money may not feel the pinch, but the pocket that pays the taxes may be hurting, for the taxes pay the subsidies. In short, food bought from agribusiness, even at low prices, costs more than people generally realize.

Environmental and social *costs*, such as pollution and hardship to farmers, are not reflected in the *prices* of products. These costs are therefore called *external costs*, or externalities. People don't pay for externalities when they buy the products: they pay in tax money used to defray these costs. Sometimes people do not pay in money at all, but in health and social stresses; and the environment pays in resource losses and deterioration. If these costs *were* included in prices, the prices of unsustainably produced products would be much higher, and people would buy fewer of these products. Instead, they would buy more products from smaller farms and ranches, produced with less technology, less pollution, and more labor.

Agribusiness is usually the kind of agricultural system that produces the most food on the smallest land area. With the help of subsidies, agribusiness also produces the cheapest food.[13] If the subsidies and other price supports were removed, the prices would rise. If the prices had to include a "tax" to pay for pollution cleanup, water protection, and land restoration, they would rise higher still. It has been suggested that the dollar prices of foods produced with so much irrigation, pesticides, fertilizers, and fossil fuel should even be high enough to pay for "the costs of unemployment when farms fail . . . national security to protect our supply of imported petroleum [for tractor fuel] . . . medical care for thousands of workers injured each year by pesticides . . . ground water contamination," and other such external costs.[14] Still other needs include education and benefits for the nation's silent slave labor force, the migrant farm workers.

PROPOSED SOLUTIONS

For each of the problems described thus far, solutions have been proposed. To put them into practice will require some new learning and the will to make changes.

Alternative Agriculture

After reviewing the problems associated with U.S. agriculture, the members of the National Research Council expressed the intent to develop an alternative mode of producing food. The goals were to conserve land, water, and energy; to exert minimal environmental impacts; and to produce abundant food profitability. They named this solution alternative agriculture.

Alternative agriculture is not a single system but a set of practices that can be matched to particular needs in local areas. It emphasizes careful use of natural processes, wherever possible, rather than chemically intensive methods. Table H20–1 contrasts alternative agriculture methods with unsustainable methods now in use. (Many of these "alternative" techniques are not really new, incidentally, and would be familiar to our great grandparents. They are superseded by high-technology methods and are now coming back into favor.)

Farming by these alternative agricultural methods produces crops reliably and lowers farmers' financial risks by reducing the effects of fluctuating prices for pesticides, fertilizers, and the like. Both large and small farms can use these practices, and many different machineries are compatible with them. Each technique has a different value for farmers of different crops in different regions. For example, corn and soybean farmers in the Midwest can relatively easily reduce or eliminate routine insecticide use, whereas fruit and vegetable growers in the hot and humid Southeast would find this harder to do. Not all crops can grow reliably without pesticides, but many can.

Alternative agriculture has some apparent disadvantages, but they are offset by advantages. For example, as chemical use falls, yields per acre also fall somewhat, but costs per acre also fall, so that the return per acre may be the same as or greater than before. More money goes to farmers and less to the fuels, fertilizers, pesticides, and irrigation that subsidies would pay for. Prices for

Table H20–1

Alternative Agricultural Techniques

Unsustainable Practice	Sustainable Practice
• Grow the same crop repeatedly on the same patch of land. This takes more and more nutrients out of the soil, making fertilizer use necessary; favors soil erosion; and invites weeds and pests to become established, making pesticide use necessary.	• Rotate crops. This increases nitrogen in the soil so there is less need to buy fertilizers. If used with appropriate plowing methods, reduces soil erosion. An acre of land planted one year in corn, the next in wheat, and the next in clover loses 2.7 tons of topsoil each year, but if it is planted only in corn three years in a row, it will lose 19.7 tons a year. Reduces problems caused by weeds and pests.
• Use fertilizers generously.	• Reduce the use of fertilizers and use livestock manure more effectively. This means storing it during the nongrowing season and applying it during the growing season. • Alternate nutrient-devouring crops with nutrient-restoring crops. • Plant legumes between grain crops (because legumes' roots leave nitrogen in the soil). • Compost on a large scale, including all plant residues not harvested. Plow the compost into the soil to improve its water-holding capacity.
• Feed livestock in feedlots where their manure produces a major water-pollution problem. Piled in heaps, it also releases methane, a global-warming gas.	• Feed livestock or buffalo on the open range where their manure will fertilize the ground on which plants grow and will release no methane. Alternatively, at least collect feedlot animals' manure and use it for fertilizer or, at the very least, treat it before release.
• Spray herbicides and pesticides over large areas to wipe out weeds and pests.	• Apply ingenuity in weed and pest control. Use rotary hoes twice instead of herbicides once. Treat when and where necessary only. Spot treat weeds by hand.[a] • Rotate crops to foil pests that lay their eggs in the soil where last year's crop was grown.[a] • Use resistant crops. Genetically improve crops so that they resist pests and diseases.[a] • Time the planting of crops so that pests that hatch at other times cannot gain access to them.[a] • Use biological controls such as predators that destroy the pests.[a]
• Plow the same way everywhere, allowing unsustainable water runoff and erosion.	• Plow in ways tailored to different areas. Conserve both soil and water by using cover crops, crop rotation, and contour plowing.
• To prevent disease in livestock, inject animals with antibiotics.	• Maintain animals' health so that they can resist disease by way of their own vigor.
• Irrigate on a large scale.	• Irrigate only during dry spells and apply only spot irrigation.

[a]These techniques, known as *integrated pest management (IPM)*, involve minimal use of poisons, less expense, and less fuel use.

Sources: Committee on the Role of Alternate Farming Methods in Modern Production Agriculture, Board on Agriculture, National Research Council, *Alternative Agriculture* (Washington, D.C.: National Academy Press, 1989); D. Pimentel, *Food, Energy and the Future of Society* (Boulder, Colo.: Associated University Press, 1980); A. B. Durning and H. B. Brough, *Taking Stock: Animal Farming and the Environment, Worldwatch Paper* 103 (Washington, D.C.: Worldwatch Institute, July 1991), p. 14; L. R. Brown, World population growth, soil erosion, and food security, *Science* 214 (1981): 995–1002.

farm products may rise, but taxes can fall, because subsidies can be eliminated. The end result is to make consumers better off financially.

Some economists and scientists have suggested that rather than subsidizing pesticide and fertilizer use, we should be taxing it. Some states are trying out that strategy with success.[15] Some are proposing to tax products such as sugar, at the grocery-store level, to raise money to repair the environmental damage it causes.[16]

Low-input agriculture works. More than 30,000 of the nation's farmers are successfully using sustainable techniques such as those described in Table H20–1. Notable among them are farmers in seven states who began pioneering these methods on a large scale in the 1980s.* Low-input agriculture has been called "an idea whose time has come."[17] It is seen as "a food production system that can indefinitely sustain a healthy food supply, restore our soil and water resources, and revitalize individual farms and rural communities, all with little reliance on fossil fuels."[18]

Increase Energy Efficiency

It need not cost 6560 kcalories to produce a can of corn or 7980 kcalories to produce a package of frozen corn (review Figure 20–5 on p.737). Much of this energy input could be reduced. Table H20–2 (on p. 754) offers many suggestions.

*In seven states, case studies were going on prior to 1990: California, Colorado, Florida, Iowa, Ohio, Pennsylvania, and Virginia. *Organic Agriculture: What the States Are Doing* (Washington, D.C.: Center for Science in the Public Interest, 1989).

The last item in the table is a suggestion that consumers center their diets on foods that require low energy inputs, a choice that is described next. In general, that means eating lots of foods derived from plants and limited amounts of foods derived from animals.

Eat Lower on the Food Chain

Studies of energy use in the U.S. food system have revealed which foods require the most and least energy to produce. The least energy is needed for grain: about one-third kcalorie is spent on fuel to produce each kcalorie of grain. Fruits and vegetables are intermediate, and most animal protein requires from 10 to 90 kcalories of fossil energy per kcalorie of usable food. Thus most animal-protein products require significantly larger inputs of energy, as well as of land and water, than do plant-protein products.[19] An exception is livestock raised on the open range; these animals require low energy inputs as do most plant foods. We raise so much more grain-fed, than range-fed, beef, however, that the average energy requirement for beef production is high. Figure H20–1 (on p. 755) shows how much less fuel vegetarian diets require than meat diets and shows that vegan diets require the least fuel of all.

To support our meat intake, we maintain several billion livestock, about four times our own weight in animals. Livestock consume ten times as much grain each day as we do. We could use much of that grain to make grain products for ourselves and share them. The shift could free up enough grain to feed 400 million people and would use less fuel, water, and land. The contrast between the Chinese, a society that lives almost entirely on plant foods, and U.S. resource use is startling (see Figure H20–2 on p. 755). Other plant-centered diets, such as the traditional Mediterranean diet, are also environmentally responsible.[20] They rely on fewer domestic animals, and therefore place fewer demands on soil, water, and energy.

Part of the solution to the livestock problem may be to cease feeding grain to animals and return to grazing them on the open range, which can be a sustainable practice. Ranchers have to manage the grazing carefully to hold the cattle's numbers to what the land can support without degradation. To accomplish this, the economic favoritism shown to livestock and feed-growing operations would have to be removed. If producers were to pay the true costs of the irrigation water, fertilizers, pesticides, fuels, and lands they use rather than paying artificially lowered prices, the prices of meats might rise to two or three times what they are now. According to classic economic theory, people would then buy less meat (reducing demand), and producers would respond by producing less meat (reducing supply). Meat production would then fall to a sustainable level.

Some individuals are taking action without waiting for prices to change. Some meat eaters are choosing to cut down on their meat portions or to eat range-fed beef or buffalo only. Livestock on the range eat grass, which people cannot eat. "Rangeburger" buffalo also offers nutrition advantages over grain-fed beef. It is lower in fat, and the fat has more polyunsaturated fatty acids, including the omega-3 type.[21]

Table H20–2

Energy-Saving Agricultural Techniques

Nonsustainable Practice	Sustainable Practice
• Use large machinery.	• Use smaller machinery scaled to the job at hand and operating at efficient speeds.
• Harrow, then plant, then fertilize.	• Combine operations—harrow, plant, and fertilize in the same operation.
• Use gasoline.	• Use diesel fuel. Use solar and wind energy on farms. Use methane from manure. Be open-minded to other alternative energy sources.
• Use as little labor as possible.	• Save on technological and chemical inputs and spend some of the savings paying people to do manual jobs. Increasing labor inputs has been considered inefficient. Reverse this thinking: more jobs are preferable to using more machinery and fuel.
• Use chemical fertilizers.	• Partially return to the organic farming techniques of using animal manure and crop rotation; this would save energy because chemical fertilizers require large energy inputs to produce.
• Transport food by trucks.	• Eliminate subsidies to truckers. Change highway funding so that the tax burden falls more heavily on truckers than on other highway users. Transport foods by rail or water (building and maintaining rail lines can add more jobs than are lost in trucking). Railways are five times more efficient than trucks. To move lettuce by truck from California to New York requires 36 kcalories for each kcalorie in the lettuce.
• Let people cook food however they wish.	• Educate people to cook food efficiently using the practices suggested in Chapter 20.
• Grow crops without regard to their energy requirements.	• Choose crops that require low energy inputs (fertilizer, pesticides, irrigation).

Source: D. Pimentel, *Food, Energy and the Future of Society* (Boulder, Colo.: Associated University Press, 1980); A. Durning. How much is enough? *Co-op America Quarterly* Winter 1991, pp. 10–15; M. Renner, *Jobs in a Sustainable Economy, Worldwatch Paper* 104, September 1991, p. 6.

Some people are switching to nonmeat, and even pure vegan, diets. Shifting to a fish diet does not appear to be a practical alternative yet, although fish farming shows promise of providing nutritious meat at a price both people and the environment could afford.[22] At present, extensive overfishing has been reducing many of the ocean's fish species for the whole last quarter of the twentieth century; ocean fishing cannot meet the world's food needs. Also, much fish production is energy-intensive, requiring large inputs of fuel for boats, refrigeration, processing, packing, and transport. Moreover, bioaccumulation of toxins in fish is becoming a serious problem in some areas; in others it rules out fish consumption altogether.

Cut the Population

Experts agree that a continuing increase in the human population can quickly defeat our best efforts to secure a viable future for our planet. If our numbers double, our food production must double, but to enlarge our food output now is costing more for each step taken. Only poor land is available now. More fertilizer, more pesticides, and more fuel are required to make such land productive. We have outstripped our environment's ability to provide a quality life for ourselves. If resources were equally shared, about 1 billion people could

Figure H20–1

Amounts of Fuel Required to Feed People Eating at Different Points on the Food Chain

Three people who eat differently are compared here. Each has the same energy intake: 3300 kcalories a day. The fossil fuel amounts necessary to produce these different diets are calculated based on U.S. conditions.

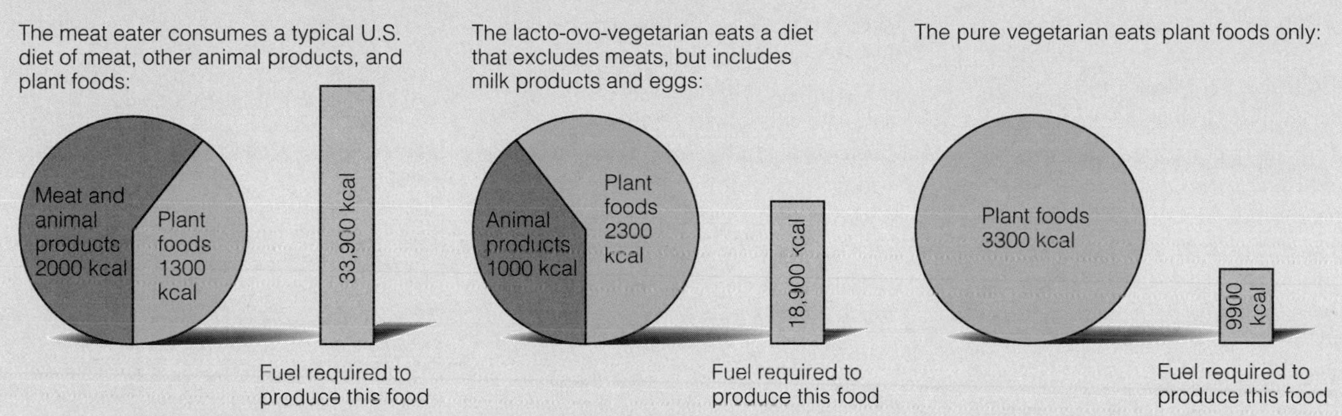

Source: Adapted from D. Pimentel, *Food, Energy and the Future of Society* (Boulder, Colo.: Associated University Press, 1980). Figure 5, p. 27.

Figure H20–2

Resource Use in the United States and China Compared

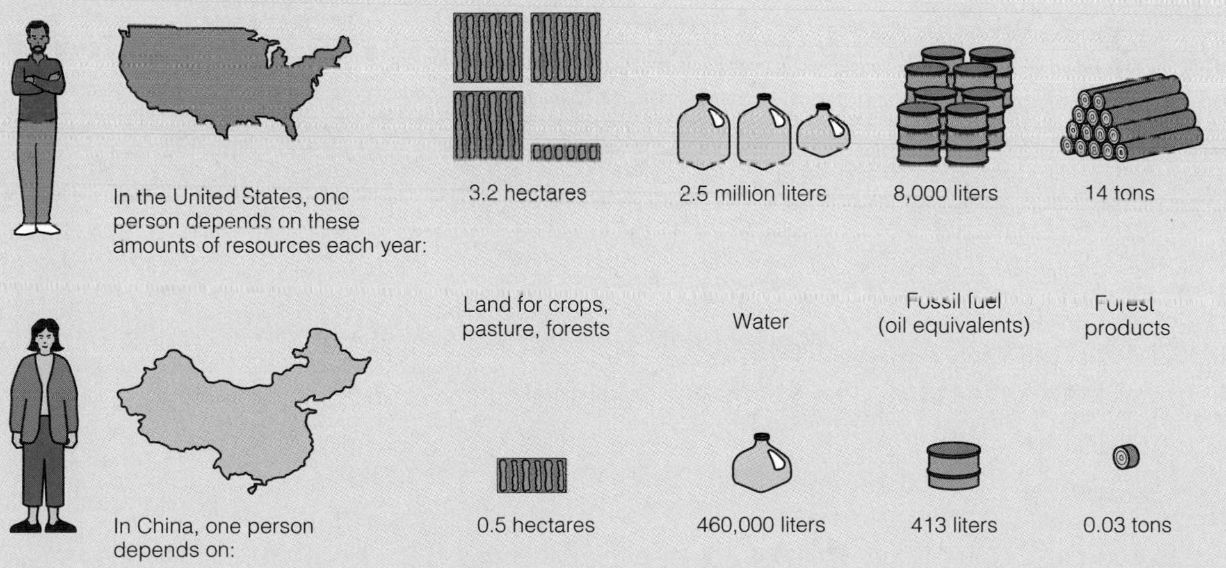

Source: D. Pimentel and M. Pimentel, Land, energy, and water: The constraints governing ideal U.S. population size. *The NPG* (Negative Population Growth) *Forum*, January 1990. Table 2, p. 2.

enjoy a relatively high-quality life, but there are more than 5 billion human beings currently on earth with resources unequally distributed. As a result, most people around the world have a low-quality life.

The hunger problem and the population problem are becoming drastically worse as we enter the twenty-first century. Meanwhile, global warming seems to be starting to contribute to the demise of agriculture. The primary agent causing global warming is carbon dioxide produced from the burning of fossil fuels. The destruction of forests is also contributing. Global warming could reduce our ability to grow many major crops where we grow them today. If the warming proceeds, the United States will cease to be a major producer of food, although for a while it may be able to produce enough to feed itself. If the polar ice caps melt and sea levels rise, river deltas now used for agriculture will disappear, and many plants and animals will become extinct. It seems, therefore, that fast progress toward producing food sustainably, and especially with reduced energy use, is imperative.

Chapter 20 and this highlight have presented many problems and have suggested that, while the problems are global in scope, the actions of individual people lie at the heart of the solutions. On learning of this, concerned people may take a perfectionist attitude, believing that they "should" be doing more than they realistically can, and so feel defeated. Yet, striving for perfection, even while falling short, is a way to achieve progress well worth celebrating. A positive attitude can bring about improvement, and improvement is enough to be proud of. Celebrate the changes that are possible today by making them a permanent part of your life; do the same with changes that become possible tomorrow and every day thereafter. The results may surprise you.

NOTES

1. Committee on the Role of Alternative Farming Methods in Modern Production Agriculture, Board on Agriculture, National Research Council, *Alternative Agriculture* (Washington, D.C.: National Academy Press, 1989).
2. World Resources Institute, *The 1992 Information Please Environmental Almanac* (Boston: Houghton Mifflin, 1992), p. 13.
3. J. Dixon, Agency warns of threats posed by plant extinction, *Tallahassee Democrat,* March 24, 1992.
4. C. B. Heiser, Jr., *Seeds to Civilization: The Story of Food* (Cambridge, Mass.: Harvard University Press, 1990), p. 13.
5. National Cattlemen's Association, *Myths and Facts about Beef Production* (Washington, D.C.: National Cattleman's Association); A. B. Durning and H. B. Brough, *Taking Stock: Animal Farming and the Environment,* Worldwatch Paper 103 (Washington, D.C.: Worldwatch Institute, July 1991), p. 14.
6. D. Pimentel, *Food, Energy and the Future of Society* (Boulder, Colo.: Associated University Press, 1980), p. 9.
7. P. H. Raven, L. R. Berg, and G. B. Johnson, *Environment* (New York: Saunders, 1993), p. 407.
8. J. D. Soule and J. K. Piper, *Farming in Nature's Image: An Ecological Approach to Agriculture* (Washington, D.C.: Island Press, 1992), p. 24.
9. U.S. Department of Commerce, *Statistical Abstract of the United States, 1994* (Washington, D.C.: Bureau of the Census, 1994), p. 668.
10. Durning and Brough, 1991, p. 35.
11. K. Mattes, Kicking the pesticide habit, *The Amicus Journal,* Fall 1989, pp. 10–17.
12. Farm subsidies: The "eyes to acres" ratio, *Rocky Mountain Institute Newsletter,* Summer 1991, p. 6.
13. A fascinating discussion of the U.S. farming community's frustration with the land-grant universities' traditional support of nonsustainable agribusiness practices is given in a newspaper series entitled "Cheap food at any cost," *High Country News,* vol. 27, May 1, 1995.
14. C. Mitlo-Shartel and the Land Stewardship Project, Regenerating American's agriculture, *Building Economic Alternatives* (a quarterly publication of Co-op America, 2100 M. Street NW, Suite 310, Washington, DC 20063), Summer 1989, pp. 9–12.
15. *Organic Agriculture: What the States Are Doing* (Washington, D.C.: Center for Science in the Public Interest, 1989), pp. 5, 14–15.
16. B. Bergstrom, Environmentalists seek penny-a-pound sugar tax, *Tallahassee Democrat,* September 30, 1993.
17. *Organic Agriculture: What the States Are Doing,* 1989. The quotation is from the assistant secretary of agriculture, Orville G. Bentley, in a USDA press release, February 1988.
18. Mitlo-Shartel and the Land Stewardship Project, 1989.
19. Pimentel, 1980, p. 11.
20. J. D. Gussow, Mediterranean diets: Are they environmentally responsible? *American Journal of Clinical Nutrition* 61 (1995): 1383S–1389S.
21. S. Smith, professor of nutrition, University of New Hampshire, Durham, NH, personal communication, August 1993.
22. C. Flavin and J. E. Young, Shaping the next industrial revolution, in L. R. Brown, *State of the World 1993* (New York: W. W. Norton, 1993), pp. 180–199.

Appendixes

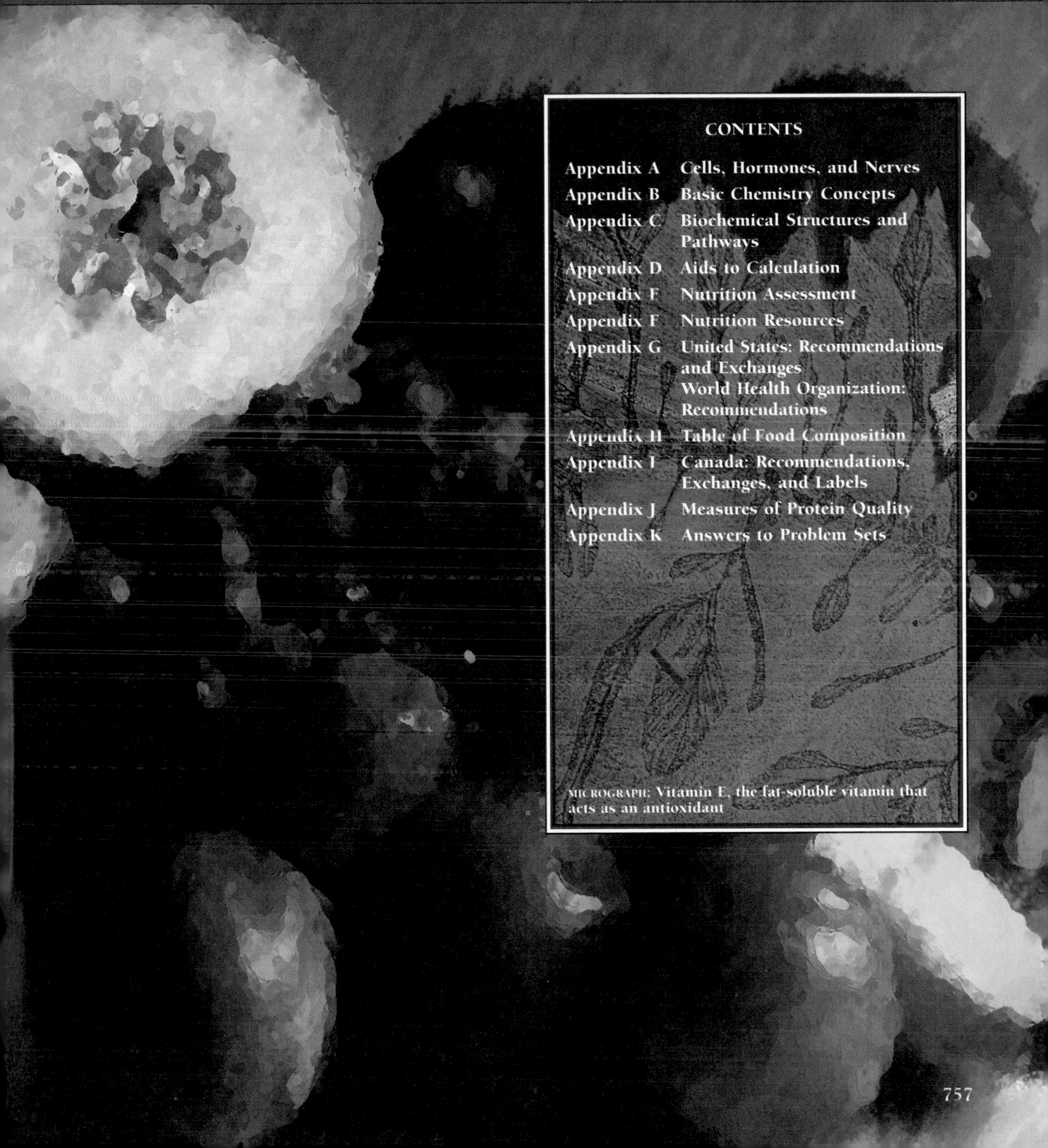

CONTENTS

MICROGRAPH: Vitamin E, the fat-soluble vitamin that acts as an antioxidant

APPENDIX A

Contents

CELLS, HORMONES, AND NERVES

This appendix is offered as an optional chapter for readers who want to enhance their understanding of the body's ways of coordinating its activities. The text presents a brief summary of the structure and function of the body's basic working unit (the cell) and of the body's two major regulatory systems (the hormonal system and the nervous system).

cell: the basic unit of life, of which all living things are composed. Every cell is surrounded by a membrane and contains cytoplasm, within which are organelles and a nucleus; the cell nucleus contains chromosomes.

cell membrane: the membrane that surrounds the cell and encloses its contents; made primarily of lipid and protein.

cytoplasm (SIGH-toe-plazm): the cell contents, except for the nucleus.
cyto = cell
plasm = a form

nucleus: a major membrane-enclosed body within every cell, which contains the cell's genetic material, DNA, embedded in chromosomes.
nucleus = a kernel

chromosomes: a set of structures within the nucleus of every cell that contain the cell's genetic material, DNA, associated with other materials (primarily proteins).

organelles: subcellular structures such as ribosomes, mitochondria, and lysosomes.
organelle = little organ

ribosomes: protein-making organelles in cells; composed of RNA and protein.
ribo = containing the sugar ribose (in RNA)
some = body

mitochondria (my-toe-KON-dree-uh); singular **mitochondrion:** the cellular organelles responsible for producing ATP aerobically; made of membranes (lipid and protein) with enzymes mounted on them.
mitos = thread (referring to their slender shape)
chondros = cartilage (referring to their external appearance)

THE CELL

The body's organs are made up of millions of cells and of materials produced by them. Each cell is specialized to perform its organ's functions, but all cells have common structures (see Figure A–1). Every cell is contained within a cell membrane. The cell membrane assists in moving materials into and out of the cell, and some of its special proteins act as "pumps" (described in Chapter 6). Some features of cell membranes, such as microvilli (Chapter 3), permit cells to interact with other cells and with their environments in highly specific ways.

Inside the membrane lies the cytoplasm, or cell "fluid." The cytoplasm contains much more than just fluid, though. It is a highly organized system of fibers, tubes, membranes, particles, and subcellular organelles as complex as a city. These parts intercommunicate, manufacture and exchange materials, package and prepare materials for export, and maintain and repair themselves.

Within each cell is another membrane-enclosed body, the nucleus. Inside the nucleus are the chromosomes, which contain the genetic material, DNA. The DNA encodes all the instructions for carrying out the cell's activities. The role of DNA in coding for cell proteins is summarized in Chapter 6, Figure 6–6. Chapter 6 also describes the variety of proteins produced by cells and the ways they perform the body's work.

Among the organelles within a cell are ribosomes, mitochondria, and lysosomes. Figure 6–6 briefly refers to the ribosomes; they assemble amino acids into proteins, following directions conveyed to them by RNA copies from the DNA in the chromosomes.

The mitochondria are made of intricately folded membranes that bear thousands of highly organized sets of enzymes on their inner and outer surfaces. Although mentioned only briefly in this book's chapters, their presence is implied whenever the enzymes of the TCA cycle and electron transport chain are mentioned because

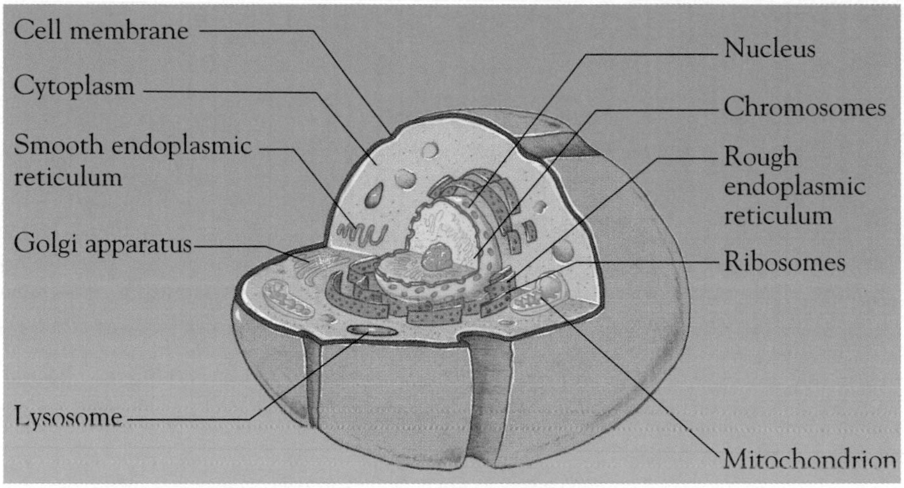

Figure A-1
The Structure of a Typical Cell

The cell shown might be one in a gland (such as the pancreas) that produces secretory products (enzymes) for export (to the intestine). The rough endoplasmic reticulum with its ribosomes produces the enzymes; the smooth reticulum conducts them to the Golgi region; the Golgi membranes merge with the cell membrane, where the enzymes can be released into the extracellular fluid.

A

the mitochondria house all these enzymes.* Mitochondria are therefore crucial to aerobic metabolism, described in Chapter 7, and muscles conditioned to work aerobically are packed with them.

The lysosomes are membranes that enclose degradative enzymes. When a cell needs to self-destruct or to digest materials in its surroundings, its lysosomes free their enzymes. Lysosomes are active when tissue repair or remodeling is taking place—for example, in cleaning up infections, healing wounds, shaping embryonic organs, and remodeling bones.

lysosomes: cellular organelles; membrane-enclosed sacs of degradative enzymes.
lysis = dissolution

Besides these and other cellular organelles, the cell's cytoplasm contains a highly organized system of membranes, the endoplasmic reticulum. The ribosomes may either float free in the cytoplasm or be mounted on these membranes. A membranous surface dotted with ribosomes looks speckled under the microscope and is called "rough" endoplasmic reticulum; such a surface without ribosomes is called "smooth." Some intracellular membranes are organized into tubules that collect cellular materials, merge with the cell membrane, and discharge their contents to the outside of the cell; these membrane systems are named the Golgi apparatus, after the scientist who first described them. The rough and smooth endoplasmic reticula and the Golgi apparatus are continuous with one another, so secretions produced deep in the interior of the cell can be efficiently transported to the outside and released. These and other cell structures enable cells to perform the multitudes of functions for which they are specialized.

rough endoplasmic reticulum (en-doh-PLAZ-mic reh-TIC-you-lum): intracellular membrane dotted with ribosomes, where protein synthesis takes place.
endo = inside
plasm = the cytoplasm

smooth endoplasmic reticulum: smooth intracellular membrane bearing no ribosomes.

Golgi (GOAL-gee) **apparatus:** a set of membranes within the cell where secretory materials are packaged for export.

The actions of cells are coordinated by both hormones and nerves, as the next sections show. Among the types of cellular organelles are receptors for the hormones delivering instructions that originate elsewhere in the body. Some hormones penetrate the cell and its nucleus and attach to receptors on chromosomes, where they activate certain genes to initiate, stop, speed up, or slow down synthesis of certain proteins as needed. Other hormones attach to receptors on the cell surface and transmit their messages from there. The hormones are described in the next section; the nerves, in the one following.

The study of hormones and their effects is **endocrinology**

*For the reactions of glycolysis, the TCA cycle, and the electron transport chain, see Chapter 7 and Appendix C. The reactions of glycolysis take place in the cytoplasm; the end product acetyl CoA moves into the mitochondria; and the TCA and electron transport reactions take place there. The mitochondria then release carbon dioxide, water, and ATP as their end products.

THE HORMONES

hormone: a chemical messenger. Hormones are secreted in response to altered conditions by a variety of endocrine glands in the body. Each hormone travels to one or more specific target tissues or organs, where it elicits a specific response.

A hormonal message originates in a gland and travels as a chemical compound—a hormone—in the bloodstream. The hormone flows everywhere in the body, but only its target organs respond to it, because only they possess the receptors to receive it.

The hormones, the glands they originate in, and their target organs and effects are described in this section. Many of the hormones you might be interested in are included, but only a few are discussed in detail. Figure A–2 identifies the glands that produce the hormones discussed in this section.

The hormonal system is a complex system in which many of the parts interact with one another. For example, several hormones are produced in the anterior pituitary gland in the brain. All of these hormones are regulated by other hormones

Figure A–2
The Endocrine System

These organs and glands release hormones that regulate body processes.

endocrine: with reference to a gland, one that secretes its product directly into (*endo*) the blood; for example, the pancreas cells that produce insulin. An **exocrine** gland secretes its product(s) out (*exo*) of the gland through a duct into a cavity; the sweat glands of the skin and the enzyme-producing glands of the pancreas are both examples. The pancreas is therefore both an endocrine and an exocrine gland.

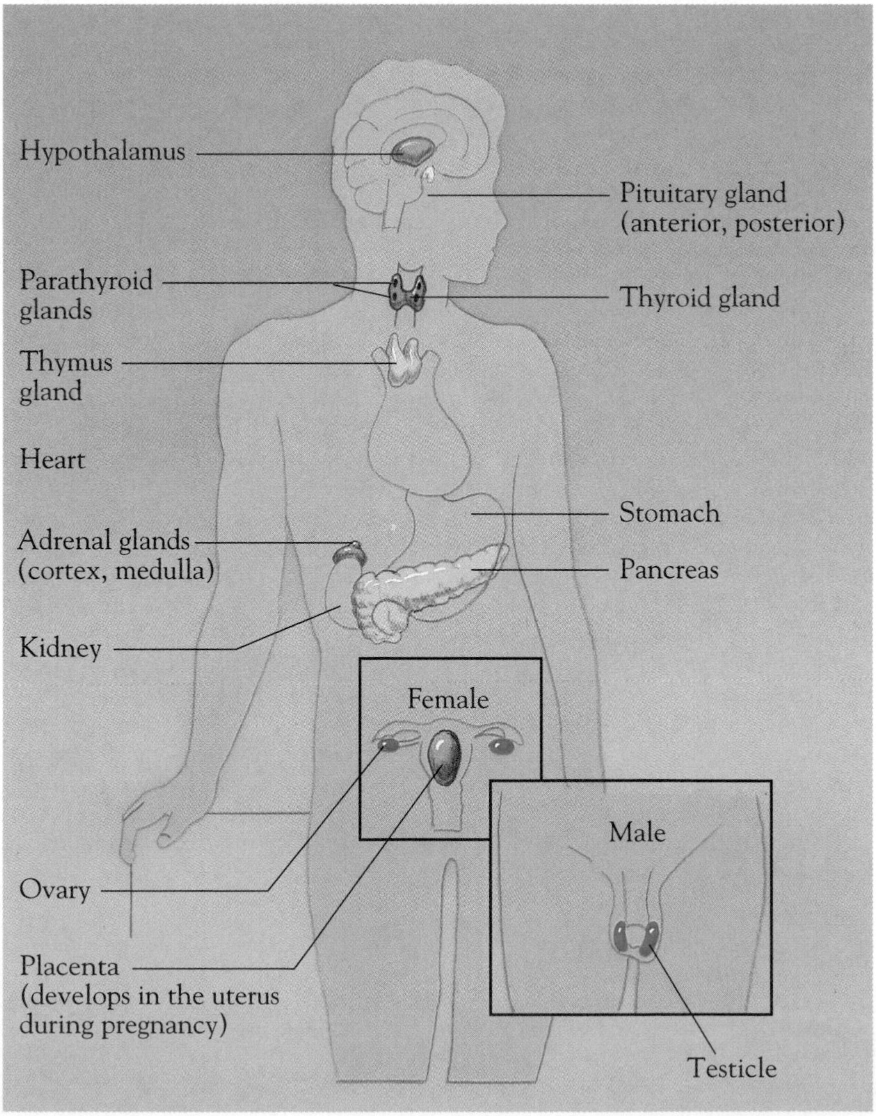

produced in another part of the brain, the hypothalamus. Furthermore, each of the pituitary gland hormones has effects on the production of compounds elsewhere in the body. Some of these compounds are also hormones that will affect still other body parts. A hormone may travel far from its point of origin and ultimately have profound, even unexpected, effects.

hypothalamus: a brain region (see Figure A–2) that is connected by a channel to the pituitary and can produce many hormones in response to signals from it or from other body conditions.
hypo = below
thalamus = another brain region

A

HORMONES OF THE PITUITARY GLAND AND HYPOTHALAMUS

The anterior pituitary gland produces the following hormones, each of which acts on one or more target organs and elicits a characteristic response:

- Adrenocorticotropin (ACTH) acts on the adrenal cortex, promoting the making and release of its hormones.
- Thyroid-stimulating hormone (TSH) acts on the thyroid gland, promoting the making and release of thyroid hormone.
- Growth hormone (GH) works on all tissues, promoting growth, fat breakdown, and the formation of antibodies.
- Follicle-stimulating hormone (FSH) works on the ovaries in the female, promoting their maturation, and on the testicles in the male, promoting sperm formation.
- Luteinizing hormone (LH) also acts on the ovaries, advancing their maturation, the making of progesterone and estrogens, and ovulation; and on the testicles, promoting the making and release of androgens (male hormones).
- Prolactin, secreted in the female during pregnancy and after she has borne a baby, acts on the mammary glands to stimulate their growth and the making of milk.
- Melanocyte-stimulating hormone (MSH) acts on the pigment cells, promoting the making and dispersal of pigment.

The **pituitary** gland in the brain has two parts—the **anterior** (front) and the **posterior** (hind) parts.

adrenocorticotropin: so named because it stimulates (*trope*) the adrenal cortex. The adrenal gland, like the pituitary, has two parts, in this case an outer portion (*cortex*) and an inner core (*medulla*).

follicle (ovarian): that part of the female reproductive system where the ovary lies and eggs are produced.

luteinizing: so called because the follicle turns orange as it matures.
lutein = an orange pigment

prolactin: so named because it promotes *(pro)* the production of milk *(lacto)*.

melanocyte (MEL-an-oh-cite): a cell containing the pigment melanin.
cyte = cell

The controls over this array of actions are sensitive and specific. Each of these seven hormones has one or more signals that turn it on and another (or others) that turns it off. Among the controlling signals are several hormones from the hypothalamus:

- Corticotropin-releasing hormone (CRH), which promotes release of ACTH, is turned on by stress and turned off by ACTH when enough has been released.
- TSH-releasing hormone (TRH), which promotes release of TSH, is turned on by large meals or low body temperature.
- GH-releasing hormone (GRH), which stimulates the release of GH, is turned on by insulin.
- GH-inhibiting hormone (GIH or somatostatin), which inhibits the release of GH and interferes with the release of TSH, is turned on by hypoglycemia and/or exercise and is rapidly destroyed by body tissues so that it does not accumulate.
- FSH/LH–releasing hormone (FSH/LH–RH) is turned on in the female by nerve messages or low estrogen and in the male by low testosterone.
- Prolactin-inhibiting hormone (PIH) is turned on by high prolactin levels and off by estrogen, testosterone, and suckling (by way of nerve messages).
- MSH-inhibiting hormone (MIH) is turned on by the hormone melatonin.

Hormones that are turned off by their own effects are said to be regulated by **negative feedback.** For example, when a pituitary gland hormone has caused the release of a substance from a target organ, that substance itself switches off the original hormone signal (that is, it feeds back negatively).

somatostatin (GIH): a hormone that inhibits the release of growth hormone; the opposite of **somatotropin (GH).**
somato = body
stat = keep the same
tropin = make more

Let's examine some of these controls. PIH, for example, responds to high prolactin levels (remember, prolactin promotes the making of milk). High prolactin levels

A

ensure that milk is made and—by calling forth PIH—ensure that prolactin levels don't get too high. But when the infant is suckling—and creating a demand for milk—PIH is not allowed to work (suckling turns off PIH). The consequence: prolactin remains high, and milk manufacture continues. Demand from the infant thus directly adjusts the infant's supply of milk. This example not only shows how the need is met but also illustrates the cooperation between nerves and hormones that achieves this effect.

As another example, consider CRH. Stress, perceived in the brain and relayed to the hypothalamus, switches on CRH. On arriving at the pituitary, CRH switches on ACTH. Then ACTH acts on its target organ, the adrenal cortex, which responds by producing and releasing stress hormones, and the stress response is under way. Events cascading from there involve every body cell and many other hormones.

The numerous steps required to set the stress response in motion make it possible for the body to fine-tune the response; control can be exerted at each step. These two examples illustrate what the body can do in response to two different stimuli—producing milk in response to an infant's need and gearing up for action in an emergency.

Two hormones produced by the posterior pituitary gland are:

antidiuretic hormone (ADH): the hormone that prevents water loss in urine (also **vasopressin**).
anti = against
di = through
ure = urine
vaso = blood vessels
pressin = pressure

oxytocin: the hormone of childbirth.
oxy = quick
tocin = childbirth

cervix: the circular muscle that guards the opening of the uterus. When a baby is about to be born, the cervix begins to stretch.
cervic = neck

- Antidiuretic hormone (ADH), or vasopressin.
- Oxytocin.

ADH promotes contraction of arteries and acts on the kidney to prevent water from being excreted. It is turned on whenever the blood volume is depleted, the blood pressure is low, or the salt concentration of the blood is too high (see Chapter 12). It is turned off by the return of these conditions to normal. Oxytocin is produced in response to reduced progesterone levels, suckling, or the stretching of the cervix and acts on two target organs. One, the uterus, contracts, thus inducing labor; the other, the mammary glands, release milk.

HORMONES THAT REGULATE ENERGY METABOLISM

Hormones produced by a number of different glands have effects on energy metabolism:

- Insulin from the pancreas beta cells.
- Glucagon from the pancreas alpha cells.
- Thyroxin from the thyroid gland.
- Norepinephrine and epinephrine from the adrenal medulla.
- Growth hormone (GH) from the anterior pituitary (already mentioned).
- Glucocorticoids from the adrenal cortex.

Norepinephrine and epinephrine were formerly called noradrenalin and adrenalin.

glucocorticoid: a hormone from the adrenal cortex that affects the body's management of glucose.
gluco = glucose
corticoid = from the cortex

Insulin is turned on by many stimuli, including raised blood glucose. It acts on cells to increase glucose and amino acid uptake into them and to promote the secretion of GRH. Glucagon responds to low blood glucose and acts on the liver to promote the breakdown of glycogen to glucose, the conversion of amino acids to glucose, and the release of glucose. Thyroxin responds to TSH and acts on many cells to increase their metabolic rate, growth, and heat production. The hormones norepinephrine and epinephrine respond to stimulation by sympathetic nerves and produce reactions in many cells that facilitate the body's readiness for fight or flight: increased heart activity, blood vessel constriction, breakdown of glycogen and glucose, raised blood glucose levels, and fat breakdown. Norepinephrine and epinephrine also influence the secretion of the many hormones from the hypothalamus that exert control on the body's other systems. The glucocorticoid hormones become active during times of stress and carbohydrate metabolism.

Every body part is affected by these hormones. Each different hormone has unique effects; and hormones that oppose each other are produced in carefully regulated amounts, so each can respond to the exact degree that is appropriate to the condition.

A

HORMONES THAT ADJUST OTHER BODY BALANCES

Hormones are involved in moving calcium into and out of the body's storage deposits in the bones:

- Calcitonin (CT) from the thyroid gland.
- Parathormone (parathyroid hormone or PTH) from the parathyroid gland.
- Vitamin D from the kidneys.

calcitonin: so called because it regulates (tones) the calcium level.

parathyroid: named for their location, the four parathyroid glands nestle in the surface layers of the two thyroid lobes in the neck.
para = beside, next to

One of calcitonin's target tissues is the bones, which respond by storing calcium from the bloodstream whenever blood calcium rises above the normal range. Calcitonin also acts on the kidneys to increase excretion of both calcium and phosphorus in the urine. Parathormone responds to the opposite condition—lowered blood calcium—and acts on three targets: the bones, which release stored calcium into the blood; the kidneys, which slow the excretion of calcium; and the intestine, which increases calcium absorption. Vitamin D acts with parathormone and is essential for the absorption of calcium in the intestine. Figure 12–9 in Chapter 12 diagrams the ways vitamin D, and the hormones calcitonin and parathormone, regulate calcium homeostasis.

Vitamin D is sometimes viewed as a hormone because it is produced in one body organ and regulates others.

Another hormone has effects on blood-making activity:

- Erythropoietin from the kidneys.

erythropoietin (eh-REE-throw-POY-eh-tin): named for its red blood cell–making function.
erythro = red (blood cell)
poiesis = creating (like poetry)

Erythropoietin is responsive to oxygen depletion of the blood and to anemia. It acts on the bone marrow to stimulate the making of red blood cells.

Another hormone, special for pregnancy, is:

- Relaxin from the ovary.

relaxin: the hormone of late pregnancy.

This hormone, which is secreted in response to the raised progesterone and estrogen levels of late pregnancy, acts on the cervix and pelvic ligaments to allow them to stretch so that they can accommodate the birth process without strain.

Other agents help regulate blood pressure:

- Renin (an enzyme), from the kidneys, in cooperation with angiotensin in the blood.
- Aldosterone, a hormone from the adrenal cortex.

renin (REN-in): an enzyme from the kidneys, which works by activating angiotensin.
ren = kidney

angiotensin: a hormone involved in blood pressure regulation.
angio = blood vessels
tensin = pressure

aldosterone: a hormone from the adrenal gland involved in blood pressure regulation.
aldo = aldehyde

Renin responds to a reduced blood supply experienced by the kidneys and acts in several ways. Encountering the inactive form of angiotensin in the bloodstream, renin converts this molecule to active angiotensin I and then to the very active angiotensin II. The angiotensins constrict the blood vessels, thus raising the blood pressure. They also stimulate thirst, leading to increased water intake, another way of raising the blood pressure. The angiotensins also cause the kidneys to retain water and salt. Thus the angiotensins increase blood pressure by several means at once.

Renin and angiotensin also stimulate the adrenal cortex to secrete the hormone aldosterone. This hormone's target is also the kidneys, which respond by excreting less sodium and with it, less water. The effect is to retain more water in the bloodstream—thus, again, raising the blood pressure. Figure 12–1 in Chapter 12 provides more details.

A

THE GASTROINTESTINAL HORMONES

Several hormones are produced in the stomach and intestines in response to the presence of food or the components of food:

- Gastrin from the stomach and duodenum.
- Cholecystokinin from the duodenum.
- Secretin from the duodenum.
- Gastric-inhibitory peptide from the duodenum and jejunum.

Gastrin stimulates the stomach to make and release its acid and digestive juices and to move and churn its contents actively. Cholecystokinin signals the gallbladder and pancreas to release their contents into the intestine to aid in digestion. Secretin calls forth acid-neutralizing bicarbonate from the pancreas into the intestine and slows the action of the stomach and its secretion of acid and digestive juices. Gastric-inhibitory peptide inhibits the secretion of gastric acid and slows the process of digestion. These hormones are presented in more detail in Chapter 3.

THE SEX HORMONES

The three major sex hormones are:

testosterone: a steroid hormone from the testicles, or testes. The steroids, as explained in Chapter 5, are chemically related to, and some are derived from, the lipid cholesterol.
sterone = a steroid hormone

estrogens: hormones responsible for the menstrual cycle and other female characteristics.
oestrus = the egg-making cycle
gen = gives rise to

progesterone: the hormone of gestation (pregnancy).
pro = promoting
gest = gestation (pregnancy)
sterone = a steroid hormone

Reminder: A *prostaglandin* is a hormonelike compound, derived from the polyunsaturated fatty acids.

- Testosterone from the testicles.
- Estrogens from the ovary.
- Progesterone from the ovary's corpus luteum in preparation for, and during, pregnancy.

In the male, testosterone is released in response to LH (described earlier). It acts on all the tissues that are involved in male sexuality and promotes their development and maintenance. Estrogens, released in response to both FSH and LH, act similarly in females. Progesterone, released in response to raised LH and prolactin, acts on the uterus and mammary glands, stimulating them to grow and develop.

THE PROSTAGLANDINS

The prostaglandins are a group of hormonelike substances produced by many different body organs. They perform a multitude of diverse functions including the regulation of blood vessel contractions, nerve impulses, and hormone responses. They don't have descriptive names but are designated by letters and numbers: E_1, E_2, and so forth. The prostaglandins are all derived from the polyunsaturated fatty acids and account in part for the necessity for these fatty acids in the diet.

This brief description of the hormones and their functions should suffice to provide an awareness of the enormous impact these compounds have on body processes. The other overall regulating agency is the nervous system.

THE NERVOUS SYSTEM

central nervous system: the central part of the nervous system, the brain and spinal cord.

peripheral (puh-RIFF-er-ul) **nervous system:** the peripheral (outermost) part of the nervous system, the vast complex of wiring that extends from the central nervous system to the body's outermost areas. It contains both somatic and autonomic components (defined next).

The nervous system has a central control system—a sort of computer—that can evaluate information about conditions within and outside the body, and a vast system of wiring that receives information and sends instructions. The control unit is the brain and spinal cord, called the central nervous system; and the vast complex of wiring between the center and the parts is the peripheral nervous system. The smooth functioning that results from the system's adjustments to changing conditions is homeostasis.

The nervous system has two general functions: it controls voluntary muscles in response to sensory stimuli from them, and it controls involuntary, internal muscles and glands in response to nerve-borne and chemical signals about their status. In fact, the nervous system is best understood as two systems that use the same or similar pathways to receive and transmit their messages. The somatic nervous system controls the voluntary muscles; the autonomic nervous system controls the internal organs.

somatic (so-MAT-ick) **nervous system:** the division of the nervous system that controls the voluntary muscles, as distinguished from the autonomic nervous system, which controls involuntary functions.
soma = body

When scientists were first studying the autonomic nervous system, they noticed that when something hurt one organ of the body, some of the other organs reacted as if in sympathy for the afflicted one. They therefore named the nerve network they were studying the sympathetic nervous system. The term is still used today to refer to that branch of the autonomic nervous system that responds to pain and stress. The other branch is called the parasympathetic nervous system. (Think of the sympathetic branch as the responder when homeostasis needs restoring and the parasympathetic branch as the commander of function during normal times.) Both systems transmit their messages through the brain and spinal cord. Nerves of the two branches travel side by side along the same pathways to transmit their messages, but they oppose each other's actions (see Figure A–3).

autonomic nervous system: the division of the nervous system that controls the body's automatic responses. Its two branches are the **sympathetic** branch, which helps the body respond to stressors from the outside environment, and the **parasympathetic** branch, which regulates normal body activities between stressful times.
autonomos = self-governing

An example will show how the sympathetic and parasympathetic nervous systems work to maintain homeostasis. When you go outside in cold weather, your skin's temperature receptors send "cold" messages to the spinal cord and brain. Your conscious mind may intervene at this point to tell you to zip your jacket, but let's say

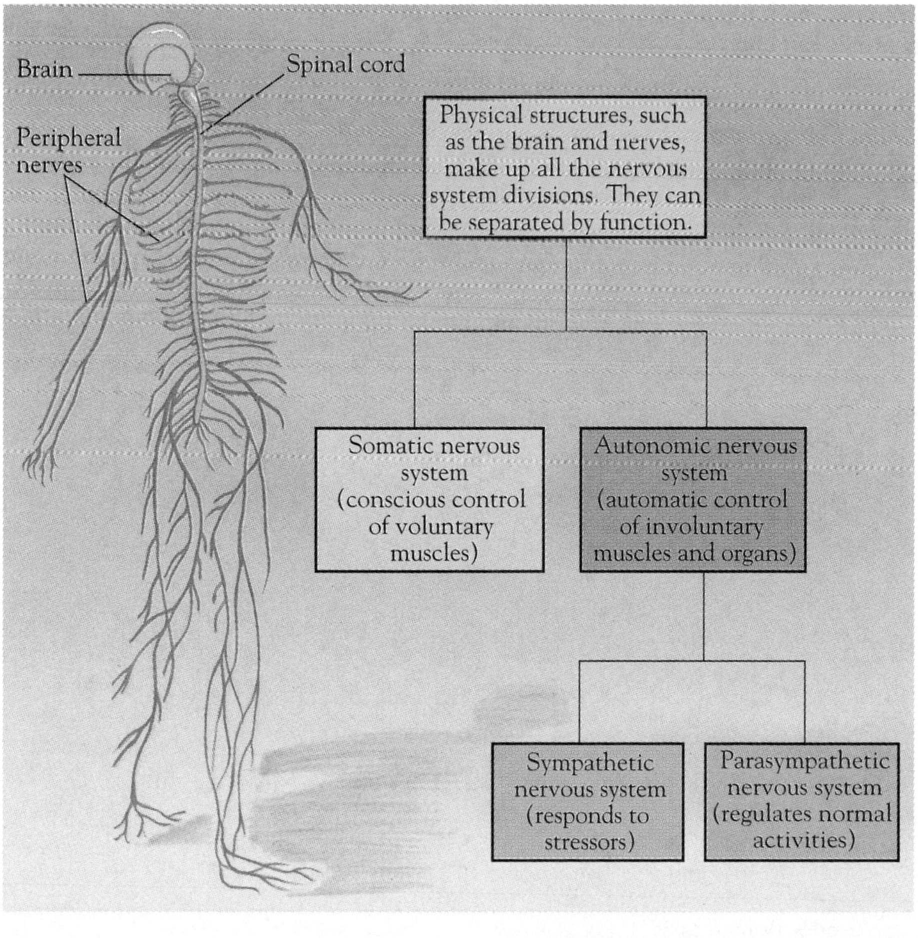

Figure A–3
The Organization of the Nervous System

The brain and spinal cord evaluate information about conditions within and outside the body, and the peripheral nerves receive information and send instructions.

A

you have no jacket. Your sympathetic nervous system reacts to the external stressor, the cold. It signals your skin-surface capillaries to shut down so your blood will circulate deeper in your tissues, where it will conserve heat. Your sympathetic nervous system also signals involuntary contractions of the small muscles just under the skin surface. The product of these muscle contractions is heat, and the visible result is goose bumps. If these measures do not raise your body temperature enough, then the sympathetic nerves signal your large muscle groups to shiver; the contractions of these large muscles produce still more heat. All of this activity adds up to a set of adjustments that maintain your homeostasis (with respect to temperature) under conditions of external extremes (cold) that would throw it off balance. The cold was a stressor; the body's response was resistance.

Now let's say you come in and sit by a fire and drink hot cocoa. You are warm and no longer need all that sympathetic activity. At this point, your parasympathetic nerves take over; they signal your skin-surface capillaries to dilate again, your goose bumps to subside, and your muscles to relax. Your body is back to normal. This is recovery.

PUTTING IT TOGETHER

The hormonal and nervous systems coordinate body functions by transmitting and receiving messages. The point-to-point messages of the nervous system travel through a central switchboard (the spinal cord and brain), whereas the messages of the hormonal system are broadcast over the airways (the bloodstream), and any organ with the appropriate receptors can pick them up. Nerve impulses travel faster than hormonal messages do—although both are remarkably swift. Whereas your brain's command to wiggle your toes reaches the toes within a fraction of a second and stops as quickly, a gland's message to alter a body condition may take several seconds or minutes to get started and may fade away equally slowly.

Together, the two systems possess every characteristic a superb communication network needs: varied speeds of transmission, along with private communication lines or public broadcasting systems, depending on the needs of the moment. The hormonal system, together with the nervous system, integrates the whole body's functioning so that all parts act smoothly together.

BASIC CHEMISTRY CONCEPTS

Contents

APPENDIX B

This appendix is intended to provide the background in basic chemistry that you need to understand the nutrition concepts presented in this book. Chemistry is the branch of natural science that is concerned with the description and classification of matter, the changes that matter undergoes, and the energy associated with these changes. Matter is anything that takes up space and has mass. Energy is the ability to do work.

MATTER: THE PROPERTIES OF ATOMS

Every substance has characteristics or properties that distinguish it from all other substances and thus give it a unique identity. These properties are both physical and chemical. The physical properties include such characteristics as color, taste, texture, and odor, as well as the temperatures at which a substance changes its state (from a solid to a liquid or from a liquid to a gas) and the weight of a unit volume (its density). The chemical properties of a substance have to do with how it reacts with other substances or responds to a change in its environment so that new substances with different sets of properties are produced.

A physical change does not change a substance's chemical composition. For example, the three states ice, water, and steam all consist of two hydrogen atoms and one oxygen atom bound together. However, a chemical change occurs if an electric current passes through water. The water disappears and two different substances are formed: hydrogen gas, which is flammable, and oxygen gas, which supports life. Chemical changes are also referred to as chemical reactions.

SUBSTANCES: ELEMENTS AND COMPOUNDS

Molecules are one or more atoms of the same element or two or more atoms of different elements joined by chemical bonds. They constitute the smallest part of a substance that can exist separately without losing its physical and chemical properties. If a molecule is composed of atoms that are alike, the substance is an element (for example, O_2). If a molecule is composed of two or more different kinds of atoms, the substance is a compound (for example, H_2O).

Just over 100 elements are known, and these are listed in Table B–1. A familiar example is hydrogen, whose molecules are composed only of hydrogen atoms linked together in pairs (H_2). On the other hand, over a million compounds are known. An example is the sugar glucose. Each of its molecules is composed of 6 carbon, 6 oxygen, and 12 hydrogen atoms linked together in a specific arrangement (as described in Chapter 4).

THE NATURE OF ATOMS

Atoms themselves are made of smaller particles. Within the atomic nucleus are protons (positively charged particles), and surrounding the nucleus are electrons (negatively charged particles). The number of protons (+) in the nucleus of an atom determines the number of electrons (−) around it. The positive charge on a proton is equal to the negative charge on an electron, so the charges cancel each other out and leave the atom neutral to its surroundings.

The nucleus may also include neutrons, subatomic particles that have no charge. Protons and neutrons are of equal mass, and together they give an atom its weight. Electrons bond atoms together to make molecules, and they are involved in chemical reactions.

Table B–1
Chemical Symbols for the Elements

Number of Protons (Atomic Number)	Element	Number of Electrons in Outer Shell	Number of Protons (Atomic Number)	Element	Number of Electrons in Outer Shell
1	Hydrogen (H)	1	52	Tellurium (Te)	6
2	Helium (He)	2	53	Iodine (I)	7
3	Lithium (Li)	1	54	Xenon (Xe)	8
4	Beryllium (Be)	2	55	Cesium (Cs)	1
5	Boron (B)	3	56	Barium (Ba)	2
6	Carbon (C)	4	57	Lanthanum (La)	2
7	Nitrogen (N)	5	58	Cerium (Ce)	2
8	Oxygen (O)	6	59	Praseodymium (Pr)	2
9	Fluorine (F)	7	60	Neodymium (Nd)	2
10	Neon (Ne)	8	61	Promethium (Pm)	2
11	Sodium (Na)	1	62	Samarium (Sm)	2
12	Magnesium (Mg)	2	63	Europium (Eu)	2
13	Aluminum (Al)	3	64	Gadolinium (Gd)	2
14	Silicon (Si)	4	65	Terbium (Tb)	2
15	Phosphorus (P)	5	66	Dysprosium (Dy)	2
16	Sulfur (S)	6	67	Holmium (Ho)	2
17	Chlorine (Cl)	7	68	Erbium (Er)	2
18	Argon (Ar)	8	69	Thulium (Tm)	2
19	Potassium (K)	1	70	Ytterbium (Yb)	2
20	Calcium (Ca)	2	71	Lutetium (Lu)	2
21	Scandium (Sc)	2	72	Hafnium (Hf)	2
22	Titanium (Ti)	2	73	Tantalum (Ta)	2
23	Vanadium (V)	2	74	Tungsten (W)	2
24	Chromium (Cr)	1	75	Rhenium (Re)	2
25	Manganese (Mn)	2	76	Osmium (Os)	2
26	Iron (Fe)	2	77	Iridium (Ir)	2
27	Cobalt (Co)	2	78	Platinum (Pt)	1
28	Nickel (Ni)	2	79	Gold (Au)	1
29	Copper (Cu)	1	80	Mercury (Hg)	2
30	Zinc (Zn)	2	81	Thallium (Tl)	3
31	Gallium (Ga)	3	82	Lead (Pb)	4
32	Germanium (Ge)	4	83	Bismuth (Bi)	5
33	Arsenic (As)	5	84	Polonium (Po)	6
34	Selenium (Se)	6	85	Astatine (At)	7
35	Bromine (Br)	7	86	Radon (Rn)	8
36	Krypton (Kr)	8	87	Francium (Fr)	1
37	Rubidium (Rb)	1	88	Radium (Ra)	2
38	Strontium (Sr)	2	89	Actinium (Ac)	2
39	Yttrium (Y)	2	90	Thorium (Th)	2
40	Zirconium (Zr)	2	91	Protactinium (Pa)	2
41	Niobium (Nb)	1	92	Uranium (U)	2
42	Molybdenum (Mo)	1	93	Neptunium (Np)	2
43	Technetium (Tc)	1	94	Plutonium (Pu)	2
44	Ruthenium (Ru)	1	95	Americium (Am)	2
45	Rhodium (Rh)	1	96	Curium (Cm)	2
46	Palladium (Pd)	—	97	Berkelium (Bk)	2
47	Silver (Ag)	1	98	Californium (Cf)	2
48	Cadmium (Cd)	2	99	Einsteinium (Es)	2
49	Indium (In)	3	100	Fermium (Fm)	2
50	Tin (Sn)	4	101	Mendelevium (Md)	2
51	Antimony (Sb)	5	102	Nobelium (No)	2

Key:
- Elements found in energy-yielding nutrients, vitamins, and water.
- Major minerals.
- Trace minerals.

Each type of atom has a characteristic number of protons in its nucleus. The hydrogen atom (symbol H) is the simplest of all. It possesses a single proton, with a single electron associated with it:

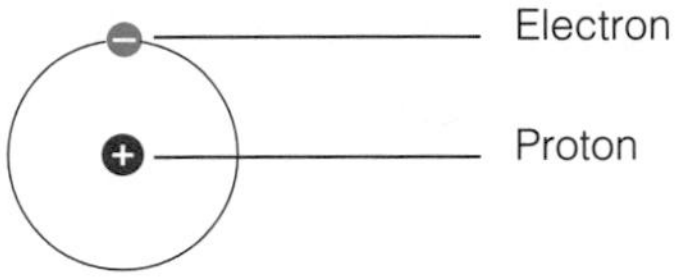

Hydrogen atom (H), atomic number 1.

Just as hydrogen always has one proton, helium always has two, lithium three, and so on. The atomic number of each element is the number of protons in the nucleus of that atom, and this never changes in a chemical reaction; it gives the atom its identity. The atomic numbers for the known elements are listed in Table B–1.

Besides hydrogen, the atoms most common in living things are carbon (C), nitrogen (N), and oxygen (O), whose atomic numbers are 6, 7, and 8, respectively. Their structures are more complicated than that of hydrogen, but each of them possesses the same number of electrons as there are protons in the nucleus. These electrons are found in orbits, or shells:

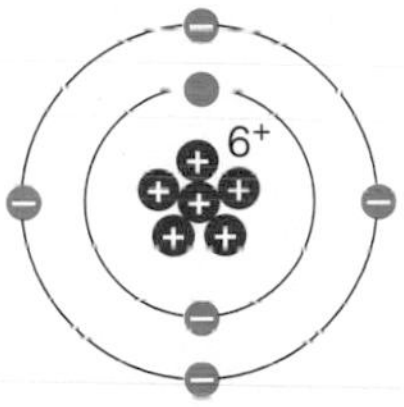

Carbon atom (C), atomic number 6.

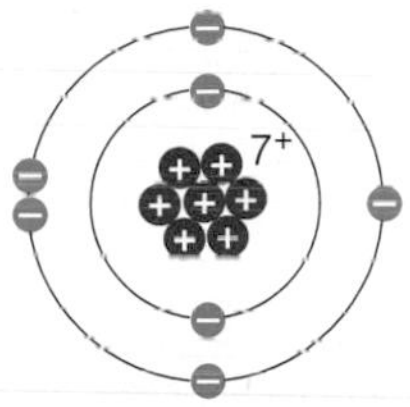

Nitrogen atom (N), atomic number 7.

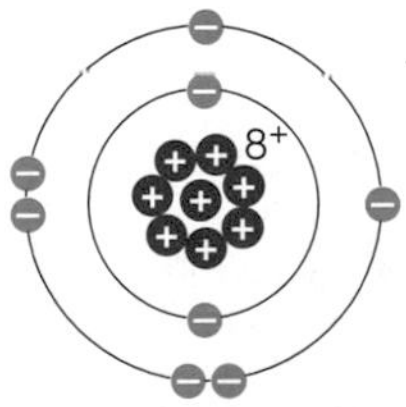

Oxygen atom (O), atomic number 8.

In these and all diagrams of atoms that follow, only the protons and electrons are shown. The neutrons, which contribute only to atomic weight, not to charge, are omitted.

The most important structural feature of an atom for determining its chemical behavior is the number of electrons in its outermost shell. The first, or innermost, shell is full when it is occupied by two electrons; so an atom with two or more electrons has a filled first shell. When the first shell is full, electrons begin to fill the second shell.

The second shell is completely full when it has eight electrons. A substance that has a full outer shell tends not to enter into chemical reactions. Atomic number 10, neon, is a chemically inert substance because its outer shell is complete. Fluorine, atomic number 9, has a great tendency to draw an electron from other substances to complete its outer shell, and thus it is highly reactive. Carbon has a half-full outer shell, which helps explain its great versatility; it can combine with other elements in a variety of ways to form a large number of compounds.

Atoms seek to reach a state of maximum stability or of lowest energy in the same way that a ball will roll down a hill until it reaches the lowest place. An atom achieves a state of maximum stability:

- By gaining or losing electrons to either fill or empty its outer shell.
- By sharing its electrons through bonding together with other atoms and thereby completing its outer shell.

The number of electrons determines how the atom will chemically react with other atoms. Hence the atomic number, not the weight, is what gives an atom its chemical nature.

CHEMICAL BONDING

Atoms often complete their outer shells by sharing electrons with other atoms. In order to complete its outer shell, a carbon atom requires four electrons. A hydrogen atom requires one. Thus, when a carbon atom shares electrons with four hydrogen atoms, each completes its outer shell (as shown on the next page).

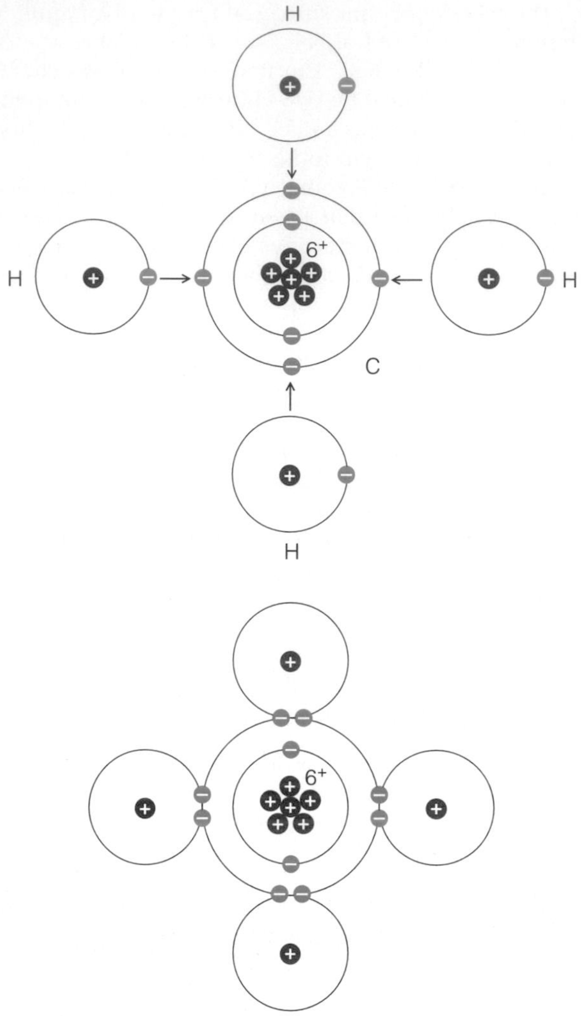

Methane molecule. The chemical formula for methane is CH_4. Note that by sharing electrons, every atom achieves a filled outer shell.

Electron sharing binds the atoms together and satisfies the conditions of maximum stability for the molecule. The outer shell of each atom is complete, since hydrogen effectively has the required two electrons in its first (outer) shell, and carbon has eight electrons in its second (outer) shell; and the molecule is electrically neutral, with a total of ten protons and ten electrons.

Bonds that involve the sharing of electrons, like the bond between carbon and hydrogen, are the most stable kind of association that atoms can form with one another. They are sometimes called covalent bonds, and the resulting combinations of atoms are called molecules. A single pair of shared electrons forms a single bond. A simplified way to represent a single bond is with a single line. Thus the structure of methane (CH_4) could be represented like this (ignoring the inner-shell electrons, which do not participate in bonding):

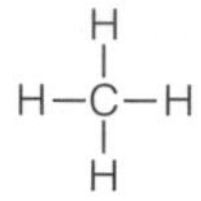

Methane (CH_4).

Similarly, one nitrogen atom and three hydrogen atoms can share electrons to form one molecule of ammonia (NH_3):

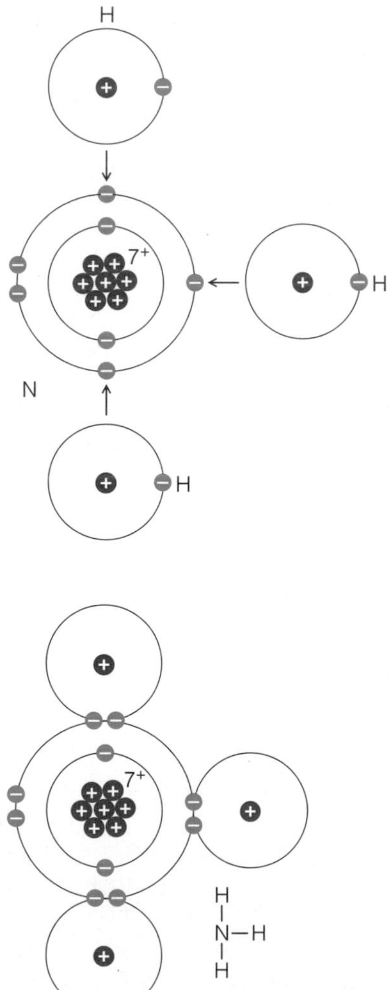

Ammonia (NH_3).

Ammonia molecule (NH_3). Count the electrons in each atom's outer shell to confirm that it is filled.

One oxygen atom may be bonded to two hydrogen atoms to form one molecule of water (H_2O):

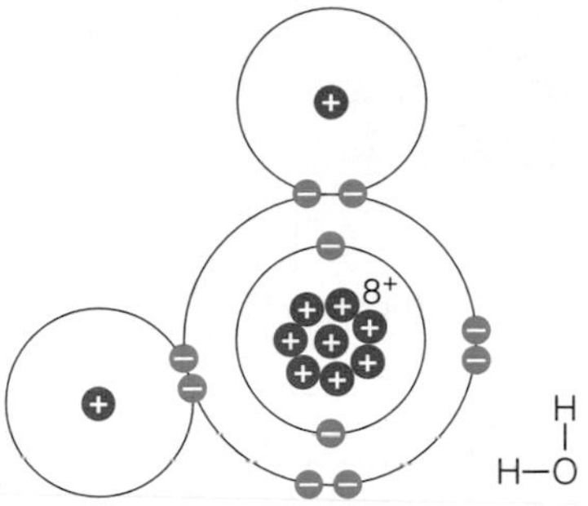

Water molecule (H_2O).

When two oxygen atoms form a molecule of oxygen, they must share two pairs of electrons. This double bond may be represented as two single lines:

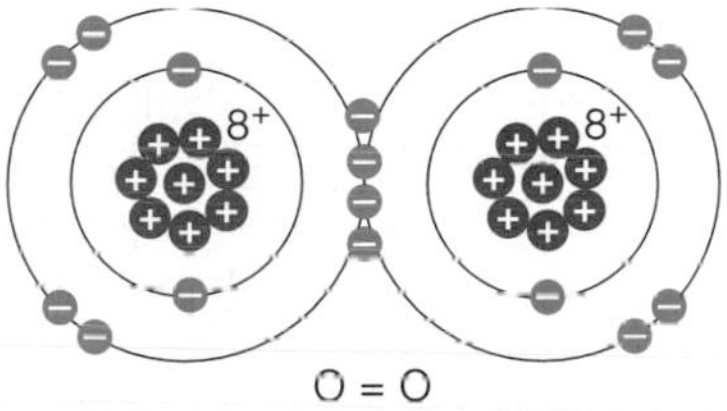

Oxygen molecule (O_2).

Small atoms form the tightest, most stable bonds. H, O, N, and C are the smallest atoms capable of forming one, two, three, and four electron-pair bonds (respectively). This is the basis for the statement in Chapter 4 that in drawings of compounds containing these atoms, hydrogen must always have one, oxygen two, nitrogen three, and carbon four bonds radiating to other atoms:

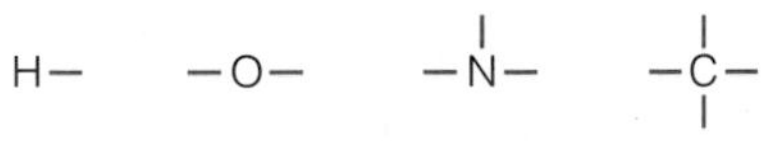

The stability of the associations between these small atoms and the versatility with which they can combine make them very common in living things. Interestingly, all cells, whether they come from animals, plants, or bacteria, contain the same elements in very nearly the same proportions. The atomic elements commonly found in living things are shown in Table B–2.

Table B–2
Elemental Composition of Living Cells

Element	Chemical Symbol	Composition by Weight (%)
Oxygen	O	65
Carbon	C	18
Hydrogen	H	10
Nitrogen	N	3
Calcium	Ca	1.5
Phosphorus	P	1.0
Sulfur	S	0.25
Sodium	Na	0.15
Magnesium	Mg	0.05
Total		99.30[a]

[a]The remaining 0.70 percent by weight is contributed by the trace elements: copper (Cu), zinc (Zn), selenium (Se), molybdenum (Mo), fluorine (F), chlorine (Cl), iodine (I), manganese (Mn), cobalt (Co), and iron (Fe). Cells may also contain variable traces of some of the following: lithium (Li), strontium (Sr), aluminum (Al), silicon (Si), lead (Pb), vanadium (V), arsenic (As), bronium (Br), and others.

FORMATION OF IONS

An atom such as sodium (Na, atomic number 11) cannot easily fill its outer shell by sharing. Sodium possesses a filled first shell of two electrons and a filled second shell of eight; there is only one electron in its outermost shell:

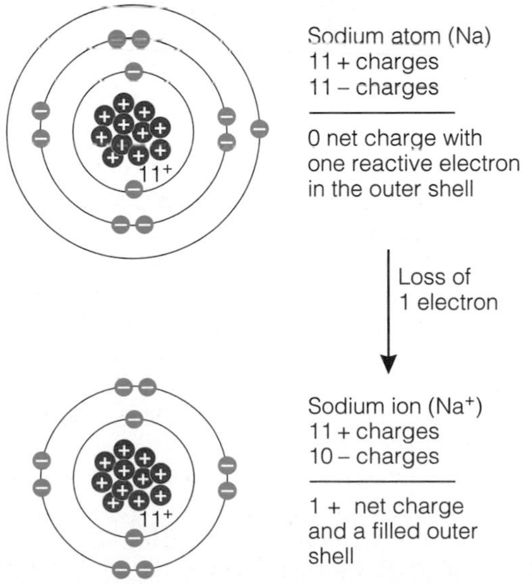

If sodium loses this electron, it satisfies one condition for stability: a filled outer shell (now its second shell counts as the outer shell). However, it is not electrically neutral. It has 11 protons (positive) and only 10 electrons (negative). It therefore has a net positive charge. An atom or molecule that has lost or gained one or more electrons and so is electrically charged is called an ion.

An atom such as chlorine (Cl, atomic number 17), with seven electrons in its outermost shell, can share electrons to fill its outer shell, or it can gain one electron to complete its outer shell and thus give it a negative charge:

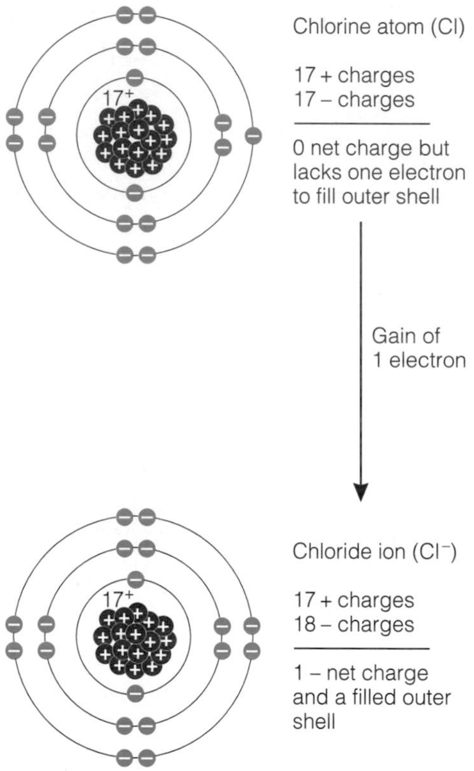

A positively charged ion such as sodium ion (Na^+) is called a cation; a negatively charged ion such as a chloride ion (Cl^-) is called an anion. Cations and anions attract one another to form salts:

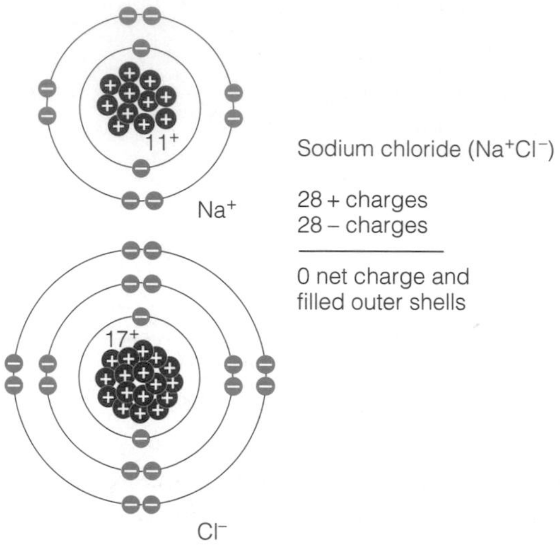

With all its electrons, sodium is a shiny, highly reactive metal; chlorine is the poisonous greenish-yellow gas that was used in World War I. But after sodium and chlorine have transferred electrons, they form the stable white salt familiar to you as table salt, or sodium chloride (Na^+Cl^-). The dramatic difference illustrates how profoundly the electron arrangement can influence the nature of a substance. The wide distribution of salt in nature attests to the stability of the union between the ions. Each meets the other's needs (a good marriage).

When dry, salt exists as crystals; its ions are stacked very regularly into a lattice, with positive and negative ions alternating in a three-dimensional checkerboard structure. In water, however, the salt quickly dissolves, and its ions separate from one another, forming an electrolyte solution in which they move about freely. Covalently bonded molecules rarely dissociate like this in a water solution. The most common exception is when they behave like acids and release H^+ ions, as discussed in the next section.

An ion can also be a group of atoms bound together in such a way that the group has a net charge and enters into reactions as a single unit. Many such groups are active in the fluids of the body. The bicarbonate ion is composed of five atoms—one H, one C, and three O—and has a net charge of -1 (HCO_3^-). Another important ion of this type is a phosphate ion with one H, one P, and four O, and a net charge of −2 (HPO_4^{-2}).

Whereas many elements have only one configuration in the outer shell and thus only one way to bond with other elements, some elements have the possibility of varied configurations. Iron is such an element. Under some conditions iron loses two electrons, and under other circumstances it loses three. If iron loses two electrons, it then has a net charge of +2, and we call it ferrous iron (Fe^{++}). If it donates three electrons to another atom, it becomes the +3 ion, or ferric iron (Fe^{+++}).

Ferrous iron (Fe^{++})	Ferric iron (Fe^{+++})
(had 2 outer-shell electrons but has lost them)	(had 3 outer-shell electrons but has lost them)
26 + charges	26 + charges
24 − charges	23 − charges
2 + net charge	3 + net charge

It is important to remember that a positive charge on an ion means that negative charges—electrons—have been lost and not that positive charges have been added to the nucleus.

WATER, ACIDS, AND BASES

Water The water molecule is electrically neutral, having equal numbers of protons and electrons. However, when a hydrogen atom shares its electron with oxygen, that electron will spend most of its time closer to the positively charged oxygen nucleus. This leaves the positive proton (nucleus of the hydrogen atom) exposed on the outer part of the water molecule. We know, too, that the two hydrogens both bond toward the same side of the oxygen. These two facts explain why water molecules are polar: they have regions of more positive and more negative charge.

Polar molecules like water are drawn to one another by the attractive forces between the positive polar areas of one and the negative poles of another. These attractive forces, sometimes known as polar bonds or hydrogen bonds, occur among many molecules and also within the different parts of single large molecules. Although very weak in comparison with covalent bonds, polar bonds may occur in such abundance that they become exceedingly important in determining the structure of such large molecules as proteins and DNA.

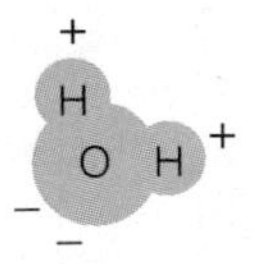

This diagram of the polar water molecule shows displacement of electrons toward the O nucleus; thus the negative region is near the O and the positive regions are near the Hs.

Water molecules have a slight tendency to ionize, separating into positive (H^+) and negative (OH^-) ions. In pure water, a small but constant number of these ions is present, and the number of positive ions exactly equals the number of negative ions.

Acids An acid is a substance that releases H^+ ions (protons) in a water solution. Hydrochloric acid (HCl) is such a substance because it dissociates in a water solution into H^+ and Cl^- ions. Acetic acid is also an acid because it dissociates in water to acetate ions and free H^+:

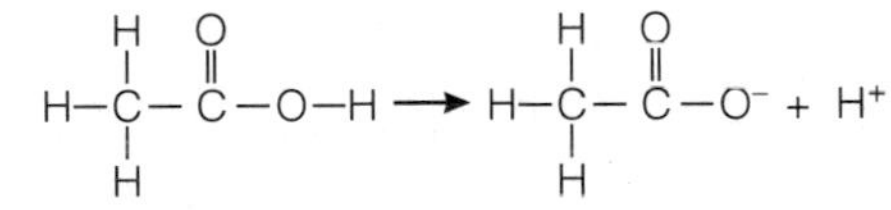

Acetic acid dissociates into an acetate ion and a hydrogen ion.

The more H^+ ions released, the stronger the acid.

pH Chemists define degrees of acidity by means of the pH scale, which runs from 0 to 14. The pH expresses the concentration of H^+ ions: a pH of 1 is extremely acidic, 7 is neutral, and 13 is very basic. There is a tenfold difference in the concentration of H^+ ions between points on this scale. A solution with pH 3, for example, has *ten times* as many H^+ ions as a solution with pH 4. At pH 7, the concentrations of free H^+ and OH^- are exactly the same—1/10,000,000 moles per liter (10^{-7} moles per liter).* At pH 4, the concentration of free H^+ ions is 1/10,000 (10^{-4}) moles per liter. This is a higher concentration of H^+ ions, and the solution is therefore acidic.

*A mole is a certain number (about 6×10^{23}) of molecules. The pH of a solution is defined as the negative logarithm of the hydrogen ion concentration of the solution. Thus, if the concentration is 10^{-2} (moles per liter), the pH is 2; if 10^{-8}, the pH is 8; and so on.

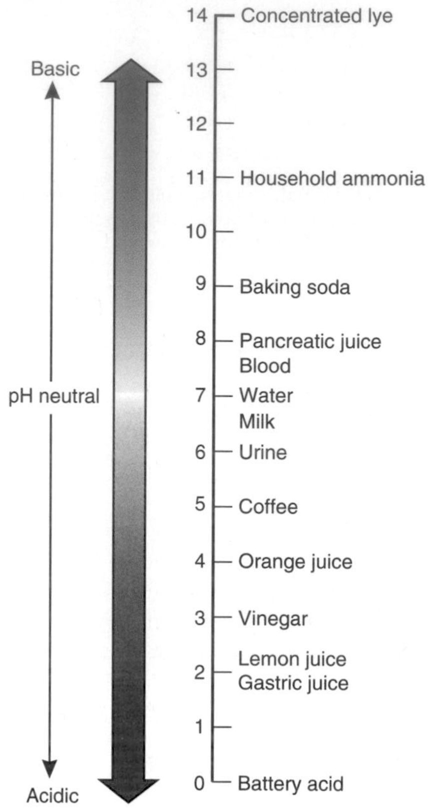

The pH scale.

Note: Each step is ten times as concentrated in base (1/10 as much acid, H^+) as the one below it.

Bases A base is a substance that can soak up, or combine with, H^+ ions, thus reducing the acidity of a solution. The compound ammonia is such a substance. The ammonia molecule has two electrons that are not shared with any other atom; a hydrogen ion (H^+) is just a naked proton with no shell of electrons at all. The proton readily combines with the ammonia molecule to form an ammonium ion; thus a free proton is withdrawn from the solution and no longer contributes to its acidity. Many compounds containing nitrogen are important bases in living systems. Acids and bases neutralize each other to produce substances that are neither acid nor base.

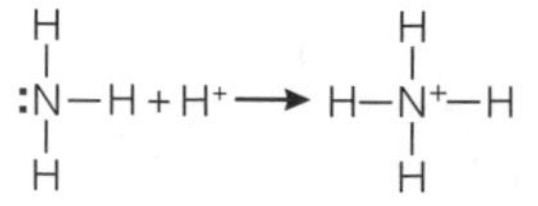

Ammonia captures a hydrogen ion from water. The two dots here represent the two electrons not shared with another atom. These are ordinarily not shown in chemical structure drawings. Compare this with the earlier diagram of an ammonia molecule (p. B–4).

CHEMICAL REACTIONS

◆

A chemical reaction, or chemical change, results in the breakdown of substances and the formation of new ones. Almost all such reactions involve a change in the bonding of atoms. Old bonds are broken, and new ones are formed. The nuclei of atoms are never involved in chemical reactions—only their outer-shell electrons take part. At the end of a chemical reaction, the number of atoms of each type is always the same as at the beginning. For example, two hydrogen molecules ($2H_2$) can react with one oxygen molecule (O_2) to form two water molecules ($2H_2O$). In this reaction two substances (hydrogen and oxygen) disappear, and a new one (water) is formed, but at the end of the reaction there are still four H atoms and two O atoms, just as there were at the beginning. Because the atoms are now linked in a different way, their characteristics or properties have changed.

In many instances chemical reactions involve not the relinking of molecules but the exchanging of electrons or protons among them. In such reactions the molecule that gains one or more electrons (or loses one or more hydrogen ions) is said to be reduced; the molecule that loses electrons (or gains protons) is oxidized. A hydrogen ion is equivalent to a proton. Oxidation and reduction take place simultaneously because an electron or proton that is lost by one molecule is accepted by another. The addition of an atom of oxygen is also oxidation because oxygen (with six electrons in the outer shell) accepts two electrons in becoming bonded. Oxidation, then, is loss of electrons, gain of protons, or addition of oxygen (with six electrons); reduction is the opposite—gain of electrons, loss of protons, or loss of oxygen. The addition of hydrogen atoms to oxygen to form water can thus be described as the reduction of oxygen *or* the oxidation of hydrogen.

If a reaction results in a net increase in the energy of a compound, it is called an endergonic, or "uphill," reaction (energy, *erg,* is added into, *endo,* the compound). An example is the chief result of photosynthesis, the making of sugar in a plant from carbon dioxide and water using the energy of sunlight. Conversely, the oxidation of sugar to carbon dioxide and water is an exergonic, or "downhill," reaction because the end products have less energy than the starting products. Oftentimes, but not always, reduction reactions are endergonic, resulting in an increase in the energy of the products. Oxidation reactions often, but not always, are exergonic.

Chemical reactions tend to occur spontaneously if the end products are in a lower energy state and therefore are more stable than the reacting compounds. These reactions often give off energy in the form of heat as they occur. The generation of heat by wood burning in a fireplace and the maintenance of human body warmth both depend on energy-

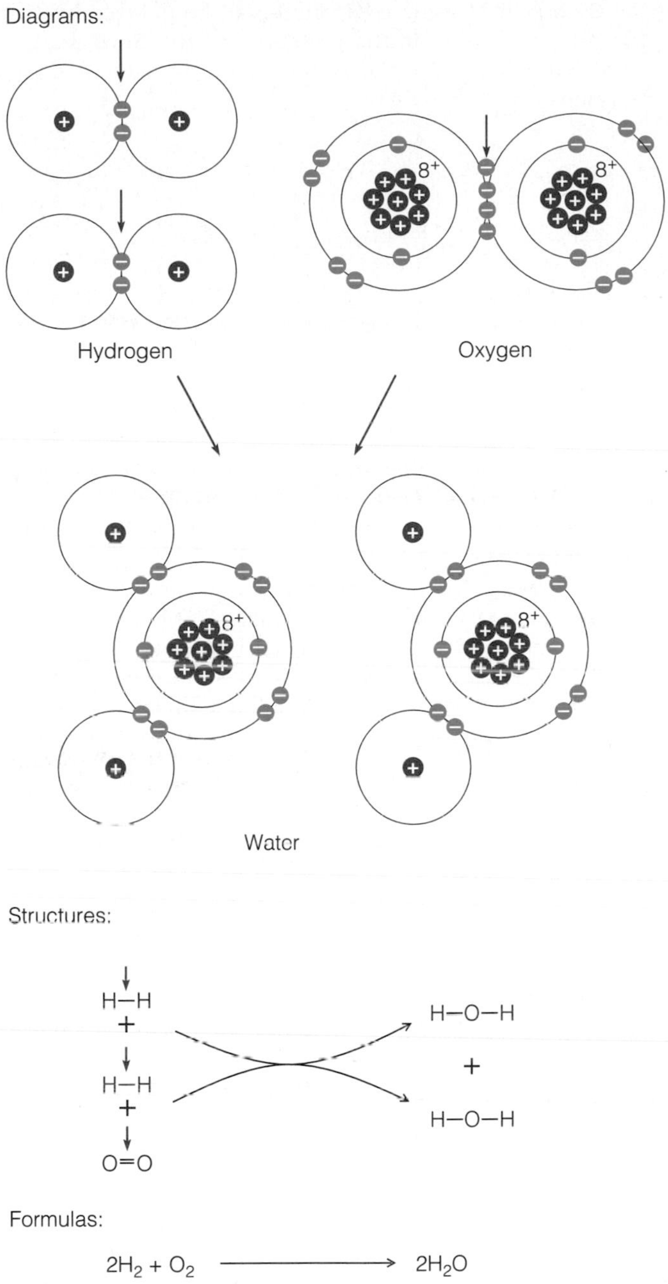

Hydrogen and oxygen react to form water.

yielding chemical reactions. These downhill reactions occur easily, although they may require some activation energy to get them started, just as a ball requires a push to start rolling downhill.

Uphill reactions, in which the products contain more energy than the reacting compounds started with, do not occur until an energy source is provided. An example of such an energy source is the sunlight used in photosynthesis, where carbon dioxide and water (low-energy compounds) are combined to form the sugar glucose (a higher-energy compound). Another example is the use of the energy in glucose to combine two low-energy compounds in the body into the high-energy compound ATP (see Chapter 7). The energy in ATP may be used to power many other energy-requiring, uphill reactions. Clearly, any of many different molecules can be used as a temporary storage place for energy.

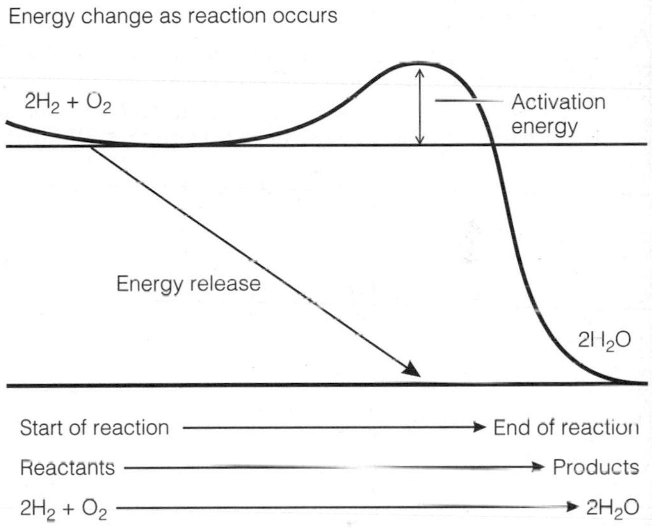

Neither downhill nor uphill reactions occur until something sets them off (activation) or until a path is provided for them to follow. The body uses enzymes as a means of providing paths and controlling chemical reactions (see Chapter 6). By controlling the availability and the action of its enzymes, the body can "decide" which chemical reactions to prevent and which to promote.

FORMATION OF FREE RADICALS

Normally, when a chemical reaction takes place, bonds break and re-form with some redistribution of atoms and rearrangement of bonds to form new, stable compounds. Normally, bonds don't split in such a way as to leave a molecule with an odd, unpaired electron. However, weak bonds can split this way, and when they do, free radicals are formed. Free radicals are highly unstable and quickly react with other compounds, forming more free radicals in a chain reaction.

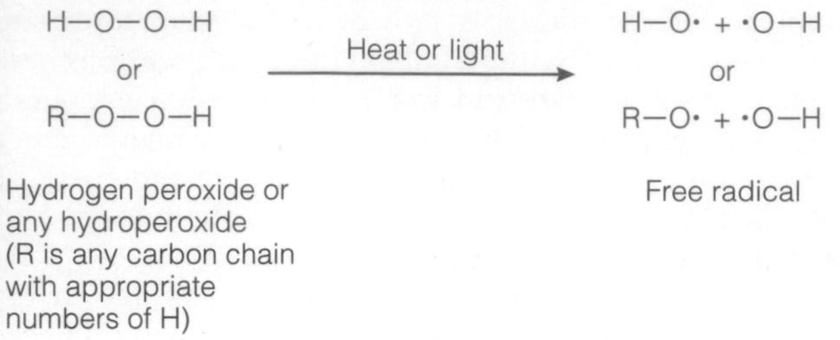

Free radicals are formed. The dots represent single electrons that are available for sharing (the atom needs another electron to fill its outer shell).

A physical event such as the arrival of an energy-carrying particle of light or other radiation starts the process by breaking a weak bond so that free radicals are formed. A cascade may ensue in which many highly reactive radicals are generated, resulting finally in the disruption of a living structure such as a cell membrane.

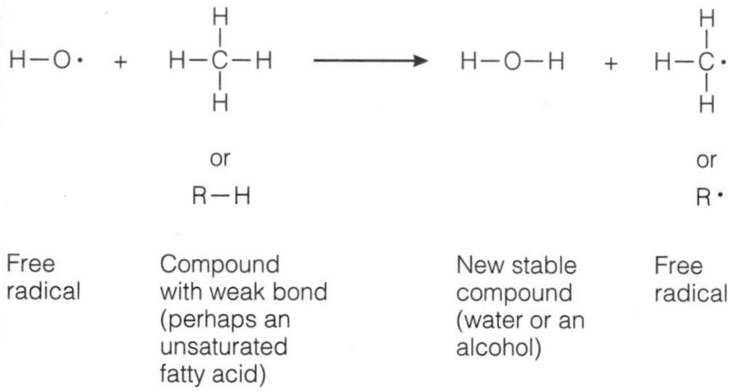

Destruction of biological compounds by free radicals. The free radical attacks a weak bond in a biological compound, disrupting it and forming a new stable molecule and another free radical. This can attack another biological compound, and so on.

Oxidation of some compounds can be induced by air at room temperature in the presence of light. Such reactions are thought to take place through the formation of compounds called peroxides:

Peroxides:

H—O—O—H	Hydrogen peroxide
R—O—O—H	Hydroperoxides (R is any carbon chain with appropriate numbers of H)
R—O—O—R	Peroxide

Some peroxides readily disintegrate into free radicals, initiating chain reactions like those just described.

Free radicals are of special interest in nutrition because the antioxidant properties of vitamins A, C, and E as well as the mineral selenium are thought to protect against the destructive effects of these free radicals (see Highlight 11). For example, vitamin E on the surface of the lungs reacts with, and is destroyed by, free radicals, thus preventing the radicals from reaching underlying cells and oxidizing the lipids in their membranes.

BIOCHEMICAL STRUCTURES AND PATHWAYS

Contents

The diagrams of nutrients presented here are meant to enhance your understanding of the most important organic molecules in the human diet. The names used are those agreed on by the American Institute of Nutrition and other scientific organizations in 1987.[1] Following the diagrams of nutrients are sections on the major metabolic pathways mentioned in Chapter 7—glycolysis, the TCA cycle, and the electron transport chain—and a description of how alcohol interferes with these pathways. Discussions of the urea cycle and the formation of ketone bodies complete the appendix.

CARBOHYDRATES

MONOSACCHARIDES

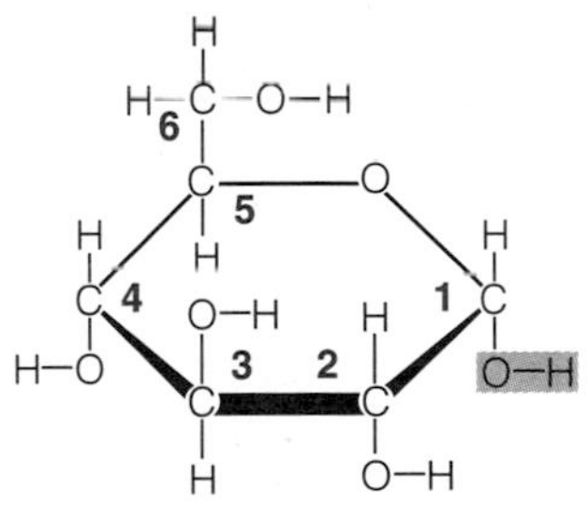

Glucose (alpha form). The ring would be at right angles to the plane of the paper. The bonds directed upward are above the plane; those directed downward are below the plane. This molecule is considered an alpha form because the OH on carbon 1 points downward.

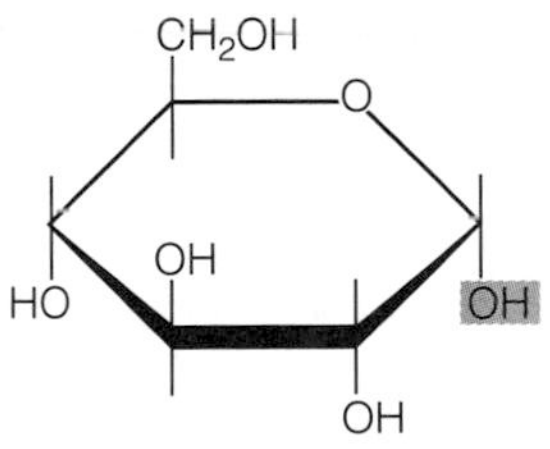

Glucose (alpha form) shorthand notation. This notation, in which the carbons in the ring and single hydrogens have been eliminated, will be used throughout this appendix.

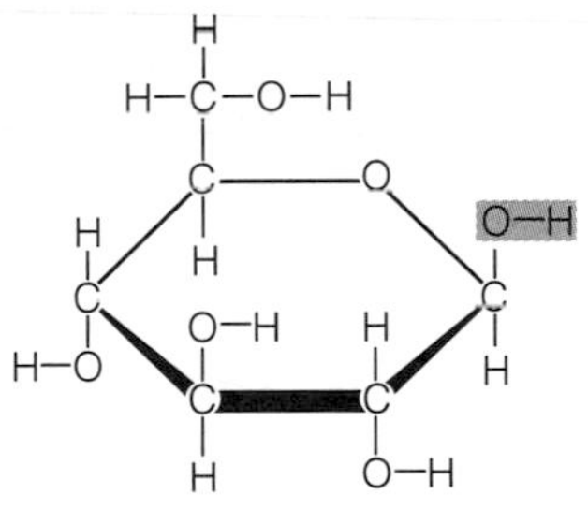

Glucose (beta form). The OH on carbon 1 points upward.
Fructose, galactose: see Chapter 4.

DISACCHARIDES

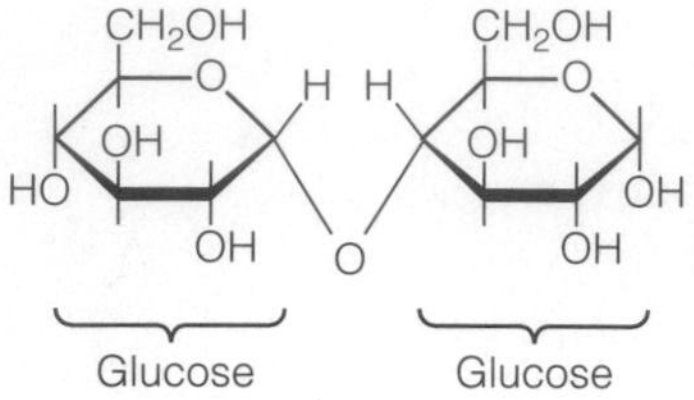

Maltose.

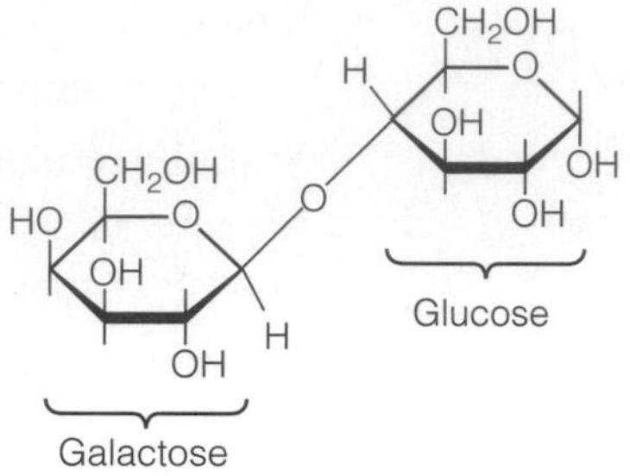

Lactose (alpha form).

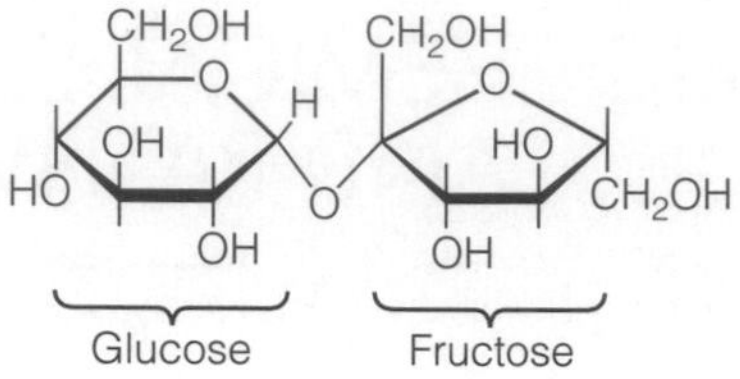

Sucrose.

POLYSACCHARIDES

As described in Chapter 4, starch, glycogen, and cellulose are all long chains of glucose molecules covalently linked together.

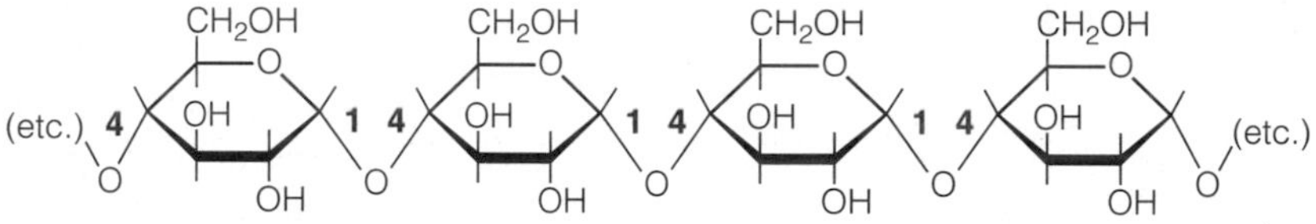

Amylose (unbranched starch)

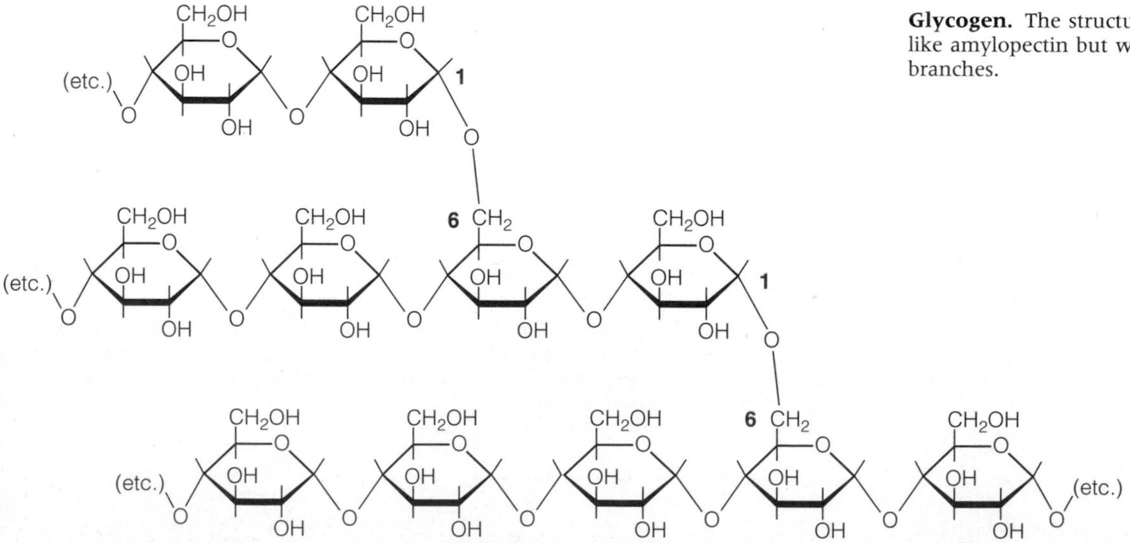

Amylopectin (branched starch)

Starch. Two kinds of covalent linkages occur between glucose molecules in starch, giving rise to two kinds of chains. Amylose is composed of straight chains, with carbon 1 of one glucose linked to carbon 4 of the next (α-1,4 linkage). Amylopectin is made up of straight chains like amylose but has occasional branches arising where the carbon 6 of a glucose is also linked to the carbon 1 of another glucose (α-1,6 linkage).

Glycogen. The structure of glycogen is like amylopectin but with many more branches.

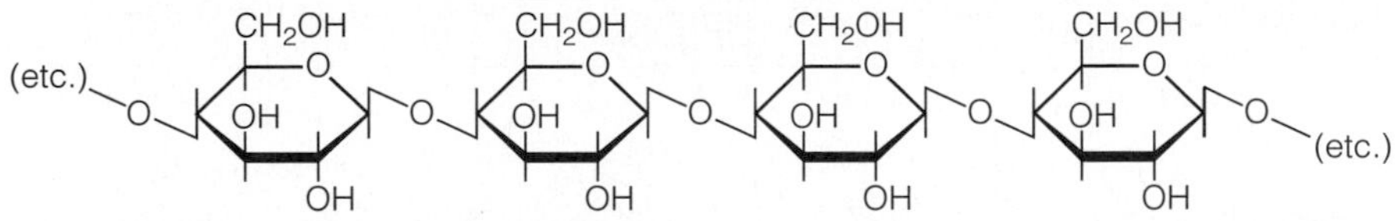

Cellulose. Like starch and glycogen, cellulose is also made of chains of glucose units, but there is an important difference: in cellulose, the OH on carbon 1 is in the beta position (see p. C-1). When carbon 1 of one glucose is linked to carbon 4 of the next, it forms a β-1, 4 linkage, which cannot be broken by digestive enzymes in the human GI tract.

Monosaccharides in backbone chain

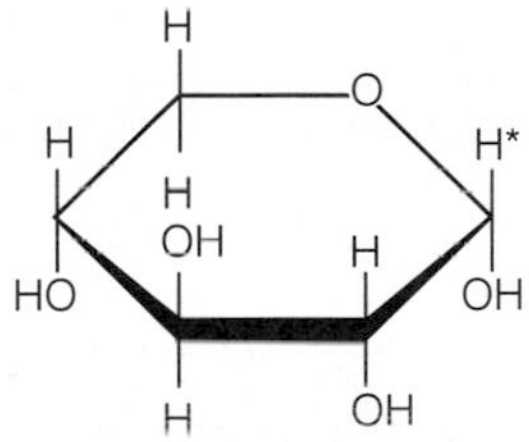

xylose

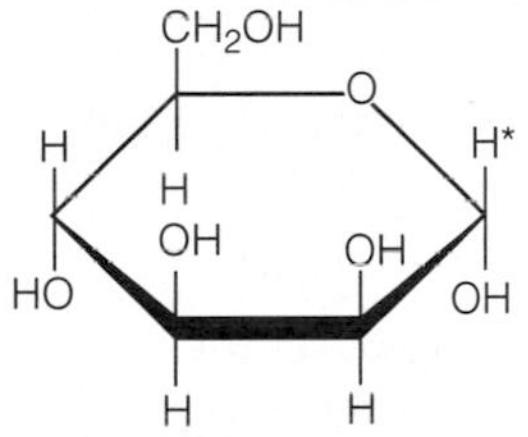

mannose

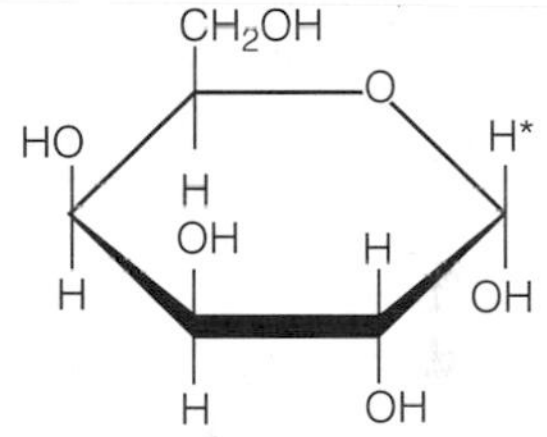

galactose

Monosaccharides in side chains

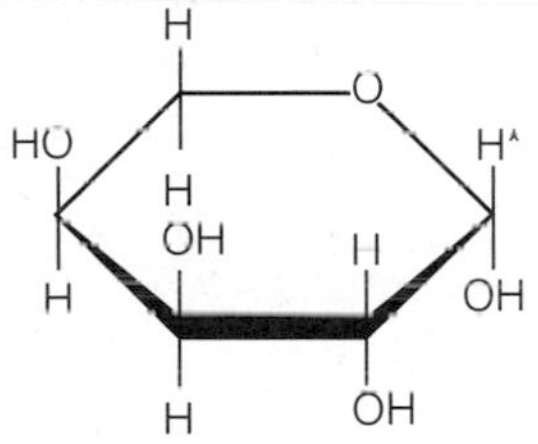

arabinose

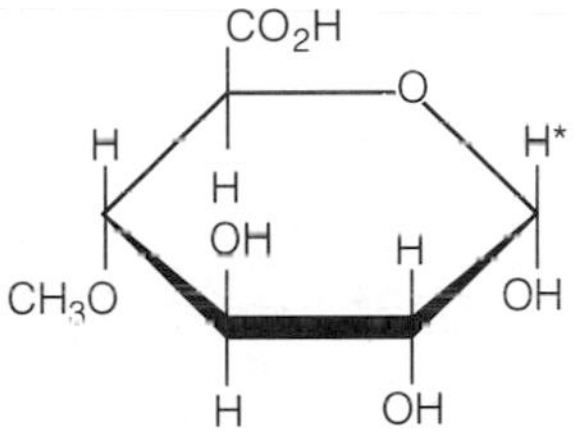

glucuronic acid

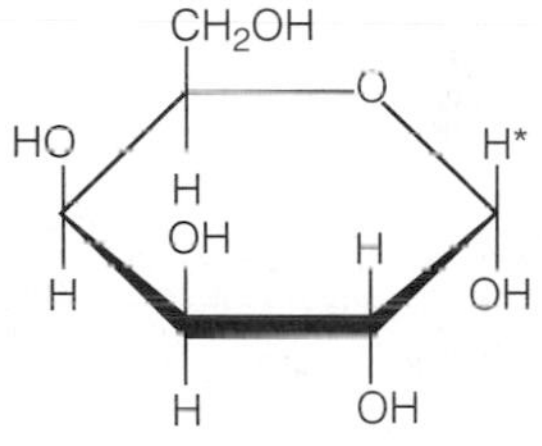

galactose

Hemicelluloses. The most common hemicelluloses are composed of a backbone chain of xylose, mannose, and galactose, with branching side chains of arabinose, glucuronic acid, and galactose.

---

*These structures are shown in the alpha form with the H on the carbon pointing upward and the OH pointing downward, but they may also appear in the beta form with the H pointing downward and the OH upward.

LIPIDS

◆

Table C-1
Saturated Fatty Acids Found in Natural Fats

Saturated Fatty Acids	Chemical Formulas	Number of Carbons	Food Source
Butyric	C_3H_7COOH	4	Butterfat
Caproic	$C_5H_{11}COOH$	6	Butterfat
Caprylic	$C_7H_{15}COOH$	8	Coconut oil
Capric	$C_9H_{19}COOH$	10	Palm oil
Lauric	$C_{11}H_{23}COOH$	12	Coconut oil
Myristic[a]	$C_{13}H_{27}COOH$	14	Coconut oil, butterfat
Palmitic[a]	$C_{15}H_{31}COOH$	16	Animal and vegetable fat
Stearic[a]	$C_{17}H_{35}COOH$	18	Animal and some vegetable fat
Arachidic	$C_{19}H_{39}COOH$	20	Peanut oil

[a]Most common saturated fatty acids.

Table C-2
Unsaturated Fatty Acids Found in Natural Fats

Unsaturated Fatty Acids	Chemical Formulas	Number of Carbons	Number of Double Bonds	Standard Notation[b]	Omega Notation[b]	Food Source
Palmitoleic	$C_{15}H_{29}COOH$	16	1	16:1;9	16:1ω7	Butterfat
Oleic	$C_{17}H_{33}COOH$	18	1	18:1;9	18:1ω9	Olive oil
Linoleic	$C_{17}H_{31}COOH$	18	2	18:2;9,12	18:2ω6	Linseed oil
Linolenic	$C_{17}H_{29}COOH$	18	3	18:3;9,12,15	18:3ω3	Linseed oil
Arachidonic	$C_{19}H_{31}COOH$	20	4	20:4;5,8,11,14	20:4ω6	Lecithin
Eicosapentanoic	$C_{18}H_{29}COOH$	20	5	20:5;5,8,11,14,17	20:5ω3	Fish oils

Note: A fatty acid has two ends; designated the methyl (CH_3) end and the carboxyl, or acid (COOH), end.

[a]Standard chemistry notation begins counting carbons at the acid end. The number of carbons the fatty acid contains comes first, followed by a colon and another number that indicates the number of double bonds; next comes a semicolon followed by a number or numbers indicating the positions of the double bonds. Thus the notation for linoleic acid, an 18-carbon fatty acid with two double bonds between carbons 9 and 10 and between carbons 12 and 13, is 18:2;9,12.

[b]Because fatty acid chains are lengthened by adding carbons at the acid end of the chain, chemists use the omega system of notation to ease the task of identifying them. The omega system begins counting carbons at the methyl end. The number of carbons the fatty acid contains comes first, followed by a colon and the number of double bonds; next comes the omega symbol (ω) and number indicating the position of the double bond nearest the methyl end. Thus linoleic acid with its first double bond at the sixth carbon from the methyl end would be noted 18:2ω6 in the omega system.

PROTEIN: AMINO ACIDS

◆

The common amino acids may be classified into the seven groups listed on the next page.[2] Amino acids marked with an asterisk (*) are essential because human beings cannot synthesize them.

1. Amino acids with aliphatic side chains, which consist of hydrogen and carbon atoms (hydrocarbons):

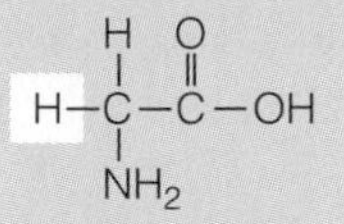

Glycine (Gly)

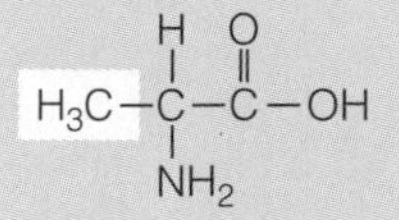

Alanine (Ala)

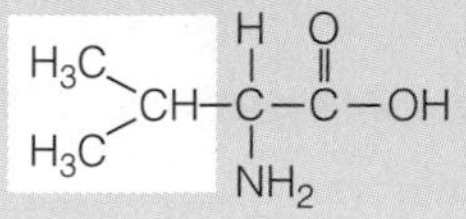

Valine* (Val)

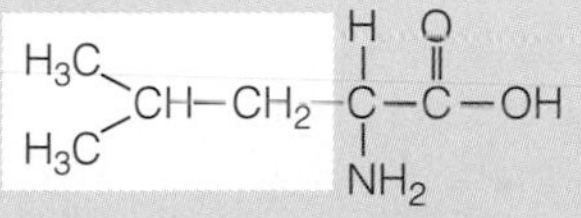

Leucine* (Leu)

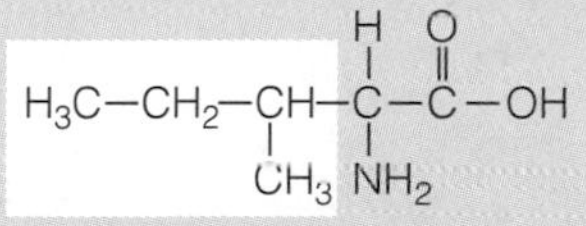

Isoleucine* (Ile)

2. Amino acids with hydroxyl (OH) side chains:

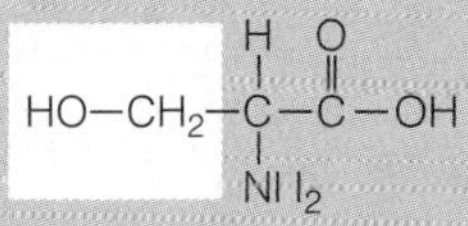

Serine (Ser)

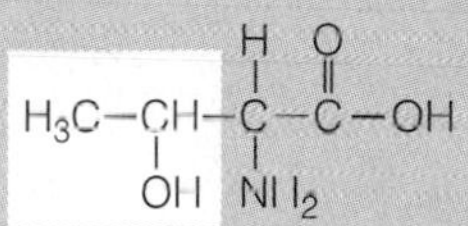

Threonine* (Thr)

3. Amino acids with side chains containing acidic groups or their amides, which contain the group NH_2:

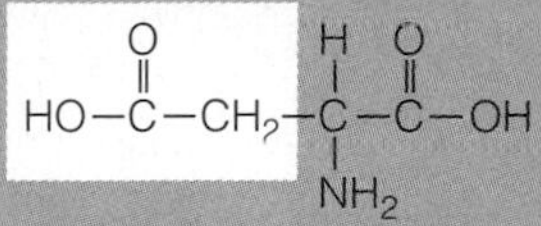

Aspartic acid (Asp)

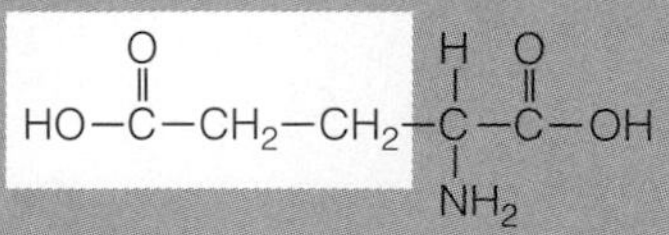

Glutamic acid (Glu)

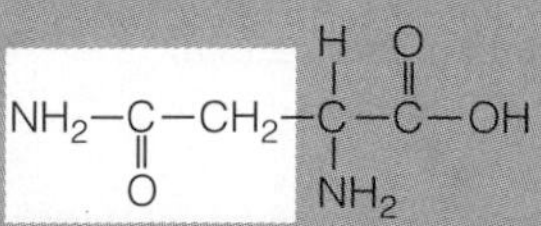

Asparagine (Asn)

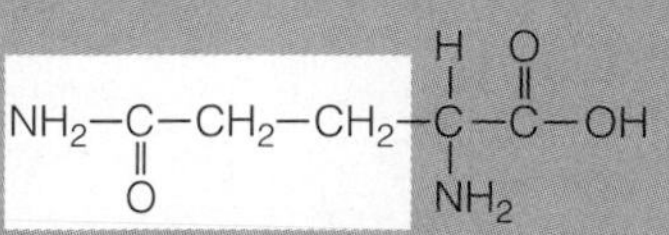

Glutamine (Gln)

4. Amino acids with basic side chains:

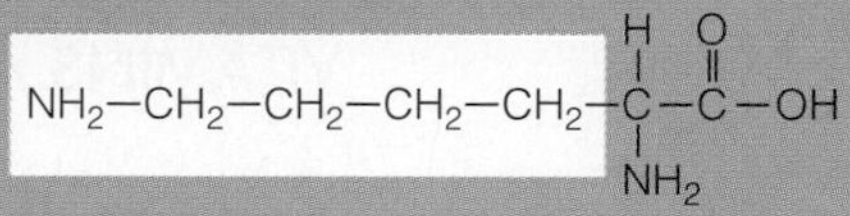

Lysine* (Lys)

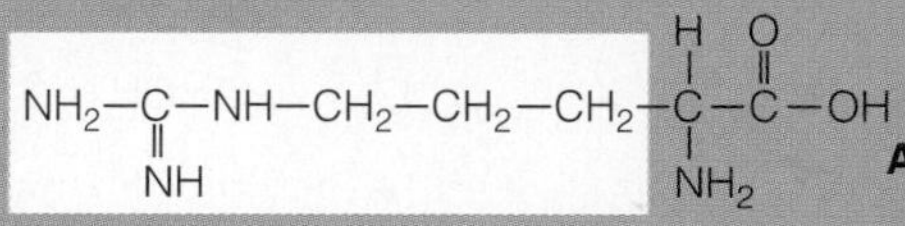

Arginine (Arg)

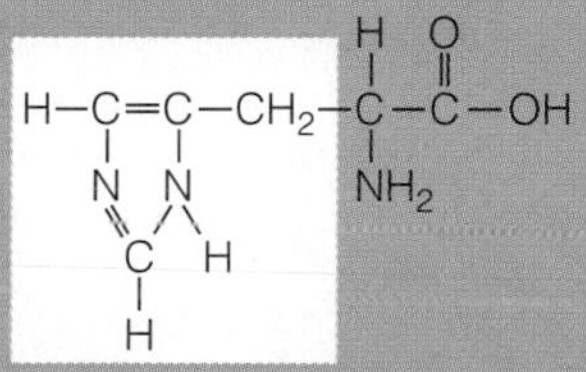

Histidine* (His)

5. Amino acids with aromatic side chains, which are characterized by the presence of at least one ring structure:

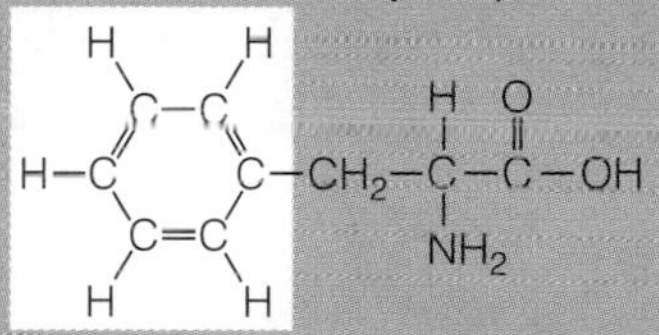

Phenylalanine* (Phe)

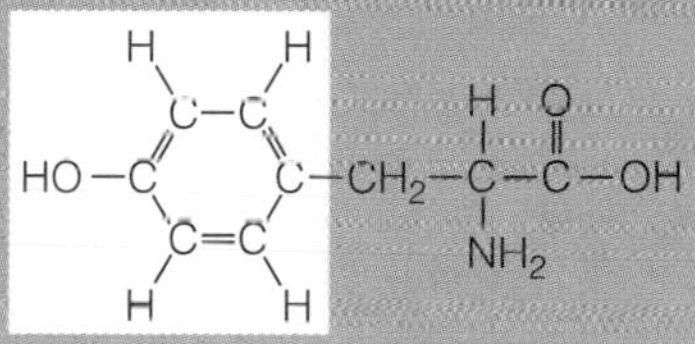

Tyrosine (Tyr)

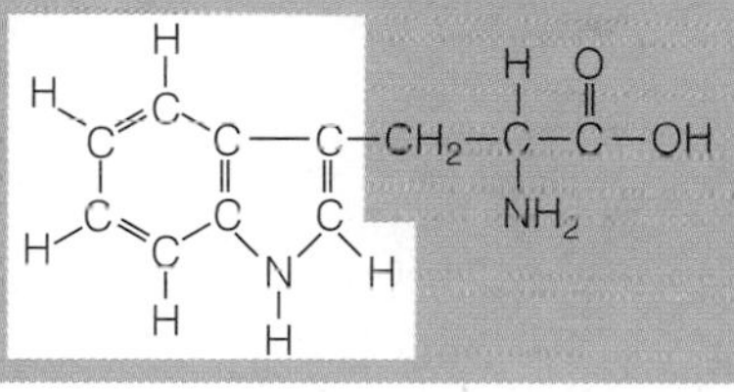

Tryptophan* (Trp)

6. Amino acids with side chains containing sulfur atoms:

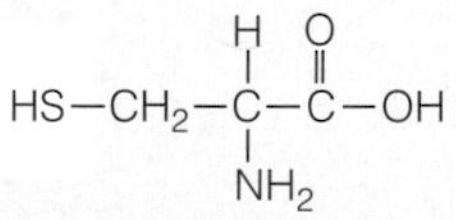

Cysteine (Cys)

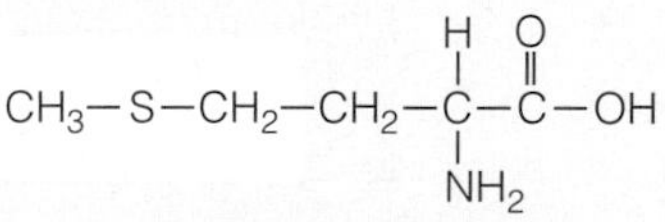

Methionine* (Met)

7. Imino acid:

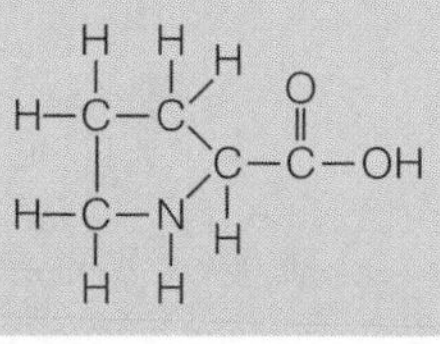

Proline (Pro) [a]

[a]Proline has the same H_2N–C–COOH structure as the other amino acids, but its amino group has given up a hydrogen to form a ring.

C

VITAMINS AND COENZYMES

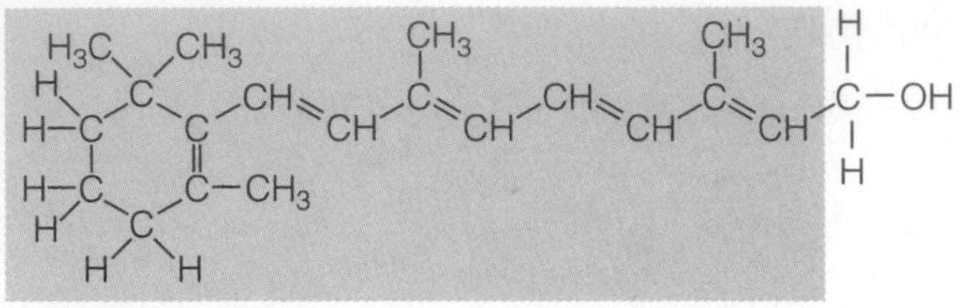

Vitamin A: retinol.

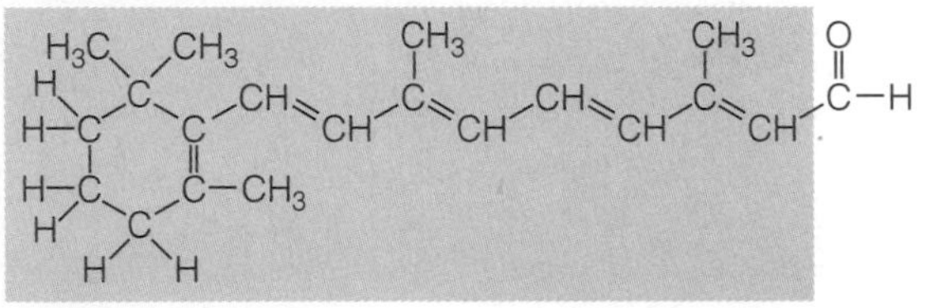

Vitamin A: retinal.

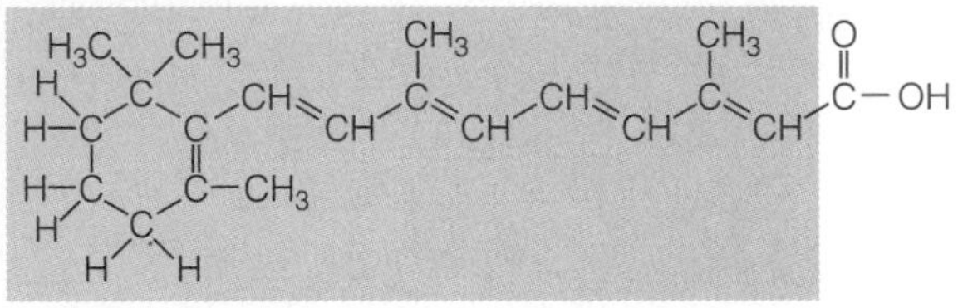

Vitamin A: retinoic acid.

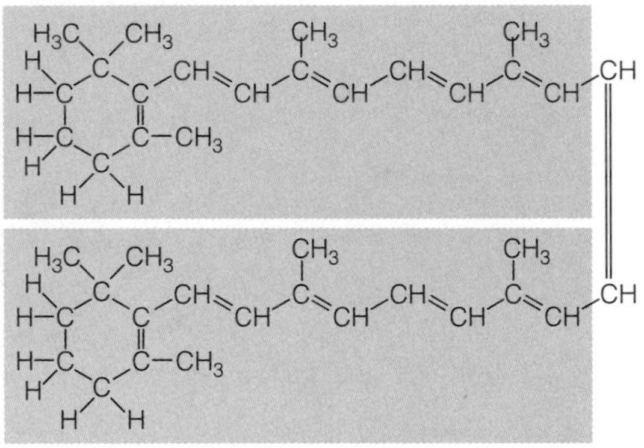

Vitamin A precursor: beta-carotene.

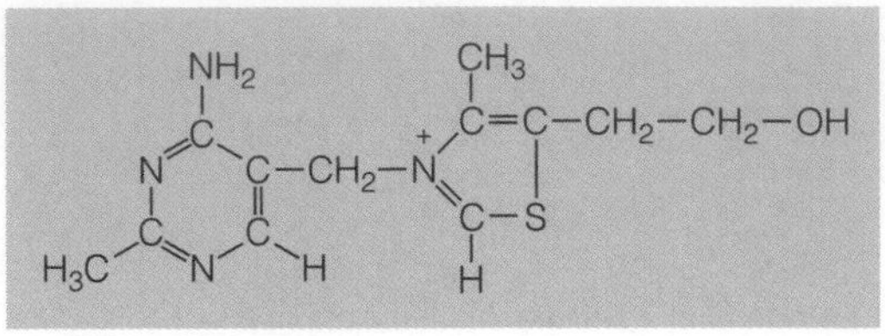

Thiamin. This molecule is part of the coenzyme thiamin pyrophosphate (TPP).

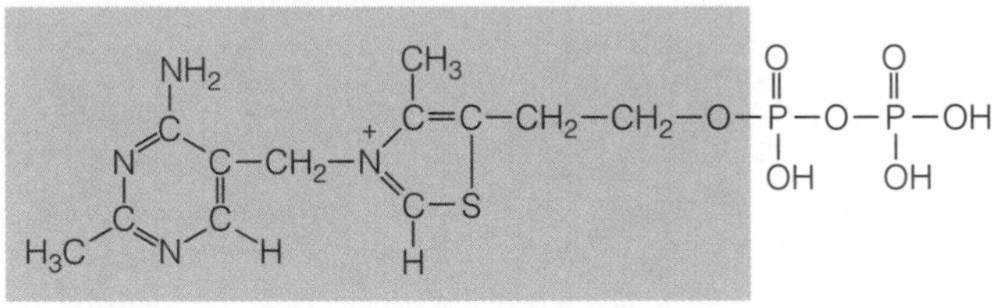

Thiamin pyrophosphate (TPP). TPP is a coenzyme that includes the thiamin molecule as part of its structure.

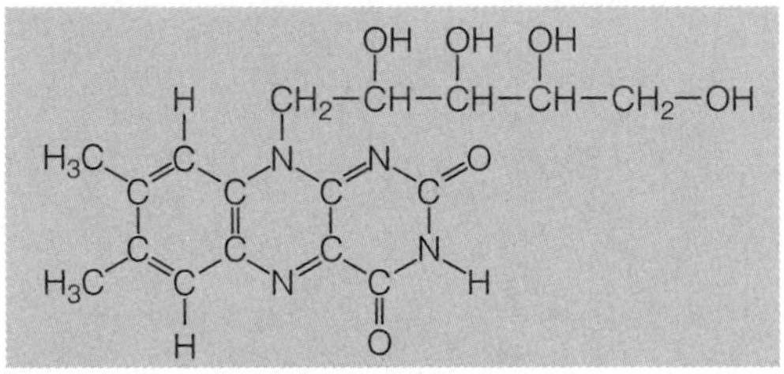

Riboflavin. This molecule is a part of two coenzymes—flavin mononucleotide (FMN) and flavin adenine dinucleotide (FAD).

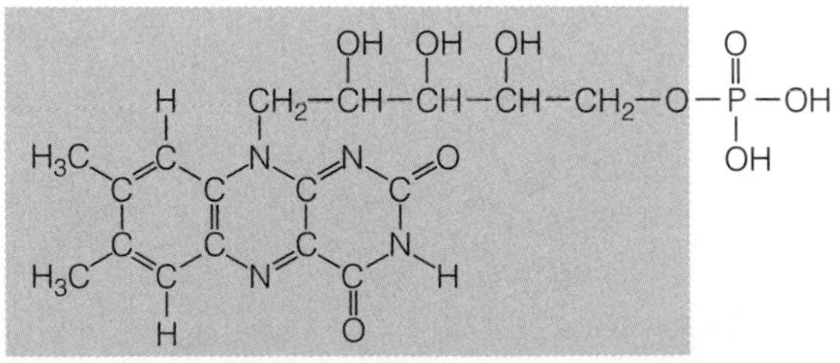

Flavin mononucleotide (FMN). FMN is a coenzyme that includes the riboflavin molecule as part of its structure.

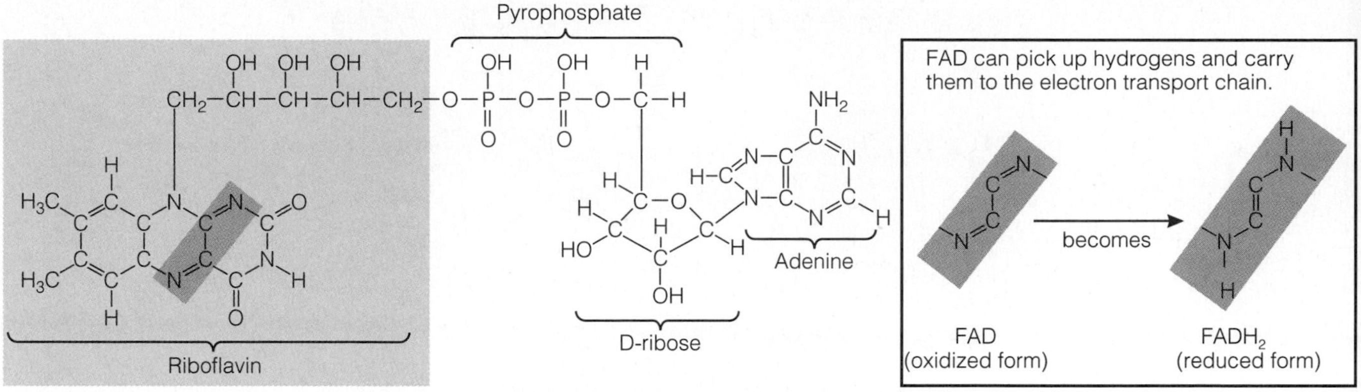

Flavin adenine dinucleotide (FAD). FAD is a coenzyme that includes the riboflavin molecule as part of its structure.

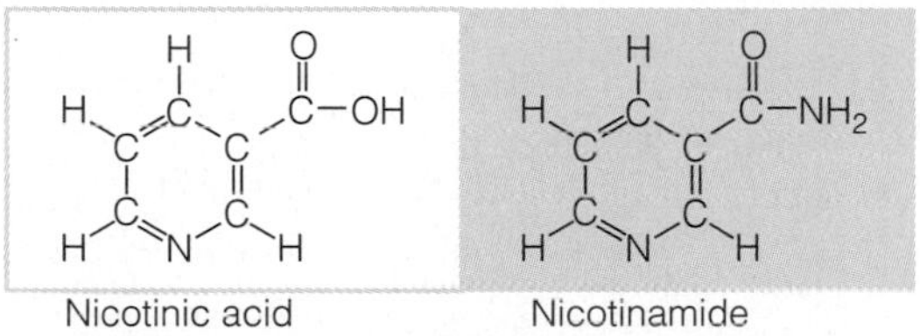

Niacin (nicotinic acid and nicotinamide). These molecules are a part of two coenzymes—nicotinamide adenine dinucleotide (NAD^+) and nicotinamide adenine dinucleotide phosphate ($NADP^+$).

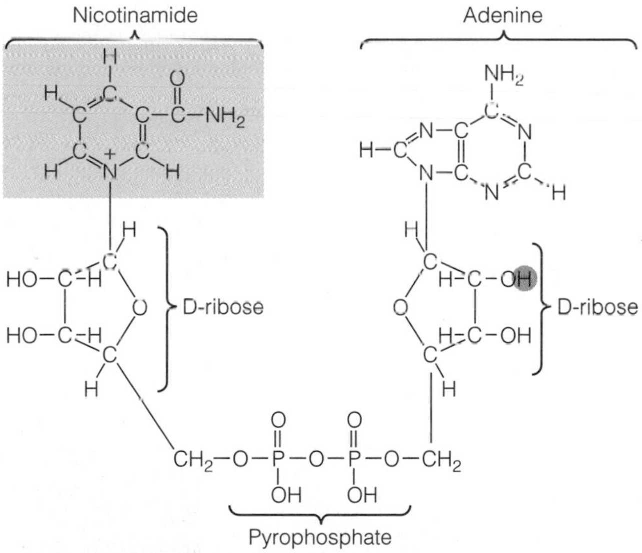

Nicotinamide adenine dinucleotide (NAD^+) and nicotinamide adenine dinucleotide phosphate ($NADP^+$). NADP has the same structure as NAD but with a phosphate group attached to the O instead of the H.

C

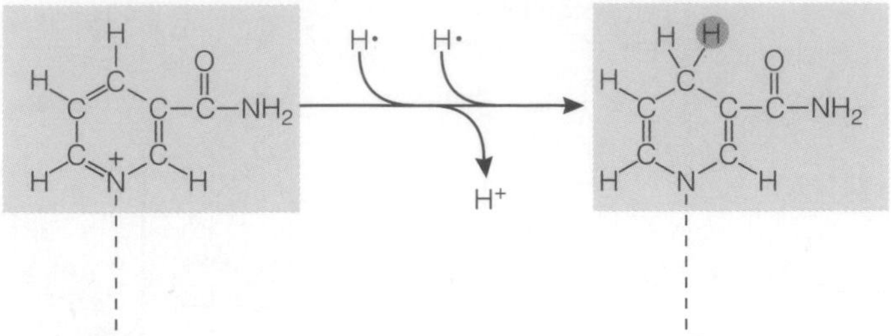

NAD⁺ NADH

Reduced NAD^+ (NADH). When NAD^+ is reduced by the addition of H^+ and two electrons, it becomes the coenzyme NADH. (The dots on the H entering this reaction represent electrons—see Appendix B.)

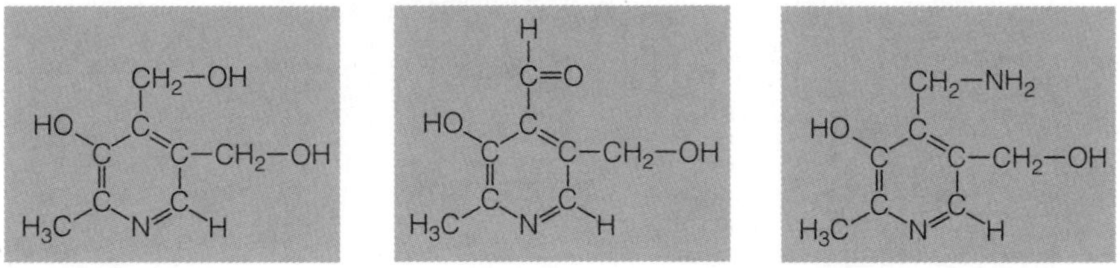

Pyridoxine Pyridoxal Pyridoxamine

Vitamin B_6 (a general name for three compounds—pyridoxine, pyridoxal, and pyridoxamine). These molecules are a part of two coenzymes—pyridoxal phosphate and pyridoxamine phosphate.

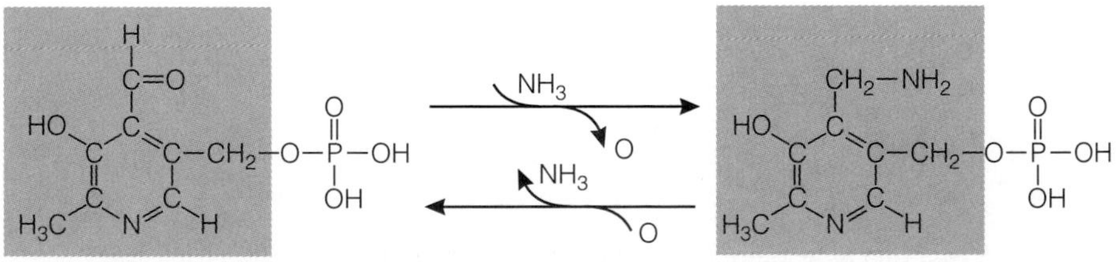

Pyridoxal phosphate Pyridoxamine phosphate

Pyridoxal phosphate (PLP) and pyridoxamine phosphate. These coenzymes are necessary for transamination and other important processes.

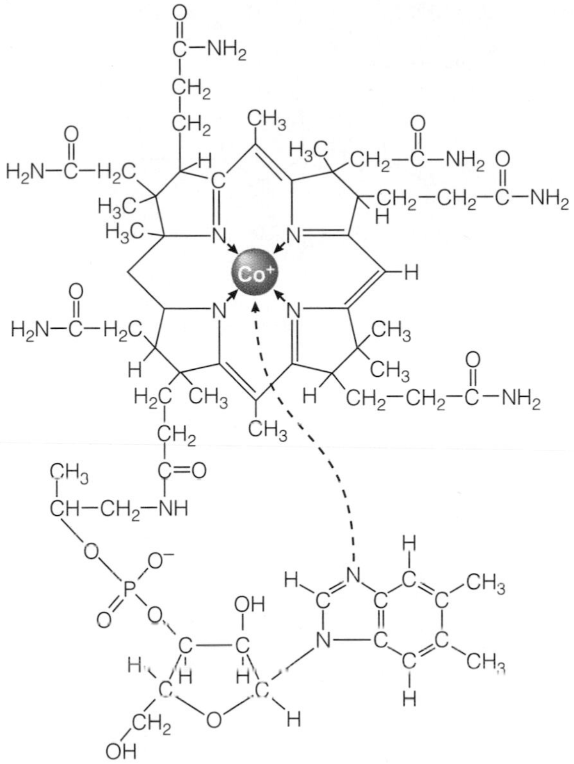

Vitamin B_{12} (cyanocobalamin). The arrows in this diagram indicate that the spare electron pairs on the nitrogens attract them to the cobalt.

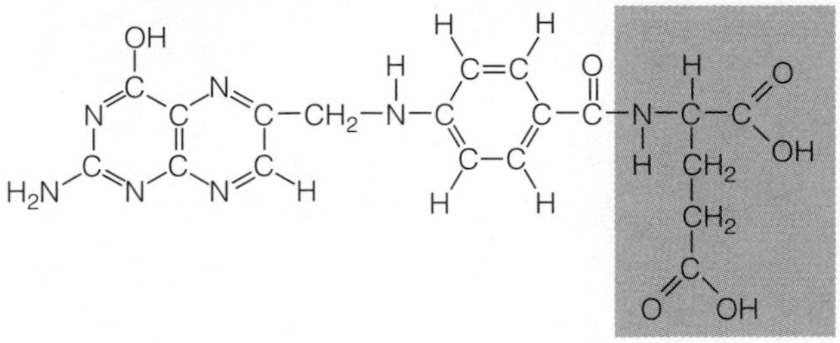

Folate (folacin or folic acid). This molecule consists of a double ring combined with a single ring and at least one glutamate (a nonessential amino acid marked in the box).

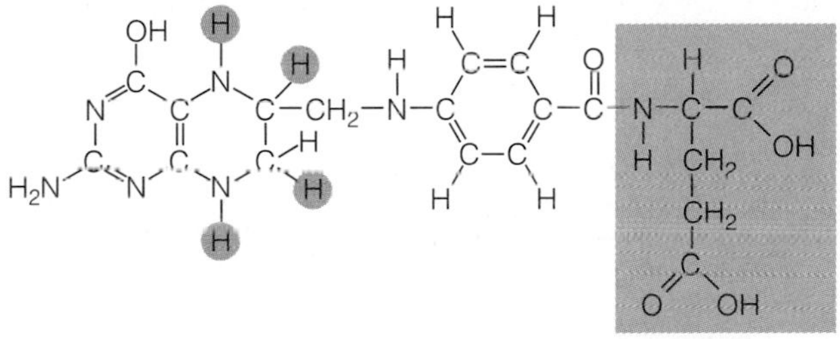

Tetrahydrofolic acid, the active coenzyme form of folate. This active form has four added hydrogens. An intermediate form, dihydrofolate, has two added hydrogens.

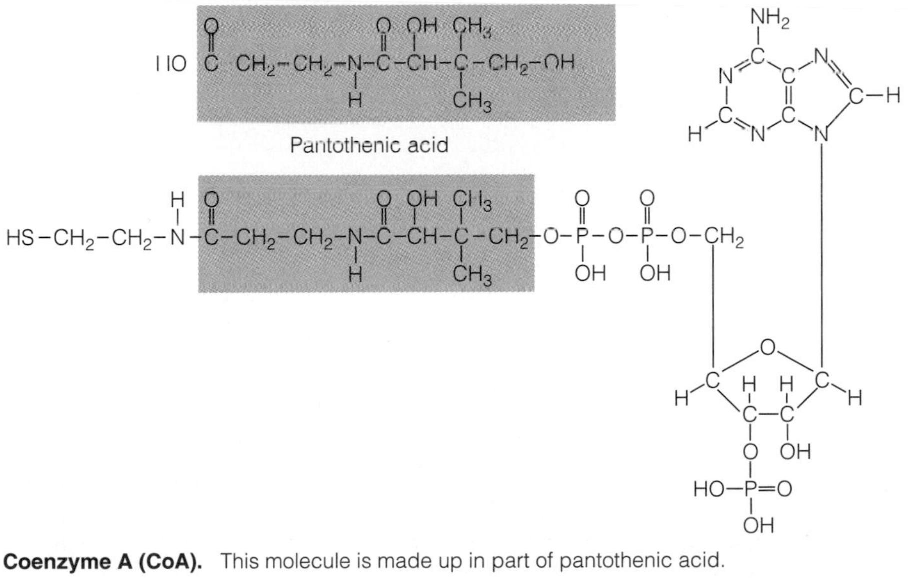

Coenzyme A (CoA). This molecule is made up in part of pantothenic acid.

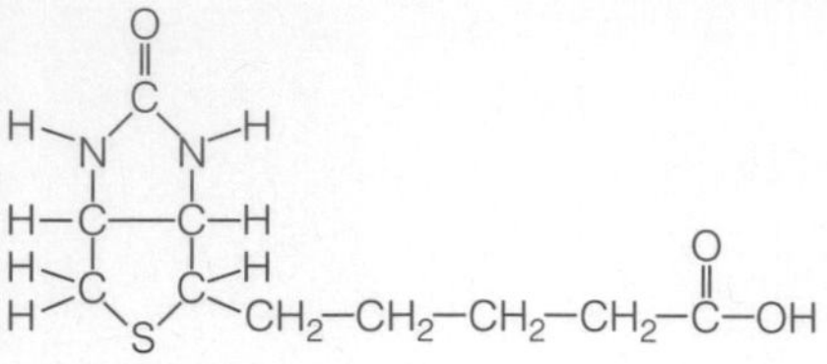

Biotin.

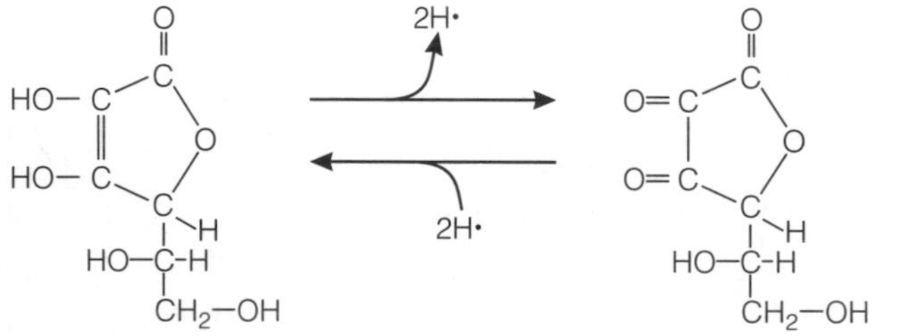

Ascorbic acid (reduced form)

Dehydroascorbic acid (oxidized form)

Vitamin C. The dots on the H indicate that two hydrogen atoms, complete with their electrons, are lost when ascorbic acid is oxidized and gained when it is reduced again.

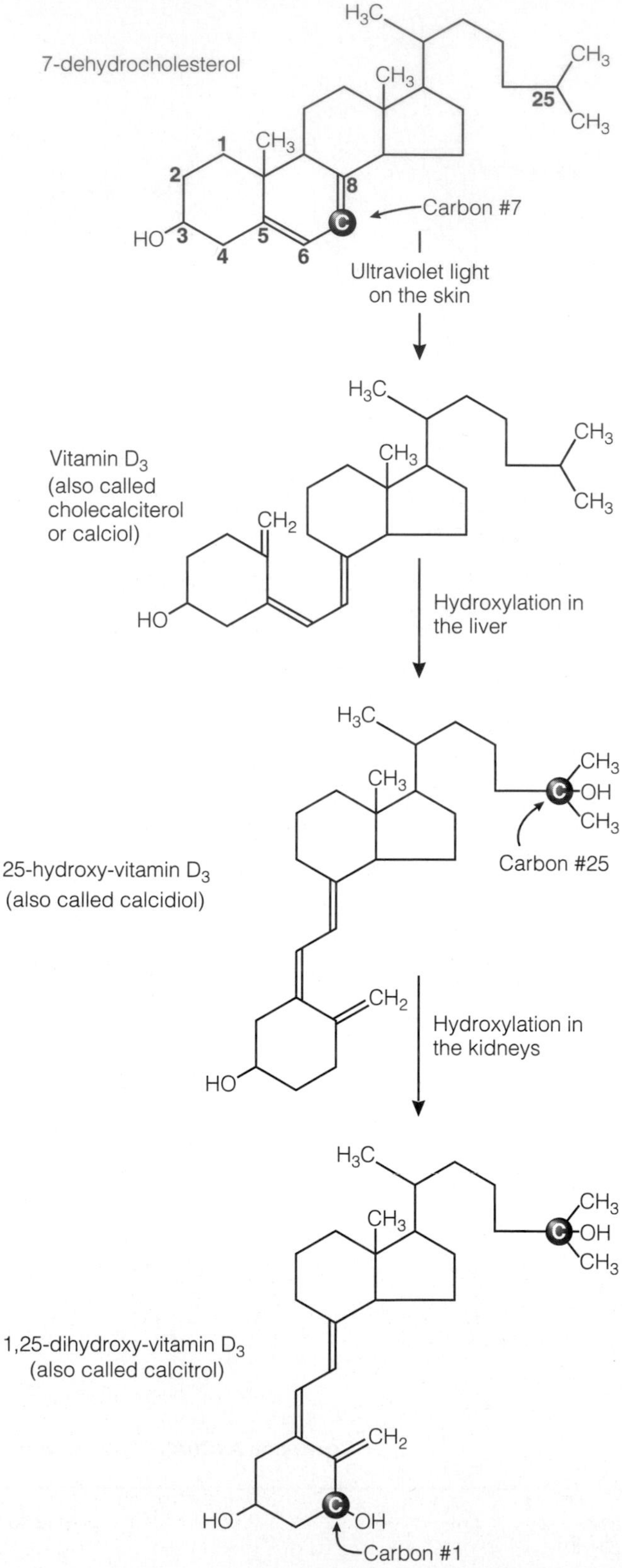

Active vitamin D and its precursors, beginning with 7-dehydrocholesterol. (The carbon atoms at which changes occur are numbered.)

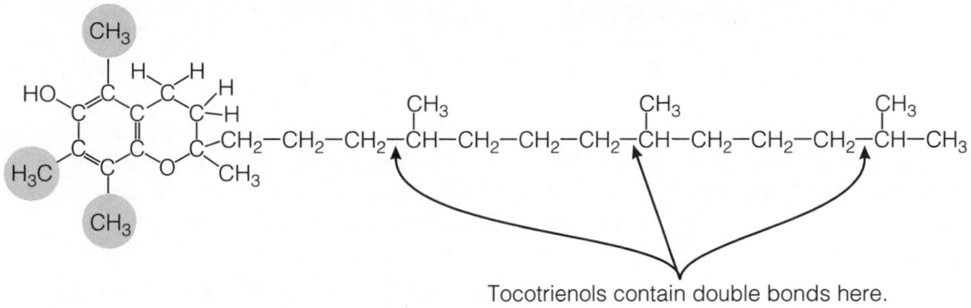

Vitamin E (alpha-tocopherol). The number and position of the methyl groups (CH_3) bonded to the ring structure differentiate among the tocopherols.

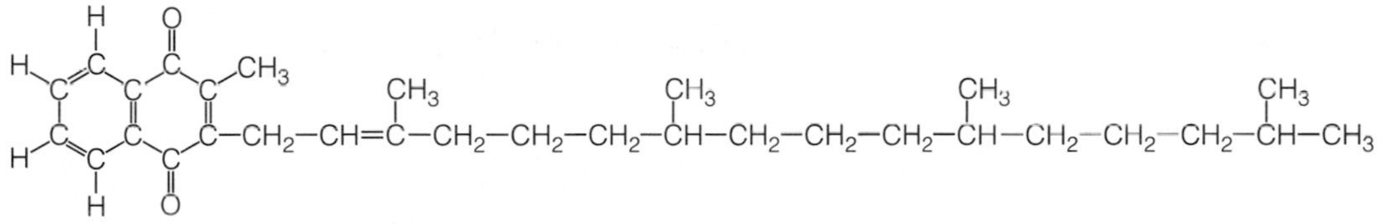

Vitamin K, a naturally occurring compound.

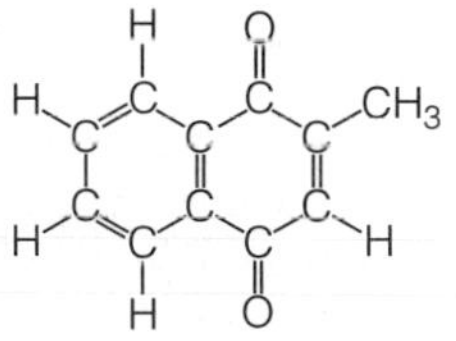

Menadione, a synthetic compound that has the same activity as natural vitamin K.

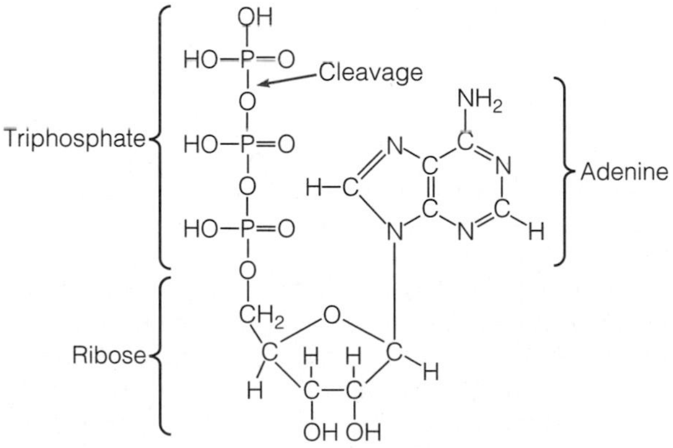

Adenosine triphosphate (ATP), the energy carrier. The cleavage point marks the bond that is broken when ATP splits to become ADP + P.

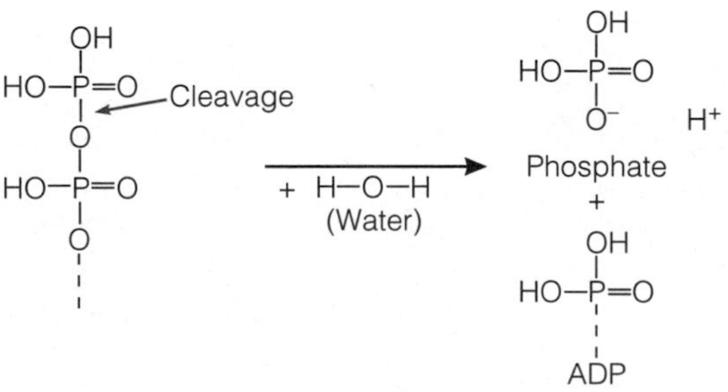

Adenosine diphosphate (ADP).

C

GLYCOLYSIS

Figure C–1 (on the next page) depicts the events of glycolysis. First, a phosphate is attached to glucose at the carbon that chemists call number 6. The product is called, logically enough, glucose-6-phosphate.

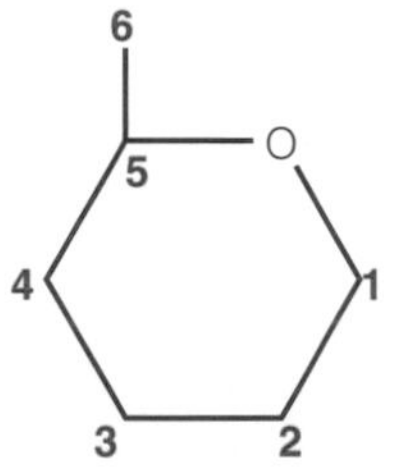

This is the way chemists number the carbons in a glucose molecule.

In the next couple of steps, glucose-6-phosphate is rearranged by an enzyme, and a phosphate is added in another coupled reaction with ATP. (A coupled reaction is a chemical event in which an enzyme complex catalyzes two reactions simultaneously. It often involves the breakdown of one compound and the synthesis of another.)

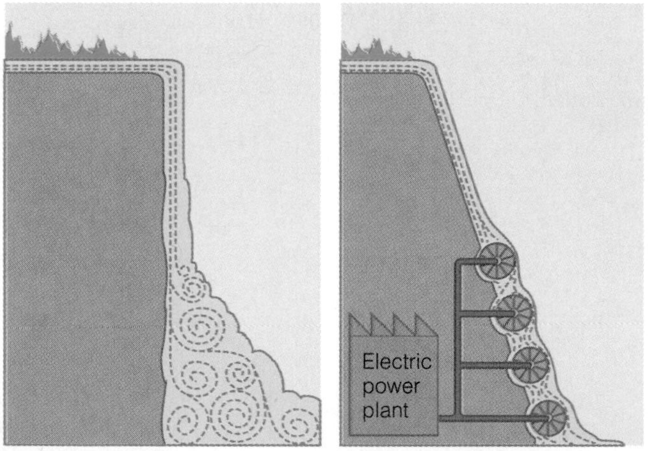

Falling water produces energy that is dissipated without doing work.

With the addition of a power plant (analogous to an enzyme), the energy of the falling water is coupled with a series of water wheels and turns them, producing energy.

A physical analogy of a coupled reaction. A coupled reaction often involves the breakdown of one compound and the synthesis of another. For example, the breakdown of glucose is coupled with the making of ATP, and the breakdown of ATP is coupled with the activation of glucose, or the making of glucose-P.

The product this time is fructose-1,6-diphosphate. At this point the six-carbon sugar has a phosphate group on its first and sixth carbons and is ready to break apart. Two ATP molecules have been used to accomplish this.

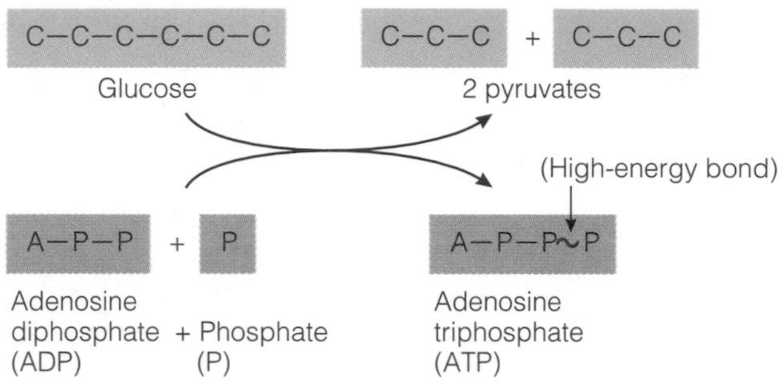

The breakdown of glucose is coupled with the making of ATP (simplified). Actually two ATP are used to prepare glucose for the reactions, and four ATP are gained in the breakdown of one glucose molecule to two molecules of pyruvate.

(From this point to the production of pyruvate, we will use letters in place of compound names. The names are in Figure C–1, for those who wish to know them.)

When fructose-1,6-diphosphate breaks in half, the two three-carbon compounds (A and A′) are not identical. Each has a phosphate group attached, but only one converts directly to pyruvate. The other compound, however, converts easily to the first. (Compound A′ is usually ignored, except for its role as the point of entry for the synthesis of glycerol; we say that two molecules of compound A are derived from one glucose molecule.)

In the step from compound A to compound B, enough energy is released to convert NAD^+ to $NADH + H^+$. Also, in the steps from B to C and from E to pyruvate, ATP is regenerated. Remember that in effect two molecules of compound A are produced from glucose; therefore, four ATP molecules are generated from each glucose molecule. Two ATP were needed to get the sequence started, so the net gain at this point is two ATP and two molecules of $NADH + H^+$.

So far, no oxygen has been used; the process has been anaerobic. But at this point, oxygen is needed. If oxygen is not immediately available, pyruvate converts to lactic acid to soak up the hydrogens from the $NADH + H^+$ that was generated. Lactic acid accumulates until oxygen becomes available. However, in the energy path from glucose to carbon dioxide, this side step usually is not necessary. As you will see later, each $NADH + H^+$ moves to the electron transport chain to unload its hydrogens onto oxygen. The associated energy produces two ATP, making a total yield of eight ATP for the process from glucose to pyruvate.

Figure C-1
Glycolysis

Notice that galactose and fructose enter at different places but all continue on the same pathway. Two molecules of compound A are produced (because compound A′ converts to A), and therefore two molecules of each succeeding compound.

- ◆ A = glyceraldehyde-3-phosphate.
- ◆ A′ = dihydroxyacetone phosphate.
- ◆ B = 1,3-diphosphoglyceric acid.
- ◆ C = 3-phosphoglyceric acid.
- ◆ D = 2-phosphoglyceric acid.
- ◆ E = phosphoenol pyruvic acid.

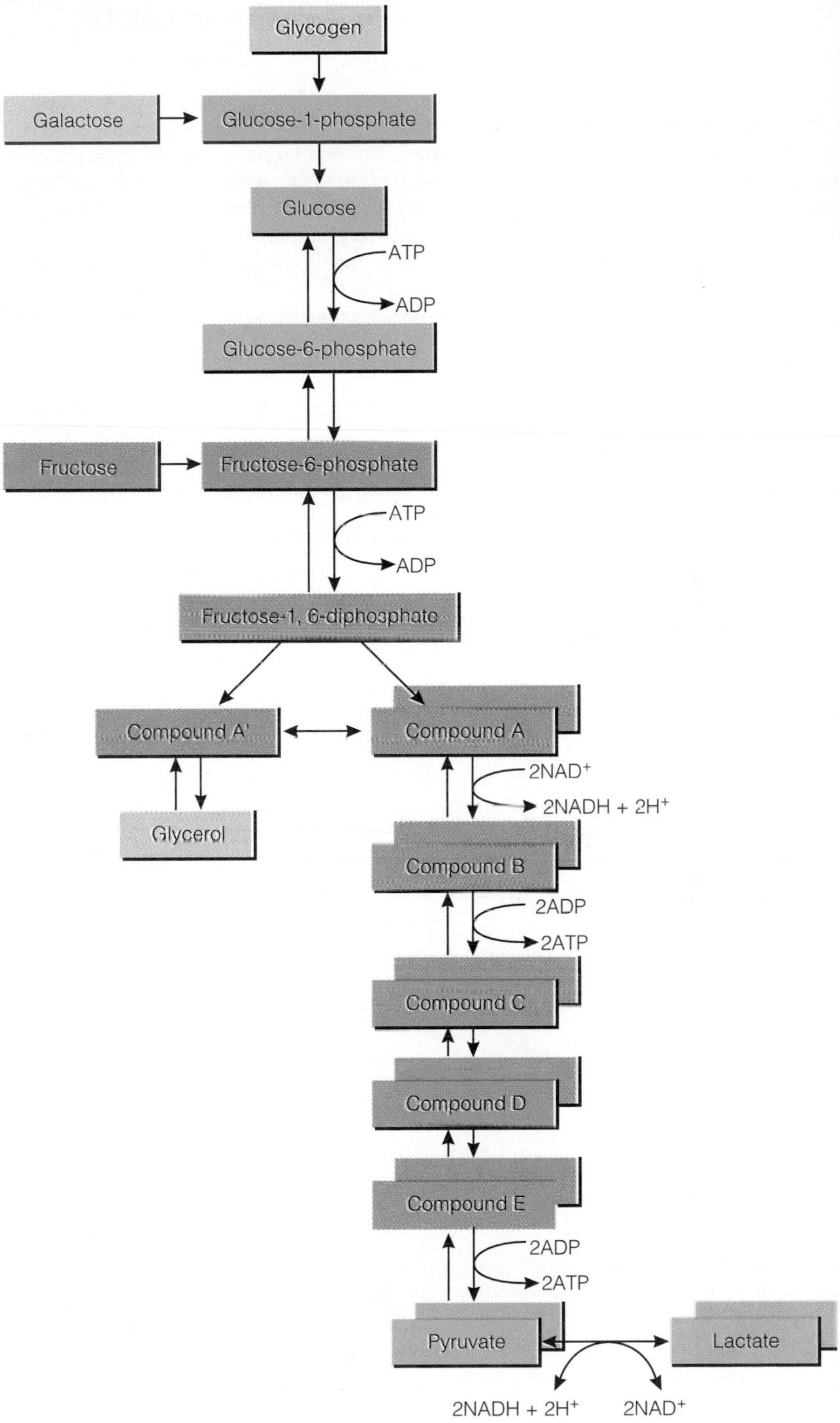

THE TCA CYCLE

The tricarboxylic acid, or TCA, cycle (Figure C–2 on p. C-15) is the name given to the set of reactions involving oxygen and leading from acetyl CoA to carbon dioxide (and water). To link glycolysis to the TCA cycle, pyruvate loses a carbon group and bonds with a molecule of CoA to become acetyl CoA. The TCA cycle is not restricted to the metabolism of carbohydrate. It also includes fat and protein. Any substance that can be converted to acetyl CoA directly, or indirectly through pyruvate, may enter the cycle.

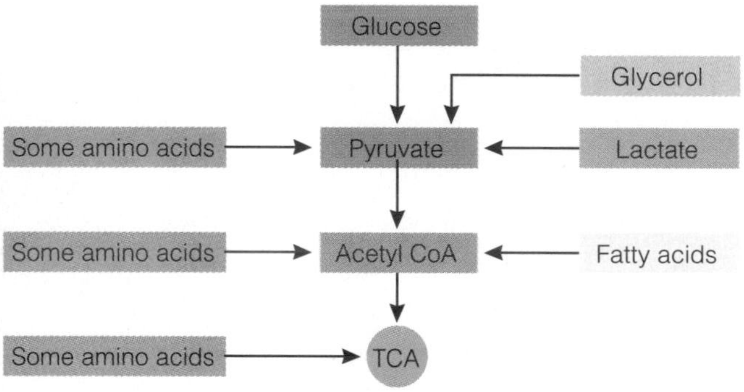

The step from pyruvate to acetyl CoA is exceedingly complex. We have included only those substances that will help you understand the transfer of energy from the nutrients. In the presence of oxygen, pyruvate loses a carbon

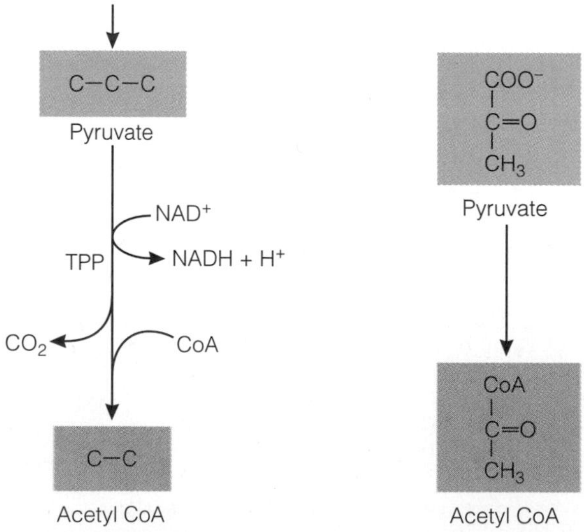

The step from pyruvate to acetyl CoA. (TPP and NAD are coenzymes containing the B vitamins thiamin and niacin, respectively.)

to carbon dioxide and is attached to a molecule of CoA. In the process, NAD^+ picks up two hydrogens with their associated energy, becoming $NADH + H^+$.

As the acetyl CoA breaks down to carbon dioxide and water, its energy is captured in ATP. Let's follow the steps by which this occurs (see Figure C–2).

1. The two-carbon acetyl CoA combines with a four-carbon compound, oxaloacetate. The CoA comes off, and the product is a six-carbon compound, citrate.
2. The atoms of citrate are rearranged to form isocitrate.
3. Now NAD^+ reacts with isocitrate. Two H and two electrons are removed from the isocitrate. One H becomes attached to the NAD^+ with the two electrons; the other H is released as H^+. Thus NAD^+ becomes $NADH + H^+$. (Remember this $NADH + H^+$. It is carrying the H and the energy released from the last reaction. But let's follow the carbons first.) A carbon is combined with two oxygens, forming carbon dioxide (which diffuses away into the blood and is exhaled). What is left is the five-carbon compound alpha-ketoglutarate.
4. Now two compounds interact with alpha-ketoglutarate —a molecule of CoA and a molecule of NAD^+. In this complex reaction, a carbon and two oxygens are removed (forming carbon dioxide); two hydrogens are removed and go to NAD^+ (forming $NADH + H^+$); and the remaining four-carbon compound is attached to the CoA, forming succinyl CoA. (Remember this $NADH + H^+$ also. You will see later what happens to it.)
5. Now two molecules react with succinyl CoA—a molecule called GDP and one of phosphate (P). The CoA comes off, the GDP and P combine to form the high-energy compound GTP (similar to ATP), and succinate remains. (Remember this GTP.)
6. In the next reaction, two H with their energy are removed from succinate and are transferred to a molecule called FAD (an electron-hydrogen receiver like NAD^+) to form $FADH_2$. The product that remains is fumarate. (Remember this $FADH_2$.)
7. Next a molecule of water is added to fumarate, forming malate.
8. A molecule of NAD^+ reacts with the malate; two H with their associated energy are removed from the malate and form $NADH + H^+$. The product that remains is the four-carbon compound oxaloacetate. (Remember this $NADH + H^+$.)

We are back where we started. The oxaloacetate formed in this process can combine with another molecule of acetyl CoA (step 1), and the cycle can begin again. The whole scheme is shown in Figure C–2.

Figure C–2
The TCA Cycle

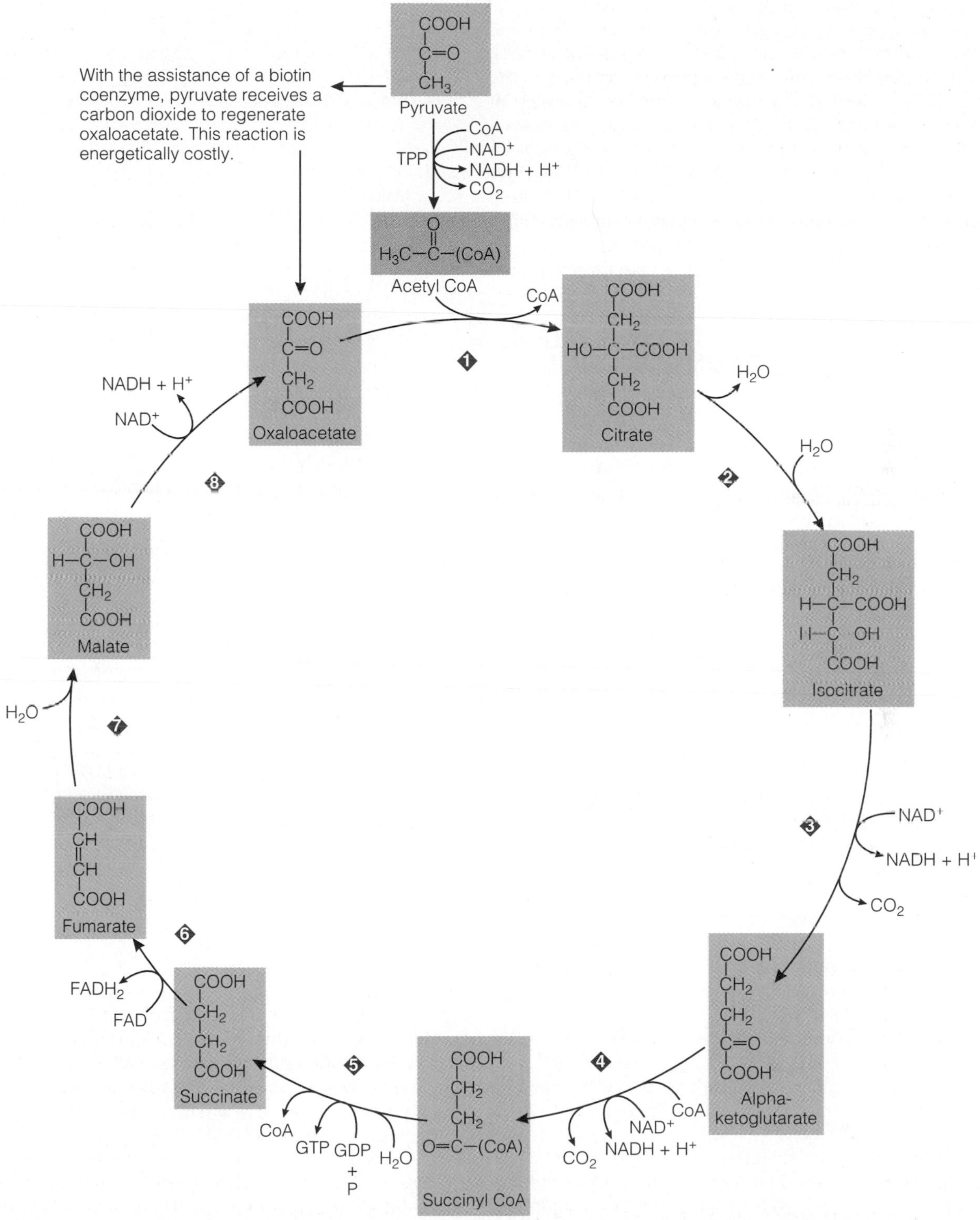

So far, we have seen two carbons brought in with acetyl CoA and two carbons ending up in carbon dioxide. But where are the energy and the ATP we promised?

Each time a pair of hydrogen atoms is removed from one of the compounds in the cycle, it includes a pair of electrons. Then the energy from this chemical bond is captured in the compound to which the H become attached. A review of the eight steps of the cycle shows that energy is transferred in this way into other compounds in steps 3, 4, 6, and 8. In step 5, energy is stored when GDP and P are bound together to form GTP. Thus the compounds NADH + H^+ (three molecules), $FADH_2$, and GTP store energy originally found in acetyl CoA. To see how this energy ends up in ATP, we must follow the electrons further. Let us take those attached to NAD^+ as an example.

THE ELECTRON TRANSPORT CHAIN

◆

The six reactions described here are those of the electron transport chain, which is shown in Figure C–3. Since oxygen is required for these reactions, and ADP and P are combined to form ATP in several of them (ADP is phosphorylated), these reactions are also called oxidative phosphorylation.

An important concept to remember at this point is that an electron is not a fixed amount of energy. The electrons that bond the H to NAD^+ in NADH have a relatively large amount of energy. In the series of reactions that follow, they lose this energy in small amounts, until at the end they are attached (with H) to oxygen (O) to make water (H_2O). In some of the steps, the energy they lose is captured into ATP in coupled reactions.

1. In the first step of the electron transport chain, NADH reacts with a molecule called a flavoprotein, losing its electrons (and their H). The products are NAD^+ and reduced flavoprotein. A little energy is lost as heat in this reaction.
2. The flavoprotein passes on the electrons to a molecule called coenzyme Q. Again they lose some energy as heat, but ADP and P bond together and form ATP, storing much of the energy. This is a coupled reaction: ADP + P → ATP.
3. Coenzyme Q passes the electrons to cytochrome *b*. Again the electrons lose energy.
4. Cytochrome *b* passes the electrons to cytochrome *c* in a coupled reaction in which ATP is formed: ADP + P → ATP.
5. Cytochrome *c* passes the electrons to cytochrome *a*.
6. Cytochrome *a* passes them (with their H) to an atom of oxygen (O), forming water (H_2O). This is a coupled reaction in which ATP is formed: ADP + P → ATP.

Figure C–3
The Electron Transport Chain

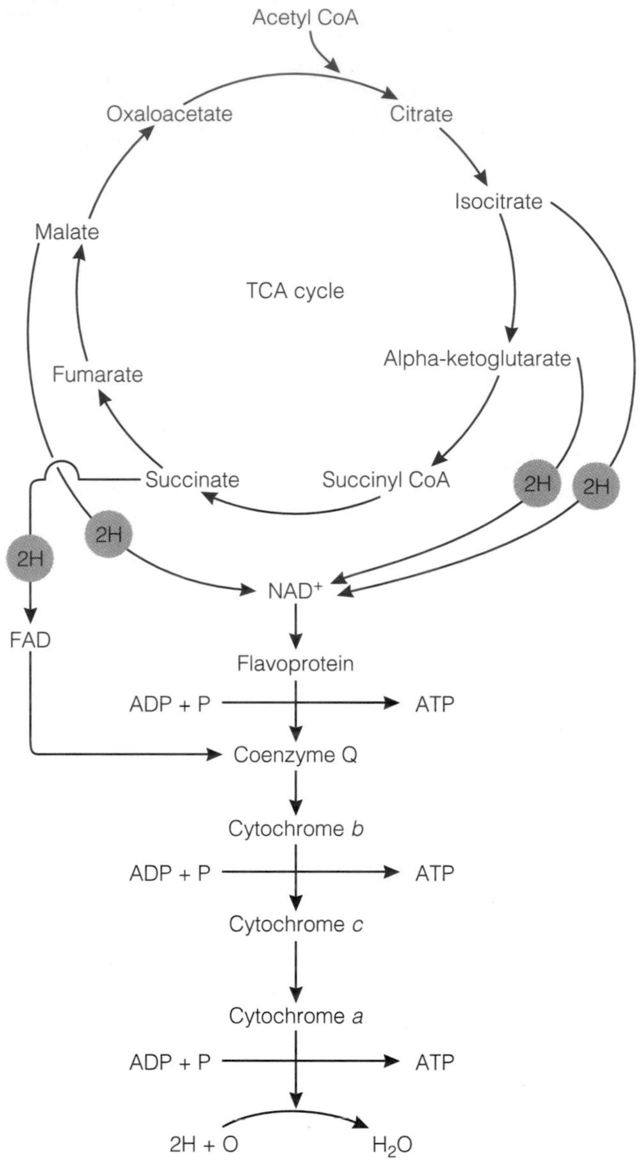

As Figure C–3 shows, each time NADH is oxidized (loses its electrons) by this means, the energy it loses is parceled out into three ATP molecules. When the electrons are passed on to water at the end, they are much lower in energy than they were originally. This completes the story of the electrons from NADH.

As for $FADH_2$, its electrons enter the electron transport chain at coenzyme Q. From coenzyme Q to water, ATP is generated in only two steps. Therefore, $FADH_2$ coming out of the TCA cycle yields just two ATP molecules.

Table C-3
Balance Sheet for Glucose Metabolism

	Expenditures	Income
Glycolysis:		
1 glucose	2 ATP	4 ATP
1 fructose-1,6-diphosphate		2 NADH + H^+
2 pyruvate		2 NADH + H^+
TCA cycle:		
2 isocitrate		2 NADH + H^+
2 alpha-ketoglutarate		2 NADH + H^+
2 succinyl CoA		2 GTP
2 succinate		2 $FADH_2$
2 malate		2 NADH + H^+
Total ATP collected:		
From glycolysis	2 ATP	4 ATP
From 2 NADH+ H^+		4–6 ATP[a]
From 8 NADH+ H^+		24 ATP
From 2 GTP		2 ATP
From 2 $FADH_2$		4 ATP
Totals:	2 ATP	38–40 ATP
Balance on hand from 1 molecule of glucose:		36–38 ATP

[a]Each NADH + H^+ from glycolysis can yield 2 or 3 ATP. See the accompanying text.

One energy-receiving compound of the TCA cycle (GTP) does not enter the electron transport chain but gives its energy directly to ADP in a simple phosphorylation reaction. This reaction yields one ATP.

It is now possible to draw up a balance sheet of glucose metabolism (see Table C–3). Glycolysis has yielded 4 NADH + H^+ and 4 ATP molecules and has spent 2 ATP. The 2 acetyl CoA going through the TCA cycle have yielded 6 NADH + H^+, 2 $FADH_2$, and 2 GTP molecules. After the NADH + H^+ and $FADH_2$ have gone through the electron transport chain, there are 34 ATP. Added to these are the 4 ATP from glycolysis and the 2 ATP from GTP, making the total 40 ATP generated from one molecule of glucose. After the expense of 2 ATP is subtracted, there is a net gain of 38 ATP.*

The TCA cycle and the electron transport chain are the body's major means of capturing the energy from nutrients in ATP molecules. Other means, such as anaerobic glycolysis, contribute, but the aerobic processes are the most efficient. Biologists and chemists understand much more about these processes than has been presented here.

*The total may sometimes be 36 or 37, rather than 38, ATP. The NADH + H^+ generated in the cytoplasm during glycolysis pass their electrons on to shuttle molecules, which move them into the mitochondria. One shuttle, malate, contributes its electrons to the electron transport chain before the first site of ATP synthesis, yielding 3 ATP. Another, glycerol phosphate, adds its electrons into the chain beyond that first site, yielding 2 ATP. Thus sometimes 3, and sometimes only 2, ATP result from the NADH + H^+ that arise from glycolysis. The amount depends on the cell.

ALCOHOL'S INTERFERENCE WITH ENERGY METABOLISM

Highlight 7 provides an overview of how alcohol interferes with energy metabolism. With an understanding of the TCA cycle, a few more details may be appreciated. During alcohol metabolism, the enzyme alcohol dehydrogenase oxidizes alcohol to acetaldehyde while it simultaneously reduces a molecule of NAD^+ to NADH + H^+. The related enzyme acetaldehyde dehydrogenase reduces another NAD^+ to NADH + H^+ while it oxidizes acetaldehyde to acetyl CoA, the compound that enters the TCA cycle to generate energy. Thus whenever alcohol is being metabolized in the body, NAD^+ diminishes, and NADH + H^+ accumulates. Chemists say that the body's "redox state" is altered, because NAD^+ can oxidize, and NADH + H^+ can reduce, many other body compounds. During alcohol metabolism, NAD^+ becomes unavailable for the multitude of reactions for which it is required.

As the previous sections just explained, for glucose to be completely metabolized, the TCA cycle must be operating, and NAD^+ must be present. If these conditions are not met (and when alcohol is present, they may not be), the pathway will be blocked, and traffic will back up—or an alternate route will be taken. Think about this as you follow the pathway shown in Figure C–4 on p. C-18.

In each step of alcohol metabolism in which NAD^+ is converted to NADH + H^+, hydrogen ions accumulate, resulting in a dangerous shift of the acid-base balance toward acid (Chapter 12 explains acid-base balance). The accumulation of NADH + H^+ depresses TCA cycle activity, so pyruvate and acetyl CoA build up. This condition favors the conversion of pyruvate to lactic acid, which serves as a temporary storage place for hydrogens from NADH + H^+. The conversion of pyruvate to lactic acid restores some NAD^+, but a lactic acid buildup has serious consequences of its own. It adds to the body's acid burden and interferes with the excretion of uric acid, causing goutlike symptoms. Molecules of acetyl CoA become building blocks for fatty acids or ketone bodies. The making of ketone bodies consumes acetyl CoA and generates NAD^+; but some ketone bodies are acids, so they push the acid-base balance further toward acid.

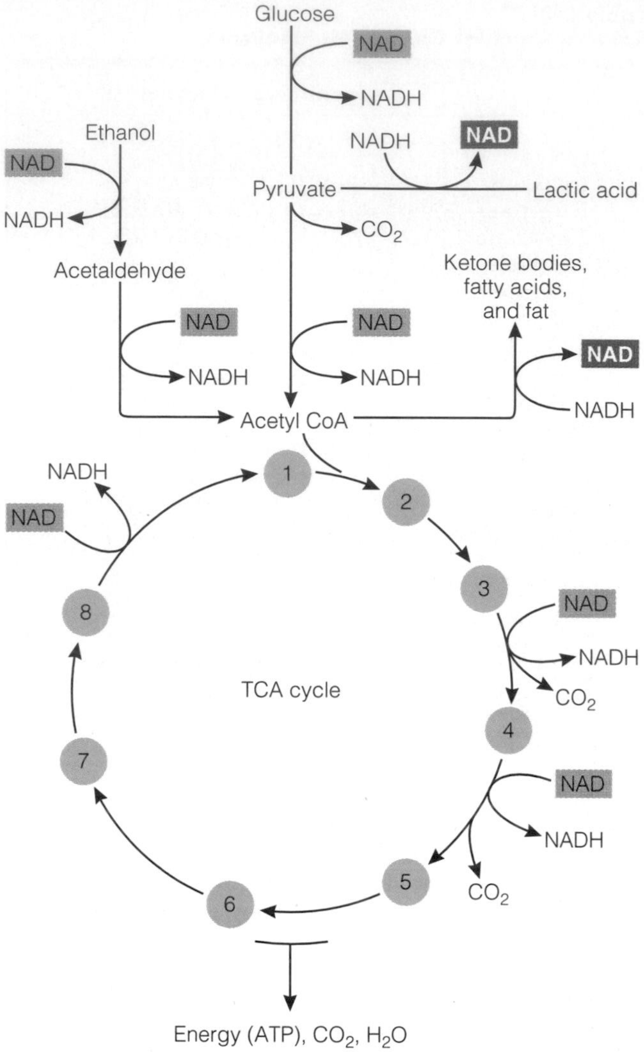

Figure C-4
Ethanol Enters the Metabolic Path

This is a simplified version of the glucose-to-energy pathway showing the entry of ethanol. The coenzyme NAD (which is the active form of the B vitamin niacin) is the only one shown here; however, many others are involved.

Thus alcohol cascades through the metabolic pathways, wreaking havoc along the way. These consequences have physical effects, which Highlight 7 describes.

THE UREA CYCLE

◆

Chapter 7 sums up the process by which waste nitrogen is eliminated from the body by stating that ammonia molecules combine with carbon dioxide to produce urea. This is true, but it is not the whole story. Urea is produced in a multistep process within the cells of the liver.

Ammonia, freed from an amino acid or other compound during metabolism anywhere in the body, arrives at the liver by way of the bloodstream and is taken into a liver cell. There, it is first combined with carbon dioxide and a phosphate group from ATP to form carbamyl phosphate:

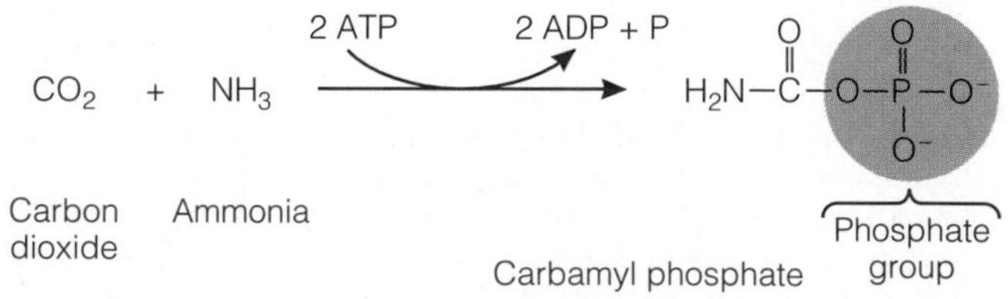

Figure C–5
The Urea Cycle

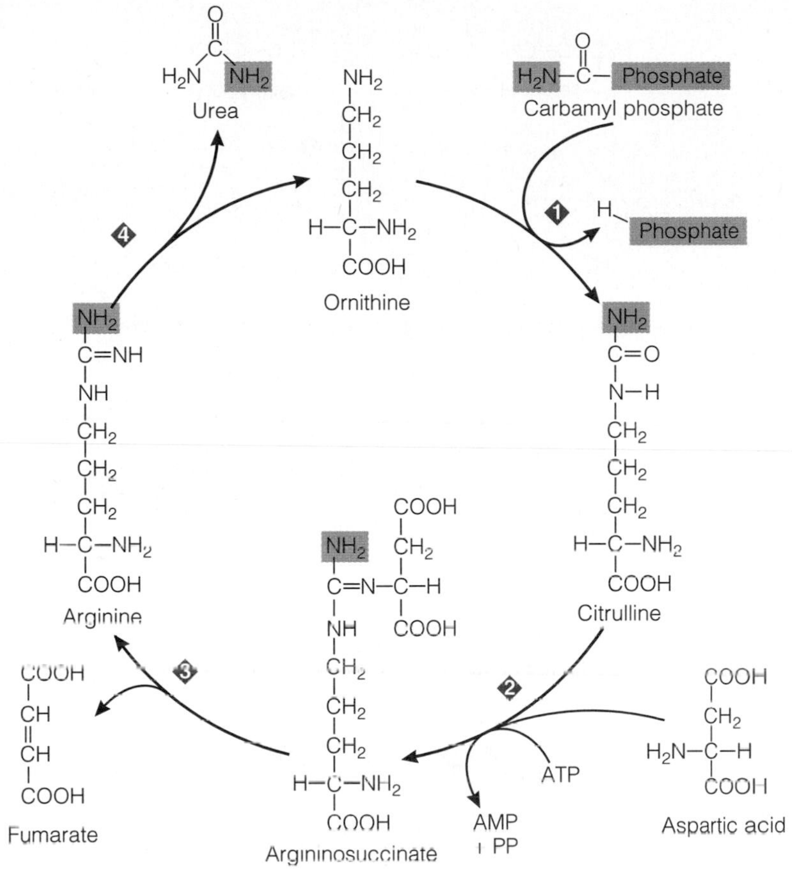

Figure C–5 shows the cycle of four reactions that follow. In the first step, carbamyl phosphate combines with the amino acid ornithine, losing its phosphate group. The compound formed is citrulline.

In the second step, citrulline combines with the amino acid aspartic acid, to form argininosuccinate. The reaction requires energy from ATP. (ATP was shown earlier losing one phosphorus atom in a phosphate group, P, to become ADP. In this reaction, it loses two phosphorus atoms joined together, PP, and becomes adenosine monophosphate, AMP.)

In the third step, argininosuccinate is split, forming another acid, fumarate, and the amino acid arginine.

In the fourth step, arginine loses its terminal carbon with two attached amino groups and picks up an oxygen from water. The end product is urea, which the kidneys excrete in the urine. The compound that remains is ornithine, identical to the ornithine with which this series of reactions began, and ready to react with another molecule of carbamyl phosphate and turn the cycle again.

FORMATION OF KETONE BODIES

Normally, fatty acid oxidation proceeds all the way to carbon dioxide and water. However, in ketosis (discussed in Chapter 7), an intermediate is formed from the condensation of two molecules of acetyl CoA: acetoacetyl CoA. Figure C–6 shows the formation of ketone bodies from that

Figure C-6
Formation of Ketone Bodies

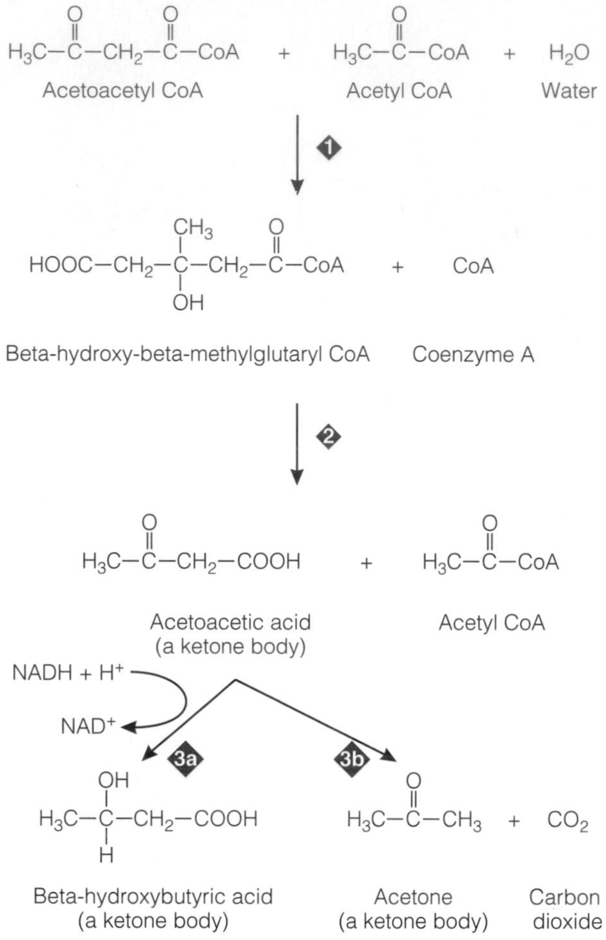

intermediate. In step 1, acetoacetyl CoA condenses with another acetyl CoA to form a six-carbon intermediate, beta-hydroxy-beta-methylglutaryl CoA. In step 2, this intermediate is cleaved to acetyl CoA and acetoacetic acid. This product can be metabolized either to beta-hydroxybutyric acid (step 3a) or to acetone (3b).

Acetoacetic acid, beta-hydroxybutyric acid, and acetone are the so-called ketone bodies of ketosis. Two are real ketones (they have a C=O group between two carbons); the other is an alcohol that has been produced during ketone formation—hence the term *ketone bodies,* rather than ketones, to describe the three of them. There are many other ketones in nature; these three are characteristic of ketosis in the body.

NOTES

◆

1. Nomenclature policy: Generic descriptors and trivial names for vitamins and related compounds, *Journal of Nutrition* 117 (1987): 7–14; Nomenclature policy: Abbreviated designations of amino acids, *Journal of Nutrition* 117 (1987): 15.
2. A discussion of the designated abbreviations for the common amino acids presented here is found in Nomenclature policy: Abbreviated designations of amino acids, *Journal of Nutrition* 117 (1987): 15.

APPENDIX D

AIDS TO CALCULATION

Contents

Many mathematical problems have been worked out as examples at appropriate places in the text. This appendix aims to help with the use of the metric system and with problems not fully explained elsewhere.

CONVERSION FACTORS

Conversion factors are useful mathematical tools in everyday calculations, including those encountered in the study of nutrition. Skill in the use of conversion factors is especially desirable as the United States "goes metric."

A conversion factor is a fraction in which the numerator (top) and the denominator (bottom) express the same quantity in different units. For example, 2.2 pounds (lb) and 1 kilogram (kg) are equivalent; they express the same weight. The conversion factor used to change pounds to kilograms or vice versa is:

$$\frac{2.2 \text{ lb}}{1 \text{ kg}} \text{ or } \frac{1 \text{ kg}}{2.2 \text{ lb}} .$$

Because both factors equal 1, measurements can be multiplied by the factor without changing the value of the measurement. Thus the units can be changed.

To perform a conversion, use the factor with the unit you are seeking in the numerator (top) of the fraction. Following are two examples of problems commonly encountered in nutrition study; they illustrate the usefulness of conversion factors.

Example 1 Convert the weight of 130 pounds to kilograms.

1. Choose the conversion factor in which the unit you are seeking is on top:

$$\frac{1 \text{ kg}}{2.2 \text{ lb}} .$$

2. Multiply 130 pounds by the factor:

$$130 \cancel{\text{lb}} \times \frac{1 \text{ kg}}{2.2 \cancel{\text{lb}}} = \frac{130 \text{ kg}}{2.2} =$$

59 kg (rounded off to the nearest whole number).

Example 2 How many grams (g) of saturated fat are contained in a 3-ounce (oz) hamburger?

1. Consider a 4-ounce hamburger that contains 7 grams of saturated fat. You are seeking grams of saturated fat; therefore, the conversion factor is:

$$\frac{7 \text{ g saturated fat}}{4 \text{ oz hamburger}} .$$

2. Multiply 3 ounces of hamburger by the conversion factor:

$$3 \cancel{\text{oz}} \text{ hamburger} \times \frac{7 \text{ g saturated fat}}{4 \cancel{\text{oz}} \text{ hamburger}} =$$

$$\frac{3 \times 7}{4} = \frac{21}{4}$$

= 5 g saturated fat (rounded off to the nearest whole number).

PERCENTAGES

A percentage is a comparison between a number of items (perhaps your intake of energy) and a standard number (perhaps the number of kcalories recommended for your age and sex—your energy RDA). The standard number is the number you divide by. The answer you get after the division must be multiplied by 100 to be stated as a percentage (*percent* means "per 100").

Example 3 What percentage of the RDA for energy is your energy intake?

1. Find your energy RDA (inside front cover, left). We'll use 2200 kcalories to demonstrate.
2. Total your energy intake for a day—for example, 1500 kcalories.
3. Divide your kcalorie intake by the RDA kcalories:

$$1500 \text{ kcal (your intake)} \div 2200 \text{ kcal (RDA)} = 0.68.$$

4. Multiply your answer by 100 to state it as a percentage:

$$0.68 \times 100 = 68 = 68\%.$$

In some problems in nutrition, the percentage may be more than 100. For example, suppose your daily intake of vitamin A is 3200 RE and your RDA (male) is 1000 RE. Your intake as a percentage of the RDA is more than 100 percent (that is, you consume more than 100 percent of your vitamin A RDA). The following calculations show your vitamin A intake as a percentage of the RDA:

$$3200 \div 1000 = 3.2.$$

$$3.2 \times 100 = 320\% \text{ of RDA.}$$

Sometimes the comparison is between a part of a whole (for example, your kcalories from protein) and the total amount (your total kcalories). In this case, the total number is the one you divide by.

Example 4 What percentages of your total kcalories for the day come from protein, fat, and carbohydrate?

1. Using Appendix H and your diet record, find the total grams of protein, fat, and carbohydrate you consumed—for example, 60 grams protein, 80 grams fat, and 310 grams carbohydrate.
2. Multiply the number of grams by the number of kcalories from 1 gram of each energy nutrient (conversion factors):

$$60 \text{ g protein} \times \frac{4 \text{ kcal}}{1 \text{ g protein}} = 240 \text{ kcal.}$$

$$80 \text{ g fat} \times \frac{9 \text{ kcal}}{1 \text{ g fat}} = 720 \text{ kcal.}$$

$$310 \text{ g carbohydrate} \times \frac{4 \text{ kcal}}{1 \text{ g carbohydrate}} = 1240 \text{ kcal.}$$

$$240 + 720 + 1240 = 2200 \text{ kcal.}$$

3. Find the percentage of total kcalories from each energy nutrient (see Example 3):

- Protein: $240 \div 2200 = 0.109 \times 100 = 10.9 = 11\%$ of kcal.
- Fat: $720 \div 2200 = 0.327 \times 100 = 32.7 = 33\%$ of kcal.
- Carbohydrate: $1240 \div 2200 = 0.563 \times 100 = 56.3 = 56\%$ of kcal.
- $11\% + 33\% + 56\% = 100\%$ of kcal (total).

The percentages total 100 percent, but sometimes they total 99 or 101 because of rounding off. This is a reasonable error.

RATIOS

A ratio is a comparison of two or three values in which one of the values is reduced to 1. A ratio compares identical units and so is expressed without units. For example, Figure 12–6 in Chapter 12 compares the milligrams of potassium to the milligrams of sodium in selected foods.

Example 5 Find the potassium-to-sodium ratio of your diet.

1. Using Appendix H and your diet record, find how many milligrams of potassium and sodium you consumed, say, 3000 milligrams potassium and 2500 milligrams sodium.
2. Divide the potassium milligrams by the sodium milligrams:

$$3000 \text{ mg potassium} \div 2500 \text{ mg sodium} = 1.2.$$

3. The potassium-to-sodium ratio is usually expressed as correct to one decimal point: 1.2.

The potassium-to-sodium ratio of your diet is 1.2:1 (read as "one point two to one" or simply "one point two"). A ratio greater than 1 means that the first value (in this case, milligrams of potassium) is greater than the second (sodium). When the second value is larger, the ratio is less than 1.

WEIGHTS AND MEASURES

◆

Length
1 inch (in) = 2.54 centimeters (cm).
1 foot (ft) = 30.48 centimeters.
1 meter (m) = 39.37 inches.

Temperature

	Celsius*	Fahrenheit	
Steam	100°C	212°F	Steam
Body temperature	37°C	98.6°F	Body temperature
Ice	0°C	32°F	Ice

To find degrees Fahrenheit (t_F) when you know degrees Celsius (t_C), multiply by 9/5 and then add 32:

$$(9/5 \times t_C) + 32 = t_F.$$

To find degrees Celsius (t_C) when you know degrees Fahrenheit (t_F), multiply by 5/9 after subtracting 32:

$$5/9\ (t_F - 32) = t_C.$$

Volume
1 liter (L) = 1.06 quarts (qt) or 0.85 imperial quart.
1 liter = 1000 milliliters (mL).
1 milliliter = 0.03 fluid ounces.
30 milliliters = 1 fluid ounce.
1 gallon = 3.79 liters.
1 quart = 0.95 liter or 32 fluid ounces.
1 cup (c) = 8 fluid ounces or about 250 milliliters.
1 tablespoon (tbs) = 15 milliliters.
3 teaspoons (tsp) = 1 tablespoon.
1 teaspoon = about 5 g or 5 mL.
16 tablespoons = 1 cup.
4 cups = 1 quart.

Weight
1 ounce (oz) = approximately 28 grams (g).
16 ounces = 1 pound (lb).
1 pound = 454 grams.
1 kilogram (kg) = 1000 grams or 2.2 pounds.
1 gram = 1000 milligrams (mg).
1 milligram = 1000 micrograms (μg).

Energy units
1 kcalorie (kcal) = 4.2 kilojoules (kJ).
1 millijoule (mJ) = 240 kcal.
1 kJ = 0.24 kcal.
1 g carbohydrate = 4 kcal = 17 kJ.
1 g fat = 9 kcal = 37 kJ.
1 g protein = 4 kcal = 17 kJ.
1 g alcohol = 7 kcal = 29 kJ.

International Units (IU)
To convert IU to:
- μg RE, divide by 3.33 for retinol and by 10 for beta-carotene.
- μg vitamin D, divide by 40 or multiply by 0.025.
- mg α-TE, divide by 1.5.

*Also known as *centigrade*.

D

APPENDIX E

Contents

NUTRITION ASSESSMENT

Nutrition assessment evaluates a person's health from a nutrition perspective. Many factors influence or reflect nutrition status. Consequently, the assessor, usually a registered dietitian assisted by other qualified health care professionals, gathers information from many sources, including:

- Historical information.
- Anthropometric measurements.
- Physical examinations.
- Biochemical analyses (laboratory tests).

Each of these methods involves collecting data in a variety of ways and interpreting each finding in relation to the others to create a total picture.

The accurate gathering of this information and its careful interpretation are the basis for a meaningful evaluation. The more information gathered about a person, the more accurate the assessment will be. Gathering information is a time-consuming process, and time is often a rare commodity in the health care setting. Nutrition care is only one part of total care. It may not be practical or essential to collect detailed information on each person.

nutrition screening: the use of preliminary nutrition assessment techniques to identify people who are malnourished or are at risk for malnutrition.

A strategic compromise is to screen clients by collecting preliminary data. Data such as height-weight and hematocrit are easy to obtain and can alert health care workers to potential problems. Nutrition screening identifies clients who will require additional nutrition assessment. This appendix provides a sample of the procedures, standards, charts, and forms commonly used in nutrition assessment.

HISTORICAL INFORMATION

Clues about present nutrition status become evident with a careful review of a person's historical data (see Table E–1). Even when the data are subjective, they reveal important facts about a person. A thorough history identifies risk factors associated with poor nutrition status (see Table E–2) and provides a sense of the whole person. Form E–1 shows the kinds of questions asked. As you can see, many

Table E–1
Historical Data Used in Nutrition Assessments

Type of History	What It Identifies
Health history	Health factors that affect nutrition status
Socioeconomic history	Personal, financial, and environmental influences on food intake, nutrient needs, and diet therapy options
Drug history	Medications and nutrient supplements that affect nutrition status
Diet history	Nutrient intake excesses or deficiencies and reasons for imbalances

E

Table E–2
Risk Factors for Poor Nutrition Status

Health History

- Acquired immune deficiency syndrome (AIDS)
- Alcoholism
- Anorexia (lack of appetite)
- Anorexia nervosa
- Bulimia nervosa
- Cancer
- Chewing or swallowing difficulties (including poorly fitted dentures, dental caries, and missing teeth)
- Chronic obstructive pulmonary disease
- Circulatory problems
- Constipation
- Crohn's disease
- Decubitus ulcers
- Dementia
- Diabetes mellitus
- Diarrhea
- Diseases of the GI tract
- Drug addiction
- Fever
- Heart disease
- Hormonal imbalance
- Hyperlipidemia
- Hypertension
- Infection
- Kidney disease
- Liver disease
- Lung disease
- Malabsorption
- Mental illness
- Mental retardation or deterioration
- Multiple pregnancies
- Nausea
- Neurologic disorders
- Organ failure
- Overweight
- Pancreatic insufficiency
- Paralysis
- Physical disability
- Pneumonia
- Pregnancy
- Radiation therapy
- Recent major illness
- Recent major surgery
- Recent weight loss or gain
- Smoking
- Surgery of the GI tract
- Trauma
- Ulcerative colitis
- Ulcers
- Underweight
- Vomiting

Socioeconomic History

- Access to groceries
- Education
- Ethnic identity
- Income
- Kitchen facilities
- Number of people in household
- Occupation
- Religious affiliation
- Social activities

Drug History

- Amphetamines
- Analgesics
- Antacids
- Antibiotics
- Anticancer agents
- Anticonvulsant agents
- Antidepressant agents
- Antidiarrheal agents
- Antihyperlipemic agents
- Antihypertensive agents
- Antiulcer agents
- Catabolic steroids
- Diuretics
- Hormonal agents
- Immunosuppressive agents
- Laxatives
- Oral contraceptives
- Sulfonylurea agents
- Vitamin and other nutrient preparations

Diet History

- Deficient or excessive food intakes
- Frequently eating out
- Intravenous fluids (other than total parenteral nutrition) for 7 or more days
- Monotonous diet (lacking variety)
- No intake for 7 or more days
- Poor appetite
- Restricted or fad diets
- Unbalanced diet (omitting any food group)

Name ______________________ Date ______________________
Address ______________________ Date of last medical checkup ______________________
______________________ Age __________ Sex __________
______________________ Height __________ Weight __________
Phone ______________________ Usual weight ______________________
Reason for admission ______________________ Ideal weight range ______________________

Health History

1. Have you been told that you have (check any that apply):
   ____ Diabetes mellitus ____ Heart disease ____ Ulcers
   ____ GI disorders ____ Lung disease ____ Cancer
   ____ High blood pressure ____ Kidney disease ____ Other
   ____ Hardening of arteries ____ Liver disease ______________
2. Do you have complaints about any of the following:
   ____ Lack of appetite ____ Diarrhea ____ Nausea
   ____ Difficulty chewing or swallowing ____ Indigestion ____ Vomiting
   ____ Constipation ____ Fever ____ Other
3. Do you use tobacco in any way? ______ How much? ______________
4. For females:
   Are you pregnant? __________ How many months? ______
   How many pregnancies have you carried to term? __________
   When was your last child born? __________
   Are your menstrual periods normal? ______ If not, please explain: ______________

Socioeconomic History

1. Last grade of school completed ______ Still in school? ______
2. Are you employed? ______ Occupation ______________
3. Does someone else live with you? ______ Who? __________
4. Do you regularly eat alone or with others? __________
5. Do you have a refrigerator? __________ Stove? __________
6. How often do you shop for food? __________ Where? ______

Drug History

1. Do you take medication, either prescribed by a doctor or over-the-counter?

Name of drug	Reason for taking	Dose	Frequency	Duration of intake

2. Have you noticed any side effects from taking these medications? ____ If so, please explain: __________
3. Do you take vitamins or any kind of supplements? ______ Which ones? __________
   How often? ________ For what reason? ______________

Diet History

1. Have you recently lost or gained more than 10 lbs? ______ If yes, explain the surrounding circumstances (including associated illness, dietary changes, and time frame): ______________
2. Do you eat at regular times each day? ________ How many times per day? __________
3. Where do you eat most of your meals? ______________
4. Do you usually eat snacks? ______ When? ______________
5. What foods do you particularly like? ______________
6. Are there foods you don't eat for other reasons? ______________
7. Do you have difficulty eating? ______________
8. How would you describe your feelings about food? ______________
9. How do your eating habits change when you are emotionally upset? ______________
10. Are you, or any member of your family, on a special diet? ____ If yes, who and what kind? __________
11. Do you drink alcohol? ________ How much? ________ How often? __________
12. How would you describe your exercise habits? __________ Type of exercise __________
    Intensity __________ Duration __________ Frequency __________
13. Are there any other facts about your lifestyle that you think might be related to your nutritional health? ______
    Explain ______________

Note: Use the appropriate form to record food intake data (Form E–2 or E–3).

aspects of a person's life influence nutrition status and provide clues to possible problems.

An adept history taker uses the interview both to gather facts and to establish a rapport with the client. This section briefly reviews the major areas of nutrition concern in a person's history: health, socioeconomic factors, drugs, and diet.

HEALTH HISTORY

The assessor can obtain health histories from records completed by the attending physician, nurse, or other health care professional. In addition, conversations with the client can uncover valuable information previously overlooked because no one thought to ask or because the client was not thinking clearly when asked.

An accurate, complete health history can reveal conditions that place a client at risk for malnutrition (review Table E–2). Diseases and their therapies can have either immediate or long-term effects on nutrition status by interfering with ingestion, digestion, absorption, metabolism, or excretion of nutrients.

health history: the medical record. Traditionally, the health history has been called the *medical history*. The term *health history* now seems more appropriate, however, since the contents describe a client's health status. Current trends in the medical profession are now emphasizing health promotion and disease prevention.

E

SOCIOECONOMIC HISTORY

Socioeconomic factors profoundly affect nutrition status. The ethnic background and educational level of both the client and the other members of the household influence food availability and food choices. An understanding of the community environment is also important in assessing nutrition status. For example, the interviewer should be familiar with the food habits of the major ethnic groups within the locale, regional food preferences, and nutrition resources and programs available in the community. Local health departments and social agencies often can provide such information.

Level of income also influences the diet. In general, the quality of the diet declines as income falls. At some point, the ability to purchase the foods required to meet nutrient needs is lost; an inadequate income puts an adequate diet out of reach. Agencies use poverty indexes to identify people at risk for poor nutrition and to qualify people for government food assistance programs.

Low income affects not only the power to purchase foods but also the ability to shop for, store, and cook them. A skilled assessor will note whether a person has transportation to a grocery store that sells a sufficient variety of low-cost foods, and whether the person has access to a refrigerator and stove.

socioeconomic history: a record of a person's social and economic background, including such factors as education, income, and ethnic identity.

DRUG HISTORY

The many interactions of foods and drugs require that health care professionals pay special attention to any client who takes drugs routinely. If a person is taking any drug, the assessor records the name of the drug; the dose, frequency, and duration of intake; the reason for taking the drug; and signs of any adverse effects on Form E–1.

The interactions of drugs and nutrients may take many forms:

- Drugs can alter food intake and the absorption, metabolism, and excretion of nutrients.
- Foods and nutrients can alter the absorption, metabolism, and excretion of drugs.

Highlight 17 discusses nutrient-drug interactions in more detail and Table H17–1 summarizes the mechanisms by which these interactions occur and provides specific examples.

drug history: a record of all the drugs, over-the-counter and prescribed, that a person takes routinely.

DIET HISTORY

diet history: a record of eating behaviors and the foods a person eats.

A diet history provides a record of a person's eating habits and food intake and can help identify possible nutrient imbalances. Food choices are an important part of lifestyle and often reflect a person's philosophy. The assessor who asks nonjudgmental questions about eating habits and food intake encourages trust and enhances the likelihood of obtaining accurate information.

Assessors evaluate food intake using various tools such as the 24-hour recall, the usual intake record, the food frequency checklist, and the food record. Food models or photos and measuring devices can help clients identify the types of foods and quantities consumed. The assessor also needs to know how the foods are prepared and when they are eaten. In addition to asking about foods, assessors will ask about beverage consumption, including beverages containing alcohol or caffeine.

Besides identifying possible nutrient imbalances, diet histories provide valuable clues about how a person will accept diet changes should they be necessary. Information about what and how a person eats provides the background for realistic and attainable nutrition goals.

24-hour recall: a record of foods eaten by a person for one 24-hour period.

24-Hour Recall The 24-hour recall provides data for one day only and is commonly used in nutrition surveys to obtain estimates of the typical food intakes for a population. The assessor asks the client to recount everything eaten or drunk in the past 24 hours or for the previous day. Form E–2 shows a typical 24-hour recall form.

An advantage of the 24-hour recall is that it is easy to obtain. It is also more likely to provide accurate data, at least about the past 24 hours, than estimates of average intakes over long periods. The usefulness of this tool is limited, however, in that it does not provide enough information to allow generalizations about an individual's usual food intake. The previous day's intake may not be typical, for example, or the person may be unable to report portion sizes accurately or may conceal or forget information about foods eaten. This limitation is partially overcome when 24-hour recalls are collected on several nonconsecutive days.

Usual Intake To obtain data about a person's usual intake, an inquiry might begin with "What is the first thing you usually eat or drink during the day?" Similar questions follow until a typical daily intake pattern emerges. This method uses the same form as the 24-hour recall (Form E–2) and can be useful, especially in verifying food intake when the past 24 hours have been atypical. It also helps the assessor verify food habits. For example, one person may always eat an afternoon snack; another may never eat breakfast. A person whose intake varies widely from day to day, however, may find it difficult to answer such general questions, and in that case, another food intake tool should be used to estimate nutrient intake.

food record: an extensive, accurate log of all foods eaten over a period of several days or weeks. A food record that includes associated information such as when, where and with whom each food is eaten is sometimes called a **food diary**.

Food Record Another tool for history taking is the food record, in which the person records food eaten, time of day, place where eaten, others present, and mood. Chapter 9 (p. 325) provides an example. A food record can help both the assessor and the client to determine factors associated with eating that may affect dietary balance and adequacy.

Food records work especially well with cooperative people but require considerable time and effort on their part. A prime advantage is that the record keeper assumes an active role and may for the first time become aware of personal food habits and assume responsibility for them. It also provides the assessor with an accurate picture of the person's lifestyle and factors that affect food intake. For these reasons, a food record can be particularly useful in outpatient counseling for such nutrition problems as overweight, underweight, or food allergy. The major disadvantages stem from poor compliance in recording the data and conscious or

Form E-2
Food Intake for a 24-Hour Recall or Usual Intake Pattern

Name and address ______________________________________

____

____

Date ____________

Did you take a vitamin mineral supplement? ______________________________________

If yes, what kind? ____________________ Dose ______________________________________

Please record the amount and type of foods and beverages consumed today. [Or: Please record the amounts and types of foods and beverages you typically consume each day.]

Time of Day	Food	Amount (c, tbs, or piece)	Description (how cooked, how served)

E

unconscious changes in eating habits that may occur while the person is keeping the record.

Food Frequency Checklist Another approach is to use a food frequency checklist to ascertain how often an individual eats a specific type of food. This information helps pinpoint food groups, and therefore nutrients, that may be excessive or deficient in the diet. That a person ate no vegetables yesterday may not seem particularly significant, but never eating vegetables is a warning of possible nutrient deficiencies. When used with the usual intake or 24-hour recall approach, the food frequency record enables the assessor to double-check the accuracy of the information obtained. Form E–3 is a food frequency checklist.

food frequency checklist: a checklist of foods on which a person can record the frequency with which he or she eats each food.

Analysis of Food Intake Data After collecting food intake data, the assessor estimates nutrient intakes, either informally by using foods guides or formally by using food composition tables. The assessor compares these intakes with standards, usually nutrient recommendations or dietary guidelines, to determine how closely the person's diet meets the standards. Are the types and amounts of proteins, carbohydrates (including fiber), and fats (including cholesterol) appropriate? Are all food groups included in appropriate amounts? Is caffeine or alcohol consumption excessive? Are intakes of any vitamins or minerals (including sodium and iron) excessive or deficient? An informal evaluation is possible only if the assessor has enough prior experience with formal calculations to "see" nutrient amounts in reported food intakes without calculations. Even then, such an informal analysis is best followed by a spot check for key nutrients by actual calculation.

Form E–3
Food Frequency Checklist

	Number of Servings	Frequency (per day, week, or month)
1. How often do you eat the following foods?[a]		
Bread, toast, rolls, muffins	______	______
Cereal (which kind?) ______	______	______
Rice or other cooked grains	______	______
Noodles (macaroni, spaghetti)	______	______
Pancakes or waffles	______	______
Crackers or pretzels	______	______
Fruits or fruit juices	______	______
Vegetables other than potatoes	______	______
Vegetable juice	______	______
Potatoes	______	______
Dried beans and peas	______	______
Beef	______	______
Pork or ham	______	______
Veal	______	______
Poultry	______	______
Fish	______	______
Organ meats (such as liver)	______	______
Bacon	______	______
Sausage	______	______
Lunch meat	______	______
Hot dogs	______	______
Other meats (which?) ______	______	______
Eggs	______	______
Peanut butter or nuts	______	______
Milk (including on cereal)	______	______
Cheese or cheese dishes	______	______
Yogurt or tofu	______	______
Other milk products (type?) ______	______	______
Butter	______	______
Margarine (type?) ______	______	______
Salt pork	______	______
Mayonnaise or salad dressing (type?) ______	______	______

[a]The assessor helps the client estimate portion sizes and frequency of use.

Formal calculations can be performed either manually (by looking up each food in a table of food composition, recording its nutrients, and adding them up) or by using a computer diet analysis program. The assessor then compares the intakes with standards such as the RDA.

Diet histories can be superbly informative, but the skillful assessor also keeps their limitations in mind. For example, a computer diet analysis tends to imply greater accuracy than is possible to obtain from data as uncertain as the starting information. Nutrient contents of foods listed in tables of food composition or stored in computer databases are averages, and for some nutrients, incomplete. In addition, the available data on nutrient contents of foods do not reflect the amounts of nutrients a person actually absorbs. Iron is a case in point: its availability from a given meal may vary from as high as 50 percent to less than 2 percent, depending on the person's iron

Form E–3
Food Frequency Checklist (continued)

	Number of Servings	Frequency (per day, week, or month)
Oil (type?) ________	____	____
Cream	____	____
Sugar, jam, jelly, syrup, honey	____	____
Sweet rolls or doughnuts	____	____
Bakery goods (cake, cookies)	____	____
Candy	____	____
Soft drinks (types?) ________	____	____
Potato or snack chips (type?) ________	____	____
Coffee or tea (type?) ________	____	____
Wine	____	____
Beer	____	____
Whiskey, vodka, rum, etc	____	____
Fast foods eaten out	____	____
TV dinners, pot pies, other prepared meals	____	____
Instant meals such as breakfast bars or diet meal beverages (which) ________	____	____

2. What specific kinds of the following foods do you eat? Include the name of the food; whether it is fresh, canned, or frozen, and how it is prepared.
   - Fruits and fruit juices ________
   - Vegetables ________
   - Milk and milk products ________
   - Meats and meat alternates ________
   - Breads and cereals ________
   - Desserts ________
   - Snack foods ________
3. Please list the names of any liquid, powder, or pill forms of vitamin or mineral products you take, and state how often you take them. Please also list any diet supplement you use (such as protein milkshakes or brewer's yeast), how much you use, and how often you use it. ________
4. Is there anything else we should know about your food/nutrient intake? ________

status; the relative amounts of heme iron, nonheme iron, vitamin C, meat, fish, and poultry eaten at the meal; and the presence of inhibitors of iron absorption such as tea, coffee, and nuts. Chapter 13 explains how to calculate iron absorption from a meal.

Furthermore, reported portion sizes may not be correct. The person who reports eating "a serving" of greens may not distinguish between 1/4 cup and 2 whole cups; only trained individuals can accurately report serving sizes. Children tend to remember the serving sizes of foods they like as being larger than serving sizes of foods they dislike.

Thus any comparison of reported nutrient intakes with nutrient needs provides many opportunities for error. Most history takers learn to use shortcut systems to obtain rough estimates of nutrient intakes and then use calculation methods to pinpoint suspected nutrient deficiencies or imbalances.

An estimate of nutrient intakes from a diet history, combined with other sources of information, allows the assessor to confirm or eliminate the possibility of suspected food intake problems. The assessor must constantly remember that nutrient intakes in adequate amounts do not guarantee adequate nutrient status for an individual. Likewise, insufficient intakes do not always indicate deficiencies, but instead alert the assessor to possible problems. Each person digests, absorbs, metabolizes, and excretes nutrients in a unique way; individual needs vary. Intakes of nutrients identified by diet histories are only pieces of a puzzle that must be put together with other indicators of nutrition status in order to extract meaning.

ANTHROPOMETRIC MEASUREMENTS

anthropometric: relating to measurement of the physical characteristics of the body, such as height and weight.
anthropos = human
metric = measuring

E

Anthropometrics are physical measurements that reflect body composition and development (see Table E–3). They serve three main purposes: first, to evaluate the progress of growth in pregnant women, infants, children, and adolescents; second, to detect undernutrition and overnutrition in all age groups; and third, to measure changes in body composition over time.

Health care professionals compare anthropometric measurements taken on an individual with population standards specific for gender and age or with previous measures of the individual. Measurements taken periodically and compared with previous measurements reveal changes in an individual's status.

Mastering the techniques for taking anthropometric measurements requires proper instruction and practice to ensure reliability. Once the correct techniques are learned, taking measurements is easy and requires minimal equipment.

Height and weight are well-recognized anthropometrics; other anthropometrics include fatfold measurements and various measures of lean tissue. Other measures are useful in specific situations. For example, a head circumference measurement may help to assess brain development in an infant, and an abdominal girth measurement supplies information about abdominal fluid retention in individuals with liver disease.

Table E–3
Anthropometric Measurements Used in Nutrition Assessments

Type of Measurement	What It Reflects
Abdominal girth measurement	Abdominal fluid retention
Height-weight	Overnutrition and undernutrition; growth in children
%IBW, %UBW,[a] recent weight change	Overnutrition and undernutrition
Head circumference	Brain growth and development in infants and children under two
Midarm circumference	Muscle mass and subcutaneous fat
Fatfold	Subcutaneous and total body fat
Midarm muscle circumference	Muscle mass (i.e., protein status)

[a]%IBW = percent ideal body weight; %UBW = percent usual body weight. These concepts are discussed in the text.

MEASURES OF GROWTH AND DEVELOPMENT

Height and weight are among the most common and useful anthropometric measurements. Length measurements for infants and children up to age three and height measurements for children over three are particularly valuable in assessing growth and therefore nutrition status. For adults, height measurements alone are not critical but help to estimate desirable weight and to interpret other assessment data. Once adult height has been reached, changes in body weight provide useful information in assessing overnutrition and undernutrition.

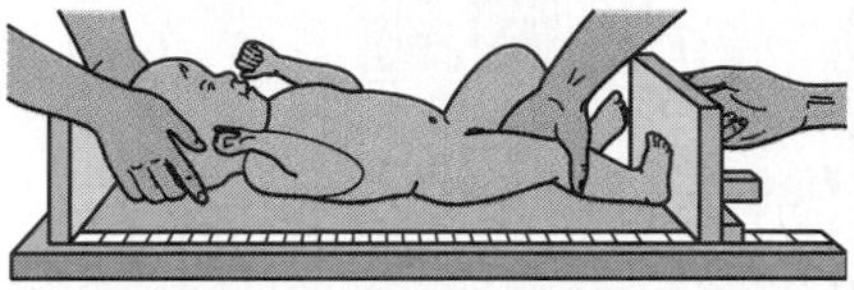

Figure E–1
Length Measurement of an Infant

An infant is measured lying down by use of a length-measuring device with a fixed headboard and a movable footboard. Note that two people are needed to measure the infant's length.

Height For infants and children younger than three, health care professionals may use special equipment to measure length. The assessor lays the barefoot infant on a measuring board that has a fixed headboard and movable footboard attached at right angles to the surface (see Figure E–1). Often two people are needed to obtain an accurate measurement: one to hold the infant's head against the headboard and keep the legs straight, and the other to do the measuring. This method provides the most accurate measure possible, but many health care professionals use a less exacting method. They may simply hold the infant straight with its head against the headboard or other vertical support, mark the blanket with a chalk or pen at the infant's heel, and then measure the distance from the headboard to the mark. Even more informally and less accurately, they may lay the infant on a flat surface and extend a nonstretchable measuring tape along the side of the infant from the top of the head to the heel of the foot.

The procedure for measuring a child who can stand erect and cooperate is the same as for an adult. The best way to measure standing height is with the person's back against a flat wall to which a nonstretchable measuring tape or stick has been fixed (see Figure E–2). The person stands erect, without shoes, with heels together. The person's line of sight should be horizontal, with the heels, buttocks, shoulders, and head touching the wall. The assessor places a block, book, or other inflexible object on top of the head at a right angle to the wall; carefully checks the height measurement; and records it immediately in either inches or centimeters. Such a practice prevents forgetting the correct measurement.

The measuring rod of a scale is commonly used, but is less accurate because it bends easily. The assessor follows the same general procedure, asking the person to face away from the scale and to take extra care to stand erect.

Unfortunately, many health care professionals merely ask clients how tall they are rather than measuring their height. Self-reported height is often inaccurate and should be used only as a last resort when measurement is impractical (in the case of an uncooperative client, an emergency admission, or the like).

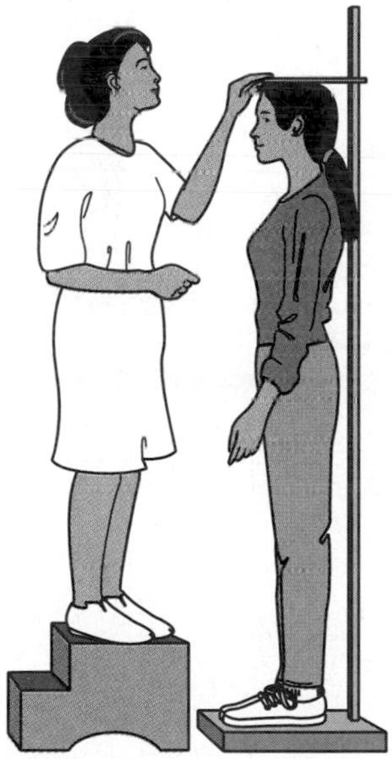

Figure E–2
Height Measurement of an Older Child or Adult

Height is measured most accurately when the person stands against a flat wall to which a measuring tape has been affixed. When the person is taller than the measurer, the measurer can stand on a stool to help ensure that the proper height measurement is obtained.

Weight Valid weight measurements require scales that have been carefully maintained, calibrated, and checked for accuracy at regular intervals. Beam balance and electronic scales are the most accurate types of scales. To measure infants' weight, assessors use special scales that allow infants to lie or sit (see Figure E–3). Weighing infants naked, without diapers, is standard procedure. Children who can stand are weighed in the same way as adults (see Figure E–4). To make repeated measures useful, standardized conditions are necessary. Each weighing should take place at the same time of day (preferably before breakfast), in the same amount of clothing (without shoes), after the person has voided, and on the same scale. Special scales and hospital beds with built-in scales are available for weighing people who are bedridden. Bathroom scales are inaccurate and inappropriate in a professional setting. As with all measurements, the assessor records the observed weight immediately in either pounds or kilograms.

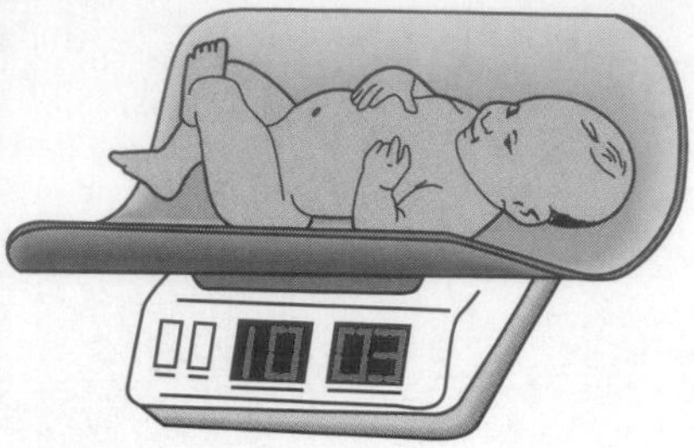

Figure E-3
Weight Measurement of an Infant

Infants sit or lie down on scales that are designed to hold them while they are being weighed.

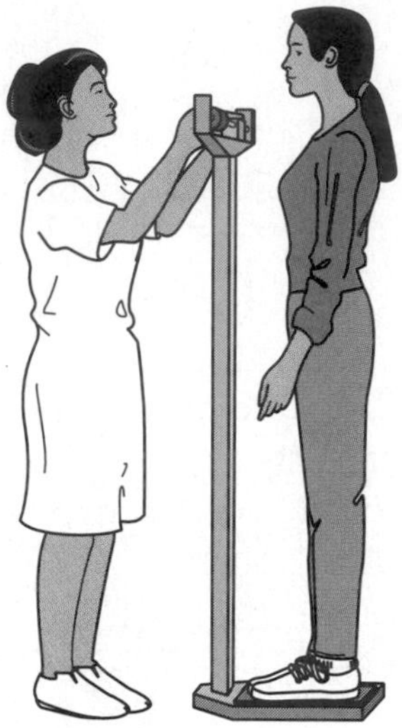

Figure E-4
Weight Measurement of an Older Child or Adult

Whenever possible, children and adults are measured on beam balance scales to ensure accuracy.

Head Circumference Assessors may also measure head circumference to confirm that infant growth is proceeding normally or to help detect protein-energy malnutrition (PEM) and evaluate the extent of its impact on brain size. To measure head circumference, the assessor places a nonstretchable tape so that it encircles the largest part of the infant's or child's head: just above the eyebrow ridges, just above the point where the ears attach, and around the occipital prominence at the back of the head. To ensure accurate recording, the assessor immediately notes the measure in either inches or centimeters.

Analysis of Measures in Infants and Children Growth retardation is an important sign of poor nutrition status. Obesity is also an important sign requiring intervention.

Health professionals generally evaluate physical development by monitoring the growth rate of a child and comparing this rate with standard charts. Standard charts compare weight to age, height to age, and weight to height; ideally, height and weight are in roughly the same percentile. Although individual growth patterns may vary, a child's growth curve will generally stay at about the same percentile throughout childhood. In children whose growth has been retarded, nutrition rehabilitation will ideally induce height and weight to increase to higher percentiles. In overweight children, the goal is for weight to remain stable as height increases, until weight becomes appropriate for height.

To evaluate growth in infants, an assessor uses charts such as E–5 (A and B), E–6 (A and B), E–7 (A and B), and E–8 (A and B). The assessor follows these steps to plot a weight measurement on a percentile graph:

- Select the appropriate chart based on age and gender. (When length is measured, use the chart for birth to 36 months; when height is measured, use the chart for 2 to 18 years.)
- Locate the child's age along the horizontal axis on the bottom or top of the chart.
- Locate the child's weight in pounds or kilograms along the vertical axis on the lower left or right side of the chart.
- Mark the chart where the age and weight lines intersect, and read off the percentile.

To assess length, height, or head circumference, the assessor follows the same procedure, using the appropriate chart. Head circumference percentile should be similar to the child's height and weight percentiles.

With height, weight, and head circumference measures plotted on growth percentile charts, a skilled clinician can begin to interpret the data. Percentile charts divide the measures of a population into 100 equal divisions. Thus half of the population falls above the 50th percentile, and half falls below. The use of percentile measures allows for comparisons among people of the same age and gender. For example, a six-month-old female infant whose weight is at the 75 percentile weighs more than 75 percent of the female infants her age.

Head circumference is generally measured in children under two years of age. Since the brain grows rapidly before birth and during early infancy, extreme and chronic malnutrition during these times can impair brain development, curtailing the number of brain cells and the size of head circumference. Nonnutritional factors, such as certain disorders and genetic variation, can also influence head circumference.

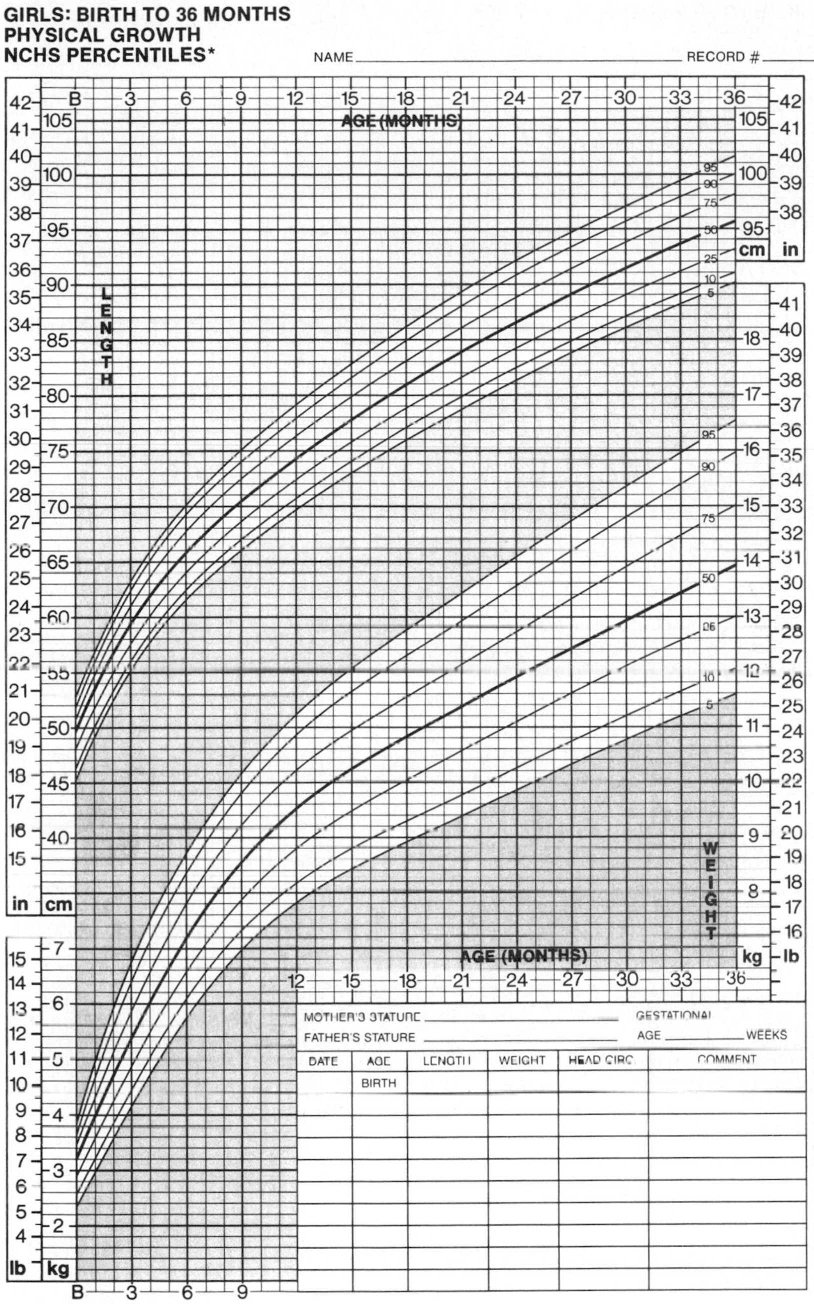

Figure E-5A
Girls: Birth to 36 Months Physical Growth National Center for Health Statistics (NCHS) Percentiles—Length and Weight for Age

*Adapted from: Hamill PVV, Drizd TA, Johnson CL, Reed RB, Roche AF, Moore WM: Physical growth: National Center for Health Statistics percentiles. AM J CLIN NUTR 32:607-629, 1979. Data from the Fels Longitudinal Study, Wright State University School of Medicine, Yellow Springs, Ohio.

Figure E-5B
Boys: Birth to 36 Months Physical Growth NCHS Percentiles—Length and Weight for Age

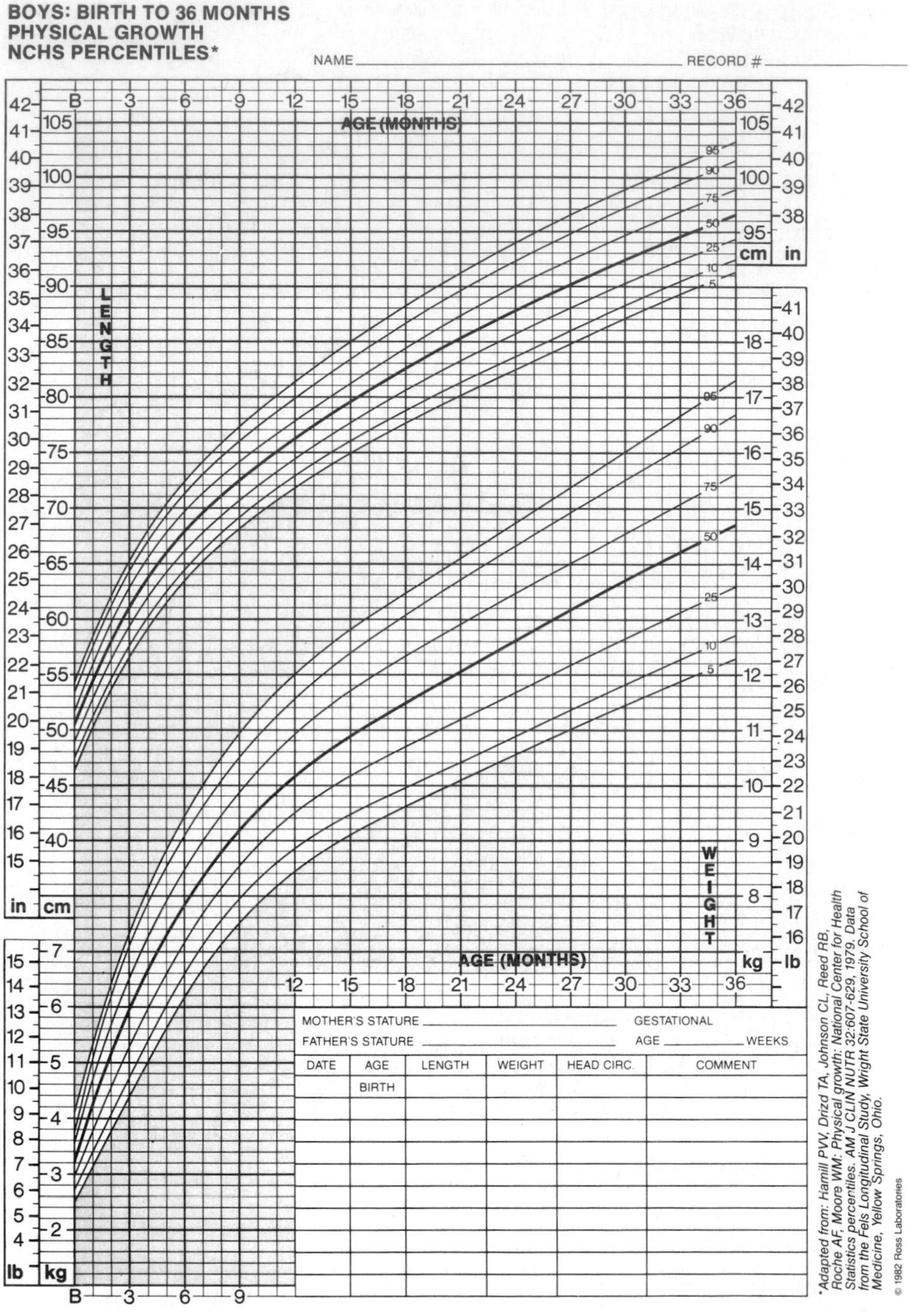

GIRLS: BIRTH TO 36 MONTHS
PHYSICAL GROWTH
NCHS PERCENTILES*

NAME ________________ RECORD # ________

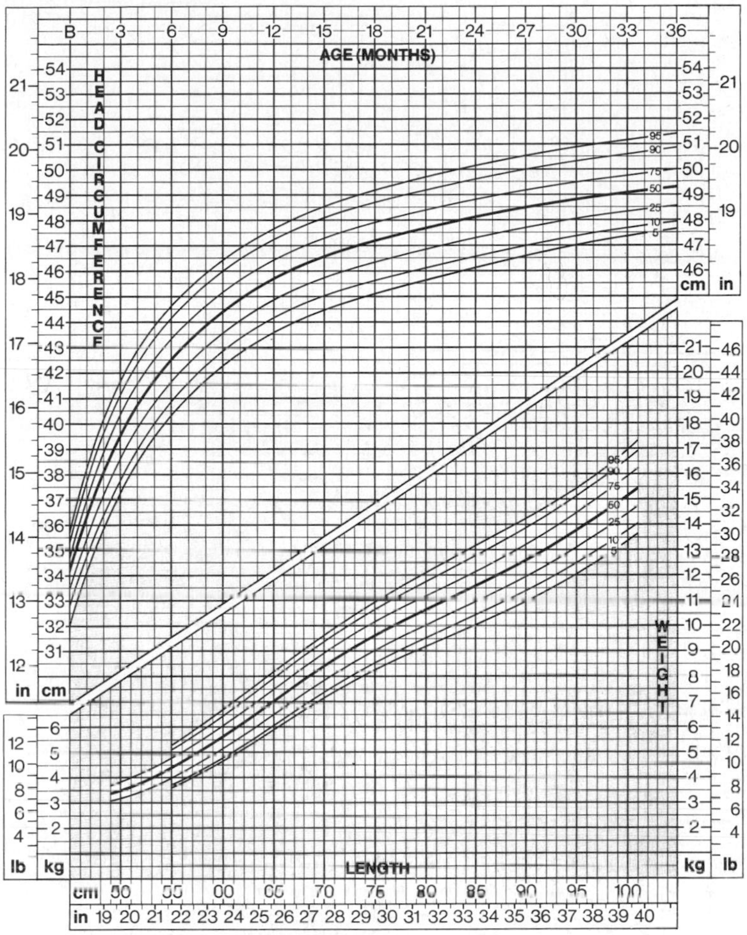

*Adapted from: Hamill PVV, Drizd TA, Johnson CL, Reed RB, Roche AF, Moore WM: Physical growth: National Center for Health Statistics percentiles. AM J CLIN NUTR 32:607-629, 1979. Data from the Fels Longitudinal Study, Wright State University School of Medicine, Yellow Springs, Ohio.

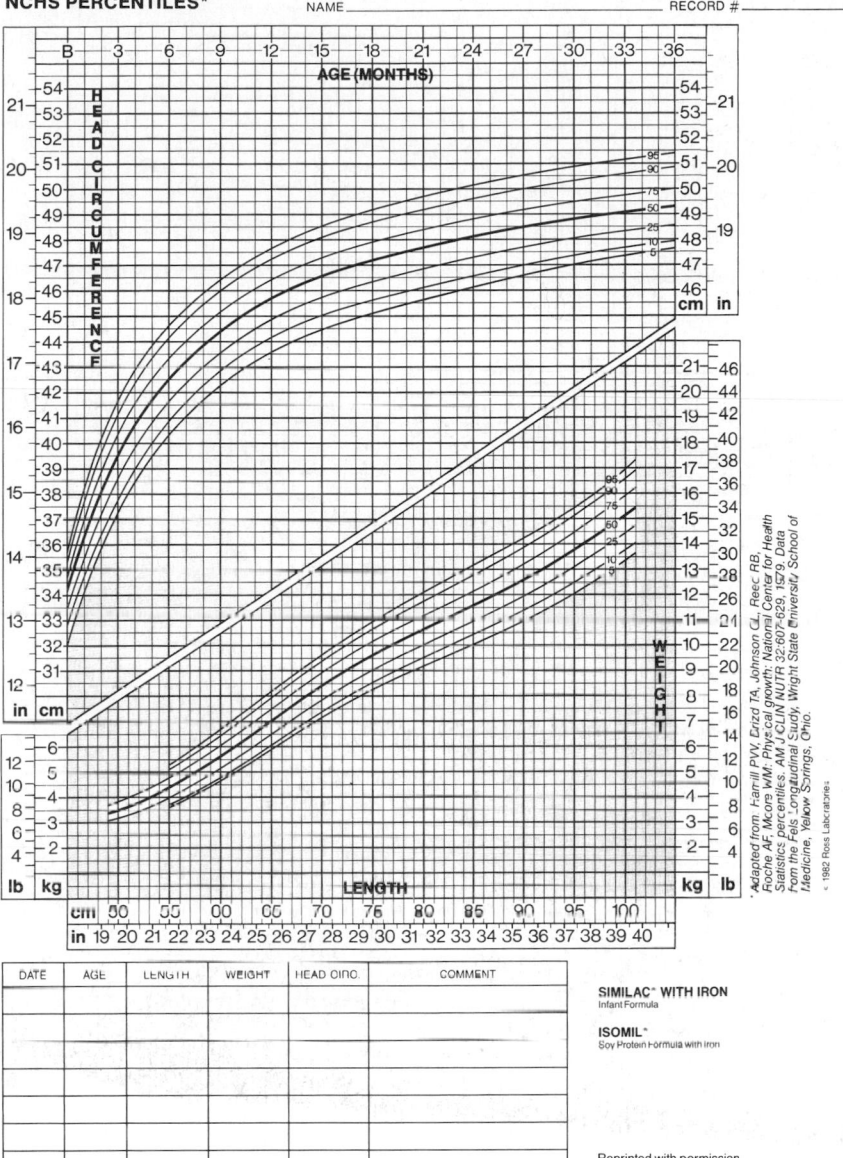

DATE	AGE	LENGTH	WEIGHT	HEAD CIRC.	COMMENT

Figure E–6A
Girls: Birth to 36 Months Physical Growth NCHS Percentiles—Head Circumference for Age and Weight for Length

E

Figure E–6B
Boys: Birth to 36 Months Physical Growth NCHS Percentiles—Head Circumference for Age and Weight for Length

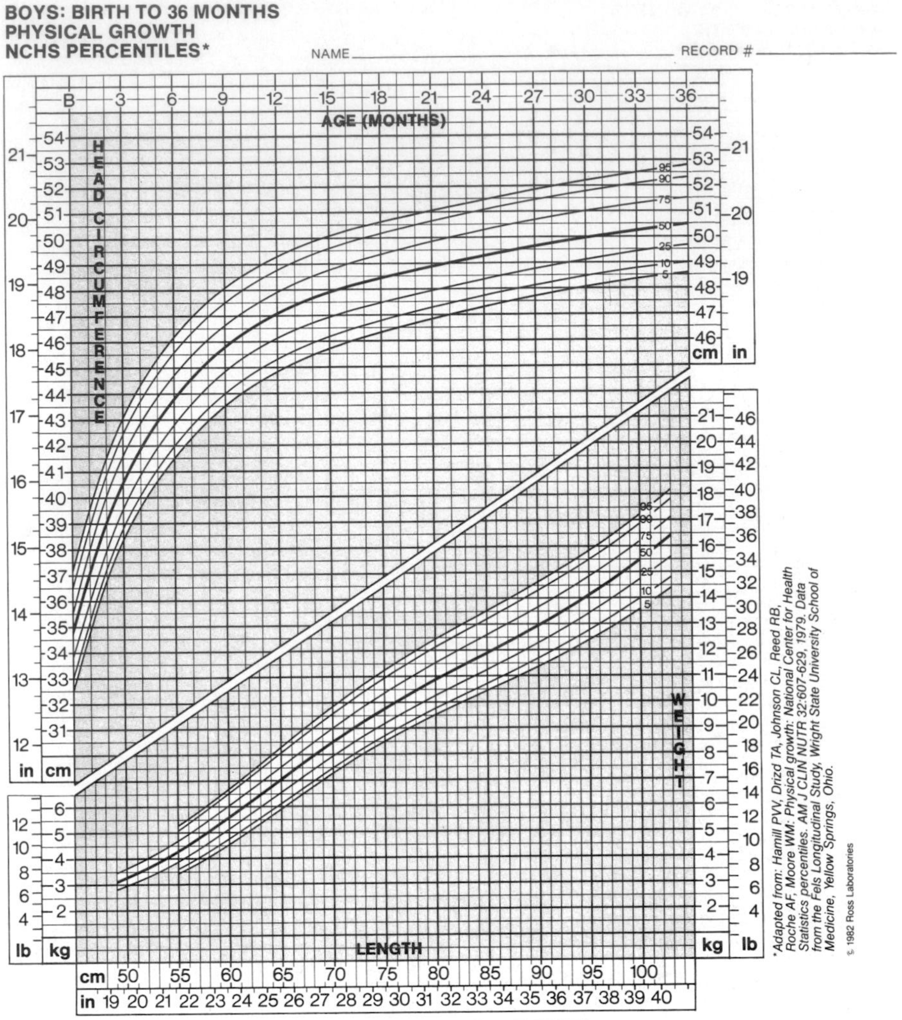

DATE	AGE	LENGTH	WEIGHT	HEAD CIRC.	COMMENT

SIMILAC® WITH IRON
Infant Formula

ISOMIL®
Soy Protein Formula with Iron

Reprinted with permission of Ross Laboratories

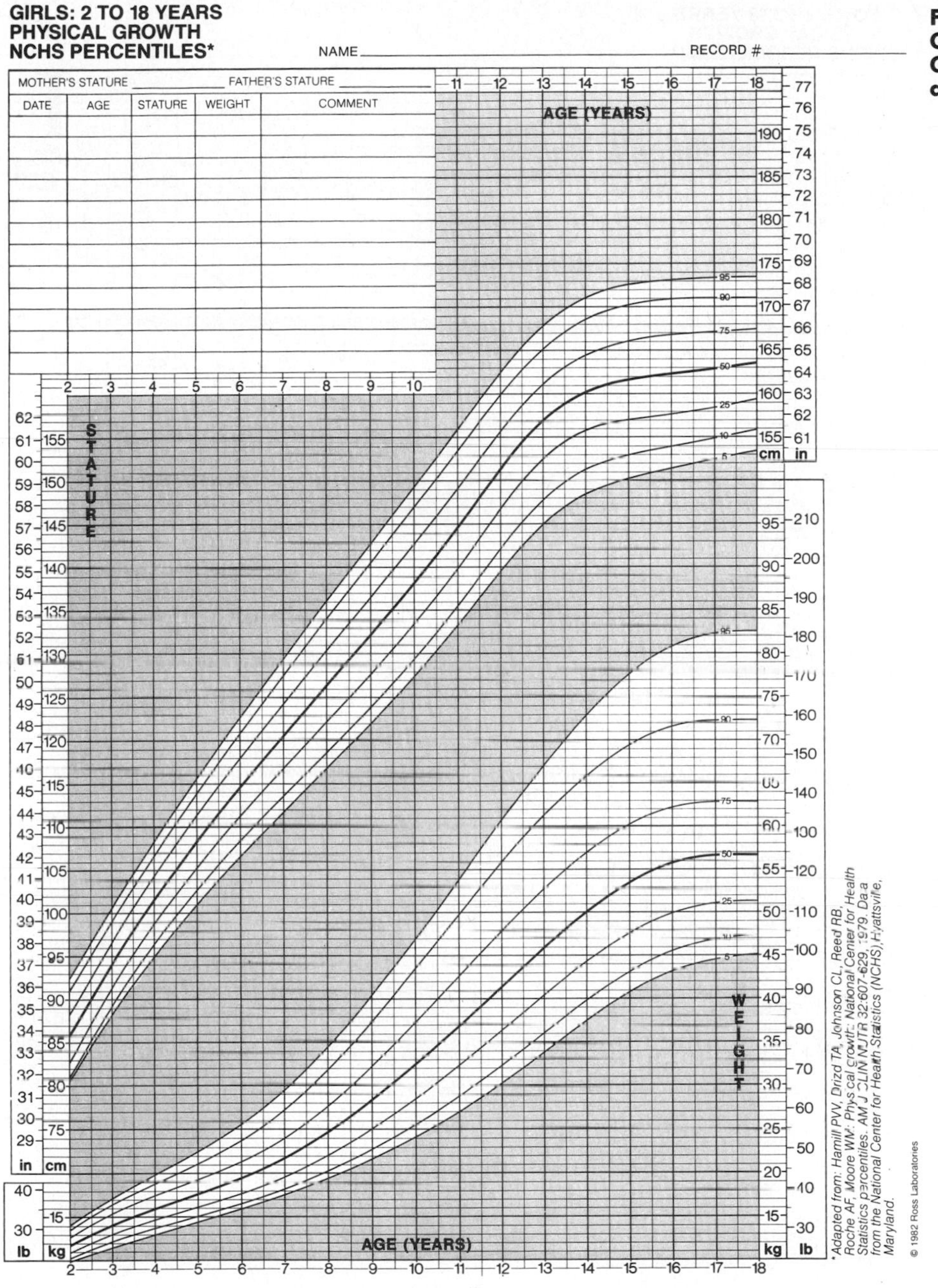

Figure E-7A
Girls: 2 to 18 Years Physical Growth NCHS Percentiles—Height and Weight for Age

Figure E–7B
Boys: 2 to 18 Years Physical Growth NCHS Percentiles—Height and Weight for Age

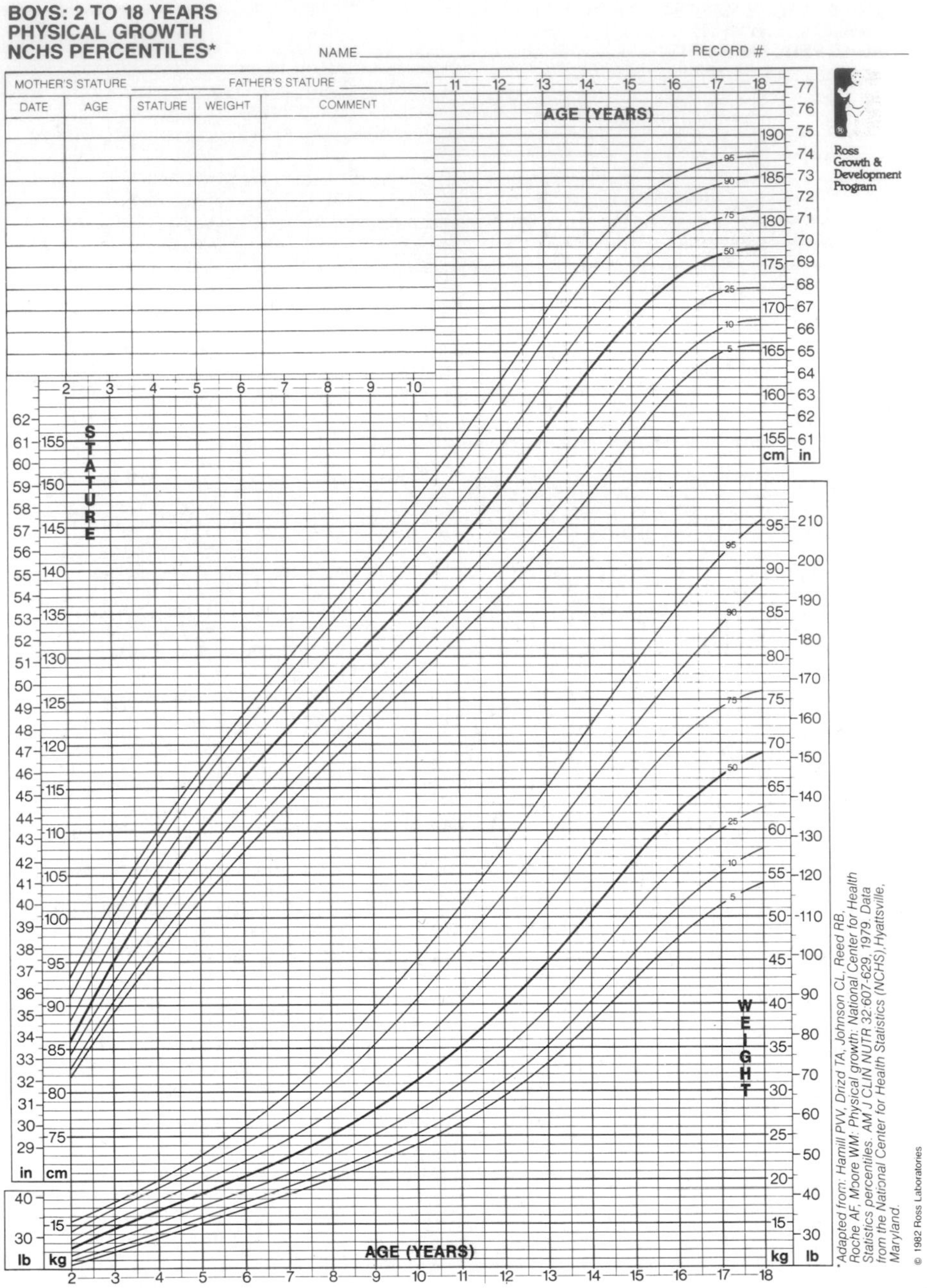

E

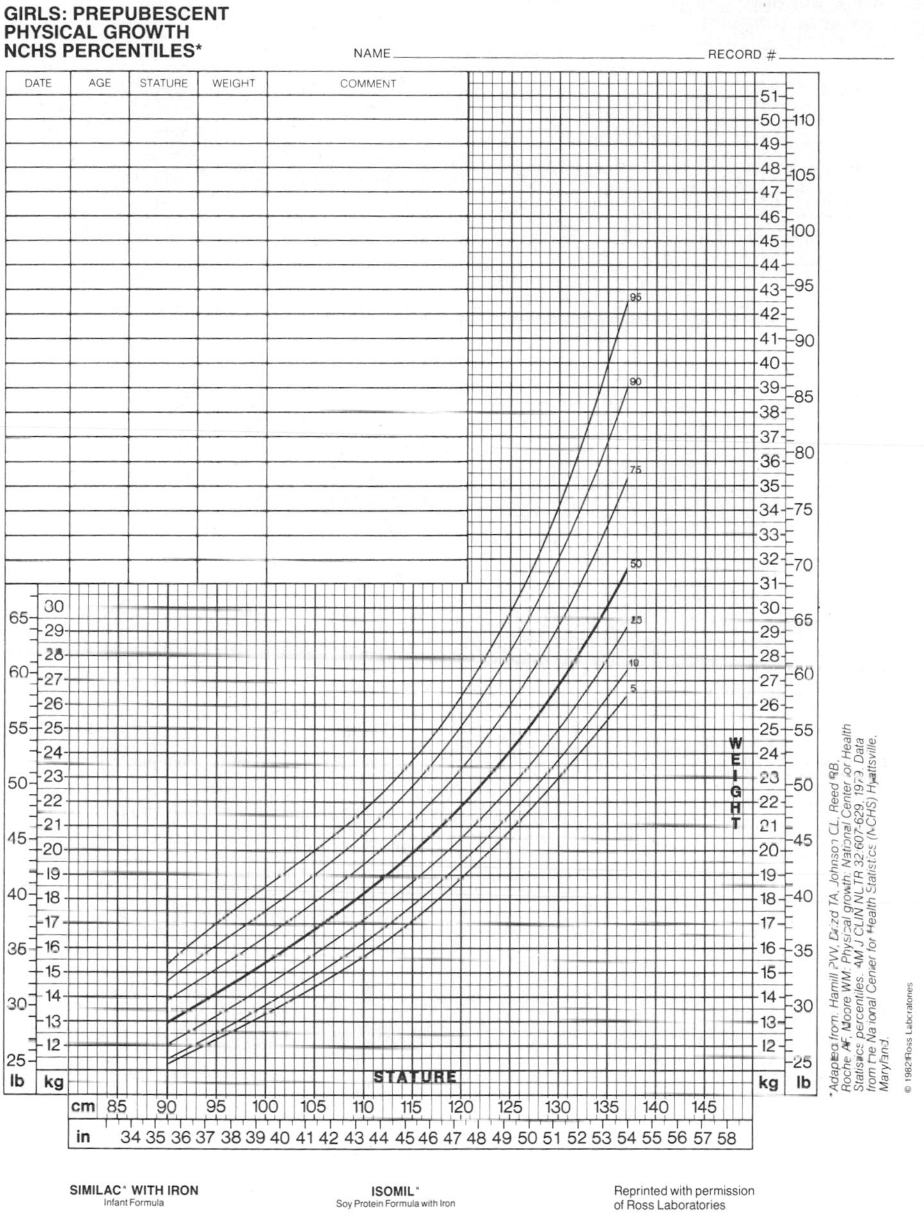

Figure E–8A
Girls: Prepubescent Physical Growth NCHS Percentiles—Weight for Height

Figure E-8B
Boys: Prepubescent Physical Growth NCHS Percentiles—Weight for Height

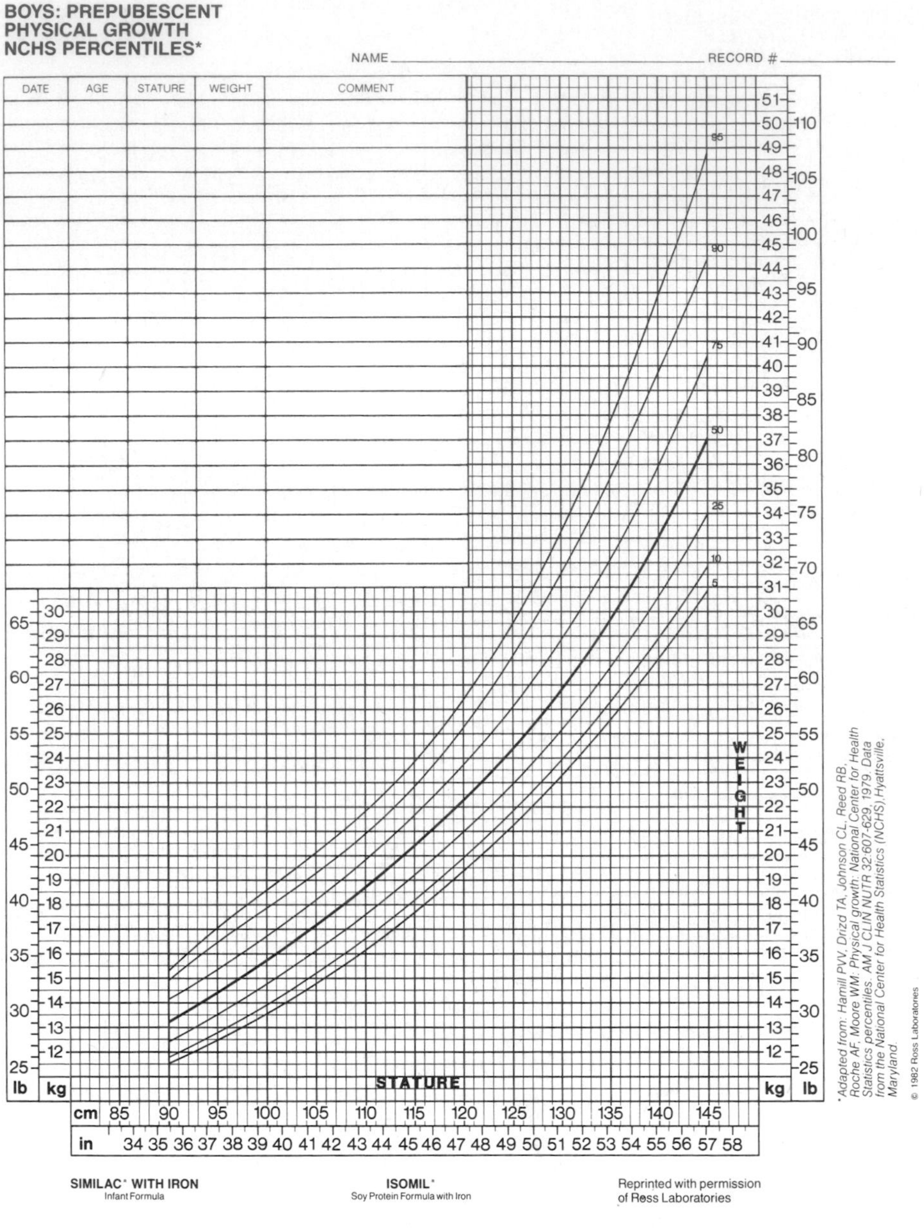

Analysis of Measures in Adults For adults, health care professionals typically compare weights with weight-for-height standards. Today, however, the standards are changing. To identify the weight most consistent with an individual's health requires good clinical judgment. One standard is the body mass index (BMI), described in Chapter 8 (pp. 290–291), which is useful for estimating the risk to health associated with overnutrition. Figure E–9 presents a nomogram for determining the BMI and the inside back covers show weight ranges for various heights based on the BMI. The weight ranges presented in Chapter 8 (Table 8–5), p. 289) are based on the BMI most consistent with health. This table presents wide ranges of weights appropriate for heights without regard to gender and allows higher weights for older people. Other weight-for-height tables, used earlier, are specific for gender and frame size and make no allowance for age. The classic example of these, the Metropolitan height-weight table, is shown in Table E–4. To determine frame size, the assessor refers to a table of frame sizes such as the one based on elbow

Reminder: The *body mass index (BMI)* is an index of a person's weight in relation to height, determined by dividing the weight in kilograms by the square of the height in meters:

$$\text{BMI} = \frac{\text{Weight (kg)}}{\text{Height}^2\ \text{(m)}}.$$

$$\%\ \text{IBW} = \frac{\text{Actual weight}}{\text{Healthy weight*}} \times 100.$$

*Use the midpoint of the healthy weight range; some assessors use the upper end of the range for people who are overweight and the lower end of the range for people who are underweight.

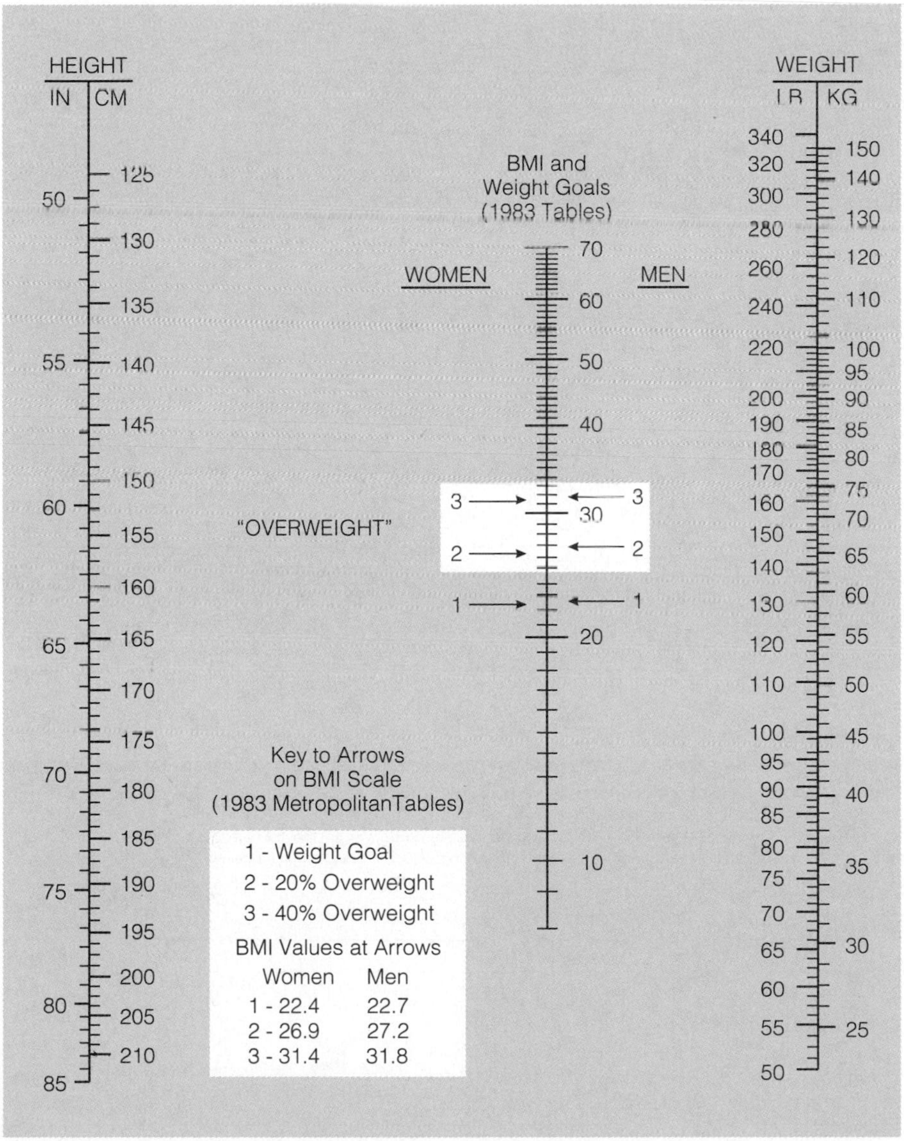

Figure E–9
Nomogram for Body Mass Index

Weights and heights are without clothing. With clothes, add 5 pounds for men or 3 pounds for women, and 1 inch in height for shoes. Draw a straight line, or place a ruler, from your height (left) to your weight (right). At the point where it crosses the BMI line, read your body mass index. The accompanying table in the margin indicates the BMI used to define the cutoff points in the graphs on the inside back covers.

	Men	Women
Underweight	<20.7	<19.1
Acceptable weight	20.7 to 27.8	19.1 to 27.3
Overweight	≥27.8	≥27.3
Severe overweight	≥31.1	≥32.3
Morbid obesity	≥45.4	≥44.8

Source: From the 1983 Metropolitan Life Insurance Company tables, designed by B. T. Burton and W. R. Foster, Health implications of obesity, an NIH Consensus Development Conference, *Journal of the American Dietetic Association* 85 (1985): 1117–1121.

breadth (Table E–5) or the one that compares wrist circumference to height (see Figure E–10 and Table E–6).

In the health care setting, the professional may bypass these tables and simply use a rule of thumb to calculate ideal weight based on height and gender (see Table E–7). While easy to use, this rule is of limited usefulness. The weights it deems ideal are low compared to the BMI standard, especially for taller and older people. Still, it offers a rough estimate of weights near the low end of the range consistent with health.

Tables of average weights for height are less useful in cases where a person has weighed much more or much less than the average throughout life. To assess such a person's weight, it may be more informative to compare the present weight not

Table E–4
1983 Metropolitan Height and Weight Tables

Men					Women				
Height		Frame			Height		Frame		
FEET	INCHES	SMALL	MEDIUM	LARGE	FEET	INCHES	SMALL	MEDIUM	LARGE
5	2	128–134	131–141	138–150	4	10	102–111	109–121	118–131
5	3	130–136	133–143	140–153	4	11	103–113	111–123	120–134
5	4	132–138	135–145	142–156	5	0	104–115	113–126	122–137
5	5	134–140	137–148	144–160	5	1	106–118	115–129	125–140
5	6	136–142	139–151	146–164	5	2	108–121	118–132	128–143
5	7	138–145	142–154	149–168	5	3	111–124	121–135	131–147
5	8	140–148	145–157	152–172	5	4	114–127	124–138	134–151
5	9	142–151	148–160	155–176	5	5	117–130	127–141	137–155
5	10	144–154	151–163	158–180	5	6	120–133	130–144	140–159
5	11	146–157	154–166	161–184	5	7	123–136	133–147	143–163
6	0	149–160	157–170	164–188	5	8	126–139	136–150	146–167
6	1	152–164	160–174	168–192	5	9	129–142	139–153	149–170
6	2	155–168	164–178	172–197	5	10	132–145	142–156	152–173
6	3	158–172	167–182	176–202	5	11	135–148	145–159	155–176
6	4	162–176	171–187	181–207	6	0	138–151	148–162	158–179

Note: To use the table, add an inch to your barefoot height (you are assumed to be wearing shoes with 1-inch heels), and adjust for clothing (the tables assume 5 pounds for clothes for men and 3 pounds for women). Weights are at age 25 to 29 based on lowest mortality, in pounds according to frame size.

Source: Reproduced courtesy of Metropolitan Life Insurance Company. Source of basic data: Society of Actuaries and Association of Life Insurance Medical Directors of America, *1979 Build Study*, 1980.

Table E–5
How to Determine Body Frame by Elbow Breadth

To make a simple approximation of frame size, do the following: Extend the arm, and bend the forearm upward at a 90° angle. Keep the fingers straight, and turn the inside of the wrist away from the body. Place the thumb and index finger on the two prominent bones on *either side* of the elbow. Measure the space between the fingers against a ruler or a tape measure.[a] Compare the measurements with the following standards.

These standards represent the elbow measurements for medium-framed men and women of various heights. Measurements smaller than those listed indicate a small frame, and larger measurements indicate a large frame.

Men		Women	
HEIGHT IN 1-INCH HEELS	ELBOW BREADTH	HEIGHT IN 1-INCH HEELS	ELBOW BREADTH
5 ft 2 in to 5 ft 3 in	$2^1/_2$ to $2^7/_8$ in	4 ft 10 in to 4 ft 11 in	$2^1/_4$ to $2^1/_2$ in
5 ft 4 in to 5 ft 7 in	$2^5/_8$ to $2^7/_8$ in	5 ft 0 in to 5 ft 3 in	$2^1/_4$ to $2^1/_2$ in
5 ft 8 in to 5 ft 11 in	$2^3/_4$ to 3 in	5 ft 4 in to 5 ft 7 in	$2^3/_8$ to $2^5/_8$ in
6 ft 0 in to 6 ft 3 in	$2^3/_4$ to $3^1/_8$ in	5 ft 8 in to 5 ft 11 in	$2^3/_8$ to $2^5/_8$ in
6 ft 4 in and over	$2^7/_8$ to $3^1/_4$ in	6 ft 0 in and over	$2^1/_2$ to $2^3/_4$ in

[a]For the most accurate measurement, measure elbow breadth with a caliper.

Source: Metropolitan Life Insurance Company.

with a population standard, but with the person's usual body weight. Calculating a person's actual weight as a percentage of ideal or usual body weight can provide a useful indicator of malnutrition (Table E–8).

To calculate the percent ideal body weight (%IBW), an assessor compares a person's actual weight and the ideal weight. This provides a rough estimate of the degree of overnutrition and undernutrition. A %IBW greater than 115 to 120 indicates obesity; less than 90 indicates undernutrition.

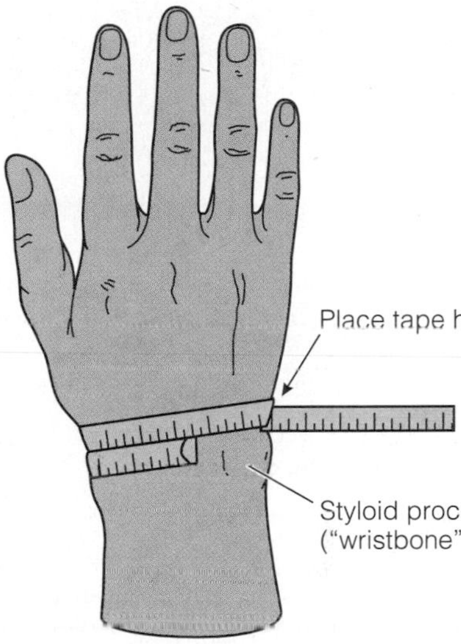

Figure E–10
Wrist Circumference

The wrist circumference is measured just above the wrist bone.

Table E–6
Frame Size from Height-Wrist Circumference Ratios (r)[a]

Frame Size	Male r Values	Female r Values
Small	>10.4	>11.0
Medium	9.6–10.4	10.1–11.0
Large	<9.6	<10.1

[a] $r = \frac{\text{height (cm)}}{\text{wrist circumference (cm)}}$. The wrist is measured where it bends (distal to the styloid process), on the right arm (see Figure E–10).

Table E–7
Quick Estimation of Ideal Body Weight

Men

For 5 feet, consider 106 pounds a reasonable weight.
For each inch over 5 feet, add 6 pounds.
Substract six pounds for each inch under 5 feet.
Add 10% for a large-framed individual; subtract 10% for a small-framed individual.
Example: A man 5 feet 8 inches tall (medium frame) would start at 106 pounds, add 48, and arrive at a reasonable weight of 154 pounds.

Women

For 5 feet, consider 100 pounds a reasonable weight.
For each inch over 5 feet, add 5 pounds.
Subtract 5 pounds for each inch under 5 feet.
Add 10% for a large-framed individual; subtract 10% for a small-framed individual.
Example: A woman 5 feet 6 inches tall (medium frame) would start at 100 pounds, add 30, and arrive at a reasonable weight of 130 pounds.

Table E–8
Weight as an Indicator of Nutrition Status

%IBW	%UBW	Nutrition Status
>120	—	Obese
110–120	—	Overweight
90–109	—	Adequate
80–89	85–95	Mildly undernourished
70–79	75–84	Moderately undernourished
<70	<75	Severely undernourished

A more valuable parameter for assessing weight measurements is the percent usual body weight (%UBW), which considers what is normal for a particular individual. The client, family, friends, and older medical records can provide such information. A health care provider may inadvertently overlook malnutrition in an obese person when using %IBW rather than %UBW.

To determine any recent weight change, the assessor compares the %UBW with the time period over which a change, if any, has occurred. A 5 percent weight loss within a month might be significant yet the same loss over five months might not be.

Weight Gain during Pregnancy One of the most important anthropometric measures predictive of an infant's birthweight is the mother's amount and pattern of weight gain or loss during pregnancy. Normal weight gains related to duration of the pregnancy in weeks are shown in Figure E–11. Patterns of weight gain that deviate from these require further investigation.

Measures of growth and development are well-recognized anthropometrics. Others include measures of body fat and lean tissue.

Figure E–11
Prenatal Weight Gain Grid

A prenatal weight gain grid plots the rate of weight gain during pregnancy. Normal weight women should gain about 3½ lb in the 1st trimester and just under 1 lb/week thereafter, achieving a total gain of 25 to 35 lb by term; underweight women should gain about 5 lb in the 1st trimester and just over 1 lb/week thereafter, achieving a total gain of 28 to 40 lb by term; and overweight women should gain about 2 lb in the 1st trimester and ⅔ lb/week thereafter, achieving a total gain of 15 to 25 lb.

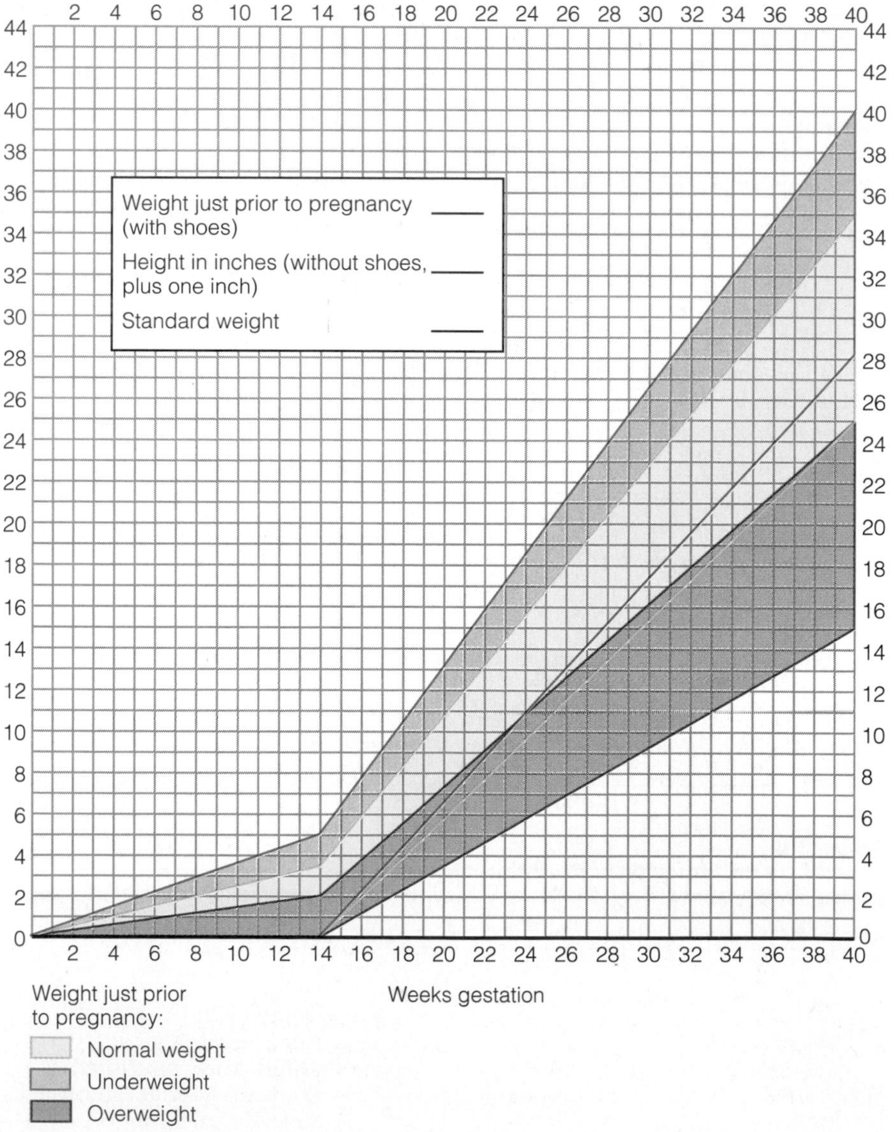

MEASURES OF BODY FAT AND LEAN TISSUE

Significant weight changes in both children and adults can reflect overnutrition and undernutrition with respect to energy and protein. To estimate the degree to which various body compartments (fat stores or lean tissues) are affected by overnutrition or malnutrition, several anthropometric measurements are useful (review Table E–3).

Fatfold Measures Approximately half the fat in the body is located directly beneath the skin, and its thickness reflects total body fat. In some parts of the body, this fat is loosely attached; a person can pull it up between the thumb and forefinger to obtain a measure of fatfold thickness. These measurements correlate well with other, more sophisticated methods of calculating total body fat. The fatfold test is therefore a valuable and practical diagnostic procedure when performed by a person trained in the use of fatfold calipers.

A major limitation of the fatfold test is that fat under the skin may be thicker in one area than in another. A pinch at the side of the waistline may not yield the same measurement as a pinch on the back of the arm. This limitation can be overcome by taking fatfold measurements at several (often three) different places on the body to obtain an accurate estimate of subcutaneous fat. Multiple measures are not always practical in clinical settings, however, and most often, the triceps fatfold measurement is used because it is easily accessible. To measure fatfold, a trained technician follows a standard procedure using reliable calipers, as illustrated in Figure E–12. Triceps fatfold percentiles are given in Table E–9.

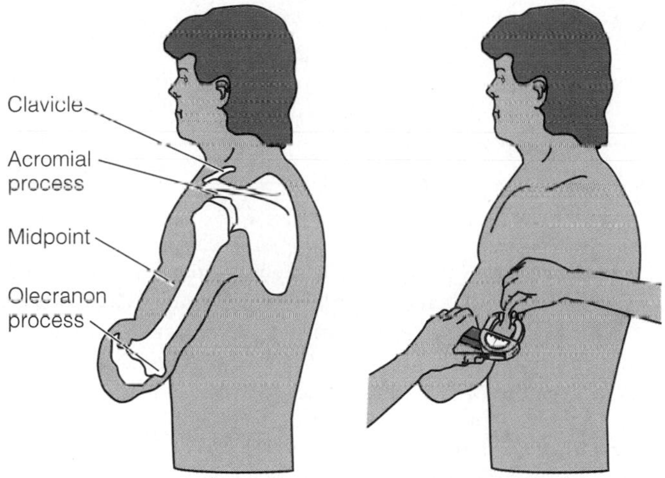

Figure E–12
How to Measure the Triceps Fatfold

A. Find the midpoint of the arm:
1. Ask the subject to bend his or her arm at the elbow and lay the hand across the stomach. (If he or she is right-handed, measure the left arm, and vice versa.)
2. Feel the shoulder to locate the acromial process. It helps to slide your fingers along the clavicle to find the acromial process. The olecranon process is the tip of the elbow.
3. Place a measuring tape from the acromial process to the tip of the elbow. Divide this measurement by 2, and mark the midpoint of the arm with a pen.

B. Measure the fatfold:
1. Ask the subject to let his or her arm hang loosely to the side.
2. Grasp a fold of skin and subcutaneous fat between the thumb and forefinger slightly above the midpoint mark. Gently pull the skin away from the underlying muscle. (This step takes a lot of practice. If you want to be sure you don't have muscle as well as fat, ask the subject to contract and relax the muscle. You should be able to feel if you are pinching muscle.)
3. Place the calipers over the fatfold at the midpoint mark, and read the measurement to the nearest 1.0 millimeter in two to three seconds. (If using plastic calipers, align pressure lines, and read the measurement to the nearest 1.0 millimeter in two to three seconds.)
4. Repeat steps 2 and 3 twice more. Add the three readings, and then divide by 3 to find the average.

Table E-9
Triceps Fatfold Percentiles (Millimeters)

Age	Male 5TH	Male 25TH	Male 50TH	Male 75TH	Male 95TH	Female 5TH	Female 25TH	Female 50TH	Female 75TH	Female 95TH
1–1.9	6	8	10	12	16	6	8	10	12	16
2–2.9	6	8	10	12	15	6	9	10	12	16
3–3.9	6	8	10	11	15	7	9	11	12	15
4–4.9	6	8	9	11	14	7	8	10	12	16
5–5.9	6	8	9	11	15	6	8	10	12	18
6–6.9	5	7	8	10	16	6	8	10	12	16
7–7.9	5	7	9	12	17	6	9	11	13	18
8–8.9	5	7	8	10	16	6	9	12	15	24
9–9.9	6	7	10	13	18	8	10	13	16	22
10–10.9	6	8	10	14	21	7	10	12	17	27
11–11.9	6	8	11	16	24	7	10	13	18	28
12–12.9	6	8	11	14	28	8	11	14	18	27
13–13.9	5	7	10	14	26	8	12	15	21	30
14–14.9	4	7	9	14	24	9	13	16	21	28
15–15.9	4	6	8	11	24	8	12	17	21	32
16–16.9	4	6	8	12	22	10	15	18	22	31
17–17.9	5	6	8	12	19	10	13	19	24	37
18–18.9	4	6	9	13	24	10	15	18	22	30
19–24.9	4	7	10	15	22	10	14	18	24	34
25–34.9	5	8	12	16	24	10	16	21	27	37
35–44.9	5	8	12	16	23	12	18	23	29	38
45–54.9	6	8	12	15	25	12	20	25	30	40
55–64.9	5	8	11	14	22	12	20	25	31	38
65–74.9	4	8	11	15	22	12	18	24	29	36

Note: If measurements fall between the percentiles shown here, the percentile can be estimated from the information in this table. For example, a measurement of 7 millimeters for a 27-year-old male would be about the 20th percentile.

Source: Adapted from A. R. Frisancho, New norms of upper limb fat and muscle areas for assessment of nutritional status. *American Journal of Clinical Nutrition* 34 (1981): 2540–2545.

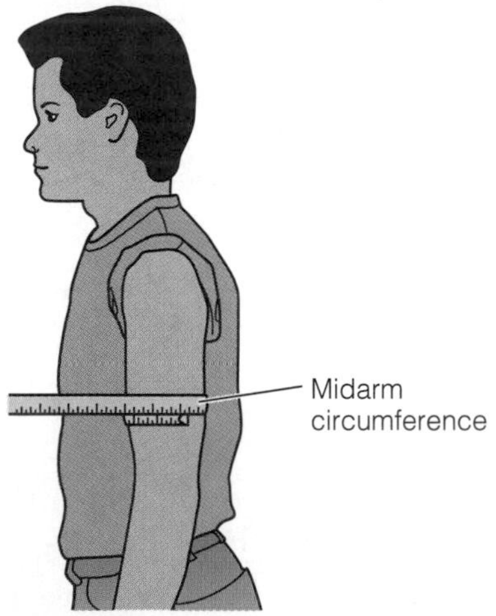

Figure E-13
How to Measure the Midarm Circumference

Ask the subject to let his or her arm hang loosely to the side. Place the measuring tape horizontally around the arm at the midpoint mark. This measurement is the midarm circumference.

Midarm Circumferences When taken together with the *midarm* circumference, the triceps fatfold measurement enables an accessor to calculate the derived midarm *muscle* circumference. The assessor measures midarm circumference with a nonstretchable tape around the arm midway between the shoulder and the elbow (see Figure E–13). The midarm circumference measures muscle mass and subcutaneous fat. This measurement is used to calculate the midarm muscle circumference. Midarm circumference percentiles are given in Table E–10.

The midarm muscle circumference derives from a mathematical equation; it is not directly measurable. The equation assumes the arm is circular and subtracts the fatfold measure from the midarm circumference (see Figure E–14). The derived midarm muscle circumference permits an estimate of muscle mass and, thus, represents protein nutrition. Midarm muscle circumference percentiles appear in Table E–11 (see p. E–26).

Waist-to-Hip Ratio Chapter 8 described how fat distribution correlates with health risks and mentioned that the waist-to-hip ratio is a valuable indicator of fat distribution. To calculate the waist-to-hip ratio, divide the number of inches (or centimeters) around the waistline by the number of inches (or centimeters) around the hips. For example, a person with a 28-inch waist and 38-inch hips would have a ratio of:

$$28 \div 38 = 0.74.$$

Table E-10
Midarm Circumference Percentiles (Centimeters)

Age	Male 5TH	Male 25TH	Male 50TH	Male 75TH	Male 95TH	Female 5TH	Female 25TH	Female 50TH	Female 75TH	Female 95TH
<1	Reliable data unavailable					Reliable data unavailable				
1–1.9	14.2	15.0	15.9	17.0	18.3	13.8	14.8	15.6	16.4	17.7
2–2.9	14.1	15.3	16.2	17.0	18.5	14.2	15.2	16.0	16.7	18.4
3–3.9	15.0	16.0	16.7	17.5	19.0	14.3	15.8	16.7	17.5	18.9
4–4.9	14.9	16.2	17.1	18.0	19.2	14.9	16.0	16.9	17.7	19.1
5–5.9	15.3	16.7	17.5	18.5	20.4	15.3	16.5	17.5	18.5	21.1
6–6.9	15.5	16.7	17.9	18.8	22.8	15.6	17.0	17.6	18.7	21.1
7–7.9	16.2	17.7	18.7	20.1	23.0	16.4	17.4	18.3	19.9	23.1
8–8.9	16.2	17.7	19.0	20.2	24.5	16.8	18.3	19.5	21.4	26.1
9–9.9	17.5	18.7	20.0	21.7	25.7	17.8	19.4	21.1	22.4	26.0
10–10.9	18.1	19.6	21.0	23.1	27.4	17.4	19.3	21.0	22.8	26.5
11–11.9	18.6	20.2	22.3	24.4	28.0	18.5	20.8	22.4	24.8	30.3
12–12.9	19.3	21.4	23.2	25.4	30.3	19.4	21.6	23.7	25.6	29.4
13–13.9	19.4	22.8	24.7	26.3	30.1	20.2	22.3	24.3	27.1	33.8
14–14.9	22.0	23.7	25.3	28.3	32.3	21.4	23.7	25.2	27.2	32.2
15–15.9	22.2	24.4	26.4	28.4	32.0	20.8	23.9	25.4	27.9	32.2
16–16.9	24.4	26.2	27.8	30.3	34.3	21.8	24.1	25.8	28.3	33.4
17–17.9	24.6	26.7	28.5	30.8	34.7	22.0	24.1	26.4	29.5	35.0
18–18.9	24.5	27.6	29.7	32.1	37.9	22.2	24.1	25.8	28.1	32.5
19–24.9	26.2	28.8	30.8	33.1	37.2	21.1	24.7	26.5	29.0	34.5
25–34.9	27.1	30.0	31.9	34.2	37.5	23.3	25.6	27.7	30.4	36.8
35–44.9	27.8	30.5	32.6	34.5	37.4	24.1	26.7	29.0	31.7	37.8
45–54.9	26.7	30.1	32.2	34.2	37.6	24.2	27.4	29.9	32.8	38.4
55–64.9	25.8	29.6	31.7	33.6	36.9	24.3	28.0	30.3	33.5	38.5
65–74.9	24.8	28.5	30.7	32.5	35.5	24.0	27.4	29.9	32.6	37.3

Source: Adapted from A. R. Frisancho, New norms of upper limb fat and muscle areas for assessment of nutritional status, *American Journal of Clinical Nutrition* 34 (1981): 2540–2545.

Figure E-14
How to Derive Midarm Muscle Circumference

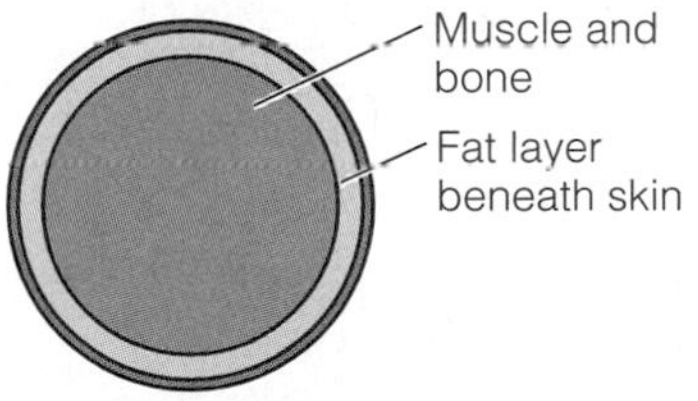

The arm is visualized as an inner circle of muscle and bone surrounded by an outer layer of fat.

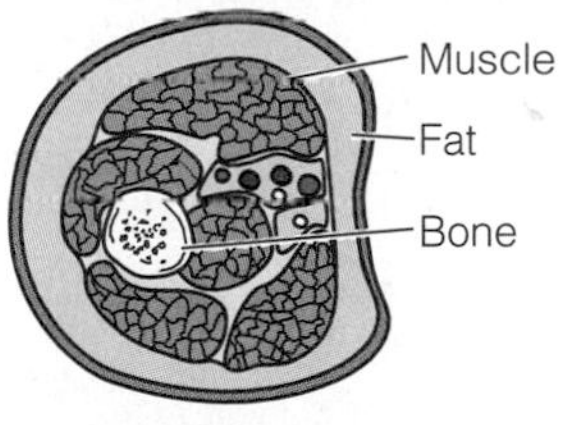

In reality, the arm is not circular, and there is some bone, but the simplified picture is approximately correct.

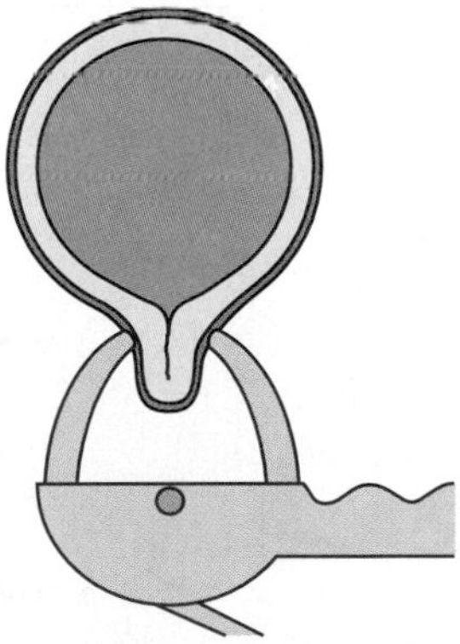

This measurement (the fatfold) equals two times the thickness of the fat.

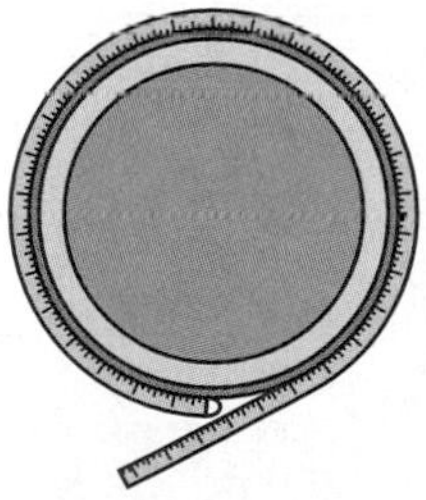

This measurement (the midarm circumference) equals muscle plus fat.

The following equation then derives the *circumference of the muscle*, an index of the body's total skeletal mass:
Midarm muscle circumference (cm) = midarm circumference (cm) – [$0.314^a \times$ triceps fatfold (mm)].

[a]This factor converts the fatfold measurement to a circumference measurement and millimeters to centimeters.

Women with a ratio of 0.8 or greater and men with a ratio of 0.95 or greater are at high risk of obesity-related health problems.

Clinicians use many other methods to estimate body fat and its distribution. Each has its advantages and disadvantages as Table E–12 summarizes.

Table E–11
Midarm Muscle Circumference Percentiles (Centimeters)

	Male					Female				
Age	5TH	25TH	50TH	75TH	95TH	5TH	25TH	50TH	75TH	95TH
1–1.9	11.0	11.9	12.7	13.5	14.7	10.5	11.7	12.4	13.9	14.3
2–2.9	11.1	12.2	13.0	14.0	15.0	11.1	11.9	12.6	13.3	14.7
3–3.9	11.7	13.1	13.7	14.3	15.3	11.3	12.4	13.2	14.0	15.2
4–4.9	12.3	13.3	14.1	14.8	15.9	11.5	12.8	13.6	14.4	15.7
5–5.9	12.8	14.0	14.7	15.4	16.9	12.5	13.4	14.2	15.1	16.5
6–6.9	13.1	14.2	15.1	16.1	17.7	13.0	13.8	14.5	15.4	17.1
7–7.9	13.7	15.1	16.0	16.8	19.0	12.9	14.2	15.1	16.0	17.6
8–8.9	14.0	15.4	16.2	17.0	18.7	13.8	15.1	16.0	17.1	19.4
9–9.9	15.1	16.1	17.0	18.3	20.2	14.7	15.8	16.7	18.0	19.8
10–10.9	15.6	16.6	18.0	19.1	22.1	14.8	15.9	17.0	18.0	19.7
11–11.9	15.9	17.3	18.3	19.5	23.0	15.0	17.1	18.1	19.6	22.3
12–12.9	16.7	18.2	19.5	21.0	24.1	16.2	18.0	19.1	20.1	22.0
13–13.9	17.2	19.6	21.1	22.6	24.5	16.9	18.3	19.8	21.1	24.0
14–14.9	18.9	21.2	22.3	24.0	26.4	17.4	19.0	20.1	21.6	24.7
15–15.0	19.9	21.8	23.7	25.4	27.2	17.5	18.9	20.2	21.5	24.4
16–16.9	21.3	23.4	24.9	26.9	29.6	17.0	19.0	20.2	21.6	24.9
17–17.9	22.4	24.5	25.8	27.3	31.2	17.5	19.4	20.5	22.1	25.7
18–18.9	22.6	25.2	26.4	28.3	32.4	17.4	19.1	20.2	21.5	24.5
19–24.9	23.8	25.7	27.3	28.9	32.1	17.9	19.5	20.7	22.1	24.9
25–34.9	24.3	26.4	27.9	29.8	32.6	18.3	19.9	21.2	22.8	26.4
35–44.9	24.7	26.9	28.6	30.2	32.7	18.6	20.5	21.8	23.6	27.2
45–54.9	23.9	26.5	28.1	30.0	32.6	18.7	20.6	22.0	23.8	27.4
55–64.9	23.6	26.0	27.8	29.5	32.0	18.7	20.9	22.5	24.4	28.0
65–74.9	22.3	25.1	26.8	28.4	30.6	18.5	20.8	22.5	24.4	27.9

Source: Adapted from A. R. Frisancho, New norms of upper limb fat and muscle areas for assessment of nutritional status, *American Journal of Clinical Nutrition* 34 (1981): 2540–2545.

Table E–12
Methods of Estimating Body Fat and Its Distribution

Method	Cost	Ease of Use	Accuracy	Measures Regional Fat
Height and weight	Low	Easy	High	No
Fatfolds	Low	Easy	Low	Yes
Circumferences	Low	Easy	Moderate	Yes
Ultrasound	Moderate	Moderate	Moderate	Yes
Hydrodensitrometry	Low	Moderate	High	No
Heavy Water Tritiated	Moderate	Moderate	High	No
Deuterium oxide, or heavy oxygen	High	Moderate	High	No
Potassium isotope (^{40}K)	Very High	Difficult	High	No
Total body electrical conductivity (TOBEC)	High	Moderate	High	No
Bioelectric impedance (BIA)	Moderate	Easy	High	No
Dual energy x-ray absorptiometry (DEXA)	High	Easy	High	No
Computed tomography (CT)	Very High	Difficult	High	Yes
Magnetic resonance imaging (MRI)	Very High	Difficult	High	Yes

Source: Adapted with permisssion from G. A. Bray, a handout presented at the North American Association for the Study of Obesity and Emory University School of Medicine conference on Obesity Update: Pathophysiology, Clinical Consequences, and Therapeutic Options, Atlanta, Georgia, August 31–September 2, 1992.

PHYSICAL EXAMINATIONS

◆

An assessor can use a physical examination to search for signs of nutrient deficiency or toxicity. Like the other assessment methods, such an examination requires knowledge and skill. Many physical signs are nonspecific; they can reflect any of several nutrient deficiencies as well as conditions not related to nutrition (see Table E–13). For example, cracked lips may be caused by sunburn, windburn, dehydration, or any of several B vitamin deficiencies, to name just a few possible causes. For this reason, physical findings by themselves are especially unreliable for diagnosis of a nutrition problem. Instead, their value is in revealing possible problems for other assessment techniques to confirm, or in confirming other assessment measures.

Table E–13
Physical Findings Used in Nutrition Assessments

Body System	Acceptable Findings	Malnutrition Findings	What the Findings Reflect
Hair	Shiny, firm in the scalp	Dull, brittle, dry, loose; falls out	PEM
Eyes	Bright, clear pink membranes; adjust easily to light	Pale membranes; spots; redness; adjust slowly to darkness	Vitamin A, the B vitamins, zinc, and iron status
Teeth and gums	No pain or caries, gums firm, teeth bright	Missing, discolored, decayed teeth; gums bleed easily and are swollen and spongy	Mineral and vitamin C status
Face	Clear complexion without dryness or scaliness	Off-color, scaly, flaky, cracked skin	PEM, vitamin A, and iron status
Glands	No lumps	Swollen at front of neck, cheeks	PEM and iodine status
Tongue	Red, bumpy, rough	Sore, smooth, purplish, swollen	B vitamin status
Skin	Smooth, firm, good color	Dry, rough, spotty; "sandpaper" feel or sores; lack of fat under skin	PEM, essential fatty acid deficiency, vitamin A, the B vitamins, and vitamin C status
Nails	Firm, pink	Spoon-shaped, brittle, ridged	Iron status
Internal systems	Regular heart rhythm, heart rate between 60 and 100, and blood pressure below 140/90; no impairment of digestive function, reflexes, or mental status	Abnormal heart rate, heart rhythm, or blood pressure; enlarged liver, spleen; abnormal digestion; burning, tingling of hands, feet; loss of balance, coordination; mental confusion, irritability, fatigue	PEM and mineral status
Muscles and bones	Muscle tone; posture, long bone development appropriate for age	"Wasted" appearance of muscles; swollen bumps on skull or ends of bones; small bumps on ribs; bowed legs or knock-knees	PEM and vitamin D status

With this limitation understood, physical symptoms can be most informative and communicate much information about nutrition health. Many tissues and organs can reflect signs of malnutrition. The signs appear most rapidly in parts of the body where cell replacement occurs at a high rate, such as in the hair, skin, and digestive tract (including the mouth and tongue). The summary tables in Chapters 10, 11, 12, and 13 list additional physical signs of vitamin and mineral malnutrition.

BIOCHEMICAL ANALYSES

The **serum** is the watery portion of the blood that remains after removal of the cells and clot-forming material; **plasma** is the fluid that remains when unclotted blood is centrifuged. In most cases, serum and plasma concentrations are similar. Lab technicians usually prefer serum samples because plasma samples occasionally clog mechanical blood analyzers.

All of the approaches to nutrition assessment discussed so far are external approaches. Biochemical analyses or laboratory tests help to determine what is happening to the body internally. Most tests are based on analysis of blood and urine samples, which contain nutrients, enzymes, and metabolites that reflect nutrition status. Other tests, such as serum glucose, help pinpoint disease-related problems with nutrition implications. Tests that define fluid and electrolyte balance, acid-base balance, and organ function also have nutrition implications. Table E–14 lists biochemical tests useful for assessing protein, vitamin, and mineral status.

The interpretation of biochemical data requires skill. Long metabolic sequences lead to the production of the end products and metabolites seen in blood and urine. No single test can reveal nutrition status because many factors influence test results. The low blood concentration of a nutrient may reflect a primary deficiency of that nutrient, but it may also be secondary to the deficiency of one or several other nutrients or to a disease. Taken together with other assessment data, however, laboratory test results help to make a total picture that becomes clear with careful interpretation. They are especially useful in helping to detect subclinical malnutrition by uncovering early signs of malnutrition before the clinical signs of a classic deficiency disease appear.

Reminder: A *subclinical deficiency* is a nutrient deficiency in the early stages before the outward signs have appeared.

Laboratory tests used to assess vitamin and mineral status (review Table E–14) are particularly useful when combined with diet histories and physical findings. Vitamin and mineral levels present in the blood and urine sometimes reflect recent rather than long-term intakes. This makes detecting subclinical deficiencies difficult. Furthermore, many nutrients interact; therefore, the amounts of other nutrients in the body can affect a lab value for a particular nutrient. It is also important to remember that nonnutrient conditions influence biochemical measures.

It is beyond the scope of this text to describe all lab tests and their relations to nutrition status. Instead, the emphasis is on lab tests used to detect protein-energy malnutrition and iron-deficiency anemia.

PROTEIN-ENERGY MALNUTRITION (PEM)

Tests available to determine protein status include serum albumin, serum transferrin, other serum proteins, and total lymphocyte count and other tests of immune function. Of these, serum albumin and total lymphocyte count are most commonly used. Physicians may also order additional tests, such as urinary creatinine, under special circumstances.

Serum Albumin Albumin accounts for over 50 percent of the total serum proteins. It helps to maintain fluid and electrolyte balance and to transport many nutrients, hormones, drugs, and other compounds. Albumin synthesis depends on the functioning liver cells and on an appropriate supply of amino acids.

Table E–14
Biochemical Tests Useful for Assessing Nutrition Status

Nutrient	Assessment Tests
Protein	Urinary creatinine excretion, serum albumin, serum prealbumin, serum transferrin, retinol-binding protein, total lymphocyte count, nitrogen balance
Vitamins	
Vitamin A	Retinol-binding protein, serum carotene
Thiamin	Erythrocyte (red blood cell) transketolase activity, urinary thiamin
Riboflavin	Erythrocyte glutathione reductase activity, urinary riboflavin
Vitamin B_6	Urinary xanthurenic acid excretion after tryptophan load test, urinary vitamin B_6, erythrocyte transaminase activity
Niacin	Urinary metabolites NMN (N-methyl nicotinamide) or 2-pyridone, or preferably both expressed as a ratio
Folate	Free folate in the blood, erythrocyte folate (reflects liver stores), urinary formiminoglutamic acid (FIGLU), vitamin B_{12} status (because folate assessment tests alone do not distinguish between the two deficiencies)
Vitamin B_{12}	Serum vitamin B_{12}, erythrocyte vitamin B_{12}, urinary methylmalonic acid synthesis or DUMP test (from the abbreviation for the chemical name of DNA's raw material, deoxyuridine monophosphate), Schilling test
Biotin	Serum biotin, urinary biotin
Vitamin C	Serum or plasma vitamin C,[a] leukocyte vitamin C, urinary vitamin C
Vitamin D	Serum alkaline phosphatase
Vitamin E	Serum tocopherol, erythrocyte hemolysis
Vitamin K	Blood clotting time (prothrombin time)
Minerals	
Potassium	Serum potassium
Magnesium	Serum magnesium
Iron	Hemoglobin, hematocrit, serum ferritin, total iron-binding capacity (TIBC), transferrin saturation, erythrocyte protoporphyrin, mean corpuscular volume (MCV), serum iron
Iodine	Serum protein-bound iodine, radioiodine uptake
Zinc	Plasma zinc, hair zinc

[a]Vitamin C shifts unpredictably between the plasma and the white blood cells known as leukocytes; thus a plasma or serum determination may not accurately reflect the body's pool. The appropriate clinical test may be a measurement of leukocyte vitamin C. A combination of both tests may be more reliable than either one alone.

Source: Adapted from A. Grant and S. DeHoog, *Nutritional Assessment and Support,* 3rd ed., 1985 (available from Anne Grant and Susan DeHoog, Box 25057, Northgate Station, Seattle, WA 98125).

Albumin concentrations reflect the protein status of the blood and internal organs. Serum albumin concentrations tend to decline slowly, in part because albumin is plentiful in the body and can shift from the cells to the blood when blood concentrations begin to fall. Additionally, because albumin breaks down slowly, it is

Table E-15
Relationship between Degree of Undernutrition and Serum Proteins

Indicator	Degree of Depletion: NORMAL	MILD	MODERATE	SEVERE
Albumin (g/100 ml)	≥3.5	2.8–3.4	2.1–2.7	<2.1
Transferrin (mg/100 ml)	≥200	150–200	100–149	<100
Prealbumin (mg/100 ml)	16–30	10–15	5–9	<5
Retinol-binding protein[a] (mg/100 ml)	2.6–7.6	—	—	—

Note: To convert albumin (g/100ml) to international standard units (nmol/L), multiply by 37.06. To convert transferrin (mg/100 ml) to standard international units (g/L), multiply by 0.01.

[a]Levels of <3 mg/100 ml suggest compromised protein status. The actual degree of depletion (mild, moderate, and severe) has not been defined.

slow to reflect changes in nutrition status.* Therefore, low serum albumin levels represent prolonged protein depletion. Conversely, albumin concentrations increase slowly with appropriate nutrition support, so measuring albumin as an indicator of response to nutrition therapy is of limited value. Table E–15 provides standards for determining the severity of low serum albumin concentrations.

Many other conditions besides malnutrition can depress albumin concentration, including liver disease, advanced kidney disease (nephrotic syndrome), infection, cancer, and burns. Therefore, as is true for all nutrition assessment measurements, albumin alone cannot determine protein status, but rather serves as one indicator among many.

Serum Transferrin Transferrin is a protein that transports iron between the intestine and sites of hemoglobin synthesis and degradation. Clinicians consider it a more sensitive indicator of protein malnutrition than albumin because it responds more promptly to changes in protein intake and has a smaller body pool.†

Most transferrin is synthesized in the liver. Transferrin levels are inversely related to iron stores; levels are high in iron deficiency and low when iron storage is excessive. Therefore, assessors may have difficulty interpreting transferrin levels when an iron deficiency is present. Liver disease, nephrotic syndrome, and burns lower the transferrin levels; pregnancy and blood loss elevate them. Standards for determining the severity of transferrin depletion are given in Table E–15.

Total Lymphocyte Count Various forms of PEM and individual nutrient deficiencies depress the immune system. The total number of lymphocytes is reduced as protein depletion occurs, so the total lymphocyte count is a useful index in nutrition assessment. White blood cell volume and red and white blood cell counts are routinely measured in hospital tests, so the total lymphocyte count can be derived:

The standard is 2500 mm^3; values below 1500 mm^3 are considered depleted.

$$\text{Total lymphocyte count } (mm^3) = \text{WBC } (mm^3) \times \%\text{lymphocytes.}$$

*The half-life of albumin is about 20 days, an indication of a slow degradation rate.

†Transferrin has a half-life of 4 to 8 days, an indication that it is sensitive to changes in protein intake.

Urinary Creatinine Excretion Creatinine is a breakdown product of the energy source phosphocreatine, or PC (described in Chapter 14). PC is present specifically in skeletal muscle. Creatinine is excreted at a constant rate determined by the amount of skeletal muscle, and the amount excreted therefore reflects skeletal muscle mass. As skeletal muscle atrophies during malnutrition, creatinine excretion decreases. Creatinine excretion is also used to determine whether other urinary lab test results are appropriate to the size of the individual's skeletal muscle mass.

Standards for creatinine excretion, based on sex and height, are given in Tables E–16 and E–17. Assessors use these standards and measured urinary creatinine concentrations to derive the creatinine-height index (CHI):

$$\text{CHI} = \frac{\text{Measured urinary creatinine (24-hr sample)}}{\text{Standard creatinine for height and sex}} \times 100.$$

The CHI is a percentage of the standard; generally, acceptable values are 90 to 100 percent. No standards are available for the elderly, which presents a problem since creatinine excretion declines with age. Standards for children are based on expected creatinine excretion of healthy children of normal height.

The measurement of urinary creatinine requires a 24-hour urine collection, which may be difficult to obtain. The test is invalid if the subject shows signs of kidney disease, since the disease may reduce the body's ability to excrete creatinine. Severe stress, infection, and fever can falsely elevate creatinine excretion.

CLASSIFICATION OF PROTEIN-ENERGY MALNUTRITION

To evaluate PEM, assessors use data from all four assessment techniques. Historical information and physical findings alert health care professionals to the possibility of

Table E–16
Creatinine-Height Index Standards for Men

Height		Small Frame			Medium Frame			Large Frame		
		Ideal Weight	Creatinine		Ideal Weight	Creatinine		Ideal Weight	Creatinine	
in	cm	(kg)	(g/24 h)	(mmol/d)	(kg)	(g/24 h)	(mmol/d)	(kg)	(g/24 h)	(mmol/d)
61	154.9	52.7	1.21	10.7	56.1	1.29	11.4	60.7	1.40	12.4
62	157.5	54.1	1.24	11.0	57.7	1.33	11.8	62.0	1.43	12.6
63	160.0	55.4	1.27	11.2	59.1	1.36	12.0	63.6	1.46	12.9
64	162.5	56.8	1.31	11.6	60.4	1.39	12.3	65.2	1.50	13.3
65	165.1	58.4	1.34	11.8	62.0	1.43	12.6	66.8	1.54	13.6
66	167.6	60.2	1.39	12.3	63.9	1.47	13.0	68.9	1.59	14.1
67	170.2	62.0	1.43	12.6	65.9	1.52	13.4	71.1	1.64	14.5
68	172.7	63.9	1.47	13.0	67.7	1.56	13.8	72.9	1.68	14.9
69	175.3	65.9	1.52	13.4	69.5	1.60	14.1	74.8	1.72	15.2
70	177.8	67.7	1.56	13.8	71.6	1.65	14.6	76.8	1.77	15.6
71	180.3	69.5	1.60	14.1	73.6	1.69	14.9	79.1	1.82	16.1
72	182.9	71.4	1.64	14.5	75.7	1.74	15.4	81.1	1.87	16.5
73	185.4	73.4	1.69	14.9	77.7	1.79	15.8	83.4	1.92	17.0
74	187.9	75.2	1.73	15.3	80.0	1.85	16.4	85.7	1.97	17.4
75	190.5	77.0	1.77	15.6	82.3	1.89	16.7	87.7	2.02	17.9

Note: To convert urinary creatinine measures (g/24 h) to standard international units (mmol/d) multiply by 8.840.

Source: A. Grant and S. DeHoog, *Nutritional Assessment and Support,* 3rd ed., 1985 (available from Anne Grant and Susan DeHoog, P.O. Box 25057, Northgate Station, Seattle, WA 98125).

Table E-17
Creatinine-Height Index Standards for Women

Height		Small Frame			Medium Frame			Large Frame		
			Creatinine			Creatinine			Creatinine	
in	cm	Ideal Weight	(g/24 h)	(mmol/d)	Ideal Weight	(g/24 h)	(mmol/d)	Ideal Weight	(g/24 h)	(mmol/d)
56	142.2	43.2	0.79	7.0	46.1	0.83	7.3	50.7	0.91	8.0
57	144.8	44.3	0.80	7.1	47.3	0.85	7.5	51.8	0.93	8.2
58	147.3	45.4	0.82	7.2	48.6	0.88	7.8	53.2	0.96	8.5
59	149.8	46.8	0.84	7.4	50.0	0.90	8.0	54.5	0.98	8.7
60	152.4	48.2	0.87	7.7	51.4	0.93	8.2	55.9	1.01	8.9
61	154.9	49.5	0.89	7.9	52.7	0.95	8.4	57.3	1.03	9.1
62	157.5	50.9	0.92	8.1	54.3	0.98	8.7	58.9	1.06	9.4
63	160.0	52.3	0.94	8.3	55.9	1.01	8.9	60.6	1.09	9.6
64	162.5	53.9	0.97	8.6	57.9	1.04	9.2	62.5	1.13	10.0
65	165.1	55.7	1.00	8.8	59.8	1.08	9.5	64.3	1.16	10.3
66	167.6	57.5	1.04	9.2	61.6	1.11	9.8	66.1	1.19	10.5
67	170.2	59.3	1.07	9.5	63.4	1.14	10.1	67.9	1.22	10.8
68	172.7	61.4	1.11	9.8	65.2	1.17	10.3	70.0	1.26	11.1
69	175.2	63.2	1.14	10.1	67.0	1.21	10.7	72.0	1.30	11.5
70	177.8	65.0	1.17	10.3	68.9	1.24	11.0	74.1	1.33	11.8

Note: To convert urinary creatinine measures (g/24 h) to standard international units (mmol/d) multiply by 8.840.

Source: A. Grant and S. DeHoog, *Nutritional Assessment and Support,* 3rd ed., 1985 (available from Anne Grant and Susan DeHoog, P.O. Box 25057, Northgate Station, Seattle, WA 98125).

Chapter 6 used the terms *kwashiorkor* and *marasmus* to classify PEM as seen in developing countries. Because PEM found in industrialized countries often develops for different reasons (as a result of illness, for example), these terms, though frequently used in clinical settings, do not denote exactly the same conditions. We use the term **acute malnutrition** to describe kwashiorkor-type malnutrition and **chronic malnutrition** to describe marasmus-type malnutrition.

malnutrition. Anthropometric measures and biochemical analyses permit classification of PEM as either acute (kwashiorkor), chronic (marasmus), or a mixture of the two. Such distinctions can be useful, but in clinical settings, these syndromes may overlap, or one may transist into another. This serves as another reminder of the need to assess nutrition status at regular intervals.

Acute Malnutrition The person with acute malnutrition typically has normal or above-standard anthropometric measurements with below-normal indices of blood and organ proteins. Because the individual may be overweight, health care workers can easily overlook malnutrition. Overweight by itself would suggest overnutrition; which again illustrates why no single parameter can be used to define nutrition status.

Chronic Malnutrition In chronic malnutrition, the individual has blood and organ protein levels that appear to be adequate, while skeletal muscle and subcutaneous fat are depleted. The emaciated appearance of the person with chronic malnutrition makes this form of malnutrition easier to notice than acute malnutrition.

Mixed PEM Mixed PEM presents signs of depleted blood, organ, and skeletal muscle proteins as well as depleted subcutaneous fat. The person with this type of malnutrition has virtually no energy reserves, has compromised organ function, and is in grave danger, especially if experiencing severe stress as well.

Energy Overnutrition Malnutrition includes both undernutrition and overnutrition. Above-normal anthropometric measures combined with normal blood protein concentrations identify a person consuming energy in excess of needs. Such a person risks obesity and the many chronic diseases associated with it (see Chapter 8).

The assessment of PEM is commonly performed because many people, including the elderly and those who are hospitalized, have this type of malnutrition and it can lead to severe consequences. The next section illustrates how biochemical tests can be used to assess nutrition-related anemias caused by iron, folate, or vitamin B_{12} deficiencies.

NUTRITIONAL ANEMIAS

Anemia, a symptom of a wide variety of nutrition- and nonnutrition-related disorders, is characterized by a reduced number of red blood cells. Iron, folate, and vitamin B_{12} deficiencies caused by inadequate intake, poor absorption, or abnormal metabolism of these nutrients are the most common nutritional anemias. Some nonnutrition-related causes of anemia include massive blood loss, infections, hereditary blood disorders such as sickle-cell anemia, and chronic liver or kidney disease.

E

ASSESSMENT OF IRON DEFICIENCY

Iron deficiency, a common mineral deficiency, develops in stages. Chapter 13 describes iron deficiency in detail. This section describes tests used to uncover iron deficiency as it progresses. Table E–18 shows which laboratory tests detect various stages of iron deficiency. Although other tests are more specific in detecting early deficiencies, hemoglobin and hematocrit are the commonly available tests.

Stages of iron deficiency:

1. Iron stores diminish.
2. Transport iron decreases.
3. Hemoglobin production falls.

Table E–18
Laboratory Tests Useful in Evaluating Nutrition-Related Anemias

Test or Test Result	What It Reflects
General Tests for Anemia	
Hemoglobin (Hg)	Total amount of hemoglobin in the red blood cells (RBC)
Hematocrit (Hct)	Percentage of RBC in the total blood volume
Red blood cell (RBC) count	Number of RBC
Mean corpuscular volume (MCV)	RBC size; helps to determine if anemia is microcytic or macrocytic
Mean corpuscular hemoglobin concentration (MCHC)	Hemoglobin concentration within the average RBC; helps to determine if anemia is hypochromic or normochromic
Bone marrow aspiration	The manufacture of blood cells in different developmental states
Iron-Deficiency Anemia	
↓ Serum ferritin	Early deficiency state with depleted iron stores
↓ Transferrin saturation	Progressing deficiency state with diminished transport iron
↑ Erythrocyte protoporphyrin	Later deficiency state with limited hemoglobin production
Folate-Deficiency Anemia	
↓ Serum Folate	Progressing deficiency state
↓ RBC Folate	Later deficiency state
Vitamin B_{12}-Deficiency Anemia	
↓ Serum vitamin B_{12}	Progressing deficiency state
Schilling test	Absorption of vitamin B_{12}

Hemoglobin Iron forms an integral part of the hemoglobin molecule that transports oxygen to the cells. In iron deficiency, the body cannot synthesize hemoglobin. Low hemoglobin values signal depleted iron stores. Table E–19 provides hemoglobin values used in nutrition assessment. Hemoglobin's usefulness in evaluating iron status is limited, however, because hemoglobin concentrations drop fairly late in the development of iron deficiency, and other nutrient deficiencies and medical conditions can also alter hemoglobin concentrations.

Hematocrit Hematocrit is commonly used to diagnose iron deficiency, even though it is an inconclusive measure of iron status. To measure the hematocrit, a clinician spins a volume of blood in a centrifuge to separate the red blood cells from the plasma. The hematocrit is the percentage of red blood cells in the total blood volume. Table E–20 provides values used to assess hematocrit status. Low values indicate incomplete hemoglobin formation, which is manifested by microcytic (abnormally small-celled), hypochromic (abnormally lacking in color) red blood cells.

Table E–19
Standards for Hemoglobin Test Results

Age (yr)	Sex	Deficient (g/100 ml)	Acceptable (g/100 ml)
<2	M–F	<9.0	10.0 or >
2–5	M–F	<10.0	11.0 or >
6–12	M–F	<10.0	11.5 or >
13–16	M	<12.0	13.0 or >
	F	<10.0	11.5 or >
>16	M	<12.0	14.0 or >
	F	<10.0	12.0 or >
Trimester 2		<9.5	11.0 or >
Trimester 3		<9.0	10.5 or >

Note: To convert hemoglobin values (g/ml) to international standard units, multiply by 10.

Table E–20
Standards for Hematocrit Test Results

Age (yr)	Sex	Deficient	Acceptable
<2	M–F	<28%	31% or >
2–5	M–F	<30%	34% or >
6–12	M–F	<30%	36% or >
13–16	M	<37%	40% or >
	F	<31%	36% or >
>16	M	<37%	44% or >
	F	<31%	38% or >
Trimester 2		<30%	35% or >
Trimester 3		<30%	33% or >

Note: To convert hematocrit values (%) to standard units, multiply by 0.01.

Low hemoglobin and hematocrit values alert the assessor to the possibility of iron deficiency. However, many nutrients and other conditions can affect hemoglobin and hematocrit. The other tests of iron status help pinpoint true iron deficiency.

Serum Ferritin In the first stage of iron deficiency, iron stores diminish. Serum ferritin measures provide a noninvasive estimate of iron stores. Such information is most valuable to iron assessment. Table E–21 shows serum ferritin cutoff values that indicate iron store depletion in children and adults. Serum ferritin is not reliable for diagnosing iron deficiency in infants, since normal serum ferritin values are often present in conjunction with iron-responsive anemia.

A decrease in transport iron characterizes the second stage of iron deficiency. This is revealed by an increase in the iron-binding capacity of the protein transferrin and a decrease in serum iron. These changes are reflected by the transferrin saturation, which is calculated from the ratio of the other two values as described in the following sections.

E

Total Iron-Binding Capacity (TIBC) Iron travels through the blood bound to the protein transferrin. TIBC is a measure of the total amount of iron that transferrin can carry. Lab technicians measure iron-binding capacity directly.

TIBC values greater than 400 μg/100 ml indicate iron deficiency.*

Serum Iron Lab technicians can also measure serum iron directly. Elevated values indicate iron overload; reduced values indicate iron deficiency. Table E–22 shows acceptable and deficient values for serum iron.

Transferrin Saturation The percentage of transferrin that is saturated with iron is an indirect measure that is derived from the serum iron and total iron-binding capacity measures as follows:

$$\%\text{Transferrin} = \frac{\text{serum iron} \times 100}{\text{total iron-binding capacity}}.$$

*To convert iron-binding capacity (μg/100 ml) to international standard units (μmol/L) multiply by 0.1791. 400 μg/100 ml = 71 μmol/L.

Table E–21
Standards for Serum Ferritin

Group	Deficient (ng/ml)
Children (3–14 years of age)	<10
Adolescents and adults	<12
Pregnant women	<10

Table E–22
Standards for Serum Iron

		Deficient		Acceptable	
Age (yr)	Sex	(μg/100 ml)	(μmol/L)	(μg/100ml)	(μmol/L)
<2	M–F	<30	<5.3	30 or >	5.3 or >
2–5	M–F	<40	<7.1	40 or >	7.1 or >
6–12	M–F	<50	<8.9	50 or >	8.9 or>
>12	M	<60	<10.7	60 or >	10.7 or>
	F	<40	<7.1	40 or >	7.1 or >

Note: To convert (μg/100 ml) to international standard units, multiply by 0.1791.

Table E–23 shows deficient and acceptable transferrin saturation values for various age groups.

The third stage of iron deficiency occurs when the supply of transport iron diminishes to the point that it limits hemoglobin production. It is characterized by increases in erythrocyte protoporphyrin, a decrease in mean corpuscular volume, and decreased hemoglobin concentration and hematocrit.

Erythrocyte Protoporphyrin The iron-containing portion of the hemoglobin molecule is heme. Heme is a combination of iron and protoporphyrin. Protoporphyrin accumulates in the blood when iron supplies are inadequate for the formation of heme. Lab technicians can measure erythrocyte protoporphyrin directly in a blood sample. The cutoffs for abnormal values of erythrocyte protoporphyrin are shown in Table E–24.

E

Mean Corpuscular Volume (MCV) A direct or calculated measure of the mean corpuscular volume (MCV) determines the average size of a red blood cell (RBC). Such a measure helps to classify the type of nutrient anemia. In iron deficiency, the red blood cells are smaller than average. The cutoffs for abnormal values of MCV that indicate iron deficiency are also shown in Table E–24.

ASSESSMENT OF FOLATE AND VITAMIN B12 ANEMIAS

Folate deficiency and vitamin B_{12} deficiency present a similar clinical picture—an anemia characterized by abnormally large red blood cell precursors (megaloblasts) in the bone marrow and abnormally large, mature red blood cells (macrocytic cells) in the blood. Distinguishing between these two deficiencies is particularly important because their treatments differ. Giving folate to a person with vitamin B_{12} deficiency improves many of the lab test results indicative of vitamin B_{12} deficiency, but this

Table E–23
Standards for Percent Transferrin Saturation

Age (yr)	Sex	Deficient	Acceptable
<2	M–F	<15%	15% or >
2–12	M–F	<20%	20% or >
≥13	M	<20%	20% or >
	F	<15%	15% or >

Table E–24
Standards for Erythrocyte Protoporphyrin and Mean Corpuscular Volume

Age (yr)	Erythrocyte Protoporphyrin (μg/dl RBC)	MCV (fL)
1–2	>80	<73
3–4	>75	<75
5–10	>70	<76
11–14	>70	<78
15–74	>70	<80

is a dangerous error because vitamin B_{12} deficiency causes nerve damage that folate cannot correct. Thus inappropriate folate administration masks vitamin B_{12}-deficiency anemia, and nerve damage worsens. For this reason, it is critical to determine whether the anemia results from a folate deficiency or from a vitamin B_{12} deficiency. The following biochemical assessment techniques help to make this distinction.

Mean Corpuscular Volume (MCV) As previously mentioned, the MCV is a measure of red blood cell size. In folate and vitamin B_{12} deficiencies, the red blood cells are larger than average (macrocytic). Additional tests must be performed to differentiate folate from vitamin B_{12}deficiency.

Folate Levels Serum folate levels fluctuate with changes in folate intake and metabolism. Thus serum folate concentrations reflect current status, but provide little information about folate stores. As folate deficiency progresses and low serum levels persist, folate stores decline, resulting in folate depletion. Folate depletion is characterized by a fall in the folate concentrations of red blood cells (erythrocytes). As erythrocyte folate levels diminish, folate-deficiency anemia develops. Because low erythrocyte folate concentrations also occur with vitamin B_{12} deficiency, serum vitamin B_{12} concentrations must also be measured. Table E–25 shows standards for folate assessment.

Vitamin B_{12} Levels Vitamin B_{12} deficiency usually arises from malabsorption. To determine whether malabsorption is the cause, a small oral dose of vitamin B_{12} is given, and urinary excretion is measured. This procedure measures vitamin B_{12} absorption and is called a Schilling test.

Early stages of vitamin B_{12} deficiency can be detected by a low percentage saturation of its transport protein, a measure similar to iron's transferrin saturation. As the deficiency progresses, serum vitamin B_{12} concentrations fall.

CAUTIONS ABOUT NUTRITION ASSESSMENT

To give all the details of nutrition assessment procedures would entail writing another textbook. Nevertheless, any student of nutrition should know the basics of a proper nutrition assessment procedure for two reasons.

First, competent medical care includes attention to nutrition. Physicians should either employ a person skilled in nutrition assessment techniques or refer all clients to such a person to ensure the sound nutrition health of their clients. Health care facilities should make nutrition assessment a routine part of the initial workup on

Table E–25
Standards for Folate Concentrations

	Deficient (ng/ml)	Borderline (ng/ml)	Acceptable (ng/ml)
Serum folate	<3.0	3.0–6.0	>6.0
Erythrocyte folate	<140	140–160	>160

Note: To convert folate values (ng/ml) to international standard units (nmol/L), multiply by 2.266.

every client so that nutritional handicaps will not hinder the response to medical treatment and the recovery from illness.

Second, because nutrition is such a popular subject today, fraudulent practices are even more abundant than they have been in the past (and they have always been rampant). The knowledgeable consumer needs to know what procedures to expect in a nutrition assessment and what kinds of information they yield. This appendix has presented the basics of nutrition assessment for these reasons.

This caution is added: the tests outlined here yield information that becomes meaningful only when integrated into a whole picture by a skilled, experienced, and educated interpreter. Potential sources of error are many, from the taking of the initial data to their reporting and analysis. Each assessment method and measure is useful only as a part of the whole to confirm or eliminate the possibility of suspected nutrition problems. For example, the assessor must constantly remember that a sufficient intake of a nutrient does not guarantee adequate nutrient status for an individual. Conversely, the apparent inadequate intake of a nutrient does not, by itself, establish that a deficiency exists.

Similarly, many uncertainties, such as the calibration of the equipment, the skills of the measurer, and the perspective of the interpreter, limit the accuracy and value of anthropometric measures. This is also true of the results of the physical examination. Physical signs suggestive of malnutrition are nonspecific: they can reflect nutrient deficiencies or may be totally unrelated to nutrition. Assessors must interpret physical findings in light of other assessment findings. Finally, the usefulness of biochemical tests is also limited; the assessor must use caution in interpreting results. Vitamin and mineral blood concentrations may reflect disease processes, abnormal hormone levels, or other aberrations rather than dietary intake. Even if concentrations do reflect dietary intake, they may reflect what the person has been eating recently and not give a true picture of the person's nutrient status. Such complications sometimes make it difficult to detect a subclinical deficiency. Furthermore, many nutrients interact. The assessor has to keep in mind that an abnormal lab value for one nutrient may reflect abnormal status of other nutrients. The final diagnosis is therefore appropriately tentative, and its confirmation comes only after careful remedial steps successfully alleviate the observed problems.

NUTRITION RESOURCES

Contents

APPENDIX F

People interested in nutrition often want to know where they can find reliable nutrition information. Wherever you live, there are several sources you can turn to:

- The Department of Health may have a nutrition expert.
- The local extension agent is often an expert.
- The food editor of your local paper may be well informed.
- The dietitian at the local hospital had to fulfill a set of qualifications before he or she became an RD (see Highlight 1).
- There may be knowledgeable professors of nutrition or biochemistry at a nearby college or university.

In addition, you may be interested in building a nutrition library of your own. Books you can buy, journals you can subscribe to, and addresses you can write to for general information are given below.

BOOKS

For students seeking to establish a personal library of nutrition references, the authors of this text recommend the following books:

- *Present Knowledge in Nutrition,* 6th ed. (Washington, D.C.: International Life Sciences Institute—Nutrition Foundation, 1990).

This 532-page paperback has a chapter on each of 59 topics, including energy, obesity, each of the nutrients, several diseases, malnutrition, growth and its assessment, immunity, alcohol, fiber, exercise, drugs, and toxins. Watch for an update; new editions come out every few years.

- M. E. Shils, J. A. Olson, and M. Shike, eds., *Modern Nutrition in Health and Disease,* 8th ed. (Philadelphia: Lea & Febiger, 1994).

This two-volume set is a major technical reference book on nutrition topics. It contains encyclopedic articles on the nutrients, foods, the diet, metabolism, malnutrition, age-related needs, and nutrition in disease.

- Food and Nutrition Board, *Recommended Dietary Allowances,* 10th ed. (Washington, D.C.: National Academy Press, 1989).

This book reviews the function of each nutrient, dietary sources, and deficiency and toxicity symptoms as well as recommendations for intakes. The Canadian equivalent is *Nutrition Recommendations,* available by mail from the Canadian Government Publishing Centre, Supply and Services Canada, Ottawa, Ontario K1A OS9, Canada.

- Food and Nutrition Board, *Diet and Health: Implications for Reducing Chronic Disease Risk* (Washington, D.C.: National Academy Press, 1989).

This 749-page book presents the integral relationship between diet and chronic disease prevention. Its nutrient chapters provide evidence on how diet influences disease development, and its disease chapters review the dietary patterns implicated in each chronic disease.

- E. M. N. Hamilton and S. A. S. Gropper, *The Biochemistry of Human Nutrition: A Desk Reference* (St. Paul, Minn.: West, 1987).

This 324-page paperback presents the biochemical concepts necessary for an understanding of nutrition. It is a handy reference book for those who have forgotten the basics of biochemistry or for those who are learning biochemistry for the first time.

We also recommend three of our own books that explore current topics in nutrition, health, and the life span:

- E. N. Whitney, C. B. Cataldo, L. K. DeBruyne, and S. R. Rolfes, *Nutrition for Health and Health Care* (St. Paul, Minn.: West, 1995).
- F. S. Sizer and E. N. Whitney, *Nutrition: Concepts and Controversies*, 6th ed. (St. Paul, Minn.: West, 1994).
- S. R. Rolfes, L. K. DeBruyne, and E. N. Whitney, *Life Span Nutrition: Conception through Life* (St. Paul, Minn.: West, 1990).

JOURNALS

Nutrition Today is an excellent magazine for the interested layperson. It makes a point of raising controversial issues and providing a forum for conflicting opinions. Six issues per year are published. Order from Williams and Wilkins, 428 East Preston Street, Baltimore, MD 21202.

The *Journal of the American Dietetic Association*, the official publication of the ADA, contains articles of interest to dietitians and nutritionists, news of legislative action on food and nutrition, and a very useful section of abstracts of articles from many other journals of nutrition and related areas. There are twelve issues per year, available from the American Dietetic Association (see "Addresses," later).

Nutrition Reviews, a publication of the International Life Sciences Institute, does much of the work for the library researcher, compiling recent evidence on current topics and presenting extensive bibliographies. Twelve issues per year are available from Springer-Verlag New York, 175 Fifth Avenue, New York, NY 10010.

Nutrition and the M.D. is a monthly newsletter that provides up-to-date, easy-to-read, practical information on nutrition for health care providers. It is available from PM, Inc., 7100 Hayven Hurst Avenue, Suite 107, Van Nuys, CA 91406.

Other journals that deserve mention here are *Food Technology*, *Journal of Nutrition*, *American Journal of Clinical Nutrition*, *Nutrition Research*, and *Journal of Nutrition Education*. *FDA Consumer*, a government publication with many articles of interest to the consumer, is available from the Food and Drug Administration (see "Addresses," below). Many other journals of value are referred to throughout this book.

ADDRESSES

Many of the organizations listed below will provide publication lists free on request.

U.S. GOVERNMENT

- Federal Trade Commission (FTC)
  Public Reference Branch
  (202) 326-2222

- Food and Drug Administration (FDA)
  Office of Consumer Affairs
  5600 Fishers Lane, HFE 88 Room 16–59
  Rockville, MD 20857
  (301) 443-3170 1 PM–3:30 PM EST

- FDA Office of Food Labeling (HFS-150)
  200 C Street SW
  Washington, DC 20204
  (202) 205-4561; fax: (202) 205-4564

- FDA Office of Plant and Dairy Foods and Beverages (HFS-300)
  200 C Street SW
  Washington, DC 20204
  (202) 205-4064; fax: (202) 205-4422

- FDA Office of Special Nutritionals (HFS-450)
  200 C Street SW
  Washington, DC 20204
  (202) 205-4168; fax: (202) 205-5295

- Food and Nutrition Information Center
  National Agricultural Library, Room 304
  10301 Baltimore Blvd.
  Beltsville, MD 20705-2351
  (301) 504-5719; fax: (301) 504-6409
  Internet e-mail: fnic@nalusda.gov

- Food Research and Action Center
  1875 Connecticut Avenue, NW, Suite 540
  Washington, DC 20009
  (202) 986-2200

- Superintendent of Documents
  P.O. Box 371954
  Pittsburgh, PA 15250-7954
  (202) 512-1800

- U.S. Department of Agriculture (USDA)
  14th Street SW and Independence Avenue
  Washington, DC 20250
  (202) 720-2791

- USDA Center for Nutrition Policy and Promotion
  1120 20th Street, NW, Suite 200, North Lobby
  Washington, DC 20036
  (202) 418-2321

- U.S. Department of Education (DOE)
  Accreditation Agency Evaluation Branch
  7th and D Street SW, Building 3, Room 336
  Washington, DC 20202
  (202) 708-7417

- U.S. Environmental Protection Agency (EPA)
  Public Information Center, 3404
  401 M Street SW
  Washington, DC 20460
  (202) 260-2080

- U.S. Public Health Service Public Affairs Office
  Hubert H. Humphrey Building, Room 725–H
  200 Independence Avenue SW
  Washington, DC 20201
  (202) 245-6867

CANADIAN GOVERNMENT

- Bureau of Nutritional Sciences, Food Directorate
  Health Protection Branch, Health Canada
  Sir Frederick Banting Research Centre
  Tunney's Pasture
  Ottawa, Ontario K1A 0L2, Canada

- Food Production and Inspection Branch
  Agriculture and Agri-Food Canada
  59 Camelot Drive
  Nepean, Ontario K1A 0Y9, Canada
  e-mail: http//aceis.agr.ca

- Nutrition Programs Unit
  Healthy Living and Disease Prevention Directorate
  Health Promotion and Services Branch
  Health Canada
  Jeanne Mance Building
  Tunney's Pasture
  Ottawa, Ontario K1A 1B4, Canada
  e-mail: http://hwc.ca

- Nutrition Specialist, Health Support Services
  Indian and Northern Health Services
  Health Canada
  11th Floor, Jeanne Mance Building
  Tunney's Pasture
  Ottawa, Ontario K1A 0L3, Canada

INTERNATIONAL AGENCIES

- Food and Agriculture Organization of the United Nations (FAO), Liaison Office for North America
  1001 22nd Street NW
  Washington, DC 20437
  (202) 653-2400

- World Health Organization (WHO)
  Regional Office
  525 23rd Street NW
  Washington, DC 20037
  (202) 861-3200

CONSUMER ORGANIZATIONS

- Center for Science in the Public Interest (CSPI)
  1875 Connecticut Avenue NW, Suite 300
  Washington, DC 20009

- Choice in Dying, Inc.
  200 Varick Street, Suite 1001
  New York, NY 10014
  (212) 366-5540; fax: (212) 366-5337

- Consumer Information Catalog
  Pueblo, CO 81009

- Consumers Union of US Inc.
  101 Truman Avenue
  Yonkers, NY 10703–1057
  (914) 378-2000

- National Council Against Health Fraud, Inc.
  P.O. Box 1276
  Loma Linda, CA 92354

FOOD SAFETY

- Alliance for Food & Fiber
  Food Safety Hotline
  (800) 266-0200

- FDA Seafood Hotline
  (800) FDA-4010

- National Lead Information Center
  (800) LEAD-FYI (532-3394)
  (800) 424-LEAD (424-5323)

- National Pesticide Telecommunications Network
  Oregon State University
  Agricultural Chemistry Extension
  Weniger Hall 333
  Corvallis, OR 97331-6502

- USDA Meat and Poultry Hotline
  (800) 535-4555

- U.S. EPA Safe Drinking Water Hotline
  (800) 426-4791

INFANCY AND CHILDHOOD

- Association of Birth Defect Children, Inc.
  827 Irma Street
  Orlando, FL 32803
  (407) 245-7035

- American Academy of Pediatrics
  141 Northwest Point Boulevard
  P.O. Box 927
  Elk Grove Village, IL 60009–0927

- Canadian Pediatric Society
  410 Smyth Road
  Ottawa, Ontario K1H 8L1, Canada

- Nurture/Center to Prevent Childhood Malnutrition
  1840 18th Street, NW
  Washington, DC 20009
  (202) 797-9244; fax: (202) 797-9257

PROFESSIONAL NUTRITION ORGANIZATIONS

- American Dietetic Association
  National Center for Nutrition and Dietetics
  216 West Jackson Boulevard, Suite 800
  Chicago, IL 60606–6995
  (312) 899-0040; (800) 366-1655
  Internet e-mail: ncndtis @ aol.com
- American Institute of Nutrition
  American Society for Clinical Nutrition
  9650 Rockville Pike
  Bethesda, MD 20814-3998
- Canadian Dietetic Association
  480 University Avenue, Suite 601
  Toronto, Ontario M5G 1V2, Canada
  (416) 596-0857
- National Academy of Sciences/National Research Council (NAS/NRC)
  2101 Constitution Avenue NW
  Washington, DC 20418
- National Institute of Nutrition
  302-265 Carling Avenue
  Ottawa, Ontario K1S 2E1, Canada
- Nutrition Foundation, Inc. (INACG)
  1126 Sixteenth Street NW, Suite 111
  Washington, DC 20036
- Nutrition Information Service
  University of Alabama at Birmingham
  Room 447 Webb Building
  UAB Station
  Birmingham, AL 35294-3360

ALCOHOL AND DRUG ABUSE

- Al-Anon Family Group Headquarters
  P.O. Box 862, Midtown Station
  New York, NY 10018–0862
  (800) 356-9996
- Alateen
  1372 Broadway
  New York, NY 10018
  (800) 356-9996
- Alcohol & Drug Abuse Information Line
  (800) 252-6465
- Alcoholics Anonymous (AA)
  475 Riverside Drive
  New York, NY 10115
  (212) 870-3400
- Narcotics Anonymous (NA)
  P.O. Box 9999
  Van Nuys, CA 91409-9999
  (818) 773-9999
- National Council on Alcoholism and Drug Dependence, Inc.
  12 West 21st Street
  New York, NY 10010
  (800) NCA-CALL
- National Clearinghouse for Alcohol and Drug Information (NCADI)
  P.O. Box 2345
  Rockville, MD 20847-2345
  (800) 729-6686

WEIGHT CONTROL AND EATING DISORDERS

- American Anorexia & Bulimia Association, Inc.
  293 Central Park West, Suite 1R
  New York, NY 10012
  (212) 501-8351
- Anorexia Nervosa and Related Eating Disorders, Inc.
  P.O. Box 5102
  Eugene, OR 97405
- National Association of Anorexia Nervosa and Associated Disorders, Inc. (ANAD)
  P.O. Box 7
  Highland Park, IL 60035
  (708) 831-3438
- National Eating Disorder Information Centre
  200 Elizabeth Street, College Wing 1-328
  Toronto, Ontario M5G 2C4, Canada
- Overeaters Anonymous (OA)
  6075 Zenith Court NE
  Rio Ranchio, NM 87124-6424
  (505) 891-2664
- TOPS (Take Off Pounds Sensibly)
  P.O. Box 07360
  Milwaukee, WI 53207
  (800) 932-8677

FITNESS

- American College of Sports Medicine
  P.O. Box 1440
  Indianapolis, IN 46204
  (317) 637-9200

PREGNANCY

- American College of Obstetricians and Gynecologists
  409 12th Street SW
  Washington, DC 20024-2188
  (202) 638-5577
- March of Dimes Birth Defects Foundation
  (National Headquarters)
  1275 Mamaroneck Avenue
  White Plains, NY 10605

TRADE AND INDUSTRY ORGANIZATIONS

- Ralcorp Holdings, Inc.
  Beech-Nut Nutrition Corporation
  800 Market Street
  St. Louis, MO 63106
  (800) 523-6633
- Borden Farm Products, Product Publicity
  180 East Broad Street
  Columbus, OH 43215
- Campbell Soup Company, Food Service Division
  Campbell Place
  Camden, NJ 08103-1799
- Elan Pharma, Nutrition Division
  2 Thurber Blvd.
  Smithfield, RI 02917
- Kraft Foods
  Consumer Response and Information Center
  One Kraft Court
  Glenview, Illinois 60025
- General Mills, Inc., Nutrition Department
  Number One General Mills Boulevard
  Minneapolis, MN 55426
- Kellogg Company
  P.O. Box CAMB
  Battle Creek, MI 49016-1986
- Mead Johnson Nutritionals
  2400 West Lloyd Expressway
  Evansville, IN 47721
- Nabisco Consumer Affairs
  100 DeForest Avenue
  East Hanover, NJ 07936
  (800) 932-7800; (800) NABISCO
- National Dairy Council
  10255 West Higgins Road, Suite 900
  Rosemond, IL 60018
- The NutraSweet Company
  P.O. Box 830
  1751 Lake Cook Road
  Deerfield, IL 60015-5239
  (800) 323-5316
- Pillsbury Company, Consumer Relations
  P.O. Box 550
  Minneapolis, MN 55440-9843
- Procter and Gamble Company
  One Procter and Gamble Plaza
  Cincinnati, OH 45202
- Ross Laboratories, Abbot Laboratory
  625 Cleveland Avenue
  Columbus, OH 43216
- Sherwood Medical
  1915 Olive Street
  St. Louis, MO 63103
- Sunkist Growers, Consumer Affairs
  P.O. Box 7888
  Van Nuys, CA 91409-7888
- United Fresh Fruit and Vegetable Association
  727 North Washington Street
  Alexandria, VA 22314
  (703) 836-3410
- USA Rice Council
  P.O. Box 740121
  Houston, TX 77274
- Vitamin Nutrition Information Service (VNIS)
  Hoffmann-LaRoche, Inc.
  340 Kingsland Street
  Nutley, NJ 07110
- Weight Watchers® Food Company
  Consumer Affairs Department
  P.O. Box 10
  Boise, ID 83707–0010

WORLD HUNGER

- Bread for the World
  1100 Wayne Ave., Ste 1000
  Silver Spring, MD 20910
- Center on Hunger, Poverty and Nutrition Policy
  Tufts University School of Nutrition
  11 Curtis Avenue
  Medford, MA 02155
  (617) 627-3956
- Freedom from Hunger
  P.O. Box 2000
  1644 DaVinci Court
  Davis, CA 95617
  (916) 758-6200
- Oxfam America
  115 Broadway
  Boston, MA 02116
- SEEDS Magazine
  P.O. Box 6170
  Waco, TX 76706
  (817) 755-7745
- Worldwatch Institute
  1776 Massachusetts Avenue NW
  Washington, DC 20036

HEALTH AND DISEASE

- Alzheimer's Association
  919 North Michigan Avenue, Suite 1000
  Chicago, IL 60611
  (800) 272-3900

- Alzheimer's Disease Education and Referral Center
P. O. Box 8250
Silver Spring, Maryland 20907-8250
(800) 438-4380
- American Academy of Allergy, Asthma, and Immunology
611 East Wells Street
Milwaukee, WI 53202
(414) 272-6071; fax: (414) 276-3349
- American Cancer Society Information Center
2200 Lake Blvd.
Atlanta, GA 30319
(800) ACS-2345
- American Council on Science and Health
1995 Broadway, 2nd Floor
New York, NY 10023-5860
- American Dental Association
Dept. of Salable Materials
211 East Chicago Avenue
Chicago, IL 60611-2678
- American Diabetes Association
1660 Duke Street
Alexandria, VA 22314
(703) 549-1500; (800) 232-3472
- American Heart Association
Box BHG, National Center
7320 Greenville Avenue
Dallas, TX 75231
(800) 242-8721
- American Institute for Cancer Research
1759 R Street NW
Washington, DC 20009
- American Medical Association
515 North State Street
Chicago, IL 60610
(312) 464-5000
- American Public Health Association
1015 Fifteenth Street NW
Washington, DC 20005
- American Red Cross AIDS Education Office
1730 D Street NW
Washington, DC 20006
(202) 737-8300
- Canadian Diabetes Association
15 Toronto Street, Suite 1001
Toronto ON M5C 2E3
(416) 363-0177; fax: (416) 363-3393
- Canadian Public Health Association
Publications, Suite 400
1565 Carling Avenue
Ottawa, Ontario K1Z 8R1, Canada
- Centers for Disease Control (CDC)
Information Hotline
(404) 332-4555
- Disease Prevention and Health Promotion's National Health Information Center
(800) 336-4797
- The Food Allergy Network
4744 Holly Avenue
Fairfax, VA 22030-5647
(703) 691-3179
- National AIDS Hotline (CDC)
(800) 342-AIDS (English)
(800) 344-SIDA (Spanish)
(800) 2437-TTY (Deaf)
(900) 820-2437
- National Cancer Institute
31 Center Drive MSC 2580
Building 31, Room 10A16
Bethesda, MD 20892-2580
(800) 4–CANCER; (800) 422-6237
- National Heart, Lung, and Blood Institute
National High Blood Pressure Education Program
P.O. Box 30105
Bethesda, MD 20824-0105
(301) 951-3260
- National Institute of Allergy and Infectious Diseases
Office of Communications, Building 31, Room 7A50
31 Center Drive, MSC 2520
Bethesda, MD 20892-2520
(301) 496-5717
- National Osteoporosis Foundation
1150 17th Street NW, Suite 500
Washington, DC 20036
(202) 223-2226
- Smoking and Health Office (CDC)
Mail Stop K-12
1600 Clifton Road NE
Atlanta, GA 30333

UNITED STATES: RECOMMENDATIONS AND EXCHANGES

WORLD HEALTH ORGANIZATION: RECOMMENDATIONS

Contents

APPENDIX G

Chapters 1 and 2 introduced Recommended Dietary Allowances (RDA), Daily Values, Healthy People 2000, and exchange systems. This appendix provides additional details. (See Appendix I for Canada's nutrition recommendations and exchange system.)

RDA

Some of the U.S. recommendations for nutrient intakes appear in the RDA table on the inside front cover, left. The remaining RDA are here, in Tables G–1, G–2, and G–3.

U.S. RDA AND DAILY VALUES

Food labels use another set of standards that derive from the RDA. From the late 1960s to the early 1990s, the set of standards used on food labels was called the U.S. RDA. The U.S. RDA were derived from the 1968 RDA and were established by the Food and Drug Administration (FDA) so that labels could express the nutrient contents of foods as percentages of those standards (see Table G–4). The intent was to help consumers evaluate the nutrient contents of foods for themselves and at the same time to spare them the burden of learning the different units in which nutrient amounts are expressed. Thus all nutrient amounts in a food, whether originally measured in micrograms, milligrams, grams, or RE, could be expressed as "percent of U.S. RDA."

With the new labeling regulations came a name change. The revised set of standards used on food labels—the Daily Values—are discussed fully in Chapter 2. With the exception of protein, the current Daily Values continue to use the same values as the old U.S. RDA. The FDA continues to consider their revision.

Table G–1
Estimated Safe and Adequate Daily Dietary Intakes of Additional Selected Vitamins and Minerals (United States)[a]

	Vitamins		Trace Elements[b]				
Age (yr)	Biotin (μg)	Pantothenic Acid (mg)	Chromium (μg)	Molybdenum (μg)	Copper (mg)	Manganese (mg)	Fluoride (mg)
Infants							
0–0.5	10	2	10–40	15–30	0.4–0.6	0.3–0.6	0.1–0.5
0.5–1	15	3	20–60	20–40	0.6–0.7	0.6–1.0	0.2–1.0
Children							
1–3	20	3	20–80	25–50	0.7–1.0	1.0–1.5	0.5–1.5
4–6	25	3–4	30–120	30–75	1.0–1.5	1.5–2.0	1.0–2.5
7–10	30	4–5	50–200	50–150	1.0–2.0	2.0–3.0	1.5–2.5
11+	30–100	4–7	50–200	75–250	1.5–2.5	2.0–5.0	1.5–2.5
Adults	30–100	4–7	50–200	75–250	1.5–3.0	2.0–5.0	1.5–4.0

[a]Less information is available on which to base allowances for these nutrients. Therefore, they are not included in the main table of the RDA, and the figures provided here are in the form of ranges of recommended intakes.
[b]The toxic levels for many trace elements may be only several times usual intakes, so the upper levels for the trace elements given in this table should not be habitually exceeded.
Source: Recommended Dietary Allowances, © 1989 by the National Academy of Sciences, National Academy Press, Washington, D.C.

G

Table G–2
Estimated Minimum Requirements of Sodium, Chloride, and Potassium

Age (yr)	Weight (kg)	Sodium[a] (mg)	Chloride (mg)	Potassium[b] (mg)
Infants				
0.0–0.5	4.5	120	180	500
0.5–1.0	8.9	200	300	700
Children				
1	11.0	225	350	1000
2–5	16.0	300	500	1400
6–9	25.0	400	600	1600
Adolescents	50.0	500	750	2000
Adults	70.0	500	750	2000

[a]Sodium requirements are based on estimates of needs for growth and for replacement of obligatory losses. They cover a wide variation of physical activity patterns and climatic exposure but do not provide for large, prolonged losses from the skin through sweat.
[b]Dietary potassium may benefit the prevention and treatment of hypertension, and recommendations to include many servings of fruits and vegetables would raise potassium intakes to about 3500 milligrams per day.
Source: Recommended Dietary Allowances, © 1989 by the National Academy of Sciences, National Academy Press, Washington, D.C.

Table G–3
Median Heights and Weights and Recommended Energy Intakes (United States)

Age (yr)	Weight		Height		Average Energy Allowance			
	kg	lb	cm	in	REE[a] (kcal/day)	MULTIPLES OF REE[b]	kcal/kg	kcal/day[c]
Infants								
0.0–0.5	6	13	60	24	320		108	650
0.5–1.0	9	20	71	28	500		98	850
Children								
1–3	13	29	90	35	740		102	1300
4–6	20	44	112	44	950		90	1800
7–10	28	62	132	52	1130		70	2000
Males								
11–14	45	99	157	62	1440	1.70	55	2500
15–18	66	145	176	69	1760	1.67	45	3000
19–24	72	160	177	70	1780	1.67	40	2900
25–50	79	174	176	70	1800	1.60	37	2900
51+	77	170	173	68	1530	1.50	30	2300
Females								
11–14	46	101	157	62	1310	1.67	47	2200
15–18	55	120	163	64	1370	1.60	40	2200
19–24	58	128	164	65	1350	1.60	38	2200
25–50	63	138	163	64	1380	1.55	36	2200
51+	65	143	160	63	1280	1.50	30	1900
Pregnant (2nd and 3rd trimesters)								+300
Lactating								+500

[a]REE (resting energy expenditure) represents the energy expended by a person at rest under normal conditions.

[b]Recommended energy allowances assume light-to-moderate activity and were calculated by multiplying the REE by an activity factor.

[c]Average energy allowances have been rounded.

Source: Recommended Dietary Allowances, © 1989 by the National Academy of Sciences, National Academy Press, Washington, D.C.

G

Table G–4
U.S. Recommended Daily Allowances (U.S. RDA)

Nutrient	Adults and Children over 4 Years	Infants	Children under 4 Years	Pregnant or Lactating Women
Protein (g)	45[a]	18[a]	20[a]	
Vitamin A (RE)	1000	300	500	1600
Vitamin D[b] (IU)	400	400	400	400
Vitamin E[b] (IU)	30	5.0	10	30
Vitamin C (mg)	60	35	40	60
Folate (mg)	0.4	0.1	0.2	0.8
Thiamin (mg)	1.5	0.5	0.7	1.7
Riboflavin (mg)	1.7	0.6	0.8	2.0
Niacin (mg)	20	8	9	20
Vitamin B_6[b] (mg)	2.0	0.4	0.7	2.5
Vitamin B_{12}[b] (μg)	6.0	2.0	3.0	8.0
Biotin[b] (mg)	0.3	0.5	0.15	0.3
Pantothenic acid[b] (mg)	10	3	5	10
Calcium (g)	1.0	0.6	0.8	1.3
Phosphorus[b] (g)	1.0	0.5	0.8	1.3
Iodine[b] (μg)	150	45	70	150
Iron (mg)	18	15	10	18
Magnesium[b] (mg)	400	70	200	450
Copper[b] (mg)	2.0	0.6	1.0	2.0
Zinc[b] (mg)	15	5	8	15

Note: Four sets of U.S. RDA were developed for different groups of people—infants, children, adults, and pregnant and lactating women. The most commonly used set was the U.S. RDA for adults. The one for infants was used for formulas. Supplements designed for children and for pregnant and lactating women used the U.S. RDA for these groups on their labels.

[a]If protein efficiency ratio of protein is equal to or better than that of casein.

[b]Optional for adults and children 4 years or over in vitamin and mineral supplements.

Source: U.S. Department of Health and Human Services, Public Health Service, Food and Drug Administration, Office of Public Affairs, 5600 Fishers Lane, Rockville, Maryland 20857, HHS publication no. (FDA) 81–2146, revised March 1981.

HEALTHY PEOPLE 2000

◆

In 1990, the U.S. Department of Health and Human Services established a set of almost 300 health objectives for the nation called *Healthy People 2000.*[1] The 21 objectives that have a nutrition component were presented throughout this text wherever their topic was discussed. Table G–5 presents them in full.

Table G–5
Healthy People 2000 Nutrition Objectives

Health-Related Objectives

- Reduce coronary heart disease deaths to no more than 100 per 100,000 people.
- Reverse the rise in cancer deaths to achieve a rate of no more than 130 per 100,000 people.
- Reduce overweight to a prevalence of no more than 20% among people aged 20 years and older and maintain prevalence at no more than 15% among adolescents aged 12 through 19 years.
- Reduce growth retardation among low-income children aged five years and younger to less than 10%.

Nutrient Intake Objectives

- Reduce dietary fat intake to an average of 30% of energy or less and average saturated fat intake to less than 10% of energy among people aged two years and older.
- Increase complex carbohydrate and fiber-containing foods in the diets of adults to five or more daily servings for vegetables (including legumes) and fruits and to six or more daily servings for grain products.
- Increase to at least 50% the proportion of overweight people aged 12 years and older who have adopted sound dietary practices combined with regular physical activity to attain an appropriate body weight.
- Increase calcium intake, so that at least 50% of youth aged 12 through 24 years and 50% of pregnant and lactating women consume three or more servings of calcium-rich foods daily and at least 50% of people aged 25 years and older consume two or more servings of calcium-rich foods daily.
- Decrease salt and sodium intake so at least 65% of home meal preparers prepare foods without adding salt, at least 80% of people avoid using salt at the table, and at least 40% of adults regularly purchase foods modified or lower in sodium.
- Reduce iron deficiency to less than 3% among children aged 1 to 4 and women of childbearing age.
- Increase to at least 75% the proportion of mothers who breastfeed their babies in the early weeks and to at least 50% the proportion who continue breastfeeding until their babies are five to six months old.
- Increase to at least 75% the proportion of parents and caregivers who use feeding practices that prevent nursing bottle tooth decay.
- Increase to at least 85% the proportion of people aged 18 and older who use food labels to make nutritious food selections.

Services and Information Objectives

- Achieve useful and informative nutrition labeling for virtually all processed foods and at least 40% of fresh meats, poultry, fish, fruits, vegetables, baked goods, and ready-to-eat carry-away foods.
- Increase to at least 5000 brand items the number of processed food products that are reduced in fat and saturated fat.
- Increase to at least 90% the proportion of restaurants and institutional foodservice operations that offer identifiable low-fat, low-kcalorie food choices, consistent with the *Dietary Guidelines for Americans.*
- Increase to at least 90% the proportion of school lunch and breakfast services and increase to at least 50% the proportion of child care foodservices with menus that are consistent with the nutrition principles in the *Dietary Guidelines for Americans.*
- Increase to at least 80% the receipt of home foodservices by people aged 65 and older who have difficulty in preparing their own meals or are otherwise in need of home-delivered meals.
- Increase to at least 75% the proportion of the nation's schools that provide nutrition education from preschool through grade 12, preferably as part of quality school health education.
- Increase to at least 50% the proportion of worksites with 50 or more employees that offer nutrition education and/or weight management programs for employees.
- Increase to at least 75% the proportion of primary care providers who provide nutrition assessment and counseling and/or referral to qualified nutritionists or dietitians.

G

U.S. EXCHANGE LISTS FOR MEAL PLANNING

The U.S. exchange system groups together foods that have about the same amount of carbohydrate, protein, fat, and kcalories. Then any food on a list can be "exchanged" for any other food on that same list. Chapter 2 introduced the exchange lists and Tables G–6 through G–14 present the lists in detail.

Table G–6

U.S. Exchange System: Starch List

1 starch exchange = 15 g carbohydrate, 3 g protein, 0–1 g fat, and 80 kcal
Note: In general, a starch serving is ½ c cereal, grain, pasta, or starchy vegetable; 1 oz of bread; ¾ to 1 oz snack food.

Serving Size	Food
Bread	
½ (1 oz)	Bagels
2 slices (1½ oz)	Bread, reduced-kcalorie
1 slice (1 oz)	Bread, white (including French and Italian), whole-wheat, pumpernickel, rye
2 (⅔ oz)	Bread sticks, crisp, 4″ x ½″
½	English muffins
½ (1 oz)	Hot dog or hamburger buns
½	Pita, 6″ across
1 (1 oz)	Plain rolls, small
1 slice (1 oz)	Raisin bread, unfrosted
1	Tortillas, corn, 6″ across
1	Tortillas, flour, 7–8″ across
1	Waffles, 4½″ square, reduced-fat
Cereals and Grains	
½ c	Bran cereals
½ c	Bulgur, cooked
½ c	Cereals, cooked
¾ c	Cereals, unsweetened, ready-to-eat
3 tbs	Cornmeal (dry)
⅓ c	Couscous
3 tbs	Flour (dry)
¼ c	Granola, low-fat
¼ c	Grape nuts
½ c	Grits, cooked
½ c	Kasha
¼ c	Millet
¼ c	Muesli
½ c	Oats
½ c	Pasta, cooked
1½ c	Puffed cereals
½ c	Rice milk
⅓ c	Rice, white or brown, cooked
½ c	Shredded wheat
½ c	Sugar-frosted cereal
3 tbs	Wheat germ
Starchy Vegetables	
⅓ c	Baked beans
½ c	Corn
1 (5 oz)	Corn on cob, medium
1 c	Mixed vegetables with corn, peas, or pasta
½ c	Peas, green
½ c	Plantains
1 small (3 oz)	Potatoes, baked or boiled
½ c	Potatoes, mashed
1 c	Squash, winter (acorn, butternut)
½ c	Yams, sweet potatoes, plain
Crackers and Snacks	
8	Animal crackers
3	Graham crackers, 2½″ square
¾ oz	Matzoh
4 slices	Melba toast
24	Oyster crackers
3 c	Popcorn (popped, no fat added or low-fat microwave)
¾ oz	Pretzels
2	Rice cakes, 4″ across
6	Saltine-type crackers
15–20 (¾ oz)	Snack chips, fat-free (tortilla, potato)
2–5 (¾ oz)	Whole-wheat crackers, no fat added
Dried Beans, Peas, and Lentils	
½ c	Beans and peas, cooked (garbanzo, lentils, pinto, kidney, white, split, black-eyed)
⅔ c	Lima beans
3 tbs	Miso
Starchy Foods Prepared with Fat	
Count as 1 starch + 1 fat exchange.	
1	Biscuit, 2½″ across
½ c	Chow mein noodles
1 (2 oz)	Corn bread, 2″ cube
6	Crackers, round butter type
1 c	Croutons
16–25 (3 oz)	French-fried potatoes
¼ c	Granola
1 (1½ oz)	Muffin, small
2	Pancake, 4″ across
3 c	Popcorn, microwave
3	Sandwich crackers, cheese or peanut butter filling
⅓ c	Stuffing, bread (prepared)
2	Taco shell, 6″ across
1	Waffle, 4½″ square
4–6 (1 oz)	Whole-wheat crackers, fat added

= 400 mg or more of sodium per serving.

Table G–7
U.S. Exchange System: Fruit List

1 fruit exchange = 15 g carbohydrate and 60 kcal
Note: In general, a fruit serving is 1 small to medium fresh fruit; ½ c canned or fresh fruit or fruit juice; ¼ c dried fruit.

Serving Size	Food	Serving Size	Food
1 (4 oz)	Apples, unpeeled, small	½ (8 oz) or 1 c cubes	Papayas
½ c	Applesauce, unsweetened	1 (6 oz)	Peaches, medium, fresh
4 rings	Apples, dried	½ c	Peaches, canned
4 whole (5½ oz)	Apricots, fresh	½ (4 oz)	Pears, large, fresh
8 halves	Apricots, dried	½ c	Pears, canned
½ c	Apricots, canned	¾ c	Pineapple, fresh
1 (4 oz)	Bananas, small	½ c	Pineapple, canned
¾ c	Blackberries	2 (5 oz)	Plums, small
¾ c	Blueberries	½ c	Plums, canned
⅓ melon (11 oz) or 1 c cubes	Cantaloupe, small	3	Prunes, dried
		2 tbs	Raisins
12 (3 oz)	Cherries, sweet, fresh	1 c	Raspberries
½ c	Cherries, sweet, canned	1¼ c whole berries	Strawberries
3	Dates	2 (8 oz)	Tangerines, small
1½ large or 2 medium (3½ oz)	Figs, fresh	1 slice (13½ oz) or 1¼ c cubes	Watermelon
1½	Figs, dried	**Fruit Juice**	
½ c	Fruit cocktail	½ c	Apple juice/cider
½ (11 oz)	Grapefruit, large	⅓ c	Cranberry juice cocktail
¾ c	Grapefruit sections, canned	1 c	Cranberry juice cocktail, reduced-kcalorie
17 (3 oz)	Grapes, small		
1 slice (10 oz) or 1 c cubes	Honeydew melon	⅓ c	Fruit juice blends, 100% juice
		⅓ c	Grape juice
1 (3½ oz)	Kiwi	½ c	Grapefruit juice
¾ c	Mandarin oranges, canned	½ c	Orange juice
½ (5½ oz) or ½ c	Mangoes, small	½ c	Pineapple juice
1 (5 oz)	Nectarines, small	⅓ c	Prune juice
1 (6½ oz)	Oranges, small		

Table G–8
U.S. Exchange System: Milk List

Serving Size	Food	Serving Size	Food
Nonfat and Very Low-Fat Milk		**Low-Fat Milk**	
1 nonfat/low-fat milk exchange = 12 g carbohydrate, 8 g protein, 0–3 g fat, 90 kcal		1 low-fat milk exchange = 12 g carbohydrate, 8 g protein, 5 g fat, 120 kcal	
1 c	Nonfat milk	1 c	2% milk
1 c	½% milk	¾ c	Plain low-fat yogurt
1 c	1% milk	1 c	Sweet acidophilus milk
1 c	Nonfat or low-fat buttermilk	**Whole Milk**	
½ c	Evaporated nonfat milk	1 whole milk exchange = 12 g carbohydrate, 8 g protein, 8 g fat, 150 kcal	
⅓ c dry	Dry nonfat milk	1 c	Whole milk
¾ c	Plain nonfat yogurt	½ c	Evaporated whole milk
1 c	Nonfat or low-fat fruit-flavored yogurt sweetened with aspartame or with a nonnutritive sweetener	1 c	Goat's milk
		1 c	Kefir

Table G–9
U.S. Exchange System: Other Carbohydrates List

1 other carbohydrate exchange = 15 g carbohydrate, or 1 starch, or 1 fruit, or 1 milk exchange

Food	Serving Size	Exchanges per Serving
Angel food cake, unfrosted	1/12 cake	2 carbohydrates
Brownies, small, unfrosted	2″ square	1 carbohydrate, 1 fat
Cake, unfrosted	2″ square	1 carbohydrate, 1 fat
Cake, frosted	2″ square	2 carbohydrates, 1 fat
Cookie, fat-free	2 small	1 carbohydrate
Cookies or sandwich cookies	2 small	1 carbohydrate, 1 fat
Cupcakes, frosted	1 small	2 carbohydrates, 1 fat
Cranberry sauce, jellied	¼ c	2 carbohydrates
Doughnuts, plain cake	1 medium (1½ oz)	1½ carbohydrates, 2 fats
Doughnuts, glazed	3¾″ across (2 oz)	2 carbohydrates, 2 fats
Fruit juice bars, frozen, 100% juice	1 bar (3 oz)	1 carbohydrate
Fruit snacks, chewy (pureed fruit concentrate)	1 roll (¾ oz)	1 carbohydrate
Fruit spreads, 100% fruit	1 tbs	1 carbohydrate
Gelatin, regular	½ c	1 carbohydrate
Gingersnaps	3	1 carbohydrate
Granola bars	1 bar	1 carbohydrate, 1 fat
Granola bars, fat-free	1 bar	2 carbohydrates
Hummus	⅓ c	1 carbohydrate, 1 fat
Ice cream	½ c	1 carbohydrate, 2 fats
Ice cream, light	½ c	1 carbohydrate, 1 fat
Ice cream, fat-free, no sugar added	½ c	1 carbohydrate
Jam or jelly, regular	1 tbs	1 carbohydrate
Milk, chocolate, whole	1 c	2 carbohydrates, 1 fat
Pie, fruit, 2 crusts	⅙ pie	3 carbohydrates, 2 fats
Pie, pumpkin or custard	⅛ pie	1 carbohydrate, 2 fats
Potato chips	12–18 (1 oz)	1 carbohydrate, 2 fats
Pudding, regular (made with low-fat milk)	½ c	2 carbohydrates
Pudding, sugar-free (made with low-fat milk)	½ c	1 carbohydrate
Salad dressing, fat-free	¼ c	1 carbohydrate
Sherbet, sorbet	½ c	2 carbohydrates
Spaghetti or pasta sauce, canned	½ c	1 carbohydrate, 1 fat
Sweet roll or danish	1 (2½ oz)	2½ carbohydrates, 2 fats
Syrup, light	2 tbs	1 carbohydrate
Syrup, regular	1 tbs	1 carbohydrate
Syrup, regular	¼ c	4 carbohydrates
Tortilla chips	6–12 (1 oz)	1 carbohydrate, 2 fats
Yogurt, frozen, low-fat, fat-free	⅓ c	1 carbohydrate, 0–1 fat
Yogurt, frozen, fat-free, no sugar added	½ c	1 carbohydrate
Yogurt, low-fat with fruit	1 c	3 carbohydrates, 0–1 fat
Vanilla wafers	5	1 carbohydrate, 1 fat

= 400 mg or more sodium per exchange.

Table G–10
U.S. Exchange System: Vegetable List

1 vegetable exchange = 5 g carbohydrate, 2 g protein, 25 kcal
Note: In general, a vegetable serving is ½ c cooked vegetables or vegetable juice; 1 c raw vegetables. Starchy vegetables such as corn, peas, and potatoes are on the starch list.

Artichokes	Mushrooms
Artichoke hearts	Okra
Asparagus	Onions
Beans (green, wax, Italian)	Pea pods
Bean sprouts	Peppers (all varieties)
Beets	Radishes
Broccoli	Salad greens (endive, escarole, lettuce, romaine, spinach)
Brussels sprouts	Sauerkraut
Cabbage	Spinach
Carrots	Summer squash (crookneck)
Cauliflower	Tomatoes
Celery	Tomatoes, canned
Cucumbers	Tomato sauce
Eggplant	Tomato/vegetable juice
Green onions or scallions	Turnips
Greens (collard, kale, mustard, turnip)	Water chestnuts
Kohlrabi	Watercress
Leeks	Zucchini
Mixed vegetables (without corn, peas, or pasta)	

= 400 mg or more sodium per exchange.

G

Table G–11

U.S. Exchange System: Meat and Meat Substitutes List

Note: In general, a meat serving is 1 oz meat, poultry, or cheese; ½ c dried beans (weigh meat and poultry and measure beans after cooking).

Serving Size	Food
Very Lean Meat and Substitutes	
1 very lean meat exchange = 7 g protein, 0–1 g fat, 35 kcal	
1 oz	Poultry: Chicken or turkey (white meat, no skin), Cornish hen (no skin)
1 oz	Fish: Fresh or frozen cod, flounder, haddock, halibut, trout; tuna, fresh or canned in water
1 oz	Shellfish: Clams, crab, lobster, scallops, shrimp, imitation shellfish
1 oz	Game: Duck or pheasant (no skin), venison, buffalo, ostrich
	Cheese with ≤ 1 g fat/oz:
¼ c	Nonfat or low-fat cottage cheese
1 oz	Fat-free cheese
	Other:
1 oz	Processed sandwich meats with ≤ 1 g fat/oz (such as deli thin, shaved meats, chipped beef 🧂, turkey ham)
2	Egg whites
¼ c	Egg substitutes, plain
1 oz	Hot dogs with ≤ 1 g fat/oz
1 oz	Kidney (high in cholesterol)
1 oz	Sausage with ≤ 1 g fat/oz 🧂
Count as one very lean meat and one starch exchange:	
½ c	Dried beans, peas, lentils (cooked)
Lean Meat and Substitutes	
1 lean meat exchange = 7 g protein, 3 g fat, 55 kcal	
1 oz	Beef: USDA Select or Choice grades of lean beef trimmed of fat (round, sirloin, and flank steak); tenderloin; roast (rib, chuck, rump); steak (T-bone, porterhouse, cubed), ground round
1 oz	Pork: Lean pork (fresh ham); canned, cured, or boiled ham; Canadian bacon 🧂; tenderloin, center loin chop
1 oz	Lamb: Roast, chop, leg
1 oz	Veal: Lean chop, roast
1 oz	Poultry: Chicken, turkey (dark meat, no skin), chicken white meat (with skin), domestic duck or goose (well-drained of fat, no skin)
	Fish:
1 oz	Herring (uncreamed or smoked)
6 medium	Oysters
1 oz	Salmon (fresh or canned), catfish
2 medium	Sardines (canned)
1 oz	Tuna (canned in oil, drained)
1 oz	Game: Goose (no skin), rabbit
	Cheese:
¼ c	4.5%-fat cottage cheese
2 tbs	Grated Parmesan
1 oz	Cheeses with ≤ 3 g fat/oz
	Other:
1½ oz	Hot dogs with ≤ 3 g fat/oz 🧂
1 oz	Processed sandwich meat with ≤ 3 g fat/oz (turkey pastrami or kielbasa)
1 oz	Liver, heart (high in cholesterol)
Medium-Fat Meat and Substitutes	
1 medium-fat meat exchange = 7 g protein, 5 g fat, and 75 kcal	
1 oz	Beef: Most beef products (ground beef, meatloaf, corned beef, short ribs, Prime grades of meat trimmed of fat, such as prime rib)
1 oz	Pork: Top loin, chop, Boston butt, cutlet
1 oz	Lamb: Rib roast, ground
1 oz	Veal: Cutlet (ground or cubed, unbreaded)
1 oz	Poultry: Chicken dark meat (with skin), ground turkey or ground chicken, fried chicken (with skin)
1 oz	Fish: Any fried fish product
	Cheese with ≤ 5 g fat/oz:
1 oz	Feta
1 oz	Mozzarella
¼ c (2 oz)	Ricotta
	Other:
1	Egg (high in cholesterol, limit to 3/week)
1 oz	Sausage with ≤ 5 g fat/oz
1 c	Soy milk
¼ c	Tempeh
4 oz or ½ c	Tofu
High-Fat Meat and Substitutes	
1 high-fat meat exchange = 7 g protein, 8 g fat, 100 kcal	
1 oz	Pork: Spareribs, ground pork, pork sausage
1 oz	Cheese: All regular cheeses (American 🧂, cheddar, Monterey Jack, swiss)
	Other:
1 oz	Processed sandwich meats with ≤ 8 g fat/oz (bologna, pimento loaf, salami)
1 oz	Sausage (bratwurst, Italian, knockwurst, Polish, smoked)
1 (10/lb)	Hot dog (turkey or chicken) 🧂
3 slices (20 slices/lb)	Bacon
Count as one high-fat meat plus one fat exchange:	
1 (10/lb)	Hot dog (beef, pork, or combination) 🧂
2 tbs	Peanut butter (contains unsaturated fat)

🧂 = 400 mg or more sodium per exchange.

Table G–12
U.S. Exchange System: Fat List

1 fat exchange = 5 g fat, 45 kcal
Note: In general, a fat serving is 1 tsp regular butter, margarine, or vegetable oil; 1 tbs regular salad dressing. Many fat-free and reduced fat foods are on the Free Foods List.

Serving Size	Food
Monounsaturated Fats	
⅛ medium (1 oz)	Avocadoes
1 tsp	Oil (canola, olive, peanut)
8 large	Olives, ripe (black)
10 large	Olives, green, stuffed
6 nuts	Almonds, cashews
6 nuts	Mixed nuts (50% peanuts)
10 nuts	Peanuts
4 halves	Pecans
2 tsp	Peanut butter, smooth or crunchy
1 tbs	Sesame seeds
2 tsp	Tahini paste
Polyunsaturated Fats	
1 tsp	Margarine, stick, tub, or squeeze
1 tbs	Margarine, lower-fat (30% to 50% vegetable oil)
1 tsp	Mayonnaise, regular
1 tbs	Mayonnaise, reduced-fat
4 halves	Nuts, walnuts, English
1 tsp	Oil (corn, safflower, soybean)
1 tbs	Salad dressing, regular
2 tbs	Salad dressing, reduced-fat
2 tsp	Mayonnaise type salad dressing, regular
1 tbs	Mayonnaise type salad dressing, reduced-fat
1 tbs	Seeds: pumpkin, sunflower
Saturated Fats*	
1 slice (20 slices/lb)	Bacon, cooked
1 tsp	Bacon, grease
1 tsp	Butter, stick
2 tsp	Butter, whipped
1 tbs	Butter, reduced-fat
2 tbs (½ oz)	Chitterlings, boiled
2 tbs	Coconut, sweetened, shredded
2 tbs	Cream, half and half
1 tbs (½ oz)	Cream cheese, regular
2 tbs (1 oz)	Cream cheese, reduced-fat
	Fatback or salt pork**
1 tsp	Shortening or lard
2 tbs	Sour cream, regular
3 tbs	Sour cream, reduced-fat

= 400 mg or more sodium per exchange
*Saturated fats can raise blood cholesterol levels.
** Use a piece 1″ × 1″ × ¼″ if you plan to eat the fatback cooked with vegetables. Use a piece 2″ × 1″ × ½″ when eating only the vegetables with the fatback removed.

G

Table G–13
U.S. Exchange System: Free Foods List

Note: A serving of free food contains less than 20 kcalories; those with serving sizes should be limited to three servings a day whereas those without serving sizes can be eaten freely.

Serving Size	Food
Fat-Free or Reduced-Fat Foods	
1 tbs	Cream cheese, fat-free
1 tbs	Creamers, nondairy, liquid
2 tsp	Creamers, nondairy, powdered
1 tbs	Mayonnaise, fat-free
1 tsp	Mayonnaise, reduced-fat
4 tbs	Margarine, fat-free
1 tsp	Margarine, reduced-fat
1 tbs	Mayonnaise type salad dressing, nonfat
1 tsp	Mayonnaise type salad dressing, reduced-fat
	Nonstick cooking spray
1 tbs	Salad dressing, fat-free
2 tbs	Salad dressing, fat-free, Italian
¼ c	Salsa
1 tbs	Sour cream, fat-free, reduced-fat
2 tbs	Whipped topping, regular or light
Sugar-Free or Low-Sugar Foods	
1 piece	Candy, hard, sugar-free
	Gelatin dessert, sugar-free
	Gelatin, unflavored
	Gum, sugar-free
2 tsp	Jam or jelly, low-sugar or light
	Sugar substitutes
2 tbs	Syrup, sugar-free
Drinks	
	Bouillon, broth, consommé
	Bouillon or broth, low-sodium
	Carbonated or mineral water
1 tbs	Cocoa powder, unsweetened
	Coffee
	Club soda
	Diet soft drinks, sugar-free
	Drink mixes, sugar-free
	Tea
	Tonic water, sugar-free
Condiments	
1 tbs	Catsup
	Horseradish
	Lemon juice
	Lime juice
	Mustard
1½ large	Pickles, dill
	Soy sauce, regular or light
1 tbs	Taco sauce
	Vinegar
Seasonings	
Flavoring extracts	
Garlic	
Herbs, fresh or dried	
Pimento	
Spices	
Hot pepper sauces	
Wine, used in cooking	
Worcestershire sauce	

= 400 mg or more sodium per exchange.

Table G–14
U.S. Exchange System: Combination Foods List

Food	Serving Size	Exchanges per Serving
Entrees		
Tuna noodle casserole, lasagna, spaghetti with meatballs, chili with beans, macaroni and cheese	1 c (8 oz)	2 carbohydrates, 2 medium-fat meats
Chow mein (without noodles or rice)	2 c (16 oz)	1 carbohydrate, 2 lean meats
Pizza, cheese, thin crust	¼ of 10″ (5 oz)	2 carbohydrates, 2 medium-fat meats, 1 fat
Pizza, meat topping, thin crust	¼ of 10″ (5 oz)	2 carbohydrates, 2 medium-fat meats, 2 fats
Pot pie	1 (7 oz)	2 carbohydrates, 1 medium-fat meat, 4 fats
Frozen entrees		
Salisbury steak with gravy, mashed potato	1 (11 oz)	2 carbohydrates, 3 medium-fat meats, 3–4 fats
Turkey with gravy, mashed potato, dressing	1 (11 oz)	2 carbohydrates, 2 medium-fat meats, 2 fats
Entree with less than 300 kcalories	1 (8 oz)	2 carbohydrates, 3 lean meats
Soups		
Bean	1 c	1 carbohydrate, 1 very lean meat
Cream (made with water)	1 c (8 oz)	1 carbohydrate, 1 fat
Split pea (made with water)	½ c (4 oz)	1 carbohydrate
Tomato (make with water)	1 c (8 oz)	1 carbohydrate
Vegetable beef, chicken noodle, or other broth-type	1 c (8 oz)	1 carbohydrate
Fast Foods		
Burritos with beef	2	4 carbohydrates, 2 medium-fat meats, 2 fats
Chicken nuggets	6	1 carbohydrate, 2 medium-fat meats, 1 fat
Chicken breast and wing, breaded and fried	1	1 carbohydrate, 4 medium-fat meats, 2 fats
Fish sandwich/tartar sauce	1	3 carbohydrates, 1 medium-fat meat, 3 fats
French fries, thin	20–25	2 carbohydrates, 2 fats
Hamburger, regular	1	2 carbohydrates, 2 medium-fat meats
Hamburger, large	1	2 carbohydrates, 3 medium-fat meats, 1 fat

Table G–14 (continued)
U.S. Exchange System: Combination Foods List

Food	Serving Size	Exchanges per Serving
Hot dog with bun	1	1 carbohydrate, 1 high-fat meat, 1 fat
Individual pan pizza	1	5 carbohydrates, 3 medium-fat meats, 3 fats
Soft serve cone	1 medium	2 carbohydrates, 1 fat
Submarine sandwich	1 (6″)	3 carbohydrates, 1 vegetable, 2 medium-fat meats, 1 fat
Taco, hard shell	1 (6 oz)	2 carbohydrates, 2 medium-fat meats, 2 fats
Taco, soft shell	1 (3 oz)	1 carbohydrate, 1 medium-fat meat, 1 fat

= 400 mg or more sodium per exchange.

NUTRITION RECOMMENDATIONS FROM WHO

Like the Committee on Diet and Health in the United States, the World Health Organization (WHO) has also assessed the relationships between diet and the development of chronic diseases.[2] Their recommendations are expressed in average daily ranges that represent the lower and upper limits:

- Total energy: sufficient to support normal growth, physical activity, and body weight (body mass index = 20–22).
- Total fat: 15 to 30 percent of total energy.
  - Saturated fatty acids: 0 to 10 percent total energy.
  - Polyunsaturated fatty acids: 3 to 7 percent total energy.
  - Dietary cholesterol: 0 to 300 milligrams per day.
- Total carbohydrate: 55 to 75 percent total energy.
  - Complex carbohydrates: 50 to 75 percent total energy.
  - Dietary fiber: 27 to 40 grams per day.
  - Refined sugars: 0 to 10 percent total energy.
- Protein: 10 to 15 percent total energy.
- Salt: upper limit of 6 grams/day (no lower limit set).

NOTES

1. *Healthy People 2000: National Health Promotion and Disease Prevention Objectives* (Washington, D.C.: U.S. Department of Health and Human Services, 1990).
2. Diet, nutrition and the prevention of chronic diseases: A report of the WHO Study Group on Diet, Nutrition and Prevention of Noncommunicable Diseases, *Nutrition Reviews* 49 (1991): 291–301.

APPENDIX H

TABLE OF FOOD COMPOSITION

This edition of the table of food composition contains more complete values for several nutrients than any comparable table.[1] These include dietary fiber; saturated, monounsaturated, and polyunsaturated fat; vitamin B_6; folate; magnesium; and zinc. The table includes a wide variety of foods from all food groups and is updated yearly to reflect current food patterns. For example, this edition includes many new nonfat items; several new ethnic items such as basmati rice, calamata olives, and gai choy chinese mustard; and a new selection of baby foods.

Sources of Data To achieve a complete and reliable listing of nutrients for all the foods, over 1000 sources of information are researched. Government sources are the primary base for all the data: the USDA *Handbook* series and its current supplemental data, as well as current data on baked goods, snacks, and sweets. In addition, provisional USDA information—both published and unpublished—is included. The data are refined through information obtained in many conversations with professional staff members at the USDA Human Nutrition Information Service in Hyattsville, Maryland.

Even with all the government sources available, however, some nutrient values are still missing; and as the USDA updates various data, it sometimes reports conflicting values for the same items. To fill in the missing values and resolve discrepancies, other reliable sources of information are used. These sources include refereed journal articles, food composition tables from Canada and England, information from other nutrient data banks and publications, unpublished scientific data, and manufacturers' data.

Accuracy of Estimates The energy and nutrients in recipes and combination foods vary widely, depending on the ingredients. The amounts of various fatty acids and cholesterol are influenced by the type of fat used (the specific type of oil, vegetable shortening, butter, margarine, etc.).

Estimates of nutrient amounts for foods and nutrients include all possible adjustments in the interest of accuracy. When multiple values are reported for a nutrient, the numbers are averaged and weighted with consideration of the original number of samples in the separate sources. Whenever water percentages are available, estimates of nutrient amounts are adjusted for water content. When no water is given, water percentage is assumed to be that shown in the table. Whenever a reported weight appeared inconsistent (cooked eggplant and collards, for example), many kitchen tests were made, and the average weight of the typical product was given as tested.

When estimates of nutrient amounts in cooked foods are derived from reported amounts in raw foods, published retention factors are applied. Some reported data for combination foods are modified in this table to include newer data available for major ingredients. For example, since the "pies" were analyzed and reported, newer data on fruits have been published. Bakery items reflect the most current data with the new enrichment levels for certain nutrients.

Considerable effort has been made to report the most accurate data available and to eliminate missing values. The table is updated annually, and the authors welcome any suggestions or comments for future editions.

Average Values It is important to know that many different nutrient values can be reported for foods, even by reliable sources. Many factors influence the amounts of

1. This food composition table has been prepared for West Publishing Company and is copyrighted by ESHA Research in Salem, Oregon—the developer and publisher of the Food Processor®, Nutrition Pro™, and Genesis™ nutrition software systems. The major sources for the data from the U.S. Department of Agriculture are supplemented by more than 1000 additional sources of information. Because the list of references is so extensive, it is not provided here, but it is available from the publisher.

nutrients in foods, including the mineral content of the soil, the method of processing, genetics, the diet of the animal or the fertilizer of the plant, the season of the year, methods of analysis, the difference in moisture content of the samples analyzed, the length and method of storage, and methods of cooking the food.

Although each nutrient from USDA government data is presented as a single number in some USDA publications, each number is actually an average of a range of data. The more detailed reports (Handbook 8 series) indicate the number of samples and the standard deviation of the data. One can also find different reported values for foods, as older USDA data are replaced with newer data in more recent publications. Therefore, nutrient data should be viewed and used only as a guide, a close approximation of nutrient content.

Dietary Fiber Dietary fiber deserves a special word. Estimates of dietary fiber are included for all the foods in this table. This information comes primarily from extensive published and unpublished data from the USDA Human Nutrition Information Service in Hyattsville, Maryland; *Composition of Foods by Southgate* (England); and many journal articles.

It is important to recognize that data for dietary fiber are still undergoing review in the scientific community. No doubt, these estimates will change as analytical techniques are refined and interpretations clarified.

Vitamin A Vitamin A is reported in retinol equivalents. The amount of this vitamin can vary by the season of the year and the maturity of the plant. Reported values in both dairy products and plants are higher in summer and early fall than in winter. The values reported here represent year-round averages. The organ meats of all animal products (liver especially) contain large amounts of vitamin A, which vary widely, depending on the background of the animal. The vitamin is also present in very small amounts in regular meat and is often reported as a trace.

Newer reported vitamin A values for some plant foods have increased significantly due to additional information and sometimes to improved plant genetics. Recent vitamin A values for canned pumpkin, for example, are 3.5 times greater than the previously reported values.

Fats Total fats, as well as the breakdown of total fats to saturated, monounsaturated, and polyunsaturated fats, are listed in the table. The fatty acids seldom add up to the total. This discrepancy is due to rounding and to the existence of small amounts of other fatty acid components that are not included in the three basic categories, including *trans*-fatty acids and glycerol.

Niacin Niacin values are for preformed niacin and do not include additional niacin that may form in the body from the conversion of tryptophan.

Using the Table The items in this table have been organized into several categories, which are listed at the head of each right-hand page. As the key shows, each group has been color-coded to make it easier to find individual items.

In an effort to conserve space, the following abbreviations have been used in the food descriptions and nutrient breakdowns:

- diam = diameter
- ea = each
- enr = enriched
- f/ = from
- g = grams
- liq = liquid
- pce = piece
- pkg = package
- w/ = with
- w/o = without
- t = trace
- 0 = zero (no nutrient value)
- — = information not available

Caffeine Sources Caffeine occurs in several plants, including the familiar coffee bean, the tea leaf, and the cocoa bean from which chocolate is made. Most human societies use caffeine regularly, most often in beverages, for its stimulant effect and flavor. Caffeine contents of beverages vary depending on the plants they are made from, the climates and soils where the plants are grown, the grind or cut size, the method and duration of brewing, and the amounts served. The accompanying table shows that in general, a cup of coffee contains the most caffeine; a cup of tea, less than half as much; and cocoa or chocolate, less still. As for cola beverages, they are made from kola nuts which contain caffeine, but most of their caffeine is added, using the purified compound obtained from decaffeinated coffee beans.

The FDA lists caffeine as a multipurpose GRAS substance that may be added to foods and beverages. Drug industries in developed countries use caffeine in many kinds of drugs: stimulants, pain relievers, cold remedies, diuretics, and weight-loss aids.

Caffeine Content of Beverages, Foods, and Over-the-Counter Drugs

Beverages and Foods	Average (mg)	Range(mg)
Coffee (5-oz cup)		
Brewed, drip method	130	110–150
Brewed, percolator	94	64–124
Instant	74	40–108
Decaffeinated, brewed or instant	3	1–5
Tea (5-oz cup)		
Brewed, major U.S. brand	40	20–90
Brewed, imported brands	60	25–110
Instant	30	25–50
Iced (12-oz can)	70	67–76
Soft drinks (12-oz can)		
Dr. Pepper		40
Colas and cherry cola		
Regular		30–46
Diet		2–58
Caffeine-free		0–trace
Jolt		72
Mountain Dew, Mello Yello		52
Fresca, Hires Root Beer, 7-Up, Sprite, Squirt, Sunkist Orange		0
Cocoa beverage (5-oz cup)	4	2–20
Chocolate milk beverage (8 oz)	5	2–7
Milk chocolate candy (1 oz)	6	1–15
Dark chocolate, semisweet (1 oz)	20	5–35
Baker's chocolate (1 oz)	26	26
Chocolate flavored syrup (1 oz)	4	4
Drugs[a]		
Cold remedies (standard dose)		
Dristan	0	
Coryban-D, Triaminicin	30	
Diuretics (standard dose)		
Aqua-ban, Permathene H_2Off	200	
Pre-Mens Forte	100	
Pain relievers (standard dose)		
Excedrin	130	
Midol, Anacin	65	
Aspirin, plain (any brand)	0	
Stimulants		
Caffedrin, NoDoz, Vivarin	200	
Weight-control aids (daily dose)		
Prolamine	280	
Dexatrim, Dietac	200	

Note: A pharmacologically active dose of caffeine is defined as 200 milligrams.

[a]Because products change, contact the manufacturer for an update on products you use regularly.

Table H–1
Food Composition

Computer Code Number	Food Description	Measure	Wt (g)	H_2O (%)	Ener (kcal)	Prot (g)	Carb (g)	Dietary Fiber (g)	Fat (g)	Fat Breakdown (g) Sat	Mono	Poly
	BEVERAGES											
	Alcoholic:											
	Beer:											
1	Regular (12 fl oz)	1½ c	356	92	146	1	13	3	0	0	0	0
2	Light (12 fl oz)	1½ c	354	95	99[1]	1	5	1	0	0	0	0
1506	Nonalcoholic (12 fl oz)	1 ea	360	98	32	1	5	0	0	0	0	0
	Gin, rum, vodka, whiskey:											
3	80 proof	1½ fl oz	42	67	97	0	0	0	0	0	0	0
4	86 proof	1½ fl oz	42	64	105	0	<1	0	0	0	0	0
5	90 proof	1½ fl oz	42	62	110	0	0	0	0	0	0	0
	Liqueur:											
1359	Coffee liqueur, 53 proof	1½ fl oz	52	31	175	<1	24	0	<1	.1	t	.1
1360	Coffee & cream liqueur, 34 proof	1½ fl oz	47	46	154	1	10	0	7	4.5	2.1	.3
1361	Crème de menthe, 72 proof	1½ fl oz	50	28	186	0	21	0	<1	t	t	.1
	Wine:											
6	Dessert (4 fl oz)	½ c	118	72	181[2]	<1	14	0	0	0	0	0
7	Red	3½ fl oz	103	88	74	<1	2	0	0	0	0	0
8	Rosé	3½ fl oz	103	89	73	<1	1	0	0	0	0	0
9	White medium	3½ fl oz	103	90	70	<1	1	0	0	0	0	0
1592	Nonalcoholic	1 c	232	98	14	1	3	0	0	0	0	0
1593	Nonalcoholic light	1 c	251	98	15	1	3	0	0	0	0	0
1409	Wine cooler, bottle (12 fl oz)	1½ c	340	90	169	<1	20	<1	<1	0	0	t
1595	Wine cooler, cup	1 c	227	90	113	<1	13	<1	<1	0	0	t
	Carbonated:[3]											
10	Club soda (12 fl oz)	1½ c	355	100	0	0	0	0	0	0	0	0
11	Cola beverage (12 fl oz)	1½ c	370	89	152	0	38	0	<1	.02	.03	.1
12	Diet cola w/aspartame (12 fl oz)	1½ c	355	100	4	<1	<1	0	0	0	0	0
13	Diet cola w/saccharin (12 fl oz)	1½ c	355	100	0	0	<1	0	0	0	0	0
14	Ginger ale (12 fl oz)	1½ c	366	91	124	0	32	0	0	0	0	0
15	Grape soda (12 fl oz)	1½ c	372	89	160	0	42	0	0	0	0	0
16	Lemon-lime (12 fl oz)	1½ c	368	90	147	0	38	0	0	0	0	0
17	Orange (12 fl oz)	1½ c	372	88	179	0	46	0	0	0	0	0
18	Pepper-type soda (12 fl oz)	1½ c	368	89	151	0	38	0	<1	.3	0	0
19	Root beer (12 fl oz)	1½ c	370	89	152	0	39	0	0	0	0	0
20	Coffee,[3] brewed	1 c	240	99	5[4]	<1	1	0	<1	0	0	0
21	Coffee,[3] prepared from instant	1 c	240	99	5[4]	<1	1	0	<1	0	0	0
	Fruit drinks, noncarbonated:[5]											
22	Fruit punch drink, canned	½ c	126	88	59	0	15	0	<1	0	0	0
1358	Gatorade	1 c	240	94	60	0	15	0	0	0	0	0
23	Grape drink, canned	½ c	125	87	63	<1	16	<1	0	0	0	0
1304	Kool-Aid, with sugar	1 c	240	90	89	0	23	0	<1	0	0	0
1356	Kool-Aid, with NutraSweet	1 c	240	95	43	0	11	0	0	0	0	0

(1) kCalories can vary from 78 to 131 for 12 fl. oz.

(2) Values are for sweet dessert wine. Dry dessert wines contain 149 kcal and 5 g of carbohydrate.

(3) Mineral content varies depending on water source.

(4) kCalorie values from USDA vary from 1 to 5 kcal per cup.

(5) Usually less than 10% fruit juice.

(Computer code number is for West Diet Analysis program)

PAGE KEY: H–4 = BEV H–6 = DAIRY H–12 = EGGS H–14 = FAT/OIL H–18 = FRUIT H–26 = BAKERY H–36 = GRAIN H–44 = FISH H–48 = MEATS H–50 = POULTRY H–54 = SAUSAGE H–56 = MIXED/FAST H–64 = NUTS/SEEDS H–68 = SWEETS H–70 = VEG/LEG H–84 = MISC H–88 = SOUPS/SAUCES H–90 = FAST H–106 = FRZN ENTREE H–112 = BABY FOODS

Chol (mg)	Calc (mg)	Iron (mg)	Magn (mg)	Phos (mg)	Pota (mg)	Sodi (mg)	Zinc (mg)	VT-A (RE)	Thia (mg)	Ribo (mg)	Niac (mg)	V-B6 (mg)	Fola (µg)	VT-C (mg)
0	18	.11	21	43	89	18	.07	0	.04	.11	1.60	.18	21	0
0	18	.14	18	42	64	11	.11	0	.04	.11	1.38	.11	15	0
0	25	.04	32	112	90	18	.04	0	.02	.09	1.63	.18	22	0
0	0	.02	0	2	1	<1	.02	0	<.01	0	0	0	0	0
0	0	.02	0	2	1	<1	.02	0	<.01	0	0	0	0	0
0	0	.02	0	2	1	<1	.02	0	<.01	0	0	0	0	0
0	1	.03	2	3	16	4	.02	0	0	.01	.07	0	0	0
7	8	.06	1	24	15	43	.08	20	0	.03	.04	.01	0	0
0	0	.04	0	0	0	2	.02	0	0	0	0	0	0	0
0	9	.28	11	11	108	11	.08	0	.02	.02	.25	0	<1	0
0	8	.44	13	14	116	5	.09	0	.01	.03	.08	.03	2	0
0	8	.39	10	15	102	5	.06	0	0	.02	.07	.02	1	0
0	9	.33	10	14	83	5	.07	0	0	.01	.07	.01	<1	0
0	21	.93	23	35	204	16	.19	0	0	.02	.23	.05	2	0
0	23	1	25	38	221	18	.2	0	0	.03	.25	.05	3	0
0	19	.92	18	22	152	29	.2	1	.02	.02	.16	.04	4	6
0	13	.61	12	15	101	19	.13	<1	.01	.02	.10	.03	3	4
0	18	.04	4	0	7	75	.36	0	0	0	0	0	0	0
0	11	.11	4	44	4	15	.04	0	0	0	0	0	0	0
0	14	.11	4	32	0	21[6]	.28	0	.02	.08	0	0	0	0
0	14	.14	4	39	7	57	.18	0	0	0	0	0	0	0
0	11	.66	4	0	4	26	.18	0	0	0	0	0	0	0
0	11	.3	4	0	4	56	.26	0	0	0	0	0	0	0
0	7	.26	4	0	4	40	.18	0	0	0	.06	0	0	0
0	19	.22	4	4	7	45	.37	0	0	0	0	0	0	0
0	11	.15	0	40	4	37	.15	0	0	0	0	0	0	0
0	19	.19	4	0	4	48	.26	0	0	0	0	0	0	0
0	5	.12	12	2	130	5	.05	0	0	0	.53	0	<1	0
0	7	.12	10	7	86	7	.07	0	0	<.01	.68	0	0	0
0	10	.26	3	1	32	28	.15	2	.03	.03	.03	0	2	37
0	0	.12	2	22	26	96	.05	0	.01	0	0	0	0	0
0	4	.13	5	5	44	1	.04	0	.01	.01	.13	.03	1	20
0	38	.12	2	48	2	34	.07	0	0	<.01	<.01	0	<1	28
0	17	.65	5	5	50	50	.26	2	.02	.05	.05	0	5	77

[6] Value for product sweetened with aspartame only; sodium is 32 mg if a blend of aspartame and sodium saccharin is used.

(For purposes of calculations, use "0" for t, <1, <.1, <.01, etc.)

H

Table H–1
Food Composition

Computer Code Number	Food Description	Measure	Wt (g)	H_2O (%)	Ener (kcal)	Prot (g)	Carb (g)	Dietary Fiber (g)	Fat (g)	Fat Breakdown (g) Sat	Mono	Poly
	BEVERAGES—Cont.											
	Fruit drinks, noncarbonated—Cont.											
26	Lemonade, frozen concentrate (6-oz can)	¾ c	219	52	396	1	103	1	<1	.1	t	.1
27	Lemonade, from concentrate	1 c	248	89	99	<1	26	<1	<1	t	t	t
28	Limeade, frozen concentrate (6-oz can)	¾ c	218	50	408	<1	107	1	<1	t	t	.1
29	Limeade, from concentrate	1 c	247	89	101	0	27	<1	<1	0	0	t
24	Pineapple grapefruit, canned	1 c	250	88	118	<1	29	<1	<1	t	t	.1
25	Pineapple orange, canned	1 c	250	87	125	3	30	<1	0	0	0	0
	Fruit and vegetable juices: see Fruit and Vegetable sections											
	Slim Fast:[1]											
1612	Chocolate malt with nonfat milk	1 c	273	82	190	14	32	2	1	.3	.1	t
1613	Strawberry with nonfat milk	1 c	273	82	190	14	32	2	1	.3	.1	t
1611	Vanilla with nonfat milk	1 c	273	82	190	14	32	2	1	.3	.1	t
	Ultra Slim Fast:[1]											
1616	Chocolate with nonfat milk	1 c	278	81	200	14	36	5	1	.3	.1	t
1614	French vanilla with nonfat milk	1 c	278	81	190	14	36	4	1	.3	.1	t
1615	Strawberry Supreme with nonfat milk	1 c	278	81	190	14	36	4	1	.3	.1	t
1357	Water, bottled: Perrier (6½ fl oz)	1 ea	192	100	0	0	0	0	0	0	0	0
1594	Water, bottled: Tonic water	1½ c	366	91	124	0	32	0	0	0	0	0
	Tea:[2]											
30	Brewed, regular	1 c	240	100	2	0	1	0	<1	0	0	t
1662	Brewed, herbal	¾ c	178	100	2	0	<1	0	t	0	0	t
32	From instant, sweetened	1 c	262	91	89	<1	22	0	<1	t	0	t
31	From instant, unsweetened	1 c	237	100	2	0	<1	0	0	0	0	0
	DAIRY											
	Butter: see Fats and Oils, #158,159,160											
	Cheese, natural:											
33	Blue	1 oz	28	42	100	6	1	0	8	5.3	2.2	.2
34	Brick	1 oz	28	41	105	7	1	0	8	5.3	2.4	.2
35	Brie	1 oz	28	48	95	6	<1	0	8	4.9	2.3	.2
36	Camembert	1 oz	28	52	85	6	<1	0	7	4.3	2	.2
37	Cheddar:	1 oz	28	37	114	7	<1	0	9	6	2.7	.3
38	1" cube	1 ea	17	37	69	4	<1	0	6	3.6	1.6	.2
39	Shredded	1 c	113	37	455	28	1	0	37	23.8	10.6	1.1
1406	Low fat, low sodium	1 oz	28	65	49	7	1	0	2	1.3	0.6	0.1
	Cottage:											
984	Low sodium, low fat	1 c	225	84	162	28	6	0	2	1.4	.6	.07
40	Creamed, large curd	1 c	225	79	232	28	6	0	10	6.4	2.9	.3
41	Creamed, small curd	1 c	210	79	216	26	6	0	9	6	2.7	.3
42	With fruit	1 c	226	72	280	22	30	0	8	4.9	2.2	.2
43	Low fat 2%	1 c	226	79	203	31	8	0	4	2.8	1.2	.1
44	Low fat 1%	1 c	226	82	164	28	6	0	2	1.5	.7	.1
46	Cream	1 oz	28	54	99	2	1	0	10	6.2	2.8	.4
983	Cream, low fat	1 oz	28	64	65	3	2	0	5	3.1	1.4	0.2
47	Edam	1 oz	28	42	101	7	<1	0	8	5	2.3	.2
48	Feta	1 oz	28	55	75	4	1	0	6	4.2	1.3	.2

(1)See Chapter 9 for healthy weight loss strategies. The formulas for these products change periodically; these data reflect nutrient values as of our publication date.

(2)Mineral content varies depending on water source.

Chol (mg)	Calc (mg)	Iron (mg)	Magn (mg)	Phos (mg)	Pota (mg)	Sodi (mg)	Zinc (mg)	VT-A (RE)	Thia (mg)	Ribo (mg)	Niac (mg)	V-B6 (mg)	Fola (μg)	VT-C (mg)
0	15	1.58	11	20	146	9	.18	21	.06	.21	.16	.05	22	39[3]
0	7	.4	5	5	37	7	.1	5	.01	.05	.04	.01	5	10[3]
0	11	.22	9	13	128	0	.09	0	.02	.02	.22	0	9	26
0	7	.07	2	2	32	5	.05	0	0	0	.05	0	2	7
0	18	.78	15	15	152	35	.15	9	.08	.04	.67	.1	26	115
0	13	.68	15	10	115	7	.15	133	.08	.05	.52	.12	27	56
4	450	6.3	140	400	690	230	5.25	350	.53	.59	7	.7	120	21
4	450	6.3	140	400	720	220	5.25	350	.53	.59	7	.7	120	21
4	450	6.31	140	401	721	220	5.24	350	.53	.59	7	.7	120	21
<1	450	6.3	140	400	800	230	5.25	350	.52	.59	7	.7	120	21
<1	450	6.3	140	400	730	250	5.25	350	.52	.59	7	.7	120	21
<1	450	6.3	140	400	710	250	5.25	350	.52	.59	7	.7	120	21
0	27	0	0	0	0	2	0	0	0	0	0	0	0	0
0	4	.04	0	0	0	15	.37	0	0	0	0	0	0	0
0	0	.05	7	2	89	7	.05	0	0	.03	0	0	12	0
0	4	.14	2	0	16	2	.07	0	.02	.01	0	0	1	0
0	5	.05	5	3	50	8	.08	0	0	.05	.09	.01	10	0
0	5	.05	5	2	47	7	.07	0	0	<.01	.09	0	1	0
21	150	.09	6	110	73	395	.75	65	.01	.11	.29	.05	10	0
27	191	.12	7	128	39	159	.74	86	0	.1	.03	.02	6	0
28	52	.14	6	53	43	178	.67	52	.02	.15	.11	.07	18	0
20	110	.09	6	98	53	239	.67	71	.01	.14	.18	.06	18	0
30	204	.19	8	145	28	176	.88	86	.01	.11	.02	.02	5	0
18	123	.12	5	87	17	106	.53	51	0	.06	.01	.01	3	0
119	815	.77	31	579	111	702	3.53	342	.03	.43	.09	.08	21	0
6	199	.2	8	137	32	6	.88	18	.01	.01	.03	.02	5	0
9	137	.32	11	302	193	29	.86	25	.05	.36	.3	.15	27	0
33	135	.32	12	297	190	911	.83	108	.05	.37	.28	.15	27	0
31	126	.29	11	277	177	851	.78	101	.04	.34	.26	.14	26	0
25	108	.25	9	237	151	915	.65	81	.04	.29	.23	.12	22	0
19	155	.36	14	341	217	918	.95	45	.05	.42	.33	.17	30	0
10	138	.32	12	303	193	918	.86	25	.05	.37	.29	.15	28	0
31	23	.34	2	29	34	84	.15	124	0	.06	.03	.01	4	0
16	32	.48	2	41	47	84	.22	63	.01	.08	.04	.02	5	0
25	207	.12	8	152	53	274	1.07	72	.01	.11	.02	.02	5	0
25	140	.18	5	96	18	316	.82	36	.04	.24	.28	.12	9	0

(3)Vitamin C can range from 5 to 72 mg in a small can of frozen concentrate, and from 1 to 18 mg in 1 c of prepared lemonade.

(For purposes of calculations, use "0" for t, <1, <.1, <.01, etc.)

Table H–1
Food Composition

Computer Code Number	Food Description	Measure	Wt (g)	H_2O (%)	Ener (kcal)	Prot (g)	Carb (g)	Dietary Fiber (g)	Fat (g)	Fat Breakdown (g) Sat	Mono	Poly
	DAIRY—Cont.											
	Cheese—Cont.											
49	Gouda	1 oz	28	42	101	7	1	0	8	5	2.2	.2
50	Gruyère	1 oz	28	33	117	8	<1	0	9	5.4	2.8	.5
51	Gorgonzola	1 oz	28	39	111	7	0	0	9	5.5	2.4	.5
52	Liederkranz	1 oz	28	53	87	5	<1	0	8	5.3	2.2	.2
1676	Limburger	1 oz	28	48	93	6	<1	0	8	4.7	2.4	.1
53	Monterey Jack	1 oz	28	41	106	7	<1	0	9	5.4	2.5	.3
54	Mozzarella, whole milk	1 oz	28	54	80	5	1	0	6	3.7	1.9	.2
55	Mozzarella, part-skim milk, low moisture	1 oz	28	49	79	8	1	0	5	3.1	1.4	.1
56	Muenster	1 oz	28	42	104	7	<1	0	9	5.4	2.5	.2
1399	Nonfat (Kraft Singles)	1 oz	28	60	45	6	4	0	0	0	0	0
	Parmesan, grated:											
57	Cup, not pressed down	1 c	100	18	456	42	4	0	30	19	8.7	.7
58	Tablespoon	1 tbs	5	18	23	2	<1	0	2	1	.4	t
59	Ounce	1 oz	28	18	129	12	1	0	9	5.4	2.5	.2
60	Provolone	1 oz	28	41	100	7	1	0	8	4.8	2.1	.2
61	Ricotta, whole milk	1 c	246	72	428	28	8	0	32	20.4	8.9	1
62	Ricotta, part-skim milk	1 c	246	74	339	28	13	0	19	12.1	5.7	.6
63	Romano	1 oz	28	31	109	9	1	0	8	4.8	2.2	.2
64	Swiss	1 oz	28	37	106	8	1	0	8	5	2.1	.3
976	Swiss, low fat	1 oz	28	60	51	8	1	0	1	.9	.4	<.1
	Pasteurized processed cheese products:											
65	American	1 oz	28	39	106	6	<1	0	9	5.6	2.5	.3
66	Swiss	1 oz	28	42	94	7	1	0	7	4.6	2	.2
67	American cheese food, jar	1 oz	28	43	93	6	2	0	7	4.4	2	.2
68	American cheese spread	1 oz	28	48	82	5	2	0	6	3.8	1.8	.2
982	Velveeta cheese spread, low fat, low sodium	1 oz	28	63	51	7	1	0	2	1.3	0.6	0.1
69	Cream, sweet:	1 c	242	81	315	7	10	0	28	17.3	8	1
	Half & half (cream & milk):											
70	Tablespoon	1 tbs	15	81	19	<1	1	0	2	1.1	.5	.1
71	Light, coffee or table:	1 c	240	74	468	6	9	0	46	28.8	13.4	1.7
72	Tablespoon	1 tbs	15	74	29	<1	1	0	3	1.8	.8	.1
73	Light whipping cream, liquid:[1]	1 c	239	64	698	5	7	0	74	46.1	21.7	2.1
74	Tablespoon	1 tbs	15	64	44	<1	<1	0	5	2.9	1.4	.1
75	Heavy whipping cream, liquid:[1]	1 c	238	58	821	5	7	0	88	54.7	25.5	3.3
76	Tablespoon	1 tbs	15	58	52	<1	<1	0	6	3.4	1.6	.2
77	Whipped cream, pressurized:	1 c	60	61	154	2	8	0	13	8.3	3.8	.5
78	Tablespoon	1 tbs	4	61	10	<1	<1	0	1	.6	.3	t
79	Cream, sour, cultured:	1 c	230	71	492	7	10	0	48	29.9	13.9	1.8
80	Tablespoon	1 tbs	14	71	30	<1	1	0	3	1.8	.8	.1
	Cream products—imitation and part dairy:											
81	Coffee whitener, frozen or liquid	1 tbs	15	77	20	<1	2	0	2	1.4	t	0
82	Coffee whitener, powdered	1 tsp	2	2	11	<1	1	0	1	.6	t	t
83	Dessert topping, frozen, nondairy:	1 c	75	50	239	1	17	0	19	16.4	1.2	.4
84	Tablespoon	1 tbs	5	50	16	<1	1	0	1	1.1	.1	t
85	Dessert topping, mix with whole milk:	1 c	80	67	151	3	13	0	10	8.6	.7	.2
86	Tablespoon	1 tbs	5	67	9	<1	1	0	1	.5	t	t

(1)For whipped cream, (non-pressurized), double the liquid cream volume of codes 73, 74 or 75, 76. One tablespoon liquid cream becomes 2 tablespoons when "whipped."

(Computer code number is for West Diet Analysis program)

PAGE KEY: H–4 = BEV H–6 = DAIRY H–12 = EGGS H–14 = FAT/OIL H–18 = FRUIT H–26 = BAKERY H–36 = GRAIN H–44 = FISH H–48 = MEATS H–50 = POULTRY H–54 = SAUSAGE H–56 = MIXED/FAST H–64 = NUTS/SEEDS H–68 = SWEETS H–70 = VEG/LEG H–84 = MISC H–88 = SOUPS/SAUCES H–90 = FAST H–106 = FRZN ENTREE H–112 = BABY FOODS

Chol (mg)	Calc (mg)	Iron (mg)	Magn (mg)	Phos (mg)	Pota (mg)	Sodi (mg)	Zinc (mg)	VT-A (RE)	Thia (mg)	Ribo (mg)	Niac (mg)	V-B6 (mg)	Fola (μg)	VT-C (mg)
32	198	.07	8	155	34	232	1.11	49	.01	.09	.02	.02	6	0
31	286	.05	10	171	23	95	1.11	85	.02	.08	.03	.02	3	0
25	149	.12	8	121	26	512	.57	103	.01	.09	.2	.04	9	0
21	110	.12	7	100	68	389	.7	91	.01	.18	.1	.04	34	0
26	141	.04	6	111	36	227	.6	90	.02	.14	.04	.02	16	0
25	211	.2	8	126	23	152	.85	72	0	.11	.03	.02	5	0
22	146	.05	5	105	19	105	.63	68	0	.07	.02	.02	2	0
15	207	.07	7	148	27	149	.89	54	.01	.1	.03	.02	3	0
27	203	.12	8	132	38	178	.8	90	0	.09	.03	.02	3	0
5	224	0	–	165	81	438	–	128	–	.10	–	–	–	0
79	1375	.95	51	807	107	1861	3.19	173	.04	.39	.31	.1	8	0
4	69	.05	3	40	5	93	.16	9	0	.02	.02	.01	<1	0
22	390	.27	14	229	30	528	.9	49	.01	.11	.09	.03	2	0
20	214	.15	8	140	39	247	.92	75	0	.09	.04	.02	3	0
124	509	.93	28	389	258	206	2.88	330	.03	.48	.26	.11	30	0
76	669	1.08	36	450	308	308	3.3	278	.05	.45	.19	.05	32	0
29	300	.22	12	215	24	340	.73	40	.01	.1	.02	.02	2	0
26	272	.05	10	171	31	74	1.11	72	.01	.1	.03	.02	2	0
10	272	.05	10	72	31	74	1.11	18	.01	.1	.03	.02	2	0
27	174	.11	6	211	46	405	.85	82	.01	.1	.02	.02	2	0
24	219	.17	8	216	61	388	1.03	65	0	.08	.01	.01	2	0
18	163	.24	9	130	79	336	.85	62	.01	.13	.04	.04	2	0
16	159	.09	8	202	69	380	.73	54	.01	.12	.04	.03	2	0
10	194	.12	7	234	51	2	.94	18	.01	.11	.02	.02	3	0
89	254	.17	25	230	315	98	1.23	259	.08	.36	.19	.09	6	2
6	16	.01	2	14	19	6	.08	16	.01	.02	.01	.01	<1	<1
158	230	.1	21	191	293	95	.65	437	.08	.35	.14	.08	6	2
10	14	.01	1	12	18	6	.04	27	.01	.02	.01	0	<1	<1
265	165	.07	17	146	231	82	.6	705	.06	.3	.1	.07	9	1
17	10	0	1	9	14	5	.04	44	.01	.02	.01	0	1	<1
326	153	.07	17	148	179	89	.55	1001	.05	.26	.09	.06	9	1
21	10	0	1	9	11	6	.03	63	0	.02	.01	0	1	<1
46	61	.03	6	54	88	78	.22	124	.02	.04	.04	.02	2	0
3	4	0	<1	4	6	5	.01	8	0	0	0	0	<1	0
102	267	.14	26	195	331	122	.62	449	.08	.34	.15	.04	25	2
6	16	.01	2	12	20	7	.04	27	0	.02	.01	0	2	<1
0	1	<.01	<1	10	29	12	0	1	0	0	0	0	0	0
0	<1	.02	<1	8	16	4	.01	<1	0	0	0	0	0	0
0	5	.09	1	6	14	19	.02	64[2]	0	0	0	0	0	0
0	<1	.01	<1	<1	1	1	0	4[2]	0	0	0	0	0	0
8	72	.03	8	69	120	53	.22	39[2]	.02	.09	.05	.02	3	1
<1	5	0	<1	4	8	3	.01	2[2]	0	.01	0	0	<1	<1

(2) Vitamin A value is from beta-carotene used for coloring.

(For purposes of calculations, use "0" for t, <1, <.1, <.01, etc.)

H

Table H–1
Food Composition

Computer Code Number	Food Description	Measure	Wt (g)	H_2O (%)	Ener (kcal)	Prot (g)	Carb (g)	Dietary Fiber (g)	Fat (g)	Fat Breakdown (g)		
										Sat	Mono	Poly
	DAIRY—Cont.											
88	Dessert topping, pressurized:	1 c	70	60	185	1	11	0	16	13.2	1.3	.2
87	Tablespoon	1 tbs	4	60	11	<1	1	0	1	.8	.1	t
91	Sour cream, imitation:	1 c	230	71	478	6	15	<1	45	40.9	1.3	.1
92	Tablespoon	1 tbs	14	71	29	<1	1	0	3	2.5	.1	t
89	Sour dressing, part dairy:	1 c	235	75	418	8	11	0	39	31.3	4.6	1.1
90	Tablespoon	1 tbs	15	75	27	<1	1	0	2	2	.3	.1
	Milk, fluid:											
93	Whole milk	1 c	244	88	150	8	11	0	8	5.1	2.3	.3
94	2% low-fat milk	1 c	244	89	121	8	12	0	5	2.9	1.3	.2
95	2% milk solids added[1]	1 c	245	89	124	9	12	0	5	2.9	1.4	.2
96	1% low-fat milk	1 c	244	90	102	8	12	–	3	1.6	.8	.1
97	1% milk solids added[1]	1 c	245	90	104	9	12	0	2	1.5	.7	.1
98	Nonfat milk, vitamin A added	1 c	245	91	86	8	12	0	<1	.3	.1	t
99	Nonfat milk solids added[1]	1 c	245	90	90	9	12	0	1	.4	.2	t
100	Buttermilk, nonfat	1 c	245	90	99	8	12	0	2	1.3	.6	.1
	Milk, canned:											
101	Sweetened condensed	1 c	306	27	982	24	166	0	27	16.8	7.4	1
102	Evaporated, whole	1 c	252	74	338	17	25	0	19	11.6	5.9	.6
103	Evaporated, nonfat	1 c	255	79	199	19	29	0	1	.3	.2	t
	Milk, dried:											
104	Buttermilk, sweet	1 c	120	3	464	41	59	0	7	4.3	2	.3
105	Instant, nonfat, envelope[2]	1 ea	91	4	325	32	47	0	1	.4	.2	t
106	Instant nonfat, cup	1 c	68	4	243	24	35	0	<1	.3	.1	t
107	Goat milk	1 c	244	87	167	9	11	0	10	6.5	2.7	.4
108	Kefir, 2% milkfat[3]	1 c	233	82	122	9	9	0	5	2.9	1.2	.1
	Milk beverages and powdered mixes:											
	Chocolate:											
109	Whole	1 c	250	82	208	8	26	3	9	5.2	2.5	.3
110	2% fat	1 c	250	83	178	8	26	3	5	3.1	1.5	.2
111	1% fat	1 c	250	85	157	8	26	3	3	1.5	.7	.1
	Chocolate-flavored beverages:											
112	Powder containing nonfat dry milk:	1 oz	28	2	102	3	22	<1	1	.7	.4	t
113	Prepared with water	¾ c	206	86	103	4	22	<1	1	.7	.4	t
114	Powder without nonfat dry milk:	¾ oz	22	1	77	1	20	1	1	.4	.2	t
115	Prepared with whole milk	1 c	266	81	226	9	31	<1	9	5.5	2.6	.3
116	Eggnog, commercial	1 c	254	74	343	10	34	0	19	11.3	5.7	.9
974	Eggnog, low fat	1 c	254	85	189	12	17	0	8	3.8	2.7	0.7
1027	Instant Breakfast, envelope, powder only:	1 ea	37	7	131	7	24	<1	1	.3	.1	t
1028	Prepared with whole milk	1 c	281	77	280	15	36	<1	9	5.4	2.5	.3
1029	Prepared with 2% milk	1 c	281	78	252	15	36	<1	5	3.3	1.5	.2
1283	Prepared with 1% milk	1 c	281	79	233	16	36	<1	3	2	.9	t
1284	Prepared with nonfat milk	1 c	281	80	215	16	36	<1	1	.6	.3	t
117	Malted milk, chocolate, powder:[4]	¾ oz	21	1	79	1	18	<1	1	.5	.2	.1
118	Prepared with whole milk	1 c	265	81	228	9	30	1	9	5.5	2.6	.4
1661	Ovaltine with whole milk	1 c	265	81	225	9	29	1	9	5.5	2.6	.4
119	Malted milk, regular, powder:[4]	¾ oz	21	2	87	2	16	<1	2	.9	.4	.3
120	Prepared with whole milk	1 c	265	81	236	10	27	<1	10	5.9	2.8	.6

(1)Milk solids added, label claims less than 10 g protein per cup.

(2)Yields 1 qt fluid milk when reconstituted according to package directions.

(3)Most values provided by product labeling.

(4)The latest USDA data from *Handbook 8–14* on beverages updates previous USDA data.

(Computer code number is for West Diet Analysis program)

PAGE KEY: H–4 = BEV H–6 = DAIRY H–12 = EGGS H–14 = FAT/OIL H–18 = FRUIT H–26 = BAKERY H–36 = GRAIN H–44 = FISH H–48 = MEATS H–50 = POULTRY H–54 = SAUSAGE H–56 = MIXED/FAST H–64 = NUTS/SEEDS H–68 = SWEETS H–70 = VEG/LEG H–84 = MISC H–88 = SOUPS/SAUCES H–90 = FAST H–106 = FRZN ENTREE H–112 = BABY FOODS

Chol (mg)	Calc (mg)	Iron (mg)	Magn (mg)	Phos (mg)	Pota (mg)	Sodi (mg)	Zinc (mg)	VT-A (RE)	Thia (mg)	Ribo (mg)	Niac (mg)	V-B6 (mg)	Fola (µg)	VT-C (mg)
0	4	.01	1	13	13	43	.01	33[2]	.0	0	0	0	0	0
0	<1	0	<1	1	1	2	0	2[2]	0	0	0	0	0	0
0	6	.9	15	102	370	235	2.74	0	0	0	0	0	0	0
0	<1	.05	1	6	23	14	.16	0	0	0	0	0	0	0
13	266	.07	23	204	381	113	.87	5[5]	.09	.38	.17	.04	28	2
1	17	0	1	13	24	7	.06	<1[5]	.01	.02	.01	0	2	<1
33	290	.12	33	228	371	120	.93	76	.09	.39	.2	.1	12	2
18	298	.12	33	232	376	122	.95	139	.09	.4	.21	.1	12	2
18	311	.12	35	244	397	128	.98	140	.1	.42	.22	.11	13	2
10	300	.12	34	235	381	123	.95	144	.09	.41	.21	.1	12	2
10	311	.12	35	244	397	128	.98	145	.1	.42	.22	.11	13	2
4	301	.1	28	247	407	126	.98	149	.09	.34	.22	.1	13	2
5	316	.12	35	255	419	129	1	149	.1	.43	.22	.11	13	2
9	284	.12	27	219	370	257	1.03	20	.08	.38	.14	.08	12	2
104	869	.58	79	774	1135	389	2.88	248	.27	1.27	.64	.16	34	8
74	658	.48	61	512	764	267	1.94	136	.12	.8	.49	.13	20	5
9	740	.74	69	497	847	293	2.29	298	.11	.79	.44	.14	22	3
83	1421	.36	132	1120	1910	620	4.84	65	.47	1.9	1.05	.41	57	7
17	1119	.28	106	896	1552	500	4.01	646[6]	.38	1.58	.81	.31	45	5
12	836	.21	80	670	1159	373	3	483[6]	.28	1.18	.61	.23	34	4
28	327	.12	34	271	498	122	.73	137	.12	.34	.68	.11	1	3
10	350	.5	28	319	205	50	.9	155	.45	.44	.3	.09	23	<1
30	280	.6	33	253	418	149	1.03	73	.09	.41	.31	.1	12	2
17	285	.6	33	255	423	151	1.03	143	.09	.41	.32	.1	12	2
7	288	.6	33	258	425	152	1.03	148	.09	.42	.32	.1	12	2
1	92	.34	24	89	202	143	.41	1	.03	.16	.17	.03	0	1
2	97	.35	25	89	202	148	.45	1	.03	.17	.18	.04	3	1
0	8	.69	22	28	129	46	.34	<1	.01	.03	.11	<.01	1	<1
32	301	.8	53	255	497	164	1.28	77	.1	.43	.32	.1	12	2
149	330	.51	47	277	419	138	1.17	203	.09	.48	.27	.13	2	4
194	269	.71	32	269	367	155	1.26	197	.11	.55	.21	.15	30	2
4	105	4.74	84	158	350	142	3.16	554	.31	.07	5.25	.42	105	28
38	396	4.86	117	356	721	262	4.09	630	.41	.47	5.46	.52	118	31
23	403	4.87	118	390	726	264	4.12	693	.41	.48	5.46	.53	118	31
14	406	4.87	118	393	731	266	4.12	698	.41	.48	5.45	.52	118	31
9	406	4.84	112	404	755	268	4.14	703	.4	.42	5.47	.52	118	31
1	13	.48	15	37	129	53	.17	4	.04	.04	.42	.03	4	<1
34	305	.61	48	265	498	172	1.09	80	.13	.44	.62	.13	16	3
34	385	4	53	313	620	244	1.17	901	.74	1.26	10.9	1.02	32	34
4	63	.15	20	75	159	104	.21	18	.11	.19	1.1	.09	10	1
37	355	.26	53	302	530	223	1.14	95	.2	.59	1.31	.19	22	3

(5)Vitamin A value is from beta-carotene used for coloring.

(6)With added vitamin A.

H

Table H–1
Food Composition

Computer Code Number	Food Description	Measure	Wt (g)	H_2O (%)	Ener (kcal)	Prot (g)	Carb (g)	Dietary Fiber (g)	Fat (g)	Fat Breakdown (g) Sat	Mono	Poly
	DAIRY—Cont.											
121	Milk shakes, chocolate (10 fl oz)	1¼ c	283	72	359	10	58	<1	10	6.5	3	.4
122	Milk shakes, vanilla (10 fl oz)	1¼ c	283	75	314	10	51	<1	8	5.3	2.4	.3
	Milk desserts:											
134	Custard, baked	1 c	265	79	278	13	28	0	12	6.2	4	1
1548	Low-fat frozen dessert bars	1 ea	81	72	90	2	18	0	1	.2	.1	.4
	Ice cream, vanilla (about 10% fat):											
123	Hardened: ½ gallon	1 ea	1064	61	2138	37	251	1	117	72.4	33.8	4.4
124	Cup	1 c	133	61	267	5	31	<1	15	9	4.2	.6
125	Fluid ounces	3 oz	50	61	101	2	12	<1	6	3.4	1.6	.2
126	Soft serve	1 c	173	60	372	7	38	<1	22	12.9	6	.8
	Ice cream, rich vanilla (16% fat):											
127	Hardened: ½ gallon	1 ea	1188	60	2554	49	264	1	154	88.9	41.5	5.5
128	Cup	1 c	148	57	357	5	33	<1	24	14.8	6.9	.9
1724	Ben & Jerry's	½ c	106	64	230	4	21	0	17	10	–	–
	Ice milk, vanilla (about 4% fat):											
129	Hardened: ½ gallon	1 ea	1048	68	1456	40	238	1	45	27.7	12.9	1.7
130	Cup	1 c	131	68	182	5	30	<1	6	3.5	1.6	.2
131	Soft serve (about 3% fat)	1 c	175	70	221	9	38	<1	5	2.8	1.3	.2
	Pudding, canned (5-oz can = .55 cup):											
135	Chocolate	1 ea	142	69	189	4	32	1	6	1	2.4	2
136	Tapioca	1 ea	142	74	169	3	27	<1	5	.9	2.2	1.9
137	Vanilla	1 ea	142	71	185	3	31	<1	5	.8	2.2	1.9
	Puddings, dry mix with whole milk:											
138	Chocolate, instant	1 c	260	75	289	8	49	3	8	4.8	2.4	.5
139	Chocolate, regular, cooked	½ c	130	74	144	4	23	1	4	2.7	1.3	.2
140	Rice, cooked	½ c	132	72	161	4	27	1	4	2.3	1.1	.2
141	Tapioca, cooked	½ c	130	74	148	4	25	<1	4	2.3	1.1	.1
142	Vanilla, instant	½ c	130	74	148	4	26	<1	4	2.3	1.1	.2
143	Vanilla, regular, cooked	½ c	130	75	144	4	24	<1	4	2.4	1.1	.2
132	Sherbet (2% fat): ½ gallon	1 ea	1542	66	2127	17	469	0	31	17.9	8.3	1.2
133	Cup	1 c	193	66	266	2	59	0	4	2.2	1	.2
144	Soy milk	1 c	240	93	79	7	4	3	5	.5	.8	2
1584	Yogurt, frozen, low-fat[1]	½ c	87	65	138	3	21	0	5	3	1.4	.2
1512	Scoop	1 ea	79	74	78	4	16	0	<1	.1	t	0
	Yogurt, low-fat:											
1172	Fruit added with low-calorie sweetener	1 c	241	86	122	11	19	1	<1	.2	.1	t
145	Fruit added[2]	1 c	227	75	232	10	43	<1	2	1.6	.7	.1
146	Plain	1 c	227	85	144	12	16	0	4	2.3	1	.1
147	Vanilla or coffee flavor	1 c	227	79	194	11	31	0	3	1.8	.8	.1
148	Yogurt, made with nonfat milk	1 c	227	85	127	13	17	0	<1	.3	.1	t
149	Yogurt, made with whole milk	1 c	227	88	139	8	11	0	7	4.8	2	.2
	EGGS[3]											
	Raw, large:											
150	Whole, without shell	1 ea	50	75	74	6	1	0	5	1.5	1.9	.7
151	White	1 ea	33	88	17	4	<1	0	0	0	0	0
152	Yolk	1 ea	17	49	59	3	<1	0	5	1.6	1.9	.7

(1)Data is from 1992 USDA data on snacks and sweets.

(2)Carbohydrate and kcalories vary widely—consult label if more precise values are needed.

(3)This data is newest revised information from the USDA with 24% less cholesterol.

(Computer code number is for West Diet Analysis program)

Chol (mg)	Calc (mg)	Iron (mg)	Magn (mg)	Phos (mg)	Pota (mg)	Sodi (mg)	Zinc (mg)	VT-A (RE)	Thia (mg)	Ribo (mg)	Niac (mg)	V-B6 (mg)	Fola (µg)	VT-C (mg)
37	320	.88	48	289	566	275	1.16	65	.16	.69	.46	.14	10	1
31	345	.25	34	289	492	232	1.02	91	.13	.52	.52	.15	9	2
231	297	.79	37	299	405	204	1.4	159	.09	.6	.22	.13	27	1
1	82	.07	10	65	111	47	.26	38	.03	.11	.06	.03	3	1
468	1362	.96	149	1117	2117	851	7.34	1245	.44	2.55	1.23	.51	53	6
59	170	.12	19	140	265	106	.92	156	.05	.32	.15	.06	7	1
22	64	.04	7	53	100	40	.34	59	.02	.12	.06	.02	3	<1
157	227	.36	21	201	306	106	.9	266	.08	.31	.16	.08	16	1
1081	1556	2.49	143	1378	2102	725	6.18	1829	.58	2.16	1.13	.57	107	10
90	173	.07	16	141	235	83	.59	272	.06	.24	.12	.06	7	1
95	150	.36	–	–	–	55	–	225	–	–	–	–	–	0
147	1456	1.05	157	1142	2211	891	4.61	493	.61	2.78	.94	.68	63	8
18	182	.13	20	143	276	111	.58	62	.08	.35	.12	.08	8	1
21	275	.1	25	212	387	123	.93	51	.09	.35	.21	.08	11	2
4	128	.72	30	114	256	183	.6	16	.04	.22	.49	.04	4	3
1	119	.33	11	112	148	168	.38	0	.03	.14	.44	.14	6	1
10	125	.18	11	97	160	192	.35	9	.03	.2	.36	.02	0	0
29	265	.75	47	621	432	738	1.09	55	.09	.37	.25	.1	10	2
16	144	.47	20	121	212	134	.58	34	.04	.23	.13	.05	5	1
15	133	.5	17	114	165	140	.6	26	.1	.18	.6	.04	5	1
16	135	.08	16	107	172	157	.44	35	.04	.18	.09	.05	5	1
14	131	.09	16	256	166	372	.43	33	.04	.18	.1	.05	5	1
16	139	.06	17	107	177	208	.45	35	.04	.18	.1	.04	5	1
77	833	2.16	123	617	1480	709	7.4	216	.39	1.03	1.48	.52	62	66
10	104	.27	15	77	185	89	.93	27	.05	.13	.18	.07	8	8
0	10	1.39	46	117	338	29	.55	7	.39	.17	.35	.1	4	0
2	124	.26	12	112	184	76	.36	50	.03	.19	.25	.07	5	1
1	137	.07	13	108	175	53	.67	1	.03	.16	.09	.04	8	1
3	369	.61	41	291	550	139	1.83	6	.1	.45	.5	.11	32	26
10	345	.16	33	270	440	133	1.68	25	.08	.4	.22	.09	21	2
14	415	.18	40	327	529	159	2.02	36	.1	.49	.26	.11	25	2
11	388	.16	37	306	497	149	1.88	30	.09	.46	.24	.1	24	2
4	452	.2	43	356	579	174	2.2	5	.11	.53	.28	.12	28	2
29	275	.11	26	215	350	105	1.34	68	.07	.32	.17	.07	17	1
213	25	.72	5	89	61	63	.55	96	.03	.25	.04	.07	24	0
0	2	.01	4	4	47	54	0	0	<.01	.15	.03	0	1	0
218	23	.59	2	83	16	7	.52	99	.03	.11	0	.06	25	0

(For purposes of calculations, use "0" for t, <1, <.1, <.01, etc.)

Table H–1
Food Composition

Computer Code Number	Food Description	Measure	Wt (g)	H_2O (%)	Ener (kcal)	Prot (g)	Carb (g)	Dietary Fiber (g)	Fat (g)	Fat Breakdown (g) Sat	Mono	Poly
	EGGS—Cont.											
	Cooked:											
153	Fried in margarine	1 ea	46	69	92	6	1	0	7	1.9	2.8	1.3
154	Hard-cooked, shell removed	1 ea	50	75	78	6	1	0	5	1.6	2	.7
155	Hard-cooked, chopped	1 c	136	75	211	17	2	0	14	4.5	5.6	1.9
156	Poached, no added salt	1 ea	50	75	75	6	1	0	5	1.6	1.9	.7
157	Scrambled with milk & margarine	1 ea	61	73	101	7	1	0	7	2.2	2.9	1.3
1681	Egg substitute, liquid	½ c	126	83	106	15	1	0	4	.8	1.1	2
1254	Egg Beaters, Fleischmann's	.25 c	61	–	30	6	1	0	0	0	0	0
1256	Eggs, scrambled, f/frozen	0.33 c	50	70	92	6	2	0	6	1.1	1.4	3.6
1262	Eggs, Second Nature, prepared	0.33 c	69	81	66	9	1	0	3	.5	.7	1.3
	FATS and OILS											
158	Butter: Stick	½ c	113	16	810	1	<1	0	92	57.1	27.6	3.4
159	Tablespoon	1 tbs	14	16	100	<1	<1	0	11	7.1	3.4	.4
160	Pat (about 1 tsp)[1]	1 ea	5	16	36	<1	<1	0	4	2.5	1.2	.2
1682	Whipped	1 tsp	3	16	22	<1	<1	0	3	1.5	.7	.1
	Fats, cooking:											
1363	Bacon fat	1 tbs	14	0	125	0	0	0	14	6.4	5.9	1.1
1362	Beef fat/tallow	1 c	205	0	1849	0	0	0	205	103	85.7	8.2
1364	Chicken fat	1 c	205	<1	1845	0	0	0	205	61.1	91.6	42.8
161	Vegetable shortening:	1 c	205	0	1812	0	0	0	205	51.5	91.2	53.5
162	Tablespoon	1 tbs	13	0	115	0	0	0	13	3.3	5.8	3.4
163	Lard:	1 c	205	0	1849	0	0	0	205	80.4	92.5	23
164	Tablespoon	1 tbs	13	0	117	0	0	0	13	5.1	5.9	1.5
	Margarine:											
165	Imitation (about 40% fat), soft:	1 c	227	58	783	1	1	0	88	14.5	33	37
166	Tablespoon	1 tbs	14	58	48	<1	<1	0	5	.9	2	2.3
167	Regular, hard (about 80% fat):	½ c	113	16	812	1	1	0	91	14.8	42	29.6
168	Tablespoon	1 tbs	14	16	101	<1	<1	0	11	1.8	5	3.6
169	Pat	1 ea	5	16	36	<1	<1	0	4	.8	1.8	1.3
170	Regular, soft (about 80% fat):	1 c	227	16	1625	2	1	0	183	30.7	83	61
171	Tablespoon	1 tbs	14	16	100	<1	<1	0	11	1.9	5.1	3.8
	Saffola:											
2056	Unsalted	1 tbs	14	20	101	0	0	0	11	1.9	4.8	4.7
2057	Reduced fat	1 tbs	14	5.27	71	0	0	0	9	1.3	2.7	4.5
172	Spread (about 60% fat), hard:	½ c	113	37	610	1	0	0	69	15.9	29.4	20.5
173	Tablespoon	1 tbs	14	37	76	<1	0	0	9	2	3.6	2.5
174	Pat[1]	1 ea	5	37	27	<1	0	0	3	.7	1.2	1
175	Spread (about 60% fat), soft:	1 c	227	37	1226	1	0	0	138	29.1	71.5	31.3
176	Tablespoon	1 tbs	14	37	76	<1	0	0	9	1.8	4.4	1.9
2160	Touch of Butter (47% fat)	1 tbs	14	36	77	<1	0	0	9	2	4.4	1.9
	Oils:											
1585	Canola:	1 c	218	0	1927	0	0	0	218	15.5	128	64.5
1586	Tablespoon	1 tbs	14	0	124	0	0	0	14	1	8.2	4.1
177	Corn:	1 c	218	0	1927	0	0	0	218	29.4	52.8	127
178	Tablespoon	1 tbs	14	0	124	0	0	0	14	1.8	3.4	8.2

(1)Pat is 1" square, ⅓" thick; about 1 tsp; 90 per lb.

Chol (mg)	Calc (mg)	Iron (mg)	Magn (mg)	Phos (mg)	Pota (mg)	Sodi (mg)	Zinc (mg)	VT-A (RE)	Thia (mg)	Ribo (mg)	Niac (mg)	V-B6 (mg)	Fola (µg)	VT-C (mg)
211	25	.72	5	89	61	162	.55	114	.03	.24	.04	.07	17	0
212	25	.59	5	86	63	62	.53	84	.03	.26	.03	.06	22	0
577	68	1.62	14	234	171	169	1.44	228	.09	.7	.09	.17	60	0
212	25	.72	5	89	60	61	.56	95	.02	.22	.03	.06	18	0
215	43	.73	7	104	84	171	.62	119	.03	.27	.05	.07	18	<1
1	67	2.65	11	152	416	223	1.65	272	.14	.38	.14	<.01	19	0
0	40	1.08	–	–	85	100	–	–	–	–	–	–	–	–
1	42	1.14	9	41	122	114	.56	77	.06	.21	.08	.07	7	<1
1	42	1.65	7	95	260	139	1.02	170	.07	.22	.08	0	9	0
247	27	.18	2	26	29	935[2]	.06	852[3]	.01	.04	.05	<.01	3	0
31	3	.02	<1	3	4	117[2]	.01	107[3]	<.01	<.01	.01	0	<1	0
11	1	.01	<1	1	1	41[2]	<.01	38[3]	0	<.01	<.01	0	<1	0
7	1	0	<1	1	1	26[2]	<.01	24[3]	0	<.01	<.01	0	<1	0
14	<1	0	<1	0	<1	76	<.01	0	0	0	0	0	0	0
223	0	0	0	0	<1	<1	0	0	0	0	0	0	0	0
174	0	0	0	0	0	0	0	351	0	0	0	0	0	0
0	0	0	0	0	0	0	0	0	0	0	0	0	0	0
0	0	0	0	0	0	0	0	0	0	0	0	0	0	0
195	<1	0	<1	0	<1	<1	.23	0	0	0	0	0	0	0
12	<1	0	<1	0	<1	<1	.01	0	0	0	0	0	0	0
0	40	0	4	31	57	800[4]	0	2254[5]	.01	.05	.03	.01	2	<1
0	2	0	<1	2	4	49[4]	0	139[5]	<.01	<.01	<.01	<.01	<1	<1
0	34	0	3	26	48	1065[4]	.23	1122[5]	.01	.04	.03	.01	1	<1
0	4	0	<1	3	6	132[4]	.03	139[5]	<.01	<.01	<.01	<.01	<1	<1
0	2	0	<1	1	2	47[4]	.01	50[5]	<.01	<.01	<.01	0	<1	<1
0	60	0	5	46	86	1678[4]	0	2254[5]	.02	.07	.04	.02	2	<1
0	4	0	<1	3	5	103[4]	0	139[5]	<.01	<.01	<.01	<.01	<1	<1
52	0	0	–	–	–	0	–	–	–	–	–	–	–	0
–	0	0	–	–	–	116	–	52	–	–	–	–	–	0
0	24	0	2	18	34	1122[4]	.17	1122[5]	.01	.03	.02	.01	1	<1
0	3	0	<1	2	4	139[4]	0	139[5]	<.01	<.01	<.01	<.01	<1	<1
0	1	0	<1	1	1	50[4]	0	50[5]	0	<.01	<.01	0	<1	<1
0	47	0	4	37	68	2256[4]	0	2254[5]	.02	.06	.04	.01	2	<1
0	3	0	<1	2	4	139[4]	0	139[5]	<.01	<.01	<.01	<.01	<1	<1
1	3	<.01	<1	2	4	140	0	152	<.01	<.01	<.01	<.01	<1	<.1
0	0	0	0	0	0	0	0	0	0	0	0	0	0	0
0	0	0	0	0	0	0	0	0	0	0	0	0	0	0
0	0	0	0	0	0	0	0	0	0	0	0	0	0	0
0	0	0	0	0	0	0	0	0	0	0	0	0	0	0

(2)For salted butter, unsalted butter contains 12 mg sodium per stick or ½ c, 1.5 mg/tbs, or .5 mg/pat.

(3)Values for vitamin A are a year-round average.

(4)For salted margarine.

(5)Based on average vitamin A content of fortified margarine. Federal specifications require a minimum of 15,000 IU/lb.

(For purposes of calculations, use "0" for t, <1, <.1, <.01, etc.)

H

Table H–1
Food Composition

Computer Code Number	Food Description	Measure	Wt (g)	H_2O (%)	Ener (kcal)	Prot (g)	Carb (g)	Dietary Fiber (g)	Fat (g)	Fat Breakdown (g) Sat	Mono	Poly
	FATS and OILS—Cont.											
	Oils—Cont.											
179	Olive:	1 c	216	0	1909	0	0	0	216	29.2	159	18.4
180	Tablespoon	1 tbs	14	0	124	0	0	0	14	1.9	10.3	1.2
1683	Olive, extra virgin	1 tbs	14	<1	126	0	0	0	14	1.96	10.8	1.3
181	Peanut:	1 c	216	0	1909	0	0	0	216	35.6	113	56.8
182	Tablespoon	1 tbs	14	0	124	0	0	0	14	2.4	7.3	3.7
183	Safflower:	1 c	218	0	1927	0	0	0	218	19.8	26.4	162
184	Tablespoon	1 tbs	14	0	124	0	0	0	14	1.3	1.7	10.4
185	Soybean:	1 c	218	0	1927	0	0	0	218	31.4	50.8	126
186	Tablespoon	1 tbs	14	0	124	0	0	0	14	2	3.3	8.1
187	Soybean/cottonseed:	1 c	218	0	1927	0	0	0	218	40	64.3	105
188	Tablespoon	1 tbs	14	0	124	0	0	0	14	2.5	4.1	6.7
189	Sunflower:	1 c	218	0	1927	0	0	0	218	25	45	144
190	Tablespoon	1 tbs	14	0	124	0	0	0	14	1.5	2.9	9.2
	Salad dressings/sandwich spreads:											
191	Blue cheese, regular	1 tbs	15	32	76	1	1	<1	8	1.5	1.9	4.4
1040	Low calorie	1 tbs	15	80	15	1	<1	<1	1	.2	.5	.4
1684	Caesar's	1 tbs	12	36	55	1	<1	<1	5	.9	3.5	.5
192	French, regular	1 tbs	16	38	69	<1	3	<1	9	1.5	1.2	3.4
193	Low calorie	1 tbs	16	69	21	<1	3	<1	1	.1	.2	.5
194	Italian, regular	1 tbs	15	38	70	<1	1	<1	9	1	1.6	4.1
195	Low calorie	1 tbs	15	82	16	<1	1	<1	1	.2	.3	.9
	Kraft, Deliciously Right											
2150	1000 Island	2 tbs	32	–	70	0	8	0	4	1	–	–
2153	Bacon & Tomato	2 tbs	31	–	60	1	3	0	5	1	–	–
2154	Cucumber Ranch	2 tbs	31	–	60	0	2	0	5	1	–	–
2151	French	2 tbs	32	–	50	0	6	0	3	.5	–	–
2152	Ranch	2 tbs	31	–	100	0	5	0	9	1.5	–	–
199	Mayo type, regular	1 tbs	15	40	58	<1	3	0	5	.7	1.4	2.7
1030	Low calorie	1 tbs	15	54	39	<1	1	0	3	.4	.8	1.4
196	Mayonnaise:											
196	Regular (soybean)	1 tbs	14	15	100	<1	<1	0	11	1.6	3.1	5.7
197	Imitation, low calorie	1 tbs	15	63	35	<1	2	0	3	.5	.7	1.6
1488	Regular, low calorie, low sodium	1 tbs	14	63	32	<1	2	0	3	.5	.6	1.4
1493	Regular, low calorie	1 tbs	16	63	37	<1	3	0	3	.5	.7	1.6
2058	Saffola Light	1 tbs	15	–	44	0	1	0	4	.5	1	2.9
198	Ranch, regular	½ c	119	35	436	4	6	0	45	6.7	19.4	17
1042	Low calorie	1 tbs	15	70	32	0	1	0	3	.5	–	1
1685	Russian	1 tbs	15	35	74	<1	2	0	8	1.1	1.8	4.5
1502	Salad dressing, low calorie, oil free	1 tbs	15	88	4	<1	1	<1	<1	0	0	0
	Salad dressing, no cholesterol											
1605	(Miracle Whip)	1 tbs	15	57	48	0	2	0	4	1.1	1.1	2.1
203	Salad dressing, from recipe, cooked[1]	1 tbs	16	69	25	1	2	<1	2	.5	.6	.3
200	Tartar sauce, regular	1 tbs	14	34	74	<1	1	<1	8	1.5	2.6	4.1
1503	Low calorie	1 tbs	14	63	31	<1	2	<1	2	.4	.6	1.3
201	Thousand island, regular	1 tbs	16	46	60	<1	2	<1	6	1	1.3	3.2
202	Low calorie	1 tbs	15	69	24	<1	2	<1	2	.2	.4	.9
204	Vinegar & oil	1 tbs	16	47	72	0	<1	0	8	1.5	2.4	3.9

[1] Fatty acid values apply to product made with regular margarine.

PAGE KEY: H–4 = BEV H–6 = DAIRY H–12 = EGGS H–14 = FAT/OIL H–18 = FRUIT H–26 = BAKERY H–36 = GRAIN H–44 = FISH H–48 = MEATS H–50 = POULTRY H–54 = SAUSAGE H–56 = MIXED/FAST H–64 = NUTS/SEEDS H–68 = SWEETS H–70 = VEG/LEG H–84 = MISC H–88 = SOUPS/SAUCES H–90 = FAST H–106 = FRZN ENTREE H–112 = BABY FOODS

Chol (mg)	Calc (mg)	Iron (mg)	Magn (mg)	Phos (mg)	Pota (mg)	Sodi (mg)	Zinc (mg)	VT-A (RE)	Thia (mg)	Ribo (mg)	Niac (mg)	V-B6 (mg)	Fola (μg)	VT-C (mg)
0	<1	.82	<1	3	0	<1	.13	0	0	0	0	0	0	0
0	<1	.05	<1	<1	0	<1	.01	0	0	0	0	0	0	0
0	–	–	–	–	–	–	–	0	0	0	0	0	0	0
0	<1	.06	<1	0	<1	<1	.02	0	0	0	0	0	0	0
0	<1	0	<1	0	0	<1	0	0	0	0	0	0	0	0
0	0	0	0	0	0	0	0	0	0	0	0	0	0	0
0	0	0	0	0	0	0	0	0	0	0	0	0	0	0
0	<1	.04	<1	1	0	0	0	0	0	0	0	0	0	0
0	<1	<.01	<1	<1	0	0	0	0	0	0	0	0	0	0
0	0	0	0	0	0	0	0	0	0	0	0	0	0	0
0	0	0	0	0	0	0	0	0	0	0	0	0	0	0
0	0	0	0	0	0	0	0	0	0	0	0	0	0	0
0	0	0	0	0	0	0	0	0	0	0	0	0	0	0
3	12	.03	0	11	6	164	0	10	<.01	.02	.02	.01	1	<1
<1	13	.08	1	12	1	180	.04	<1	<.01	.02	.01	<.01	<1	<1
12	22	.19	3	19	20	202	.12	6	<.01	.02	.49	.01	2	1
9	2	.06	0	2	13	219	.01	3	<.01	<.01	<.01	<.01	1	0
1	2	.06	0	2	13	126	.03	0	0	0	0	0	0	0
0	2	.03	<1	1	2	118	.02	4	<.01	<.01	0	<.01	1	0
1	<1	.03	0	1	2	118	.02	0	0	0	0	0	0	0
5	0	0	–	–	55	320	–	0	–	–	–	–	–	0
3	0	0	–	–	40	300	–	0	–	–	–	–	–	0
0	0	0	–	–	20	450	–	0	–	–	–	–	–	0
0	0	0	–	–	15	260	–	100	–	–	–	–	–	0
0	0	0	–	–	0	320	–	0	–	–	–	–	–	0
4	2	.03	<1	4	1	107	.03	13	<.01	<.01	<.01	<.01	1	0
4	2	.03	<1	4	1	107	.03	10	<.01	<.01	0	0	1	0
8	3	.07	<1	4	5	80	.02	12	0	0	<.01	.08	1	0
4	<1	0	<1	<1	2	75	.02	0	0	0	0	0	0	0
3	0	0	0	0	1	15	.02	1	0	<.01	0	0	<1	0
4	<1	0	<1	<1	2	80	02	0	0	0	0	0	0	0
–	0	0	–	–	–	103	–	0	–	–	–	–	–	0
47	119	.31	12	100	158	522	.44	86	.04	.17	.08	.05	6	1
5	11	0	–	–	5	150	–	0	–	–	–	–	–	0
3	3	.1	.23	6	24	130	.06	31	.01	.01	.1	<.01	1.59	1
0	1	.04	2	1	7	256	<.01	<1	0	0	<.01	<.01	<1	<1
0	0	<.01	0	0	0	102	0	2	0	0	0	0	0	0
9	13	.08	0	14	19	117	0	20	.01	.02	.04	0	0	<1
7	3	.13	<1	4	11	99	.02	9	<.01	<.01	0	.01	1	<1
3	2	.09	<1	1	5	83	.02	2	<.01	<.01	.01	<.01	<1	<1
4	2	.09	<1	3	18	112	.02	15	<.01	<.01	<.01	<.01	1	0
2	2	.09	<1	3	17	150	.02	14	<.01	<.01	<.01	<.01	1	0
0	0	0	0	0	1	<1	0	0	0	0	0	0	0	0

(2)Sodium bisulfite used to preserve color; unsulfured product would contain lower levels of sodium.

(For purposes of calculations, use "0" for t, <1, <.1, <.01, etc.)

H

Table H–1
Food Composition

Computer Code Number	Food Description	Measure	Wt (g)	H_2O (%)	Ener (kcal)	Prot (g)	Carb (g)	Dietary Fiber (g)	Fat (g)	Fat Breakdown (g) Sat	Mono	Poly
	FATS and OILS—Cont.											
	Salad dressings/sandwich spreads—Cont.											
	Wishbone											
2179	Fat Free French	1 tbs	16	–	6	0	1	–	0	0	–	.1
2180	Lite Creamy Italian	1 tbs	15	–	26	<1	2	–	2	.4	–	.7
2166	Lite Italian	1 tbs	16	77	6	0	1	7	–	0	–	.1
2167	Lite Ranch	1 tbs	15	–	42	<1	3	0	4	.7	–	2.3
	FRUITS and FRUIT JUICES											
	Apples:											
	Fresh, raw, with peel:											
205	2 ¾" diam (about 3 per lb w/cores)	1 ea	138	84	81	<1	21	3	<1	.1	t	.1
206	3 ¾" diam (about 2 per lb w/cores)	1 ea	212	84	125	<1	32	4	1	.1	t	.2
207	Raw, peeled slices	1 c	110	85	63	<1	16	2	<1	.1	t	.1
208	Dried, sulfured	10 ea	64	32	155	1	42	6	<1	t	t	.1
209	Apple juice, bottled or canned	1 c	248	88	116	<1	29	<1	<1	<1	t	<.1
210	Applesauce, sweetened	1 c	255	80	193	<1	51	3	<1	.1	t	.1
211	Applesauce, unsweetened	1 c	244	88	104	<1	28	3	<1	<1	t	t
	Apricots:											
212	Raw, w/o pits (about 12 per lb w/ pits)	3 ea	106	86	51	1	12	2	<1	t	.2	.1
	Canned (fruit and liquid):											
213	Heavy syrup	1 c	258	78	214	1	55	3	<1	t	.1	t
214	Halves	3 ea	85	78	70	<1	18	1	<1	t	t	t
215	Juice pack	1 c	248	87	119	2	30	3	<1	t	t	t
216	Halves	3 ea	84	87	40	1	10	1	<1	t	t	t
217	Dried, halves	10 ea	35	31	83	1	22	3	<1	t	.1	t
218	Dried, cooked, unsweetened, w/liquid	1 c	250	76	212	3	55	9	<1	t	.2	.1
219	Apricot nectar, canned	1 c	251	85	140	1	36	2	<1	t	.1	t
	Avocados, raw, edible part only:											
220	California (2 lb with refuse)	1 ea	173	73	306	4	12	6	30	4.5	19.4	3.5
221	Florida (1 lb with refuse)	1 ea	304	80	340	5	27	8	27	5.3	14.8	4.5
222	Mashed, fresh, average	1 c	230	74	370	5	17	9	35	5.6	22.1	4.5
	Bananas, raw, without peel:											
223	Whole, 8¾" long (175 g w/peel)	1 ea	114	74	104	1	27	2	1	.2	t	.1
224	Slices	1 c	150	74	137	2	35	3	1	.3	.1	.1
1285	Bananas, dehydrated slices	1 oz	28	3	98	1	25	2	1	.2	t	.1
225	Blackberries, raw	1 c	144	86	75	1	18	6	1	.3	.1	.1
	Blueberries:											
226	Fresh	1 c	145	85	81	1	20	4	1	t	.2	.3
227	Frozen, sweetened	10 oz	284	77	230	1	62	6	<1	.1	.1	.2
228	Frozen, thawed	1 c	230	77	186	1	50	5	<1	.1	.1	.2
	Cherries:											
229	Sour, red pitted, canned water pack	1 c	244	90	88	2	22	2	<1	.1	.1	.1
230	Sweet, red pitted, raw	10 ea	68	81	49	1	11	<1	1	.1	.2	.2
231	Cranberry juice cocktail[1]	1 c	253	85	144	0[2]	36	<1	<1	.1	t	.1
1411	Cranberry juice, low calorie	¾ c	178	95	34	0	8	1	0	0	0	0
232	Cranberry-apple juice	1 c	253	83	169	<1	43	<1	<1[3]	t	t	.1

(1) Data here are from the newest USDA *Handbook 8–14* on beverages. These data are somewhat different from that presented in *Handbook 8–9* on fruits and fruit juices.

(2) The newest USDA *Handbook 8–14* data on beverages indicates "0" for protein.

(3) The newest USDA *Handbook 8–14* data on beverages indicates "0" for fat.

(Computer code number is for West Diet Analysis program)

PAGE KEY: H–4 = BEV H–6 = DAIRY H–12 = EGGS H–14 = FAT/OIL H–18 = FRUIT H–26 = BAKERY H–36 = GRAIN H–44 = FISH H–48 = MEATS H–50 = POULTRY H–54 = SAUSAGE H–56 = MIXED/FAST H–64 = NUTS/SEEDS H–68 = SWEETS H–70 = VEG/LEG H–84 = MISC H–88 = SOUPS/SAUCES H–90 = FAST H–106 = FRZN ENTREE H–112 = BABY FOODS

Chol (mg)	Calc (mg)	Iron (mg)	Magn (mg)	Phos (mg)	Pota (mg)	Sodi (mg)	Zinc (mg)	VT-A (RE)	Thia (mg)	Ribo (mg)	Niac (mg)	V-B6 (mg)	Fola (μg)	VT-C (mg)
0	–	–	–	–	–	249	–	–	–	–	–	–	–	–
<1	0	0	–	–	–	148	–	–	0	0	0	–	–	0
0	1	0	–	–	–	249	–	–	0	0	0	–	–	–
5	0	0	0	0	0	148	0	–	0	0	0	–	–	0
0	10	.25	7	10	159	0	.05	7	.02	.02	.11	.07	4	8
0	15	.38	11	15	244	0	.08	11	.04	.03	.16	.1	6	12
0	4	.08	3	8	124	0	.04	5	.02	.01	.1	.05	<1	4
0	9	.9	10	24	288	56[2]	.13	6	0	.1	.59	.08	0	2
0	17	.92	7	17	295	7	.07	<1	.05	.04	.25	.07	<1	2
0	10	.89	8	18	155	8	.1	3	.03	.07	.48	.07	2	4[4]
0	7	.29	7	17	183	5	.07	7	.03	.06	.46	.06	1	3[4]
0	15	.57	8	20	313	1	.28	277	.03	.04	.64	.06	9	11
0	23	.77	18	31	361	10	.28	317	.05	.06	.97	.14	4	8
0	8	.25	6	10	119	3	.09	105	.02	.02	.32	.05	1	3
0	30	.74	25	50	409	10	.27	419	.04	.05	.85	.13	4	12
0	10	.25	8	17	139	3	.09	142	.01	.02	.29	.04	1	4
0	16	1.65	16	41	482	4	.26	253	<.01	.05	1.05	.05	4	1
0	40	4.18	42	102	1222	8	.66	590	.01	.07	2.36	.28	0	4
0	18	.95	13	23	286	8	.23	331	.02	.03	.65	.05	3	2[5]
0	19	2.04	71	73	1096	21	.73	106	.19	.21	3.32	.48	113	14
0	33	1.61	103	118	1483	15	1.28	185	.33	.37	5.84	.85	162	24
0	25	2.37	90	94	1377	23	.97	140	.25	.28	4.42	.64	142	18
0	7	.35	33	23	451	1	.18	9	.05	.11	.62	.66	22	10
0	9	.46	43	30	594	2	.24	12	.07	.15	.81	.87	29	14
0	6	.33	31	21	417	1	.17	9	.05	.07	.79	.15	11	2
0	46	.82	29	30	282	0	.39	24	.04	.06	.58	.08	49	30
0	9	.25	7	14	129	9	.16	15	.07	.07	.52	.05	9	19
0	17	1.11	6	20	170	3	.17	13	.06	.15	.72	.17	19	3
0	14	.9	5	16	138	2	.14	10	.05	.12	.58	.14	15	2
0	27	3.37	15	24	239	17	.17	183	.04	.1	.43	.11	19	5
0	10	.26	7	13	152	0	.04	14	.03	.04	.27	.02	3	5
0	8	.38	5	5	45	5	.18	1	.02	.02	.09	.05	1	90[6]
0	16	.07	4	2	39	5	.04	1	.02	.02	.06	.03	<1	57
0	18	.15	5	8	68	5	.1	1	.01	.05	.15	.05	1	81[6]

(4)Value based on products without added vitamin C. Bottled apple juice with added vitamin C usually contains 41.6 mg/100 g, or 103 mg per cup. Check label for specific vitamin C values.

(5)Without added vitamin C. Products with added vitamin C contain 136 mg per cup. Check label.

(6)Nutrient added.

(For purposes of calculations, use "0" for t, <1, <.1, <.01, etc.)

H

Table H–1
Food Composition

Computer Code Number	Food Description	Measure	Wt (g)	H_2O (%)	Ener (kcal)	Prot (g)	Carb (g)	Dietary Fiber (g)	Fat (g)	Fat Breakdown (g) Sat	Mono	Poly
	FRUITS and FRUIT JUICES—Cont.											
233	Cranberry sauce, canned, strained	1 c	277	61	418	1	107	3	<1	t	.1	.2
234	Dates, whole, without pits	10 ea	83	22	228	2	61	6	<1	.2	.1	t
235	Dates, chopped	1 c	178	22	490	4	130	13	1	.3	.2	t
236	Figs, dried	10 ea	187	28	477	6	122	17	2	.4	.5	1
	Fruit cocktail, canned, fruit and liq:											
237	Heavy syrup pack	1 c	255	80	186	1	48	3	<1	t	t	.1
238	Juice pack	1 c	248	87	114	1	29	3	<1	t	t	t
	Grapefruit:											
	Raw 3¾" diam (half w/rind = 241 g)											
239	Pink/red, half fruit, edible part	1 ea	123	91	37	1	9	2	<1	t	t	t
240	White, half fruit, edible part	1 ea	118	90	39	1	10	2	<1	t	t	t
241	Canned sections with light syrup	1 c	254	84	152	1	39	1	<1	t	t	.1
	Grapefruit juice:											
242	Fresh, raw	1 c	247	90	96	1	23	<1	<1	t	t	.1
243	Canned, unsweetened	1 c	247	90	94	1	22	<1	<1	t	t	.1
244	Sweetened	1 c	250	87	115	1	28	<1	<1	t	t	.1
	Frozen concentrate, unsweetened:											
245	Undiluted, 6-fl-oz can	¾ c	207	62	302	4	71	1	1	.1	.1	.2
246	Diluted with 3 cans water	1 c	247	89	101	1	24	<1	<1	.1	t	.1
	Grapes, raw European (adherent skin):											
247	Thompson seedless	10 ea	50	81	35	<1	9	<1	<1	.1	t	.1
248	Tokay/Emperor, seeded types	10 ea	57	81	40	<1	10	<1	<1	.1	t	.1
	Grape juice:											
249	Bottled or canned	1 c	253	84	154	1	38	2	<1	.1	t	.1
	Frozen concentrate, sweetened:											
250	Undiluted, 6-fl-oz can	¾ c	216	54	387	1	96	<1	1	.2	t	.2
251	Diluted with 3 cans water	1 c	250	87	127	<1	32	<1	<1	.1	t	.1
1410	Low calorie	1 c	250	84	153	1	37	<1	<1	.1	t	.1
252	Kiwi fruit, raw, peeled (88 g with peel)	1 ea	76	83	46	1	11	1	<1	t	.1	.1
253	Lemons, raw, without peel and seeds (about 4 per lb whole)	1 ea	58	89	17	1	5	2	<1	t	t	.1
	Lemon juice:											
254	Fresh:	1 c	244	91	61	1	21	1	<1	.1	t	.2
255	Tablespoon	1 tbs	15	91	4	<1	1	<1	<1	t	t	t
256	Canned or bottled, unsweetened:	1 c	244	93	51	1	16	1	1	.1	t	.2
257	Tablespoon	1 tbs	15	93	3	<1	1	<1	<1	t	t	t
258	Frozen, single strength, unsweetened:	1 c	244	92	54	1	16	1	1	.1	t	.2
259	Tablespoon	1 tbs	15	92	3	<1	1	<1	<1	t	t	t
	Lime juice:											
260	Fresh:	1 c	246	90	66	1	22	1	<1	t	t	.1
261	Tablespoon	1 tbs	15	90	4	<1	1	<1	<1	t	t	t
262	Canned or bottled, unsweetened	1 c	246	93	52	1	16	1	1	.1	.1	.2
263	Mangoes, raw, edible part (300 g w/skin & seeds)	1 ea	207	82	134	1	35	6	1	.1	.2	.1

(Computer code number is for West Diet Analysis program)

H

PAGE KEY: H–4 = BEV H–6 = DAIRY H–12 = EGGS H–14 = FAT/OIL H–18 = FRUIT H–26 = BAKERY H–36 = GRAIN H–44 = FISH H–48 = MEATS H–50 = POULTRY H–54 = SAUSAGE H–56 = MIXED/FAST H–64 = NUTS/SEEDS H–68 = SWEETS H–70 = VEG/LEG H–84 = MISC H–88 = SOUPS/SAUCES H–90 = FAST H–106 = FRZN ENTREE H–112 = BABY FOODS

Chol (mg)	Calc (mg)	Iron (mg)	Magn (mg)	Phos (mg)	Pota (mg)	Sodi (mg)	Zinc (mg)	VT-A (RE)	Thia (mg)	Ribo (mg)	Niac (mg)	V-B6 (mg)	Fola (µg)	VT-C (mg)
0	11	.61	8	17	72	80	.14	6	.04	.06	.28	.04	2	6
0	27	.95	29	33	541	2	.24	4	.07	.08	1.83	.16	10	0
0	57	2.05	62	71	1160	5	.52	9	.16	.18	3.92	.34	22	0
0	269	4.19	110	127	1331	21	.95	24	.13	.16	1.3	.42	14	2
0	15	.74	13	28	224	15	.2	51	.05	.05	.95	.13	7	5
0	20	.52	17	35	235	10	.22	77	.03	.04	1	.13	6	7
0	13	.15	10	11	159	0	.09	32[1]	.04	.02	.23	.05	15	47
0	14	.07	11	9	175	0	.08	1	.04	.02	.32	.05	12	39
0	36	1.02	25	25	328	5	.2	2	.1	.05	.62	.05	22	54
0	22	.49	30	37	400	2	.12	2[2]	.1	.05	.49	.11	25	94
0	17	.49	25	27	378	2	.22	2	.1	.05	.57	.05	26	72
0	20	.9	25	27	405	5	.15	2	.1	.06	.8	.05	26	67
0	56	1.01	79	101	1001	6	.37	6	.3	.16	1.6	.32	26	248
0	20	.35	27	35	336	2	.12	2	.1	.05	.54	.11	9	83
0	6	.13	3	7	92	1	.03	3	.05	.03	.15	.05	2	5
0	6	.15	3	7	105	1	.03	4	.05	.03	.17	.06	2	6
0	23	.61	25	28	334	8	.13	3	.07	.09	.66	.16	7	<1
0	28	.78	32	32	159	15	.28	6	.11	.2	.93	.32	9	179[3]
0	10	.25	10	10	52	5	.1	2	.04	.06	.31	.1	3	60[3]
0	22	.6	25	27	330	8	.12	2	.06	.09	.65	.16	6	<1
0	20	.31	23	30	252	4	.08[4]	13	.01	.04	.38	.04	17	74
0	15	.35	5	9	80	1	.03	2	.02	.01	.06	.05	6	31
0	17	.07	15	15	303	2	.12	5	.07	.02	.24	.12	31	112
0	1	0	1	1	19	<1	.01	<1	0	0	.01	.01	2	7
0	27	.32	19	22	249	51	.15	4	.1	.02	.48	.1	25	60
0	2	.02	1	1	15	3	.01	<1	.01	0	.03	.01	2	4
0	19	.29	19	19	217	2	.12	3	.14	.03	.33	.15	23	77
0	1	.02	1	1	13	<1	.01	<1	.01	0	.02	.01	1	5
0	22	.07	15	17	268	2	.15	2	.05	.02	.25	.11	20	72
0	1	0	1	1	16	<1	.01	<1	0	0	.01	.01	1	4
0	29	.57	17	25	184	39[5]	.15	4	.08	.01	.4	.07	19	16
0	21	.27	19	23	323	4	.08	805	.12	.12	1.21	.28	39	57

(1) Vitamin A in Texas red grapefruit would be 74 RE.

(2) This is vitamin A for white grapefruit juice; pink or red grapefruit juice = 109 RE per cup.

(3) With added vitamin C (ascorbic acid).

(4) Data are estimated from other fruit data.

(5) Sodium benzoate and sodium bisulfite added as preservatives.

(For purposes of calculations, use "0" for t, <1, <.1, <.01, etc.)

H

Table H–1
Food Composition

Computer Code Number	Food Description	Measure	Wt (g)	H_2O (%)	Ener (kcal)	Prot (g)	Carb (g)	Dietary Fiber (g)	Fat (g)	Fat Breakdown (g) Sat	Mono	Poly
	FRUITS and FRUIT JUICES—Cont.											
	Melons, raw, without rind and contents:											
264	Cantaloupe, 5" diam (2 ⅓ lb whole with refuse), orange flesh	½ ea	267	90	93	2	22	2	1	.1	.1	.2
265	Honeydew, 6½" diam (5¼ lb whole with refuse), slice = ⅒ melon	1 pce	129	90	45	1	12	1	<1	t	t	t
266	Nectarines, raw, w/o pits, 2½" diam	1 ea	136	86	67	1	16	2	1	.1	.2	.3
	Oranges, raw:											
267	Whole w/o peel and seeds, 2 ⅝" diam (180 g with peel and seeds)	1 ea	131	87	62	1	15	3	<1	t	t	t
268	Sections, without membranes	1 c	180	87	85	2	21	4	<1	t	t	t
	Orange juice:											
269	Fresh, all varieties	1 c	248	88	112	2	26	<1	<1	.1	.1	.1
270	Canned, unsweetened	1 c	249	89	105	1	24	<1	<1	t	.1	.1
271	Chilled	1 c	249	88	110	2	25	<1	1	.1	.1	.2
	Frozen concentrate:											
272	Undiluted (6-oz can)	¾ c	213	58	339	5	81	2	<1	.1	.1	.1
273	Diluted w/3 parts water by volume	1 c	249	88	112	2	27	<1	<1	t	t	t
1345	Orange juice, from dry crystals	1 c	248	88	114	0	29	0	<1	t	t	t
274	Orange and grapefruit juice, canned	1 c	247	89	106	1	25	<1	<1	t	t	t
	Papayas, raw:											
275	½" slices	1 c	140	89	54	1	14	3	<1	.1	.1	t
276	Whole, 3½" diam by 5⅛" w/o seeds and skin (1 lb w/refuse)	1 ea	304	89	118	2	30	5	<1	.1	.1	.1
1031	Papaya nectar, canned	1 c	250	85	142	<1	36	2	<1	.1	.1	.1
	Peaches:											
277	Raw, whole, 2½" diam, peeled, pitted (about 4 per lb whole)	1 ea	87	88	37	1	10	2	<1	t	t	t
278	Raw, sliced	1 c	170	88	73	1	19	3	<1	t	.1	.1
	Canned, fruit and liquid:											
279	Heavy syrup pack:	1 c	256	79	189	1	51	3	<1	t	.1	.1
280	Half	1 ea	81	79	60	<1	16	1	<1	t	t	t
281	Juice pack:	1 c	248	88	109	2	29	4	<1	t	t	t
282	Half	1 ea	77	88	34	<1	9	1	<1	t	t	t
283	Dried, uncooked	10 ea	130	32	311	5	80	12	1	.1	.4	.5
284	Dried, cooked, fruit and liquid	1 c	258	78	198	3	51	7	1	.1	.2	.3
	Frozen, slice, sweetened:											
285	10-oz package	1 ea	284	75	266	2	68	4	<1	t	.1	.2
286	Cup, thawed measure	1 c	250	75	235	2	60	4	<1	t	.1	.2
1032	Peach nectar, canned	1 c	249	86	134	1	35	1	<1	t	t	t
	Pears:											
	Fresh, with skin, cored:											
287	Bartlett, 2½" diam (about 2½ per lb)	1 ea	166	84	98	1	25	4[1]	1	t	.1	.2
288	Bosc, 2 1/5" diam (about 3 per lb)	1 ea	141	84	83	1	21	3[1]	1	t	.1	.1
289	D'Anjou, 3" diam (about 2 per lb)	1 ea	200	84	118	1	30	5[1]	1	t	.2	.2
	Canned, fruit and liquid:											
290	Heavy syrup pack:	1 c	255	80	188	1	49	5[1]	<1	t	.1	.1
291	Half	1 ea	79	80	58	<1	15	2[1]	<1	t	t	t
292	Juice pack:	1 c	248	86	124	1	32	5[1]	<1	t	t	t
293	Half	1 ea	77	86	38	<1	10	2[1]	<1	t	t	t

(1)Dietary fiber data vary 2.4 to 3.4 g/100 g for fresh pears; 1.6 to 2.6 g/100 g for canned pears.

(Computer code number is for West Diet Analysis program)

Chol (mg)	Calc (mg)	Iron (mg)	Magn (mg)	Phos (mg)	Pota (mg)	Sodi (mg)	Zinc (mg)	VT-A (RE)	Thia (mg)	Ribo (mg)	Niac (mg)	V-B6 (mg)	Fola (µg)	VT-C (mg)
0	29	.56	29	45	825	24	.43	860	.1	.06	1.53	.31	45	113
0	8	.09	9	13	350	13	.11	5	.1	.02	.77	.08	39	32
0	7	.2	11	22	288	0	.12	101	.02	.06	1.35	.03	5	7
0	52	.13	13	18	237	0	.09	27	.11	.05	.37	.08	40	70
0	72	.18	18	25	326	0	.13	38	.16	.07	.51	.11	54	96
0	27	.5	27	42	496	2	.12	50	.22	.07	.99	.1	75	124
0	20	1.1	27	35	436	5	.17	45	.15	.07	.78	.22	45	86
0	25	.42	27	27	473	3	.1	20[2]	.19	.28	.05	.7	45[2]	82[2]
0	68	.75	72	121	1435	6	.38	59	.6	.14	1.53	.33	330	294
0	22	.25	25	40	473	3	.12	20	.2	.04	.5	.11	109	97
0	62	.2	2	37	50	12	.1	551	0	.04	0	0	142	121
0	20	1.14	25	35	390	7	.17	30	.14	.07	.83	.06	35	72
0	34	.14	14	7	360	4	.1	39	.04	.04	.47	.03	53	86
0	73	.3	30	15	781	9	.21	85	.08	.1	1.03	.06	115	187
0	25	.85	7	0	77	13	.37	27	.01	.01	.37	.02	5	8
0	4	.1	6	10	171	0	.12	47	.01	.04	.86	.02	3	6
0	8	.19	12	20	335	0	.24	92	.03	.07	1.68	.03	6	11
0	8	.69	13	28	235	15	.23	84	.03	.06	1.57	.05	8	7
0	2	.22	4	9	74	5	.07	27	.01	.02	.5	.01	3	2
0	15	.67	17	42	317	10	.27	94	.02	.04	1.44	.05	8	9
0	5	.21	5	13	99	3	.08	29	.01	.01	.45	.01	3	3
0	36	5.28	55	153	1293	9	.74	281	<.01	.28	5.69	.09	<1	6
0	23	3.38	33	98	826	5	.46	52	.01	.05	3.92	.1	<1	10
0	9	1.05	14	31	369	17	.14	81	.04	.1	1.85	.05	9	267[3]
0	8	.92	12	27	325	15	.12	71	.03	.09	1.63	.04	8	236[3]
0	12	.47	10	15	100	17	.2	64	.01	.03	.72	.02	3	13
0	18	.41	10	18	208	0	.2	3	.03	.07	.17	.03	12	7
0	16	.35	8	16	176	0	.17	3	.03	.06	.14	.02	10	6
0	22	.5	12	22	250	0	.24	4	.04	.08	.2	.04	15	8
0	13	.56	10	18	165	13	.2	1	.03	.06	.62	.04	3	3
0	4	.17	3	6	51	4	.06	<1	.01	.02	.19	.01	1	1
0	22	.72	17	30	238	10	.22	2	.03	.03	.5	.03	3	4
0	7	.22	5	9	74	3	.07	1	.01	.01	.15	.01	1	1

(2) Values for juice from California oranges indicate the following values for 1 c: 36 RE of vitamin A, 72 µg of folate, and 106 mg of vitamin C.

(3) With added vitamin C (ascorbic acid).

(For purposes of calculations, use "0" for t, <1, <.1, <.01, etc.)

H

Table H-1
Food Composition

Computer Code Number	Food Description	Measure	Wt (g)	H_2O (%)	Ener (kcal)	Prot (g)	Carb (g)	Dietary Fiber (g)	Fat (g)	Fat Breakdown (g) Sat	Mono	Poly
	FRUITS and FRUIT JUICES—Cont.											
294	Dried halves	10 ea	175	27	459	3	121	13	1	.1	.2	.3
1033	Pear nectar, canned	1 c	250	84	150	<1	39	2	<1	t	t	t
	Pineapple:											
295	Fresh chunks, diced	1 c	155	87	76	1	19	2	1	t	.1	.2
	Canned, fruit and liquid:											
	Heavy syrup pack:											
296	Crushed, chunks, tidbits	⅓ c	84	79	65	<1	17	1	<1	t	t	t
297	Slices	1 ea	58	79	45	<1	12	<1	<1	t	t	t
	Pineapple, canned—Cont.											
298	Juice pack, crushed, chunks, tidbits	1 c	250	84	150	1	39	2	<1	t	t	.1
299	Juice pack, slices	1 ea	58	84	35	<1	9	<1	<1	t	t	t
300	Pineapple juice, canned, unsweetened	1 c	250	86	140	1	35	<1	<1	t	t	.1
	Plantains, without peel:											
301	Raw slices (whole = 179 g w/o peel)	1 c	148	65	181	2	47	3[1]	1	.3	.1	.1
302	Cooked, boiled, sliced	1 c	154	67	179	1	48	4	<1	.1	t	.1
	Plums:											
303	Fresh, medium, 2⅛" diam	1 ea	66	85	36	1	9	1	<1	t	.3	.1
304	Fresh, small, 1½" diam	1 ea	28	85	15	<1	4	<1	<1	t	.1	t
	Canned, purple, with liquid:											
305	Heavy syrup pack:	1 c	258	76	229	1	60	3	<1	t	.2	.1
306	Plums	3 ea	110	76	98	<1	26	1	<1	t	.1	t
307	Juice pack:	1 c	252	84	146	1	38	3	<1	t	t	t
308	Plums	3 ea	95	84	55	<1	14	1	<1	t	t	t
1698	Pomegranate, fresh	1 ea	154	81	105	1	27	5	<1	–	–	–
	Prunes, dried, pitted:											
309	Uncooked (10 = 97 g w/pits, 84 g w/o pits)	10 ea	84	32	200	2	53	8[2]	<1	t	.3	.1
310	Cooked, unsweetened, fruit & liq (250 g w/pits)	1c	212	70	227	3	60	14	<1	t	.3	.1
311	Prune juice, bottled or canned	1c	256	81	182	2	45	3	1	t	.5	t
	Raisins, seedless:											
312	Cup, not pressed down	1 c	145	15	435	5	115	5	1	.2	t	.2
313	One packet, ½ oz	½ oz	14	15	42	<1	11	1	<1	t	t	t
	Raspberries:											
314	Fresh	1 c	123	87	60	1	14	5	1	t	.1	.4
315	Frozen, sweetened:	10 oz	284	73	293	2	74	13	<1	t	t	.3
316	Cup, thawed measure	1 c	250	73	258	2	66	11	<1	t	t	.2
317	Rhubarb, cooked, added sugar	1 c	240	68	278	1	75	5	<1	t	t	.1
	Strawberries:											
318	Fresh, whole, capped	1 c	149	92	45	1	10	2	1	t	.1	.3
	Frozen, sliced, sweetened:											
319	10-oz container	10 oz	284	73	272	2	74	5	<1	t	.1	.2
320	Cup, thawed measure	1 c	255	73	244	1	66	5	<1	t	t	.2
	Tangerines, without peel and seeds:											
321	Fresh (2⅜" whole) 116 g w/refuse	1 ea	84	88	37	1	9	1	<1	t	t	t
322	Canned, light syrup, fruit and liquid	1 c	252	83	153	1	41	2	<1	t	t	t
323	Tangerine juice, canned, sweetened	1 c	249	87	124	1	30	<1	<1	t	t	.1

(1)Dietary fiber value partially derived from data for bananas.

(2)Dietary fiber data can vary between 6 and 13 g for 10 prunes.

Chol (mg)	Calc (mg)	Iron (mg)	Magn (mg)	Phos (mg)	Pota (mg)	Sodi (mg)	Zinc (mg)	VT-A (RE)	Thia (mg)	Ribo (mg)	Niac (mg)	V-B6 (mg)	Fola (μg)	VT-C (mg)
0	59	3.68	58	103	933	10	.68	1	.01	.25	2.4	.13	0	12
0	12	.65	7	7	32	10	.17	<1	<.01	.03	.32	.03	3	3
0	11	.57	22	11	175	2	.12	4	.14	.06	.65	.13	16	24
0	12	.32	13	6	87	1	.1	1	.08	.02	.24	.06	4	6
0	8	.22	9	4	60	1	.07	1	.05	.01	.17	.04	3	4
0	35	.7	35	15	305	3	.25	10	.24	.05	.71	.18	12	24
0	8	.16	8	3	71	1	.06	2	.05	.01	.16	.04	3	6
0	42	.65	32	20	335	3	.27	1	.14	.05	.64	.24	58	27[3]
0	4	.89	55	50	739	6	.21	167[4]	.08	.08	1.02	.44	33	27
0	3	.89	49	43	716	8	.2	140	.07	.08	1.16	.37	40	17
0	3	.07	5	7	113	0	.07	21	.03	.06	.33	.05	1	6
0	1	.03	2	3	48	0	.03	9	.01	.03	.14	.02	1	3
0	23	2.17	13	33	234	49	.18	67	.04	.1	.75	.07	6	1
0	10	.92	5	14	100	21	.08	29	.02	.04	.32	.03	3	<1
0	25	.86	20	38	388	3	.28	255	.06	.15	1.19	.07	7	7
0	10	.32	8	14	146	1	.1	96	.02	.06	.45	.03	2	3
0	5	.46	5	12	399	5	–	0	.05	.05	.46	.16	–	9
0	43	2.08	38	66	625	3	.44	167	.07	.14	1.65	.22	3	3
0	49	2.35	42	74	708	4	.51	65	.05	.21	1.53	.46	<1	6
0	31	3	36	64	707	10	.54	1	.04	.18	2	.56	1	11
0	71	3.02	48	141	1088	17	.39	1	.23	.13	1.19	.36	5	5
0	7	.29	5	14	105	2	.04	<1	.02	.01	.11	.03	<1	<1
0	27	.7	22	15	186	0	.57	16	.04	.11	1.11	.07	32	31
0	43	1.85	37	48	324	3	.51	17	.05	.13	.65	.1	74	47
0	37	1.63	32	42	285	3	.45	15	.05	.11	.57	.08	65	41
0	348	.5	29	19	230	2	.19	17	.04	.05	.48	.05	13	8
0	21	.57	15	28	247	1	.19	4	.03	.1	.34	.09	26	84
0	31	1.68	20	37	278	9	.17	7	.04	.14	1.14	.08	42	117
0	28	1.51	18	33	250	8	.15	6	.04	.13	1.02	.08	38	105
0	12	.08	10	8	131	1	.2	77	.09	.02	.13	.06	17	26
0	18	.93	20	25	196	15	.6	212	.13	.11	1.12	.11	12	50
0	45	.5	20	35	443	3	.07	105	.15	.05	.25	.08	11	55

[3] If vitamin C is added, it contains 96 mg per cup.

[4] Vitamin A values range from 1.5 RE for white-fleshed varieties to 178 RE for yellow-fleshed varieties.

(For purposes of calculations, use "0" for t, <1, <.1, <.01, etc.)

H

Table H–1
Food Composition

Computer Code Number	Food Description	Measure	Wt (g)	H_2O (%)	Ener (kcal)	Prot (g)	Carb (g)	Dietary Fiber (g)	Fat (g)	Fat Breakdown (g) Sat	Mono	Poly
	FRUITS and FRUIT JUICES—Cont.											
	Watermelon, raw, without rind & seeds:											
324	Piece, 1" by 10" diam (2 lb w/refuse or 926 g)	1 pce	482	91	154	3	35	1	2	.6	.4	1.1
325	Diced	1 c	160	91	51	1	11	1	1	.2	.1	.4
	BAKED GOODS: BREADS, CAKES, COOKIES, CRACKERS, PIES											
326	Bagels, plain, enriched, 3½" diam	1 ea	68	33	187	7	36	2	1	.1	.1	.5
1663	Bagel, oat bran	1 ea	68	33	173	7	36	8	1	.1	.2	.3
	Biscuits:											
327	From home recipe	1 ea	28	29	100	2	13	<1	5	1.2	2	1.2
328	From mix	1 ea	28	29	94	2	14	1	3	.8	1.2	1.2
329	From refrigerated dough	1 ea	20	27	75	1	9	<1	4	2	1	.1
330	Bread crumbs, dry, grated (see #364, 365 for soft crumbs)	1 c	100	6	395	12	72	4	5	1.3	2.1	2
	Breads:											
331	Boston brown, canned, 3¼" slice	1 pce	45	47	88	2	19	2	1	.1	.1	.3
332	Cracked wheat (¼ cracked-wheat & ¾ enr wheat flour): 1-lb loaf	1 ea	454	36	1180	39	225	27	18	4.2	8.6	3.1
333	Slice (18 per loaf)	1 pce	25	36	65	2	12	2	1	.2	.5	.2
334	Slice, toasted	1 pce	21	30	59	2	11	1	1	.2	.4	.2
335	French/Vienna, enriched: 1-lb loaf	1 ea	454	34	1243	40	236	13	14	2.9	5.5	3.1
337	Slice, 4¾ x 4 x ½"	1 pce	25	34	68	2	13	1	1	.2	.3	.2
336	French, slice, 5 x 2½"	1 pce	35	34	96	3	18	1	1	.2	.4	.2
	French toast: see Mixed Dishes, and Fast Foods, #691											
2083	Honey Wheatberry	1 pce	38	2	100	3	18	2	2	0	.5	0
338	Italian, enriched: 1-lb loaf	1 ea	454	36	1230	40	227	14	16	3.9	3.7	6.3
339	Slice, 4½ x 3¼ x ¾"	1 pce	30	36	81	3	15	1	1	.3	.2	.4
340	Mixed grain, enriched: 1-lb loaf	1 ea	454	38	1135	45	211	32	17	3.7	6.9	4.2
341	Slice (18 per loaf)	1 pce	25	38	62	3	12	2	1	.2	.4	.2
342	Slice, toasted	1 pce	23	32	63	3	12	2	1	.2	.4	.2
343	Oatmeal, enriched: 1-lb loaf	1 ea	454	37	1221	38	220	18	20	3.2	7.2	7.7
344	Slice (18 per loaf)	1 pce	25	37	67	2	12	1	1	.2	.4	.4
345	Slice, toasted	1 pce	23	31	67	2	12	1	1	.2	.4	.4
346	Pita pocket bread, enr, 6½" round	1 ea	60	32	165	5	33	1	1	.1	.1	.3
347	Pumpernickel (⅔ rye & ⅓ enr wheat flour): 1-lb loaf	1 ea	454	38	1135	39	216	33	14	2	4.2	5.6
348	Slice, 5 x 4 x ⅜"	1 pce	32	38	80	3	15	2	1	.1	.3	.4
349	Slice, toasted	1 pce	29	32	80	3	15	2	1	.1	.3	.4
350	Raisin, enriched: 1-lb loaf	1 ea	454	34	1243	36	237	20	20	4.9	10.4	3.1
351	Slice (18 per loaf)	1 pce	25	34	68	2	13	1	1	.3	.6	.2
352	Slice, toasted	1 pce	21	28	62	2	12	1	1	.2	.5	.2
353	Rye, light (⅓ rye & ⅔ enr wheat flour): 1-lb loaf	1 ea	454	37	1177	39	219	28	15	2.8	6	3.6
354	Slice, 4¾ x 3¾ x 7/16"	1 pce	25	37	65	2	12	2	1	.2	.3	.2
355	Slice, toasted	1 pce	22	31	62	2	12	2	1	.2	.3	.2

(1)A blend of white and whole-wheat flour—no official ratio specified.

(Computer code number is for West Diet Analysis program)

H

PAGE KEY: H–4 = BEV H–6 = DAIRY H–12 = EGGS H–14 = FAT/OIL H–18 = FRUIT H–26 = BAKERY H–36 = GRAIN H–44 = FISH H–48 = MEATS H–50 = POULTRY H–54 = SAUSAGE H–56 = MIXED/FAST H–64 = NUTS/SEEDS H–68 = SWEETS H–70 = VEG/LEG H–84 = MISC H–88 = SOUPS/SAUCES H–90 = FAST H–106 = FRZN ENTREE H–112 = BABY FOODS

Chol (mg)	Calc (mg)	Iron (mg)	Magn (mg)	Phos (mg)	Pota (mg)	Sodi (mg)	Zinc (mg)	VT-A (RE)	Thia (mg)	Ribo (mg)	Niac (mg)	V-B6 (mg)	Fola (μg)	VT-C (mg)
0	39	.82	53	43	559	10	.34	178	.39	.1	.96	.69	11	46
0	13	.27	18	14	186	3	.11	59	.13	.03	.32	.23	4	15
0	50	2.43	20	65	69	363	.6	0	.37	.21	3.1	.03	15	0
0	8	2.1	39	112	139	345	1.42	<1	.23	.23	2.01	.14	31	<1
1	67	.81	5	46	34	163	.15	6	.1	.09	.84	.01	3	<1
1	52	.58	7	131	53	267	.17	7	.1	.1	.86	.02	2	<1
1	24	.44	2	70	23	158	.08	7	.07	.05	.44	.01	2	0
0	227	6.13	46	147	221	862	1.23	.1	.76	.43	6.85	.1	25	0
<1	31	.95	28	50	143	284	.22	5	.01	.05	.5	.04	3	0
0	195	12.8	236	695	804	2452	5.68	0	1.63	1.09	16.7	1.38	177	0
0	11	.7	13	38	44	135	.31	0	.09	.06	.92	.08	10	0
0	10	.64	12	35	40	123	.29	0	.07	.05	.75	.06	6	0
0	341	11.5	123	477	513	2764	3.95	0	2.36	1.49	21.6	.19	141	0
0	19	.63	7	26	28	152	.22	0	.13	.08	1.19	.01	8	0
0	26	.89	9	37	40	213	.3	0	.18	.11	1.66	.01	11	0
0	20	.72	–	–	–	200	–	0	.12	.07	.8	–	–	0
0	354	13.4	123	468	499	2648	3.9	0	2.15	1.33	19.9	.22	136	0
0	23	.88	8	31	33	175	.26	0	.14	.09	1.31	.01	9	0
0	413	15.8	241	799	926	2216	5.81	0	1.85	1.55	19.8	1.51	218	1
0	23	.87	13	44	51	122	.32	0	.1	.09	1.09	.08	12	<1
0	23	.87	13	44	51	122	.32	0	.08	.08	.98	.07	9	<1
0	300	12.3	168	572	645	2724	4.68	9	1.81	1.09	14.3	.31	123	2
0	16	.68	9	32	36	150	.26	<1	.1	.06	.78	.02	7	<1
0	17	.68	9	32	35	150	.26	<1	.08	.05	.71	.01	5	<1
0	52	1.58	16	58	72	322	.5	0	.36	.2	2.78	.02	14	0
0	309	13.1	245	808	944	3050	6.76	0	1.48	1.38	14	.57	155	0
0	22	.92	17	57	67	215	.48	0	.1	.1	.99	.04	11	0
0	22	.92	17	57	66	214	.47	0	.08	.09	.89	.04	8	0
0	300	13.2	118	495	1030	1770	3.27	.9	1.54	1.81	15.8	.31	154	2
0	17	.73	7	27	57	97	.18	.05	.08	.1	.87	.02	9	<1
0	15	.66	6	25	52	89	.16	.42	.06	.08	.71	.01	5	<1
0	331	12.9	182	568	754	2996	5.22	0	1.97	1.52	17.3	.34	232	0
0	18	.71	10	31	42	165	.29	0	.11	.08	.95	.02	13	0
0	18	.68	9	30	40	160	.28	0	.08	.07	.83	.02	9	<1

(For purposes of calculations, use "0" for t, <1, <.1, <.01, etc.)

Table H–1
Food Composition

Computer Code Number	Food Description	Measure	Wt (g)	H_2O (%)	Ener (kcal)	Prot (g)	Carb (g)	Dietary Fiber (g)	Fat (g)	Fat Breakdown (g) Sat	Mono	Poly
	BAKED GOODS: BREADS, CAKES, COOKIES, CRACKERS, PIES—Cont.											
356	Wheat (enr wheat & whole-wheat flour):[1] 1-lb loaf	1 ea	454	37	1180	41	213	25	19	3.9	7.3	4.5
357	Slice (18 per loaf)	1 pce	25	37	64	2	12	1	1	.2	.4	.2
358	Slice, toasted	1 pce	23	32	65	2	12	1	1	.2	.4	.2
359	White, enriched: 1-lb loaf	1 ea	454	37	1213	38	225	12	16	3.7	7.3	3.4
360	Slice (18 per loaf)	1 pce	25	37	67	2	12	1	1	.2	.4	.2
361	Slice, toasted	1 pce	22	30	64	2	12	1	1	.2	.4	.2
362	Slice (22 per loaf)	1 pce	20	37	53	2	10	1	1	.2	.3	.2
363	Slice, toasted	1 pce	17	30	50	2	9	<1	1	.2	.3	.1
364	White bread cubes, soft	1 c	30	36	81	3	15	1	1	.2	.5	.2
365	White bread crumbs, soft	1 c	45	36	120	4	23	1	1	.3	.6	.4
366	Whole-wheat: 1-lb loaf	1 ea	454	38	1116	44	209	28	19	4.2	7.6	4.5
367	Slice (16 per loaf)	1 pce	28	38	69	3	13	2	1	.3	.5	.3
368	Slice, toasted	1 pce	25	30	69	3	13	2	1	.3	.5	.3
	Bread stuffing, prepared from mix:											
369	Dry type	1 c	140	65	249	4	30	4	12	2.4	5.3	3.6
370	Moist type, with egg and margarine	1 c	203	65	341	8	45	4	15	3	6.5	4.3
	Cakes, prepared from mixes:[1]											
	Angel food:											
371	Whole cake, 9¾" diam tube	1 ea	635	33	1641	38	367	10	5	.8	.5	2.3
372	Piece, 1/12 of cake	1 pce	53	33	137	3	31	1	<1	.1	t	.2
373	Boston cream pie, ⅛ of cake	1 pce	120	45	302	3	52	2	10	3	5.3	1.2
	Coffee cake:											
374	Whole cake, 7¾ x 5⅝ x 1¼"	1 ea	430	31	1368	24	227	7	41	8	16.6	13.6
375	Piece, ⅙ of cake	1 pce	72	31	229	4	38	1	7	1.3	2.8	2.3
	Devil's food, chocolate frosting:											
376	Whole cake, 2 layer, 8 or 9" diam	1 ea	1107	23	4059	45	605	31	182	51.4	99.6	21.1
377	Piece, 1/16 of cake	1 pce	69	23	253	3	38	2	11	3.2	6.2	1.3
378	Cupcake, 2½" diam	1 ea	42	23	154	2	23	1	7	1.9	3.8	.8
	Gingerbread:											
379	Whole cake, 8" square	1 ea	570	33	1764	23	289	18	58	14.8	21.9	7.6
380	Piece, ⅑ of cake	1 pce	63	33	195	3	32	2	6	1.6	3.5	.8
	Yellow, chocolate frosting, 2 layer:											
381	Whole cake, 8 or 9" diam	1 ea	1108	22	4207	42	613	20	193	52.4	107	23.2
382	Piece, 1/16 of cake	1 pce	69	22	262	3	38	1	12	3.3	6.7	1.4
	Cakes from recipes w/enr flour:											
	Carrot cake, cream cheese frosting:[2]											
383	Whole, 9 x 13" cake	1 ea	1536	21	6693	71	725	20	406	75.1	100	208
384	Piece, 1/16 of cake, 2¼ x 3¼" slice	1 pce	112	23	488	5	53	1	30	5.5	7.3	15.2
	Fruitcake, dark:											
385	Whole cake, 7½" diam tube, 2¼" high	1 ea	1361	25	4409	39	838	48	124	15.2	56.8	44.1
386	Piece, 1/32 of cake, ⅔" arc	1 pce	43	25	139	1	26	2	4	.5	1.8	1.4
	Sheet, plain, no frosting:[3]											
387	Whole cake, 9" square	1 ea	777	23	2773	42	444	6	96	25	41.3	24.5
388	Piece, ⅑ of cake	1 pce	86	23	307	5	48	<1	11	3.3	5	2.8

(1)Excepting angel food cake, cakes were made from mixes containing vegetable shortening, and frostings were made with margarine. All mixes use enriched flour.

(2)Made with vegetable oil.

(3)Cake made with vegetable shortening.

PAGE KEY: H–4 = BEV H–6 = DAIRY H–12 = EGGS H–14 = FAT/OIL H–18 = FRUIT H–26 = BAKERY H–36 = GRAIN H–44 = FISH H–48 = MEATS H–50 = POULTRY H–54 = SAUSAGE H–56 = MIXED/FAST H–64 = NUTS/SEEDS H–68 = SWEETS H–70 = VEG/LEG H–84 = MISC H–88 = SOUPS/SAUCES H–90 = FAST H–106 = FRZN ENTREE H–112 = BABY FOODS

Chol (mg)	Calc (mg)	Iron (mg)	Magn (mg)	Phos (mg)	Pota (mg)	Sodi (mg)	Zinc (mg)	VT-A (RE)	Thia (mg)	Ribo (mg)	Niac (mg)	V-B6 (mg)	Fola (μg)	VT-C (mg)
0	476	15	209	681	913	2414	4.77	0	2	1.28	18.7	.49	185	0
0	26	.83	12	38	50	133	.26	0	.11	.08	1.13	.03	11	0
0	26	.83	12	38	50	132	.26	0	.08	.06	.93	.02	7	0
5	490	12.9	109	427	541	2452	2.81	0	2.13	1.5	17	.29	154	0
<1	27	.71	6	24	30	135	.15	0	.12	.09	.99	.01	9	0
<1	26	.73	6	23	29	130	.15	0	.09	.08	.86	.01	6	0
<1	22	.57	5	19	24	108	.12	0	.09	.07	.75	.01	7	0
<1	20	.57	4	18	22	101	.12	0	.07	.06	.67	.01	4	0
<1	25	.84	6	28	32	151	.19	0	.14	.1	1.19	.02	10	0
<1	38	1.3	9	44	48	227	.28	0	.18	.11	1.5	.15	16	0
0	327	15	390	1039	1144	2382	8.85	0	1.59	.93	17.4	.81	227	0
0	20	.94	24	64	72	147	.55	0	.1	.06	1.09	.05	14	0
0	20	.93	24	65	71	148	.55	0	.08	.05	.97	.05	10	0
0	45	1.54	17	59	104	760	.39	113	.19	.15	2.07	.06	24	0
0	130	3.35	30	99	266	936	.65	140	.34	.29	3.23	.11	35	3
0	889	3.3	76	1473	591	4756	.44	0	.65	3.12	5.61	.2	19	0
0	74	.28	6	123	49	397	.04	0	.05	.26	.47	.02	2	0
44	28	.46	7	59	47	173	.19	28	.49	.32	.23	.03	10	<1
211	585	6.19	77	925	482	1810	1.94	172	.72	.75	6.54	.21	52	1
35	98	1.04	13	155	81	303	.32	29	.12	.13	1.09	.04	9	<1
509	476	24.5	376	1350	2214	3690	7.64	310	.3	1.47	6.39	.41	89	1
32	30	1.52	23	84	138	230	.48	19	.02	.09	.4	.03	6	<1
19	18	.93	14	51	84	140	.29	12	.01	.06	.24	.02	3	<1
200	393	18.9	91	958	1375	2615	2.34	91	1.08	1.06	8.89	.22	57	1
22	43	2.09	10	106	152	289	.26	10	.12	.12	.98	.02	6	<1
609	410	23.2	332	1783	1975	3742	6.87	299	1.33	1.74	13.9	.32	89	1
38	25	1.44	21	111	123	233	.43	19	.08	.11	.86	.02	6	<1
829	384	19.4	276	1090	1714	3	7.53	5897	2.09	2.4	15.5	1.17	184	17
60	28	1.41	20	79	125	276	.55	480	.15	.17	1.13	.08	13	1
68	449	28.3	218	708	2082	3674	3.67	475	.68	1.35	10.8	.63	41	5
2	14	.89	7	22	66	116	.12	15	.02	.04	.34	.02	1	<1
505	497	11.7	108	793	613	2331	2.75	130	1.24	1.4	10.1	.26	54	2
56	55	1.3	12	88	68	258	.3	14	.14	.15	1.12	.03	6	<1

H

Table H–1
Food Composition

Computer Code Number	Food Description	Measure	Wt (g)	H_2O (%)	Ener (kcal)	Prot (g)	Carb (g)	Dietary Fiber (g)	Fat (g)	Fat Breakdown (g) Sat	Mono	Poly
	BAKED GOODS: BREADS, CAKES, COOKIES, CRACKERS, PIES—Cont.											
	Sheet, plain, uncooked white frosting:											
389	Whole cake, 9" square	1 ea	1096	22	4085	38	644	10	159	26.1	67	56.1
390	Piece, 1/6 of cake	1 pce	121	22	451	4	71	1	18	2.9	7.4	6.2
	Pound cake:											
391	Loaf, 8½ x 3½ x 3¼"	1 ea	478	25	1863	26	234	4	95	53	26.7	5.21
392	Piece, 1/17 of loaf, ½" slice	1 pce	28	25	109	2	14	<1	6	3	1.5	.31
	Cakes, commercial:											
	Cheesecake:											
401	Whole cake, 9" diam	1 ea	1110	46	3559	61	283	23	250	128	86	15.3
402	Piece, 1/12 of cake	1 pce	92	46	295	5	23	2	21	10.6	7.1	1.3
	Pound cake:											
393	Loaf, 8½ x 3½ x 3"	1 ea	500	25	1948	27	244	3	99	55.5	27.9	5.4
394	Slice, 1/17 of loaf, 2" slice	1 pce	29	25	113	2	14	<1	6	3.2	1.6	.3
	Snack: 2 small cakes per package											
395	Chocolate w/creme filling (Ding Dong)	1 ea	28	20	105	1	17	<1	4	.9	1.5	1.2
396	Sponge w/creme filling (Twinkie)	1 ea	42	20	153	1	27	<1	5	1.1	1.9	1.5
1677	Sponge cake, 1/12 of 12" cake	1 pce	65	30	188	4	40	<1	2	.5	.6	.3
1678	Strawberry shortcake, fresh	1 ea	254	74	327	5	40	4	17	10.1	4.9	1
	White, white frosting, 2 layer:											
397	Whole cake, 8 or 9" diam	1 ea	1140	20	4271	38	718	11	154	45.7	68.1	39.8
398	Piece, 1/16 of cake	1 pce	71	20	266	2	45	1	10	2.8	4.2	2.5
	Yellow, chocolate frosting, 2 layer:											
399	Whole cake, 8 or 9" diam	1 ea	1108	22	4207	42	614	20	193	52.4	107	23.2
400	Piece, 1/16 of cake	1 pce	69	22	262	3	38	1	12	3.3	6.7	1.4
1332	Bagel chips	5 pce	70	4	298	6	52	6	7	1.2	1.9	3.3
2225	Bagel chips, Onion Garlic, Toasted	0.5 oz	14	–	70	2	9	–	2	0	2	0
1035	Cheese puffs/Cheetos	1 oz	28	1	155	2	15	<1	10	1.9	5.8	1.3
	Cookies made with enriched flour:											
	Brownies with nuts:											
403	Commercial w/frosting, 1½ x 1¾ x ⅞"	1 ea	25	14	101	1	16	1	4	1.1	2.1	.6
404	Home recipe, 1¾ x 1¾ x ⅞"[1]	1 ea	20	13	93	1	10	<1	6	1.5	2.2	1.9
1902	Fat Free, Entenmann's	1 pce	40	24	110	2	27	1	0	0	0	0
	Chocolate chip:											
405	Commercial, 2¼" diam	4 ea	42	12	192	1	25	1	10	3.1	5.5	1.1
406	Home recipe, 2¼" diam	4 ea	40	6	195	2	23	1	11	3.2	4.2	3.4
407	From refrigerated dough, 2¼" diam	4 ea	48	13	213	2	29	1	10	3.3	4.8	1
408	Fig bars	4 ea	56	16	195	2	40	3	4	.7	2.2	.7
2052	Fruit Bar, No Fat	1 ea	28	–	90	2	21	0	0	0	0	0
2162	Fudge, Fat Free, Snackwell	16 g	16	14	53	1	12	<1	<1	.1	.1	<.1
2002	Granola Cookie, Fat Free	3 ea	28	17	85	2	19	2	0	0	0	0
409	Oatmeal raisin, 2⅝" diam	4 ea	52	6	226	3	36	2	8	1.7	3.6	2.6
410	Peanut butter, home recipe, 2⅝" diam[2]	4 ea	48	6	228	4	28	1	11	2.1	5.2	3.5
411	Sandwich-type, all	4 ea	40	2	189	2	28	1	8	1.7	4.7	1.1
412	Shortbread, commercial, small	4 ea	32	4	161	2	21	1	8	2	4.3	1
413	Shortbread, home recipe, large[3]	2 ea	28	3	153	2	16	1	9	5.8	2.7	.4

(1)Made with vegetable oil.

(2)Made with vegetable shortening.

(3)Made with margarine.

(Computer code number is for West Diet Analysis program)

Chol (mg)	Calc (mg)	Iron (mg)	Magn (mg)	Phos (mg)	Pota (mg)	Sodi (mg)	Zinc (mg)	VT-A (RE)	Thia (mg)	Ribo (mg)	Niac (mg)	V-B6 (mg)	Fola (µg)	VT-C (mg)
614	680	11.8	66	1567	581	3770	2.74	208	1.1	.77	5.48	.38	99	2
68	75	1.31	7	173	64	416	.3	23	.12	.08	.6	.04	11	<1
0	85	1.71	–	–	324	1502	–	745	0	.51	6.26	.07	53	0
0	5	.1	–	–	19	88	–	44	0	.03	.4	<.01	3	0
611	566	6.99	122	1032	999	2297	5.66	1787	.31	2.14	2.16	.58	167	7
51	47	.58	10	86	83	190	.47	148	.03	.18	.18	.05	14	1
1105	175	6.95	55	685	595	1983	2.3	779	.68	1.15	6.55	.17	55	1
64	10	.4	3	40	34	115	.13	45	.04	.07	.38	.01	3	<1
5	21	.94	12	26	35	119	.16	1	.06	.08	.69	.01	2	<1
7	19	.55	3	32	38	153	.13	2	.06	.06	.51	.01	2	<1
66	46	1.77	7	89	64	158	.33	30	.16	.18	1.25	.03	8	0
53	209	2.33	29	289	359	510	.57	172	.29	.33	2.26	.13	40	95
91	547	9.12	60	742	661	2665	1.77	369	1.14	1.48	10.3	.16	64	1
6	34	.57	4	46	41	166	.11	23	.07	.09	.64	.01	4	<1
609	410	23.2	332	1783	1975	3742	6.87	299	1.33	1.74	13.9	.32	89	1
38	25	1.44	21	111	123	233	.43	19	.08	.11	.86	.02	6	<1
0	9	1.38	41	145	137	418	.88	0	.1	.12	1.57	.1	58	0
0	–	–	–	–	–	80	–	–	.09	.03	1.20	–	–	–
1	16	.67	5	31	47	294	.11	10	.07	.1	.92	.04	34	<1
4	7	.56	8	25	37	78	.18	5	.06	.05	.43	.01	3	<1
15	11	.37	11	26	35	69	.19	40	.03	.04	.2	.02	3	<1
0	0	1.08	–	–	90	140	–	0	–	–	–	–	–	0
0	6	1.02	15	21	39	137	.19	21	.05	.08	.68	.07	2	0
13	16	.99	22	40	90	144	.37	66	.07	.07	.54	.03	5	<1
11	12	1.08	11	33	86	100	.24	8	.09	.09	.95	.02	4	0
0	36	1.63	15	35	116	196	.22	2	.09	.12	1.05	.04	6	<1
0	0	.36	–	–	–	95	–	0	–	–	–	–	–	0
0	3	.29	5	11	26	71	.08	–	.02	.02	.26	0	–	0
0	–	.72	–	–	85	80	–	–	.09	.03	.40	–	–	4
17	52	1.38	22	84	124	280	.45	85	.13	.09	.65	.04	6	<1
15	19	1.08	19	56	111	249	.39	75	.11	.1	1.68	.04	9	<1
0	10	1.56	18	39	70	242	.32	.04	.03	.07	.83	.01	2	0
6	11	.88	5	35	32	146	.17	4	.11	.1	1.07	.01	3	0
25	5	.75	4	20	20	132	.12	85	.1	.07	.83	.01	3	0

(For purposes of calculations, use "0" for t, <1, <.1, <.01, etc.)

Table H–1
Food Composition

Computer Code Number	Food Description	Measure	Wt (g)	H_2O (%)	Ener (kcal)	Prot (g)	Carb (g)	Dietary Fiber (g)	Fat (g)	Fat Breakdown (g) Sat	Mono	Poly
	BAKED GOODS: BREADS, CAKES, COOKIES, CRACKERS, PIES—Cont.											
414	Sugar, from refrigerated dough, 2" diam	4 ea	48	5	232	2	31	<1	11	2.8	6.2	1.4
1874	Vanilla Sandwich, Snackwell's	26 g	26	3	109	1	21	1	2	.5	.8	.2
415	Vanilla wafers	10 ea	40	5	176	2	29	8	6	1.4	2.4	1.5
416	Corn chips	1 oz	28	1	151	2	16	1	9	1.3	2.7	4.7
	Crackers:[1]											
1034	Armenian cracker bread	4 pce	28	4	110	3	23	1	.3	<.1	<.1	<.1
417	Cheese	10 ea	10	3	50	1	6	<1	3	.9	.9	.5
418	Cheese with peanut butter	4 ea	30	4	145	4	17	<1	7	1.5	3.6	1.3
	Fat Free:											
2161	Cracked Pepper, Snackwell	15 g	15	2	60	2	13	<1	<1	.1	.1	.2
2159	Wheat, Snackwell	7 ea	15	1	60	2	12	1	<1	.1	.1	.1
2075	Whole Wheat, Herb seasoned	.5 oz	14	.709	45	2	9	2	0	0	0	0
2077	Whole Wheat, Onion	.5 oz	14	.709	45	2	9	2	0	0	0	0
419	Graham	2 ea	14	4	59	1	11	<1	1	.4	.7	.2
420	Melba toast, plain	1 pce	5	5	19	1	4	<1	<1	<.1	<.1	<.1
1514	Rice cakes, unsalted	2 ea	18	6	69	1	14	<1	1	.2	.2	.2
421	Rye wafer, whole grain	2 ea	14	5	47	1	11	2	<1	<.1	<.1	<.1
422	Saltine®[2]	4 ea	12	4	52	1	9	<1	1	.3	.8	.2
1971	Saltine®, Unsalted Tops	2 ea	6	–	25	1	4	0	1	0	0	0
423	Snack-type, round like Ritz	3 ea	9	3	45	1	5	<1	2	.4	1	.8
424	Wheat, thin	4 ea	8	3	38	1	5	1	2	.7	.8	.2
425	Whole-wheat wafers	2 ea	8	3	35	1	5	1	1	.2	.8	.2
426	Croissants, 4½ x 4 x 1¾"	1 ea	57	23	231	5	26	1	12	6.7	3.2	.7
1699	Croutons, seasoned	½ c	15	4	70	2	10	<1	3	.8	1.4	.4
	Danish pastry:											
427	Packaged ring, plain, 12 oz	1 ea	340	21	1349	19	181	1	65	13.5	40.8	6.4
428	Round piece, plain, 4¼" diam, 1" high	1 ea	57	21	226	3	30	<1	11	2.3	6.8	1.1
429	Ounce, plain	1 oz	28	21	111	2	15	<1	5	1.1	3.4	.5
430	Round piece with fruit	1 ea	65	29	231	3	31	–	11	2.3	7	1.1
	Desserts, 3 x 3" piece:											
1348	Apple crisp	1 pce	78	61	127	1	25	–	3	.6	1.2	.8
1353	Apple cobbler	1 pce	104	57	199	2	35	1	6	1.3	2.7	1.9
1349	Cherry crisp	1 pce	138	75	158	2	27	1	5	1	2.4	1.7
1352	Cherry cobbler	1 pce	129	66	198	2	34	1	6	1.3	2.7	1.9
1350	Peach crisp	1 pce	139	73	166	1	30	1	5	1	2.3	1.6
1351	Peach cobbler	1 pce	130	65	204	2	36	1	6	1.3	2.7	1.9
	Doughnuts:											
431	Cake type, plain, 3¼" diam	1 ea	50	21	211	3	25	1	11	1.9	4.8	4.1
432	Yeast-leavened, glazed, 3¾" diam	1 ea	60	25	242	4	27	1	14	3.5	7.7	1.7
	English muffins:											
433	Plain, enriched	1 ea	57	42	134	4	26	2	1	.1	.2	.5
434	Toasted	1 ea	50	37	128	4	25	2	1	.1	.2	5
1504	Whole wheat	1 ea	50	46	102	4	20	5	1	.2	.3	.4
2010	Fruit & Fitness bar, fat free	1 ea	38	20	110	2	27	1	0	0	0	0
1414	Granola bar, soft	1 ea	42	6	188	3	29	2	7	3.1	1.6	2.3
1415	Granola bar, hard	1 ea	28	4	132	3	18	2	6	.7	1.2	3.4

(1)Crackers made with enriched white (wheat) flour except for rye wafers and whole-wheat wafers.

(2)Made with lard.

(Computer code number is for West Diet Analysis program)

Chol (mg)	Calc (mg)	Iron (mg)	Magn (mg)	Phos (mg)	Pota (mg)	Sodi (mg)	Zinc (mg)	VT-A (RE)	Thia (mg)	Ribo (mg)	Niac (mg)	V-B6 (mg)	Fola (μg)	VT-C (mg)
15	43	.89	4	90	78	225	.13	5	.09	.06	1.16	.01	3	0
<1	17	.61	5	36	28	95	.16	–	.05	.07	.69	.01	–	0
23	19	.96	6	42	39	125	.14	7	.11	.13	1.24	.03	4	0
0	36	.37	21	52	40	179	.36	3	.01	.04	.33	.07[3]	6[4]	<1
0	5	1.4	7	32	32	140	.2	0	.19	.13	1.6	.01	5	0
1	15	.48	4	22	14	99	.11	9	.06	.04	.47	.05	3	0
2	24	.88	17	97	73	298	.33	3	.12	.1	1.96	.45	8	0
<1	26	.73	4	51	19	148	.14	–	.05	.06	.78	.01	–	<1
<1	28	.58	7	61	43	169	.21	–	.04	.07	.73	.02	–	0
0	.36	–	–	–	70	80	–	–	.06	–	.4	–	–	–
0	.36	–	–	–	70	80	–	–	.06		.4	–	–	–
0	3	.52	4	15	19	85	.11	0	.03	.04	.58	.01	2	0
0	5	.19	3	10	10	41	.1	0	.02	.01	.21	<.01	1	0
0	2	.37	25	63	52	5	.54	1	0	.03	1.4	.02	4	0
0	6	.83	17	47	69	111	.39	<1	.06	.04	.22	.04	6	<1
0	14	.65	3	13	15	156	.09	0	.07	.05	.63	<.01	4	0
0	–	.36	–	–	5	50	–	–	–	–	–	–	–	–
0	11	.32	2	21	12	76	.06	0	.03	.03	.36	<.01	1	0
2	3	.25	6[5]	15	17	69	.24[5]	0	.04	.03	.4	.01	1	0
0	4	.25	8[5]	24	24	53	.17	0	.02	.01	.36	.01	2	0
43	21	1.16	9	60	67	424	.43	78	.22	.14	1.25	.03	16	<1
<1	14	.42	6	21	27	186	.14	1	.08	.06	.7	.01	6	0
105	143	6.94	54	286	371	1261	1.87	20	.99	.75	8.5	.2	54	10
18	24	1.16	9	48	62	211	.31	3	.16	.12	1.43	.03	9	2
9	12	.58	4	24	31	105	.16	2	.08	.06	.71	.02	5	1
13	15	.97	10	47	76	230	.33	17	.2	.14	1.24	.04	10	1
0	22	.58	5	19	76	142	.12	24	.07	.06	.6	.03	4	2
1	31	.78	6	44	87	304	.16	76	.1	.09	.74	.04	3	<1
0	29	2.15	12	23	164	73	.15	145	.07	.08	.59	.06	10	3
1	37	1.81	10	48	114	311	.2	135	.1	.11	.85	.05	9	2
0	23	.95	13	31	198	69	.2	104	.05	.05	1.03	.03	6	5
1	33	.91	10	54	140	308	.23	105	.09	.09	1.18	.03	6	3
18	22	.98	10	135	63	273	.27	9	.11	.12	.92	.03	4	<1
4	26	1.23	13	56	65	205	.46	6	.22	.13	1.71	.03	13	0
0	99	1.43	12	76	75	264	.4	0	.25	.16	2.21	.02	21	<1
0	94	1.37	11	72	71	252	.38	0	.19	.14	1.9	.02	14	<1
0	133	1.23	35	141	105	319	.8	0	.15	.07	1.71	.08	24	0
0	–	1.08	–	–	120	35	–	–	.12	.07	.8	–	–	6
<1	45	1.09	31	98	136	118	.64	0	.12	.07	.22	.04	10	0
0	17	.84	27	79	95	83	.58	4	.07	.03	.45	.02	7	<1

(3)Vitamin B_6 values vary between brands. Check the label.

(4)Values from 1992 USDA data for snacks and sweets.

(5)Values derived from whole-wheat recipes and retention values.

Table H–1
Food Composition

Computer Code Number	Food Description	Measure	Wt (g)	H_2O (%)	Ener (kcal)	Prot (g)	Carb (g)	Dietary Fiber (g)	Fat (g)	Fat Breakdown (g) Sat	Mono	Poly
	BAKED GOODS: BREADS, CAKES, COOKIES, CRACKERS, PIES—Cont.											
	Granola bar, Fat free:											
1985	Blueberry	1 ea	43	7	140	3	33	3	0	0	0	0
2012	Chocolate	1 ea	43	7	140	3	33	3	0	0	0	0
1983	Date Almond	1 ea	43	7	140	3	33	3	0	0	0	0
1984	Raisin	1 ea	43	7	140	3	33	3	0	0	0	0
2011	Strawberry	1 ea	43	7	140	3	33	3	0	0	0	0
	Muffins, 2½" diam, 1½" high:											
	From home recipe											
435	Blueberry[1]	1 ea	45	39	131	3	18	7	5	1.1	1.2	2.4
436	Bran, wheat[2]	1 ea	45	35	130	3	19	3	6	1.2	1.4	2.8
437	Cornmeal	1 ea	45	32	144	3	20	2	6	1.2	1.4	2.8
	From commercial mix:											
438	Blueberry	1 ea	45	36	135	2	22	1	4	.7	1.6	1.4
439	Bran, wheat	1 ea	45	35	124	3	21	4	4	1.1	2.1	.6
440	Cornmeal	1 ea	45	30	144	3	22	2	5	1.3	2.4	.6
	Nabisco Newtons, Fat free:											
1864	Cranberry	1 ea	23	–	68	1	16	–	0	0	0	0
1867	Fig	1 ea	23	–	68	1	16	–	0	0	0	0
1865	Raspberry	1 ea	23	–	68	1	16	–	0	0	0	0
1868	Strawberry	1 ea	23	–	68	1	16	–	0	0	0	0
	Pancakes, 4" diam:											
441	Buckwheat, from mix w/ egg and milk	1 ea	27	54	56	2	8	1	2	.5	.5	.8
442	Plain, from home recipe	1 ea	27	53	61	2	8	<1	3	.6	.7	1.2
443	Plain, from mix; egg, milk, oil added	1 ea	27	53	52	1	10	<1	1	.1	.2	.2
1468	Pan Dulce, Sweet roll w/topping	1 ea	79	21	291	5	48	1	9	2	3.9	2.7
	Piecrust, with enriched flour, vegetable shortening, baked:											
444	Home recipe, 9" shell	1 ea	180	10	949	11	85	3	62	15.5	27.4	16.4
	From mix:											
445	For 2-crust pie	1 ea	320	10	1686	20	152	6	111	27.6	48.6	29.2
446	1 pie shell	1 ea	180	11	902	12	91	3	55	13.9	31.1	6.9
	Pies, 9" diam; crust made with vegetable shortening, enriched flour:											
447	Apple:[3] Whole pie	1 ea	945	52	2239	18	321	16	104	19.9	56.1	19.8
448	Piece, ⅙ of pie	1 pce	158	52	374	3	54	3	17	3.3	9.4	3.3
449	Banana cream: Whole pie	1 ea	1188	48	3195	52	391	–	162	44.7	68	39.2
450	Piece, ⅙ of pie	1 pce	198	48	533	9	65	–	27	7.4	11.3	6.5
451	Blueberry:[3] Whole pie	1 ea	945	51	2315	25	317	13	112	27.6	48.4	29.1
452	Piece, ⅙ of pie	1 pce	158	51	387	4	53	2	19	4.6	8.1	4.9
453	Cherry:[3] Whole pie	1 ea	945	46	2551	26	364	14	115	28.3	50.2	30.7
454	Piece, ⅙ of pie	1 pce	158	46	427	4	61	2	19	4.7	8.4	5.1
455	Chocolate cream:[4] Whole pie	1 ea	1194	46	3367	57	372	6	192	62	78	40
456	Piece, ⅙ of pie	1 pce	199	46	561	10	62	1	32	10	13	6.7
457	Custard:[3] Whole pie	1 ea	910	61	1911	50	189	11	106	25.3	52.4	17.5
458	Piece, ⅙ of pie	1 pce	152	61	319	8	32	2	18	4.2	8.8	2.9
459	Lemon meringue:[3] Whole pie	1 ea	840	42	2251	13	396	10	73	13.1	30.5	24.3
460	Piece, ⅙ of pie	1 pce	140	42	375	2	66	2	12	2.2	5.1	4

(1)Made with vegetable shortening.
(2)Made with vegetable oil
(3)Values from latest USDA data for Baked Goods.
(4)Values based on recipe: pie crust, cooked chocolate pudding, whipped cream topping.

(Computer code number is for West Diet Analysis program)

Chol (mg)	Calc (mg)	Iron (mg)	Magn (mg)	Phos (mg)	Pota (mg)	Sodi (mg)	Zinc (mg)	VT-A (RE)	Thia (mg)	Ribo (mg)	Niac (mg)	V-B6 (mg)	Fola (µg)	VT-C (mg)
0	20	3.6	–	–	120	10	–	–	.03	.07	.4	–	–	–
0	20	3.6	–	–	120	10	–	–	.03	.07	.4	–	–	–
0	20	3.6	–	–	120	10	–	–	.03	.07	.4	–	–	–
0	20	3.6	–	–	120	10	–	–	.03	.07	.4	–	–	–
0	20	3.6	–	–	120	10	–	–	.03	.07	.4	–	–	–
18	85	1.03	7	65	55	198	.24	13	.12	.13	.99	.02	5	1
16	84	1.89	35	128	143	265	1.24	108	.15	.2	1.81	.14	23	4
20	116	1.18	10	79	65	263	.27	18	.14	.14	1.07	.04	8	<1
21	11	.51	5	85	35	197	.17	10	.07	.14	1.01	.03	5	<1
31	14	1.14	26	150	66	210	.52	14	.09	.11	1.29	.08	7	0
28	34	.88	9	173	59	358	.29	20	.11	.12	.94	.05	5	<1
–	–	–	–	–		76	–	–	–	–	–	–	–	–
–	–	–	–	–	–	76	–	–	–	–	–	–	–	–
–	–	–	–	–	–	76	–	–	–	–	–	–	–	–
–	–	–	–	–	–	76	–	–	–	–	–	–	–	–
18	69	.51	15	110	63	144	.32	18	.05	.07	.36	.04	5	<1
16	59	.49	4	43	36	119	.15	15	.05	.08	.42	.01	3	<1
3	34	.42	5	90	47	170	.1	2	.06	.06	.46	.03	2	<1
26	13	1.82	10	56	57	140	.35	88	.23	.21	1.98	.04	22	<1
0	18	5.22	25	121	121	976	.79	0	.7	.5	5.96	.04	20	0
0	32	9.28	45	214	214	1734	1.41	0	1.25	.89	10.6	.08	35	0
0	108	3.89	27	151	112	1312	.7	0	.54	.33	4.27	.1	22	0
0	104	4.25	66	227	614	2513	1.51	284	.26	.25	2.49	.36	38	30
0	17	.71	11	38	103	420	.25	47	.04	.04	.42	.06	6	5
606	891	12.5	190	1092	1960	2851	5.7	832	1.65	2.46	12.5	1.58	131	19
101	149	2.08	32	182	327	475	.95	139	.27	.41	2.08	.26	22	3
0	66	11.7	76	284	473	1748	1.89	38	1.45	1.25	11.2	.32	47	7
0	11	1.96	13	47	79	292	.32	6	.24	.21	1.88	.05	8	1
0	94	17.6	85	284	728	1804	1.89	454	1.4	1.18	12.1	.32	66	9
0	16	2.94	14	47	122	302	.32	76	.23	.2	2.02	.05	11	2
632	967	15.3	311	1313	1755	2924	7.6	872	1.6	2.4	12	.56	119	6
105	161	2.04	52	219	292	487	1.3	145	.27	.4	2	.09	20	1
300	728	5.28	100	1019	965	2184	4.73	456	.35	1.89	2.66	.44	182	3
50	122	.88	17	170	161	365	.79	76	.06	.32	.44	.07	30	<1
378	470	5.12	126	882	748	1226	4.12	437	.52	1.76	5.45	.25	67	27
63	78	.85	21	147	125	204	.69	73	.09	.29	.91	.04	11	4

(For purposes of calculations, use "0" for t, <1, <.1, <.01, etc.)

Table H–1
Food Composition

Computer Code Number	Food Description	Measure	Wt (g)	H_2O (%)	Ener (kcal)	Prot (g)	Carb (g)	Dietary Fiber (g)	Fat (g)	Fat Breakdown (g) Sat	Mono	Poly
	BAKED GOODS: BREADS, CAKES, COOKIES, CRACKERS, PIES—Cont.											
461	Peach: Whole pie	1 ea	945	45	2603	22	377	13	108	26.4	49	31.8
462	Piece, ⅙ of pie	1 pce	158	45	435	4	63	2	18	4.4	8.2	5.3
463	Pecan:[1] Whole pie	1 ea	825	19	3300	33	472	29	153	31	88	24.5
464	Piece, ⅙ of pie	1 pce	138	19	552	6	79	5	25	5.2	14.9	4.1
465	Pumpkin:[1] Whole pie	1 ea	1240	58	2604	48	339	33	118	25	62.1	19.8
466	Piece, ⅙ of pie	1 pce	206	58	433	8	56	6	20	4.2	10.3	3.3
467	Pies, fried, commercial: Apple	1 ea	85	40	266	2	33	2	14	6.5	5.8	1.2
468	Pies, fried, commercial: Cherry	1 ea	85	40	269	3	36	2	14	2	6	4.6
	Pretzels, made with enriched flour:											
469	Thin sticks, 2¼" long	10 ea	3	3	11	<1	2	<1	<1	t	t	t
470	Dutch twists, 2¾ x 2⅝"	1 ea	16	3	61	1	13	<1	1	.1	.2	.2
471	Thin twists, 3¼ x 2¼ x ¼"	10 ea	60	3	229	5	47	2	2	.4	.8	.7
	Rolls & buns, enriched, commercial:											
472	Cloverleaf rolls, 2½" diam, 2" high	1 ea	28	32	85	2	14	1	2	.5	1.1	.3
473	Hot dog buns	1 ea	40	34	114	3	20	1	2	.5	1	.4
474	Hamburger buns	1 ea	45	34	129	4	23	1	2	.5	1.1	.4
475	Hard roll, white, 3¾" diam, 2" high	1 ea	50	31	147	5	26	1	2	.3	.6	.9
476	Submarine rolls/hoagies, 11½ x 3 x 2½"	1 ea	135	31	392	12	75	4	4	.9	1.3	1.4
	Rolls & buns, enriched, home recipe:											
477	Dinner rolls 2½" diam, 2" high	1 ea	35	29	112	3	19	1	3	.7	1.1	.7
478	Toaster pastries, fortified (Poptarts)	1 ea	54	12	212	3	38	1	6	.8	2.2	2.1
2132	Toaster Strudel pastry—Cream Cheese	1 ea	53	32	184	3	28	<1	9	2.8	–	–
2134	Toaster Strudel pastry—French Toast	1 ea	53	31	177	3	27	1	7	2.8	–	–
	Tortilla chips:											
1271	Plain	1 oz	28	7	140	2	18	2	6	2	4.4	1
1036	Nacho flavor	1 oz	28	2	139	2	18	1	7	1.4	4.3	1
1037	Taco flavor	1 oz	28	2	134	2	18	2	7	1.3	4	1
	Tortillas:											
479	Corn, enriched, 6" diam	1 ea	30	44	67	2	14	2	1	.1	.2	.3
480	Flour, 8" diam	1 ea	35	27	115	3	20	1	2	.4	1	1
1301	Flour, 10" diam	1 ea	57	27	185	5	32	1	4	.6	1.6	1.6
481	Taco shells	1 ea	14	4	66	1	9	1	3	.4	1.5	.6
	Waffles, 7" diam:											
482	From home recipe	1 ea	75	42	218	6	25	1	11	2.1	2.6	5.1
483	From mix, egg/milk added	1 ea	75	42	218	5	26	1	10	1.7	2.7	5.2
1510	Whole grain, prepared from frozen	1 ea	39	44	106	4	12	1	5	1.6	1.9	1
	GRAIN PRODUCTS: CEREAL, FLOUR, GRAIN, PASTA and NOODLES, POPCORN											
484	Barley, pearled, dry, uncooked	1 c	200	10	704	20	155	27	2	.5	.3	1.1
485	Barley, pearled, cooked	1 c	157	69	193	4	44	8	1	.1	.1	.3
	Breakfast bars, fat free:											
2009	Apple	1 ea	38	21	110	2	24	3	0	0	0	0
2005	Chocolate	1 ea	38	21	110	2	24	3	0	0	0	0
2003	Strawberry	1 ea	38	21	110	2	24	3	0	0	0	0

(1)Values from latest USDA data for Baked Goods.

(Computer code number is for West Diet Analysis program)

PAGE KEY: H–4 = BEV H–6 = DAIRY H–12 = EGGS H–14 = FAT/OIL H–18 = FRUIT H–26 = BAKERY H–36 = GRAIN H–44 = FISH H–48 = MEATS H–50 = POULTRY H–54 = SAUSAGE H–56 = MIXED/FAST H–64 = NUTS/SEEDS H–68 = SWEETS H–70 = VEG/LEG H–84 = MISC H–88 = SOUPS/SAUCES H–90 = FAST H–106 = FRZN ENTREE H–112 = BABY FOODS

Chol (mg)	Calc (mg)	Iron (mg)	Magn (mg)	Phos (mg)	Pota (mg)	Sodi (mg)	Zinc (mg)	VT-A (RE)	Thia (mg)	Ribo (mg)	Niac (mg)	V-B6 (mg)	Fola (µg)	VT-C (mg)
17	79	3	68	256	1132	2660	1.59	187	.28	.5	1	.42	49	11
3	13	.57	11	43	789	445	.27	31	.05	.09	.2	.07	8	2
264	140	8.66	149	635	611	3498	4.7	388	.75	1.01	2.05	.17	49	9
44	23	1.45	25	106	102	585	.79	65	.13	.17	.34	.03	8	2
248	744	9.8	186	880	1909	3496	5.58	5951[2]	.68	1.9	2.32	.71	186	19
41	124	1.63	31	146	317	581	.93	989[2]	.11	.31	.38	.12	31	3
13	13	.88	8	37	51	325	.17	8	.1	.08	.98	.03	4	2
13	19	.88	9	37	55	318	.17	15	.1	.08	.98	.03	3	1
0	1	.13	1	3	4	51	.03	0	.01	.02	.16	<.01	2	0
0	6	.69	6	18	23	274	.14	0	.07	.1	.84	.02	13	0
0	22	2.59	21	68	88	1029	.51	0	.28	.37	3.15	.07	50	0
<1	34	.89	6	33	38	148	.22	0	.14	.09	1.14	.01	8	<1
0	56	1.27	8	35	56	224	.25	0	.19	.12	1.57	.02	11	0
0	63	1.43	9	40	63	252	.28	0	.22	.14	1.77	.02	12	0
0	47	1.65	14	50	54	272	.47	0	.24	.17	2.12	.03	8	0
0	122	3.78	27	115	122	783	.85	0	.54	.33	4.47	.05	41	0
13	21	1.04	7	44	53	145	.24	28	.14	.14	1.21	.02	15	<1
0	14	1.89	10	60	60	226	.36	57[3]	.16	.2	2.13	.21	43	<1
12	12	.95	–	–	–	–	–	17	–	–	–	–	–	0
6	6	.84	–	–	–	191	–	2	–	–	–	–	–	0
0	0	0	25	58	65	135	.43	0	.02	.05	.36	.08	3	0
1	42	.4	23	69	61	198	.34	12	.04	.05	.4	.08	4	1
1	44	.57	25	68	61	221	.36	25	.07	.06	.57	.08	6	<1
0	52	.42	19	94	46	48	.28	8	.03	.02	.45	.07	5	0
0	44	1.17	9	44	46	169	.25	0	.19	.1	1.26	.02	4	0
0	71	1.88	15	70	74	272	.4	0	.3	.17	2.03	.03	7	0
0	22	.35	15	35	25	51	.18	5	.04	.02	.23	.04	1	0
52	191	1.74	14	143	119	383	.51	49	.2	.26	1.55	.04	11	<1
52	91	1.23	14	143	119	383	.5	49	.15	.3	1.55	.04	11	<1
39	84	.7	15	83	91	150	.41	25	.08	.12	.75	.05	7	<1
0	58	5	158	442	560	18	4.26	4	.38	.23	9.22	.52	46	0
0	17	2.09	34	85	146	5	1.29	2	.13	.1	3.23	.18	25	0
0	20	.72	–	–	160	65	–	–	.09	.03	.4	–	–	2
0	20	.72	–	–	160	65	–	–	.09	.03	.4	–	–	2
0	20	.72	–	–	160	65	–	–	.09	.03	.4	–	–	2

(2)Latest USDA values of vitamin A for canned pumpkin are almost 3.5 times greater than previously published values. Canned pumpkin is usually a blend of pumpkin and winter squash.

(3)Vitamin A values from label declarations vary.

Table H-1
Food Composition

Computer Code Number	Food Description	Measure	Wt (g)	H_2O (%)	Ener (kcal)	Prot (g)	Carb (g)	Dietary Fiber (g)	Fat (g)	Fat Breakdown (g) Sat	Mono	Poly
	GRAIN PRODUCTS: CEREAL, FLOUR, GRAIN, PASTA and NOODLES, POPCORN—Cont.											
	Breakfast cereals, hot, cooked:											
	Corn grits (hominy) enriched:											
486	Regular and quick, prepared, yellow	1 c	242	85	145	3	31	5	<1	.1	.1	.2
487	Instant, prepared from packet, white	1 ea	137	85	82	2	18	<1	<1	t	t	<.1
	Cream of wheat:											
488	Regular, quick, instant	1 c	244	87	131	4	27	1	<1	.1	.1	.2
489	Mix and eat, plain, packet	1 ea	142	82	102	3	21	<1	<1	t	t	.1
1664	Farina cereal, cooked	½ c	117	87	58	2	12	2	<1	t	t	t
490	Malt-O-Meal	1 c	240	88	122	4	26	1	<1	t	t	.1
494	Maypo	1 c	242	83	172	6	32	6	2	.4	.8	.1
	Oatmeal or rolled oats:											
491	Regular, quick, instant, nonfort	1 c	234	85	145	6	25	4	2	.4	.7	.9
	Instant, fortified:											
492	Plain, from packet	¾ c	177	85	104	4	18	3	2	.3	.6	.7
493	Flavored, from packet	¾ c	164	76	167	4	33	2	2	.3	.6	.7
	Breakfast cereals, ready to eat:											
495	All-Bran	⅓ c	28	3	70	4	21	10	1	.1	.1	.3
1306	Alpha Bits	1 c	28	1	109	2	24	1	1	.1	.2	.3
1307	Apple Jacks	1 c	28	2	109	2	25	1	<1	t	t	t
1308	Bran Buds	1 c	84	3	217	12	64	31	2	.4	.3	1.1
1305	Bran Chex	1 c	49	2	156	5	39	8	1	.2	.2	.8
1309	Honey BucWheat Crisp	¾ c	28	5	109	3	23	2	1	.2	.2	.4
1310	C. W. Post, plain	1 c	97	2	432	9	70	7	15	11.3	1.7	1.4
1311	C. W. Post, with raisins	1 c	103	4	446	9	74	14	15	11	1.7	1.4
496	Cap'n Crunch	1 c	37	2	156	2	30	1	3	2.2	.4	.5
1312	Cap'n Crunchberries	1 c	38	3	160	2	31	1	3	2.1	.4	.5
1313	Cap'n Crunch, peanut butter	1 c	38	2	167	3	29	<1	5	2.1	1.5	1.1
497	Cheerios	1 c	23	5	90	3	16	2	1	.3	.5	.6
1314	Cocoa Krispies	1 c	36	2	139	2	32	<1	1	.1	.1	.2
1316	Cocoa Pebbles	1 c	31	2	127	1	27	<1	2	t	t	t
1315	Corn Bran	1 c	36	2	125	2	30	7	1	.2	.3	.7
1317	Corn Chex	1 c	28	2	110	2	25	<1	1	.1	.2	.6
498	Corn Flakes, Kellogg's	1¼ c	28	3	109	2	24	1	<1	t	t	t
499	Corn Flakes, Post Toasties	1¼ c	28	3	108	2	24	1	<1	t	t	t
1340	Corn Pops	1 c	28	3	107	1	25	<1	<1	t	t	.1
1318	Cracklin' Oat Bran	1 c	60	4	229	6	41	10	9	2.1	2.3	3.5
1038	Crispy Wheat `N Raisins	1 c	43	7	150	3	35	3	1	.1	.1	.4
1319	Fortified Oat Flakes	1 c	48	3	177	9	35	1	1	.1	.3	.3
500	40% Bran Flakes, Kellogg's	1 c	39	3	127	5	31	6	1	.1	.1	.4
501	40% Bran Flakes, Post	1 c	47	3	152	5	37	9	1	.2	.2	.3
502	Froot Loops	1 c	28	3	111	2	25	1	1	.2	.1	.1
518	Frosted Flakes	1 c	35	3	133	2	32	1	<1	t	t	t
1320	Frosted Mini-Wheats	4 ea	31	5	111	3	26	2	<1	.1	t	.2
1321	Frosted Rice Krispies	1 c	28	3	108	1	26	<1	<1	t	t	t
1324	Fruit & Fibre w/dates	½ c	28	9	95	2	21	4	1	.2	.6	.5
1325	Fruitful Bran	¾ c	34	1	144	3	37	6	<1	.1	.1	.2

(Computer code number is for West Diet Analysis program)

Chol (mg)	Calc (mg)	Iron (mg)	Magn (mg)	Phos (mg)	Pota (mg)	Sodi (mg)	Zinc (mg)	VT-A (RE)	Thia (mg)	Ribo (mg)	Niac (mg)	V-B6 (mg)	Fola (µg)	VT-C (mg)
0	0	1.55[1]	10	29	53	0[2]	.17	14[3]	.24[1]	.14[1]	1.96[1]	.06	2	0
0	7	1.01[1]	5	16	29	343	.08	0	.18[1]	.08[1]	1.3[1]	.03	1	0
0	51[1]	10.5[1]	12	102[4]	46	141[4]	.34	0	.24[1]	0[1]	1.46[1]	.03	10	0
0	20[1]	8.09[1]	7	20[1]	38	241	.24	376[1]	.43[1]	.28[1]	4.97[1]	.57	101	0
0	2	.58	2	14	15	0[5]	.08	0	.09	.06	.64	.01	2	0
0	5	9.6[1]	5	24[1]	31	2[5]	.17	0	.48[1]	.24[1]	5.76[1]	.02	5	0
0	126	8.47	51	249	213	9.7	1.5	709	.73	.73	9.44	.97	10	29
0	19	1.59	56	177	131	2[5]	1.15	4	.26	.05	.3	.05	9	0
0	162[1]	6.3[1]	42	132	99	283[1]	.87	453[1]	.53[1]	.28[1]	5.47[1]	.74	150	0
0	172[1]	7[1]	38	138	156	235[1]	1	458[1]	.53[1]	.38[1]	5.9[1]	.76	156	0
0	23	4.52[1]	105	261	345	315	3.75	371[1]	.37[1]	.43[1]	5[1]	.51	100	15[1]
0	8	2.7	17	51	108	177	1.51	371	.37	.43	5	.51	100	0
0	3	4.52	6	30	23	124	3.75	370	.37	.43	5	.51	100	15
0	56	13.4	267	729	1403	515	11.1	1111	1.09	1.26	14.8	1.51	296	44
0	29	7.79	125	326	393	454	2.14	11	.64	.26	8.62	.88	172	26
0	40	8.12	32	80	106	266	.51	673	.68	.77	9	1.4	9	27
<1	47	15.4	67	224	197	166	1.64	1283	1.26	1.46	17.1	1.75	342	0
<1	50	16.4	74	231	260	160	1.64	1362	1.34	1.55	18.1	1.85	363	0
0	6	9.81[1]	15	47	48	278	4	5[1]	.66[1]	.71[1]	8.62[1]	1	238	0
<1	12	9.8	15	51	54	265	3.88	5	.65	.74	8.92	1.02	140	0
0	8	10	20	53	62	291	4.15	6	.66	.77	9.73	1.14	265	0
0	39	3.66[1]	32	109	82	249	.64	304[1]	.3[1]	.34[1]	4.05[1]	.41	5	12[1]
<1	6	2.27	12	47	53	275	1.91	476	.47	.54	6.34	.65	127	19
0	5	1.97	13	24	52	148	1.66	411	.41	.47	5.52	.56	109	0
0	41	12.2	18	52	70	310	4	8	.37	.7	10.9	.86	232	0
0	3	1.8	4	11	23	268	.1	14	.37	.07	5	.51	100	15
0	1	1.8[1]	3	18	26	286	.08	370[1]	.36[1]	.42[1]	4.93[1]	.5	99	15[1]
0	1	.74[1]	4	12	32	293	.08	370[1]	.36[1]	.42[1]	4.93[1]	.5	99	0
0	1	1.8	2	28	17	103	1.51	370	.37	.43	5	.51	100	15
0	40	3.78	116	241	355	487	3.18	794	.78	.9	10.6	1.08	212	32
0	71	6.84	34	117	173	204	.51	569	.56	.64	7.57	.77	15	0
0	68	13.7	58	176	343	429	1.5	635	.62	.72	8.45	.86	169	0
0	19	24.8[1]	71	191	247	302	5.15	516[1]	.51[1]	.58[1]	6.86[1]	.7	137	0
0	21	7.47[1]	101	296	250	430	2.49	622[1]	.61[1]	.7[1]	8.27[1]	.85	165	0
0	3	4.52[1]	7	24	26	144	3.75	370[1]	.37[1]	.43[1]	5[1]	.51	100	15[1]
0	1	2.21[1]	3	26	22	283	.05	463[1]	.45[1]	.52[1]	6.16[1]	.63	123	19[1]
0	10	1.95	25	81	105	9	1.64	410	.4	.46	5.46	.56	109	16
0	1	1.79	5	27	21	237	.31	370	.37	.43	5	.51	100	15
0	15	5	40	108	167	132	1.51	356	.37	.43	5	.5	100	0
0	23	5	67	152	276	264	1.3	270	.46	.43	6	.5	100	<1

(1)Nutrient added (values sometimes based on label declaration).

(2)Cooked without salt. If salt is added according to label recommendation, sodium content is 540 mg.

(3)Value for yellow corn grits; cooked white corn grits contain 0 RE of vitamin A.

(4)Values for quick cereal.

(5)Cooked without salt. If added according to label recommendations, sodium content is 390 mg for Cream of Wheat; 324 mg for Malt-O-Meal; 374 mg for oatmeal; 385 mg for Farina.

(For purposes of calculations, use "0" for t, <1, <.1, <.01, etc.)

Table H–1
Food Composition

Computer Code Number	Food Description	Measure	Wt (g)	H_2O (%)	Ener (kcal)	Prot (g)	Carb (g)	Dietary Fiber (g)	Fat (g)	Fat Breakdown (g) Sat	Mono	Poly
	GRAIN PRODUCTS: CEREAL, FLOUR, GRAIN, PASTA and NOODLES, POPCORN—Cont.											
	Breakfast cereals, ready to eat—Cont.											
1322	Fruity Pebbles	1 c	32	3	131	1	28	1	2	.4	.3	.4
503	Golden Grahams	1 c	39	2	150	2	33	1	1	1	.1	.2
504	Granola, homemade	½ c	61	3	297	8	34	6	17	2.9	4.7	8.6
1670	Granola, low fat, commercial	½ c	47	3	179	4	36	3	3	0	–	–
505	Grape Nuts	½ c	57	3	203	7	47	6	<1	t	t	.2
1326	Grape Nuts Flakes	1 c	32	3	116	3	26	3	<1	.1	t	.1
1665	Heartland Natural with raisins	1 c	101	5	430	10	70	6	14	–	–	–
1327	Honey & Nut Corn Flakes	1 c	38	4	151	2	31	1	2	.3	.7	1
506	Honey Nut Cheerios	1 c	33	3	126	4	27	1	1	.1	.3	.3
1328	HoneyBran	1 c	35	2	119	3	29	4	1	.1	.1	.4
1329	HoneyComb	1 c	22	1	86	1	20	<1	<1	.1	.1	.2
1330	King Vitaman	1 c	19	2	77	1	16	1	1	.7	.1	.2
1039	Kix	1 c	19	3	74	2	16	<1	<1	.1	.1	.2
1331	Life	1 c	43	5	158	8	31	3	1	.1	.2	.4
507	Lucky Charms	1 c	32	3	125	3	26	1	1	.2	.4	.5
1323	Mueslix Five Grain	1 c	82	5	279	7	63	7	3	.5	1	1.2
1416	Granola, low-fat	⅓ c	31	3	119	3	25	2	2	0	–	–
	Health Valley Granola, fat-free:											
2081	Date & Almond	1 oz	28	7	90	2	21	3	0	0	0	0
2080	Raisin Cinnamon	1 oz	28	7	90	2	21	3	0	0	0	0
2082	Tropical Fruit	1 oz	28	7	90	21	2	3	0	0	0	0
508	Nature Valley Granola	1 c	113	4	502	12	75	6	20	13	2.9	2.8
1666	Nutri Grain Almond Raisin	⅔ c	40	9	140	3	31	3	2	0	–	–
1333	Nutri-Grain—corn	1 c	42	3	160	3	35	3	1	.1	.2	.6
1335	Nutri-Grain—wheat	1 c	44	3	158	4	37	3	<1	.1	.1	.3
1336	100% Bran	1 c	66	3	177	8	48	20	3	.6	.6	1.9
509	100% Natural cereal, plain	½ c	57	2	267	7	36	5	12	8.2	2.3	1.1
1337	100% Natural with apples & cinnamon	1 c	104	2	478	11	70	7	20	15.4	1.8	1.3
1338	100% Natural with raisins & dates	1 c	110	3	496	11	72	7	20	13.6	3.7	1.7
510	Product 19	1 c	33	3	125	3	27	1	<1	t	t	.1
1339	Quisp	1 c	30	2	124	2	25	<1	2	1.5	.3	.3
511	Raisin Bran, Kellogg's	1 c	49	8	152	5	37	5	1	.2	.1	.4
512	Raisin Bran, Post	1 c	56	9	171	5	42	8	1	.2	.2	.4
1667	Raisin Squares	½ c	28	8	90	2	23	2	0	0	0	0
1041	Rice Chex	¾ c	19	3	75	1	17	<1	1	.2	.2	.3
513	Rice Krispies, Kellogg's	1 c	29	2	114	2	25	<1	<1	t	t	.1
514	Rice, puffed	1 c	14	3	56	1	13	<1	<1	t	t	t
515	Shredded Wheat	1 c	43	5	155	5	34	4	1	.2	.2	.5
516	Special K	1 c	21	2	83	4	16	1	<1	t	t	t
517	Super Golden Crisp	1 c	33	1	123	2	30	1	<1	t	t	.1
519	Honey Smacks	1 c	38	3	142	3	33	<1	1	.1	.1	.3
1341	Tasteeos	1 c	24	2	94	3	19	3	1	.2	.2	.3
1342	Team	1 c	42	4	164	3	36	<1	1	.2	.2	.3
520	Total, wheat, with added calcium	1 c	33	4	116	3	26	4	1	.1	.1	.3
521	Trix	1 c	28	2	109	2	25	<1	<1	.2	.1	.1
1344	Wheat Chex	1 c	46	2	168	5	38	4	1	.2	.2	.6

H

Chol (mg)	Calc (mg)	Iron (mg)	Magn (mg)	Phos (mg)	Pota (mg)	Sodi (mg)	Zinc (mg)	VT-A (RE)	Thia (mg)	Ribo (mg)	Niac (mg)	V-B6 (mg)	Fola (μg)	VT-C (mg)
0	4	2.04	9	19	25	178	1.73	424	.42	.49	5.6	.58	114	0
<1	24	6.21[1]	16	56	86	386	.34	517[1]	.51[1]	.59[1]	6.87[1]	.7	6	21[1]
0	38	2.42	71	247	306	6	2.23	2	.37	.15	1.07	.21	49	1
0	19	7	38	108	136	47	5.66	329	.55	.64	7.55	.76	146	–
0	5	2.47[1]	38	143	190	396	1.25	755[1]	.74[1]	.85[1]	9.98[1]	1.03	201	0
0	13	9.28	36	95	113	181	.65	423	.42	.49	5.71	.58	114	0
0	61	3.7	130	346	382	207	2.61	6	.29	.13	1.43	.18	41	1
0	5	2.39	8	17	48	302	.14	503	.49	.57	6.67	.68	133	20
0	23	5.3[1]	39	122	116	299	.87	437[1]	.43[1]	.5[1]	5.87[1]	.6	22	18[1]
0	16	5.57	46	131	150	202	.9	463	.45	.52	6.16	.63	23	19
0	4	2.09	7	22	70	123	1.17	291	.29	.33	3.87	.4	78	0
0	2	11.4	6	24	23	145	.15	644	.83	.95	11.6	1.06	259	30
0	24	5.44	8	26	30	194	.16	252	.25	.28	3.35	.34	67	10
0	150	11.3	14	232	192	224	1.42	9	.93	.97	11.3	.08	36	0
0	36	5.09[1]	27	89	66	227	.56	424[1]	.42[1]	.48[1]	5.63[1]	.58	6	17[1]
0	38	8.94	82	215	369	107	7.46	747	.75	.84	9.84	.99	197	1
0	–	1.8	24	80	95	60	3.74	150	.37	.42	4.99	.5	100	–
0	–	.36	–	–	85	35	–	–	.06	–	.4	–	–	–
0	–	.36	–	–	85	35	–	–	.06	–	.4	–	–	–
0	–	.36	–	–	85	35	–	–	.06	–	.4	–	–	–
0	71	3.77	115	353	388	232	2.19	7	.4	.19	.82	.09	85	0
0	16	.8	11	77	130	220	3.75	–	.38	.43	5	.5	100	–
0	1	.89	27	120	98	276	5.54	556	.55	.63	7.39	.76	148	22
0	12	1.24	34	164	119	299	5.81	583	.57	.66	7.74	.79	155	23
0	46	8.12	312	801	824	457	5.74	0	1.58	1.78	20.9	2.11	47	63
<1	99	1.68	68	209	281	24	1.28	3	.17	.31	1.3	.1	17	0
1	157	2.9	72	351	515	52	2	6	.33	.57	1.88	.11	17	1
1	159	3.12	124	347	537	47	2.11	6	.31	.65	2.09	.16	45	0
0	4	21[1]	12	46	51	378	.49	1746[1]	1.75[1]	1.98[1]	23.3[1]	2.34	465	70[1]
0	9	6.33	12	25	45	240	.18	5	.54	.76	5.79	.91	8	0
0	17	22.2[1]	63	182	254	271	5	498[1]	.49[1]	.59[1]	6.66[1]	.69	132	0
0	26	8.9[1]	95	234	344	365	2.97	741[1]	.73[1]	.84[1]	9.86[1]	1.01	197	0
0	10	8.1	26	84	110	0	1.5	0	.38	.43	5	.5	100	–
0	3	1.2	5	19	22	158	.26	1	.25	.01	3.34	.34	67	10
0	5	1.83[1]	12	32	28	213	.49	0[1]	.12[1]	.03[1]	.2[1]	.05	3	15[1]
0	1	.15[1]	4	14	16	<1	.14	0	.01[1]	.01[1]	.42[1]	.01	3	0
0	16	1.8	57	152	156	4	1.41	0	.11	.12	2.24	.11	21	0
<1	6	3.39[1]	12	41	37	196	2.82	275[1]	.28[1]	.32[1]	3.75[1]	.38	75	11[1]
0	7	2.08[1]	20	60	123	29	1.75	437[1]	.43[1]	.49[1]	5.81[1]	.59	116	0
0	4	2.39[1]	18	41	56	100	.38	503[1]	.49[1]	.57[1]	6.67[1]	.68	133	20[1]
0	11	3.82	26	96	71	182	.69	318	.31	.36	4.22	.43	9	13
0	6	2.57	19	65	71	259	.58	556	.55	.63	7.39	.76	7	22
0	282	21[1]	37	136	123	326	.78	1746[1]	1.75[1]	1.98[1]	23.3[1]	2.34	465	70[1]
0	6	4.52[1]	6	19	27	179	.13	371[1]	.37[1]	.43[1]	5[1]	.51	3	15[1]
0	18	7.31	58	181	173	308	1.23	0	.6	.17	8.1	.83	162	24

(1)Nutrient added (values sometimes based on label declaration).

(For purposes of calculations, use "0" for t, <1, <.1, <.01, etc.)

Table H–1
Food Composition

Computer Code Number	Food Description	Measure	Wt (g)	H_2O (%)	Ener (kcal)	Prot (g)	Carb (g)	Dietary Fiber (g)	Fat (g)	Fat Breakdown (g) Sat	Mono	Poly
	GRAIN PRODUCTS: CEREAL, FLOUR, GRAIN, PASTA and NOODLES, POPCORN—Cont.											
1043	Wheat cereal, puffed, fortified	1 c	12	3	44	2	10	1	<1	t	t	.1
522	Wheaties	1 c	29	5	101	3	23	3	<1	.1	t	.2
	Buckwheat flour:											
523	Dark	1 c	98	11	328	12	69	8	3	.7	.9	.9
524	Light	1 c	98	12	340	6	78	6	1	.2	.4	.4
525	Buckwheat, whole grain, dry	1 c	175	10	600	23	125	18	6	1.3	1.8	1.8
526	Bulgar, dry, uncooked	1 c	140	9	479	17	106	26	2	.3	.2	.8
527	Bulgar, cooked	1 c	182	78	151	6	34	8	<1	<.1	<.1	.2
	Cereal bar, Snackwell											
2165	Apple-Cinnamon	37 g	37	16	119	1	29	1	0	0.1	<.1	.1
2164	Blueberry	37 g	37	16	121	1	29	1	0	0.1	<.1	.1
2163	Strawberry	37 g	37	16	120	1	29	1	0	<.1	<.1	.1
	Cornmeal:											
528	Whole-ground, unbolted, dry	1 c	122	10	442	10	94	9	4	.6	1.2	2
529	Bolted, nearly whole, dry	1 c	122	10	441	10	94	12	4	.6	1.2	2
530	Degermed, enriched, dry	1 c	138	12	505	12	107	10	2	.3	.6	1
531	Degermed, enriched, cooked	1 c	240	78	209	5	44	4	1	.1	.2	.4
	Macaroni, cooked:											
532	Enriched	1 c	140	66	197	7	40	2	1	.1	.1	.4
533	Whole wheat	1 c	140	67	174	7	37	5	1	.1	.1	.3
534	Vegetable, enriched	1 c	134	68	172	6	36	6	<1	t	t	.1
535	Millet, cooked	½ c	120	71	143	4	28	2	1	.2	.2	.6
	Noodles (see also Pasta and Spaghetti)											
1507	Cellophane noodles	1 c	190	79	160	<1	39	<1	<1	t	t	t
1995	Cellophane noodles, dry	½ c	70	13	246	<1	60	<1	<1	<.1	<.1	<.1
537	Chow mein, dry	1 c	45	1	237	4	26	2	14	2	3.5	7.8
536	Egg noodles, cooked, enriched	1 c	160	69	213	8	40	2	2	.5	.7	.7
538	Spinach noodles, dry	3½ oz	100	8	372	13	75	11	2	.2	.2	.6
1343	Oat bran, dry	¼ c	23	7	57	4	16	4	2	.3	.6	.7
	Pasta, cooked (see also #953–956):											
1418	Fresh	2 oz	57	69	74	3	14	1	1	.1	.1	.2
1417	Linguini	1 c	140	66	197	7	40	2	1	.1	.1	.4
1598	Rotini	1 c	140	66	197	7	40	2	1	.1	.1	.4
	Popcorn:											
539	Air popped, plain	1 c	8	4	31	1	6	1	<1	<.1	.1	.2
1042	Microwaved, low fat, low sodium	1 c	6	3	24	1	4	1	1	.1	.2	.3
540	Popped in vegetable oil/salted	1 c	11	2	55	1	6	1	3	.5	.9	1.5
541	Sugar-syrup coated	1 c	35	2	151	1	28	2	4	1.3	1	1.6
	Rice:											
542	Brown rice, cooked	1 c	195	73	216	5	45	4	2	.4	.6	.6
2215	Mexican rice	½ c	113	–	410	8	90	3	15	2	.1	.1
2216	Spanish rice	½ c	123	85	65	2	14	1	1	–	–	–
	White, enriched, all types:											
543	Regular/long grain, dry	1 c	185	11	675	13	148	2	1	.3	.4	.3
544	Regular/long grain, cooked	1 c	205	68	267	6	58	1	<1	.2	.2	.2
545	Instant, prepared without salt	1 c	165	76	161	3	35	1	<1	.1	.1	.1

(Computer code number is for West Diet Analysis program)

PAGE KEY: H–4 = BEV H–6 = DAIRY H–12 = EGGS H–14 = FAT/OIL H–18 = FRUIT H–26 = BAKERY H–36 = GRAIN H–44 = FISH H–48 = MEATS H–50 = POULTRY H–54 = SAUSAGE H–56 = MIXED/FAST H–64 = NUTS/SEEDS H–68 = SWEETS H–70 = VEG/LEG H–84 = MISC H–88 = SOUPS/SAUCES H–90 = FAST H–106 = FRZN ENTREE H–112 = BABY FOODS

Chol (mg)	Calc (mg)	Iron (mg)	Magn (mg)	Phos (mg)	Pota (mg)	Sodi (mg)	Zinc (mg)	VT-A (RE)	Thia (mg)	Ribo (mg)	Niac (mg)	V-B6 (mg)	Fola (μg)	VT-C (mg)
0	3	.57	17	43	42	<1	.28	0	.02	.03	1.3	.02	4	0
0	44	4.61[1]	32	100	108	276	.65	384[1]	.38[1]	.43[1]	5.1[1]	.52	102	15[1]
0	40	3.98	246	330	565	11	3.06	0	.41	.19	6.03	.57	53	0
0	11	1	47	86	314	1	2.56	0	.09	.05	.47	.09	100	0
0	32	3.85	405	606	805	2	4.2	0	.18	.74	12.3	.37	52	0
0	49	3.44	230	420	574	24	2.7	0	.32	.16	7.15	.48	38	0
0	18	1.75	58	73	123	9	1.04	0	.1	.05	1.82	.15	33	0
<1	17	5	6	37	68	103	3.88	–	.39	.44	5.2	.52	–	<1
<1	14	4.83	5	35	44	107	3.85	–	.39	.44	5.2	.52	–	<1
<1	14	4.82	6	35	47	102	3.83	–	.39	.44	5.2	.52	–	2
0	7	4.21	155	294	350	43	2.22	57	.47	.24	4.43	.37	31	0
0	7	4.21	154	294	350	43	2.22	57	.37	.1	2.3	.37	31	0
0	7	5.7	55	115	224	4	.99	57	.99	.56	6.96	.35	66	0
0	3	2.35	22	48	91	1	.41	23	.3	.21	2.42	.12	22	0
0	10	1.96	25	76	43	1	.74	0	.29	.14	2.34	.05	10	0
0	21	1.48	42	124	62	4	1.13	0	.15	.06	.99	.11	7	0
0	15	.66	26	67	41	8	.59	7	.15	.08	1.43	.03	8	0
0	4	.76	53	120	74	2	1.09	0	.13	.1	1.6	.13	23	0
0	14	1	3	15	5	9	.23	0	.07	0	.09	.02	1	0
0	18	1.53	2	22	7	7	.29	0	.11	.0	.14	.04	1	0
0	18	1.53	2	22	7	7	.29	0	.11	0	.14	.04	1	0
53	19	2.54	30	110	45	11	.99	10	.3	.13	2.38	.06	11	0
0	58	2.13	174	332	376	36	2.76	46	.37	.2	4.55	.32	48	0
0	13	1.27	55	169	130	1	.73	0	.27	.05	.22	.04	12	0
19	3	.65	10	36	14	3	.32	3	.12	.09	.56	.02	4	0
0	10	1.96	25	76	43	1	.74	0	.29	.14	2.34	.05	10	0
0	10	1.96	25	76	43	1	.74	0	.29	.14	2.34	.05	10	0
0	1	.21	11	24	24	<1	.27	2	.02	.02	.15	.02	2	0
0	1	.13	9	15	14	28	.22	1	.02	.01	.12	.01	1	0
0	1	.31	12	27	25	97	.29	2	.01	.01	.17	.02	2	<1
2	15	.61	12	29	38	72	.2	4	.02	.02	.77	.01	1	0
0	19	.82	84	162	84	10	1.23	0	.19	.05	2.98	.28	8	0
0	150	4.5	–	–	–	1350	–	–	–	–	–	–	–	48
0	–	.36	–	–	–	670	–	–	–	–	–	–	–	–
0	52	8	46	213	213	9	2.02	0	1.07	.09	7.75	.3	15	0
0	20	2.48	25	88	72	2	1	0	.33	.03	3.03	.19	6	0
0	13	1.04	8	23	7	5[2]	.4	0	.12	.08	1.45	.02	7	0

(1)Nutrient added (values sometimes based on label declaration).

(2)If prepared with salt according to label recommendation, sodium would be 608 mg.

(Computer code number is for West Diet Analysis program)

Table H-1
Food Composition

Computer Code Number	Food Description	Measure	Wt (g)	H_2O (%)	Ener (kcal)	Prot (g)	Carb (g)	Dietary Fiber (g)	Fat (g)	Fat Breakdown (g) Sat	Mono	Poly
	GRAIN PRODUCTS: CEREAL, FLOUR, GRAIN, PASTA and NOODLES, POPCORN—Cont.											
	Parboiled/converted rice:											
546	Raw, dry	1 c	185	10	686	13	151	3	1	.3	.3	.3
547	Cooked	1 c	175	73	200	4	43	1	<1	.1	.1	.1
1486	Sticky rice (glutinous), cooked	1 c	241	76	234	5	51	2	<1	.1	.2	.2
548	Wild rice, cooked	1 c	164	73	166	7	35	2	1	.1	.1	.4
1700	Rice and pasta (Rice-a-Roni), cooked	½ c	109	71	133	3	23	4	3	.6	1.2	1
549	Rye flour, medium	1 c	102	10	361	10	79	15	2	.2	.2	.8
1044	Soy flour, low-fat	1 c	88	2	324	45	30	1	6	.9	1.3	3.3
	Spaghetti pasta:											
550	Without salt, enriched	1 c	140	66	197	7	40	2	1	.1	.1	.4
551	With salt, enriched	1 c	140	66	197	7	40	2	1	.1	.1	.4
552	Whole-wheat spaghetti, cooked	1 c	140	67	174	7	37	6	1	.1	.1	.3
1302	Tapioca, pearl, dry	1 c	152	11	518	<1	134	2	<1	.01	.01	.01
553	Wheat bran, crude	½ c	30	10	65	5	19	13	1	.2	.2	.7
554	Wheat germ, raw	1 c	100	11	360	23	52	15	10	1.7	1.4	6
555	Wheat germ, toasted	1 c	113	5	432	33	56	16	12	2.1	1.7	7.5
1669	Wheat germ, with brown sugar & honey	½ c	57	5	215	12	35	3	5	.8	.7	2.8
556	Rolled wheat, cooked	1 c	240	83	149	5	33	4	1	.2	.2	.4
557	Whole-grain wheat, cooked	⅓ c	50	86	28	1	7	1	<1	t	t	.1
	Wheat flour (unbleached):											
	All-purpose white, enriched:											
558	Sifted	1 c	115	11	419	12	88	3	1	.2	.1	.5
559	Unsifted	1 c	125	11	455	13	95	3	1	.2	.1	.5
560	Cake or pastry, enriched, sifted	1 c	96	12	348	8	75	2	1	.1	.1	.4
561	Self-rising, enriched, unsifted	1 c	125	11	443	12	93	3	1	.2	.1	.5
562	Whole wheat, from hard wheats	1 c	120	10	406	16	87	15	2	.4	.3	.9
	MEATS: FISH and SHELLFISH											
1045	Bass, baked or broiled	4 oz	113	68	166	27	0	0	5	1.1	2.1	1.5
1046	Bluefish, baked or broiled	4 oz	113	62	180	29	0	0	6	1.3	2.6	1.5
1047	Bluefish, fried in bread crumbs	4 oz	113	61	232	26	5	<1	11	2.4	4.9	2.8
1686	Catfish, breaded/flour fried	4 oz	113	48	325	21	14	1	20	5	9	5
	Clams:											
563	Raw meat only	4 oz	113	81	84	14	3	0	1	.1	.1	.3
564	Canned, drained	4 oz	113	72	168	29	6	0	2	.2	.2	.6
1290	Steamed, meat only	20 ea	90	71	133	23	5	0	2	.2	.2	.5
	Cod:											
565	Baked with butter	4 oz	113	75	150	26	0	0	4	.4	.3	.6
566	Batter fried	4 oz	113	76	196	20	8	<1	9	2.2	3.6	2.6
567	Poached, no added fat	4 oz	113	77	116	25	0	0	1	.2	.1	.3
	Crab, meat only:											
1048	Blue crab, cooked	4 oz	113	77	115	23	0	0	2	.3	.3	.8
1049	Dungeness crab, cooked	4 oz	113	73	124	25	1	0	1	.2	.2	.5
568	Blue crab, canned	4 oz	113	76	112	23	0	0	1	.3	.2	.5
1587	Crab, imitation, from surimi	4 oz	113	74	115	14	12	0	1	.3	.2	.8
569	Fish sticks, breaded pollock	2 ea	57	46	155	9	14	<1	7	1.8	2.9	1.8
	Flounder/sole, baked w/lemon juice:											
570	With butter	4 oz	113	73	160	21	<1	0	8	4.3	2	.7
571	With margarine	4 oz	113	73	160	21	<1	0	8	1.6	3.1	2.5

(Computer code number is for West Diet Analysis program)

PAGE KEY: H–4 = BEV H–6 = DAIRY H–12 = EGGS H–14 = FAT/OIL H–18 = FRUIT H–26 = BAKERY H–36 = GRAIN H–44 = FISH H–48 = MEATS H–50 = POULTRY H–54 = SAUSAGE H–56 = MIXED/FAST H–64 = NUTS/SEEDS H–68 = SWEETS H–70 = VEG/LEG H–84 = MISC H–88 = SOUPS/SAUCES H–90 = FAST H–106 = FRZN ENTREE H–112 = BABY FOODS

Chol (mg)	Calc (mg)	Iron (mg)	Magn (mg)	Phos (mg)	Pota (mg)	Sodi (mg)	Zinc (mg)	VT-A (RE)	Thia (mg)	Ribo (mg)	Niac (mg)	V-B6 (mg)	Fola (µg)	VT-C (mg)
0	111	6.6	57	252	222	9	1.78	0	1.1	.13	6.72	.65	31	0
0	33	1.98	21	73	65	5	.54	0	.44	.03	2.45	.03	7	0
0	5	.34	12	19	24	12	.99	0	.05	.03	.7	.06	2	0
0	5	.98	52	134	166	5	2.2	0	.08	.14	2.12	.22	43	0
1	9	1.02	13	40	46	619	.31	0	.13	.08	1.94	.11	8	<1
0	24	2.16	76	211	347	3	2.03	0	.29	.12	1.76	.27	19	0
0	165	5.27	201	521	2260	16	1.04	4	.33	.25	1.9	.46	360	0
0	10	1.96	25	76	43	1	.74	0	.29	.14	2.34	.05	10	0
0	10	1.96	25	76	43	140	.74	0	.29	.14	2.34	.05	10	0
0	21	1.48	42	125	62	4	1.13	0	.15	.06	.99	.11	7	0
0	30	2.4	2	11	17	2	.18	0	.01	0	0	.01	6	0
0	22	3.18	183	304	355	1	2.18	0	.16	.17	4.08	.39	24	0
0	39	6.26	239	842	892	12	12.3	0	1.88	.5	6.81	1.3	281	0
0	51	10.3	362	1294	1070	5	18.8	0	1.89	.93	6.32	1.11	398	7
0	19	3.86	136	490	405	2	7.06	0	.71	.35	2.37	.42	150	7
0	17	1.49	53	166	170	0	1.15	0	.17	.12	2.14	.17	26	0
0	3	.29	12	26	33	<1	.24	0	.04	.01	.5	.03	4	0
0	17	5.34	25	124	122	2	.8	0	.9	.57	6.79	.05	30	0
0	19	5.8	27	135	133	2	.87	0	.98	.62	7.38	.05	32	0
0	13	7	15	82	101	2	.6	15	.36	.4	6.5	.03	18	0
0	423	5.84	24	743	155	1586	.77	0	.84	.52	7.29	.06	52	0
0	41	4.66	166	415	486	6	3.52	0	.54	.26	7.64	.41	53	0
98	116	2.17	43	290	517	102	.94	40	.1	.1	1.72	.16	19	2
86	10	.7	48	328	539	87	1.19	155	.08	.11	8.22	.53	2	0
68	9	.6	42	323	468	76	1.02	136	.07	.09	6.24	.41	2	<1
92	40	1.44	34	270	576	597	1.03	32	.4	.22	3.2	.22	19	<1
38	52	15.9	10	191	355	63	1.54	102	.09	.24	2	.07	18	15
76	104	31.6	20	383	707	127	3.1	194	.17	.48	3.81	.12	33	25
60	83	25.2	16	304	565	101	2.46	154	.13	.38	3.02	.1	26	20
68	23	.56	48	159	278	254	.66	34	.1	.09	2.85	.32	11	<1
64	43	.9	36	230	443	124	.61	17	.12	.12	2.54	.23	10	1
61	23	.54	41	259	496	69	.64	14	.09	.08	2.48	.28	8	1
113	118	1.03	37	234	367	316	4.79	2	.11	.06	3.74	.2	57	4
86	67	.49	66	198	461	427	6.21	35	.06	.23	4.11	.2	48	4
100	114	.95	44	295	423	378	4.56	2	.09	.09	1.55	.17	48	3
23	15	.44	49	320	102	951	.37	23	.04	.03	.2	.03	2	0
64	11	.42	14	103	148	331	.38	18	.07	.1	1.21	.03	10	0
91	21	.37	67	249	363	193	.71	72	.09	.13	2.47	.27	13	1
73	21	.37	67	249	364	201	.71	92	.09	.13	2.47	.27	13	1

(For purposes of calculations, use "0" for t, <1, <.1, <.01, etc.)

Table H–1
Food Composition

Computer Code Number	Food Description	Measure	Wt (g)	H_2O (%)	Ener (kcal)	Prot (g)	Carb (g)	Dietary Fiber (g)	Fat (g)	Fat Breakdown (g) Sat	Mono	Poly
	MEATS: FISH and SHELLFISH—Cont.											
572	Without added fat	4 oz	113	73	133	27	0	0	2	.4	.3	.5
1599	Grouper, baked or broiled	4 oz	113	73	133	28	0	0	1	.3	.3	.5
573	Haddoc, breaded, fried[1]	4 oz	113	55	264	22	14	1	13	3.2	5.4	3.3
1050	Haddock, smoked	4 oz	113	72	131	29	0	0	1	.2	.2	.4
	Halibut:											
1600	Baked or broiled	4 oz	113	72	158	30	0	0	3	.5	1.1	1.1
574	Baked with butter & lemon juice	4 oz	113	69	186	29	0	0	7	2.7	2.1	1.1
1051	Smoked	1 oz	28	49	63	6	0	0	4	.7	1.3	1.9
1054	Raw	4 oz	113	78	124	24	0	0	3	.4	.7	.9
575	Herring, pickled	3 oz	85	55	223	12	8	0	15	2	10.1	1.4
1052	Lobster meat, cooked w/moist heat	1 c	145	76	142	30	2	0	1	.2	.2	.1
1687	Ocean perch, baked/broiled	4 oz	113	73	137	27	0	0	2	.4	.9	.6
576	Ocean perch, breaded/fried	4 oz	113	59	249	22	9	1	13	3.2	5.7	3.4
1056	Octopus, raw	4 oz	113	80	93	17	3	0	1	.3	.2	.3
	Oysters:											
577	Raw, Eastern	1 c	248	85	169	18	10	0	6	1.9	.8	2.4
578	Raw, Pacific	1 c	248	82	201	23	12	0	6	1.3	.9	2.2
	Cooked:											
579	Eastern, breaded, fried, medium	6 ea	88	65	173	8	10	<1	11	2.8	4.1	2.9
580	Western, simmered	4 oz	113	64	184	21	11	0	5	1.2	.8	2
581	Pollock, baked or broiled	4 oz	113	74	128	27	0	0	1	.3	.2	.6
1055	Pollock, moist heat, poached	4 oz	113	74	128	27	0	0	1	.3	.2	.6
	Salmon:											
582	Canned pink, solids and liquid	4 oz	113	69	157	22	0	0	7	1.7	2.1	2.3
583	Broiled or baked	4 oz	113	62	244	31	0	0	13	2.2	6	2.7
584	Smoked	4 oz	113	72	132	21	0	0	5	1	2.3	1.1
585	Atlantic sardines, canned, drained, 2 = 24 g	4 oz	113	60	235	28	0	0	13	1.7	4.4	5.8
586	Scallops, breaded, cooked from frozen	6 ea	93	58	199	17	9	<1	10	2.5	4.2	2.7
1588	Scallops, imitation, from surimi	4 oz	113	74	112	14	12	0	<1	.1	.1	.2
1688	Scallops, steamed/boiled	½ c	60	81	64	10	1	0	2	.3	.7	.6
	Shrimp:											
587	Cooked, boiled, 2 large = 11 g	16 ea	86	77	85	18	0	0	1	.2	.2	.4
588	Canned, drained	½ c	64	73	77	15	1	0	1	.2	.2	.5
589	Fried, 2 large = 15 g[1]	12 ea	90	53	218	19	10	<1	11	1.9	3.6	4.6
1057	Raw, large, about 7 g each	14 ea	100	76	106	20	1	0	2	.3	.3	.7
1589	Shrimp, imitation, from surimi	4 oz	113	75	114	14	10	0	2	.3	.2	.9
1053	Snapper, baked or broiled	4 oz	113	70	145	30	0	0	2	.4	.4	.7
1060	Squid, fried in flour[2]	4 oz	113	65	198	20	9	<1	8	2.1	3.1	2.4
1590	Surimi[3]	4 oz	113	76	112	17	8	0	1	.2	.2	.5
1058	Swordfish, raw	4 oz	113	76	137	22	0	0	5	1.2	1.8	1
1059	Swordfish, baked or broiled	4 oz	113	69	176	29	0	0	6	1.6	2.2	1.3
590	Trout, baked or broiled	4 oz	113	71	170	26	0	0	7	1.8	2	2.1
	Tuna, light, canned, drained solids:											
591	Oil pack	3 oz	85	60	168	25	0	0	7	1.3	2.5	2.4
592	Water pack	3 oz	85	74	98	22	0	0	1	.2	.1	.3
1061	Bluefin tuna, fresh	4 oz	113	68	163	26	0	0	6	1.4	1.8	1.9

(1)Dipped in egg, bread crumbs, and flour; fried in vegetable shortening.

(2)Recipe is 94.6% squid, 4.9% flour, and 0.6% salt.

(3)Surimi is processed from Walleye (Alaska) pollock. Also see Imitation crab, shrimp, scallops.

(Computer code number is for West Diet Analysis program)

PAGE KEY: H–4 = BEV H–6 = DAIRY H–12 = EGGS H–14 = FAT/OIL H–18 = FRUIT H–26 = BAKERY H–36 = GRAIN H–44 = FISH H–48 = MEATS H–50 = POULTRY H–54 = SAUSAGE H–56 = MIXED/FAST H–64 = NUTS/SEEDS H–68 = SWEETS H–70 = VEG/LEG H–84 = MISC H–88 = SOUPS/SAUCES H–90 = FAST H–106 = FRZN ENTREE H–112 = BABY FOODS

Chol (mg)	Calc (mg)	Iron (mg)	Magn (mg)	Phos (mg)	Pota (mg)	Sodi (mg)	Zinc (mg)	VT-A (RE)	Thia (mg)	Ribo (mg)	Niac (mg)	V-B6 (mg)	Fola (µg)	VT-C (mg)
77	20	.39	66	327	390	119	.72	13	.09	.13	2.47	.27	10	2
53	24	1.29	42	162	537	60	.58	57	.09	.01	.43	.4	12	0
96	63	1.93	46	228	346	524	.59	33	.08	.14	4.51	.28	19	<1
87	56	1.59	61	285	469	862	.57	25	.05	.06	5.75	.45	17	0
47	68	1.21	121	323	652	78	.6	61	.08	.1	8.07	.45	16	0
54	66	1.17	116	308	636	112	.57	93	.08	.1	7.69	.43	16	5
28	14	.24	23	63	128	136	.12	13	.01	.02	1.64	.09	1	<1
36	53	.95	94	252	510	61	.48	53	.07	.08	6.62	.39	14	0
11	65	1.04	7	76	59	740	.45	219	.03	.12	2.81	.14	2	0
104	88	.57	51	268	510	551	4.23	38	.01	.1	1.55	.11	16	0
61	155	1	44	314	395	109	.7	16	.15	.15	2.77	.31	12	1
71	136	1.58	38	263	324	432	.67	23	.14	.18	2.69	.24	15	1
54	60	6.01	34	211	395	261	1.91	51	.03	.04	2.38	.41	18	6
131	112	16.5	117	335	387	523	225	74	.25	.24	3.42	.15	25	9
124	20	12.6	55	402	417	263	41.2	201	.17	.58	4.98	.12	25	20
71	55	6.12	51	139	214	366	76.7	79	.13	.18	1.45	.06	12	3
113	18	10.4	50	276	342	240	37.6	169	.14	.5	4.11	.1	17	15
108	7	.32	83	544	437	132	.68	26	.08	.09	1.87	.08	4	0
108	7	.32	83	544	437	132	.68	26	.08	.09	1.87	.08	4	0
62	242[4]	.95	38	373	368	626	1.04	19	.03	.21	7.42	.34	17	0
99	8	.62	35	312	425	75	.58	71	.24	.19	7.56	.25	6	0
26	12	.96	20	185	197	885	.35	29	.03	.11	5.35	.31	2	0
160	433[4]	3.31	44	553	450	572	1.5	76	.09	.26	5.95	.19	13	0
57	39	.76	55	219	309	431	.99	20	.04	.1	1.4	.13	17	2
25	9	.35	49	320	117	899	.37	23	.01	.02	.35	.03	2	0
19	15	.15	33	95	168	246	.55	31	.01	.04	.6	.08	7	1
167	33	2.65	29	117	156	192	1.34	57	.03	.03	2.22	.11	3	2
110	38	1.75	26	148	135	108	.8	11	.02	.02	1.76	.07	1	1
159	60	1.13	36	196	202	309	1.24	50	.12	.12	2.76	.09	7	1
152	52	2.41	37	205	185	148	1.11	54	.03	.03	2.55	.1	3	2
41	21	.68	49	320	101	797	.37	23	.03	.04	.19	.03	2	0
53	45	.27	42	228	590	65	.5	40	.06	<.01	.39	.52	7	2
295	44	1.15	43	285	316	347	1.97	12	.06	.52	2.95	.07	6	5
34	10	.29	49	319	127	162	.37	22	.02	.02	.25	.03	2	0
44	5	.92	31	297	326	102	1.3	41	.04	.11	11	.37	2	1
57	7	1.18	38	381	417	130	1.67	46	.05	.13	13.3	.43	3	1
78	97	.43	35	304	507	63	.58	17	.17	.11	6.54	.39	22	2
15	11	1.18	26	264	175	301	.77	20	.03	.1	10.5	.09	5	0
25	9	1.3	23	139	201	287	.65	14	.03	.06	11.3	.3	3	0
43	9	1.16	57	288	286	44	.68	740	.27	.28	9.81	.52	2	0

[4] If bones are discarded, calcium value is greatly reduced.

(For purposes of calculations, use "0" for t, <1, <.1, <.01, etc.)

Table H–1
Food Composition

Computer Code Number	Food Description	Measure	Wt (g)	H_2O (%)	Ener (kcal)	Prot (g)	Carb (g)	Dietary Fiber (g)	Fat (g)	Fat Breakdown (g)		
										Sat	Mono	Poly
	MEATS: BEEF, LAMB, PORK, and others											
	BEEF, cooked:[1]											
	Braised, simmered, pot roasted:											
	Relatively fat, choice chuck blade:											
593	Lean and fat, piece 2½ x 2½ x ¾"	4 oz	113	47	393	30	0	0	29	11.6	12.6	1.1
594	Lean only	4 oz	113	55	297	35	0	0	16	6.3	7	.5
	Relatively lean, like choice round:											
595	Lean and fat, pce 4⅛ x 2½ x ¾"	4 oz	113	52	311	32	0	0	19	7.2	8.3	.7
596	Lean only	4 oz	113	57	249	36	0	0	11	3.6	4.7	.4
	Ground beef, broiled, patty 3 x ⅝":											
597	Extra lean, about 16% fat	4 oz	113	54	299	32	0	0	18	7	7.8	.7
598	Lean, 21% fat	4 oz	113	53	316	32	0	0	20	7.9	8.7	.7
	Roasts, oven cooked, no added liquid:											
	Relatively fat, prime rib:											
601	Lean and fat, pce 4⅛ x 2¼ x ½"	4 oz	113	46	425	25	0	0	35	14.3	15.2	1.3
602	Lean only	4 oz	113	58	274	31	0	0	16	6.6	6.8	.5
	Relatively lean, choice round:											
603	Lean and fat, pce 2½ x 2½ x ¾"	4 oz	113	59	273	30	0	0	16	6.2	6.9	.6
604	Lean only	4 oz	113	65	198	33	0	0	6	2.3	2.7	.2
1701	Steak, rib, broiled, lean	4 oz	113	58	250	32	0	0	13	5	5	.4
	Steak, broiled, relatively lean, choice sirloin:											
605	Lean and fat, pce 2½ x 2½ x ¾"	4 oz	113	52	320	31	0	0	21	8.7	9.3	.8
606	Lean only	4 oz	113	62	228	34	0	0	9	3.5	3.9	.4
	Steak, broiled, relatively fat, choice T-bone:											
1063	Lean and fat	4 oz	113	53	337	28	0	0	24	9.7	10.1	.9
1064	Lean only	4 oz	113	60	242	32	0	0	12	4.7	4.7	.4
	Variety meats:											
1086	Brains, panfried	4 oz	113	71	221	15	0	0	18	4.2	4.5	2.6
599	Heart, simmered	4 oz	113	64	197	33	<1	0	6	1.9	1.4	1.5
600	Liver, fried	4 oz	113	56	245	30	9	0	9	3	1.8	1.9
1062	Tongue, cooked	4 oz	113	56	320	25	<1	0	23	10.3	11	.9
607	Beef, canned, corned	4 oz	113	58	282	31	0	0	17	7	6.8	.7
608	Beef, dried, cured	1 oz	28	57	46	8	<1	0	1	.5	.5	.1
	LAMB, domestic, cooked:											
	Chop, arm, braised (5.6 oz raw w/bone):											
609	Lean and fat	1 ea	70	44	242	21	0	0	17	6.9	7.1	1.2
610	Lean only	1 ea	55	49	153	20	0	0	8	2.8	3.4	.5
	Chop, loin, broiled (4.2 oz. raw w/bone):											
611	Lean and fat	1 ea	64	52	202	16	0	0	15	6.3	6.2	1.1
612	Lean only	1 ea	46	61	99	14	0	0	4	1.6	2	.3
1067	Cutlet, avg of lean cuts, cooked	4 oz	113	54	330	28	0	0	23	9.9	9.9	1.7
	Leg, roasted, 3 oz = 4⅛ x 2¼ x ½":											
613	Lean and fat	4 oz	113	57	292	29	0	0	19	7.8	7.9	1.3
614	Lean only	4 oz	113	64	216	32	0	0	9	3.1	3.8	.6
615	Rib, roasted, lean and fat	4 oz	113	48	406	24	0	0	34	14.5	14.2	2.5
616	Rib, roasted, lean only	4 oz	113	60	262	30	0	0	15	5.4	6.6	1
1065	Shoulder, roasted, lean and fat	4 oz	113	56	312	25	0	0	23	9.6	9.2	1.8

(1)Outer layer of fat removed to about ½" of the lean. Deposits of fat within the cut remain.

(Computer code number is for West Diet Analysis program)

PAGE KEY: H–4 = BEV H–6 = DAIRY H–12 = EGGS H–14 = FAT/OIL H–18 = FRUIT H–26 = BAKERY H–36 = GRAIN H–44 = FISH H–48 = MEATS H–50 = POULTRY H–54 = SAUSAGE H–56 = MIXED/FAST H–64 = NUTS/SEEDS H–68 = SWEETS H–70 = VEG/LEG H–84 = MISC H–88 = SOUPS/SAUCES H–90 = FAST H–106 = FRZN ENTREE H–112 = BABY FOODS

Chol (mg)	Calc (mg)	Iron (mg)	Magn (mg)	Phos (mg)	Pota (mg)	Sodi (mg)	Zinc (mg)	VT-A (RE)	Thia (mg)	Ribo (mg)	Niac (mg)	V-B6 (mg)	Fola (µg)	VT-C (mg)
112	11	3.46	22	244	274	67	7.61	0	.08	.27	3.55	.32	10	0
120	15	4.17	26	265	297	81	11.7	0	.09	.32	3.03	.33	7	0
109	7	3.54	25	278	319	57	5.57	0	.08	.27	4.23	.37	11	0
109	6	3.92	28	308	348	58	6.21	0	.08	.29	4.63	.41	12	0
112	10	3.14	28	214	418	93	7.29	0	.08	.36	6.63	.36	12	0
114	14	2.78	27	205	396	101	7.03	0	.07	.27	6.77	.34	12	0
96	12	2.62	22	195	334	71	5.94	0	.08	.19	3.81	.26	8	0
90	11	2.96	28	242	422	81	7.87	0	.09	.24	4.67	.34	9	0
81	7	2.09	27	234	405	67	4.89	0	.09	.18	3.93	.4	7	0
78	6	2.21	31	256	447	70	5.38	0	.1	.19	4.25	.43	8	0
90	15	3	31	235	445	78	8	0	.11	.25	5.92	.45	9	0
102	12	3.4	32	247	407	70	6.5	0	.13	.3	4.38	.45	10	0
101	12	3.81	36	277	456	75	7.39	0	.15	.33	4.85	.51	11	0
94	9	3.01	28	208	401	69	5.31	0	.11	.25	4.63	.39	8	0
91	8	3.4	33	235	460	74	6.12	0	.13	.28	5.26	.44	9	0
2253	10	2.52	17	436	400	178	1.53	0	.15	.29	4.29	.44	7	4
219	7	8.52	28	282	264	71	3.55	0	.16	1.75	4.62	.24	2	2
545	12	7.12	26	522	411	120	6.18	12123[2]	.24	4.69	16.4	1.63	249	26
121	8	3.84	19	160	204	68	5.44	0	.03	.4	2.44	.18	6	1
97	14	2.36	16	126	153	1136	4.04	0	.02	.17	2.77	.15	10	2
12	2	1.28	9	49	126	972	1.49	0	.02	.06	1.55	.1	3	4
84	18	1.68	18	144	214	50	4.26	0	.05	.18	4.67	.08	13	0
67	14	1.49	16	127	186	42	4.01	0	.04	.15	3.48	.07	12	0
64	13	1.16	15	125	209	49	2.23	0	.06	.16	4.54	.08	12	0
44	9	.92	13	104	173	39	1.9	0	.05	.13	3.15	.07	11	0
110	12	2.27	25	206	340	77	4.68	0	.13	.32	7.51	.16	19	0
105	12	2.25	27	217	355	75	4.99	0	.11	.31	7.47	.17	23	0
101	9	2.4	29	234	383	77	5.6	0	.13	.33	7.19	.19	26	0
110	25	1.81	23	188	307	83	3.96	0	.1	.24	7.65	.13	17	0
100	24	2.01	26	221	356	92	5.07	0	.1	.26	6.99	.17	25	0
104	23	2.22	26	209	285	75	5.94	0	.1	.27	6.97	.15	24	0

(2)Value varies widely.

(For purposes of calculations, use "0" for t, <1, <.1, <.01, etc.)

H

Table H–1
Food Composition

Computer Code Number	Food Description	Measure	Wt (g)	H_2O (%)	Ener (kcal)	Prot (g)	Carb (g)	Dietary Fiber (g)	Fat (g)	Fat Breakdown (g) Sat	Mono	Poly
	MEATS: BEEF, LAMB, PORK, and others—Cont.											
1066	Shoulder, roasted, lean only	4 oz	113	63	231	28	0	0	12	4.6	4.9	1.1
	Variety meats:											
1069	Brains, panfried	4 oz	113	76	164	14	0	0	12	2.9	2.1	1.2
1068	Heart, braised	4 oz	113	64	209	28	2	0	9	3.6	2.5	.9
1070	Sweetbreads, cooked	4 oz	113	60	264	26	0	0	17	7.8	6.2	.8
1071	Tongue, cooked	4 oz	113	58	311	24	0	0	23	8.9	11.3	1.4
	PORK, cured, cooked (see also #669–672):											
617	Bacon, medium slices	3 pce	19	13	109	6	<1	0	9	3.3	4.5	1.1
1087	Breakfast strips, cooked	2 pce	23	27	106	7	<1	0	8	2.9	3.7	1.3
618	Canadian-style bacon	2 pce	47	62	87	11	1	0	4	1.3	1.9	.4
	Ham, roasted:											
619	Lean and fat, 2 pces 4⅛ x 2¼ x ¼"	4 oz	113	65	275	24	0	0	19	6.8	8.9	2.1
620	Lean only	4 oz	113	68	177	24	0	0	6	2	3	.7
621	Ham, canned, roasted, 8% fat	4 oz	113	69	189	24	1	0	10	3.2	4.6	1
	PORK, fresh, cooked:											
	Chops, loin (cut 3 per lb with bone):											
1291	Braised, lean and fat	1 ea	71	44	170	19	0	0	10	3.6	4.3	1
1292	Braised, lean only	1 ea	55	51	112	16	0	0	5	1.9	2.3	1
622	Broiled, lean and fat	1 ea	87	50	211	24	0	0	12	4.6	5.4	1
623	Broiled, lean only	1 ea	72	57	151	21	0	0	7	2.6	3.4	1
624	Panfried, lean and fat	1 ea	89	45	247	27	0	0	15	5.4	6.3	1.7
625	Panfried, lean only	1 ea	67	53	161	17	0	0	10	3.5	4	1.7
626	Leg, roasted, lean and fat	4 oz	113	53	308	30	0	0	20	7	9	2
627	Leg, roasted, lean only	4 oz	113	59	233	35	0	0	9	3	4	1
628	Rib, roasted, lean and fat	4 oz	113	51	288	31	0	0	17	6.7	7.9	1
629	Rib, roasted, lean only	4 oz	113	57	252	32	0	0	13	4.9	5.9	.96
630	Shoulder, braised, lean and fat	4 oz	113	47	391	32	0	0	26	9.6	11.8	2.6
631	Shoulder, braised, lean only	4 oz	113	54	281	37	0	0	14	4.8	6.5	1.3
1088	Spareribs, cooked, yield from 1 lb raw with bone	4 oz	113	40	450	33	0	0	34	12.5	15	3
1095	Rabbit, roasted (1 cup meat = 140 g)	4 oz	113	61	223	33	0	0	9	2.7	2.5	1.8
	VEAL, cooked:											
632	Cutlet, braised or broiled, 4⅛ x 2¼ x ½"	4 oz	113	52	322	34	0	0	19	7.6	7.6	1.3
633	Rib roasted, lean, 2 pieces 4⅛ x 2¼ x ¼"	4 oz	113	60	257	27	0	0	16	6.1	6.2	1.1
634	Liver, panfried	4 oz	113	67	187	24	3	0	8	2.9	1.7	1.2
1096	Venison (deer meat), roasted	4 oz	113	65	179	34	0	0	4	1.4	1	.7
	MEATS: POULTRY and POULTRY PRODUCTS											
	CHICKEN, cooked:											
	Fried, batter dipped:[1]											
635	Breast (5.6 oz with bones)	1 ea	140	52	364	35	13	<1	18	4.9	7.6	4.3
636	Drumstick (3.4 oz with bones)	1 ea	72	53	192	16	6	<1	11	3	4.6	2.7
637	Thigh	1 ea	86	51	238	19	8	<1	14	3.8	5.8	3.3
638	Wing	1 ea	49	46	158	10	5	<1	11	2.9	4.4	2.5
	Fried, flour coated:[1]											
639	Breast (4.2 oz with bones)	1 ea	98	57	217	31	2	<1	9	2.4	3.4	1.9

(1)Fried in vegetable shortening.

(Computer code number is for West Diet Analysis program)

Chol (mg)	Calc (mg)	Iron (mg)	Magn (mg)	Phos (mg)	Pota (mg)	Sodi (mg)	Zinc (mg)	VT-A (RE)	Thia (mg)	Ribo (mg)	Niac (mg)	V-B6 (mg)	Fola (µg)	VT-C (mg)
99	21	2.42	28	227	301	77	6.48	0	.1	.29	6.53	.17	28	0
2309	14	1.91	16	381	232	152	1.54	0	.12	.27	2.8	.12	6	14
281	16	6.26	27	288	213	71	4.17	0	.19	1.35	4.94	.34	2	8
452	14	2.4	21	489	328	59	3.04	0	.02	.24	2.9	.06	15	23
213	11	2.99	18	151	179	76	3.39	0	.09	.48	4.18	.19	3	8
16	2	.31	5	64	92	303	.62	0	.13	.05	1.39	.05	1	6[2]
24	3	.45	6	61	107	483	.83	0	.17	.08	1.72	.08	1	10
27	5	.38	10	139	183	726	.8	0	.39	.09	3.25	.21	2	10[2]
70	8	1	21	242	323	1341	2.6	0	.68	.25	5.04	.43	3	0
62	8	1	25	257	357	1500	2.9	0	.77	.29	5.67	.53	5	0
46	8	1	23	250	397	1207	2.6	0	1.09	.28	5.68	.45	6	26[2]
57	15	.77	13	129	266	34	1.7	2	.43	.18	3	.26	2	<1
43	15	.77	13	129	266	34	1.7	1	.38	.2	3	.25	2	<1
70	17	.76	24	214	368	54	2	3	.76	.28	4.37	.35	4	<1
57	12	.66	21	182	315	46	1.8	1	.66	.22	3.99	.34	4	<1
82	24	.81	26	231	378	71	2	3	.91	.27	5	.35	5	<1
55	15	.7	17	148	245	52	2.6	1	.49	.25	3.03	.27	3	<1
106	16	1.15	25	297	398	68	3.36	3	.72	.35	5.16	.45	11	<1
108	8	1.29	33	322	442	73	3.41	3	.91	.4	5.56	.38	3	<1
82	32	1.01	24	261	476	52	2.34	2	.82	.34	7	.34	3	<1
80	29	1.13	25	268	494	53	2.4	2	.86	.35	7	.39	3	<1
123	20	1.83	21	240	417	99	4.7	3	.61	.35	6	.4	5	<1
129	9	2.22	25	255	458	115	5.64	2	.68	.41	6.74	.46	6	<1
137	53	2.1	27	295	362	105	5.22	3	.46	.43	6.2	.4	5	0
93	21	2.57	24	297	433	53	2.59	0	.1	.24	9.56	.53	12	0
134	32	1.24	27	249	316	91	4.13	0	.04	.34	10.3	.29	16	0
125	12	1.1	25	222	333	104	4.64	0	.06	.31	7.92	.28	15	0
635	8	2.97	22	360	232	60	10.8	9095[3]	.15	2.2	9.62	.56	858	35
127	8	5.07	27	256	379	61	3.12	0	.2	.68	7.61	.43[4]	5[4]	0
119	28	1.75	34	259	281	385	1.33	28	.16	.2	14.7	.6	8	0
62	12	.97	14	105	133	193	1.68	19	.08	.15	3.67	.19	6	0
80	15	1.25	18	133	165	247	1.75	25	.1	.19	4.91	.22	8	0
39	10	.63	8	59	68	156	.68	17	.05	.07	2.58	.15	3	0
87	16	1.17	29	228	253	74	1.08	15	.08	.13	13.5	.57	4	0

(2)Values based on products containing added ascorbic acid or sodium ascorbate. If none added, ascorbic acid content would be negligible.

(3)Value varies widely.

(4)Values estimated from other game meat.

(For purposes of calculations, use "0" for t, <1, <.1, <.01, etc.)

H

Table H–1
Food Composition

Computer Code Number	Food Description	Measure	Wt (g)	H_2O (%)	Ener (kcal)	Prot (g)	Carb (g)	Dietary Fiber (g)	Fat (g)	Fat Breakdown (g) Sat	Mono	Poly
MEATS:	POULTRY and POULTRY PRODUCTS—Cont.											
	CHICKEN—Cont.											
1212	Breast, without skin	1 ea	86	60	160	29	<1	.02	4	1.1	1.5	.9
640	Drumstick (2.6 oz with bones)	1 ea	49	57	120	13	1	<1	7	1.8	2.7	1.6
641	Thigh	1 ea	62	54	162	17	2	<1	9	2.5	3.6	2.1
1099	Thigh, without skin	1 ea	52	59	113	15	1	<1	5	1.4	2	1.3
642	Wing	1 ea	32	49	102	8	1	<1	7	1.9	2.8	1.6
	Roasted:											
643	All types of meat	1 c	140	64	266	40	0	0	10	2.9	3.7	2.4
644	Dark meat	1 c	140	63	287	38	0	0	14	3.7	5	3.2
645	Light meat	1 c	140	65	242	43	0	0	6	1.8	2.2	1.4
646	Breast, without skin	1 ea	86	65	141	27	0	0	3	.9	1.1	.7
647	Drumstick	1 ea	44	67	95	12	0	0	5	1.4	2	1
1703	Leg, without skin	1 ea	95	65	163	26	0	0	5	1.4	2	1
648	Thigh	1 ea	62	59	153	15	0	0	10	2.7	3.8	2.1
1100	Thigh, without skin	1 ea	52	63	108	13	0	0	6	1.6	2.2	1.3
649	Stewed, all types:	1 c	140	67	248	38	0	0	9	2.6	3.3	2.2
656	Canned, boneless chicken	4 oz	113	69	187	25	0	0	9	2.5	3.6	2
1102	Gizzards, simmered	3 ea	66	67	101	18	1	0	2	.7	.6	.7
1101	Hearts, simmered	8 ea	25	65	45	6	<1	0	2	.6	.5	.6
650	Liver, simmered: Ounce	3 oz	85	68	133	21	1	0	5	1.6	1.1	.8
1098	Liver, simmered: Piece = 20 g	6 ea	120	68	187	29	1	0	7	2.2	1.6	1.1
	DUCK, roasted:											
1293	Meat with skin, about 2.7 cups	½ ea	382	52	1287	73	0	0	108	36.9	49.3	13.9
651	Meat only, about 1.5 cups	½ ea	221	64	444	52	0	0	25	9.2	8.2	3.2
	GOOSE, domesticated, roasted:											
1294	Meat only, 4.2 cups	½ ea	591	57	1406	171	0	0	75	26.9	25.6	9.1
1295	Meat with skin, about 5.5 cups	½ ea	774	52	2360	194	0	0	169	53.2	78.9	19.5
	TURKEY:											
	Roasted, meat only:											
652	Dark meat	4 oz	113	63	250	31	0	0	13	4	4	3.5
653	Light meat	4 oz	113	66	223	32	0	0	9	2.7	3.8	2.3
	Roasted, meat only—Cont.											
654	All types, chopped or diced	1 c	140	65	238	41	0	0	7	2.3	1.5	2
655	All types, sliced	4 oz	113	65	193	33	0	0	6	1.9	1.2	1.6
1103	Ground, cooked	4 oz	113	59	266	31	0	0	15	3.8	5.5	3.7
1104	Breast, barbecued	2 oz	57	69	72	11	2	0	2	.6	.6	.4
1105	Breast, hickory smoked	2 oz	57	72	62	13	0	0	1	.3	.3	.2
1106	Gizzard, cooked	2 ea	134	65	218	39	1	0	5	1.5	1	1.5
1107	Heart, cooked	4 ea	64	64	113	17	1	0	4	1.1	.8	1.1
1108	Liver, cooked	1 ea	75	66	126	18	3	0	4	1.4	1.1	.8
	POULTRY FOOD PRODUCTS (see also items in Sausages and Lunchmeats section):											
658	Chicken roll, light meat	2 pce	57	69	91	11	1	0	4	1.1	1.7	.9
1567	Chicken patty, breaded, cooked	1 ea	75	49	213	12	11	<1	13	4	6	1.7
659	Turkey and gravy, frozen package	3 oz	85	85	57	5	4	<1	2	.7	.8	.4
	Turkey breast, Louis Rich											
1943	Hickory Smoked	1 pce	80	–	80	16	2	0	1	0	–	–

(Computer code number is for West Diet Analysis program)

PAGE KEY: H–4 = BEV H–6 = DAIRY H–12 = EGGS H–14 = FAT/OIL H–18 = FRUIT H–26 = BAKERY H–36 = GRAIN H–44 = FISH H–48 = MEATS H–50 = POULTRY H–54 = SAUSAGE H–56 = MIXED/FAST H–64 = NUTS/SEEDS H–68 = SWEETS H–70 = VEG/LEG H–84 = MISC H–88 = SOUPS/SAUCES H–90 = FAST H–106 = FRZN ENTREE H–112 = BABY FOODS

Chol (mg)	Calc (mg)	Iron (mg)	Magn (mg)	Phos (mg)	Pota (mg)	Sodi (mg)	Zinc (mg)	VT-A (RE)	Thia (mg)	Ribo (mg)	Niac (mg)	V-B6 (mg)	Fola (μg)	VT-C (mg)
78	14	.98	27	211	237	68	.93	6	.07	.11	12.7	.55	3	0
44	6	.66	11	86	112	44	1.42	12	.04	.11	2.96	.17	4	0
60	9	.92	16	115	146	55	1.56	18	.06	.15	4.31	.2	5	0
53	7	.76	14	103	134	49	1.45	11	.05	.13	3.7	.2	5	0
26	5	.4	6	48	57	25	.56	12	.02	.04	2.14	.13	1	0
124	21	1.69	35	273	340	120	2.94	22	.1	.25	12.8	.66	8	0
130	21	1.86	32	251	336	130	3.92	31	.1	.32	9.17	.5	11	0
119	21	1.48	38	302	346	107	1.72	13	.09	.16	17.4	.84	6	0
73	13	.89	25	196	220	64	.86	5	.06	.1	11.8	.52	3	0
41	5	.57	10	77	101	40	1.4	8	.03	.1	2.67	.15	4	0
88	11	1.26	23	174	234	90	3.03	18	.07	.22	5.8	.35	9	0
58	7	.83	14	107	137	52	1.46	30	.04	.13	3.95	.19	4	0
49	6	.68	12	95	123	46	1.34	10	.04	.12	3.39	.18	4	0
116	20	1.64	29	210	252	98	2.79	21	.07	.23	8.55	.36	8	0
70	16	1.79	14	126	155	570	1.6	39	.02	.15	7.18	.4	5	2
128	7	2.74	13	102	118	44	2.89	37	.02	.16	2.63	.08	35	1
61	5	2.22	5	49	33	12	1.8	2	.01	.18	.69	.08	20	<1
536	12	7.23	18	264	119	42	3.68	4177	.13	1.49	3.78	.5	655	13
757	17	10.2	25	373	168	61	5.21	5894	.18	2.1	5.34	.7	924	19
320	42	10.3	61	596	779	225	7.11	241	.66	1.03	18.4	.69	23	0
196	26	5.97	44	449	557	143	5.75	51	.57	1.04	11.3	.55	22	0
567	83	17	147	1826	2293	449	18.7	71	.54	2.3	24.1	2.78	71	0
704	100	21.9	170	2089	2546	541	20.3	163	.6	2.5	32.3	2.86	15	0
101	37	2.64	27	221	310	86	4.7	0	.07	.28	3.99	.36	10	0
86	24	1.53	29	235	322	71	2.31	0	.07	.15	7.11	.53	7	0
106	35	2.49	36	298	417	98	4.34	0	.09	.25	7.62	.64	10	0
86	28	2.02	29	242	338	79	3.52	0	.07	.21	6.17	.52	8	0
116	28	2.2	27	222	306	121	3.25	0	.06	.19	5.47	.44	8	0
22	10	.4	12	184	166	609	.5	0	.02	.06	5.45	.22	2	<1
23	4	.23	11	130	158	816	.64	0	.02	.06	4.72	.2	2	0
310	20	7.28	25	172	281	72	5.57	75	.04	.44	4.11	.16	69	2
145	8	4.4	14	131	117	35	3.37	5	.04	.56	2.08	.2	50	1
469	8	5.85	11	204	145	48	2.32	2805	.04	1.07	4.46	.39	500	1
28	24	.55	11	89	129	332	.41	14	.04	.07	3.02	.12	1	0
45	7	.86	18	195	208	352	.61	21	.11	.1	5.18	.26	8	<1
15	12	.79	7	69	52	471	.59	11	.02	.11	1.53	.08	3	0
35	0	.72	–	–	–	1060	–	0	–	–	–	–	–	0

[1]If sodium ascorbate is added, product contains 11 mg ascorbic acid.

(For purposes of calculations, use "0" for t, <1, <.1, <.01, etc.)

H

Table H–1
Food Composition

Computer Code Number	Food Description	Measure	Wt (g)	H_2O (%)	Ener (kcal)	Prot (g)	Carb (g)	Dietary Fiber (g)	Fat (g)	Fat Breakdown (g) Sat	Mono	Poly
MEATS:	POULTRY and POULTRY PRODUCTS											
	TURKEY—Cont.											
1947	Honey roasted	1 pce	80	–	80	16	3	0	1	.5	–	–
1945	Oven roasted	1 pce	80	–	70	16	–	0	1	0	–	–
660	Turkey loaf, breast meat	4 oz	113	72	125	25	0	0	2	.5	.5	.3
661	Turkey patty, breaded, fried	2 oz	57	50	160	8	9	<1	10	2.7	4.2	2.7
662	Turkey, frozen, roasted, seasoned	4 oz	113	68	175	24	3	0	7	2.2	1.4	1.9
1704	Turkey roll, light meat	1 pce	28	72	42	5	<1	0	2	.6	.7	.5
MEATS:	SAUSAGES and LUNCHMEATS (see also Poultry Food Products)											
1072	Beerwurst/beer salami, beef	1 oz	28	53	93	4	<1	0	8	3.7	4	.3
1074	Beerwurst/beer salami, pork	1 oz	28	61	67	4	1	0	5	1.8	2.5	.7
1075	Berliner sausage	1 oz	28	61	65	4	1	0	5	1.7	2.3	.4
	Bologna:											
1297	Beef	1 pce	23	55	72	3	<1	0	7	2.8	3.2	.3
663	Beef & pork	1 pce	28	54	88	3	1	0	8	3	3.8	.7
2155	Healthy Favorites	2 ea	46	–	45	7	2	0	1	0	–	–
1298	Pork	1 pce	23	61	57	4	<1	0	5	1.6	2.2	.5
664	Turkey	1 pce	28	65	56	4	<1	0	4	1.4	1.4	1.2
	Bologna, Oscar Mayer											
2115	Beef, light	1 pce	28	–	60	3	2	0	4	1.5	–	–
2114	Regular, light	1 pce	28	–	60	3	2	0	4	1.5	–	–
665	Braunschweiger sausage	2 pce	57	48	205	8	2	0	18	6.2	8.5	2.1
1073	Bratwurst, link	1 ea	70	51	226	10	2	0	19	6.9	9.3	2
666	Brown & serve sausage links, cooked	2 ea	26	45	102	4	1	0	10	3.4	4.4	1
1089	Cheesefurter/cheese smokie	2 ea	86	52	280	12	1	0	25	9	11.8	2.6
2157	Chicken breast, Healthy Favorites	4 pce	52	–	40	9	1	0	0	0	0	0
1556	Chorizo, pork & beef	3 oz	85	32	387	20	2	0	33	12.2	15.6	2.9
1950	Coldcuts, Louis Rich, Deli Thin	1 pce	13	–	10	2	1	0	0	0	0	0
1090	Corned beef loaf, jellied	1 pce	28	69	43	6	0	0	2	.7	.8	.1
	Frankfurters (see also #657):											
1077	Beef, large link, 8/package	1 ea	57	55	180	7	1	0	16	6.9	7.7	.8
1078	Beef and pork, large link, 8/package	1 ea	57	54	182	6	1	0	17	6.2	7.8	1.6
667	Beef and pork, small link, 10/pkg	1 ea	45	54	144	5	1	0	13	4.9	6.2	1.2
657	Chicken frankfurter, 10/package	1 ea	45	57	115	6	3	0	9	2.5	3.8	1.8
668	Turkey frankfurter, 10/package	1 ea	45	63	101	6	1	0	8	2.7	2.5	2.2
1968	Turkey/Chicken frank 8/pkg	1 ea	43	–	80	6	1	0	6	2	–	–
	Ham:											
669	Ham lunchmeat, canned, 3 x 2 x ½"	1 pce	21	52	70	3	<1	0	6	2.3	3	.7
670	Chopped ham, packaged	2 pce	42	64	76	7	1.3	0	4.5	1.4	2.1	.5
671	Ham lunchmeat, regular	2 pce	57	65	103	10	2	0	6	1.9	2.8	.7
672	Ham lunchmeat, extra lean	2 pce	57	71	74	11	1	0	3	.9	1.3	.3
2156	Honey ham, Healthy Favorites	4 pce	52	–	50	9	2	0	2	.5	–	–
2113	Oscar Mayer Lower Sodium Ham	1 pce	21	–	23	3	1	0	1	0.3	–	–
673	Turkey ham lunchmeat	2 pce	57	71	73	11	<1	0	3	1	.7	.9
1091	Kielbasa sausage	1 pce	26	54	81	3	1	0	7	2.6	3.4	.8
1092	Knockwurst sausage, link	1 ea	68	55	209	8	1	0	19	6.9	8.7	2
1093	Mortadella lunchmeat	2 pce	30	52	93	5	1	0	8	2.9	3.4	.9
1097	Olive loaf lunchmeat	2 pce	57	58	134	7	5	<1	9	3.3	4.5	1.1
1970	Turkey Bologna, Louis Rich	1 pce	28	–	50	3	1	0	4	1	–	–

(Computer code number is for West Diet Analysis program)

Chol (mg)	Calc (mg)	Iron (mg)	Magn (mg)	Phos (mg)	Pota (mg)	Sodi (mg)	Zinc (mg)	VT-A (RE)	Thia (mg)	Ribo (mg)	Niac (mg)	V-B6 (mg)	Fola (µg)	VT-C (mg)
35	0	.72	–	–	–	940	–	0	–	–	–	–	–	0
35	0	–	–	–	–	910	–	0	–	–	–	–	–	0
46	8	.45	23	260	315	1617	1.28	0	.04	.12	9.45	.41	5	0[1]
35	8	1.25	9	153	156	456	.82	6	.06	.11	1.3	.11	5	0
60	6	1.86	25	277	338	768	2.88	0	.05	.19	7.11	.31	6	0
12	11	.37	4	52	71	137	.45	0	.03	.06	1.98	.09	1	0
17	3	.43	3	27	49	288	.69	0	.02	.03	.96	.05	1	4
17	2	.22	4	29	72	347	.49	0	.16	.05	.92	.1	1	8
13	3	.33	4	37	80	363	.7	0	.11	.06	.88	.06	1	2
13	3	.38	3	20	36	226	.5	0	.01	.02	.55	.03	1	5
15	3	.43	3	26	51	288	.55	0	.05	.04	.73	.05	1	6[2]
15	–	.36	–	–	–	510	–	–	–	–	–	–	–	–
14	3	.18	3	32	65	272	.47	0	.12	.04	.9	.06	1	8
28	24	.43	4	37	56	246	.49	0	.02	.05	1	.06	2	0
10	–	–	–	–	–	310	–	–	–	–	–	–	–	–
15	–	–	–	–	–	310	–	–	–	–	–	–	–	–
89	5	5.34	6	96	113	652	1.6	2405	.14	.87	4.77	.19	25	6[2]
44	34	.72	11	94	196	778	1.47	0	.17	.16	2.31	.09	4	20
16	2	.62	4	42	70	248	3	0	.21	.09	.96	.06	1	0
58	50	.93	11	153	177	930	1.94	33	.21	.14	2.5	.11	3	17
25		.72	–	–	–	620	–	–	–	–	–	–	–	–
75	7	1.35	15	128	338	1049	2.9	0	.54	.25	4.36	.45	2	0
4	0	.18	–	–	–	153	–	0	–	–	–	–	–	0
13	3	.58	3	20	29	267	1.16	0	0	.03	.5	.03	2	2
35	11	.81	2	50	95	585	1.24	0	.03	.06	1.38	.07	2	14
28	6	.66	6	49	95	638	1.05	0	.11	.07	1.5	.07	2	15
22	5	.52	4	39	75	504	.83	0	.09	.05	1.18	.06	2	12[2]
45	43	.9	6	48	38	616	.47	17	.03	.05	1.39	.14	2	0
39	48	.83	6	60	81	641	1.4	0	.02	.08	1.86	.1	4	0
40	60	1.08	–	–	–	480	–	0	–	–	–	–	–	0
13	1	.15	2	17	45	270	.31	0	.08	.04	.65	.04	1	<1
21	3	.35	7	65	134	576	.9	0	.36	.09	2.2	.15	1	12[2]
32	4	.56	11	140	188	746	1.21	0	.49	.14	2.98	.19	2	16[2]
27	4	.43	10	124	198	810	1.09	0	.53	.13	2.74	.26	2	15[2]
25	–	.72	–	–	–	630	–	–	–	–	–	–	–	–
10	–	.24	–	–	–	173	–	–	–	–	–	–	–	–
32	6	1.57	9	108	185	567	1.68	0	.03	.14	2.01	.14	3	0
17	11	.38	4	38	70	279	.52	0	.06	.06	.75	.05	1	5
39	7	.62	7	67	135	687	1.13	0	.23	.09	1.86	.12	1	18
17	5	.42	3	29	49	374	.63	0	.04	.05	.8	.04	1	8
22	62	.31	11	72	169	846	.79	11	.17	.15	1.05	.13	1	5
20	20	.36	–	–	–	250	–	0	–	–	–	–	–	0

(2)Values based on products containing added ascorbic acid or sodium ascorbate. If none added, ascorbic acid content would be negligible.

H

Table H–1
Food Composition

Computer Code Number	Food Description	Measure	Wt (g)	H_2O (%)	Ener (kcal)	Prot (g)	Carb (g)	Dietary Fiber (g)	Fat (g)	Fat Breakdown (g) Sat	Mono	Poly
	MEATS: SAUSAGES and LUNCHMEATS (see also Poultry Food Products)—Cont.											
1952	Turkey breast, fat free	1 pce	28	–	25	4	1	0	0	0	0	0
1080	Turkey pastrami	2 pce	57	71	80	10	1	0	4	1	1.2	.9
1969	Turkey salami	1 pce	28	–	45	5	0	0	3	1	–	–
1081	Pepperoni sausage	2 pce	11	27	54	2	<1	0	5	1.8	2.3	.5
1094	Pickle & pimento loaf	2 pce	57	57	149	7	3	<1	12	4.5	5.5	1.5
1082	Polish sausage	1 oz	28	53	92	4	<1	0	8	2.9	3.9	.9
674	Pork sausage, cooked,[1] link, small	2 ea	26	45	96	5	<1	0	8	2.8	3.6	1
1079	Pork sausage, cooked, patty	4 oz	113	45	418	22	1	0	35	12.2	15.8	4.3
675	Salami, pork and beef	2 pce	57	60	143	8	1	0	11	4.6	5.2	1.1
676	Salami, turkey	2 pce	57	66	111	9	<1	0	8	2.3	2.6	2
677	Beef & pork, dry	3 pce	30	35	125	7	1	0	10	3.7	5.1	1
	Sandwich spreads:											
1300	Ham salad spread	1 c	240	63	518	21	26	0	37	12.2	17.3	6.5
678	Pork and beef	2 tbs	30	60	70	2	4	<1	5	1.8	2.3	.8
1296	Chicken/turkey	2 tbs	26	66	52	3	2	0	4	.9	.8	1.6
1084	Smoked link sausage, beef and pork	1 ea	68	52	228	9	1	0	21	7.2	9.7	2.2
1083	Smoked link sausage, pork	1 ea	68	39	265	15	1	0	22	7.7	9.9	2.6
1085	Summer sausage	2 pce	46	51	154	7	<1	0	14	5.5	6	.6
1076	Turkey breakfast sausage	1 pce	28	60	65	6	0	0	5	1.6	1.8	1.2
679	Vienna sausage, canned	2 ea	32	60	89	3	1	0	8	3	4	.5
	MIXED DISHES and FAST FOODS											
	MIXED DISHES:											
1445	Almond chicken	1 c	242	77	275	20	18	4	14	2	5.3	5.8
1454	Bean cake	1 ea	32	23	130	2	16	1	7	1	2.9	2.6
680	Beef stew w/ vegetables, homemade	1 c	245	82	218	16	15	2	10	4.9	4.5	.5
1109	Beef stew w/ vegetables, canned	1 c	245	82	194	14	17	2	8	2.4	3.1	.3
1116	Beef, macaroni, tomato sauce casserole	1 c	226	73	284	21	25	3	11	4.2	4.7	.6
1452	Beef fajita	1 ea	189	63	347	15	39	3	15	4.3	6.4	1
1265	Beef flauta	1 ea	113	49	360	17	13	2	27	4.9	11.6	9.1
681	Beef pot pie, homemade[2]	1 pce	210	55	517	21	39	3	31	8.4	14.9	7.4
1898	Broccoli, batter fried	1 c	85	74	123	3	9	2	9	1.3	2.2	4.9
1462	Buffalo wings/spicy chicken wings	2 ea	32	53	98	8	<1	<1	7	1.8	2.8	1.6
1675	Carrot raisin salad	½c	88	58	202	1	21	3	14	2.1	3.9	7.1
682	Chicken à la king, homemade	1 c	245	68	468	27	12	1	34	12.7	14.3	6.2
683	Chicken & noodles, homemade	1 c	240	71	367	22	26	2	18	5.9	7.1	3.5
684	Chicken chow mein, canned	1 c	250	89	95	6	18	2	1	0	.1	.8
685	Chicken chow mein, homemade	1 c	250	78	255	31	10	1	10	2.4	4.3	3.1
1451	Chicken fajitas	1 ea	189	61	344	17	43	4	11	2	5	1
1264	Chicken flauta	1 ea	113	53	343	14	13	2	27	4.3	11.1	9.6
686	Chicken pot pie, homemade (⅓)	1 pce	232	57	545	23	42	3	33	10.9	15.5	6.6
1672	Chili con carne	½ c	127	77	128	12	11	2	4	1.7	1.7	.3
1112	Chicken salad with celery	2 c	78	53	268	11	1	<1	25	4	7.2	12.1
1382	Chicken teriyaki-breast	1 pce	128	67	176	26	7	<1	4	.9	1.0	0.9
687	Chili with beans, canned	1 c	255	76	286	15	30	11	14	6	5.9	.9
1479	Chinese pastry	1 oz	28	46	67	1	13	<1	1	.2	.4	.8
688	Chop suey with beef & pork	1 c	250	63	483	26	35	4	25	5.7	9.8	3.9

(1)Cooked weight is half the weight of raw sausage.

(2)Crust made with vegetable shortening and enriched flour.

(Computer code number is for West Diet Analysis program)

H

PAGE KEY: H–4 = BEV H–6 = DAIRY H–12 = EGGS H–14 = FAT/OIL H–18 = FRUIT H–26 = BAKERY H–36 = GRAIN H–44 = FISH H–48 = MEATS H–50 = POULTRY H–54 = SAUSAGE H–56 = MIXED/FAST H–64 = NUTS/SEEDS H–68 = SWEETS H–70 = VEG/LEG H–84 = MISC H–88 = SOUPS/SAUCES H–90 = FAST H–106 = FRZN ENTREE H–112 = BABY FOODS

Chol (mg)	Calc (mg)	Iron (mg)	Magn (mg)	Phos (mg)	Pota (mg)	Sodi (mg)	Zinc (mg)	VT-A (RE)	Thia (mg)	Ribo (mg)	Niac (mg)	V-B6 (mg)	Fola (µg)	VT-C (mg)
10	0	0	–	–	–	310	–	0	–	–	–	–	–	0
31	5	.95	8	114	148	595	1.23	0	.03	.14	2.01	.15	3	0
20	0	0	–	–	–	290	–	0	–	–	–	–	–	0
9	1	.15	2	13	38	224	.27	0	.03	.03	.54	.03	<1	0
21	54	.58	10	80	194	792	.8	4	.17	.14	1.17	.11	3	8
20	3	.41	4	39	67	245	.55	0	.14	.04	.97	.05	1	<1
22	8	.32	4	48	94	336	.65	0	.19	.07	1.18	.09	1	<1
94	36	1.42	19	209	409	1462	2.84	0	.84	.29	5.13	.37	2	2
37	7	1.51	9	65	112	607	1.21	0	.14	.21	2.01	.12	1	7[8]
47	11	.92	9	60	139	572	1.03	0	.04	.1	2.01	.14	2	0
24	2	.45	5	43	113	558	.97	0	.18	.09	1.46	.15	1	8[8]
89	19	1.42	24	288	360	2188	2.64	0	1.04	.29	5.04	.36	2	14
11	4	.24	2	18	33	304	.31	3	.05	.04	.52	.04	1	0
8	3	.16	3	9	48	98	.27	11	.01	.02	.43	.03	1	<1
48	7	.99	8	73	128	642	1.43	0	.18	.12	2.19	.12	1	13
46	20	.79	13	110	228	1020	1.92	0	.48	.17	3.08	.24	3	1
33	6	1.17	6	51	125	571	1.18	0	.07	.15	1.98	.12	1	9
23	5	.52	6	52	76	188	.97	0	.03	.08	1.42	.08	1	0
17	3	.28	2	16	32	304	.51	0	.03	.03	.51	.04	1	0
35	81	2.12	59	238	550	615	1.56	75	.08	.19	8.59	.4	31	10
0	3	.65	6	21	56	55	.15	0	.06	.04	.49	.02	9	0
64	29	2.94	40	184	613	292	5.29	568	.15	.17	4.66	.28	37	17
34	29	2.21	39	110	426	1006	4.24	262	.07	.12	2.45	.2	31	7
57	28	3.11	42	161	559	841	4.3	93	.23	.25	5.22	.33	22	13
22	64	3	32	170	362	721	2	44	.3	.26	4	.27	21	24
45	50	2.15	29	199	292	187	4.18	15	.07	.15	2.13	.25	10	14
44	29	3.78	6	149	334	596	3.17	519	.29	.29	4.83	.24	29	6
16	67	.94	20	71	242	62	.38	102	.08	.13	.75	.11	43	53
26	5	.4	6	47	59	61	.56	17	.01	.04	2.06	.13	1	<1
10	26	.74	14	46	317	117	.18	1462	.08	.05	.63	.22	9	5
186	127	2.45	20	358	404	760	1.8	272	.1	.42	5.39	.23	11	12
96	26	2.16	26	247	149	600	1.53	10	.05	.17	4.32	.19	10	0
8	45	1.25	14	85	418	725	1.3	28	.05	.1	1	.09	12	12
78	57	2.5	28	293	473	718	2.12	50	.07	.22	4.25	.41	19	10
35	71	3	43	174	451	372	1.5	47	.41	.34	5.6	.03	35	19
37	52	.97	28	146	243	189	1.18	21	.05	.1	3.21	.22	8	14
72	70	3.02	25	232	343	594	2	735	.32	.32	4.87	.46	29	5
67	34	2.62	23	99	347	506	1.8	84	.06	.57	1.25	.17	15	<1
47	16	.62	11	80	138	201	.8	31	.03	.07	3.27	.34	8	1
80	27	1.75	36	199	309	1866	1.94	16	.08	.2	8.69	.46	13	3
43	120	8.75	115	393	931	1331	5.1	87	.12	.27	.91	.34	58	4
0	7	.55	6	16	28	3	.2	<1	.04	<.01	.35	.02	1	0
52	44	4.45	61	284	586	930	3.9	152	.42	.42	6.4	.47	50	23

(8)Values based on products containing added ascorbic acid or sodium ascorbate. If none added, ascorbic acid content would be negligible.

(For purposes of calculations, use "0" for t, <1, <.1, <.01, etc.)

H

Table H–1
Food Composition

Computer Code Number	Food Description	Measure	Wt (g)	H_2O (%)	Ener (kcal)	Prot (g)	Carb (g)	Dietary Fiber (g)	Fat (g)	Fat Breakdown (g) Sat	Mono	Poly
	MIXED DISHES and FAST FOOD—Cont.											
	MIXED DISHES—Cont.											
690	Coleslaw[1]	1 c	120	74	178	2	15	2	13	2	2.9	7.7
689	Corn pudding[2]	1 c	250	76	273	11	32	4	13	6.3	4.3	1.7
1110	Corned beef hash, canned	1 c	220	67	398	19	24	1	25	11.9	10.9	.9
1255	Deviled egg (½ egg + filling)	1 ea	31	69	63	4	<1	0	5	1.2	1.7	1.5
	Egg foo yung patty:											
1467	Meatless	1 ea	86	94	26	3	<1	0	1	.4	.5	.2
1458	With beef	1 ea	86	74	129	9	3	<1	9	2.2	3.2	2.4
1465	With chicken	1 ea	86	74	130	9	4	<1	9	2.1	3.1	2.5
1602	Egg roll, meatless	1 ea	64	70	101	3	10	1	6	1.2	2.5	1.6
1550	Egg roll, with meat	1 ea	64	66	114	5	9	1	6	1.6	2.9	1.6
1113	Egg salad	1 c	183	57	586	17	3	0	56	10.6	17.5	24.2
691	French toast w/wheat bread, homemade[3]	1 pce	65	54	151	5	16	<1	7	2	3	1.7
1355	Green pepper, stuffed	1 ea	172	74	236	11	20	2	12	5.3	5.3	.6
1487	Hot & sour soup (Chinese)	1 c	244	88	133	12	5	<1	6	2	2.9	1.2
1997	Hummous/Hummus	¼ c	62	64	105	3	12	2	5	0.8	2.2	2.0
	Lasagna:											
1346	With meat, homemade	1 pce	245	66	382	22	39	3	15	7.7	5	.8
1111	Without meat, homemade	1 pce	218	68	298	15	39	3	9	5.4	2.4	.6
1117	Frozen entree	1 pce	205	74	235	15	25	3	9	4	3.3	.5
1606	Lo mein, meatless	1 c	200	83	123	6	23	3	1	.3	.3	.4
1607	Lo mein, with meat	1 c	200	71	284	16	27	3	13	2.9	4.2	4.7
692	Macaroni & cheese, canned[4]	1 c	240	80	228	9	26	1	10	4.2	3.1	1.4
693	Macaroni & cheese, homemade[5]	1 c	200	58	430	17	40	1	22	8.9	8.8	3.6
1115	Macaroni salad, no cheese	1 c	141	60	363	3	21	3	30	4.4	8.5	15.5
1120	Meat loaf, beef	1 pce	87	62	185	14	5	<1	11	4	4.8	.6
1119	Meat loaf, beef and pork (⅓)	1 pce	87	57	221	17	4	<1	15	5.4	6.4	1.2
1303	Moussaka (lamb & eggplant)	1 c	250	83	209	18	14	3	9	2.7	3.7	1.5
1899	Mushrooms, batter fried	5 ea	70	66	148	2	8	1	12	2.1	3.0	6.4
715	Potato salad with mayonnaise and eggs[6]	½ c	125	76	179	3	14	2	10	1.8	3.1	4.7
1674	Pizza, combination, 1/12 of 12" round	1 pce	53	48	123	9	14	–	4	1	1.7	.6
1673	Pizza, pepperoni, 1/12 of 12" round	1 pce	47	46	121	7	13	–	5	1.5	2.1	.8
694	Quiche Lorraine, ⅛ of 8" quiche[7]	1 pce	176	54	508	20	20	1	39	18	13.8	4.9
1449	Ramen noodles, cooked	1 c	227	83	156	5	29	3	2	.4	.4	.4
1671	Ravioli, meat	½ c	125	68	194	11	18	1	9	3	3.6	1
1597	Fried rice (meatless)	1 c	166	68	264	5	34	1	11	1.7	2.9	6.2
2142	Roast beef hash	½ c	95	68	158	11	10	1	8	2.5	2.9	1.7
	Spaghetti (enriched) in tomato sauce:											
	With cheese:											
695	Canned	1 c	250	80	190	5	38	2	1	0	.4	.5
696	Homemade	1 c	250	77	260	9	37	2	9	2	5.4	1.2

(1)Recipe: 41% cabbage; 12% celery; 12% table cream; 12% sugar; 7% green pepper; 6% lemon juice; 4% onion; 3% pimento; 3% vinegar; 2% each for salt, dry mustard, and white pepper.

(2)Recipe: 55% yellow corn, 23% whole milk, 14% egg, 4% sugar, 3% salt, and 1% pepper.

(3)Recipe: 35% whole milk, 32% white bread, 29% egg, and cooked in 4% margarine.

(4)Made with corn oil.

(5)Made with margarine.

(6)Recipe: 62% potatoes; 12% egg; 8% mayonnaise; 7% celery; 6% sweet pickle relish; 2% onion; 1% each for green pepper, pimento, salt, and dry mustard.

(7)Crust made with vegetable shortening and enriched flour.

(Computer code number is for West Diet Analysis program)

PAGE KEY: H–4 = BEV H–6 = DAIRY H–12 = EGGS H–14 = FAT/OIL H–18 = FRUIT H–26 = BAKERY H–36 = GRAIN H–44 = FISH H–48 = MEATS H–50 = POULTRY H–54 = SAUSAGE H–56 = MIXED/FAST H–64 = NUTS/SEEDS H–68 = SWEETS H–70 = VEG/LEG H–84 = MISC H–88 = SOUPS/SAUCES H–90 = FAST H–106 = FRZN ENTREE H–112 = BABY FOODS

Chol (mg)	Calc (mg)	Iron (mg)	Magn (mg)	Phos (mg)	Pota (mg)	Sodi (mg)	Zinc (mg)	VT-A (RE)	Thia (mg)	Ribo (mg)	Niac (mg)	V-B6 (mg)	Fola (µg)	VT-C (mg)
6[9]	41	.88	11	43	215	324	.24	60	.05	.04	.1	.13	47	10
250	100	1.4	37	143	403	138	1.25	90	1.03	.32	2.47	.29	63	7
73	29	4.4	36	147	440	1188	3.3	0	.02	.2	4.62	.43	20	0
121	15	.35	3	49	37	94	.3	49	.02	.14	.02	.05	13	0
37	7	.26	2	38	77	257	.17	14	.01	.07	1.07	.02	5	0
180	26	1.1	11	112	143	185	1.16	92	.05	.24	.73	.16	22	3
182	28	.85	12	102	143	188	.81	95	.05	.24	.95	.13	22	3
30	12	.74	9	39	97	307	.25	15	.07	.1	.75	.05	13	3
38	12	.77	10	58	124	305	.5	14	.13	.12	1.31	.09	8	2
574	74	1.8	13	236	180	666	1.44	262	.08	.66	.08	.47	61	0
76	64	1.09	11	76	86	311	.44	81	.13	.21	1.06	.05	15	<1
38	17	1.88	20	89	230	203	2.2	44	.14	.09	2.91	.31	17	55
22	29	1.87	27	160	351	1562	1.15	2	.19	.22	4.56	.15	12	1
0	31	.97	18	69	107	150	.68	2	.06	.03	.25	.24	37	5
56	258	3.43	50	289	461	745	3.19	158	.21	.33	4	.21	19	16
31	252	2.5	44	239	375	714	1.7	156	.2	.28	2.49	.17	17	15
33	158	2.17	39	185	453	496	2.19	149	.16	.24	3.06	.19	17	25
22	48	2.18	30	115	396	624	.91	163	.18	.23	2.48	.18	41	13
61	25	2.2	34	177	260	276	1.85	38	.42	.27	3.4	.26	39	9
24	199	.96	31	182	139	730	1.2	73	.12	.24	.96	.02	8	<1
42	362	1.8	37	322	240	1086	1.2	234	.2	.4	1.8	.05	10	1
22	27	.67	16	51	137	289	.38	39	.08	.05	.75	.26	16	3
72	35	1.61	18	129	236	329	2.92	14	.07	.22	3.36	.11	10	1
91	35	1.55	16	129	236	389	3.12	23	.2	.22	3.18	.19	11	1
101	104	2.2	38	204	578	400	2.84	105	.21	.31	4.01	.26	45	6
14	54	.77	8	103	180	121	.42	10	.07	.22	1.65	.05	8	1
85	24	.81	19	65	318	661	.39	41	.1	.07	1.11	.18	8	13
14	68	1.03	12	88	119	255	.75	68	.14	.12	1.31	.06	18	1
10	43	.63	6	50	102	178	.35	36	.09	.16	2.04	.04	35	1
205	201	1.9	27	271	271	549	1.48	243	.22	.45	4.71	.1	17	3
38	20	1.78	24	82	51	1349	.61	204	.22	.09	1.42	.07	8	<1
84	33	1.99	20	109	259	619	1.67	94	.13	.20	2.85	.15	13	11
42	30	1.84	24	94	134	286	.84	62	.21	.11	2.25	.1	22	4
29	10	1.24	18	103	294	427	2.53	<1	.08	.1	1.89	.25	8	4
8	40	2.75	21	87	303	955	1.12	120	.35	.27	4.5	.13	6	10
8	80	2.25	26	135	408	955	1.3	140	.25	.17	2.25	.2	8	12

(9)From dairy cream in recipe.

H

Table H-1
Food Composition

Computer Code Number	Food Description	Measure	Wt (g)	H_2O (%)	Ener (kcal)	Prot (g)	Carb (g)	Dietary Fiber (g)	Fat (g)	Fat Breakdown (g) Sat	Mono	Poly
	MIXED DISHES and FAST FOODS—Cont.											
	MIXED DISHES—Cont.											
	With meatballs:											
697	Canned	1 c	250	78	258	12	28	6	10	2.1	3.9	3.9
698	Homemade	1 c	248	70	332	19	39	8	12	3.3	6.3	2.2
716	Spinach soufflé[1]	1 c	136	74	219	11	3	4	18	7.1	6.8	3.1
1553	Sweet & sour pork	1 c	226	76	231	14	25	1	8	2.8	3.8	2.9
1263	Sweet & sour chicken breast	1 ea	131	79	117	8	15	1	3	0.6	0.8	1.5
1515	Three bean salad	1 ea	340	82	316	9	30	7	19	2.8	4.3	11.1
717	Tuna salad[2]	1 c	205	63	383	33	19	1	19	3.2	5.9	8.4
1121	Tuna noodle casserole, homemade	1 c	202	75	238	17	25	2	7	1.9	1.5	3.2
1270	Waldorf salad	1 c	142	59	411	3	13	2	41	5.4	10.9	22.2
	FAST FOODS and SANDWICHES (see end of this appendix for additional Fast Foods):											
699	Burrito,[3] beef & bean	1 ea	175	52	385	17	50	4	14	6.3	5.3	.9
700	Burrito, bean	1 ea	174	53	358	11	57	7	11	5.5	3.8	1
2106	Burrito, chicken con queso	1 ea	306	77	280	12	53	5	6	1.5	–	–
701	Cheeseburger with bun, regular	1 ea	112	55	261	13	20	–	14	6.7	5.2	1.1
702	Cheeseburger with bun, 4-oz patty	1 ea	194	51	487	25	41	–	25	10.2	9.1	3.1
703	Chicken patty sandwich	1 ea	157	47	444	21	33	1	25	7.4	9	7.2
704	Corndog	1 ea	111	47	292	11	35	–	12	3.3	5.8	2.2
1922	Corndog, chicken	1 ea	113	59	272	13	26	–	13	–	–	–
705	Enchilada	1 ea	230	63	451	14	40	–	27	15	8.9	1.1
706	English muffin with egg, cheese, bacon	1 ea	138	49	362	19	30	1	19	8.6	6.4	1.9
	Fish sandwich:											
707	Regular, with cheese	1 ea	140	45	400	16	36	<1	22	6.2	6.8	7.2
708	Large, no cheese	1 ea	170	47	464	18	44	<1	24	5.6	8.3	8.9
709	Hamburger with bun, regular	1 ea	98	45	252	12	30	1	9	3.2	3.4	1.6
710	Hamburger with bun, 4-oz patty	1 ea	174	51	466	26	31	–	26	9.7	11.4	2.2
711	Hot dog/frankfurter with bun	1 ea	85	54	210	9	16	–	13	4.4	5.9	1.5
	Lunchables											
2129	Bologna & American cheese	1 ea	128	–	450	18	19	0	34	15	–	–
2130	Ham & swiss cheese	1 ea	128	–	320	22	19	0	17	8	–	–
2117	Honey ham & Amer. w/choc pudding	1 ea	176	–	390	18	34	1	20	9	–	–
2118	Honey turkey & cheddar w/Jello	1 ea	163	–	320	17	27	1	16	9	–	–
2131	Pepperoni & American cheese	1 ea	128	–	480	20	19	0	36	17	–	–
2125	Salami & American cheese	1 ea	128	–	430	18	18	0	32	15	–	–
2127	Turkey & cheddar	1 ea	128	–	360	20	20	1	22	11	–	–
712	Pizza, cheese, ⅛ of 15" round[4]	1 pce	120	49	268	15	39	2	6	2.9	1.9	.9
	SANDWICHES:											
	Avocado, cheese, tomato, & lettuce:											
1276	On white bread, firm	1 ea	205	57	489	15	40	4	32	9	12.7	8
1278	On part whole wheat	1 ea	195	58	454	14	33	5	31	9	12.6	8
1277	On whole wheat	1 ea	209	57	481	16	39	7	32	9	12.9	8

(1)Recipe: 29% whole milk, 26% spinach, 13% egg white, 13% cheddar cheese, 7% egg yolk, 7% butter, 4% flour, 1% salt and pepper.

(2)Made with drained chunk light tuna, celery, onion, pickle relish, and mayonnaise-type salad dressing.

(3)Made with a 10½"-diameter flour tortilla.

(4)Crust made with vegetable shortening and enriched flour.

PAGE KEY: H–4 = BEV H–6 = DAIRY H–12 = EGGS H–14 = FAT/OIL H–18 = FRUIT H–26 = BAKERY H–36 = GRAIN H–44 = FISH H–48 = MEATS H–50 = POULTRY H–54 = SAUSAGE H–56 = MIXED/FAST H–64 = NUTS/SEEDS H–68 = SWEETS H–70 = VEG/LEG H–84 = MISC H–88 = SOUPS/SAUCES H–90 = FAST H–106 = FRZN ENTREE H–112 = BABY FOODS

Chol (mg)	Calc (mg)	Iron (mg)	Magn (mg)	Phos (mg)	Pota (mg)	Sodi (mg)	Zinc (mg)	VT-A (RE)	Thia (mg)	Ribo (mg)	Niac (mg)	V-B6 (mg)	Fola (μg)	VT-C (mg)
22	52	3.25	20	113	245	1220	2.39	100	.15	.17	2.25	.12	5	5
74	124	3.72	40	236	665	1009	2.45	159	.25	.3	3.97	.2	10	22
184	230	1.35	38	231	201	763	1.29	676	.09	.3	.48	.12	62	3
38	28	1.49	34	148	390	1220	1.7	27	.55	.22	3.62	.35	11	23
23	16	.8	21	75	187	732	.66	20	.06	.08	3.06	.18	6	12
0	80	3.21	57	147	508	1164	1.22	52	.16	.21	.91	.1	120	10
27	35	2.05	39	365	365	824	1.15	55	.06	.14	13.7	.17	15	5
41	34	2.3	31	156	182	775	1.21	13	.18	.15	7.81	.2	10	1
22	42	.85	36	78	268	250	.59	41	.09	.05	.35	.37	27	6
37	80	3.71	63	107	497	1011	2.91	49	.4	.63	4.1	.28	56	1
3	90	3.62	70	78	524	790	1.22	26	.5	.49	3.25	.24	94	2
10	40	.72	–	–	–	600		40	–	–	–	–	–	15
38	132	1.93	19	157	167	710	1.9	51	.23	.17	4.64	.11	16	2
70	200	4	35	283	392	1228	4.07	76	.41	.33	9.41	.21	27	2
52	52	4.03	30	201	305	826	1.62	27	.28	.2	5.87	.17	25	8
50	64	3.92	11	105	167	617	.83	23	.18	.44	2.64	.06	38	0
65	–	–	–	–	–	670	–	–	–	–	–	–	–	–
62	458	1.86	71	189	338	1106	3.54	262	.11	.6	2.69	.55	48	1
221	196	3.11	32	302	201	741	1.71	149	.45	.5	3.71	.15	41	1
52	141	2.67	28	238	270	718	.9	74	.35	.32	3.23	.08	24	2
60	90	2.81	36	228	366	661	1.07	32	.36	.24	3.66	.12	48	3
39	47	2.25	21	101	197	516	1.88	12	.23	.29	4.3	.12	16	2
84	75	4.49	37	230	426	600	4.7	3	.28	.33	5.45	.3	37	1
38	20	2.01	11	84	124	581	1.72	0	.2	.24	3.16	.04	26	<1
85	300	2.70		–	–	1620	–	60		–	–	–	–	0
60	300	1.80	–	–	–	1770	–	80	–	–	–	–	–	–
55	250	2.7	–	–	–	1540	–	–	–	–	–	–	–	–
50	20	6	–	–	–	1360	–	–	–	–	–	–	–	–
95	250	2.70	–	–	–	1840	–	–	–	–	–	–	–	–
80	250	2.70	–	–	–	1740	–	60	–	–	–	–	–	–
70	300	1.80	–	–	–	1650	–	60	–	–	–	–	–	–
18	222	1.1	30	215	209	640	1.56	140	.35	.31	4.73	.08	112	2
35	282	2.98	52	232	554	552	1.67	146	.36	.38	3.59	.3	77	11
32	277	3.01	64	248	584	525	1.85	136	.33	.37	3.73	.36	76	11
33	269	3.45	97	323	648	594	2.63	137	.34	.36	4.18	.41	88	11

H

Table H–1
Food Composition

Computer Code Number	Food Description	Measure	Wt (g)	H_2O (%)	Ener (kcal)	Prot (g)	Carb (g)	Dietary Fiber (g)	Fat (g)	Fat Breakdown (g) Sat	Mono	Poly
	FAST FOODS and SANDWICHES (see end of this appendix for additional Fast Foods)—Cont.											
	SANDWICHES—Cont.											
	Bacon, lettuce & tomato:											
1137	On white bread, soft	1 ea	135	46	401	12	34	2	24	6	9	8
1139	On part whole wheat	1 ea	136	47	398	13	32	3	25	6	9.5	8
1138	On whole wheat	1 ea	149	47	421	14	37	6	26	6	9.6	8
	Cheese, grilled:											
1140	On white bread, soft	1 ea	117	37	393	17	29	1	23	12.2	7.6	2.1
1142	On part whole wheat	1 ea	117	37	389	18	27	2	24	12.3	7.7	2.2
1141	On whole wheat	1 ea	131	38	416	19	33	5	24	12.5	8	2.4
1596	Chicken fillet	1 ea	182	47	515	24	39	1	29	8.5	10.4	8.4
	Chicken salad:											
1143	On white bread, soft	1 ea	105	39	371	10	28	1	24	4	7.3	12
1145	On part whole wheat	1 ea	105	40	366	10	27	2	25	4	7	12
1144	On whole wheat	1 ea	118	40	389	12	32	5	25	4	7.6	12
1146	Corned beef & swiss on rye	1 ea	147	45	457	28	25	3	28	9.8	9	6.4
	Egg salad:											
1147	On white bread, soft	1 ea	111	42	380	9	29	1	26	4.5	8	11.8
1149	On part whole wheat	1 ea	111	42	375	9	27	2	26	4.5	8	11.8
1148	On whole wheat	1 ea	125	42	403	11	33	5	27	4.7	8	12
	Ham:											
1279	On rye bread	1 ea	116	56	241	16	20	3	10	2.2	3.8	3.6
1151	On white bread, soft	1 ea	122	55	260	17	23	1	11	2.3	4.1	3.6
1153	On part whole wheat	1 ea	122	55	257	17	22	2	11	2.3	4.1	3.7
1152	On whole wheat	1 ea	136	54	284	19	27	4	12	2.5	4.4	3.9
	Ham & cheese:											
1280	On white bread, soft	1 ea	151	49	388	21	29	1	20	7.8	6.8	4.6
1282	On part whole wheat	1 ea	151	50	384	22	27	3	21	7.8	6.9	4.7
1281	On whole wheat	1 ea	165	49	411	24	33	5	22	8	7.1	4.9
1150	Ham & swiss on rye	1 ea	145	50	368	23	25	3	19	7.2	6.2	4.6
	Ham salad:											
1154	On white bread, soft	1 ea	125	46	365	10	34	1	21	5	8	7.5
1156	On part whole wheat	1 ea	125	46	360	10	33	2	22	5	8	7.5
1155	On whole wheat	1 ea	139	46	387	12	38	5	22	5	8	7.8
1157	Patty melt: Ground beef & cheese on rye	1 ea	177	42	600	36	24	3	40	13.8	14.5	7.9
	Peanut butter & jelly:											
1158	On white bread, soft	1 ea	100	27	345	10	47	3	14	2.7	6.6	3.9
1160	On part whole wheat	1 ea	100	27	341	11	46	4	14	2.8	6.6	4
1159	On whole wheat	1 ea	114	28	368	13	51	7	15	2.9	6.9	4.2
1161	Reuben, grilled: Corned beef, swiss cheese, sauerkraut on rye	1 ea	233	51	639	29	40	5	40	13.7	12.8	9.7
	Roast beef:											
713	On a bun	1 ea	150	49	374	23	36	–	15	3.9	7.3	1.8
1162	On white bread, soft	1 ea	122	46	315	23	27	1	13	2.7	4.3	4.9
1164	On part whole wheat	1 ea	122	47	311	23	25	2	13	2.8	4.3	5
1163	On whole wheat	1 ea	136	46	339	25	30	4	14	3	4.6	5.3
	Tuna salad:											
1165	On white bread, soft	1 ea	116	45	331	13	32	2	17	3	5	8
1167	On part whole wheat	1 ea	116	46	326	13	30	3	17	3	5	8

(Computer code number is for West Diet Analysis program)

Chol (mg)	Calc (mg)	Iron (mg)	Magn (mg)	Phos (mg)	Pota (mg)	Sodi (mg)	Zinc (mg)	VT-A (RE)	Thia (mg)	Ribo (mg)	Niac (mg)	V-B6 (mg)	Fola (μg)	VT-C (mg)
28	60	2.33	22	144	252	731	1.16	35	.4	.23	3.8	.19	31	13
27	73	2.6	38	177	313	753	1.43	35	.4	.25	4.3	.23	35	14
26	62	3.18	75	257	378	818	2.29	35	.4	.23	4.6	.29	47	13
55	393	1.79	26	473	152	1129	2.03	209	.28	.39	2.27	.08	24	<1
53	405	2.08	38	502	206	1143	2.27	209	.25	.36	2.35	.09	27	<1
53	398	2.53	73	581	269	1219	3.05	211	.26	.34	2.72	.16	39	<1
60	60	4.68	35	233	353	957	1.87	31	.33	.24	6.81	.2	29	9
32	56	1.98	17	95	129	447	.73	26	.23	.17	3.36	.25	24	<1
31	67	2.13	30	124	181	461	.98	26	.24	.18	3.78	.29	27	<1
31	58	2.58	63	196	240	526	1.72	26	.25	.17	4.17	.34	39	<1
79	307	2.75	39	290	193	1064	3.69	80	.23	.35	3.26	.19	32	1
147	65	2.21	15	112	106	507	.69	73	.24	.29	1.82	.2	34	0
146	77	2.36	29	141	161	521	.93	73	.26	.32	2.25	.24	38	0
147	69	2.81	61	215	217	592	1.68	74	.27	.31	2.61	.3	49	0
35	38	1.72	29	197	303	1289	1.76	6	.78	.28	4.66	.38	23	17
36	47	1.86	24	193	287	1263	1.59	6	.8	.25	4.67	.36	19	17
35	56	2.09	34	216	329	1274	1.79	6	.8	.27	5.03	.39	21	17
36	50	2.5	62	283	389	1364	2.45	6	.83	.27	5.45	.46	31	18
59	224	2.2	29	381	304	1564	2.26	87	.78	.35	4.47	.34	24	14
57	236	2.49	43	412	356	1578	2.5	87	.75	.37	4.92	.38	27	14
57	228	2.93	77	488	419	1655	3.27	88	.76	.36	5.29	.45	39	14
56	309	1.99	41	353	313	1289	2.74	77	.73	.38	4.52	.37	29	14
31	53	1.93	17	125	148	872	.98	11	.47	.26	3	.18	20	3
29	64	2.2	31	154	200	886	1.22	11	.48	.23	3.45	.2	24	3
28	57	2.65	64	228	262	961	1.98	11	.49	.21	3.82	.29	36	3
116	219	3.76	43	407	369	895	6.79	137	.28	.47	6.39	.35	39	<1
2	61	2.23	51	132	256	290	1.02	<1	.3	.17	5.17	.13	43	<1
0	73	2.52	65	162	309	305	1.26	<1	.27	.19	5.63	.17	47	<1
0	64	2.97	99	238	374	375	2.04	<1	.28	.18	6.03	.24	59	<1
114	411	3.68	47	413	318	1685	5.44	130	.25	.41	4	.3	39	15
55	58	4.56	33	258	341	855	3.66	22	.4	.33	6.33	.28	43	2
34	47	3.21	23	157	335	1243	2.95	9	.26	.28	5	.32	23	10
34	56	3.33	33	182	377	1254	3.14	9	.24	.25	5.36	.33	26	10
34	50	3.77	61	247	438	1343	3.85	9	.25	.25	5.78	.4	36	10
16	56	2	21	143	149	543	.62	24	.23	.17	5	.13	23	1
14	67	2.35	34	172	200	557	.86	24	.25	.19	5	.17	27	1

(For purposes of calculations, use "0" for t, <1, <.1, <.01, etc.)

Table H–1
Food Composition

Computer Code Number	Food Description	Measure	Wt (g)	H_2O (%)	Ener (kcal)	Prot (g)	Carb (g)	Dietary Fiber (g)	Fat (g)	Fat Breakdown (g) Sat	Mono	Poly
	FAST FOODS and SANDWICHES (see end of this appendix for additional Fast Foods)—Cont.											
1166	On whole wheat	1 ea	130	45	353	15	36	5	18	3	5	8
	Turkey:											
1168	On white bread, soft	1 ea	122	54	270	19	22	1	11	2	3.5	5
1170	On part whole wheat	1 ea	122	54	267	19	21	2	11	2	3.5	5
1169	On whole wheat	1 ea	136	53	294	21	26	4	12	2.2	3.8	5.3
	Turkey ham:											
1272	On rye bread	1 ea	116	57	239	16	19	3	10	2.2	3.1	4.3
1273	On white bread, soft	1 ea	122	55	259	17	23	1	11	2.3	3.3	4.4
1275	On part whole wheat	1 ea	122	56	255	17	22	2	11	2.4	3.3	4.4
1274	On whole wheat	1 ea	136	55	282	19	27	4	12	2.6	3.6	4.7
714	Taco	1 ea	78	58	168	9	12	–	9	5.2	3	.4
	Tostada:											
1114	With refried beans	1 ea	157	66	243	10	29	8	11	5.9	3.3	.8
1118	With beans & beef	1 ea	192	70	284	14	25	3	14	9.8	3	.5
1354	With beans & chicken	1 ea	157	67	253	19	19	3	11	4.5	4.4	1.6
	Vegetarian foods:											
1511	Baked beans, canned	½ c	127	73	118	6	26	6	1	.1	t	.2
1175	Breakfast links	1 ea	34	50	87	6	3	1	6	1	2	3.2
1171	Nuteena	1 pce	67	58	160	8	5	2	12	1.7	4.6	3.7
1173	Redi-burger	1 pce	68	57	130	14	5	1	6	.7	1.3	3.3
1174	Vege-burger	½ c	108	73	110	22	4	1	1	.1	.1	.4
	Vegetarian Foods, Worthington											
1854	Burger, no salt added	½ c	113	–	150	22	7	–	4	–	–	–
1846	Chik slices, canned	2 pce	60	–	90	4	2	–	8	–	–	–
1833	Chili, canned	½ c	106	–	144	8	11	–	8	–	–	–
1835	Choplets	2 pce	92	–	100	18	4	–	2	–	–	–
1831	Country stew	9.5 oz	269	–	219	1	23	–	10	–	–	–
1836	Non-meat balls	3 ea	54	–	100	6	5	–	6	–	–	–
1838	Numete, slices	1 pce	68	–	150	7	7	–	11	–	–	–
1839	Prime steaks, canned	1 pce	92	–	160	10	7	–	10	–	–	–
1840	Protose, slices	1 pce	76	–	180	17	9	–	8	–	–	–
1842	Saucettes, canned links	2 pce	67	–	150	10	3	–	11	–	–	–
1844	Savory slices	2 pce	56	–	100	8	4	–	6	–	–	–
1849	Skallops, no salt added	½ c	85	–	80	13	4	–	1	–	–	–
1847	Turkee slices	2 pce	63	–	130	9	3	–	9	–	–	–
	NUTS, SEEDS, and PRODUCTS											
	Almonds:											
1365	Dry roasted, salted	1 c	138	3	810	22	33	14	71	6.7	46.2	14.9
718	Slivered, packed, unsalted	1 c	135	4	795	27	27	13[1]	70	6.7	45.8	14.9
719	Whole, dried, unsalted:	1 c	142	4	836	28	29	13[1]	74	7	48.1	15.6
720	Ounce	1 oz	28	4	165	6	6	3[1]	15	1.4	9.6	3.1
721	Almond butter	1 tbs	16	1	101	2	3	1	9	.9	6.1	2
722	Brazil nuts, dry (about 7)	1 oz	28	3	184	4	4	2	19	4.6	6.5	6.8
	Cashew nuts, salted:											
723	Dry roasted:	1 c	137	2	786	21	45	4	64	12.5	37.4	10.7
724	Ounce	1 oz	28	2	161	4	9	1	13	2.6	7.7	2.2

(1)Values reported for dietary fiber in almonds vary from 7.0 to 14.3 g/100 g.

PAGE KEY: H–4 = BEV H–6 = DAIRY H–12 = EGGS H–14 = FAT/OIL H–18 = FRUIT H–26 = BAKERY H–36 = GRAIN H–44 = FISH H–48 = MEATS H–50 = POULTRY H–54 = SAUSAGE H–56 = MIXED/FAST H–64 = NUTS/SEEDS H–68 = SWEETS H–70 = VEG/LEG H–84 = MISC H–88 = SOUPS/SAUCES H–90 = FAST H–106 = FRZN ENTREE H–112 = BABY FOODS

Chol (mg)	Calc (mg)	Iron (mg)	Magn (mg)	Phos (mg)	Pota (mg)	Sodi (mg)	Zinc (mg)	VT-A (RE)	Thia (mg)	Ribo (mg)	Niac (mg)	V-B6 (mg)	Fola (µg)	VT-C (mg)
14	59	2.79	67	246	262	629	1.66	24	.26	.18	6	.22	39	1
34	44	1.57	24	198	236	1238	1.05	9	.2	.18	7	.33	19	0
34	53	1.8	34	223	279	1249	1.24	9	.21	.19	7.39	.35	22	0
35	47	2.19	62	289	336	1339	1.89	9	.22	.19	7.88	.41	32	0
41	40	3.03	28	178	287	1004	2.43	6	.2	.29	3.81	.23	24	0
43	49	3.29	23	172	271	976	2.27	6	.21	.27	3.81	.23	20	0
41	58	3.42	33	197	313	987	2.46	6	.22	.29	4.17	.25	23	0
43	52	3.86	61	263	371	1069	3.15	6	.23	.28	4.57	.31	33	0
26	101	1.1	32	93	216	366	1.79	67	.07	.2	1.47	.11	11	1
33	229	2.06	64	127	440	592	2.07	93	.11	.36	1.44	.17	82	1
63	161	2.09	58	148	419	743	2.71	148	.08	.42	2.44	.21	83	3
53	171	1.81	49	240	367	435	2.29	87	.11	.2	4.49	.32	54	3
0	63	.37	41	132	376	504	1.78	22	.19	.08	.54	.17	30	4
0	21	1.27	12	77	79	302	.5	22	.8	.14	3.8	.2	9	0
0	21	1.2	40	111	200	120	.87	10	.47	.58	.14	.45	60	<1
0	19	1.4	13	56	120	370	1.2	10	.6	.4	6.7	.8	17	<1
0	32	2.7	24	105	110	190	1.1	10	.53	.68	5	.56	27	<1
–	–	1.80	–	–	40	170	–	–	.30	.10	8	.50	–	–
–	–	.72	–	–	20	330	–	–	.03	.03	.80	.12	–	–
–	–	.82	–	–	136	417	–	–	.11	.05	3.79	.15	–	–
–	–	.36	–	–	10	440	–	–	–	–	–	–	–	–
–	40	2.69	–	–	299	758	–	–	.38	.34	7.98	.30	–	–
–	20	.72	–	–	30	210	–	–	.90	.03	.20	–	–	–
–	20	–	–	–	150	410	–	–	.09	–	6	.04	–	–
–	–	1.08	–	–	35	410	–	–	.15	.17	3	.12	–	–
–	20	1.80	–	–	120	470	–	–	.23	.17	8	.30	–	–
–	–	–	–	–	15	430	–	–	.03	.03	.14	.12	–	–
–	–	.36	–	–	35	340	–	–	.03	.07	.20	.08	–	–
–	–	.72	–	–	5	80	–	–	–	–	–	–	–	–
–	–	.72	–	–	25	430	–	–	.90	.07	3	.16	–	–
0	389	5.24	420	756	1062	1076	6.76	0	.18	.83	3.89	.1	88	1
0	359	4.94	400	702	988	15	3.94	0	.28	1.05	4.54	.15	79	1
0	378	5.2	420	738	1039	16[3]	4.15	0	.3	1.11	4.77	.16	83	1
0	75	1.04	84	147	205	3[3]	.83	0	.06	.22	.95	.03	17	<1
0	43	.59	48	84	121	2[4]	.49	0	.02	.1	.46	.01	10	<1
0	50	.96	64	168	170	1	1.3	0	.28	.03	.46	.07	1	<1
0	62	8.22	356	671	774	877[5]	7.67	0	.27	.27	1.92	.35	95	0
0	13	1.7	74	137	158	179[5]	1.59	0	.06	.06	.4	.07	19	0

(3)Salted almonds contain 1108 mg sodium per cup, 221 mg per ounce.

(4)Salted almond butter contains 72 mg sodium per tablespoon.

(5)Dry-roasted cashews without salt contain 21 mg sodium per cup, or 4 mg per ounce.

(For purposes of calculations, use "0" for t, <1, <.1, <.01, etc.)

H

Table H–1
Food Composition

Computer Code Number	Food Description	Measure	Wt (g)	H_2O (%)	Ener (kcal)	Prot (g)	Carb (g)	Dietary Fiber (g)	Fat (g)	Fat Breakdown (g) Sat	Mono	Poly
	NUTS, SEEDS, and PRODUCTS—Cont.											
725	Oil roasted:	1 c	130	4	748	21	37	4	63	12.4	36.9	10.6
726	Ounce	1 oz	28	4	161	5	8	1	14	2.7	8	2.3
1366	Cashew nuts, unsalted, dry roasted	1 c	137	2	786	21	45	4	64	12.5	37.4	10.7
1367	Cashew nuts, unsalted, oil roasted	1 c	130	4	748	21	37	4	63	12.4	36.9	10.6
727	Cashew butter, unsalted	1 tbs	16	3	94	3	4	1	8	1.6	4.7	1.3
728	Chestnuts, European, roasted (1 cup = approx 17 kernels)	1 c	143	40	350	5	76	9	3	.6	1.1	1.2
	Coconut, raw:											
729	Piece 2 x 2 x ½"	1 pce	45	47	159	2	7	4	15	13.4	.6	.2
730	Shredded/grated, unpacked[1]	½ c	40	47	142	1	6	4	13	11.9	.6	.2
	Coconut, dried, shredded/grated:											
731	Unsweetened	1 c	78	3	514	5	19	13	50	44.6	2.1	.6
732	Sweetened	1 c	93	13	465	3	44	4	33	29.3	1.4	.4
733	Filberts/hazelnuts, chopped:	1 c	115	5	726	15	18	9	72	5.3	56.4	6.9
734	Ounce	1 oz	28	5	177	4	4	2	18	1.3	13.9	1.7
735	Macadamias, oil roasted, salted:	1 c	134	2	962	10	17	12	102	15.3	80.9	1.8
736	Ounce	1 oz	28	2	201	2	4	3	21	3.2	16.9	.4
1368	Macadamias, oil roasted, unsalted	1 c	134	2	962	10	17	12	102	15.3	80.9	1.8
	Mixed nuts:											
737	Dry roasted, salted	1 c	137	2	814	24	35	12	71	9.4	43	14.7
738	Oil roasted, salted	1 c	142	2	876	24	30	13	80	12.4	45	18.9
1369	Oil roasted, unsalted	1 c	142	2	876	24	30	13	80	12.4	45	18.9
	Peanuts:											
739	Oil roasted, salted:	1 c	144	2	837	38	27	10	71	9.8	35.3	22.5
740	Ounce	1 oz	28	2	163	7	5	2	14	1.9	6.9	4.4
1370	Oil roasted, unsalted	1 c	144	2	837	38	27	9	71	9.8	35.3	22.5
741	Dried, unsalted:	1 c	146	2	854	35	31	10	73	10.1	36.1	22.9
742	Ounce	1 oz	28	2	166	7	6	2	14	2	7	4.4
743	Peanut butter:	½ c	129	1	759	32	27	8	64	12.3	30.4	18.6
1371	Tablespoon	2 tbs	32	1	188	8	7	2	16	3.1	7.6	4.6
744	Pecan halves, dried, unsalted:	1 c	108	5	720	8	20	5[2]	73	5.8	45.5	18.1
745	Ounce	1 oz	28	5	187	2	5	1[2]	19	1.5	11.9	4.8
1372	Pecan halves, dry roasted, salted	¼ c	28	1	185	2	6	1	18	1.5	11.4	4.5
746	Pine nuts/piñons, dried	1 oz	28	6	159	3	5	3	17	2.7	6.5	7.3
747	Pistachios, dried, shelled	1 oz	28	4	162	6	7	3	14	1.7	9.3	2.1
1373	Pistachios, dry roasted, salted, shelled	1 c	128	2	776	19	35	14	68	8.6	45.6	10.2
748	Pumpkin kernels, dried, unsalted	1 oz	28	7	151	7	5	4	13	2.5	4	5.9
1374	Pumpkin kernels, roasted, salted	1 c	227	7	1184	75	30	15	96	18.1	29.7	43.6
749	Sesame seeds, hulled, dried	¼ c	38	5	223	10	4	3	21	2.9	7.9	9.1
	Sunflower seed kernels:											
750	Dry	¼ c	36	5	205	8	7	2	18	1.9	3.4	11.8
751	Oil roasted	¼ c	34	3	209	7	5	2	19	2	3.7	12.9
752	Tahini (sesame butter)	1 tbs	15	3	91	3	3	1	8	1.2	3.2	3.7
1334	Trail Mix w/chocolate chips	1 c	146	7	707	21	66	–	47	8.9	19.8	16.5
753	Black walnuts, chopped:	1 c	125	4	758	30	15	6	71	4.5	15.9	46.9

(1)½ cup packed = 65 g.

(2)Dietary fiber data calculated/derived from data on other nuts.

(Computer code number is for West Diet Analysis program)

PAGE KEY: H–4 = BEV H–6 = DAIRY H–12 = EGGS H–14 = FAT/OIL H–18 = FRUIT H–26 = BAKERY H–36 = GRAIN H–44 = FISH H–48 = MEATS H–50 = POULTRY H–54 = SAUSAGE H–56 = MIXED/FAST H–64 = NUTS/SEEDS H–68 = SWEETS H–70 = VEG/LEG H–84 = MISC H–88 = SOUPS/SAUCES H–90 = FAST H–106 = FRZN ENTREE H–112 = BABY FOODS

Chol (mg)	Calc (mg)	Iron (mg)	Magn (mg)	Phos (mg)	Pota (mg)	Sodi (mg)	Zinc (mg)	VT-A (RE)	Thia (mg)	Ribo (mg)	Niac (mg)	V-B6 (mg)	Fola (µg)	VT-C (mg)
0	53	5.33	332	553	689	813[3]	6.18	0	.55	.23	2.34	.32	88	0
0	11	1.16	72	120	148	175[3]	1.35	0	.12	.05	.51	.07	19	0
0	62	8.22	356	671	774	22	7.67	0	.27	.27	1.92	.35	95	0
0	53	5.33	332	553	689	22	6.18	0	.55	.23	2.34	.32	88	0
0	7	.8	41	73	87	2[4]	.83	0	.05	.03	.26	.04	11	0
0	41	1.3	47	153	847	3	.81	3	.35	.25	1.92	.71	100	37
0	6	1.09	14	51	160	9	.49	0	.03	.01	.24	.02	12	1
0	6	.97	13	45	142	8	.44	0	.03	.01	.22	.02	11	1
0	20	2.59	70	160	423	29	1.57	0	.05	.08	.47	.23	7	1
0	14	1.79	46	99	313	243	1.69	0	.03	.02	.44	.25	8	1
0	216	3.76	327	358	511	3	2.76	8	.57	.13	1.31	.7	83	1
0	53	.93	80	88	126	1	.68	2	.14	.03	.32	.17	20	<1
0	60	2.41	157	268	440	348[5]	1.47	1	.28	.15	2.71	.26	21	0
0	13	.5	32	56	92	73[5]	.31	<1	.06	.03	.57	.05	4	0
0	60	2.41	155	268	440	9	1.47	1	.28	.15	2.71	.26	21	0
0	96	5.07	308	596	817	917[6]	5.21	1	.27	.27	6.44	.41	69	1
0	153	4.56	334	659	825	926[6]	7.21	3	.71	.31	7.19	.34	118	1
0	153	4.56	334	659	825	16	7.21	3	.71	.31	7.19	.34	118	1
0	126	2.64	266	744	982	624[7]	9.55	0	.36	.16	20.4	.37	181	0
0	25	.52	52	147	193	123[7]	1.88	0	.07	.03	4.03	.07	36	0
0	126	2.64	266	744	982	9	9.55	0	.36	.16	20.4	.37	181	0
0	79	3.3	256	523	961	9	4.83	0	.64	.14	19.7	.37	212	0
0	15	.64	49	101	187	2	.94	0	.12	.03	3.83	.07	41	0
0	44	2.15	203	417	930	617[8]	3.24	0	.18	.13	16.9	.48	101	0
0	11	.54	50	104	232	153[8]	.81	0	.04	.03	4.22	.12	25	0
0	39	2.3	138	314	423	1[9]	5.91	14	.92	.14	.96	.2	42	2
0	10	.6	36	82	111	<1[9]	1.55	4	.24	.04	.25	.05	11	1
0	10	.62	38	86	105	218	1.61	4	.09	.03	.26	.05	11	1
0	2	.87	66	10	176	20	1.22	1	.35	.06	1.24	.03	16	1
0	38	1.92	45	142	306	2[10]	.38	7	.23	.05	.31	.07	16	2
0	90	4.06	166	609	1241	998	1.74	31	.54	.31	1.8	.33	76	9
0	12	4.24	152	332	226	5[11]	2.12	11	.06	.09	.49	.06	16	1
0	98	33.8	1212	2658	1829	1305	16.9	86	.48	.72	3.95	.2	130	4
0	50	2.96	132	295	155	15	3.91	3	.27	.03	1.78	.05	36	0
0	42	2.44	127	253	248	1[12]	1.82	2	.82	.09	1.62	.28	82	1
0	19	2.28	43	387	164	1[12]	1.77	2	.11	.09	1.4	.27	80	<1
0	21	.95	53	118	69	<1	1.58	1	.24	.02	.85	.02	15	0
5.84	159	4.96	253	565	946	177	4.28	6	.6	.33	6.44	.38	95	2
0	73	3.85	253	580	655	1	4.58	37	.27	.14	.26	.69	82	4

(3)Oil-roasted cashews without salt contain 22 mg sodium per cup, or 5 mg per ounce.

(4)Salted cashew butter contains 98 mg sodium per tablespoon.

(5)Macadamia nuts without salt contain 9 mg sodium per cup, or 2 mg per ounce.

(6)Mixed nuts without salt contain about 15 mg sodium per cup.

(7)Peanuts without salt contain 22 mg sodium per cup, or 4 mg per ounce.

(8)Peanut butter without added salt contains 3 mg sodium per tablespoon.

(9)Salted pecans contain 816 mg sodium per cup, or 214 mg per ounce.

(10)Salted pistachios contain approx 221 mg sodium per ounce.

(11)Salted pumpkin/squash kernels contain approximately 163 mg sodium per ounce.

(12)Unsalted sunflower seeds contain 1 mg sodium per ¼ cup.

(For purposes of calculations, use "0" for t, <1, <.1, <.01, etc.)

Table H–1
Food Composition

Computer Code Number	Food Description	Measure	Wt (g)	H_2O (%)	Ener (kcal)	Prot (g)	Carb (g)	Dietary Fiber (g)	Fat (g)	Fat Breakdown (g) Sat	Mono	Poly
	NUTS, SEEDS, and PRODUCTS—Cont.											
754	Ounce	1 oz	28	4	170	7	3	1	16	1	3.6	10.6
755	English walnuts, chopped:	1 c	120	4	770	17	22	5	74	6.7	17	47
756	Ounce	1 oz	28	4	180	4	5	1	17	1.6	4	11.1
	SWEETENERS and SWEETS (see also Dairy [milk desserts] and Baked Goods)											
757	Apple butter	2 tbs	35	52	64	<1	17	<1	<1	t	t	.1
1124	Butterscotch topping	2 tbs	41	32	103	1	27	<1	<1	t	t	0
1125	Caramel topping	2 tbs	41	32	103	1	27	<1	<1	t	t	0
	Cake frosting, creamy vanilla:											
1127	Canned	2 tbs	31	13	131	<1	22	0	5	1.5	2.7	.7
1123	From mix	2 tbs	31	12	132	<1	22	0	5	1	2.1	1.8
	Cake frosting, lite:											
2061	Milk chocolate	1 tbs	29	18	105	0	21	1	2	.7	–	–
2062	Vanilla	1 tbs	29	15	110	0	22	<1	2	.6	–	–
	Candy:											
1128	Almond Joy candy bar	1 oz	28	8	130	1	16	2	8	4.7	1.5	.7
2069	Butterscotch morsels	¼ c	43	1	243	0	29	0	12	12.3	–	–
758	Caramel, plain or chocolate	1 oz	28	8	107	1	22	<1	2	1.9	.2	.1
1961	Chewing gum, sugarless	1 pce	3	–	5	0	2	–	0	–	0	0
	Chocolate (see also #784, 785, 971):											
	Milk chocolate:											
759	Plain	1 oz	28	1	143	2	17	1	9	5.2	2.8	.3
760	With almonds	1 oz	28	2	147	3	15	2	10	4.8	3.8	.6
761	With peanuts	1 oz	28	5	155	5	11	2	12	3.4	5.1	2.6
762	With rice cereal	1 oz	28	2	139	2	18	1	7	4.5	2.4	.2
763	Semisweet chocolate chips	1 c	170	1	811	7	108	10	50	29.8	16.9	1.6
764	Sweet dark chocolate (candy bar)	1 oz	28	1	133	1	17	2	8	5.9	3.3	.3
1133	SKOR English toffee candy bar	1 ea	32	4	169	1	18	<1	11	7	2.5	2
765	Fondant candy, uncoated (mints, candy corn, other)	1 oz	28	7	100	0	26	0	<1	.1	0	–
1697	Fruit Roll-up (small)	1 ea	14	21	41	<1	11	<1	<1	t	t	.1
766	Fudge, chocolate	1 oz	28	10	107	<1	22	<1	2	1.5	.7	.1
767	Gumdrops	1 oz	28	1	108	0	28	0	<1	0	t	.1
768	Hard candy, all flavors	1 oz	28	1	104	0	28	0	0	0	0	0
769	Jellybeans	1 oz	28	6	104	0	26	0	<1	0	t	.1
1134	M&M's plain chocolate candy	1 pkg	48	1	228	3	33	1	11	5	3	.3
1135	M&M's peanut chocolate candy	1 pkg	47	2	234	5	28	2	13	5	5.1	2
1130	Mars almond bar	1 ea	50	5	234	4	31	1	11	4.8	4.4	.8
1129	Milky Way candy bar	1 ea	60	2	251	3	43	1	9	4.7	3.3	.3
1708	Milk chocolate-coated peanuts	½ c	85	2	441	11	42	4	29	12.4	11	3.7
1709	Peanut brittle, recipe	½ c	74	2	335	6	51	1	14	3.7	6.2	3.5
1132	Reese's peanut butter cup	2 ea	45	8	218	5	21	2	14	10.4	.9	.9
1131	Snickers candy bar (2.2oz)	1 ea	61	6	278	6	37	2	14	7.3	4.1	.5
1482	Fruit juice bar (2.5 fl oz)	1 ea	77	78	63	1	16	–	<1	–	–	–
771	Gelatin dessert/Jello, prepared	½ c	120	85	71	1	17	0	0	0	0	0
1702	SugarFree	½ c	113	98	8	1	1	0	0	0	0	0
772	Honey:	1 c	339	17	1030	1	279	0	0	0	0	0
773	Tablespoon	1 tbs	21	17	64	<1	17	<1	0	0	0	0

(Computer code number is for West Diet Analysis program)

Chol (mg)	Calc (mg)	Iron (mg)	Magn (mg)	Phos (mg)	Pota (mg)	Sodi (mg)	Zinc (mg)	VT-A (RE)	Thia (mg)	Ribo (mg)	Niac (mg)	V-B6 (mg)	Fola (µg)	VT-C (mg)
0	16	.87	57	132	149	<1	.97	9	.06	.03	.2	.16	18	1
0	113	2.93	203	380	602	12	3.28	15	.46	.18	1.25	.67	79	4
0	27	.69	48	90	142	3	.77	4	.11	.04	.29	.16	18	1
0	2	.05	1	2	32	0	.02	0	0	<.01	.03	.01	0	1
<1	22	.07	3	19	34	143	.08	11	0	.04	.02	.01	1	<1
<1	22	.07	3	19	34	143	.08	11	0	.04	.02	.01	1	<1
0	1	.03	<1	12	11	28	0	70	0	<.01	<.01	0	0	0
0	3	.07	1	8	7	69	.03	33	.01	.01	.11	<.01	0	0
0	3	.43	–	–	–	72	–	0	–	–	–	–	–	0
0	1	.03	–	–	–	53	–	0	–	–	–	–	–	0
1	22	.34	19	40	105	38	.23	3	.01	.04	.13	.02	2	<1
0	0	0	–	–	79	45	–	0	.03	.04	.03	–	–	0
2	39	.04	5	32	61	69	.12	2	<.01	.05	.07	.01	1	<1
–	–	–	–	–	0	0	–	–	–	–	–	–	–	–
6	54	.39	17	61	109	23	.39	14	.02	.08	.09	.01	2	<1
5	63	.46	25	75	124	21	.38	4	.02	.12	.21	.01	3	<1
3	33	.53	35	83	150	11	.69	6	.08	.05	2.14	.04	23	0
5	48	.21	14	55	97	41	.32	3	.02	.08	.13	.02	3	<1
0	54	5.32	196	224	621	19	2.75	3	.09	.15	.73	.08	5	0
0	5	.59	33	45	96	3	.42	1	.01	.07	.19	.01	1	0
19	36	.13	11	48	76	74	.24	22	.01	.11	.03	.01	2	<1
0	1	.02	<1	1	4	11	.01	0	<.01	<.01	<.01	<.01	0	0
0	6	.55	13	6	12	2	.01	<1	<.01	.01	.2	.03	0	<1
4	12	.14	7	16	29	18	.11	13	<.01	.02	.03	<.01	1	<1
0	1	.11	<1	<1	1	12	0	0	0	<.01	<.01	0	0	0
0	1	.08	1	1	1	11	<.01	0	<.01	<.01	<.01	<.01	0	0
0	1	.31	1	1	10	7	.01	0	0	0	0	0	0	0
0	81	.73	32	94	188	49	.61	12	.03	.12	.26	.03	4	0
0	63	.7	39	130	184	44	.72	5	.03	.1	1.51	.08	26	0
4	84	.55	36	114	163	85	.55	22	.02	.16	.47	.03	7	1
12	78	.46	20	98	145	144	.43	28	.02	.13	.21	.03	5	1
8	88	1.12	77	180	427	35	1.61	0	.1	.15	3.61	.18	7	0
10	22	1.02	37	82	153	334	.71	35	.14	.04	2.57	.08	52	0
7	35	.49	38	108	180	131	.63	9	.02	.09	1.79	.04	13	0
7	70	.48	37	129	200	164	.7	19	.03	.11	1.83	.11	24	<1
0	4	.15	3	5	41	3	.04	2	.01	.01	.12	.02	5	7
0	2	.04	1	26	1	50	.04	0	0	<.01	<.01	<.01	0	0
0	2	.01	1	31	0	54	.03	0	0	<.01	<.01	<.01	0	0
0	20	1.42	7	14	176	14	.75	0	0	.13	.41	.08	7	8
0	1	.09	<1	1	11	1	.05	0	0	.01	.03	.01	<1	<1

H

Table H–1
Food Composition

Computer Code Number	Food Description	Measure	Wt (g)	H_2O (%)	Ener (kcal)	Prot (g)	Carb (g)	Dietary Fiber (g)	Fat (g)	Fat Breakdown (g)		
										Sat	Mono	Poly
	SWEETENERS and SWEETS (see also Dairy [milk desserts] and Baked Goods)—Cont.											
774	Jams or preserves:	1 tbs	20	35	48	<1	13	<1	<1	0	t	0
775	Packet	1 ea	14	34	34	<1	9	<1	<1	t	t	0
776	Jellies:	1 tbs	18	28	49	<1	13	<1	<1	t	t	t
777	Packet	1 ea	14	28	38	<1	10	<1	<1	t	t	t
1136	Marmalade	2 tbs	40	33	98	<1	26	<1	0	0	0	0
770	Marshmallows	4 ea	28	16	90	1	23	<1	<1	0	0	0
1126	Marshmallow creme topping	3 tbs	50	18	155	1	40	0	<1	0	0	0
778	Popsicle/ice pops	1 ea	95	80	68	0	18	0	0	0	0	0
	Sugars:											
779	Brown sugar	1 c	220	2	827	0	214	0	0	0	0	0
780	White sugar, granulated:	1 c	200	<1	774	0	200	0	0	0	0	0
781	Tablespoon	1 tbs	12	<1	46	0	12	0	0	0	0	0
782	Packet	1 ea	6	<1	23	0	6	0	0	0	0	0
783	White sugar, powdered, sifted	1 c	100	<1	389	0	100	0	<1	0	0	0
	Sweeteners:											
1711	Equal, packet	1 ea	1	5	4	1	0	0	0	0	0	0
1712	Sweet 'N Low, packet	1 ea	1	<1	4	0	1	0	0	0	0	0
	Syrups:											
	Chocolate:											
785	Hot fudge type	2 tbs	38	22	131	2	22	<1	5	2.2	1.4	1.2
784	Thin type	2 tbs	38	37	83	1	22	1	<1	.2	.1	<.1
786	Molasses, blackstrap[1]	2 tbs	40	29	94	0	24	0	0	0	0	0
1710	Light cane	1 tbs	21	26	56	0	14	0	<1	0	0	0
787	Pancake table syrup (corn and maple)	¼ c	79	24	227	0	60	0	0	0	0	0
	VEGETABLES and LEGUMES											
788	Alfalfa sprouts	1 c	33	91	10	1	1	1	<1	t	t	.1
1815	Amaranth leaves, raw, chopped	1 c	28	93	7	1	1	<1	<1	<.1	<.1	<.1
1816	Amaranth leaves, raw, each	1 ea	14	93	4	0	1	<1	<1	<.1	<.1	<.1
1817	Amaranth leaves, cooked	1 c	132	92	28	3	5	2	<1	.1	.1	.1
1987	Argula, raw, chopped	5 ea	10	92	3	0	0	–	0	–	–	–
789	Artichokes, cooked globe (300 g w/refuse)	1 ea	120	84	60	4	13	6	<1	t	t	.1
1177	Artichoke hearts, cooked from frozen	9 oz	240	86	108	7	22	13	1	.3	t	.5
1176	Artichoke hearts, marinated	6 oz	170	59	168	4	13	8	14	2	3	7.7
2021	Artichoke hearts in water	.6 c	101	86	44	2	10	6	0	<.1	<.1	.1
	Asparagus, green, cooked:											
	From fresh:											
790	Cuts and tips	½ c	90	92	22	2	4	2	<1	.1	t	.1
791	Spears, ½" diam at base	6 ea	90	92	22	2	4	2	<1	.1	t	.1
	From frozen:											
792	Cuts and tips	½ c	90	91	25	3	4	2	<1	.1	t	.2
793	Spears, ½" diam at base	6 ea	90	91	25	3	4	2	<1	.1	t	.2
794	Canned, spears, ½" diam at base	6 ea	120	94	23	3	3	2	1	.2	t	.3
795	Bamboo shoots, canned, drained slices	1 c	131	94	25	2	4	3	1	.1	t	.2
1795	Bamboo shoots, raw	1 c	151	91	41	4	8	3	<1	.1	0	.2
1798	Bamboo shoots, cooked	1 c	120	96	14	2	2	1	0	.1	<.1	.1

(1)Light molasses would contain about 66 mg calcium, 2.1 mg iron, 18 mg magnesium, and 366 mg potassium for 2 tbsp.

PAGE KEY: H–4 = BEV H–6 = DAIRY H–12 = EGGS H–14 = FAT/OIL H–18 = FRUIT H–26 = BAKERY H–36 = GRAIN H–44 = FISH H–48 = MEATS H–50 = POULTRY H–54 = SAUSAGE H–56 = MIXED/FAST H–64 = NUTS/SEEDS H–68 = SWEETS H–70 = VEG/LEG H–84 = MISC H–88 = SOUPS/SAUCES H–90 = FAST H–106 = FRZN ENTREE H–112 = BABY FOODS

Chol (mg)	Calc (mg)	Iron (mg)	Magn (mg)	Phos (mg)	Pota (mg)	Sodi (mg)	Zinc (mg)	VT-A (RE)	Thia (mg)	Ribo (mg)	Niac (mg)	V-B6 (mg)	Fola (μg)	VT-C (mg)
0	4	.2	1	2	15	8	.01	<1	0	<.01	.01	<.01	7	2
0	3	.07	1	2	11	6	.01	<1	0	<.01	.01	<.01	5	1
0	1	.04	1	1	12	6	.01	<1	<.01	<.01	.01	<.01	<1	<1
0	1	.03	1	1	9	5	.01	<1	<.01	<.01	.01	<.01	<1	<1
0	15	.06	1	2	15	22	.02	2	<.01	<.01	.02	.01	14	2
0	1	.06	1	2	1	13	.01	<1	<.01	<.01	.02	<.01	<1	0
0	2	.11	1	4	3	23	.02	<1	<.01	<.01	.04	<.01	1	0
0	0	0	1	0	4	11	.02	0	0	0	0	0	0	0
0	187	4.2	64	48	761	86	.4	0	.02	.01	.18	.06	2	0
0	2	.13	0	4	4	2	.07	0	0	.04	0	0	0	0
0	<1	.01	0	<1	<1	<1	<.01	0	0	<.01	0	0	0	0
0	<1	<.01	0	<1	<1	<1	<.01	0	0	<.01	0	0	0	0
0	1	.06	1	2	2	1	.03	0	0	0	0	0	0	0
0	<1	.02	–	0	<1	<1	–	0	0	0	0		–	0
0	<1	–	<1	–	1	1	–	–	–	–	–	–	–	–
5	38	.46	18	65	82	49	.3	8	.01	.08	.08	.01	2	<1
0	5	.81	25	49	85	36	.28	1	<.01	.02	.12	<.01	2	<1
0	344[2]	7[1]	86[1]	16	997[1]	22	.4	0	.01	.02	.43	.28	<1	0
0	43	.99	51	7	307	8	.06	0	.01	<.01	.2	.14	0	0
0	1	.07	2	7	2	66	.03	0	.01	.01	.02	0	0	0
0	11	.32	9	23	26	2	.3	5	.03	.04	.16	.01	12	3
0	61	.66	16	14	174	6	.26	83	.01	.04	.19	.05	24	12
0	30	.32	8	7	86	3	.13	41	0	.02	.09	.03	12	6
0	276	2.98	73	95	846	28	1.16	366	.03	.18	.74	.23	75	54
0	16	.15	5	5	37	3	.05	24	0	.01	.03	.01	10	2
0	54	1.55	72	103	425	114	.59	21	.08	.08	1.2	.13	61	12
0	50	1.34	74	146	634	127	.86	39	.15	.38	2.2	.21	286	12
0	39	1.62	48	102	439	899	.54	28	.06	.17	1.38	.15	149	52
0	40	1.36	40	60	265	66	.3	15	.06	.05	.59	.09	45	7
0	18	.66	9	49	144	10	.38	49	.11	.11	.97	.11	131	10
0	18	.66	9	49	144	10	.38	49	.11	.11	.97	.11	131	10
0	21	.58	12	49	196	4	.5	74	.06	.09	.94	.02	122	22
0	21	.58	12	49	196	4	.5	74	.06	.09	.94	.02	122	22
0	19	2.2	12	52	206	468[2]	.48	64	.07	.12	1.14	.13	115	22
0	10	.42	5	33	105	9	.85	1	.03	.03	.18	.18	4	1
0	20	.76	5	89	805	6	1.68	3	.23	.11	.91	.36	11	6
0	14	.29	4	24	640	5	.56	0	.02	.06	.36	.12	3	0

(2)Low sodium pack contains 3 mg sodium.

(For purposes of calculations, use "0" for t, <1, <.1, <.01, etc.)

Table H–1
Food Composition

Computer Code Number	Food Description	Measure	Wt (g)	H_2O (%)	Ener (kcal)	Prot (g)	Carb (g)	Dietary Fiber (g)	Fat (g)	Fat Breakdown (g) Sat	Mono	Poly
	VEGETABLES AND LEGUMES—Cont.											
	Beans (see also alphabetical listing in this section):											
796	Black beans, cooked	½ c	86	66	114	8	20	7	<1	.1	t	.2
	Canned beans (white/navy):											
803	With pork and tomato sauce	½ c	126	73	123	7	24	6	1	.5	.6	.2
804	With sweet sauce	1 c	253	71	281	13	53	11	4	1.4	1.6	.5
805	With frankfurters	1 c	257	69	365	17	40	18	17	6	7.3	2.2
	Lima beans:											
797	Thick seeded (Fordhooks), cooked from frozen	½ c	85	74	85	5	16	6	<1	.1	t	.1
798	Thin seeded (Baby), cooked from frozen	½ c	90	72	95	6	18	6	<1	.1	t	.1
799	Cooked from dry, drained	½ c	94	70	108	7	20	7	<1	.1	t	.2
1998	Red Mexican, cooked f/dry	1 c	224	70	252	15	47	18	1	.2	.2	.3
	Snap bean/green string beans cuts and french style:											
800	Cooked from fresh	½ c	62	89	22	1	5	2	<1	t	t	.1
801	Cooked from frozen	½ c	67	92	17	1	4	2	<1	t	t	.1
802	Canned, drained	½ c	67	93	13	1	3	1	<1	t	t	t
1713	Snap bean, yellow, cooked f/fresh	½ c	63	89	22	1	5	1	<1	t	t	.1
	Bean sprouts (mung):											
806	Raw	1 c	104	90	31	3	6	2	<1	.1	t	.1
807	Cooked, stir-fried	1 c	124	84	62	5	13	4	<1	.1	.1	.1
808	Cooked, boiled, drained	1 c	124	93	26	3	5	1	<1	t	t	t
1788	Canned, drained	1 c	125	96	15	2	3	1	0	<.1	<.1	<.1
	Beets, cooked from fresh:											
809	Sliced or diced	½ c	85	87	37	1	8	1	<1	t	t	.1
810	Whole beets, 2" diam	2 ea	100	87	44	2	10	2	<1	t	t	.1
	Beets, canned:											
811	Sliced or diced	½ c	85	91	26	1	6	2	<1	t	t	t
812	Pickled slices	½ c	114	82	74	1	19	2	<1	t	t	t
813	Beet greens, cooked, drained	½ c	72	89	19	2	4	2	<1	t	t	.1
	Broccoli, raw:											
817	Chopped	1 c	88	91	25	3	5	3	<1	.1	t	.2
818	Spears	1 ea	151	91	42	4	8	5	1	.1	t	.3
	Broccoli, cooked from fresh:											
819	Spears	1 ea	180	91	50	5	9	5	1	.1	t	.3
820	Chopped	1 c	156	91	44	5	8	5	1	.1	t	.3
	Broccoli, cooked from frozen:											
821	Spear, small piece	3 ea	90	91	25	3	5	2	<1	t	t	.1
822	Chopped	1 c	184	91	51	6	10	5	<1	t	t	.1
1603	Broccoflower, steamed	3½ oz	100	90	32	3	6	3	<1	t	t	.1
823	Brussels sprouts, cooked from fresh	½ c	78	87	30	2	7	4	<1	.1	t	.2
824	Brussels sprouts, cooked from frozen	½ c	77	87	33	3	6	3	<1	.1	t	.2
	Cabbage, common varieties:											
825	Raw, shredded or chopped	1 c	70	92	17	1	4	1	<1	t	t	.1

H

Chol (mg)	Calc (mg)	Iron (mg)	Magn (mg)	Phos (mg)	Pota (mg)	Sodi (mg)	Zinc (mg)	VT-A (RE)	Thia (mg)	Ribo (mg)	Niac (mg)	V-B6 (mg)	Fola (µg)	VT-C (mg)
0	23	1.81	60	120	305	1	.97	1	.21	.05	.43	.06	128	0
9	71	4.15	44	148	378	554	7.4	16	.07	.06	.63	.09	28	4
18	154	4.23	86	266	673	850	3.82	29	.12	.15	.89	.22	95	8
15	123	4.47	72	267	604	1105	4.83	40	.15	.14	2.32	.12	77	6
0	19	1.16	29	54	347	45	.37	16	.06	.05	.91	.1	18	11
0	25	1.76	50	101	370	26	.5	15	.06	.05	.69	.1	14	5
0	16	2.26	40	104	478	2	.89	0	.15	.05	.4	.15	78	0
0	84	3.72	96	279	738	481	1.74	1	.27	.13	.75	.23	188	4
0	29	.79	16	24	185	2	.22	41[1]	.05	.06	.38	.03	21	6
0	30	.55	14	16	75	9	.42	35[2]	.03	.05	.28	.04	5	5
0	17	.6	9	13	73	168[3]	.19	23[4]	.01	.04	.13	.02	21	3
0	29	.8	16	25	188	2	.23	5	.05	.06	.39	.04	21	6
0	14	.95	22	56	154	6	.43	2	.09	.13	.78	.09	63	14
0	16	2.36	41	98	272	11	1.12	4	.17	.22	1.49	.16	86	20
0	15	.81	17	35	125	12	.58	2	.06	.13	1.01	.07	36	14
0	18	.54	11	40	34	175	.35	3	.04	.09	.28	.04	12	<1
0	14	.67	20	32	259	65	.3	3	.02	.03	.28	.06	68	3
0	16	.79	23	38	305	77	.35	4	.03	.04	.33	.07	80	4
0	13	1.55	14	14	125	232[5]	.18	1	.01	.03	.13	.05	26	3
0	13	.47	17	19	168	301	.3	1	.01	.05	.29	.06	30	3
0	82	1.37	49	29	654	174	.36	367	.08	.21	.36	.09	10	18
0	42	.77	22	58	286	24	.35	136[6]	.06	.1	.56	.14	62	82
0	72	1.33	38	100	491	41	.6	233[6]	.1	.18	.96	.24	107	141
0	83	1.51	43	106	526	47	.68	250[6]	.1	.2	1.03	.26	90	134
0	72	1.31	37	92	456	41	.59	217[6]	.09	.18	.89	.22	78	116
0	46	.55	18	49	162	22	.27	170[6]	.05	.07	.41	.12	27	36
0	94	1.12	37	101	331	44	.55	348[6]	.1	.15	.84	.24	103	74
0	32	.7	20	64	322	23	.5	67	.07	.09	.76	.18	48	63
0	28	.94	16	44	247	16	.26	56	.08	.06	.47	.14	47	48
0	19	.57	19	42	252	18	.28	46	.08	.09	.42	.22	78	35
0	33	.41	10	16	172	13	.13	9	.03	.03	.21	.07	30	22

(1)Data is for green varieties; yellow beans contain 10 RE per cup.

(2)Data is for green varieties; yellow beans contain 15 RE per cup.

(3)Low sodium pack contains 3 mg sodium per cup.

(4)For green varieties; yellow beans contain 14 RE per cup.

(5)Low sodium pack contains 39 mg sodium.

(6)Vitamin A for whole plant: leaves are 1600 RE/100 g raw; flower clusters are 300/100 g raw; stalks are 40 RE/100 g raw.

(For purposes of calculations, use "0" for t, <1, <.1, <.01, etc.)

H

Table H–1
Food Composition

Computer Code Number	Food Description	Measure	Wt (g)	H_2O (%)	Ener (kcal)	Prot (g)	Carb (g)	Dietary Fiber (g)	Fat (g)	Fat Breakdown (g)		
										Sat	Mono	Poly
	VEGETABLES AND LEGUMES—Cont.											
826	Cooked, drained	1 c	150	94	33	2	7	4	1	.1	t	.3
	Cabbage, Chinese:											
1178	Bok choy, raw, shredded	1 c	70	95	9	1	2	1	<1	t	t	.1
827	Bok choy, cooked, drained	1 c	170	96	20	3	3	3	<1	t	t	.1
828	Pe tsai, raw, chopped	1 c	76	94	12	1	2	1	<1	t	t	.1
1796	Pe Tsai, cooked	1 c	119	95	17	2	3	2	0	<.1	<.1	.1
1937	Cabbage, Kim Chee style	1 c	150	92	31	2	6	2	0	<.1	<.1	.2
	Cabbage, red, coarsely chopped:											
829	Raw	1 c	70	92	19	1	4	2	<1	t	t	.1
830	Cooked, drained	½ c	75	94	16	1	3	2	<1	t	t	.1
831	Cabbage, savoy, coarsely chopped, raw	1 c	70	91	19	1	4	2	<1	t	t	t
1785	Cabbage, savoy, cooked	1 c	145	92	35	3	8	4	0	<.1	<.1	.1
1896	Capers	5 g	5	86	0	0	0	0	0	–	–	–
	Carrots, raw:											
832	Whole, 7 ½ x 1 ⅛"	1 ea	72	88	31	1	7	2	<1	t	t	.1
833	Grated	½ c	55	88	24	1	6	2	<1	t	t	t
	Carrots, cooked, sliced, drained:											
834	From fresh	½ c	78	87	35	1	8	2	<1	t	t	.1
835	From frozen	½ c	73	90	26	1	6	3	<1	t	t	t
836	Carrots, canned, sliced, drained	½ c	73	93	17	<1	4	2	<1	t	t	.1
837	Carrot juice, canned	½ c	123	89	49	1	11	2	<1	t	t	.1
	Cauliflower, flowerets:											
838	Raw	½ c	50	92	12	1	3	1	<1	t	t	.1
839	Cooked from fresh, drained	½ c	62	93	14	1	3	1	<1	.1	t	.1
840	Cooked, from frozen, drained	½ c	90	94	17	1	3	2	<1	t	t	.1
	Celery, pascal type, raw:											
841	Large outer stalk, 8 x 1½" (root end)	1 ea	40	95	6	<1	1	1	<1	t	t	t
842	Diced	1 c	120	95	19	1	4	2	<1	t	t	.1
1789	Celery/Celeric root, cooked	3.5 oz	99	93	25	1	6	4	<1	<.1	<.1	.1
1179	Chard, swiss, raw, chopped	1 c	36	93	7	1	1	1	<1	t	t	t
1180	Chard, swiss, cooked	1 c	175	93	35	3	7	4	<1	t	t	.1
1855	Chayote fruit, raw	1 ea	203	93	49	2	11	6	1	–	–	–
1856	Chayote fruit, cooked	1 c	160	93	38	1	8	1	1	–	–	–
	Chickpeas (see Garbanzo Beans #854)											
	Collards, cooked, drained:											
843	From fresh	½ c	64	95	17	1	4	2	<1	t	t	.1
844	From frozen	½ c	85	88	31	3	6	3	<1	.1	t	.1
	Corn, cooked, drained:											
845	From fresh, on cob, 5" long	1 ea	77	70	83	3	19	2	1	.2	.3	.5
846	From frozen, on cob, 3½" long	1 ea	63	73	59	2	14	2	<1	.1	.1	.2
847	Kernels, cooked from frozen	½ c	82	76	66	2	17	2	<1	t	t	t
	Corn, canned:											
848	Cream style	½ c	128	79	92	2	23	2	1	.1	.2	.3
849	Whole kernel, vacuum pack	½ c	105	77	83	3	20	6	1	.1	.2	.3
	Cowpeas (see Black-eyed peas #814–816)											
850	Cucumber slices with peel	7 pce	28	96	4	<1	1	<1	<1	t	t	t
1948	Cucumber, Kim Chee style	1 c	150	91	32	2	7	2	<1	.1	0	.1

(Computer code number is for West Diet Analysis program)

Chol (mg)	Calc (mg)	Iron (mg)	Magn (mg)	Phos (mg)	Pota (mg)	Sodi (mg)	Zinc (mg)	VT-A (RE)	Thia (mg)	Ribo (mg)	Niac (mg)	V-B6 (mg)	Fola (µg)	VT-C (mg)
0	46	.25	12	22	146	12	.13	19	.09	.08	.42	.17	30	30
0	73	.56	13	26	176	45	.13	210	.03	.05	.35	.14	46	31
0	158	1.77	19	49	631	58	.29	437	.05	.11	.73	.28	69	44
0	58	.24	10	22	180	7	.17	91	.03	.04	.3	.18	60	20
0	38	.36	12	46	268	11	.21	115	.05	.05	.6	.21	64	19
0	145	1.28	28	59	375	995	.35	426	.07	.1	.75	.34	88	80
0	36	.34	11	29	144	8	.15	3	.03	.02	.21	.15	14	40
0	28	.26	8	22	105	6	.11	2	.03	.01	.15	.1	9	26
0	24	.28	20	29	161	20	.19	70	.05	.02	.21	.13	56	22
0	44	.55	35	48	267	35	.33	129	.07	.03	.03	.22	67	25
0	2	.05	–	–	–	105	–	1	–	–	–	–	–	0
0	19	.36	11	32	232	25	.14	2024	.07	.04	.67	.11	10	7
0	15	.27	8	24	177	19	.11	1546	.05	.03	.51	.08	8	5
0	24	.48	10	23	177	51	.23	1913	.03	.04	.39	.19	11	2
0	20	.34	7	19	115	43	.17	1291	.02	.03	.32	.09	8	2
0	18	.47	6	17	130	175[1]	.19	1004	.01	.02	.4	.08	7	2
0	29	.57	17	52	359	36	.22	3166	.11	.07	.47	.27	5	10
0	11	.22	7	22	152	15	.14	1	.03	.03	.26	.11	28	23
0	10	.2	6	20	88	9	.11	1	.03	.03	.25	.11	27	27
0	15	.37	8	22	125	16	.12	2	.03	.05	.28	.08	37	28
0	16	.16	4	10	115	35	.05	5	.02	.02	.13	.03	11	3
0	48	.48	13	30	344	104	.16	16	.06	.05	.39	.1	34	8
0	26	.43	12	65	172	61	.2	0	.03	.04	.42	.1	3	4
0	18	.65	29	17	136	77	.13	119	.01	.03	.14	.04	5	11
0	101	3.96	150	58	961	313	.58	550	.06	.15	.63	.15	15	31
0	39	.81	28	53	305	8	.71	11	.06	.08	1.02	.27	56	22
0	21	.35	19	46	277	2	.5	8	.04	.06	.67	.19	29	13
0	15	.1	4	5	83	10	.07	175	.01	.03	.19	.03	4	8
0	179	.95	25	23	213	42	.23	508	.04	.1	.54	.1	64	22
0	2	.47	25	79	193	13	.37	17[2]	.17	.06	1.24	.05	36	5
0	2	.38	18	47	158	3	.4	13[2]	.11	.04	.96	.14	19	3
0	2	.25	15	38	113	4	.29	20[2]	.06	.06	1.05	.08	19	2
0	4	.49	22	65	172	364[3]	.68	12[2]	.03	.07	1.23	.08	57	6
0	5	.44	24	67	195	286[4]	.48	25[2]	.04	.08	1.23	.06	51	9
0	4	.07	3	6	41	1	.06	6	.01	.01	.06	.01	4	2
0	14	7.23	12	20	176	1532	.77	50	.05	.05	.69	.17	35	5

(1) Low sodium pack contains 31 mg sodium.

(2) For yellow varieties; white varieties contain only a trace of vitamin A.

(3) Low sodium pack contains 4 mg sodium per ½ cup.

(4) Low sodium pack contains 6 mg sodium per cup.

(For purposes of calculations, use "0" for t, <1, <.1, <.01, etc.)

H

Table H–1
Food Composition

Computer Code Number	Food Description	Measure	Wt (g)	H_2O (%)	Ener (kcal)	Prot (g)	Carb (g)	Dietary Fiber (g)	Fat (g)	Fat Breakdown (g) Sat	Mono	Poly
	VEGETABLES AND LEGUMES—Cont.											
	Dandelion greens:											
851	Raw	1 c	55	86	25	1	5	2	<1	.1	t	.2
852	Chopped, cooked, drained	1 c	105	90	35	2	7	3	1	.1	.1	.4
853	Eggplant, cooked	1 c	160	92	45	1	11	4	<1	.1	t	.2
1714	Endive, fresh, chopped	¼ c	13	94	2	<1	<1	<1	<1	t	t	t
856	Escarole/curly endive, chopped	1 c	50	94	8	1	2	1	<1	t	t	t
854	Garbanzo beans (chickpeas), cooked	1 c	164	60	269	15	45	8	4	.4	1	1.9
1939	Grape leaves, raw	10 g	10	79	7	0	1	–	0	–	–	–
855	Great northern beans, cooked	1 c	177	69	209	15	37	10	1	.3	t	.3
857	Jerusalem artichoke, raw slices	1 c	150	78	114	3	26	2	<1	0	t	t
1016	Jicama	1 c	120	90	46	1	11	6	0	<.1	0	.1
	Kale, cooked, drained:											
858	From fresh	½ c	65	91	21	1	4	1	<1	t	t	.1
859	From frozen	½ c	65	90	19	2	3	1	<1	t	t	.2
860	Kidney beans, canned	1 c	256	77	217	13	40	16	1	.1	.1	.5
1181	Kohlrabi, raw slices	1 c	140	91	38	2	9	5	<1	t	t	.1
861	Kohlrabi, cooked	1 c	165	90	48	3	11	3	<1	t	t	.1
1183	Leeks, raw, chopped	1 c	104	83	63	2	15	3	<1	t	t	.2
1182	Leeks, cooked, chopped	½ c	52	91	16	<1	4	2	<1	t	t	.1
862	Lentils, cooked from dry	½ c	99	70	115	9	20	5	<1	.1	.1	.2
1288	Lentils, sprouted, stir-fried	4 oz	113	69	115	10	24	4	1	.1	.1	.2
1289	Lentils, sprouted, raw	1 c	77	67	82	7	17	3	<1	t	.1	.2
	Lettuce:											
	Butterhead/Boston types:											
863	Head, 5" diameter	¼ ea	41	96	5	1	1	1	<1	t	t	.1
864	Leaves, inner or outer	4 ea	30	96	4	<1	1	<1	<1	t	t	t
	Iceberg/crisphead:											
865	Head, 6" diameter	¼ ea	135	96	17	1	3	1	<1	t	t	.1
866	Wedge, ¼ head	1 ea	135	96	18	1	3	1	<1	t	t	.1
867	Chopped or shredded	1 c	56	96	7	1	1	1	<1	t	t	.1
868	Looseleaf, chopped	½ c	28	94	5	<1	1	<1	<1	t	t	t
869	Romaine, chopped	½ c	28	95	4	<1	1	<1	<1	t	t	t
870	Romaine, inner leaf	3 ea	30	95	5	<1	1	<1	<1	t	t	t
1930	Luffa, cooked	1 c	178	89	57	3	13	6	0	.1	<.1	.1
	Mushrooms:											
871	Raw, sliced	½ c	35	92	9	1	2	<1	<1	t	t	.1
872	Cooked from fresh, pieces	½ c	78	91	21	2	4	2	<1	t	t	.1
1962	Stir fried, shitake	1 c	145	84	80	2	21	3	<1	.1	.1	<.1
873	Canned, drained	½ c	78	91	19	1	4	2	<1	t	t	.1
1951	Mushroom caps, pickled	8 ea	47	92	11	1	2	1	<1	<.1	0	.1
	Mustard greens:											
874	Cooked from fresh	½ c	70	95	11	2	1	1	<1	t	.1	t
875	Cooked from frozen	½ c	75	94	14	2	2	2	<1	t	.1	t
876	Navy beans, cooked from dry	1 c	182	63	258	16	48	16	1	.3	.1	.4
	Okra, cooked:											
877	From fresh pods	8 ea	85	90	27	2	6	2	<1	t	t	t
878	From frozen slices	½ c	92	91	34	2	8	3	<1	.1	t	.1
1236	Batter fried from fresh	1 c	92	69	175	3	12	2	13	2.1	3.4	7.1
1930	Chinese, (Luffa), cooked	1 c	178	89	57	3	13	6	0	.1	<.1	.1

(Computer code number is for West Diet Analysis program)

PAGE KEY: H–4 = BEV H–6 = DAIRY H–12 = EGGS H–14 = FAT/OIL H–18 = FRUIT H–26 = BAKERY H–36 = GRAIN H–44 = FISH H–48 = MEATS H–50 = POULTRY H–54 = SAUSAGE H–56 = MIXED/FAST H–64 = NUTS/SEEDS H–68 = SWEETS H–70 = VEG/LEG H–84 = MISC H–88 = SOUPS/SAUCES H–90 = FAST H–106 = FRZN ENTREE H–112 = BABY FOODS

Chol (mg)	Calc (mg)	Iron (mg)	Magn (mg)	Phos (mg)	Pota (mg)	Sodi (mg)	Zinc (mg)	VT-A (RE)	Thia (mg)	Ribo (mg)	Niac (mg)	V-B6 (mg)	Fola (µg)	VT-C (mg)
0	102	1.71	20	36	218	42	.23	770	.1	.14	.44	.14	15	19
0	147	1.89	25	44	243	46	.29	1229	.14	.18	.54	.17	13	19
0	10	.56	21	35	397	5	.24	10	.12	.03	.96	.14	23	2
0	7	.10	2	4	41	3	.1	27	.01	.01	.05	<.01	18	1
0	26	.41	8	14	157	11	.39	103	.04	.04	.2	.01	71	3
0	80	4.74	79	276	477	11	2.51	4	.19	.1	.86	.23	282	2
0	72	.69	–	4	26	2	–	86	.02	.01	.12	–	–	3
0	120	3.77	88	292	692	4	1.56	<1	.28	.1	1.21	.21	181	2
0	21	5.1	25	117	644	6	.18	3	.3	.09	1.95	.12	20	6
0	14	.72	14	22	180	5	.19	2	.02	.03	.24	.05	14	24
0	47	.58	12	18	148	15	.16	481	.03	.05	.32	.09	9	27
0	90	.61	12	18	209	10	.12	413	.03	.07	.44	.06	9	16
0	61	3.23	72	240	658	873	1.41	<1	.27	.22	1.17	.06	129	3
0	34	.56	27	64	490	28	.04	5	.07	.03	.56	.21	22	87
0	41	.66	31	74	561	35	.51	6	.07	.03	.64	.25	20	89
0	61	2.18	29	36	187	21	.12	10	.06	.03	.42	.24	67	12
0	16	.57	7	9	45	5	.03	2	.01	.01	.1	.06	13	2
0	19	3.3	36	178	365	2	1.26	1	.17	.07	1.05	.18	178	1
0	16	3.52	40	174	322	11	1.81	5	.25	.1	1.36	.19	76	14
0	19	2.47	28	133	247	8	1.16	3	.18	.1	.87	.15	77	13
0	13	.12	5	9	104	2	.07	40	.02	.02	.12	.02	30	3
0	10	.09	4	7	76	2	.05	29	.02	.02	.09	.01	22	2
0	25	.67	12	27	213	12	.3	45	.06	.04	.25	.05	76	5
0	25	.67	12	27	213	12	.3	45	.06	.04	.25	.05	76	5
0	11	.28	5	11	88	5	.12	18	.03	.02	.1	.02	31	2
0	19	.39	3	7	74	3	.08	53	.01	.02	.11	.01	14	5
0	10	.31	2	13	81	2	.07	73	.03	.03	.14	.01	38	7
0	11	.33	2	14	87	2	.07	78	.03	.03	.15	.01	41	7
0	112	.8	101	99	570	420	.97	103	.23	.1	1.54	.33	81	29
0	2	.43	3	36	129	1	.26	0	.04	.16	1.44	.03	7	1
0	5	1.36	9	68	277	2	.68	0	.06	.23	3.48	.07	14	3
0	4	.64	20	42	170	6	1.94	0	.05	.25	2.18	.23	30	.44
0	9	.62	12	51	101	331	.56	0	.07	.02	1.24	.05	10	0
0	2	.5	5	38	139	95	.28	0	.03	.16	1.42	.03	6	1
0	51	.49	11	29	141	11	.08	212	.03	.04	.3	.07	51	18
0	76	.84	10	18	104	19	.15	335	.03	.04	.19	.08	52	10
0	127	4.51	107	286	670	2	1.93	<1	.37	.11	.97	.3	255	2
0	54	.38	48	48	273	4	.47	49	.11	.05	.74	.16	39	14
0	88	.62	47	42	215	3	.57	47	.09	.11	.72	.04	133	11
15	104	.77	37	106	214	137	.5	43	.13	.1	.75	.13	37	10
0	112	.8	101	99	570	420	.97	103	.23	.1	1.54	.33	81	29

(For purposes of calculations, use "0" for t, <1, <.1, <.01, etc.)

H

Table H–1
Food Composition

Computer Code Number	Food Description	Measure	Wt (g)	H_2O (%)	Ener (kcal)	Prot (g)	Carb (g)	Dietary Fiber (g)	Fat (g)	Fat Breakdown (g) Sat	Mono	Poly
	VEGETABLES AND LEGUMES—Cont.											
	Onions:											
879	Raw, chopped	1 c	160	90	61	2	14	3	<1	t	t	.1
880	Raw, sliced	1 c	115	90	44	1	10	2	<1	t	t	.1
881	Cooked, drained, chopped	½ c	105	88	46	1	11	1	<1	t	t	.1
882	Dehydrated flakes	¼ c	14	4	45	1	12	1	<1	t	t	t
1934	Onions, pearl, cooked	1 c	185	87	81	3	19	3	<1	.1	.1	.1
	Spring/green onions, chopped:											
883	Bulb and top	½ c	50	90	16	1	4	1	<1	t	t	t
1185	Green tops only	1 c	100	92	34	2	6	3	<1	.1	.1	.2
1184	White part only	½ c	50	92	25	1	5	1	<1	t	t	t
884	Onion rings, breaded, heated f/frozen	2 ea	20	28	81	1	8	<1	5	1.7	2.2	1
1917	Palm Hearts, cooked slices	1 c	146	70	150	4	39	2	<1	.1	.1	<.1
	Parsley:											
885	Raw, chopped	½ c	30	88	11	1	2	1	<1	t	.1	t
886	Raw, sprigs	5 ea	5	88	2	<1	<1	<1	<1	t	t	t
887	Freeze dried	¼ c	1	2	3	<1	<1	<1	<1	t	t	t
888	Parsnips, sliced, cooked	½ c	78	78	63	1	15	3	<1	t	.1	t
	Peas:											
	Black-eyed, cooked:											
814	From dry, drained	½ c	85	70	99	7	18	6	<1	.1	t	.2
815	From fresh, drained	½ c	82	76	80	3	17	4	<1	.1	t	.1
816	From frozen, drained	½ c	85	66	112	7	20	7	1	.2	.1	.2
889	Edible pod peas, cooked	1 c	160	89	67	5	11	4	<1	.1	t	.2
890	Green, canned, drained	½ c	85	82	59	4	11	3	<1	.1	t	.1
891	Green, cooked from frozen	½ c	80	80	62	4	11	4	<1	t	t	.1
1786	Snow peas, raw, cup	1 c	145	89	61	4	11	4	0	.1	<.1	.1
1787	Snow peas, raw each	10 ea	29	89	12	1	2	1	0	<.1	<.1	<.1
892	Split, green, cooked from dry	½ c	98	70	116	8	21	3	<1	.1	.1	.2
1187	Peas & carrots, cooked from frozen	½ c	80	86	38	2	8	3	<1	.1	t	.2
1186	Peas & carrots, canned w/liquid	½ c	128	88	49	3	11	4	<1	.1	t	.2
	Peppers, hot:											
893	Hot green chili, canned	½ c	68	93	17	1	4	1	<1	t	t	t
894	Hot green chili, raw	1 ea	45	88	18	1	4	1	<1	t	t	.1
1715	Hot red chili, raw, diced	1 tbs	9	88	4	<1	1	<1	<1	t	t	t
1988	Jalapeno, raw	2 oz	57	90	25	–	–	–	–	–	–	–
895	Jalapeno, chopped, canned	½ c	68	89	16	1	3	2	<1	t	t	.2
1918	Wheels in brine (Ortega)	2 tbs	29	–	10	0	2	–	0	0	0	0
	Peppers, sweet, green:											
896	Whole pod (90 g with refuse), raw	1 ea	74	92	20	1	5	1	<1	t	t	.1
897	Cooked, chopped (1 pod cooked = 73 g)	½ c	68	92	19	1	5	1	<1	t	t	.1
	Peppers, sweet, red:											
1286	Raw, chopped	1 c	100	92	27	1	6	2	<1	t	t	.1
1807	Raw, each	1 ea	74	92	20	1	5	1	<1	<.1	<.1	.1
1287	Cooked, chopped	½ c	68	92	19	1	5	1	<1	t	t	.1
	Peppers, sweet, yellow:											
1872	Raw, large	1 ea	186	92	50	2	12	4	<1	.1	.1	2.1
1873	Strips (pieces)	10 pce	52	92	14	1	3	1	<1	0	<.1	.6
898	Pinto beans, cooked from dry	½ c	85	64	116	7	22	7	<1	t	.1	.2

(Computer code number is for West Diet Analysis program)

PAGE KEY: H–4 = BEV H–6 = DAIRY H–12 = EGGS H–14 = FAT/OIL H–18 = FRUIT H–26 = BAKERY H–36 = GRAIN H–44 = FISH H–48 = MEATS H–50 = POULTRY H–54 = SAUSAGE H–56 = MIXED/FAST H–64 = NUTS/SEEDS H–68 = SWEETS H–70 = VEG/LEG H–84 = MISC H–88 = SOUPS/SAUCES H–90 = FAST H–106 = FRZN ENTREE H–112 = BABY FOODS

Chol (mg)	Calc (mg)	Iron (mg)	Magn (mg)	Phos (mg)	Pota (mg)	Sodi (mg)	Zinc (mg)	VT-A (RE)	Thia (mg)	Ribo (mg)	Niac (mg)	V-B6 (mg)	Fola (μg)	VT-C (mg)
0	32	.35	16	53	251	5	.3	0	.07	.03	.24	.19	30	10
0	23	.25	12	38	181	3	.22	0	.05	.02	.17	.13	22	7
0	23	.25	12	37	174	3	.22	0	.04	.02	.17	.13	16	5
0	36	.22	13	42	227	3	.26	0	.07	.01	.14	.22	23	10
0	41	.44	20	64	305	433	.39	0	.08	.04	.30	.24	28	10
0	36	.74	10	19	138	8	.19	19	.03	.04	.26	.03	32	9
0	56	2.2	21	39	260	7	.22	40	.07	.1	.6	0	80	51
0	20	.44	8	20	115	3	.12	<1	.03	.02	.17	.05	18	13
0	6	.34	4	16	26	75	.08	5	.06	.03	.72	.01	3	<1
0	26	2.47	15	204	2637	20	5.45	10	.07	.25	1.25	1.06	30	10
0	41	1.86	15	17	166	17	.32	156	.03	.03	.39	.03	46	40
0	6	.31	3	3	27	3	.04	26	<.01	<.01	.02	<.01	8	7
0	2	.54	4	5	63	4	.06	63	.01	.03	.15	.02	21	1
0	29	.45	23	53	286	8	.2	0	.06	.04	.56	.07	45	10[1]
0	20	2.15	45	133	238	3	1.1	1	.17	.05	.42	.09	177	<1
0	106	.92	43	42	343	3	.85	65	.08	.12	1.16	.05	104	2
0	20	1.8	43	104	319	4	1.21	6	.22	.05	.62	.08	120	2
0	67	3.15	42	88	384	6	.59	21	.2	.12	.86	.23	47	77
0	17	.81	14	57	147	186[2]	.6	65	.1	.07	.62	.05	38	8
0	19	1.26	23	72	134	70	.75	54	.23	.08	1.18	.09	47	8
0	62	3.02	35	77	290	6	.39	21	.22	.12	.87	.23	60	87
0	12	.6	7	15	58	1	.08	4	.04	.02	.17	.05	12	17
0	14	1.26	35	97	355	2	.98	1	.19	.05	.87	.05	64	<1
0	18	.75	13	39	126	54	.36	621	.18	.05	.92	.07	21	6
0	29	.96	18	59	128	332	.74	739	.09	.07	.74	.11	23	8
0	5	.34	10	12	127	797	.12	41[3]	.01	.03	.54	.1	7	46
0	8	.54	11	21	153	3	.13	35[3]	.04	.04	.43	.13	11	109
0	2	.11	2	4	32	1	.03	101	.01	.01	.09	.03	2	22
—	—	—	—	—	3	3	—	38	—	—	—	—	—	66
0	18	1.9	8	12	92	995	.13	116	.02	.03	.34	.14	9	9
0	—	—	—	—	55	390	—	—	—	—	—	—	—	21
0	7	.34	7	14	131	1	.09	47	.05	.02	.38	.18	16	66
0	6	.31	7	12	113	1	.08	40	.04	.02	.32	.16	11	51
0	9	.46	10	19	177	2	.12	570	.07	.03	.51	.25	22	190
0	7	.34	7	14	131	1	.09	422	.05	.02	.38	.18	16	141
0	6	.31	7	12	112	1	.08	256	.04	.02	.32	.16	11	116
0	20	.86	22	45	394	4	.32	44	.05	.05	1.66	.31	48	342
0	6	.24	6	12	110	1	.09	12	.01	.01	.46	.09	14	96
0	41	2.23	47	137	398	2	.92	<1	.16	.08	.34	.13	147	2

(1)Value for Vitamin C is highest right after harvest and drops after that.

(2)Low sodium pack contains 1.7 mg sodium.

(3)Data is for green chili peppers; red varieties contain 809 RE vitamin A per ½ cup; 484 RE per whole pepper.

(For purposes of calculations, use "0" for t, <1, <.1, <.01, etc.)

Table H–1
Food Composition

Computer Code Number	Food Description	Measure	Wt (g)	H_2O (%)	Ener (kcal)	Prot (g)	Carb (g)	Dietary Fiber (g)	Fat (g)	Fat Breakdown (g) Sat	Mono	Poly
VEGETABLES AND LEGUMES—Cont.												
1191	Poi, two finger	¼ c	60	72	67	<1	16	<1	<1	t	t	t
	Potatoes:[1]											
	Baked in oven, 4¾" x 2⅓" diam:											
899	With skin	1 ea	202	71	220	5	51	5	<1	.1	1	.1
900	Flesh only	1 ea	156	75	145	3	34	2	<1	t	t	.1
901	Skin only	1 ea	58	47	115	2	27	2	<1	t	t	t
	Baked in microwave, 4¾" x 2⅓" diam:											
902	With skin	1 ea	202	72	212	5	49	5	<1	.1	t	.1
903	Flesh only	1 ea	156	74	156	3	36	2	<1	t	t	.1
904	Skin only	1 ea	58	64	77	3	17	2	<1	t	t	t
	Boiled, about 2½" diam:											
905	Peeled after boiling	1 ea	136	77	118	3	27	2	<1	t	t	.1
906	Peeled before boiling	1 ea	135	78	116	2	27	2	<1	t	t	.1
	French fried, strips 2–3½" long:											
907	Oven heated	10 pce	50	35	163	2	19	1	9	3.8	4.2	.9
908	Fried in vegetable oil	10 ea	50	40	155	2	19	2	8	2.5	4	1.2
1188	Fried in veg and animal oil	10 ea	50	38	158	2	20	2	8	3.4	4	.5
909	Hashed browns from frozen	1 c	156	56	340	5	44	3	18	7	8	2.1
	Mashed:											
910	Home recipe with whole milk[2]	½ c	105	79	81	2	18	2	1	.3	.2	.1
911	Home recipe with milk and marg	½ c	105	76	111	2	18	2	4	1.1	1.9	1.3
912	Prepared from flakes; water, milk, margarine, salt added	½ c	110	76	124	2	17	1	6	1.6	2.5	1.7
	Potato products, prepared:											
	Au gratin:											
913	From dry mix	½ c	122	79	114	3	16	2	5	3.2	1.4	.2
914	From home recipe[3]	½ c	122	74	162	6	14	2	9	4.3	3.2	1.3
	Scalloped:											
915	From dry mix	½ c	122	79	114	3	16	1	5	3.2	1.5	.2
916	From home recipe[4]	½ c	122	81	105	4	13	1	5	1.7	1.6	.9
	Potato salad (see Mixed Dishes #715)											
1192	Potato puffs, cooked from frozen	½ c	62	61	107	1	16	1	6	1.1	1.9	0
917	Potato chips	14 ea	28	2	150	2	15	1	10	3.1	2.8	3.5
918	Pumpkin, cooked from fresh, mashed	1 c	245	94	49	2	12	2	<1	.1	t	t
919	Pumpkin, canned	½ c	123	90	42	1	10	3	<1	.2	.1	t
1891	Radicchio, raw, shredded	0.5 c	20	93	5	0	1	–	<1	–	–	–
1894	Radicchio leaf, raw	10 ea	80	93	18	1	4	–	<1	–	–	–
920	Red radishes	10 ea	45	95	8	<1	2	<1	<1	t	t	t
1793	Daikon radishes (Chinese) raw	0.5 c	44	95	8	<1	2	1	<.1	<.1	<.1	<.1
921	Refried beans, canned	½ c	126	72	135	8	23	7	1	.5	.6	.2
1375	Rutabaga, cooked cubes	½ c	85	89	33	1	7	2	<1	t	t	.1
922	Sauerkraut, canned with liquid	½ c	118	93	22	1	5	3	<1	t	t	.1
923	Seaweed, kelp, raw	1 oz	28	82	12	<1	3	<1	<1	.1	t	t
924	Seaweed, spirulina, dried	1 oz	28	5	31	16	7	1	2	.8	.2	.6
1866	Shallots, raw, chopped	1 tbs	10	80	7	0	2	0	<1	0	0	0

(1) Vitamin C varies with length of storage. After 3 months of storage approximately two-thirds of the ascorbic acid remains; after 6 to 7 months, about one-third remains.

(2) Recipe: 84% potatoes, 15% whole milk, 1% salt.

(3) Recipe: 55% potatoes, 30% whole milk, 9% cheddar cheese, 3% butter, 2% flour, 1% salt.

(4) Recipe: 59% potatoes, 36% whole milk, 2% butter, 2% flour, 1% salt.

(Computer code number is for West Diet Analysis program)

H

PAGE KEY: H–4 = BEV H–6 = DAIRY H–12 = EGGS H–14 = FAT/OIL H–18 = FRUIT H–26 = BAKERY H–36 = GRAIN H–44 = FISH H–48 = MEATS H–50 = POULTRY H–54 = SAUSAGE H–56 = MIXED/FAST H–64 = NUTS/SEEDS H–68 = SWEETS H–70 = VEG/LEG H–84 = MISC H–88 = SOUPS/SAUCES H–90 = FAST H–106 = FRZN ENTREE H–112 = BABY FOODS

Chol (mg)	Calc (mg)	Iron (mg)	Magn (mg)	Phos (mg)	Pota (mg)	Sodi (mg)	Zinc (mg)	VT-A (RE)	Thia (mg)	Ribo (mg)	Niac (mg)	V-B6 (mg)	Fola (μg)	VT-C (mg)
0	10	.53	14	23	110	7	.13	1	.08	.02	.66	.16	13	2
0	20	2.75	55	115	844	16	.65	0	.22	.07	3.31	.7	22	26[1]
0	8	.55	39	78	610	8	.45	0	.16	.03	2.18	.47	14	20[1]
0	20	4.08	25	59	332	12	.28	0	.07	.06	1.78	.36	13	8[1]
0	22	2.5	55	212	903	16	.73	0	.24	.06	3.45	.69	24	30[1]
0	8	.64	39	170	641	11	.51	0	.2	.04	2.54	.5	19	24[1]
0	27	3.45	21	48	377	9	.3	0	.04	.04	1.29	.28	10	9[1]
0	7	.42	30	60	515	5	.41	0	.14	.03	1.96	.41	14	18[1]
0	11	.42	27	54	443	7	.36	0	.13	.03	1.77	.36	12	10[1]
0	6	.83	11	48	270	306	.2	0	.04	.02	1.33	.11	11	3
0	8	.68	17	67	356	82	.26	1	07	.02	1.14	.12	17	3
6	10	.38	17	47	366	108	.19	0	.09	.01	1.63	.12	15	5
0	23	2.36	26	112	680	53	.5	0	.17	.03	3.78	.2	10	10
2	27	.28	19	50	314	318	.3	6	.09	.04	1.18	.24	9	7[1]
2[5]	27	.27	19	48	303	310	.28	57	.09	.04	1.13	.23	8	6[1]
4[5]	54	.24	20	62	256	365	.2	59	.12	.05	.73	.01	8	11
6	102	.39	18	116	268	536	.29	38	.02	.1	1.15	.05	8	4
18[6]	146	.78	24	138	483	528	.84	47	.08	.14	1.22	.21	10	12
13	44	.47	17	68	249	416	.31	54	.02	.07	1.26	.05	12	4
7[7]	70	.7	23	77	463	410	.49	38	.08	.11	1.29	.22	11	13
0	19	0	12	30	162	251	.19	1	12	.01	1.05	.14	10	1
0	7	.46	19	46	357	166[8]	.31	0	.05	.06	1.07	.19	13	9
0	37	1.4	22	74	564	2	.56	2651	.08	.19	1.01	.11	21	12
0	32	1.71	28	43	253	6	.21	2712	.03	.07	.45	.07	15	5
0	4	.11	3	8	60	4	.12	1	0	.01	.05	.01	12	2
0	15	.45	10	32	242	18	.50	2	.01	.02	.20	.05	48	6
0	9	.13	4	8	104	11	.13	<1	<.01	.02	.13	.03	12	10
0	12	.18	7	10	100	9	.07	0	.01	.01	.09	.02	12	10
0	58	2.24	49	106	495	534	1.73	<1	.06	.07	.61	.13	105	8
0	41	.45	20	48	277	17	.3	48	.07	.03	.61	.09	13	16
0	35	1.73	15	24	201	780	.22	2	.02	.03	.17	.15	28	17
0	48	.81	34	12	25	66	.35	3	.01	.04	.13	<.01	50	<1
0	34	8.08	55	33	382	293	.57	16	.67	1.04	3.63	.1	26	3
0	4	.12	2	6	33	1	.04	0	.01	0	.02	.03	3	1

(5)Data is for margarine; if butter is used, cholesterol = 25 mg for 29 total mg.

(6)Data is for butter; if margarine is used, cholesterol = 37 mg.

(7)Data is for butter; if margarine is used cholesterol = 15 mg.

(8)If no salt added, sodium = 2 mg.

(For purposes of calculations, use "0" for t, <1, <.1, <.01, etc.)

H

Table H–1
Food Composition

Computer Code Number	Food Description	Measure	Wt (g)	H_2O (%)	Ener (kcal)	Prot (g)	Carb (g)	Dietary Fiber (g)	Fat (g)	Fat Breakdown (g) Sat	Mono	Poly
	VEGETABLES AND LEGUMES—Cont.											
1557	Snow peas, stir-fried	1 c	165	89	69	5	12	4	<1	.1	t	.1
925	Soybeans, cooked from dry	½ c	86	63	149	14	9	5	8	1.1	1.7	4.4
1996	Soybeans, dry roasted	½ c	86	–	387	34	28	7	19	2.7	4.1	10.5
	Soybean products:											
926	Miso	½ c	138	42	284	16	39	7	8	1.2	1.8	4.7
927	Tofu (soybean curd, regular)	½ c	124	85	94	10	2	1	6	.9	1.3	3.3
	Spinach:											
928	Raw, chopped	1 c	56	92	12	2	2	2	<1	t	t	.1
929	Cooked, from fresh, drained	½ c	90	91	21	3	3	2	<1	t	t	.1
930	Cooked from frozen (leaf)	½ c	95	90	27	3	5	2	<1	t	t	.1
931	Canned, drained solids	½ c	107	92	25	3	4	3	1	.1	t	.2
	Spinach soufflé (see Mixed Dishes)											
	Squash, summer varieties, cooked:											
932	Varieties averaged	½ c	90	94	18	1	4	1	<1	.1	t	.1
933	Crookneck	½ c	90	94	18	1	4	1	<1	.1	t	.1
934	Zucchini	½ c	90	95	14	1	4	1	<1	t	t	t
	Squash, winter varieties, cooked:											
	Average of all varieties, baked:											
935	Mashed	1 c	245	89	96	2	21	7	2	.3	.1	.7
936	Cubes	1 c	205	89	80	2	18	6	1	.3	.1	.5
937	Acorn, baked, mashed	½ c	122	83	68	1	18	5	<1	t	t	.1
1218	Acorn, boiled, mashed	½ c	122	90	41	1	11	3	<1	t	t	t
	Butternut:											
938	Baked cubes	1 c	205	88	82	2	22	6	<1	t	t	.1
1219	Baked, mashed	½ c	122	88	49	1	13	3	<1	t	t	t
1193	Cooked from frozen	½ c	120	88	47	1	12	3	<1	t	t	t
1194	Hubbard, baked, mashed	½ c	120	85	60	3	13	3	1	.2	.1	.3
1195	Hubbard, boiled, mashed	½ c	118	91	35	2	8	3	<1	.1	t	.2
1196	Spaghetti, baked or boiled	½ c	77	92	22	1	5	1	<1	t	t	.1
1189	Succotash, cooked from frozen	½ c	85	74	79	4	17	5	1	.1	.1	.4
	Sweet potatoes:											
939	Baked in skin, peeled, 5 x 2" diam	1 ea	114	67	140	3	28	4	<1	t	t	.1
940	Boiled without skin, 5 x 2" diam	1 ea	151	73	159	3	37	3	<1	.1	t	.2
941	Candied, 2½ x 2"	1 pce	105	67	143	1	29	2	3	1.4	.7	.2
	Canned:											
942	Solid pack	½ c	128	74	129	3	30	2	<1	.1	t	.1
943	Vacuum pack, mashed	½ c	127	76	116	2	27	4	<1	.1	t	.1
944	Vacuum pack, 3¾ x 1"	2 pce	80	76	73	1	17	2	<1	t	t	.1
1940	Taro shoots, cooked	1 c	140	95	20	1	4	–	0	<.1	<.1	<.1
	Tomatillos:											
1877	Raw, each	1 ea	34	92	11	0	2	1	<1	–	–	–
1875	Raw, chopped	0.5 c	66	92	21	1	4	1	1	–	–	–
	Tomatoes:											
945	Raw, whole, 2⅗" diam	1 ea	123	94	26	1	6	1	<1	.1	.1	.2
946	Raw, chopped	1 c	180	94	38	2	8	2	1	.1	.1	.2

(Computer code number is for West Diet Analysis program)

Chol (mg)	Calc (mg)	Iron (mg)	Magn (mg)	Phos (mg)	Pota (mg)	Sodi (mg)	Zinc (mg)	VT-A (RE)	Thia (mg)	Ribo (mg)	Niac (mg)	V-B6 (mg)	Fola (μg)	VT-C (mg)
0	71	3.43	40	87	330	7	.45	21	.22	.12	.94	.25	55	84
0	88	4.42	74	211	443	1	.99	1	.13	.24	.34	.2	46	1
0	232	3.41	196	558	1173	2	4.11	2	.37	.65	.91	.19	176	4
0	92	3.76	58	211	226	5033	4.57	12	.13	.34	1.19	.3	46	0
0	130	6.65	126	120	150	9	.99	11	.1	.06	.24	.06	19	<1
0	55	1.52	44	27	312	44	.3	376	.04	.11	.4	.11	109	16
0	122	3.21	78	50	419	63	.68	737	.09	.21	.44	.22	131	9
0	139	1.44	65	46	283	82	.66	739	.06	.16	.4	.14	103	12
0	136	2.46	81	47	370	29[1]	.49	939	.02	.15	.41	.11	105	15
0	24	.32	22	35	173	1	.35	26[2]	.04	.04	.46	.06	18	5
0	24	.32	22	35	173	1	.35	26[2]	.04	.04	.46	.08	18	5
0	12	.31	20	36	228	3	.16	22[2]	.04	.04	.38	.07	15	4
0	34	.81	20	49	1070	2	.64	871	.21	.06	1.72	.18	69	24
0	29	.68	16	41	896	2	.53	729	.17	.05	1.44	.15	57	20
0	54	1.14	52	55	535	5	.21	52	.2	.02	1.08	.24	23	13
0	32	.68	32	33	322	4	.13	31	.12	.01	.65	.14	14	8
0	84	1.23	59	55	582	8	.27	1435	.15	.03	1.99	.25	39	31
0	50	.73	35	33	348	5	.16	854	.09	.02	1.19	.15	23	18
0	23	.69	11	17	160	2	.14	401	.06	.05	.56	.08	20	4
0	20	.56	26	28	430	10	.18	725	.09	.06	.67	.21	19	11
0	12	.33	15	16	253	6	.12	473	.05	.03	.39	.12	11	8
0	16	.26	8	11	91	14	.15	8	.03	.02	.63	.08	6	3
0	13	.75	20	60	225	38	.38	20	.06	.06	1.11	.08	28	5
0	32	2	28	74	396	11	.33	1928	.08	.14	.69	.27	26	25
0	32	.85	15	41	276	20	.41	2575	.08	.21	.97	.37	17	26
8[3]	27	1.19	12	27	198	73	.16	440	.02	.04	.41	.04	12	7
0	38	1.7	31	67	268	96	.27	1937	.03	.11	1.22	.3	14	7
0	28	1.13	28	62	398	67	.23	1013	.05	.07	.94	.24	21	34
0	18	.71	18	39	250	42	.14	638	.03	.05	.59	.15	13	21
0	20	.57	11	36	482	3	.76	7	.05	.07	1.13	.16	4	26
0	2	.21	7	13	91	<1	.07	4	.01	.01	.63	.02	2	4
0	5	.41	13	26	177	1	.15	8	.03	.02	1.22	.04	5	8
0	6	.55	13	29	273	11	.11	76	.07	.06	.77	.1	18	23[4]
0	9	.81	20	43	400	16	.16	112	.11	.09	1.13	.14	27	34[4]

(1)Dietary pack contains 58 mg sodium.

(2)Applies to squash including skin; flesh has no appreciable vitamin A value.

(3)For recipe using butter.

(4)Year-round average. From June through October, ascorbic acid is approximately 32 mg and 47 mg, respectively, for one tomato and 1 c chopped tomato. From November through May, market samples average around 12 and 18 mg, respectively.

(For purposes of calculations, use "0" for t, <1, <.1, <.01, etc.)

Table H-1
Food Composition

Computer Code Number	Food Description	Measure	Wt (g)	H_2O (%)	Ener (kcal)	Prot (g)	Carb (g)	Dietary Fiber (g)	Fat (g)	Fat Breakdown (g) Sat	Mono	Poly
	VEGETABLES AND LEGUMES—Cont.											
	Tomatoes—Cont.:											
947	Cooked from raw	1 c	240	92	65	3	14	2	1	.1	.2	.4
948	Canned, solids and liquid	1 c	240	94	48	2	10	2	1	.1	.1	.2
	Tomatoes, sundried:											
1879	Cup measure	1 c	54	15	139	8	30	7	2	.2	.3	.6
1881	Pieces	10 pce	20	15	52	3	11	2	1	.1	.1	.2
1885	Oil pack, drained	33 ea	100	54	213	5	23	7	14	1.9	8.7	2.1
2020	Tomato, Roma, fresh	1 ea	123	94	26	1	6	1	<1	.1	.1	.2
949	Tomato juice, canned	1 c	244	94	41	2	10	1	<1	t	t	.1
	Tomato products, canned:											
950	Paste	1 c	262	80	220	10	49	11	2	.3	.4	.9
951	Puree	1 c	250	87	102	4	25	6	<1	t	t	.1
952	Sauce	1 c	245	89	73	3	18	3	<1	.1	.1	.2
953	Turnips, cubes, cooked from fresh	½ c	78	94	14	1	4	2	<1	t	t	t
	Turnip greens, cooked:											
954	From fresh, leaves and stems	1 c	144	93	29	2	6	4	<1	.1	t	.1
955	From frozen, chopped	1 c	164	90	49	6	8	7	1	.2	.1	.3
956	Vegetable juice cocktail, canned	½ c	121	93	23	1	6	1	<1	t	t	t
	Vegetables, mixed:											
957	Canned, drained	½ c	81	87	38	2	8	3	<1	t	t	.1
958	Frozen, cooked, drained	½ c	91	83	53	3	12	5	<1	t	t	.1
1888	Water chestnuts, Chinese, raw	½ c	62	74	66	1	15	2	0	<.1	<.1	<.1
959	Water chestnuts, canned, slices	½ c	70	86	35	1	9	2	<1	t	t	t
960	Water chestnuts, canned, whole	4 ea	28	86	14	<1	3	1	<1	t	t	t
1190	Watercress, fresh, chopped	½ c	17	95	2	<1	<1	<1	<1	t	t	t
	MISCELLANEOUS											
	Baking powders for home use:											
	Sodium aluminum sulfate:											
962	With monocalcium phosphate monohydrate	1 tsp	3	2	4	<1	1	0	0	0	0	0
963	With monocalcium phosphate monohydrate, calcium sulfate	1 tsp	3	5	2	0	1	0	0	0	0	0
964	Straight phosphate	1 tsp	4	4	2	<1	1	0	0	0	0	0
965	Low sodium	1 tsp	4	6	4	<1	2	0	<1	0	0	0
1204	Baking soda	1 tsp	3	<1	0	0	0	0	0	0	0	0
966	Basil, dried	1 tbs	4	6	10	1	2	1	<1	–	–	–
2068	Cajun Seasoning	1 tsp	3	.5	6	<1	1	<1	<1	–	–	–
961	Carob flour	1 c	103	4	394	5	92	41	1	.1	.2	.2
967	Catsup:	¼ c	61	67	64	1	17	1	<1	t	t	.1
968	Tablespoon	1 tbs	15	67	16	<1	4	<1	<1	t	t	t
1200	Cayenne/red pepper	1 tbs	5	8	16	1	3	1	1	.2	.1	.4
969	Celery seed	1 tsp	2	6	8	<1	1	<1	1	t	.3	.1
1203	Chili powder:	1 tbs	8	8	25	1	4	3	1	.3	.3	.6
970	Teaspoon	1 tsp	3	8	8	<1	2	1	<1	.1	.1	.2
	Chocolate:											
971	Baking, unsweetened, square	1 oz	28	1	146	3	8	4	15	9.2	5.2	.5

(Computer code number is for West Diet Analysis program)

PAGE KEY: H–4 = BEV H–6 = DAIRY H–12 = EGGS H–14 = FAT/OIL H–18 = FRUIT H–26 = BAKERY H–36 = GRAIN H–44 = FISH H–48 = MEATS H–50 = POULTRY H–54 = SAUSAGE H–56 = MIXED/FAST H–64 = NUTS/SEEDS H–68 = SWEETS H–70 = VEG/LEG H–84 = MISC H–88 = SOUPS/SAUCES H–90 = FAST H–106 = FRZN ENTREE H–112 = BABY FOODS

Chol (mg)	Calc (mg)	Iron (mg)	Magn (mg)	Phos (mg)	Pota (mg)	Sodi (mg)	Zinc (mg)	VT-A (RE)	Thia (mg)	Ribo (mg)	Niac (mg)	V-B6 (mg)	Fola (μg)	VT-C (mg)
0	14	1.34	34	74	670	26	.26	178	.17	.14	1.8	.23	31	55
0	62[1]	1.46	29	46	530	391[2]	.38	144	.11	.07	1.76	.22	19	36
0	59	4.91	105	192	1851	1131	1.08	47	.29	.26	4.89	.18	37	21
0	22	1.82	39	71	685	419	.40	17	.11	.10	1.81	.07	14	8
0	47	2.68	81	139	1565	266	.78	129	.19	.38	3.63	.32	23	102
0	6	.55	14	30	273	11	.11	77	.07	.06	.77	.10	18	23
0	22	1.42	27	46	537	881[3]	.34	137	.11	.08	1.64	.27	49	45
0	92	7.83	133	206	2441	2070[4]	2.1	647	.41	.5	8.44	1	59	110
0	37	2.33	60	100	1050	998[5]	.55	340	.18	.13	4.3	.38	27	88
0	34	1.89	47	78	909	1482[6]	.61	240	.16	.14	2.82	.38	23	32
0	17	.17	6	15	105	39	.16	0	.02	.02	.23	.05	7	9
0	197	1.15	32	42	292	42	.2	792	.06	.1	.59	.26	170	39
0	248	3.18	43	56	366	25	.67	1308	.09	.12	.77	.11	65	36
0	13	.51	13	21	234	442	.24	142	.05	.03	.88	.17	25	33
0	22	.86	13	34	237	121	.33	944	.04	.04	.47	.06	19	4
0	23	.74	20	46	154	32	.45	389	.06	.11	.77	.07	17	3
0	7	.04	14	39	362	9	.31	0	.09	.12	.62	.20	10	2
0	3	.61	3	13	83	6	.27	<1	.01	.02	.25	.11	4	1
0	1	.25	1	5	33	2	.11	<1	<.01	.01	.1	.04	2	<1
0	20	.03	4	10	56	7	.02	80	.01	.02	.03	.02	2	7
0	58	0	<1	87	4	328	0	0	0	0	0	0	0	0
0	176	.32	1	63	1	318	<.01	0	0	0	0	0	0	0
0	295	.43	1	377	<1	316	<.01	0	0	0	0	0	0	0
0	173	.35	1	295	434	4	.03	0	0	0	0	0	0	0
0	0	0	0	0	0	821	0	0	0	0	0	0	0	0
0	85	1.68	19	22	154	2	.26	38	.01	.01	.31	–	–	2
–	–	–	–	–	30	474	–	–	–	–	–	–	–	–
0	358	3.04	56	81	852	36	.95	1	.05	.47	1.96	.38	30	<1
0	12	.43	13	24	295	723	.14	62	.05	.04	.84	.11	9	9
0	3	.1	3	6	72	178	.03	15	.01	.01	.21	.03	2	2
0	8	.41	8	15	106	2	.13	209	.02	.05	.44	–	–	4
0	35	.9	9	11	28	3	.14	<1	.01	.01	.1	–	–	<1
0	22	1.12	14	24	149	81	.21	279	.03	.06	.61	–	4	5
0	7	.43	5	8	50	30	.07	105	.01	.02	.2	–	2	2
0	21	1.79	88	117	233	4	1.14	3	.02	.05	.31	.03	2	0

(1) Calcium is added as a firming agent.

(2) Dietary pack contains 31 mg sodium.

(3) If no salt is added, sodium content is 24 mg.

(4) If salt is added, sodium content is 2070 mg.

(5) If salt is added, sodium content is 998 mg.

(6) With salt added.

(For purposes of calculations, use "0" for t, <1, <.1, <.01, etc.)

H

Table H–1
Food Composition

Computer Code Number	Food Description	Measure	Wt (g)	H_2O (%)	Ener (kcal)	Prot (g)	Carb (g)	Dietary Fiber (g)	Fat (g)	Fat Breakdown (g) Sat	Mono	Poly
	MISCELLANEOUS—Cont.											
	For other chocolate items, see Sweeteners & Sweets											
972	Cilantro/coriander, fresh	1 tbs	1	93	<1	<1	<1	<1	<1	t	t	t
1197	Cornstarch	1 tbs	8	8	30	<1	7	<1	<1	t	t	t
973	Cinnamon	1 tsp	2	10	5	<1	2	1	<1	t	t	t
974	Curry powder	1 tsp	2	10	7	<1	1	1	<1	t	.2	t
1202	Dill weed, dried	1 tbs	3	7	8	1	2	1	<1	–	–	–
1705	Dip, french onion	1 tbs	14	70	31	<1	<1	<1	3	1.9	.9	.1
975	Garlic cloves	1 ea	3	59	4	<1	1	<1	<1	t	0	t
976	Garlic powder	1 tsp	3	6	10	1	2	<1	<1	t	t	t
977	Gelatin, dry, unsweetened: Envelope	1 ea	7	13	23	6	0	0	<1	t	t	t
978	Ginger root, slices, raw	2 pce	4	81	3	<1	1	<1	<1	t	t	t
1198	Horseradish, prepared	1 tbs	15	87	6	<1	1	<1	<1	t	t	t
1199	Hummous/hummus	1 c	246	65	421	12	50	10	21	3	9	8
1909	Mustard, country dijon	1 tsp	5	–	5	0	0	0	0	0	0	0
979	Mustard, prepared (1 packet = 1 tsp)	1 tsp	5	80	4	<1	<1	<1	<1	t	.2	t
	Miso (see #926 under Vegetables and Legumes, Soybean products)											
2067	No msg seasoning blend	1 tsp	5	.5	3	<1	1	<1	<1	–	–	–
980	Olives, green	5 ea	19	78	22	<1	<1	<1	2	.3	1.9	.2
981	Olives, ripe, pitted	5 ea	22	80	25	<1	1	1	2	.3	1.8	.2
982	Onion powder	1 tsp	2	5	7	<1	2	<1	<1	t	t	t
983	Oregano, ground	1 tsp	1	7	3	<1	1	<1	<1	t	t	.1
2066	Oriental seasoning blend	1 tsp	3	.5	10	<1	2	<1	<1	–	–	–
984	Paprika	1 tsp	2	10	6	<1	1	<1	<1	t	t	.2
985	Black pepper	1 tsp	2	11	5	<1	1	1	<1	t	t	t
	Pickles:											
986	Dill, medium, 3¾ x 1¼" diam	1 ea	65	92	12	<1	3	1	<1	t	t	.1
987	Fresh pack, slices, 1½" diam x ¼"	2 pce	15	92	3	<1	3	<1	<1	t	t	t
988	Sweet, medium	1 ea	35	65	41	<1	11	<1	<1	t	t	t
989	Pickle relish, sweet	2 tbs	30	63	41	<1	10	1	<1	.1	t	.1
	Popcorn (see Grain Products #539–541)											
1201	Sage, ground	1 tsp	1	8	3	<1	1	<1	<1	.1	t	t
1347	Salsa, from recipe	1 tbs	14	93	3	<1	1	<1	<1	t	t	t
2118	Salsa, pico de Gallo-med	2 tbs	30	92	5	0	2	.5	0	0	0	0
990	Salt	1 tsp	5	<1	0	0	0	0	0	0	0	0
	Salt substitutes:											
1205	Morton, salt substitute	1 tsp	2	2	<1	0	<1	0	0	0	0	0
1207	Morton, Light Salt	1 tsp	6	0	0	0	0	0	0	0	0	0
1206	Norcliff Thayer, No Salt, packet	1 ea	1	0	0	0	0	0	0	0	0	0
	Sports/Fitness bar:											
2043	Forza energy bar	1 ea	70	18	231	11	45	4	1	–	–	–
2042	Power bar	1 ea	65	21	225	10	40	3	1	–	–	–
2041	Tiger sports bar	1 ea	65	17	230	11	40	4	2	–	–	–
991	Vinegar, cider	½ c	120	94	17	0	7	0	0	0	0	0
	Vinegar, Fleischmann's											
2172	Balsamic	1 tbs	15	64	21	0	5	0	0	0	0	0
2176	Malt	1 tbs	15	90	5	0	<1	0	0	0	0	0
2182	Tarragon	1 tbs	15	95	3	0	<1	0	0	0	0	0
2181	White wine	1 tbs	15	89	5	0	<1	0	0	0	0	0

(Computer code number is for West Diet Analysis program)

H

PAGE KEY: H–4 = BEV H–6 = DAIRY H–12 = EGGS H–14 = FAT/OIL H–18 = FRUIT H–26 = BAKERY H–36 = GRAIN H–44 = FISH H–48 = MEATS H–50 = POULTRY H–54 = SAUSAGE H–56 = MIXED/FAST H–64 = NUTS/SEEDS H–68 = SWEETS H–70 = VEG/LEG H–84 = MISC H–88 = SOUPS/SAUCES H–90 = FAST H–106 = FRZN ENTREE H–112 = BABY FOODS

Chol (mg)	Calc (mg)	Iron (mg)	Magn (mg)	Phos (mg)	Pota (mg)	Sodi (mg)	Zinc (mg)	VT-A (RE)	Thia (mg)	Ribo (mg)	Niac (mg)	V-B6 (mg)	Fola (μg)	VT-C (mg)
0	1	.02	<1	<1	5	<1	<.01	3	<.01	<.01	.01	<.01	<1	<1
0	<1	.04	<1	1	<1	1	<.01	0	0	0	0	0	0	0
0	25	.76	1	1	10	1	.04	1	<.01	<.01	.03	.02	–	1
0	10	.59	5	7	31	1	.08	2	<.01	.01	.07	–	–	<1
0	54	1.46	14	17	99	6	.1	0	.01	.01	.09	.04	–	–
6	17	.01	2	13	22	27	.04	28	.01	.02	.02	<.01	2	<1
0	5	.05	1	5	12	1	.03	0	.01	<.01	.02	.04	<1	1
0	2	.08	2	13	33	1	.07	0	.01	<.01	.02	.61	2	<1
0	4	.08	2	3	1	14	.01	0	<.01	.02	.01	<.01	2	0
0	1	.02	2	1	17	1	.01	0	<.01	<.01	.03	.01	<1	<1
0	9	.13	4	5	44	14	.18	0	0	0	0	.01	2	0
0	123	4	71	276	428	600	2.7	6	.23	.13	1	.98	146	19
0	–	–		–	10	120	–	–	–	–	–	–	–	–
0	4	.1	2	4	6	63	.03	0	0	0	0	<.01	0	0
–	–	–	–	–	13	1390	–	–	–	–	–	–	–	–
0	12	.31	4	3	10	456	.01	6	0	0	0	<.01	<1	0
0	19	.74	1	1	2	192	.05	9	<.01	0	.01	<.01	0	<1
0	8	.06	2	7	19	1	.05	0	.01	<.01	.01	.03	3	<1
0	16	.44	3	2	17	<1	.04	7	<.01	<.01	.06	–	–	1
–	–	–	–	–	12	107	–	–	–	–	–	–	–	–
0	4	.5	4	7	47	1	.08	121	.01	.04	.32			1
0	9	.58	4	3	25	1	.03	<1	<.01	<.01	.02	0	–	0
0	6	.34	7	14	75	833	.09	21	.01	.02	.04	.01	1	1
0	5	.08	2	3	17	192	.02	5	<.01	<.01	.01	<.01	<1	<1
0	1	.21	1	4	11	328	.03	4	<.01	.01	.06	.01	<1	<1
0	6	.24	1	4	60	214	.02	3	0	.01	0	<.01	0	2
0	17	.28	4	1	11	<1	.05	6	.01	<.01	.06	–	–	<1
0	1	.06	1	3	23	55	.02	21	.01	<.01	.06	.01	2	5
0	–	–	–	–	–	260	–	–	–	–	–	–	–	–
0	1	.01	<1	0	<1	1938	0	0	0	0	0	0	0	0
0	11	–	<1	10	1006	<1	–	0	–	–	–	–	–	–
0	3	0	4	0	1500	1099	0	0	0	0	0	0	0	0
0	–	–	–	–	385	0	–	0	0	0	0	0	0	0
0	300	6.3	160	350	220	65	5.25	–	1.5	1.7	20	2	400	60
–	300	5.4	140	350	120	20	5.25	–	1.5	1.7	20	2	400	60
–	350	4.5	140	400	280	100	–	50	1.5	1.7	20	2	400	60
0	7	.7	26	11	120	1	0	0	0	0	0	0	0	0
–	2	.07	–	3	11	3	–	–	.07	.07	.07	–	–	<1
–	2	.07	–	2	14	5	–	–	.07	.07	.07	–	–	2
–	<1	.07	–	<1	2	1	–	–	.07	.07	.07	–	–	<1
–	1	.07	–	15	12	1	–	–	.07	.07	.07	–	–	<1

(For purposes of calculations, use "0" for t, <1, <.1, <.01, etc.)

H

Table H-1
Food Composition

Computer Code Number	Food Description	Measure	Wt (g)	H_2O (%)	Ener (kcal)	Prot (g)	Carb (g)	Dietary Fiber (g)	Fat (g)	Fat Breakdown (g) Sat	Mono	Poly
	MISCELLANEOUS—Cont.											
	Yeast:											
992	Baker's, dry, active, package	1 ea	7	8	21	3	3	2	<1	t	.2	t
993	Brewer's, dry	1 tbs	8	5	23	3	3	3	<1	t	t	0
	SOUPS, SAUCES, AND GRAVIES											
	SOUPS, canned, condensed:											
	Unprepared, condensed:											
1210	Cream of celery	1 c	251	85	181	3	18	2	11	2.8	2.6	5
1215	Cream of chicken	1 c	251	82	233	7	19	1	15	4.2	6.5	3
1216	Cream of mushroom	1 c	251	81	259	4	19	1	19	5.1	3.6	8.9
1220	Onion	1 c	246	86	113	8	16	2	4	.5	1.5	1.3
	Prepared w/equal volume whole milk:											
994	Clam chowder, New England	1 c	248	85	164	9	17	1	7	2.9	2.3	1.1
1209	Cream of celery	1 c	248	87	164	6	15	1	10	3.9	2.5	2.6
995	Cream of chicken	1 c	248	85	191	7	15	<1	11	4.6	4.5	1.6
996	Cream of mushroom	1 c	248	85	203	6	15	1	14	5.1	3	4.6
1214	Cream of potato	1 c	248	87	149	6	17	1	6	3.8	1.7	.6
1213	Oyster stew	1 c	245	89	135	6	10	0	8	5	2.1	.3
997	Tomato	1 c	248	85	161	6	22	1	6	2.9	1.6	1.1
	Prepared with equal volume of water:											
998	Bean with bacon	1 c	253	84	172	8	23	9	6	1.5	2.2	1.8
999	Beef broth/bouillon/consommé	1 c	240	98	17	3	<1	0	1	.3	.2	t
1000	Beef noodle	1 c	244	92	83	5	9	1	3	1.1	1.2	.5
1001	Chicken noodle	1 c	241	92	75	4	9	1	2	.7	1.1	.6
1002	Chicken rice	1 c	241	94	60	4	7	1	2	.5	.9	.4
1208	Chili beef	1 c	250	85	170	7	21	9	7	3.3	2.8	.3
1003	Clam chowder, Manhatten	1 c	244	92	78	2	12	1	2	.4	.4	1.3
1004	Cream of chicken	1 c	244	91	117	3	9	<1	7	2.1	3.3	1.5
1005	Cream of mushroom	1 c	244	90	129	2	9	<1	9	2.4	1.7	4.2
1006	Minestrone	1 c	241	91	82	4	11	1	3	.6	.7	1.1
1211	Onion	1 c	241	93	58	4	8	1	2	.3	.8	.7
1007	Split pea & ham	1 c	253	82	190	10	28	5	4	1.8	1.8	.6
1008	Tomato	1 c	244	90	85	2	17	<1	2	.4	.4	1
1009	Vegetable beef	1 c	244	92	78	6	10	<1	2	.9	.8	.1
1010	Vegetarian vegetable	1 c	241	92	72	2	12	<1	2	.3	.8	.7
1707	Ready to serve											
	Chunky chicken soup	½ c	126	84	89	6	9	<1	3	1	1.5	.7
	SOUPS, dehydrated:											
	Unprepared, dry products:											
1011	Beef bouillon, packet	1 ea	6	3	14	1	1	<1	1	.3	.2	t
1012	Onion soup, packet	1 ea	34	4	100	4	18	4	2	.5	1.2	.2
	Prepared with water:											
1299	Beef broth/bouillon	1 c	244	97	20	1	2	0	1	.3	.3	t
1376	Chicken broth	1 c	244	97	22	1	1	0	1	.3	.4	.4
1013	Chicken noodle	1 c	251	94	53	3	8	<1	1	.3	.5	.4
1122	Cream of chicken	1 c	261	91	107	2	13	1	5	3.4	1.2	.4
1014	Onion	1 c	246	96	27	1	5	<1	1	.1	.3	.1
1217	Split pea	1 c	255	87	125	7	21	3	1	.4	.7	.3
1015	Tomato vegetable	1 c	252	93	55	2	10	1	1	.4	.3	.1

(Computer code number is for West Diet Analysis program)

Chol (mg)	Calc (mg)	Iron (mg)	Magn (mg)	Phos (mg)	Pota (mg)	Sodi (mg)	Zinc (mg)	VT-A (RE)	Thia (mg)	Ribo (mg)	Niac (mg)	V-B6 (mg)	Fola (μg)	VT-C (mg)
0	4	1.16	7	90	140	4	.45	<1	.16	.38	2.79	.11	164	<1
0	17[1]	1.38	18	140	151	10	.63	0	1.25	.34	3.03	.4	313	0
28	80	1.26	13	75	245	1900	.3	60	.06	.1	.66	.02	5	1
20	68	1.2	5	75	175	1972	1.26	113	.06	.12	1.64	.03	3	<1
3	65	1.05	10	85	168	2033	1.19	0	.06	.17	1.62	.02	8	2
0	54	1.35	5	22	137	2115	1.23	0	.07	.05	1.21	.1	30	2
22	186	1.49	22	156	300	992	.8	40	.07	.24	1.03	.13	10	3
32	186	.69	22	151	310	1009	.2	67	.07	.25	.44	.06	8	1
27	181	.67	17	151	273	1047	.67	94	.07	.26	.92	.07	8	1
20	179	.59	20	156	270	1076	.64	37	.08	.28	.91	.06	10	2
22	166	.55	17	161	322	1061	.67	67	.08	.24	.64	.09	9	1
32	166	1.05	20	162	235	1041	10.3	44	.07	.23	.34	.06	10	4
17	159	1.81	22	149	449	932	.29	109	.13	.25	1.52	.16	21	68
3	81	2.05	46	132	402	951	1.03	89	.09	.03	.57	.04	32	2
0	14	.41	5	31	130	782	0	0	<.01	.05	1.87	.02	5	0
5	15	1.1	5	46	100	952	1.54	63	.07	.06	1.07	.04	4	<1
7	17	.77	5	36	55	1106	.39	71	.05	.06	1.39	.03	2	<1
7	17	.75	0	22	101	815	.26	66	.02	.02	1.13	.02	1	<1
13	43	2.13	30	148	525	1035	1.4	151	.06	.07	1.07	.16	18	4
2	27	1.63	12	41	187	578	.98	96	.03	.04	.82	.1	10	4
10	34	.61	2	37	88	986	.63	56	.03	.06	.82	.02	2	<1
2	46	.51	5	49	100	1032	.59	0	.05	.09	.72	.01	5	1
2	34	.92	7	55	313	911	.73	234	.05	.04	.94	.1	16	1
0	27	.67	2	12	67	1053	.61	0	.03	.02	.6	.05	15	1
8	23	2.28	48	213	400	1006	1.32	45	.15	.08	1.47	.07	3	2
0	12	1.76	7	34	264	871	.24	69	.09	.05	1.42	.11	15	66
5	17	1.12	5	41	173	956	1.54	189	.04	.05	1.03	.08	10	2
0	22	1.08	7	34	210	822	.46	301	.05	.05	.92	.05	11	1
15	13	.87	4	57	88	446	.5	65	.04	.09	2.21	.03	2	1
1	4	.06	3	19	27	1019	0	<1	<.01	.01	.27	.01	2	0
2	48	.51	22	110	226	3044	.2	1	.1	.21	1.73	.03	6	1
0	10	.02	7	24	37	1362	.07	1	<.01	.02	.36	0	0	0
0	15	.07	5	12	24	1484	.01	12	.01	.03	.19	0	2	0
3	32	.5	7	32	31	1278	.2	6	.07	.06	.88	.01	2	<1
3	76	.26	5	97	214	1185	1.57	123	.1	.2	2.61	.05	5	1
0	12	.15	5	29	64	849	.06	<1	.03	.06	.48	0	1	<1
3	20	.94	43	124	224	1148	.56	5	.21	.14	1.26	.05	40	0
0	8	.63	20	31	104	1142	.17	19	.06	.04	.79	.05	10	7

(For purposes of calculations, use "0" for t, <1, <.1, <.01, etc.)

H

Table H–1
Food Composition

Computer Code Number	Food Description	Measure	Wt (g)	H_2O (%)	Ener (kcal)	Prot (g)	Carb (g)	Dietary Fiber (g)	Fat (g)	Fat Breakdown (g) Sat	Mono	Poly
	SAUCES											
	From dry mixes, prepared with milk:											
1016	Cheese sauce	1 c	279	77	307	16	23	1	17	9.3	5.3	1.6
1017	Hollandaise	1 c	259	84	240	5	14	<1	20	11.6	5.9	.9
1018	White sauce	1 c	264	82	240	10	21	<1	13	6.4	4.7	1.7
	From home recipe:											
1019	White sauce, medium[1]	1 c	250	77	355	9	20	<1	27	7.8	9.1	8.8
1206	Lofat cheese sauce	¼ c	61	73	85	6	4	0	5	2.1	1.9	.9
	Ready to serve:											
2202	Alfredo sauce	¼ c	69	–	170	5	16	0	10	6	–	–
1020	Barbeque sauce	1 tbs	16	81	10	<1	1	<1	<1	t	.1	.1
1706	Chili sauce, tomato base	1 tbs	17	68	18	<1	4	<1	<1	t	t	t
2126	Creole sauce	¼ c	62	–	25	1	4	1	1	0	–	–
2124	Hoison sauce	2 tbs	34	48	70	1	14	0	2	0	–	–
2199	Pesto sauce	2 tbs	29	21	155	5	2	<1	14	3.6	9.1	1.1
1021	Soy sauce	1 tbs	18	71	10	<1	2	0	<1	t	t	t
2123	Szechuan sauce	2 tbs	31	82	23	1	4	<1	1	.1	.2	.2
1380	Teriyaki sauce	1 tbs	18	68	15	<1	3	0	0	0	0	0
	Spaghetti sauce, canned:											
1377	Plain	1 c	249	75	271	5	40	8	12	1.7	6.1	3.3
1378	With meat	1 c	257	74	309	9	39	8	15	2.8	7.2	3.3
1379	With mushrooms	½ c	123	75	108	2	13	1	3	.4	1.5	.8
	GRAVIES											
	Canned:											
1022	Beef	1 c	233	88	123	9	11	1	6	2.7	2	.2
1023	Chicken	1 c	238	85	188	5	13	<1	14	3.4	6.1	3.5
1024	Mushroom	1 c	238	89	119	3	13	<1	6	1	2.8	2.4
1025	From dry mix, brown	1 c	258	92	75	2	13	<1	2	.8	.7	.1
1026	From dry mix, chicken	1 c	260	91	83	3	14	<1	2	.5	.9	.4
	FAST FOOD RESTAURANTS											
	ARBY'S											
1402	Bac'n cheddar deluxe	1 ea	226	59	501	21	38	<1	31	8.5	12.4	11.2
	Roast beef sandwiches:											
1403	Regular	1 ea	147	47	363	21	34	1	17	6.6	7.6	2.4
1404	Junior	1 ea	86	48	275	11	22	<1	10	3.9	5	1.7
1405	Super	1 ea	234	58	509	22	50	1	26	7	11	5.4
1407	Beef 'n cheddar	1 ea	197	34	516	25	44	1	27	7.6	12.1	7.1
1408	Chicken breast sandwich	1 ea	184	52	401	20	47	1	20	3	8.8	10.3
1412	Ham'n cheese sandwich	1 ea	156	54	328	23	32	<1	13	4.7	5.4	2.7
1726	Italian sub sandwich	1 ea	297	–	671	34	47	–	39	12.8	15.7	8.5
1413	Turkey sandwich, deluxe	1 ea	197	61	263	20	33	<1	6	1.6	2.3	7.8
1680	Turkey sub sandwich	1 ea	277	62	486	33	47	–	19	5.3	6	7
	Milk shakes:											
1419	Chocolate	1 ea	340	74	451	10	77	<1	12	2.8	7	1.7
1420	Jamocha	1 ea	326	75	368	9	59	0	11	2.5	6.4	1.6
1421	Vanilla	1 ea	312	75	330	11	46	0	12	3.9	5.3	2.3
1728	Salad, roast chicken	1 ea	400	89	204	24	12	–	7	3.3	.9	.9
1729	Sports drink, Upper Ten, svg	1 ea	358	88	169	0	42	–	0	0	0	0

Source: Arby's Inc. for the basic nutrients. Values for some nutrients from known values of major ingredients.

[1]Made with enriched flour, margarine, and whole milk.

(Computer code number is for West Diet Analysis program)

Chol (mg)	Calc (mg)	Iron (mg)	Magn (mg)	Phos (mg)	Pota (mg)	Sodi (mg)	Zinc (mg)	VT-A (RE)	Thia (mg)	Ribo (mg)	Niac (mg)	V-B6 (mg)	Fola (μg)	VT-C (mg)
53	569	.28	47	438	552	1565	.97	117	.15	.56	.32	.14	13	2
52	124	.9	8	127	124	1564	.7	220	.04	.18	.06	.5	22	<1
34	425	.26	264	256	444	797	.55	92	.08	.45	.53	.07	16	3
29	261	.73	32	217	344	369	.94	310	.19	.42	.98	.1	14	2
11	165	.25	10	181	99	387	.73	58	.03	.14	.16	.03	4	0
30	150	0	–	100	80	600	–	80	0	.1	0	–	–	0
0	3	.12	1	3	27	128	.03	14	<.01	<.01	.06	.01	1	1
0	3	.14	2	9	63	227	.05	24	.02	.01	.27	.02	1	3
0	20	0	–	–	–	340	–	40	–	–	–	–	–	0
0	0	0	–	–	–	500	–	0	–	–	–	–	–	0
9	209	1.22	17	104	103	211	.52	43	.01	.05	.22	.04	8	3
0	3	.36	6	20	32	1029	.07	0	.01	.02	.6	.03	3	3
0	6	.28	6	6	54	255	.06	27	.01	.01	.28	.02	1	2
0	4	.31	11	28	41	690	.02	0	.01	.01	.23	.02	4	0
0	70	1.62	60	90	956	1235	.52	306	.14	.15	3.76	.88	54	28
16	69	2	61	117	978	1213	1.41	299	.14	.17	4.64	.9	54	27
0	15	1	15	30	333	494	.34	242	.08	.08	.93	.16	13	9
7	14	1.63	5	70	188	1304	2.33	0	.07	.08	1.54	.02	5	0
5	48	1.12	5	69	259	1373	1.9	264	.04	.1	1.05	.02	5	0
0	17	1.57	5	36	252	1356	1.67	0	.08	.15	1.6	.05	29	0
3	67	.23	10	44	57	1075	.31	0	.04	.08	.81	0	0	0
3	39	.26	10	47	62	1133	.32	0	.05	.15	.78	.03	3	3
37	108	4.5	–	–	422	1672	3	39	.34	.45	9.4	–	–	11
41	57	4.6	15	114	400	888	3.56	1	.28	.46	10.4	.2	13	1
21	39	2.6	8	58	194	502	1.5	–	.17	.25	6.4	.1	7	–
40	83	6	23	175	491	1082	3.45	28	.36	.5	11.4	.3	19	8
53	152	6.2	24	260	326	1184	3.05	–	.43	.64	10	–	19	1
41	54	2.6	27	162	298	919	.14	–	.2	.51	8	.34	16	5
51	157	2.7	29	374	353	1292	.83	37	.77	.34	7	.31	24	22
69	410	4.32	–	–	565	2062	–	100	.92	.49	8.2	–	–	11
33	131	2.7	30	253	357	1275	1.5	40	.08	.43	15.6	.52	20	12
51	400	4.68	–	–	500	2033	–	–	13.2	.54	18.8	–	–	–
36	250	2.7	48	350	410	341	1.5	40	.06	.85	.8	.14	14	5
35	250	2.7	36	350	525	262	1.5	60	.06	.77	5	.14	14	2
32	300	2.7	36	350	686	281	1.5	100	.23	.85	4	.14	37	2
43	170	1.98	–	–	877	508	–	485	.33	.54	5.6	–	–	51
0	–	–	–	–	0	40	–	–	–	–	–	–	–	–

(For purposes of calculations, use "0" for t, <1, <.1, <.01, etc.)

H

Table H–1
Food Composition

Computer Code Number	Food Description	Measure	Wt (g)	H_2O (%)	Ener (kcal)	Prot (g)	Carb (g)	Dietary Fiber (g)	Fat (g)	Fat Breakdown (g) Sat	Mono	Poly
	BURGER KING											
	Croissant sandwiches:											
1422	Egg, bacon, & cheese	1 ea	119	50	353	15	18	<1	24	8.1	12.1	3
1423	Egg, sausage, & cheese	1 ea	163	47	543	21	22	1	42	14	20.5	5.1
1424	Egg, ham, & cheese	1 ea	145	57	352	18	19	<1	22	7	11.1	2
	Whopper sandwiches:											
1425	Whopper	1 ea	265	58	618	27	44	3	38	10.8	10.8	12.8
1426	Whopper with cheese	1 ea	289	57	708	32	44	3	45	15.7	12.8	12.8
1427	Double beef	1 ea	351	57	860	46	45	3	56	19	19	13
1428	Double beef & cheese	1 ea	374	57	947	52	45	3	63	23.9	21.9	14
1429	Hamburger deluxe	1 ea	136	53	339	15	28	<1	19	5.9	5.9	6.9
1430	Cheeseburger deluxe	1 ea	158	52	408	19	30	<1	24	8.4	7.3	7.3
1431	Hamburger	1 ea	109	47	275	15	30	1	11	4	5	1
1432	Cheeseburger	1 ea	120	49	313	18	29	1	15	6.3	6.3	1
1433	Double cheeseburger with bacon	1 ea	159	49	460	32	20	1	28	13	12.9	2
1434	Chicken sandwich	1 ea	230	45	703	26	54	2	43	8	11	20.1
1629	BK broiler chicken sandwich	1 ea	248	59	540	30	41	2	29	6	–	–
1739	Chicken caesar pita sandwich	1 ea	237	59	520	27	44	4	26	6	–	–
1435	Chicken tenders	1 ea	95	50	270	17	15	2	13	3.2	5.3	3.2
1436	Ham & cheese sandwich	1 ea	230	59	471	24	44	<1	23	10	8	4
1437	Ocean catch fish fillet	1 ea	189	47	534	19	44	1	36	6	5.8	12.7
1740	Monterey roast beef sandwhich	1 ea	238	57	540	30	40	3	30	9	–	–
1439	French fries (salted)	1 ea	74	38	255	3	27	2	13	3	6	1
1630	French toast sticks-svg	1 ea	141	33	500	4	60	1	27	–	–	–
1440	Onion rings	1 ea	79	51	198	3	26	3	9	1.3	5.1	2.6
1441	Milk shakes, chocolate	1 ea	273	75	298	9	52	3	7	3.9	3.9	0
1442	Milk shakes, vanilla	1 ea	273	75	298	9	51	1	7	3.9	2.9	0
1443	Fried apple pie	1 ea	125	47	343	3	43	2	17	3.3	8.9	1
	Source: Burger King Corporation.											
	DAIRY QUEEN											
	Ice cream cones:											
1446	Small vanilla	1 ea	85	64	140	4	22	0	4	3	1	–
1447	Regular vanilla	1 ea	142	65	230	6	36	0	7	5	1	1
1448	Large vanilla	1 ea	213	66	340	9	53	0	10	7	1	1
1450	Chocolate dipped	1 ea	156	60	330	6	40	<1	16	8	4	3
1453	Chocolate sundae	1 ea	177	62	300	6	54	<1	7	5	1	1
1455	Banana split	1 ea	383	68	529	9	97	2	11	8.3	3.1	.4
1456	Peanut Buster Parfait	1 ea	305	53	710	16	94	1	32	10	10	9
1457	Hot Fudge Brownie Delight	1 ea	266	53	619	10	89	1	25	12.2	10.5	1.7
1459	Buster bar	1 ea	149	45	450	11	40	<1	29	9	10	8
1645	Breeze, strawberry, regular	1 ea	354	70	420	12	90	–	1	–	–	–
1460	Dilly bar	1 ea	85	55	210	3	21	<1	13	6	3	3
1461	DQ ice cream sandwich	1 ea	60	48	138	3	24	<1	4	2	1	1
1463	Milk shakes, regular	1 ea	418	71	548	13	93	<1	15	8.4	2.1	2.1
1464	Milk shakes, large	1 ea	489	72	636	14	107	<1	17	10.6	2.1	2.1
1466	Malted milkshake	1 ea	418	68	610	13	106	<1	14	8	2	2
1468	Float	1 ea	397	76	410	5	82	0	7	5	1	1
1469	Freeze	1 ea	397	72	500	9	89	0	12	7.5	3.4	.4
1640	Sundae, waffle cone, strawberry	1 ea	173	–	173	8	56	–	12	5	3	3

PAGE KEY: H–4 = BEV H–6 = DAIRY H–12 = EGGS H–14 = FAT/OIL H–18 = FRUIT H–26 = BAKERY H–36 = GRAIN H–44 = FISH H–48 = MEATS H–50 = POULTRY H–54 = SAUSAGE H–56 = MIXED/FAST H–64 = NUTS/SEEDS H–68 = SWEETS H–70 = VEG/LEG H–84 = MISC H–88 = SOUPS/SAUCES H–90 = FAST H–106 = FRZN ENTREE H–112 = BABY FOODS

Chol (mg)	Calc (mg)	Iron (mg)	Magn (mg)	Phos (mg)	Pota (mg)	Sodi (mg)	Zinc (mg)	VT-A (RE)	Thia (mg)	Ribo (mg)	Niac (mg)	V-B6 (mg)	Fola (µg)	VT-C (mg)
227	151	1.8	–	–	–	797	–	81	.32	.3	2.02	.11	–	2
261	154	2.97	–	–	–	1025	–	82	.37	.33	4.1	.12	–	<1
232	151	1.8	–	–	–	1400	–	81	.49	.32	3.02	.22	–	10
88	59	4.4	–	–	–	834	–	98	.32	.4	6.87	.34	–	9
113	246	4.4	–	–	–	1248	–	147	.33	.47	6.88	.32	–	9
169	80	7.3	–	–	–	920	–	100	.34	.56	10	–	–	9
193	249	7.28	–	–	–	1336	–	150	.35	.63	9.97	–	–	9
42	39	2.76	–	–	–	489	–	30	.23	.25	3.94	.14	–	6
59	110	2.93	–	–	–	682	–	89	.24	.3	4.19	–	–	6
32	42	1.9	–	–	–	529	–	21	.23	.25	4.23	–	–	3
47	104	1.88	–	–	–	741	–	63	.23	.29	4.17	–	–	3
104	144	3.24	–	–	–	863	–	58	.22	.3	4.32	–	–	1
60	100	3.62	–	–	–	1406	–	13	.45	.31	10	–	–	1
80	40	5.4	–	–	–	480	–	40	–	–	–	–	–	6
55	250	2.7	–	–	490	1050	–	80	–	–	–	–	–	2
38	19	.78	–	–	–	571	–	5	.08	.08	7.56	–	–	<1
70	195	3.2	–	–	–	1534	–	85	.87	.42	6	–	–	7
45	44	2.67	–	–	–	808	–	15	.21	.2	2.96	–	–	1
75	300	3.6	–	–	500	1270		80	–	–	–	–	–	5
0	6	.69	–	–	–	153	–	0	.06	.2	5	–	–	2
0	60	2.7	–	–	–	490	–	–	–	–	–	–	–	–
0	79	.51	–	–	–	516	–	0	.04	.03	.46	–	–	<1
19	192	1.73	–	–	–	221	–	58	.12	.53	.12	–	–	0
19	288	–	–	–	–	221	–	58	.11	.55	.12	–	–	3
0	17	1.6	–	–	–	254	–	4	.27	.18	.6	–	–	7
15	100	.4	–	100	150	60	–	20	.03	.17	.06	–	–	<1
20	150	.7	–	150	260	95	–	40	.06	.26	.11	.09	–	0
30	200	1.4	–	200	380	140	–	60	.12	.34	.17	–	–	0
20	300	.7	–	150	290	100	–	40	.06	.26	.11	.09	–	0
20	150	1.1	–	150	290	140	–	40	.06	.26	.3	.14	–	0
31	311	3.74	–	42	893	259	–	156	.16	.27	.41	.21	–	16
30	350	3.6	–	450	660	410	–	60	.15	.51	3	.22	–	2
30	262	4.71	–	523	445	297	–	70	.1	.6	.26	.16	–	1
15	300	1.1	–	250	400	220	–	20	.12	.17	3	.08	–	1
–	500	1.8	–	350	490	170	–	–	.12	.68	–	–	–	24
10	250	.72	–	80	170	50	–	20	.03	.14	–	.06	–	1
5	59	.71	–	59	103	133	–	15	.03	.26	.39	.05	–	<1
47	421	1.52	–	369	600	242	–	84	.24	.63	.84	.2	–	0
53	477	1.53	–	477	700	276	–	212	.16	.72	.85	–	–	0
45	400	1.44	–	350	570	230	–	80	.12	.66	.8	.19	–	0
20	200	1.1	–	200	–	85	–	40	.06	.26	.05	.09	–	<1
30	300	1.8	–	350	–	180	–	98	.15	.51	–	.15	–	2
20	150	1.44	–	200	330	220	–	40	.09	.26	–	–	–	6

(For purposes of calculations, use "0" for t, <1, <.1, <.01, etc.)

H

Table H–1
Food Composition

Computer Code Number	Food Description	Measure	Wt (g)	H_2O (%)	Ener (kcal)	Prot (g)	Carb (g)	Dietary Fiber (g)	Fat (g)	Fat Breakdown (g) Sat	Mono	Poly
	DAIRY QUEEN—Cont.											
	Mr. Misty:											
1470	Regular	1 ea	330	81	250	0	63	0	0	0	0	0
1471	Kiss	1 ea	89	81	70	0	17	0	0	0	0	0
1472	Freeze	1 ea	411	72	500	9	91	0	12	7.4	3.4	.4
1473	Float	1 ea	411	78	390	5	74	0	7	4.3	2	.3
	Yogurt											
1641	Yogurt cone	1 ea	142	67	180	6	38	–	1	–	–	–
1643	Yogurt sundae-strawberry	1 ea	170	70	200	6	43	–	1	–	–	–
	Sandwiches:											
1474	Chicken	1 ea	202	56	455	25	39	<1	21	4.2	7.4	8.5
1647	Grilled chicken fillet	1 ea	184	63	300	25	33	–	8	2	2	3
1475	Fish fillet	1 ea	177	58	385	17	41	<1	17	3.1	5.2	8.3
1476	Fish fillet with cheese	1 ea	191	56	436	20	42	<1	22	6.2	7.3	8.3
1477	Hamburger, single	1 ea	148	55	323	18	30	<1	17	6.2	6.2	1
1478	Hamburger, double	1 ea	210	57	488	33	31	<1	26	12.7	11.7	2.1
1480	Cheeseburger, single	1 ea	162	55	379	21	31	<1	19	9.3	7.3	1
1481	Cheeseburger, double	1 ea	239	54	603	39	33	<1	36	19	13.7	2.1
	Hot dog:											
1483	Regular	1 ea	100	51	283	9	23	<1	16	6.1	7.1	2
1484	With cheese	1 ea	114	49	333	12	24	<1	21	9.1	8.1	2
1485	With chili	1 ea	128	53	323	11	26	2	19	7.1	8.1	2
1489	French fries, small	1 ea	71	38	210	3	29	1	10	2	5	3
1490	French fries, large	1 ea	113	50	344	4	46	2	16	3.5	7.1	5.3
1491	Onion rings	1 ea	85	46	240	4	29	<1	12	3	5	4
	Source: International Dairy Queen.											
	HARDEE'S											
1734	Frisco burger hamburger	1 ea	242	–	760	36	43	–	50	18	–	–
1735	Frisco grilled chicken sandwich	1 ea	244	–	620	35	44	–	34	10	–	–
1736	Frisco grilled chicken salad	1 ea	278	–	120	18	2	–	4	1	–	–
1737	Peach shake	1 ea	345	–	390	10	77	–	4	3	–	–
	JACK IN THE BOX											
	Breakfast items:											
1492	Breakfast Jack sandwich	1 ea	126	50	312	19	31	–	13	5.2	5	2.5
1494	Sausage crescent	1 ea	156	39	580	22	28	–	43	15.5	21.5	5.7
1495	Supreme crescent	1 ea	146	39	506	22	32	–	31	13.2	18.9	7.8
1496	Pancake platter	1 ea	231	45	610	15	87	–	22	8.6	7.6	3.5
1497	Scrambled egg platter	1 ea	249	52	655	21	58	–	37	10.2	19.4	5.1
	Sandwiches:											
1654	Bacon bacon cheeseburger	1 ea	242	49	710	35	41	0	45	15	15.7	8.7
1498	Hamburger	1 ea	98	39	283	13	31	0	11	4.1	4.9	2
1499	Cheeseburger	1 ea	113	39	339	16	33	0	14	6	6	2.3
1500	Jumbo Jack burger	1 ea	205	55	501	23	37	0	31	9	11.6	7.4
1501	Jumbo Jack burger with cheese	1 ea	246	55	620	29	42	0	37	12	15.2	9.1
1655	Chicken sandwich	1 ea	160	52	400	20	38	0	18	4	–	–
1505	Chicken supreme	1 ea	228	55	577	23	45	0	34	10	13.8	10.6

PAGE KEY: H–4 = BEV H–6 = DAIRY H–12 = EGGS H–14 = FAT/OIL H–18 = FRUIT H–26 = BAKERY H–36 = GRAIN H–44 = FISH H–48 = MEATS H–50 = POULTRY H–54 = SAUSAGE H–56 = MIXED/FAST H–64 = NUTS/SEEDS H–68 = SWEETS H–70 = VEG/LEG H–84 = MISC H–88 = SOUPS/SAUCES H–90 = FAST H–106 = FRZN ENTREE H–112 = BABY FOODS

Chol (mg)	Calc (mg)	Iron (mg)	Magn (mg)	Phos (mg)	Pota (mg)	Sodi (mg)	Zinc (mg)	VT-A (RE)	Thia (mg)	Ribo (mg)	Niac (mg)	V-B6 (mg)	Fola (µg)	VT-C (mg)
0	0	0	–	–	–	10	–	0	0	0	–	0	–	2
0	0	0	–	–	–	10	–	0	0	0	–	0	–	0
30	300	1.4	–	200	–	140	–	98	.12	.51	–	.18	–	2
20	200	.7	–	200	–	95	–	49	.06	.26	–	.09	–	1
–	200	.72	–	150	190	80	–	–	.06	.26	–	–	–	–
–	250	.72	–	150	240	80	–	–	.06	.34	–	–	–	12
58	42	1.9	–	370	370	804	–	21	.4	.36	12	–	–	3
50	60	3.6	–	350	330	800	–	20	.3	1.02	12	–	–	2
47	42	1.9	–	156	292	656	–	16	.3	.24	3	–	–	–
62	104	1.9	–	260	301	882	–	83	.3	.27	5	–	–	–
47	104	3.75	–	156	271	605	–	21	.31	.27	4	–	–	1
101	42	5.7	–	265	440	668	–	21	.3	.46	7	–	–	1
62	156	3.74	–	260	280	831	–	83	.31	.35	4	–	–	1
127	212	5.7	–	423	465	1132	–	159	.3	.54	7.4	–	–	1
25	40	1.41	–	61	172	707	–	0	.23	.14	2	–	–	<1
35	101	1.41	–	151	182	928	–	89	.23	.17	2	–	–	<1
30	40	1.45	–	60	262	726	–	60	.23	.14	3	–	–	<1
0	10	.72	–	100	430	115		0	.09	.02	2	–	–	5
0	13	1.27	–	132	689	177	–	0	.13	.03	2.65	–	–	8
0	20	.72	–	60	90	135		15	.09	.05	.4	–	–	2
70	–	–	–	–	–	1280	–	–	–	–	–	–	–	–
95	–	–	–	–	–	1730	–	–	–	–	–	–	–	–
60	–	–	–	–	–	520	–	–	–	–	–	–	–	–
25	–	–	–	–	–	290	–	–	–	–				
193	208	2.8	–	–	229	927	–	83	.47	.41	3	–	–	9
185	150	2.7	–	–	260	1010	–	100	.6	.51	4.6	–	–	0
200	143	3.4	–	–	258	887	–	143	.65	.54	4.2	–	–	11
100	100	1.8	–	–	310	890	–	80	.03	.85	7	–	–	6
444	175	5.73	–	–	526	1239	–	175	–	.77	5.85	–	–	11
110	250	5.4	–	–	540	1240	–	80	.24	.48	8.8	.39	–	9
26	101	1.8	–	–	–	556	–	–	.15	.26	2	–	–	–
41	205	2.72	–	–	–	753	–	40	.23	.23	3.03	–	–	–
67	80	2.86	–	–	–	677	–	–	.33	.27	1.66	–	–	–
104	203	3.86	–	–	–	1108	–	–	.37	.45	1.63	–	–	–
45	150	1.8	–	–	180	1290	–	40	–	–	–	–	–	0
79	186	2.7	–	–	–	1368	–	74	.36	.3	10.2	–	–	6

(For purposes of calculations, use "0" for t, <1, <.1, <.01, etc.)

Table H–1
Food Composition

Computer Code Number	Food Description	Measure	Wt (g)	H_2O (%)	Ener (kcal)	Prot (g)	Carb (g)	Dietary Fiber (g)	Fat (g)	Fat Breakdown (g) Sat	Mono	Poly
	JACK IN THE BOX—Cont.											
1656	Chicken sandwich, Sourdough ranch	1 ea	225	73	205	14	41	7	0	0	0	0
1583	Double cheeseburger	1 ea	149	41	441	24	34	0	27	11.8	11.6	3.1
1651	Grilled Sourdough burger	1 ea	223	48	670	32	39	0	43	16	17.8	7.9
1508	Tacos, regular	1 ea	81	58	191	7	16	2	11	4.2	–	–
1509	Tacos, super	1 ea	135	59	300	13	24	3	17	6.4	–	–
1513	Taco salad	1 ea	402	76	503	34	28	–	31	13.4	11.9	1.6
	Teriyaki bowl:											
1668	Chicken	1 ea	440	62	580	28	115	6	2	–	–	–
1679	Beef	1 ea	440	62	640	28	124	7	3	1	–	–
1516	French fries	1 ea	109	37	351	5	45	5	17	4	11	.6
1517	Hash browns	1 ea	62	51	174	1	15	1	12	2.8	7.4	.3
1518	Onion rings	1 ea	108	34	398	5	40	0	24	6.3	15.9	.9
	Milk shakes:											
1519	Chocolate	1 ea	322	72	390	9	74	0	6	3.5	2.1	–
1520	Strawberry	1 ea	328	67	363	10	66	0	8	4.3	2	–
1521	Vanilla	1 ea	317	73	365	9	65	0	7	4.2	1.8	–
1522	Apple turnover	1 ea	119	34	379	3	52	0	21	4.3	11.5	1.8
	Source: Jack in the Box Restaurant, Inc.											
	KENTUCKY FRIED CHICKEN											
	Rotisserie Gold:											
1472	Dark Qtr–no skin	1 ea	117	60	217	27	0	–	12	3.5	–	–
1473	Dark Qtr–w/skin	1 ea	146	54	333	30	1	–	24	6.6	–	–
1513	White Qtr with wing w/skin	1 ea	176	59	335	40	1	–	19	5.4	–	–
1525	White Qtr with wing–no skin	1 ea	117	20	199	37	0	–	6	1.7	–	–
	Original recipe:											
1253	Center breast	1 ea	95	52	240	23	8	<1	13	3.5	7.2	1.8
1251	Side breast	1 ea	69	47	204	14	7	<1	12	3.5	7.3	1.7
1250	Drumstick	1 ea	47	51	125	11	2	<1	7	1.8	3.4	1.1
1252	Thigh	1 ea	88	49	266	17	7	<1	19	4.9	8.7	2.6
1249	Wing	1 ea	42	41	136	9	4	<1	9	2.3	4.6	1.4
	Dinners:											
1254	2-pce dinner, white	1 ea	322	59	702	32	56	2	39	9.5	18.4	7.9
1255	2-pce dinner, dark	1 ea	346	71	721	33	57	1	40	10.1	17.9	8.5
1256	2-pce dinner, combo	1 ea	341	47	741	32	58	1	42	10.7	19.3	8.8
	Hot & Spicy											
1451	Chicken Center breast	1 ea	125	48	360	28	13	–	22	5	–	–
1452	Chicken Side breast	1 ea	120	43	400	22	16	–	28	6	–	–
1430	Chicken Thigh	1 ea	119	47	370	24	10	–	27	6	–	–
1471	Chicken Whole Wing	1 ea	61	38	220	14	5	–	16	4	–	–
	Extra crispy recipe:											
1261	Center breast	1 ea	104	48	291	25	9	<1	17	4	9.5	1.9
1259	Side breast	1 ea	84	40	290	17	11	<1	20	4.2	9.3	1.7
1258	Drumstick	1 ea	58	48	170	11	5	<1	11	3	6.8	1.5
1260	Thigh	1 ea	107	43	373	18	13	<1	29	7.6	15.7	4
1257	Wing	1 ea	53	32	216	10	8	<1	15	4	9.6	2
	Dinners:											
1262	2-pce dinner, white	1 ea	348	57	829	34	62	1	49	11.8	25.6	8.6
1263	2-pce dinner, dark	1 ea	375	59	878	36	62	1	54	13.3	26.9	9.9

PAGE KEY: H–4 = BEV H–6 = DAIRY H–12 = EGGS H–14 = FAT/OIL H–18 = FRUIT H–26 = BAKERY H–36 = GRAIN H–44 = FISH H–48 = MEATS H–50 = POULTRY H–54 = SAUSAGE H–56 = MIXED/FAST H–64 = NUTS/SEEDS H–68 = SWEETS H–70 = VEG/LEG H–84 = MISC H–88 = SOUPS/SAUCES H–90 = FAST H–106 = FRZN ENTREE H–112 = BABY FOODS

Chol (mg)	Calc (mg)	Iron (mg)	Magn (mg)	Phos (mg)	Pota (mg)	Sodi (mg)	Zinc (mg)	VT-A (RE)	Thia (mg)	Ribo (mg)	Niac (mg)	V-B6 (mg)	Fola (μg)	VT-C (mg)
0	0	4.91	–	–	–	136	–	341	–	–	–	–	–	82
72	245	2.7	–	–	–	842	–	98	.15	.34	6	–	–	–
110	200	4.5	–	–	510	1140	–	150	.65	.48	8	.33	–	6
21	104	1.1	35	152	249	426	1.2	0	.07	.17	1	.13	–	0
37	161	1.6	45	212	316	771	1.8	0	.12	.08	1.4	.18	–	3
92	410	3.8	–	–	–	1600	–	270	.29	.53	5.8	–	–	9
30	100	1.8	–	–	380	1220	–	1100	–	–	–	–	–	9
25	150	4.5	–	–	430	930	–	1000	–	–	–	–	–	6
0	0	1.3	–	–	–	194	–	–	.18	.03	3.8	–	–	29
0	0	.39	–	–	–	339	–	0	.05	–	1.09	–	–	7
0	31	2.31	–	–	–	473	–	–	.3	.18	2.73	–	–	3
25	300	.72	–	–	680	210			.15	.6	.4	–	–	0
33	330	.36	–	–	605	198	–	–	.15	.43	.4	–	–	0
31	313	–	–	–	594	188	–	–	.15	.34	.4	–	–	0
0	0	2.12	–	–	87	498	–	–	.24	.14	2.12			10
128	10	.18	–	–	–	772	–	15	–	–	–	–	–	1
163	10	.18	–	–	–	980	–	15	–	–	–	–	–	1
157	10	.18	–	–	–	1104	–	15	–	–	–			1
97	10	.18	–	–	–	667	–	15	–	–	–	–	–	1
85	28	.83	–	–	–	562	–	14	.07	.14	9.5	–	–	–
65	57	.92	–	–	–	502	–	12	.05	.1	5.29	–	–	–
62	17	.91	–	–	–	222	–	12	.04	.1	2.64	–	–	–
104	37	1.1	–	–	–	547	–	29	.07	.25	4.65	–	–	–
47	24	.92	–	–	–	304	–	12	.02	.06	2.83	–	–	–
119	215	3.71	–	–	–	1854	–	76	.22	.38	11.8	.5	–	36
164	197	3.84	–	–	–	1738	–	76	.25	.57	10.6	.46	–	37
160	217	3.88	–	–	–	1801	–	57	.24	.53	10.9	.47	–	38
80	20	.72	–	–	–	750	–	15			–	–	–	6
80	40	1.08	–	–	–	850	–	15	–	–	–	–	–	6
100	20	1.08	–	–	–	670	–	15	–	–	–	–	–	6
65	20	.72	–	–	–	440	–	65	30	–	–	–	–	–
66	29	.62	–	–	–	652	–	13	.08	.1	11.5	–	–	–
54	14	.61	–	–	–	514	–	11	.07	.08	6.49	–	–	–
58	12	.59	–	–	–	277	–	27	.05	.1	3.11	–	–	–
88	48	1.08	–	–	–	510	–	29	.09	.19	6.38	–	–	–
58	18	.05	–	–	–	287	–	27	–	.03	.05	2.69	–	–
125	161	2.51	–	–	–	1915	–	76	.31	.34	12.8	.56	–	36
176	180	3.48	–	–	–	1869	–	77	.32	.5	12	.53	–	36

(For purposes of calculations, use "0" for t, <1, <.1, <.01, etc.)

H

Table H–1
Food Composition

Computer Code Number	Food Description	Measure	Wt (g)	H_2O (%)	Ener (kcal)	Prot (g)	Carb (g)	Dietary Fiber (g)	Fat (g)	Fat Breakdown (g) Sat	Mono	Poly
	KENTUCKY FRIED CHICKEN—Cont.											
1264	2-pce dinner, combo	1 ea	371	57	919	35	65	1	58	14.1	29.4	10.6
1265	Mashed potatoes	⅓ c	80	81	60	2	12	1	1	.2	.4	t
1526	Breadstick	1 ea	33	10	110	3	17	0	3	0	–	–
1268	Corn-on-the-cob	1 ea	143	70	210	5	32	8	11	.5	1	1.5
1527	Cornbread	1 pce	56	26	228	3	25	1	13	2	–	–
1269	Coleslaw	⅓ c	79	75	100	1	12	<1	5	.9	1.5	3
1429	Chicken Hot Wings	1 ea	119	38	415	24	16	–	29	–	–	–
1381	Kentucky nuggets	6 ea	96	41	287	16	15	<1	18	4	8.7	2.2
	Kentucky nugget sauce:											
1382	Barbeque	2 tsp	30	68	37	<1	8	–	1	.1	–	.3
1383	Sweet & sour	2 tbs	30	48	61	<1	14	–	1	.1	–	.3
1384	Honey	2 tbs	30	8	104	0	26	–	–	–	–	–
1385	Mustard	2 tbs	30	69	38	1	6	–	1	.1	–	1.2
1386	Kentucky fries	1 ea	119	42	352	5	40	5	18	5	12.5	1.1
1534	Macaroni & Cheese	1 ea	114	71	162	7	15	0	8	3	–	–
1387	Mashed potatoes & gravy	⅓ c	86	80	74	1	11	<1	4	.4	.4	.2
1388	Buttermilk biscuit	1 ea	75	28	270	6	32	<1	15	3.7	6.7	2.5
1530	Pasta Salad	1 ea	108	78	135	2	14	1	8	1	–	–
1389	Potato salad	⅓ c	90	74	130	2	13	1	8	1.4	2.8	3.5
1383	Potato Wedges	1 ea	92	55	192	3	25	3	9	3	–	–
1390	Baked beans	⅓ c	89	70	107	4	19	3	2	.4	.5	.2
1391	Chicken Little sandwich	1 ea	57	32	205	7	17	1	12	2.4	–	4.1
1535	Red Beans & Rice	1 ea	111	76	113	4	18	3	3	1	–	–
1529	Vegetable Medley Salad	1 ea	114	77	126	1	21	3	4	1	–	–
	Source: Kentucky Fried Chicken Corporation.											
	LONG JOHN SILVER'S											
	Fish, batter fried:											
1523	Fish & Fryes (fries), 3 piece	1 ea	350	54	893	28	84	–	46	10	26	9
1524	Fish & Fryes, 2 piece	1 ea	260	54	608	27	52	–	37	8	23	5
1525	Fish dinner, 3 piece	1 ea	540	60	1180	47	93	–	70	–	–	–
	Fish, breaded & fried:											
1526	Fish dinner, 3 piece	1 ea	450	60	940	35	84	–	52	–	–	–
1527	Fish dinner, 2 piece	1 ea	400	60	818	26	76	–	46	–	–	–
	Chicken:											
1528	Chicken Plank dinner, 3 piece	1 ea	370	56	825	30	94	–	41	9	23	9
1529	Chicken Plank dinner, 4 piece	1 ea	440	60	1037	41	82	–	59	–	–	–
1530	Chicken Nugget dinner, 6 piece	1 ea	300	60	699	23	54	–	45	–	–	–
1531	Clam chowder	1 ea	185	86	131	10	9	1	6	2	2	2
1532	Clam dinner	1 ea	460	47	1262	31	145	–	66	14	40	13
1533	Fish & chicken dinner	1 ea	460	52	1014	38	109	–	52	11	31	10
1534	Oyster dinner	1 ea	360	60	789	17	78	–	45	–	–	–
1535	Scallop dinner	1 ea	320	60	747	17	66	–	45	–	–	–
1536	Seafood platter	1 ea	410	60	976	29	85	–	58	–	–	–
1537	Shrimp dinner, batter fried	1 ea	300	54	761	16	80	–	43	9	25	8
1538	Fish sandwich platter	1 ea	400	59	835	30	84	–	42	–	–	–
	Salads:											
1539	Ocean chef salad	1 ea	320	89	150	16	18	3	1	6	6	3
1540	Seafood salad	1 ea	480	89	656	26	21	3	54	9	14	30

H

PAGE KEY: H–4 = BEV H–6 = DAIRY H–12 = EGGS H–14 = FAT/OIL H–18 = FRUIT H–26 = BAKERY H–36 = GRAIN H–44 = FISH H–48 = MEATS H–50 = POULTRY H–54 = SAUSAGE H–56 = MIXED/FAST H–64 = NUTS/SEEDS H–68 = SWEETS H–70 = VEG/LEG H–84 = MISC H–88 = SOUPS/SAUCES H–90 = FAST H–106 = FRZN ENTREE H–112 = BABY FOODS

Chol (mg)	Calc (mg)	Iron (mg)	Magn (mg)	Phos (mg)	Pota (mg)	Sodi (mg)	Zinc (mg)	VT-A (RE)	Thia (mg)	Ribo (mg)	Niac (mg)	V-B6 (mg)	Fola (μg)	VT-C (mg)
172	183	2.96	–	–	–	1949	–	76	.31	.45	11.7	.49	–	36
<1	21	.28	14	41	218	228	.16	5	.01	.04	.96	.11	7	4
0	30	.18	–	–	–	15	–	0	–	–	–	–	–	0
688	0	.34	–	–	72	–	–	19	.14	.11	1.8	–	–	2
42	60	.72	–	–	–	194	–	10	–	–	–	–	–	–
4	26	.32	–	–	–	155	–	28	.03	.03	.17	–	–	24
132	35	2.86	–	–	–	1084	–	13	–	–	–	–	–	5
67	2	.1	–	–		874	–	15	.02	.02	1	.05	–	<1
–	6	.21	–	–	–	477	–	39	–	.01	.2	–	–	–
–	5	.21	–	–	–	157	–	60	–	.02	.04	–	–	–
–	1	.21	–	–	–	–	–	0	–	.01	.08	–	–	–
–	11	.32	–	–	–	367	–	1	–	.01	.17	–	–	–
7	17	1.5	–	–	–	826	–	0	.23	.08	3.09	–	–	0
16	120	.72	–	–	–	531	–	–	–	–	–	–	–	0
<1	14	.3	–	–	–	278	–	11	–	.03	.86	–	–	–
3	49	2.2	–	–	–	652	–	32	.28	.22	3	–	–	–
1	20	1.08	–	–	–	663	–	110					–	7
8	7	1.6	11	23	184	305	.29	58	.05	.02	.4	.14	5	–
3	–	–	–	–	–	428	–	–	–	–	–	–	–	–
2	32	1.2	23	73	185	433	1.29	40	.05	.04	.4	.07	26	2
21	27	2.05	–		–	401	–	6	.19	.14	2.65	–	–	–
4	10	.71	–	–	–	312	–	–	–	–	–	–	–	–
0	20	.36	–	–	–	240	–	375				–	–	5
64	182	4	–	–	1021	1395	2.7	36	.41	.39	7.3	–	–	14
60	40	2	–	–	897	1474	1.2	–	.38	.34	8	–	–	9
119	–	–	–	–	–	2797	–	–	–	–		–	–	–
101	–	–	–	–	–	1900	–	–	–	–	–	–	–	–
76	–	–	–	–	–	1526	–	–	–	–	–	–	–	–
51	185	4	–	–	1085	1855	2.78	37	.49	.47	14.8	–	–	8
25	–	–	–	–	–	2433	–	–	–		–	–	–	–
25	–	–	–	–	–	853	–	–	–	–	–	–	–	–
19	187	1.68	–	–	355	551	1.56	140	.1	.24	1.87	–	–	–
96	255	5.73	–	–	1160	2332	3.8	51	.96	.55	15	–	–	15
80	213	4.8	–	–	1366	2231	3	43	.64	.64	15	–	–	10
55	–	–	–	–	–	763	–	–	–	–	–	–	–	–
37	–	–	–	–	–	1579	–	–	–	–	–	–	–	–
95	–	–	–	–	–	2161	–	–	–	–	–	–	–	–
91	181	3.26	–	–	761	1477	2.7	36	.41	.4	8	–	–	8
75	–	–	–	–	–	1402	–	–	–	–	–	–	–	–
55	137	5	–	–	130	998	.4	684	1.6	.2	4	–	–	29
95	259	8	–	–	224	1692	1.5	345	.26	.45	5	–	–	36

(For purposes of calculations, use "0" for t, <1, <.1, <.01, etc.)

H

Table H–1
Food Composition

Computer Code Number	Food Description	Measure	Wt (g)	H_2O (%)	Ener (kcal)	Prot (g)	Carb (g)	Dietary Fiber (g)	Fat (g)	Fat Breakdown (g) Sat	Mono	Poly
	LONG JOHN SILVER'S—Cont.											
1541	Coleslaw	1 ea	98	70	140	1	20	1	6	1	1.5	3.5
1542	Fryes (fries) serving	1 ea	85	43	250	3	28	1	15	2.5	7.4	5
1543	Hush puppies	1 ea	47	38	137	4	20	<1	4	1.8	2.6	1.4
	Source: Long John Silver's, Lexington, KY.											
	McDONALD'S											
	Sandwiches:											
1221	Big Mac	1 ea	215	53	508	25	46	3	26	9	7.4	4.1
1444	McChicken	1 ea	187	52	486	17	41	2	28	5	8.4	10
1591	McLean Deluxe	1 ea	206	64	332	23	36	2	11	4	3.5	1
	Sandwiches—Cont.											
1438	McLean Deluxe with Cheese	1 ea	219	63	382	25	37	2	15	7	4	1.3
1222	Quarter-Pounder	1 ea	166	52	403	22	34	2	20	8	7	1
1223	Quarter-Pounder with Cheese	1 ea	194	50	507	27	34	2	28	12	1	2
1224	Filet-O-Fish	1 ea	142	49	357	13	40	2	16	3.6	4	5
1225	Hamburger	1 ea	102	49	251	12	33	2	8	3	2.7	9
1226	Cheeseburger	1 ea	116	55	302	14	34	2	12	5	3.6	1
1227	French fries, small serving	1 ea	68	40	207	3	26	2	10	1.7	3.1	2.5
1228	Chicken McNuggets	6 ea	112	51	1224	19	16	0	18	3.8	5.7	3.7
	Sauces (packet):											
1229	Hot mustard	1 ea	30	60	63	5	8	<1	4	.47	1.1	2
1230	Barbecue	1 ea	32	58	53	<1	12	<1	<1	.05	.13	2.4
1231	Sweet & sour	1 ea	32	57	55	<1	14	<1	<1	.1	.1	.3
	Low-fat (frozen yogurt) milk shakes:											
1232	Chocolate	1 ea	293	71	346	13	66	<1	5	3.5	.1	.7
1233	Strawberry	1 ea	293	72	342	12	63	<1	5	3.4	.1	.6
1234	Vanilla	1 ea	293	75	308	12	54	<1	5	3.3	.1	.6
	Low-fat (frozen yogurt) sundaes:											
1237	Hot caramel	1 ea	168	56	283	6	58	<1	3	2	.5	1.5
1235	Hot fudge	1 ea	168	60	275	8	50	2	5	4.5	.5	2
1267	Strawberry	1 ea	168	65	226	6	49	1	1	.7	.2	.5
1238	Vanilla	1 ea	80	65	100	4	21	<1	1	.3	.2	.5
1239	Pie, apple	1 ea	83	35	286	3	34	1	14	3.7	4.5	2.8
	Muffins (fat-free)											
1266	Blueberry	1 ea	75	41	170	3	40	–	0	0	0	0
1240	Apple bran	1 ea	85	39	206	4	46	2	.77	.2	.14	.4
1241	Cookies, McDonaldland	1 ea	56	3	258	.03	41	<1	9	4.5	.9	.9
1242	Cookies, Chocolaty chip	1 ea	56	3	282	3	36	1	14	.7	.9	3.6
	Breakfast items:											
1243	English muffin with spread	1 ea	59	41	146	5	27	2	2	2.3	.6	.6
1244	Egg McMuffin	1 ea	138	57	292	18	29	1	13	6.1	1	4.1
1245	Hotcakes with marg & syrup	1 ea	176	44	442	8	80	2	11	1.9	4	4.6
1246	Scrambled eggs	1 ea	100	73	166	12	1	0	12	2	5	2
1247	Pork sausage	1 ea	48	45	193	8	<1	0	18	6	7	2
1248	Hashbrown potatoes	1 ea	53	55	130	1	15	1	7	1.4	7.3	2
1392	Sausage McMuffin	1 ea	117	42	377	13	28	2	24	8.6	8.5	3
1393	Sausage McMuffin with egg	1 ea	167	53	452	22	28	2	29	10.0	13.9	4
1394	Biscuit with biscuit spread	1 ea	75	32	257	5	32	1	13	9	1	3

(Computer code number is for West Diet Analysis program)

PAGE KEY: H–4 = BEV H–6 = DAIRY H–12 = EGGS H–14 = FAT/OIL H–18 = FRUIT H–26 = BAKERY H–36 = GRAIN H–44 = FISH H–48 = MEATS H–50 = POULTRY H–54 = SAUSAGE H–56 = MIXED/FAST H–64 = NUTS/SEEDS H–68 = SWEETS H–70 = VEG/LEG H–84 = MISC H–88 = SOUPS/SAUCES H–90 = FAST H–106 = FRZN ENTREE H–112 = BABY FOODS

Chol (mg)	Calc (mg)	Iron (mg)	Magn (mg)	Phos (mg)	Pota (mg)	Sodi (mg)	Zinc (mg)	VT-A (RE)	Thia (mg)	Ribo (mg)	Niac (mg)	V-B6 (mg)	Fola (µg)	VT-C (mg)
15	60	.72	–	–	190	260	.6	40	.06	.07	2	–	–	–
0	200	.72	–	–	370	500	.4	–	.09	–	1.6	–	–	6
–	78	1.4	–	–	127	49	.6	–	.12	.06	1.6	–	–	–
76	201	4.3	45	266	454	928	4.8	–	.49	.43	6	.25	49	3
52	127	2.5	32	220	316	789	1	–	.9	.24	7.6	.39	36	1
57	126	4	38	218	517	780	4.7	–	.38	.34	7	.28	42	8
70	134	4	42	280	537	1005	–	150	.38	.34	7	–	–	6
68	123	4	33	281	394	672	–	40	.38	.26	7	.32	–	4
94	139	4	–	–	–	1132	–	150	.38	.34	7	.32	–	4
36	121	1.81	31	179	260	735	–	20	.3	.14	9.06	.1	–	<1
27	119	2.7	23	106	245	490	–	40	.3	.17	4	–	–	2
40	127	2.7	26	169	267	725	–	80	.3	.26	4	–	–	2
0	9	.53	26	88	469	110	–	0	.15	0	2	.18	–	9
65	15	1.08	26	306	323	580	–	0	.12	.14	8	.36	–	0
3	7	.8	–	18	29	85	–	2	.01	.01	.15	–	–	<1
0	4	0	–	7	51	277	–	40	.01	.01	.17	–	–	2
0	2	.17	–	7	8	158	–	60	0	.01	.08	–	–	1
24	369	.84	–	352	539	240	–	60	.12	.51	.4	.1	–	0
24	365	.29	–	327	540	169	–	60	.12	.51	.4	.11	–	0
24	360	.1	–	326	533	171	–	60	.12	.51	.31	–	–	0
7	227	.14	–	199	318	180	–	60	.09	.34	.27	–	–	0
5	242	.55	–	223	414	170	–	40	.09	.34	.29	–	–	0
5	209	.16	–	162	307	109	–	40	.06	.34	.25	–	–	1
3	95	.23	–	–	–	76	–	19	.03	.16	.38	–	–	0
0	17	1.2	7	37	68	175	.16	10	.12	.09	1.02	.03	3	1
0	80	.72	–	114	–	220	.37	–	.12	.14	.8	–	–	1
0	39	1.22	15	70	–	227	–	1	.17	.19	2.27	–	–	1
0	10	1.63	11	83	–	271	–	0	.13	.15	1.81	.03	–	0
3	28	1.6	4	–	–	249	–	0	.13	.15	1.78	–	–	0
6	126	2	13	67	65	362	.39	31	.24	.29	2.45	.03	16	1
235	152	2.76	4	272	–	726	–	102	.48	.34	3.79	.08	–	0
9	86	1.57	22	399	–	693	–	40	.3	.34	3.03	.11	–	0
416	49	1.8	10	169	–	290	–	100	.07	.26	.05	–	–	0
36	8	.6	7	66	–	346	–	0	.26	.11	2.23	–	–	0
0	7	.27	11	51	–	330	–	0	.06	.02	.8	–	–	1
49	138	2.34	23	163	–	667	–	35	.46	.22	4.33	.13	–	0
264	160	3.78	27	282	–	966	–	105	.56	.45	5.25	.21	–	0
0	67	1.44	9	349	–	730	–	0	.23	.1	1.65	.03	–	0

(For purposes of calculations, use "0" for t, <1, <.1, <.01, etc.)

Table H–1
Food Composition

Computer Code Number	Food Description	Measure	Wt (g)	H_2O (%)	Ener (kcal)	Prot (g)	Carb (g)	Dietary Fiber (g)	Fat (g)	Fat Breakdown (g) Sat	Mono	Poly
	McDONALD'S—Cont.											
	Breakfast items—Cont.:											
1395	Biscuit with sausage	1 ea	123	37	448	12	33	1	30	9	10	3
1396	Biscuit with sausage & egg	1 ea	180	48	548	19	34	1	37	11	14	4
1397	Biscuit with bacon, egg, cheese	1 ea	156	46	462	15	34	1	28	9	9	3
	Salads:											
1398	Chef salad	1 ea	283	86	186	18	8	3	10	4	3	1
1400	Garden salad	1 ea	213	92	77	5	6	2	4	1	1	1
1401	Chunky chicken salad	1 ea	250	86	138	24	7	3	4	1	1	1
	Source: McDonald's Corporation.											
	PIZZA HUT											
	Pan Pizza:											
1657	Cheese	2 pce	205	48	492	30	57	5	18	8.6	5.5	2.7
1658	Pepperoni	2 pce	211	45	540	29	62	5	22	9.2	9.3	3.4
1659	Supreme	2 pce	255	54	589	32	53	7	30	13.8	11.9	4.3
1660	Super Supreme	2 pce	257	55	563	33	53	6	26	12	–	–
	Thin 'N Crispy:											
1649	Cheese Pizza	2 pce	148	43	398	28	37	4	17	10	4.6	2.3
1623	Pepperoni Pizza	2 pce	146	42	413	26	36	4	20	11	–	–
1622	Supreme Pizza	2 pce	200	53	459	28	41	5	22	11	–	–
1620	Super Supreme Pizza	2 pce	203	52	463	29	44	5	21	10	–	–
	Hand Tossed:											
1619	Cheese Pizza	2 pce	220	50	518	34	55	7	20	13.6	–	–
1618	Pepperoni Pizza	2 pce	197	47	500	28	50	6	23	12.9	–	–
1648	Supreme Pizza	2 pce	239	54	540	32	50	7	26	13.8	–	–
1617	Super Supreme Pizza	2 pce	243	53	556	33	54	7	25	13	–	–
	Personal Pan Pizza:											
1610	Pepperoni	1 ea	256	43	675	37	76	8	29	12.5	12.1	4.5
1609	Supreme	1 ea	264	47	647	33	76	9	28	11.2	12.4	4.4
	Source: Pizza Hut.											
	TACO BELL											
	Breakfast burrito:											
1601	Bacon breakfast burrito	1 ea	99	48	291	11	23	–	17	4	–	–
1627	Country breakfast burrito	1 ea	113	53	281	10	26	–	16	5	–	–
1626	Fiesta breakfast burrito	1 ea	92	47	275	9	23	–	16	6	–	–
1625	Grande breakfast burrito	1 ea	177	52	457	14	46	–	24	8	–	–
1604	Sausage breakfast burrito	1 ea	106	49	303	11	23	–	19	6	–	–
	Burritos:											
1544	Bean with red sauce	1 ea	191	54	414	14	58	11	13	6.4	4.4	1.1
1545	Beef with red sauce	1 ea	191	53	457	23	44	4	19	9.7	6.9	.8
1546	Beef & bean with red sauce	1 ea	191	59	393	17	44	5	15	4.8	5.8	1.9
1552	Chicken burrito	1 ea	171	58	345	17	41	–	13	5	–	–
1547	Supreme with red sauce	1 ea	241	61	475	19	52	5	21	7.3	7.5	1.9
1569	Big beef burrito supreme	1 ea	298	64	525	25	51	–	25	11	–	–
1571	7 layer burrito	1 ea	234	60	458	14	55	8	20	5.9	–	–
1538	Chilito	1 ea	156	49	391	17	41	–	18	9	–	–
1549	Chilito, steak	1 ea	257	62	496	26	47	–	23	10	–	–

(Computer code number is for West Diet Analysis program)

PAGE KEY: H–4 = BEV H–6 = DAIRY H–12 = EGGS H–14 = FAT/OIL H–18 = FRUIT H–26 = BAKERY H–36 = GRAIN H–44 = FISH H–48 = MEATS H–50 = POULTRY H–54 = SAUSAGE H–56 = MIXED/FAST H–64 = NUTS/SEEDS H–68 = SWEETS H–70 = VEG/LEG H–84 = MISC H–88 = SOUPS/SAUCES H–90 = FAST H–106 = FRZN ENTREE H–112 = BABY FOODS

Chol (mg)	Calc (mg)	Iron (mg)	Magn (mg)	Phos (mg)	Pota (mg)	Sodi (mg)	Zinc (mg)	VT-A (RE)	Thia (mg)	Ribo (mg)	Niac (mg)	V-B6 (mg)	Fola (µg)	VT-C (mg)
34	78	1.88	16	424	–	1084	–	0	.47	.18	4.17	.21	–	0
259	106	3	22	528	–	1244	–	62	.46	.36	4.1	.21	–	0
244	105	2.75	21	569	–	1238	–	102	.39	.35	2.04	.13	–	0
161	142	1.54	36	302	–	427	–	1067	.32	.28	4.27	–	–	22
27	48	1.62	22	370	–	79	–	1014	.1	.11	.45	–	–	24
64	45	1.06	37	569	–	225	–	1666	.22	.17	8.82	–	–	26
34	630	5.4	60	470	320	940	4.1	90	.56	.6	5.2	.17	–	7
42	520	6.3	56	440	405	1127	4.2	100	.63	.49	5.4	.17	0	8
48	500	5	76	460	580	1363	5.6	120	.81	.8	6	.31	–	10
55	540	6.7	72	470	532	1447	5.4	120	.75	.66	6.4	–	–	11
33	660	3.2	48	470	261	867	3.6	70	.39	.39	4.8	.16	–	5
46	450	3.2	44	370	287	986	3.5	70	.42	.43	5.2	–	–	6
42	430	5.9	68	400	544	1328	4.7	100	.6	.49	5.4	–	–	10
56	460	4.9	60	420	463	1336	4.5	100	.59	.44	5.4	–	–	8
55	750	5.4	72	550	396	1276	4.7	100	.48	.49	5.4	–	–	10
50	440	5	60	390	415	1267	3.8	100	.54	.53	5.6	–	–	7
55	480	8.1	80	460	578	1470	5.7	110	.69	.53	7.2	–	–	12
54	440	6.8	76	420	516	1648	4.8	110	.71	.58	7.4	–	–	12
53	730	5.8	60	450	408	1335	3.8	120	.56	.66	8.2	.2	–	10
49	520	6.7	60	400	487	1313	3.8	120	.59	.66	8	.32	–	11
181	80	1.8	–	–	–	652	–	310	–	–	–	–	–	–
173	80	3.42	–	–	–	627	–	310	–	–	–	–	–	–
27	60	1.44	–	–	–	680	–	260	–	–	–	–	–	–
183	200	3.6	–	–	–	1053	–	630	–	–	–	–	–	1
183	80	1.8	–	–	–	661	–	320	–	–	–	–	–	–
9	136	3.22	–	–	459	1064	–	46	.03	1.87	1.84	.29	–	49
53	106	3.46	–	–	352	1215	–	67	.37	1.98	3.19	.3	–	2
32	107	2.07	48	212	426	1095	2.58	77	.47	.4	2.98	.57	37	2
57	140	2.52	–	–	–	854	–	440	–	–	–	–	–	1
31	145	3.4	47	215	473	1116	–	118	.39	2	2.73	.33	–	24
72	200	4.5	–	–	–	1418	–	840	–	–	–	–	–	8
17	85	2.29	–	–	–	983	–	297	–	–	–	–	–	5
47	300	3.06	–	–	–	980	–	950	–	–	–	–	–	–
78	200	2.70	–	–	–	1313	–	970	–	–	–	–	–	2

(For purposes of calculations, use "0" for t, <1, <.1, <.01, etc.)

H

Table H–1
Food Composition

Computer Code Number	Food Description	Measure	Wt (g)	H_2O (%)	Ener (kcal)	Prot (g)	Carb (g)	Dietary Fiber (g)	Fat (g)	Fat Breakdown (g) Sat	Mono	Poly
	TACO BELL—Cont											
1549	Enchirito with red sauce	1 ea	213	62	382	20	31	5	20	9.3	4.9	1.5
	Tacos:											
1551	Taco	1 ea	78	59	183	10	11	1	11	4.6	4.5	.8
1552	Taco Bellgrande	1 ea	163	63	355	18	18	1	23	10.9	9	1.3
1554	Soft taco	1 ea	92	54	225	12	18	1	12	5.4	4.3	1.2
1536	Soft taco supreme	1 ea	124	60	262	13	20	2	15	7.3	–	–
1568	Soft taco, chicken	1 ea	128	65	223	14	20	–	10	4	–	–
1572	Soft taco, steak	1 ea	100	56	217	12	21	–	9	4	–	–
1555	Tostada with red sauce	1 ea	156	69	243	9	27	5	11	4.1	5.5	.8
1558	Mexican pizza	1 ea	223	55	575	21	40	2	37	11.4	14	9.7
1559	Taco salad with salsa	1 ea	595	73	939	36	60	8	62	19	26.6	12.3
1560	Nachos, regular	1 ea	107	39	349	8	38	3	19	6.1	7.6	2.1
1561	Nachos, Bellgrande	1 ea	287	58	649	22	61	–	35	12.3	–	2.6
1562	Pintos & cheese with red sauce	1 ea	128	69	190	9	19	7	9	3.6	4	.8
1563	Taco sauce, packet	1 ea	4	96	1	<1	<1	<1	<1	0	0	0
1564	Salsa	1 ea	10	42	18	1	4	–	<1	0	0	0
1565	Cinnamon twists	1 ea	47	3	231	3	32	1	11	5.4	3.5	1.2
1628	Caramel roll	1 ea	85	19	353	6	46	–	16	4	–	–
	Border Light menu:											
1749	Bean burrito	1 ea	198	–	330	14	55	8	6	2	–	–
1750	Burrito supreme	1 ea	248	–	350	20	50	4	8	3	–	–
1744	7 layer burrito	1 ea	276	–	440	19	67	10	9	3.5	–	–
1745	Taco	1 ea	78	–	140	11	11	2	5	1.5	–	–
1746	Taco supreme	1 ea	106	–	160	13	14	2	5	1.5	–	–
1747	Soft taco	1 ea	99	–	180	13	19	2	5	2.5	–	–
1748	Soft taco supreme	1 ea	128	–	200	14	23	2	5	2.5	–	–
1742	Taco salad without chips	1 ea	464	–	330	30	35	10	9	4.5	–	–
1743	Taco salad with chips	1 ea	535	–	680	35	81	10	25	8	–	–
	Source: Taco Bell Corporation.											
	WENDY'S											
	Hamburgers:											
1566	Single on white bun, no toppings	1 ea	119	44	350	21	29	<1	16	–	–	–
1568	Double on white bun, no toppings	1 ea	197	44	560	41	32	<1	34	7.4	12.5	8
1569	Big Classic	1 ea	241	63	470	26	36	–	25	–	–	–
	Cheeseburgers:											
1570	Bacon cheeseburger	1 ea	147	46	460	29	23	<1	28	13	13	2
1571	Double with lettuce & tomato	1 ea	215	50	548	30	32	2	33	12.9	11.8	5.4
1572	Double with all toppings	1 ea	291	50	735	48	27	2	47	18.4	18	5.9
1730	Chicken sandwich, grilled	1 ea	177	62	290	24	35	2	7	1.5	–	–
	Baked potatoes:											
1573	Plain	1 ea	250	75	250	6	52	4	<1	t	t	.1
1574	With bacon & cheese	1 ea	350	71	570	19	57	4	30	11.8	11.4	5.6
1575	With broccoli & cheese	1 ea	365	74	500	13	54	5	25	9.2	8.3	4.5
1576	With cheese	1 ea	350	71	590	16	55	4	34	12.5	12.7	7.1
1577	With chili & cheese	1 ea	400	72	510	22	63	8	20	13	6.8	.9
1578	With sour cream & chives	1 ea	310	71	460	6	53	4	24	10	7.9	3.3
1579	Chili	1ea	256	81	230	21	16	–	9	–	–	–

Chol (mg)	Calc (mg)	Iron (mg)	Magn (mg)	Phos (mg)	Pota (mg)	Sodi (mg)	Zinc (mg)	VT-A (RE)	Thia (mg)	Ribo (mg)	Niac (mg)	V-B6 (mg)	Fola (μg)	VT-C (mg)
54	269	2.84	–	–	423	1243	–	100	.26	.42	2.3	1	–	28
32	84	1.07	–	–	159	276	–	24	.05	.14	1.2	.12	–	1
56	182	1.9	–	–	334	472	–	40	.11	.29	2.02	.21	–	5
32	116	2.27	–	–	196	554	–	30	.39	.22	2.74	.1	–	1
44	78	1.74	–	–	–	533	–	291	–	–	–	–	–	2
58	60	1.44	–	–	–	553	–	540	–	–	–	–	–	2
31	50	1.08	–	–	–	569	–	130	–	–	–	–	–	–
16	179	1.53	–	–	401	596	–	95	.06	.17	.63	.26	–	45
52	257	3.74	80	400	408	1031	5.4	215	.32	.33	2.96	1.11	60	31
82	405	7.22	–	–	1066	1307	–	407	.52	.77	4.88	.57	–	78
9	193	.91	52	262	161	403	1.7	88	.17	.16	.69	.19	10	2
36	297	3.48	–	–	674	997	–	40	.1	.34	2.17	–	–	58
16	156	1.42	110	156	384	642	2.17	87	.05	.15	.4	.21	68	52
0	1	.02	–	–	4	42	–	6	0	<.01	.02	<.01	–	<1
0	36	.6	–	–	376	376	–	7	.02	.14	0	–	–	2
1	37	.49	–	–	36	316	–	0	.14	.05	.96	.05	–	1
15	60	1.44	–	–	–	312	–	330	–	–	–	–	–	4
5	100	3.6	–	–	–	1340	–	400	–	–	–	–	–	2
25	80	2.7	–	–	–	1300	–	600	–	–	–	–	–	9
5	250	4.5	–	–	–	1430	–	350	–	–	–	–	–	5
20	0	0	–	–	–	280	–	40	–	–	–	–	–	0
20	0	0	–	–	–	340	–	100	–	–	–	–	–	2
25	40	1.08	–	–	–	550	–	40	–	–	–	–	–	0
25	40	1.08	–	–	–	610	–	100	–	–	–	–	–	2
50	100	2.7	–	–	–	1610	–	1200	–	–	–	–	–	27
50	250	3.6	–	–	–	1620	–	1800	–	–	–	–	–	27
65	100	4.5	–	–	265	420	–	0	.38	.34	6	–	–	–
125	48	6.3	42	339	431	575	8.35	0	.22	.43	9	.47	29	<1
80	40	4.5	–	–	470	900	–	60	.3	.25	5	–	–	12
65	136	3.6	33	296	332	860	5.14	82	.26	.28	5.7	.23	25	1
84	177	4	33	339	430	864	4.41	111	.34	.35	5.29	.25	28	5
165	180	5.4	50	470	620	883	8.8	112	.36	.53	10	.46	31	5
55	100	2.8	–	–	–	720	–	20	–	–	–	–	–	6
0	40	2.7	66	169	1360	60	.65	0	.27	.1	3.82	.7	67	36
22	200	3.7	80	406	1380	180	2.53	150	.22	.17	4.64	.87	33	36
22	250	3.6	83	373	1550	430	.86	350	.3	.25	4	.86	66	90
22	350	3.6	78	50	1380	450	.61	200	.22	.25	3.3	.8	33	36
22	250	6.13	111	498	1590	810	3.78	172	.3	.26	4.1	.9	50	36
15	40	2.7	70	185	1420	230	.9	100	.22	.14	3	.79	32	36
–	60	4.5	–	–	565	960	–	200	.12	.17	3	–	–	9

Table H–1
Food Composition

Computer Code Number	Food Description	Measure	Wt (g)	H_2O (%)	Ener (kcal)	Prot (g)	Carb (g)	Dietary Fiber (g)	Fat (g)	Fat Breakdown (g) Sat	Mono	Poly
	WENDY'S—Cont.											
1580	French fries	1 ea	106	43	306	4	38	1	15	7	5	2
1581	Frosty dairy dessert	1 c	216	35	354	7	53	0	13	5	3	2
1582	Chocolate chip cookies	1 ea	64	4	320	3	40	1	17	5.5	5.8	4.9
	Source: Wendy's International.											
	CONVENIENCE FOODS & MEALS											
	ALPINE LACE											
	Cheese spread, free'n lean:											
1926	Cheddar	1 oz	28	–	30	5	1	–	0	0	0	0
1928	Cream cheese	1 oz	28	–	30	5	1	–	0	0	0	0
1929	Garden vegetable	1 oz	28	–	30	5	1	–	0	0	0	0
1932	Garlic herb	1 oz	28	–	30	5	1	–	0	0	0	0
1933	Horseradish	1 oz	28	–	30	5	1	–	0	0	0	0
	BUDGET GOURMET											
1695	Chicken cacciatore	1 ea	312	80	300	20	27	–	13	–	–	–
1694	Sweet & sour chicken with rice	1 ea	284	72	350	18	53	–	7	–	–	–
1689	Teriyaki chicken	1 ea	340	77	360	20	44	–	12	–	–	–
1692	Linguini & shrimp	1 ea	284	77	330	15	33	–	15	–	–	–
1691	Scallops & shrimp	1 ea	326	79	320	16	43	–	9	–	–	–
1693	Sirloin tips with country gravy	1 ea	284	80	310	16	21	–	18	–	–	–
1690	Veal parmigiana	1 ea	340	75	440	26	39	–	20	–	–	–
1696	Yankee pot roast	1 ea	312	77	380	27	22	–	21	–	–	–
	Source: The All American Gourmet Company.											
	HAAGEN DAZS											
	Sorbet:											
1758	Lemon	½ c	113	–	140	0	35	–	0	0	0	0
1760	Orange	½ c	113	–	140	0	36	–	0	0	0	0
1759	Raspberry	½ c	113	–	110	0	27	–	0	0	0	0
	Yogurt, frozen:											
1753	Chocolate	½ c	98	–	170	8	26	–	4	2	2	0
1754	Strawberry	½ c	98	–	170	6	27	–	4	2	2	0
1755	Vanilla almond	1 ea	107	–	370	6	26	–	27	14	10	3
	Yogurt extra, frozen:											
1752	Brownie nut	½ c	101	–	220	8	29	–	9	4	4	1
1751	Raspberry rendezvous	½ c	101	–	132	4	26	–	2	1	1	0
	HEALTHY CHOICE											
	Entrees:											
1628	Chicken Chow Mein	1 ea	241	78	220	18	31	–	3	.8	–	.8
1630	Fillet of Fish Florentine	1 ea	273	80	220	26	13	–	7	3	–	2
2112	Fish, lemon pepper	1 ea	303	78	290	14	47	7	5	1	–	–
1624	Lasagna	1 ea	284	78	260	18	37	–	5	–	–	–
2111	Meatloaf, traditional	1 ea	340	79	320	16	46	7	8	4	–	–
1629	Seafood Newburg	1 ea	227	80	200	13	30	–	3	.8	–	.8
1625	Spaghetti	1 ea	284	77	280	14	42	–	6	–	–	–
2104	Zucchini lasagna	1 ea	397	80	330	20	58	11	2	1	–	–

(Computer code number is for West Diet Analysis program)

PAGE KEY: H–4 = BEV H–6 = DAIRY H–12 = EGGS H–14 = FAT/OIL H–18 = FRUIT H–26 = BAKERY H–36 = GRAIN H–44 = FISH H–48 = MEATS H–50 = POULTRY H–54 = SAUSAGE H–56 = MIXED/FAST H–64 = NUTS/SEEDS H–68 = SWEETS H–70 = VEG/LEG H–84 = MISC H–88 = SOUPS/SAUCES H–90 = FAST H–106 = FRZN ENTREE H–112 = BABY FOODS

Chol (mg)	Calc (mg)	Iron (mg)	Magn (mg)	Phos (mg)	Pota (mg)	Sodi (mg)	Zinc (mg)	VT-A (RE)	Thia (mg)	Ribo (mg)	Niac (mg)	V-B6 (mg)	Fola (µg)	VT-C (mg)
15	13	1.02	45	197	689	105	.51	0	.15	.04	2.96	.26	33	12
44	257	.86	43	238	518	194	.92	143	.11	.45	.31	.12	17	<1
5	10	1.09	15	62	100	235	.46	0	.06	.07	.4	.03	6	0
5	100	–	–	–	30	165	–	–	–	–	–	–	–	–
5	100	–	–	–	30	165	–	–	–	–	–	–	–	–
5	100	–	–	–	30	165	–	–	–	–	–	–	–	–
5	100	–	–	–	30	165	–	–	–	–	–	–	–	–
5	100	–	–	–	30	165	–	–	–	–	–	–	–	–
60	150	1.8	–	–	–	810	–	40	.23	.51	5	–	–	21
40	60	.72	–	–	–	640	–	80	.12	.34	3	–	–	2
55	80	1.4	–	–	–	610	–	300	.15	.34	6	–	–	12
75	10	3.6	–	–	–	1250	–	1000	.3	.17	3	–	–	2
70	150	.72	–	–	–	690	–	150	–	.26	3	–	–	12
40	60	.36	–	–	–	570	–	150	.15	.17	4	–	–	2
165	30	4.5	–	–	–	1160	–	1000	.45	.6	6	–	–	6
70	150	1.8	–	–	–	690	–	600	.15	.43	7	–	–	6
0	–	–	–	–	30	20	–	–	–	–	–	–	–	7
0	–	–	–	–	80	20	–	–	–	–	–	–	–	20
0	–	–	–	–	60	15	–	–	–	–	–	–	–	7
40	146	.7	–	146	240	45	–	20	–	.17	–	–	–	–
50	146	–	–	146	140	45	–	20	.03	.17	–	–	–	–
90	160	.38	–	107	220	85	–	160	–	.18	–	–	–	–
55	152	.73	–	152	250	60	–	20	–	.14	–	–	–	–
20	81	–	–	61	97	25	–	0	–	.1	–	–	–	5
45	20	1.4	–	290	290	440	–	81	.15	.14	4	–	–	4
65	150	.72	58	–	780	590	1.2	500	.15	.34	2	.14	<1	1
25	20	1.08	–	–	–	360	–	100	–	–	–	–	–	30
20	100	2.7	–	210	500	420	–	150	.3	.26	2	–	–	2
35	40	1.8	–	–	–	460	–	150	–	–	–	–	–	54
55	60	1.1	–	160	270	440	–	3	.12	.14	1.2	–	–	4
20	6	3.6	–	160	540	480	–	250	.38	.26	2	–	–	5
10	200	2.7	–	–	–	310	–	250	–	–	–	–	–	0

(For purposes of calculations, use "0" for t, <1, <.1, <.01, etc.)

H

Table H–1
Food Composition

Computer Code Number	Food Description	Measure	Wt (g)	H_2O (%)	Ener (kcal)	Prot (g)	Carb (g)	Dietary Fiber (g)	Fat (g)	Fat Breakdown (g) Sat	Mono	Poly
	HEALTHY CHOICE—Cont.											
	Dinners:											
2110	Pasta shells marinara	1 ea	340	74	360	25	59	5	3	1.5	–	–
1627	Sirloin Tips	1 ea	334	81	280	23	30	–	8	–	–	–
1626	Sole Au Gratin	1 ea	312	80	270	16	40	–	5	–	–	–
	Low-fat ice milk:											
1601	Berry	½ c	113	–	120	3	23	–	2	1	–	0
1604	Chocolate	½ c	113	–	130	3	24	–	2	1	–	0
1608	Cookie & Cream	½ c	113	–	130	4	24	–	2	–	–	0
1621	Vanilla	½ c	113	–	120	4	21	–	2	1	–	0
	Low-fat ice cream:											
973	Brownie	½ c	71	61	120	3	22	2	2	1	–	.7
650	Chocolate chip	½ c	71	62	120	3	21	1	2	1	–	0
259	Butter pecan	½ c	71	61	120	3	22	1	2	1	–	.7
45	Rocky road	½ c	71	53	140	3	28	2	2	1	–	0
391	Vanilla fudge	½ c	71	62	120	3	21	1	2	1.5	–	.7
	Source: ConAgra Frozen Foods, Omaha, NE.											
	HEALTH VALLEY											
	Soups, fat-free:											
2001	Beef broth, no salt added	6.9 oz	196	98	15	4	0	0	0	0	0	0
2073	Beef broth, w/salt	6.9 oz	196	98	15	4	0	0	0	0	0	0
2016	Black bean & vegetable	7.5 oz	213	93	70	7	12	11	0	0	0	0
2017	Chicken broth	7.5 oz	213	97	22	4	1	0	0	0	0	0
2018	14 garden vegetable	7.5 oz	213	92	50	5	6	5	0	0	0	0
2015	Lentil & carrot	7.5 oz	213	86	90	8	14	7	0	0	0	0
2014	Split pea & carrot	7.5 oz	213	86	90	8	14	7	0	0	0	0
2013	Tomato vegetable	7.5 oz	213	90	50	5	8	6	0	0	0	0
	LA CHOY											
2100	Egg rolls, mini, chicken	1 ea	106	53	220	8	35	3	6	1.5	–	–
2099	Egg roles, mini, shrimp	1 ea	106	56	210	7	35	3	4	1	–	–
	LEAN CUISINE											
	Dinners:											
1639	Baked Cheese Ravioli	1 ea	241	77	240	13	30	3	8	3	3	.5
1640	Chicken Cacciatore	1 ea	308	80	280	22	31	4	7	2	–	1
1632	Chicken Chow Mein	1 ea	255	78	240	14	34	–	5	1	–	1
1633	Lasagna	1 ea	291	79	260	19	34	2	5	2	2	.5
1634	Macaroni & Cheese	1 ea	255	74	290	15	37	–	9	4	–	.5
1631	Spaghetti w/Meatballs	1 ea	269	75	280	19	35	11	7	2	2.6	1
	Pizza:											
1635	French Bread Cheese Pizza	1 ea	145	52	300	17	38	<1	9	3	5	.5
1638	French Bread Deluxe Pizza	1 ea	174	56	320	22	39	2	8	3	3	.5
1637	French Bread Pepperoni Pizza	1 ea	149	51	330	19	38	2	11	3	5.4	1
1636	French Bread Sausage Pizza	1 ea	170	55	330	22	40	2	9	3	4.3	.5
	Source: Stouffer's Foods Corp, Solon, OH.											
	TASTE ADVENTURE SOUPS											
1905	Black bean	8 oz	227	–	130	6	26	6	1	–	–	–
1903	Curry lentil	8 oz	227	–	130	6	28	5	1	–	–	–
1906	Lentil chili	8 oz	227	–	170	10	31	6	1	–	–	–
1903	Split pea	8 oz	227	–	130	5	25	5	1	–	–	–

(Computer code number is for West Diet Analysis program)

PAGE KEY: H–4 = BEV H–6 = DAIRY H–12 = EGGS H–14 = FAT/OIL H–18 = FRUIT H–26 = BAKERY H–36 = GRAIN H–44 = FISH H–48 = MEATS H–50 = POULTRY H–54 = SAUSAGE H–56 = MIXED/FAST H–64 = NUTS/SEEDS H–68 = SWEETS H–70 = VEG/LEG H–84 = MISC H–88 = SOUPS/SAUCES H–90 = FAST H–106 = FRZN ENTREE H–112 = BABY FOODS

Chol (mg)	Calc (mg)	Iron (mg)	Magn (mg)	Phos (mg)	Pota (mg)	Sodi (mg)	Zinc (mg)	VT-A (RE)	Thia (mg)	Ribo (mg)	Niac (mg)	V-B6 (mg)	Fola (μg)	VT-C (mg)
25	400	1.8	–	–	–	390	–	100	–	–	–	–	–	4
65	20	2.7	–	190	540	370	–	700	.15	.17	5	.35	–	42
55	80	1.1	–	260	430	470	–	–	.23	.17	1.6	–	–	6
5	100	–	–	10	160	60	–	–	.03	.17	–	–	–	–
5	100	–	–	10	191	70	–	–	.03	.17	–	–	–	–
5	150	–	–	10	180	80	–	–	.03	.17	–	–	–	–
5	150	–	–	10	180	60	–	–	.06	.25	–	–	–	–
3	80	0	–	113	268	55	–	40	–	–	–	–	–	0
3	100	0	–	141	240	50	–	40	–	–	–	–	–	0
3	100	0	–	113	212	60	–	40	–	–	–	–	–	0
3	100	0	–	9	168	60	–	40	.03	.15	–	–	–	0
3	100	0	–	141	296	50	–	40	–	–	–	–	–	0
0	–	–	–	–	160	60	–	–	–	–	.8	–	–	–
0	–	–	–	–	160	290	–	–	–	–	.8	–	–	–
0	60	4.5	–	–	600	290	–	1000	.3	.1	1.2	.2	120	0
0	–	.39	–	43	130	315	–	–	–	.03	2.17	–	–	–
0	40	1.08	–	–	360	250	–	1000	.23	.07	2	.16	24	6
0	60	4.5	–	–	390	270	–	1000	.09	.14	5	.4	24	0
0	60	4.5	–	–	390	270	–	1000	.09	.14	5	.4	–	0
0	40	.72	–	–	540	230	–	1000	.09	.07	2	.12	32	9
5	20	1.44	–	–	–	460	–	20	–	–	–	–	–	0
5	20	1.44	–	–	–	510	–	20	–	–	–	–	–	0
55	200	1.44	42	168	380	590	1.5	60	.06	.25	1.2	.2	48	36
45	40	1.44	47	–	560	570	.97	100	.22	.17	6	–	–	9
30	40	1.08	30	–	350	530	1.1	60	.15	.17	5	–	–	6
25	150	1.8	44	–	700	590	2.9	100	.15	.25	3	.32		6
30	250	.72	–	–	160	550	–	20	.12	.25	1.2	–	–	0
35	100	1.8	47	–	500	490	2.5	60	.15	.25	3	.2	–	4
15	250	2.7	34	–	320	590	1.6	60	.37	.34	4	.1	–	6
40	200	1.44	38	–	440	860	2.08	150	.45	.51	5	.16	–	6
25	200	3.6	34	–	390	790	1.8	100	.45	.42	5	.07	–	6
40	250	2.7	39	–	440	860	2.2	80	.45	.51	5	.07	–	6
–	–	–	–	–	609	530	–	–	–	–	–	–	–	–
–	–	–	–	–	440	550	–	–	–	–	–	–	–	–
–	–	–	–	–	609	420	–	–	–	–	–	–	–	–
–	–	–	–	–	450	550	–	–	–	–	–	–	–	–

(For purposes of calculations, use "0" for t, <1, <.1, <.01, etc.)

H

Table H–1
Food Composition

Computer Code Number	Food Description	Measure	Wt (g)	H_2O (%)	Ener (kcal)	Prot (g)	Carb (g)	Dietary Fiber (g)	Fat (g)	Fat Breakdown (g) Sat	Mono	Poly
	WEIGHT WATCHERS											
1981	Baked beans	5 oz	142	74	100	9	18	9	0	0	0	0
	Cheese, fat free:											
1978	Cheddar, sharp	2 pce	21	60	30	5	2	0	0	0	0	0
1980	Swiss	2 pce	21	59	30	5	2	0	0	0	0	0
1977	White	2 pce	21	59	30	5	2	0	0	0	0	0
1979	Yellow	2 pce	21	59	30	5	2	0	0	0	0	0
	Dinners:											
1641	Beef Stroganoff	1 ea	238	73	290	22	26	3	9	4	3	2
1646	Oven Fried Fish	1 ea	198	79	240	20	23	–	7	–	5	2
1647	Fried Chicken Patty	1 pce	184	73	270	16	14	–	16	8	6	2
1654	Chicken Burrito w/Vegetable	1 ea	216	68	330	15	36	–	14	4	6	3
2029	Chicken chow mein	1 ea	255	81	200	12	34	3	2	.5	–	–
1656	Pasta Primavera	1 ea	238	75	260	15	22	2	11	.8	8	3
1972	Margarine, reduced fat	1 tbs	14	50	60	0	0	0	7	1.5	–	–
	Pizza:											
1653	Cheese Pizza	1 ea	164	56	300	22	37	2	7	3	3	1
1650	Deluxe Combination Pizza	1 ea	200	64	330	26	35	3	10	3	5	2
1651	Sausage Pizza	1 ea	175	60	320	24	35	2	10	2	6	2
1652	Pepperoni Pizza	1 ea	171	56	320	26	31	–	10	3	5	2
	Desserts:											
1645	Apple pie	1 ea	98	49	200	2	39	–	5	1	2	2
1643	Boston cream pie	1 ea	85	48	170	4	35	1	4	1	1	2
1644	Chocolate brownie	1 ea	35	29	100	3	17	<1	4	1	2	1
2024	Chocolate eclair	1 ea	60	45	150	3	24	2	5	1.5	–	–
1642	Strawberry cheesecake	1 ea	109	62	180	7	28	–	5	1	1	2
2027	Triple chocolate cheesecake	1 ea	89	52	200	7	32	1	5	2.5	–	–
1655	Chocolate mousse	1 ea	70	46	170	6	24	<1	6	–	4	2
	Sweet Success:											
	Drinks, prepared:											
1776	Chocolate chip	1 c	265	81	180	15	30	6	3	1.6	–	–
1777	Chocolate fudge	1 c	265	81	180	15	30	6	2	–	–	–
1774	Chocolate mocha	1 c	265	81	180	15	30	6	1	1	–	–
1778	Milk chocolate	1 c	265	81	180	15	30	6	2	1	–	–
1775	Vanilla	1 c	265	81	180	15	33	6	1	.6	–	–
	Drinks, ready to drink:											
2147	Chocolate mint	10 oz	284	82	179	11	34	5	3	0	–	–
2148	Strawberry	10 oz	284	82	179	11	34	5	3	0	–	–
	Shakes:											
1771	Chocolate almond	1¼ c	313	82	200	12	38	6	3	1.1	1.6	.3
1773	Chocolate fudge	1¼ c	313	82	200	12	38	6	5	1.1	1.6	.3
1768	Chocolate mocha	1¼ c	313	82	200	12	38	6	3	.8	.8	1.3
1769	Chocolate raspberry truffle	1¼ c	313	82	200	12	38	6	3	1.1	1.6	.3
1770	Vanilla creme	1¼ c	313	82	200	12	38	6	3	.8	1.8	.4
	Snack bars:											
1767	Chocolate brownie	1 ea	33	8	120	2	23	3	4	2	.5	.6
1766	Chocolate chip	1 ea	33	8	120	2	23	3	4	2	.4	.5
1765	Peanut butter	1 ea	33	8	120	2	23	3	4	2	.6	.6
1921	Oatmeal raisin	1 ea	33	7	120	2	23	3	4	2	–	–

Source: Foodway National Inc., Boise, ID.

(Computer code number is for West Diet Analysis program)

PAGE KEY: H–4 = BEV H–6 = DAIRY H–12 = EGGS H–14 = FAT/OIL H–18 = FRUIT H–26 = BAKERY H–36 = GRAIN H–44 = FISH H–48 = MEATS H–50 = POULTRY H–54 = SAUSAGE H–56 = MIXED/FAST H–64 = NUTS/SEEDS H–68 = SWEETS H–70 = VEG/LEG H–84 = MISC H–88 = SOUPS/SAUCES H–90 = FAST H–106 = FRZN ENTREE H–112 = BABY FOODS

Chol (mg)	Calc (mg)	Iron (mg)	Magn (mg)	Phos (mg)	Pota (mg)	Sodi (mg)	Zinc (mg)	VT-A (RE)	Thia (mg)	Ribo (mg)	Niac (mg)	V-B6 (mg)	Fola (μg)	VT-C (mg)
0	60	2.7	–	–	329	190	–	–	.2	.1	1.2	–	–	12
0	100	0	–	–	65	310	–	57	–	–	–	–	–	0
0	100	0	–	–	75	280	–	57	–	–	–	–	–	0
0	100	0	–	–	65	310	–	57	–	–	–	–	–	0
0	100	0	–	–	65	310	–	57	–	–	–	–	–	0
25	80	2.7	–	–	350	600	–	60	.23	.26	4	.32	–	4
15	20	.72	–	–	340	380	–	100	.09	.14	1.6	–	–	5
70	39	1.7	–	–	350	610	–	75	.19	.18	4	–	–	6
65	56	2.3	–	–	390	800	–	38	.52	.39	5.9	–	–	3
25	40	.72	–	–	360	430	–	300	–	–	–	–	–	36
5	300	1.8	–	–	260	800	–	350	.23	.26	3	.18	–	18
0	0	0	–	–	5	130	–	50	–	–	–	–	–	0
35	450	1.4	–	–	420	630	–	200	.3	.51	3	.06	–	12
25	350	1.8	–	–	490	650	–	350	.3	.51	3	.2	–	21
35	300	1.8	–	–	470	630	–	250	.3	.51	3	.06	–	18
35	400	1.8	–	–	420	710	–	200	.23	.51	3	–	–	15
5	20	1.1	–	–	80	280	–	–	.06	.07	.4	–	–	1
5	65	.6	–	–	120	290	–	14	.03	.02	.3	.08	–	1
10	19	.9	–	–	120	150	–	14	.06	.03	.2	.03	–	1
0	40	0	–	–	65	150	–	0	–	–	–	–	–	0
20	80	.36	–	–	140	210	–	40	.06	.07	1.6	–	–	2
10	80	1.08	–	–	170	200	–	0	–	–	–	–	–	0
5	60	1.1	–	–	210	190	–	–	.03	.03	.4	.06	–	5
6	500	6.3	140	350	600	288	5.25	–	.53	.6	7	.7	140	21
6	500	6.3	140	350	750	336	5.25	–	.53	.6	7	.7	140	21
6	500	6.3	140	350	800	336	5.25	–	.53	.6	7	.7	140	21
6	500	6.3	140	350	750	336	5.25	–	.53	.6	7	.7	140	21
6	500	6.3	140	350	830	312	5.25	–	.53	.6	7	.7	140	21
6	449	5.67	125	315	502	215	4.82	314	.48	.54	6.24	.62	125	19
6	449	5.67	125	315	502	188	4.82	314	.48	.54	6.24	.62	125	19
5	500	6.3	140	350	540	240	5.25	–	.53	.6	7	.7	140	21
4	500	6.3	140	350	520	220	5.25	–	.53	.6	7	.7	140	21
5	500	6.3	140	350	1490	220	5.25	–	.53	.6	7	.7	140	21
5	500	6.3	140	350	520	220	5.25	–	.53	.6	7	.7	140	21
5	500	6.3	140	350	350	220	5.25	–	.53	.6	7	.7	140	21
5	150	2.71	8	50	140	35	.01	–	.22	.25	3	.3	60	9
5	150	2.71	8	150	110	40	.01	–	.22	.25	3	.3	60	9
5	150	2.71	8	150	125	35	.01	–	.22	.25	3	.3	60	9
5	2	2.71	–	–	–	30	–	–	–	–	–	–	–	9

(For purposes of calculations, use "0" for t, <1, <.1, <.01, etc.)

Table H–1
Food Composition

Computer Code Number	Food Description	Measure	Wt (g)	H_2O (%)	Ener (kcal)	Prot (g)	Carb (g)	Dietary Fiber (g)	Fat (g)	Fat Breakdown (g) Sat	Mono	Poly
BABY FOODS												
1720	Apple juice	4 fl oz	125	88	59	0	15	–	<1	–	–	–
1721	Applesauce, strained	1 tbs	14	89	6	<1	2	–	<1	–	–	–
1716	Carrots, strained	1 tbs	14	92	4	<1	1	–	<1	–	–	–
1718	Cereal, mixed, millk added	1 tbs	14	75	16	1	2	–	<1	–	–	–
1719	Cereal, rice, milk added	1 tbs	14	75	16	1	2	–	<1	–	–	–
1723	Chicken and noodles, strained	1 tbs	14	88	7	<1	1	–	<1	–	–	–
1722	Peas, strained	1 tbs	14	88	6	1	1	–	<1	–	–	–
1717	Teething biscuits	1 ea	11	6	43	1	8	–	<1	–	–	–

(Computer code number is for West Diet Analysis program)

PAGE KEY: H–4 = BEV H–6 = DAIRY H–12 = EGGS H–14 = FAT/OIL H–18 = FRUIT H–26 = BAKERY H–36 = GRAIN H–44 = FISH H–48 = MEATS H–50 = POULTRY H–54 = SAUSAGE H–56 = MIXED/FAST H–64 = NUTS/SEEDS H–68 = SWEETS H–70 = VEG/LEG H–84 = MISC H–88 = SOUPS/SAUCES H–90 = FAST H–106 = FRZN ENTREE H–112 = BABY FOODS

Chol (mg)	Calc (mg)	Iron (mg)	Magn (mg)	Phos (mg)	Pota (mg)	Sodi (mg)	Zinc (mg)	VT-A (RE)	Thia (mg)	Ribo (mg)	Niac (mg)	V-B6 (mg)	Fola (μg)	VT-C (mg)
_	5	.71	4	6	114	4	.04	3	.01	.02	.1	.04	<1	72
_	1	.03	<1	1	10	<1	<.01	<1	<.01	<.01	.01	<.01	<1	6
_	3	.05	1	3	28	5	.02	164	<.01	.01	.07	.01	2	1
_	31	1.49	4	20	28	7	.1	3	.06	.08	.82	.01	2	_
_	34	1.73	6	25	27	7	.09	4	.07	.07	.74	.02	1	_
_	3	.06	1	3	6	2	.04	16	<.01	.01	.07	.01	1	<1
_	3	.14	2	6	16	<1	.05	8	.01	.01	.14	.01	4	1
_	29	.39	4	18	36	40	.1	1	.03	.06	.48	.01	2	1

(For purposes of calculations, use "0" for t, <1, <.1, <.01, etc.)

H

Contents

CANADA: RECOMMENDATIONS, EXCHANGES, AND LABELS

Chapter 2 introduced Recommended Nutrient Intakes (RNI), exchange systems, and food labels. This appendix presents details for Canadians. Appendix F includes addresses of Canadian governmental agencies and professional organizations that may provide additional information.

Table I–1
Recommended Nutrient Intakes for Canadians, 1990

Age	Sex	Weight (kg)	Protein (g/day)[a]	Fat-Soluble Vitamins: VITAMIN A (RE/day)[b]	VITAMIN D (μg/day)[c]	VITAMIN E (mg/day)[d]
Infants (months)						
0–4	Both	6	12[f]	400	10	3
5–12	Both	9	12	400	10	3
Children and Adults (years)						
1	Both	11	13	400	10	3
2–3	Both	14	16	400	5	4
4–6	Both	18	19	500	5	5
7–9	M	25	26	700	2.5	7
	F	25	26	700	2.5	6
10–12	M	34	34	800	2.5	8
	F	36	36	800	5	7
13–15	M	50	49	900	5	9
	F	48	46	800	5	7
16–18	M	62	58	1000	5	10
	F	53	47	800	2.5	7
19–24	M	71	61	1000	2.5	10
	F	58	50	800	2.5	7
25–49	M	74	64	1000	2.5	9
	F	59	51	800	2.5	6
50–74	M	73	63	1000	5	7
	F	63	54	800	5	6
75+	M	69	59	1000	5	6
	F	64	55	800	5	5
Pregnancy (additional amount needed)						
1st trimester			5	0	2.5	2
2nd trimester			20	0	2.5	2
3rd trimester			24	0	2.5	2
Lactation (additional amount needed)			20	400	2.5	3

Note: Recommended intakes of energy and of certain nutrients are not listed in this table because of the nature of the variables upon which they are based. The figures for energy are estimates of average requirements for expected patterns of activity (see Table I–2). For nutrients not shown, the following amounts are recommended based on at least 2000 kcalories per day and body weights as given: thiamin, 0.4 milligrams per 1000 kcalories (0.48 milligrams/5000 kilojoules); riboflavin, 0.5 milligrams per 1000 kcalories (0.6 milligrams/5000 kilojoules); niacin, 7.2 niacin equivalents per 1000 kcalories (8.6 niacin equivalents/5000 kilojoules); vitamin B_6, 15 micrograms, as pyridoxine, per gram of protein. Recommended intakes during periods of growth are taken as appropriate for individuals representative of the midpoint in each age group. All recommended intakes are designed to cover individual variations in essentially all of a healthy population subsisting upon a variety of common foods available in Canada.

Source: Health and Welfare Canada, *Nutrition Recommendations: The Report of the Scientific Review Committee* (Ottawa: Canadian Government Publishing Centre, 1990), Table 20, p. 204.

RNI

◆

The Canadian equivalent of the RDA is the Recommended Nutrient Intakes (RNI). The Canadian RNI are presented in Tables I–1 and I–2.

Table I–1 (continued)
Recommended Nutrient Intakes for Canadians, 1990

Water-Soluble Vitamins			Minerals					
VITAMIN C (mg/day)[e]	FOLATE (µg/day)	VITAMIN B_{12} (µg/day)	CALCIUM (mg/day)	PHOSPHORUS (mg/day)	MAGNESIUM (mg/day)	IRON (mg/day)	IODINE (µg/day)	ZINC (mg/day)
20	25	0.3	250	150	20	0.3[g]	30	2[h]
20	40	0.4	400	200	32	7	40	3
20	40	0.5	500	300	40	6	55	4
20	50	0.6	550	350	50	6	65	4
25	70	0.8	600	400	65	8	85	5
25	90	1.0	700	500	100	8	110	7
25	90	1.0	700	500	100	8	95	7
25	120	1.0	900	700	130	8	125	9
25	130	1.0	1100	800	135	8	110	9
30	175	1.0	1100	900	185	10	160	12
30	170	1.0	1000	850	180	13	160	9
40	220	1.0	900	1000	230	10	160	12
30	190	1.0	700	850	200	12	160	9
40	220	1.0	800	1000	240	9	160	12
30	180	1.0	700	850	200	13	160	9
40	230	1.0	800	1000	250	9	160	12
30	185	1.0	700	850	200	13[i]	160	9
40	230	1.0	800	1000	250	9	160	12
30	195	1.0	800	850	210	8	160	9
40	215	1.0	800	1000	230	9	160	12
30	200	1.0	800	850	210	8	160	9
0	200	0.2	500	200	15	0	25	6
10	200	0.2	500	200	45	5	25	6
10	200	0.2	500	200	45	10	25	6
25	100	0.2	500	200	65	0	50	6

[a]The primary units are expressed per kilogram of body weight. The figures shown here are examples.

[b]One retinol equivalent (RE) corresponds to the biological activity of 1 microgram of retinol, 6 micrograms of beta-carotene, or 12 micrograms of other carotenes.

[c]Expressed as cholecalciferol or ergocalciferol.

[d]Expressed as δ-α-tocopherol equivalents, relative to which β- and γ-tocopherol and α-tocotrienol have activities of 0.5, 0.1, and 0.3, respectively.

[e]Cigarette smokers should increase intake by 50 percent.

[f]The assumption is made that the protein is from breast milk or has the same biological value as breast milk and that, between 3 and 9 months, adjustment for the quality of the protein is made.

[g]Based on the assumption that breast milk is the source of iron.

[h]Based on the assumption that breast milk is the source of zinc.

[i]After menopause, the recommended intake is 8 milligrams per day.

Table I-2
Average Energy Requirements for Canadians

Age	Sex	Average Height (cm)	Average Weight (kg)	Requirements[a] (kcal/kg)[b]	(MJ/kg)[b]	(kcal/day)	(MJ/day)	(kcal/cm)	(MJ/cm)
Infants (months)									
0–2	Both	55	4.5	120–100	0.50–0.42	500	2.0	9	0.04
3–5	Both	63	7.0	100–95	0.42–0.40	700	2.8	11	0.05
6–8	Both	69	8.5	95–97	0.40–0.41	800	3.4	11.5	0.05
9–11	Both	73	9.5	97–99	0.41	950	3.8	12.5	0.05
Children and Adults (years)									
1	Both	82	11	101	0.42	1100	4.8	13.5	0.06
2–3	Both	95	14	94	0.39	1300	5.6	13.5	0.06
4–6	Both	107	18	100	0.42	1800	7.6	17	0.07
7–9	M	126	25	88	0.37	2200	9.2	17.5	0.07
	F	125	25	76	0.32	1900	8.0	15	0.06
10–12	M	141	34	73	0.30	2500	10.4	17.5	0.07
	F	143	36	61	0.25	2200	9.2	15.5	0.06
13–15	M	159	50	57	0.24	2800	12.0	17.5	0.07
	F	157	48	46	0.19	2200	9.2	14	0.06
16–18	M	172	62	51	0.21	3200	13.2	18.5	0.08
	F	160	53	40	0.17	2100	8.8	13	0.05
19–24	M	175	71	42	0.18	3000	12.6		
	F	160	58	36	0.15	2100	8.8		
25–49	M	172	74	36	0.15	2700	11.3		
	F	160	59	32	0.13	1900	8.0		
50–74	M	170	73	31	0.13	2300	9.7		
	F	158	63	29	0.12	1800	7.6		
75+	M	168	69	29	0.12	2000	8.4		
	F	155	64	23	0.10	1500	6.3		

[a]Requirements can be expected to vary within a range of ±30 percent.

[b]First and last figures are averages at the beginning and end of the three-month period.

Source: Health and Welfare Canada, *Nutrition Recommendations: The Report of the Scientific Review Committee* (Ottawa: Canadian Government Publishing Centre, 1990), Tables 5 and 6, pp. 25, 27.

THE CANADIAN EXCHANGE SYSTEM

◆

The *Good Health Eating Guide* is the Canadian exchange system of meal planning.[1] It contains several features similar to those of the U.S. exchange system including the following:

- Foods are divided into lists according to carbohydrate, protein, and fat content.
- Foods are interchangeable within a group.
- Most foods are eaten in measured amounts.
- An energy value is given for each food group.

Tables I–3 through I–10 present the Canadian exchange system.

[1] The tables for the Canadian exchange system are adapted from the *Good Health Eating Guide Resource,* copyright 1994, with permission of the Canadian Diabetes Association.

Table I–3
Canadian Exchange System: Starch Foods

1 starch choice = 15 g carbohydrate (starch), 2 g protein, 290 kJ (68 kcal)

Food	Measure	Mass (Weight)
Breads		
Bagels	½	30 g
Bread crumbs	50 mL (¼ c)	30 g
Bread cubes	250 mL (1 c)	30 g
Bread sticks	2	20 g
Brewis, cooked	50 mL (¼ c)	45 g
Chapati	1	20 g
Cookies, plain	2	20 g
English muffins, crumpets	½	30 g
Flour	40 mL (2 ½ tbs)	20 g
Hamburger buns	½	30 g
Hot dog buns	½	30 g
Kaiser rolls	½	30 g
Matzo, 15 cm	1	20 g
Melba toast, rectangular	4	15 g
Melba toast, rounds	7	15 g
Pita, 20-cm (8″) diameter	¼	30 g
Pita, 15-cm (6″) diameter	½	30 g
Plain rolls	1 small	30 g
Pretzels	7	20 g
Raisin bread	1 slice	30 g
Rice cakes	2	30 g
Roti	1	20 g
Rusks	2	20 g
Rye, coarse or pumpernickel	½ slice	30 g
Soda crackers	6	20 g
Tortillas, corn (taco shell)	1	30 g
Tortilla, flour	1	30 g
White (French and Italian)	1 slice	25 g
Whole-wheat, cracked-wheat, rye, white enriched	1 slice	30 g
Cereals		
Bran flakes, 100% bran	125 mL (½ c)	30 g
Cooked cereals, cooked	125 mL (½ c)	125 g
Dry	30 mL (2 tbs)	20 g
Cornmeal, cooked	125 mL (½ c)	125 g
Dry	30 mL (2 tbs)	20 g
Ready-to-eat unsweetened cereals	125 mL (½ c)	20 g
Shredded wheat biscuits, rectangular or round	1	20 g
Shredded wheat, bite size	125 mL (½ c)	20 g
Wheat germ	75 mL (⅓ c)	30 g
Cornflakes	175 mL (⅔ c)	20 g
Rice Krispies	175 mL (⅔ c)	20 g
Cheerios	200 mL (¾ c)	20 g
Muffets	1	20 g
Puffed rice	300 mL (1¼ c)	15 g
Puffed wheat	425 mL (1⅔ c)	20 g

(continued on the next page)

Table I–3 (continued)
Canadian Exchange System: Starch Foods

Food	Measure	Mass (Weight)
Grains		
Barley, cooked	125 mL (½ c)	120 g
Dry	30 mL (2 tbs)	20 g
Bulgur, kasha, cooked, moist	125 mL (½ c)	70 g
Cooked, crumbly	75 mL (⅓ c)	40 g
Dry	30 mL (2 tbs)	20 g
Rice, cooked, brown & white (short & long grain)	125 mL (½ c)	70 g
Rice, cooked, wild	75 mL (⅓ c)	70 g
Tapioca, pearl and granulated, quick cooking, dry	30 mL (2 tbs)	15 g
Couscous, cooked moist	125 mL (½ c)	70 g
Dry	30 mL (tbs)	20 g
Quinoa, cooked moist	125 mL (½ c)	70 g
Dry	30 mL (2 tbs)	20 g
Pastas		
Macaroni, cooked	125 mL (½ c)	70 g
Noodles, cooked	125 mL (½ c)	80 g
Spaghetti, cooked	125 mL (½ c)	70 g
Starchy Vegetables		
Beans and peas, dried, cooked	125 mL (½ c)	80 g
Breadfruit	1 slice	75 g
Corn, canned, whole kernel	125 mL (½ c)	85 g
Corn on the cob	½ medium cob	140 g
Cornstarch	30 mL (2 tbs)	15 g
Plantains	⅓ small	50 g
Popcorn, air-popped, unbuttered	750 mL (3 c)	20 g
Potatoes, whole (with or without skin)	½ medium	95 g
Yams, sweet potatoes, (with or without skin)	½	75 g

Food	Exchanges per serving	Measure	Mass (Weight)
Note: Food items found in this category provide more than 1 starch exchange:			
Bran flakes	1 starch + ½ sugar	150 mL (⅔ c)	24 g
Croissant, small	1 starch + 1½ fats	1 small	35 g
Large	1 starch + 1½ fats	½ large	30 g
Corn, canned creamed	1 starch + ½ fruits and vegetables	12 mL (½ c)	113 g
Potato chips	1 starch + 2 fats	15 chips	30 g
Tortilla chips (nachos)	1 starch + 1½ fats	13 chips	20 g
Corn chips	1 starch + 2 fats	30 chips	30 g
Cheese twists	1 starch + 1½ fats	30 chips	30 g
Cheese puffs	1 starch + 2 fats	27 chips	30 g
Tea biscuit	1 starch + 2 fats	1	30 g
Pancakes, homemade using 50 mL (¼ c) batter (6″ diameter)	1 ½ starches + 1 fat	1 medium	50 g
Potatoes, french fried (homemade or frozen)	1 starch + 1 fat	10 regular size	35 g
Soup, canned*, (prepared with equal volume of water)	1 starch	250 mL (1 c)	260 g
Waffles, packaged	1 starch + 1 fat	1	35 g

*Soup can vary according to brand and type. Check the label for Food Choice Values and Symbols or the core nutrient listing.

Table I-4
Canadian Exchange System: Fruits and Vegetables

1 fruits and vegetables choice = 10 g carbohydrate, 1 g protein, 190 kJ (44 kcal)

Food	Measure	Mass (Weight)
Fruits (fresh, frozen, without sugar, canned in water)		
Apples, raw (with or without skin)	½ medium	75 g
Sauce unsweetened	125 mL (½ c)	120 g
Sweetened	see *Combined Food Choices*	
Apple butter	20 mL (4 tsp)	20 g
Apricots, raw	2 medium	115 g
Canned, in water	4 halves, plus 30 mL (2 tbs) liquid	110 g
Bake-apples (cloudberries), raw	125 mL (½ c)	120 g
Bananas, with peel	½ small	75 g
Peeled	½ small	50 g
Berries (blackberries, blueberries, boysenberries, huckleberries, loganberries, raspberries)		
Raw	125 mL (½ c)	70 g
Canned, in water	125 mL (½ c), plus 30 mL (2 tbs) liquid	100 g
Cantaloupe, wedge with rind	¼	240 g
Cubed or diced	250 mL (1 c)	160 g
Cherries, raw, with pits	10	75 g
Raw, without pits	10	70 g
Canned, in water, with pits	75 mL (⅓ c), plus 30 mL (2 tbs) liquid	90 g
Canned, in water, without pits	75 mL (⅓ c), plus 30 mL (2 tbs) liquid	85 g
Crabapples, raw	1 small	55 g
Cranberries, raw	250 mL (1 c)	100 g
Figs, raw	1 medium	50 g
Canned, in water	3 medium, plus 30 mL (2 tbs) liquid	100 g
Foxberries, raw	250 mL (1 c)	100 g
Fruit cocktail, canned, in water	125 mL (½ c), plus 30 mL (2 tbs) liquid	120 g
Fruit, mixed, cut-up	125 mL (½ c)	120 g
Gooseberries, raw	250 mL (1 c)	150 g
Canned, in water	250 mL (1 c), plus 30 mL (2 tbs) liquid	230 g
Grapefruit, raw, with rind	½ small	185 g
Raw, sectioned	125 mL (½ c)	100 g
Canned, in water	125 mL (½ c), plus 30 mL (2 tbs) liquid	120 g
Grapes, raw, slip skin	125 mL (½ c)	75 g
Raw, seedless	125 mL (½ c)	75 g
Canned, in water	75 mL (⅓ c), plus 30 mL (2 tbs) liquid	115 g
Guavas, raw	½	50 g
Honeydew melon, raw, with rind	½	225 g
Cubed or diced	250 mL (1 c)	170 g
Kiwis, raw, with skin	2	155 g
Kumquats, raw	3	60 g
Loquats, raw	8	130 g
Lychee fruit, raw	8	120 g
Mandarin oranges, raw, with rind	1	135 g
Raw, sectioned	125 mL (½ c)	100 g
Canned, in water	125 mL (½ c), plus 30 mL (2 tbs) liquid	100 g
Mangoes, raw, without skin and seed	⅓	65 g
Diced	75 mL (⅓ c)	65 g
Nectarines	½ medium	75 g
Oranges, raw, with rind	1 small	130 g
Raw, sectioned	125 mL (½ c)	95 g

(continued on the next page)

Table I-4 (continued)
Canadian Exchange System: Fruits and Vegetables

1 fruits and vegetables choice = 10 g carbohydrate, 1 g protein, 190 kJ (44 kcal)

Food	Measure	Mass (Weight)
Papayas, raw, with skin and seeds	¼ medium	150 g
Raw, without skin and seeds	¼ medium	100 g
Cubed or diced	125 mL (½ c)	100 g
Peaches, raw, with seed and skin	1 large	100 g
Raw, sliced or diced	125 mL (½ c)	100 g
Canned in water, halves or slices	125 mL (½ c), plus 30 mL (2 tbs) liquid	120 g
Pears, raw, with skin and core	½	90 g
Raw, without skin and core	½	85 g
Canned, in water, halves	1 half plus 30 mL (2 tbs) liquid	90 g
Persimmons, raw, native	1	30 g
Raw, Japanese	¼	50 g
Pineapple, raw	1 slice	75 g
Raw, diced	125 mL (½ c)	75 g
Canned, in juice, diced	75 mL (⅓ c), plus 15 mL (1 tbs) liquid	55 g
Canned, in juice, sliced	1 slice, plus 15 mL (1 tbs) liquid	55 g
Canned, in water, diced	125 mL (½ c), plus 30 mL (2 tbs) liquid	100 g
Canned, in water, sliced	2 slices, plus 15 mL (1 tbs) liquid	100 g
Plums, raw	2 small	60 g
Damson	6	65 g
Japanese	1	70 g
Canned, in apple juice	2, plus 30 mL (2 tbs) liquid	70 g
Canned, in water	3, plus 30 mL (2 tbs) liquid	100 g
Pomegranates, raw	½	140 g
Strawberries, raw	250 mL (1 c)	150 g
Frozen/canned, in water	250 mL (1 c), plus 30 mL (2 tbs) liquid	240 g
Rhubarb	250 mL (1 c)	150 g
Tangelos, raw	1	205 g
Tangerines, raw	1 medium	115 g
Raw, sectioned	125 mL (½ c)	100 g
Watermelon, raw, with rind	1 wedge	310 g
Cubed or diced	250 mL (1 c)	160 g
Dried Fruit		
Apples	5 pieces	15 g
Apricots	4 halves	15 g
Banana flakes	30 mL (2 tbs)	15 g
Currants	30 mL (2 tbs)	15 g
Dates, without pits	2	15 g
Peaches	½	15 g
Pears	½	15 g
Prunes, raw, with pits	2	15 g
Raw, without pits	2	10 g
Stewed, no liquid	2	20 g
Stewed, with liquid	2, plus 15 mL (1 tbs) liquid	35 g
Raisins	30 mL (2 tbs)	15 g
Juices (no sugar added or unsweetened)		
Apricot, grape, guava, mango, prune	50 mL (¼ c)	55 g
Apple, carrot, papaya, pear, pineapple, pomegranate	75 mL (⅓ c)	80 g
Cranberry (see Sugars Section)		
Clamato (see Sugars Section)		
Grapefruit, loganberry, orange, raspberry, tangelo, tangerine	125 mL (½ c)	130 g

Table I-4 (continued)
Canadian Exchange System: Fruits and Vegetables

1 fruits and vegetables choice = 10 g carbohydrate, 1 g protein, 190 kJ (44 kcal)

Food	Measure	Mass (Weight)
Tomato, tomato-based mixed vegetables	250 mL (1 c)	255 g
Vegetables (fresh, frozen, or canned)		
Artichokes, French, globe	2 small	50 g
Beets, diced or sliced	125 mL (½ c)	85 g
Carrots, diced, cooked or uncooked	125 mL (½ c)	75 g
Chestnuts, fresh	5	20 g
Parsnips, mashed	125 mL (½ c)	80 g
Peas, fresh or frozen	125 mL (½ c)	80 g
Canned	75 mL (⅓ c)	55 g
Pumpkin, mashed	125 mL (½ c)	45 g
Rutabagas, mashed	125 mL (½ c)	85 g
Sauerkraut	250 mL (1 c)	235 g
Snow peas	250 mL (1 c)	135 g
Squash, yellow or winter, mashed	125 mL (½ c)	115 g
Succotash	75 mL (⅓ c)	55 g
Tomatoes, canned	250 mL (1 c)	240 g
Tomato paste	50 mL (¼ c)	55 g
Tomato sauce*	75 mL (⅓ c)	100 g
Turnips, mashed	125 mL (½ c)	115 g
Vegetables, mixed	125 mL (½ c)	90 g
Water chestnuts	8 medium	50 g

*Tomato sauce varies according to brand name. Check the label or discuss with your dietitian.

Table I-5
Canadian Exchange System: Milk

Type of Milk	Carbohydrate (g)	Protein (g)	Fat (g)	Energy
Nonfat (0%)	6	4	0	170 kJ (40 kcal)
1%	6	4	1	206 kJ (49 kcal)
2%	6	4	2	244 kJ (58 kcal)
Whole (4%)	6	4	4	319 kJ (76 kcal)

Food	Measure	Mass (Weight)
Buttermilk (higher in salt)	125 mL (½ c)	125 g
Evaporated milk	50 mL (¼ c)	50 g
Milk	125 mL (½ c)	125 g
Powdered milk, regular	30 mL (2 tbs)	15 g
Instant	50 mL (¼ c)	15 g
Plain yogurt	125 mL (½ c)	125 g

Note: Food items found in this category provide more than 1 milk exchange:

Food	Exchanges per serving	Measure	Mass (Weight)
Milkshake	1 milk + 3 sugars + ½ protein	250 mL (1 c)	300 g
Chocolate milk, 2%	2 milks 2% + 1 sugar	250 mL (1 c)	300 g
Frozen yogurt	1 milk + 1 sugar	125 mL (½ c)	125 g

Table I–6
Canadian Exchange System: Sugars

1 sugar choice = 10 g carbohydrate (sugar), 167 kJ (40 kcal)

Food	Measure	Mass (Weight)
Beverages		
Condensed milk	15 mL (1 tbs)	
Flavoured fruit crystals*	75 mL (⅓ c)	
Iced tea mixes*	75 mL (⅓ c)	
Regular soft drinks	125 mL (½ c)	
Sweet drink mixes*	75 mL (⅓ c)	
Tonic water	125 mL (½ c)	
*These beverages have been made with water.		
Miscellaneous		
Bubble gum (large square)	1 piece	5 g
Cranberry cocktail	75 mL (⅓ c)	80 g
Cranberry cocktail, light	350 mL (1⅓ c)	260 g
Cranberry sauce	30 mL (2 tbs)	
Hard candy mints	2	5 g
Honey, molasses, corn & cane syrup	10 mL (2 tsp)	15 g
Jelly bean	4	10 g
Licorice	1 short stick	10 g
Marshmallows	2 large	15 g
Popsicle	1 stick (½ popsicle)	
Powdered gelatin mix (Jello®) (reconstituted)	50 mL (¼ c)	
Regular jam, jelly, marmalade	15 mL (1 tbs)	
Sugar, white, brown, icing, maple	10 mL (2 tsp)	10 g
Sweet pickles	2 small	100 g
Sweet relish	30 mL (2 tbs)	

Food	Exchanges per Serving	Measures	Mass (Weight)
The following food items provide more than 1 sugar exchange:			
Brownie	1 sugar + 1 fat	1	20 g
Clamato juice	1½ sugars	175 mL (⅔ c)	
Fruit salad, light syrup	1 sugar + 1 fruits & vegetables	125 mL (½ c)	130 g
Aero® bar	2½ sugars + 2½ fats	1 bar	43 g
Smarties®	4½ sugars + 2 fats	1 box	60 g
Sherbet	3 sugars + ½ fat	125 mL (½ c)	95 g

Table I–7
Canadian Exchange System: Protein Foods

1 protein choice = 7 g protein, 3 g fat, 230 kJ (55 kcal)

Food	Measure	Mass (Weight)
Cheese		
Low-fat cheese, about 7% milk fat	1 slice	30 g
Cottage cheese, 2% milkfat or less	50 mL (¼ c)	55 g
Ricotta, about 7% milkfat	50 mL (¼ c)	60 g
Fish		
Anchovies (see *Extras*, Table I–9)		
Canned, drained (e.g., mackerel, salmon, tuna packed in water)	(⅓ of 6.5 oz can)	30 g
Cod tongues, cheeks	75 mL (⅓ c)	50 g
Fillet or steak (e.g., Boston blue, cod, flounder, haddock, halibut, mackerel, orange roughy, perch, pickerel, pike, salmon, shad, snapper, sole, swordfish, trout, tuna, whitefish)	1 piece	30 g
Herring	⅓ fish	30 g
Sardines, smelts	2 medium or 3 small	30 g
Squid, octopus	50 mL (¼ c)	40 g
Shellfish		
Clams, mussels, oysters, scallops, snails	3 medium	30 g
Crab, lobster, flaked	50 mL (¼ c)	30 g
Shrimp, fresh	5 large	30 g
Frozen	10 medium	30 g
Canned	18 small	30 g
Dry pack	50 mL (¼ c)	30 g
Meat and Poultry (e.g., beef, chicken, goat, ham, lamb, pork, turkey, veal, wild game)		
Back, peameal bacon	3 slices, thin	30 g
Chop	½ chop, with bone	40 g
Minced or ground, lean or extra-lean	30 mL (2 tbs)	30 g
Sliced, lean	1 slice	30 g
Steak, lean	1 piece	30 g
Organ Meats		
Hearts, liver	1 slice	30 g
Kidneys, sweetbreads, chopped	50 mL (¼ c)	30 g
Tongue	1 slice	30 g
Tripe	5 pieces	60 g
Soyabean		
Bean curd or tofu	½ block	70 g
Eggs		
In shell, raw or cooked	1 medium	50 g
Without shell, cooked or poached in water	1 medium	45 g
Scrambled	50 mL (¼ c)	55 g

(continued on the next page)

Table I–7 (continued)
Canadian Exchange System: Protein Foods

1 protein choice = 7 g protein, 3 g fat, 230 kJ (55 kcal)			
Food	**Exchanges per Serving**	**Measures**	**Mass (Weight)**
Note: The following choices provide more than 1 protein exchange:			
Cheese			
Cheeses	1 protein + 1 fat	1 piece	25 g
Cheese, coarsely grated (e.g., Cheddar)	1 protein + 1 fat	50 mL (¼ c)	25 g
Cheese, dry, finely grated (e.g., parmesan)	1 protein + 1 fat	45 mL	15 g
Cheese, ricotta, high fat	1 protein + 1 fat	50 mL (¼ c)	55 g
Fish			
Eel	1 protein + 1 fat	1 slice	50 g
Meat			
Bologna	1 protein + 1 fat	1 slice	20 g
Canned lunch meats	1 protein + 1 fat	1 slice	20 g
Corned beef, canned	1 protein + 1 fat	1 slice	25 g
Corned beef, fresh	1 protein + 1 fat	1 slice	25 g
Ground beef, medium-fat	1 protein + 1 fat	30 mL (2 tbs)	25 g
Meat spreads, canned	1 protein + 1 fat	45 mL	35 g
Mutton chop	1 protein + 1 fat	½ chop, with bone	35 g
Paté (see *Fats and Oils* group, Table I–8)			
Sausages, garlic, Polish or knockwurst	1 protein + 1 fat	1 slice	50 g
Sausages, pork, links	1 protein + 1 fat	1 link	25 g
Spareribs or shortribs, with bone	1 protein + 1 fat	1 large	65 g
Stewing beef	1 protein + 1 fat	1 cube	25 g
Summer sausage or salami	1 protein + 1 fat	1 slice	40 g
Weiners, hot dog	1 protein + 1 fat	½ medium	25 g
Miscellaneous			
Blood pudding	1 protein + 1 fat	1 slice	25 g
Peanut butter	1 protein + 1 fat	15 mL (1 tbs)	15 g

I

Table I-8
Canadian Exchange System: Fats and Oils

1 fat choice = 5 g fat, 190 kJ (45 kcal)

Food	Measure	Mass (Weight)
Avocado*	⅛	30 g
Bacon, side, crisp*	1 slice	5 g
Butter*	5 mL (1 tsp)	5 g
Cheese spread	15 mL (1 tbs)	15 g
Coconut, fresh*	45 mL (3 tbs)	15 g
Coconut, dried*	15 mL (1 tbs)	10 g
Cream, Half and half		
(cereal), 10%*	30 mL (2 tbs)	30 g
Light (coffee), 20%*	15 mL (1 tbs)	15 g
Whipping, 32 to 37%*	15 mL (1 tbs)	15 g
Cream cheese*	15 mL (1 tbs)	15 g
Gravy*	30 mL (2 tbs)	30 g
Lard*	5 mL (1 tsp)	5 g
Margarine	5 mL (1 tsp)	5 g
Nuts, shelled:		
Almonds	8	5 g
Brazil nuts	2	10 g
Cashews	5	10 g
Filberts, hazelnuts	5	10 g
Macadamia	3	5 g
Peanuts	10	10g
Pecans	5 halves	5 g
Pignolias, pine nuts	25 mL (5 tsp)	10 g
Pistachios, shelled	20	10 g
Pistachios, in shell	20	20 g
Pumpkin and squash seeds	20 mL (4 tsp)	10 g
Nuts (continued):		
Sesame seeds	15 mL (1 tbs)	10 g
Sunflower seeds		
Shelled	15 mL (1 tbs)	10 g
In shell	45 mL (3 tbs)	15 g
Walnuts	4 halves	10 g
Oil, cooking and salad	5 mL (1 tsp)	5 g
Olives, green	10	45 g
Ripe black	7	57 g
Pâté, liverwurst, meat spreads	15 mL (1 tbs)	15 g
Salad dressing: blue,	10 mL (2 tsp)	10 g
French, Italian, mayonnaise, Thousand Island	5 mL (1 tsp)	5 g
Salad dressing, low-caloric	30 mL (2 tbs)	30 g
Salt pork, raw or cooked*	5 mL (1 tsp)	5 g
Sesame oil	5 mL (1 tsp)	5 g
Sour cream		
12% milkfat	30 mL (2 tbs)	30 g
7% milkfat	60 mL (4 tbs)	60 g
Shortening*	5 mL (1 tsp)	

*These items contain higher amounts of saturated fat.

Table I–9
Canadian Exchange System: Extras

Extras have no more than 2.5 g carbohydrate, 60 kJ (14 kcal)

Vegetables 125 mL (½ c)
Artichokes
Asparagus
Bamboo shoots
Bean sprouts, mung or soya
Beans, string, green, or yellow
Bitter melon (balsam pear)
Bok choy
Broccoli
Brussels sprouts
Cabbage
Cauliflower
Celery
Chard
Cucumbers
Eggplant
Endive
Fiddleheads
Greens: beet, collard, dandelion, mustard, turnip, etc.
Kale
Kohlrabi
Leeks
Lettuce
Mushrooms
Okra
Onions, green or mature
Parsley
Peppers, green, yellow or red
Radishes
Rapini
Rhubarb
Sauerkraut
Shallots
Spinach
Sprouts: alfalfa, radish, etc.
Tomato wedges
Watercress
Zucchini

Free Foods (may be used without measuring)
Artificial sweetener, such as cyclamate or aspartame
Baking powder, baking soda
Bouillon from cube, powder, or liquid
Bouillon or clear broth
Chowchow, unsweetened
Coffee, clear
Consommé
Dulse
Flavorings and extracts
Garlic
Gelatin, unsweetened
Ginger root
Herbal teas, unsweetened
Horseradish, uncreamed
Lemon juice or lemon wedges
Lime juice or lime wedges
Marjoram, cinnamon, etc.
Mineral water
Mustard
Parsley
Pimentos
Salt, pepper, thyme
Soda water, club soda
Soya sauce
Sugar-free Crystal Drink
Sugar-free Jelly Powder
Sugar-free soft drinks
Tea, clear
Vinegar
Water
Worcestershire sauce

Condiments

Food	**Measure**
Anchovies	2 fillets
Barbecue sauce	15 mL (1 tbs)
Bran, natural	30 mL (2 tbs)
Brewer's yeast	5 mL (1 tsp)
Carob powder	5 mL (1 tsp)
Catsup	5 mL (1 tsp)
Chili sauce	5 mL (1 tsp)
Cocoa powder	5 mL (1 tsp)
Cranberry sauce, unsweetened	15 mL (1 tbs)
Dietetic fruit spreads	5 mL (1 tsp)
Maraschino cherries	1
Nondairy coffee whitener	5 mL (1 tsp)
Nuts, chopped pieces	5 mL (1 tsp)
Pickles	
unsweetened dill	2
sour mixed	11
Sugar substitutes, granular	5 mL (1 tsp)
Whipped toppings	15 mL (1 tbs)

Table I-10
Canadian Exchange System: Combined Food Choices

Food	Exchanges per serving	Measure	Mass (Weight)
Angel food cake	½ starch + 2½ sugars	1/12 cake	50 g
Apple crisp	½ starch + 1½ fruits & vegetables + 1 sugar + 1–2 fats	125 mL (½ c)	
Applesauce, sweetened	1 fruits & vegetables + 1 sugar	125 mL (½ c)	
Beans and pork in tomato sauce	1 starch + ½ fruits & vegetables + ½ sugar + 1 protein	125 mL (½ c)	135 g
Beef burrito	2 starches + 3 proteins + 3 fats		110 g
Brownie	1 sugar + 1 fat	1	20 g
Cabbage rolls*	1 starch + 2 proteins	3	310 g
Caesar salad	2–4 fats	20 mL dressing (4 tsp)	
Cheesecake	½ starch + 2 sugars + ½ protein + 5 fats	1 piece	80 g
Chicken fingers	1 starch + 2 proteins + 2 fats	6 small	100 g
Chicken and snow pea Oriental	2 starches + ½ fruits & vegetables + 3 proteins + 1 fat	500 mL (2 c)	
Chili	1½ starches + ½ fruits & vegetables + 3½ protein	300 mL (1¼ c)	325 g
Chips			
Potato chips	1 starch + 2 fats	15 chips	30 g
Corn chips	1 starch + 2 fats	30 chips	30 g
Tortilla chips	1 starch + 1½ fats	13 chips	
Cheese twist	1 starch + 1½ fats	30 chips	30 g
Chocolate bar			
Aero®	2½ sugars + 2½ fats	bar	43 g
Smarties®	4½ sugars + 2 fats	package	60 g
Chocolate cake (without icing)	1 starch + 2 sugars + 3 fats	1/10 of a 8″ pan	
Chocolate devil's food cake (without icing)	2 starches + 2 sugars + 3 fats	1/12 of a 9″ pan	
Chocolate milk	2 milks 2% + 1 sugar	250 mL (1 c)	300 g
Clubhouse (triple-decker) sandwich	3 starches + 3 proteins + 4 fats		
Cookies			
chocolate chip	½ starch + ½ sugar + 1½ fats	2	22 g
oatmeal	1 starch + 1 sugar + 1 fat	2	40 g
Donut (chocolate glazed)	1 starch + 1½ sugars + 2 fats	1	65 g
Egg roll	1 starch + ½ protein + 1 fat		75 g
Four bean salad	1 starch + ½ protein + 1 fat	125 mL (½ c)	
French toast	1 starch + ½ protein + 2 fats	1 slice	65 g
Fruit in heavy syrup	1 fruits & vegetables + 1½ sugars	125 mL (½ c)	
Granola bar	½ starch + 1 sugar + 1–2 fats		30 g
Granola cereal	1 starch + 1 sugar + 2 fats	125 mL (½ c)	45 g
Hamburger	2 starches + 3 proteins + 2 fats	junior size	
Ice cream and cone, plain flavour			
Ice cream	½ milk + 2–3 sugars + 1–2 fats		100 g
Cone	½ sugar		4 g
Lasagna			
regular cheese	1 starch + 1 fruits & vegetables + 3 proteins + 2 fats	3″ x 4″ piece	
low-fat cheese	1 starch + 1 fruits & vegetables + 3 proteins	3″ x 4″ piece	

* If eaten with sauce, add ½ fruits & vegetables exchange.

(continued on the next page)

Table I–10 (continued)
Canadian Exchange System: Combined Food Choices

Food	Exchanges per serving	Measure	Mass (Weight)
Legumes			
Dried beans (kidney, navy, pinto, fava, chick peas)	2 starches + 1 protein	250 mL (1 c)	180 g
Dried peas	2 starches + 1 protein	250 mL (1 c)	210 g
Lentils	2 starches + 1 protein	250 mL (1 c)	210 g
Macaroni and cheese	2 starches + 2 proteins + 2 fats	250 mL (1 c)	210 g
Minestrone soup	1½ starches + ½ fruits & vegetables + ½ fat	250 mL (1 c)	
Muffin	1 starch + ½ sugar + 1 fat	1 small	45 g
Nuts (dry or roasted without any oil added).			
Almonds, dried sliced	½ protein + 2 fats	50 mL (¼ c)	22 g
Brazil nuts, dried unblanched	½ protein + 2½ fats	5 large	23 g
Cashew nuts, dry roasted	½ starch + ½ protein + 2 fats	50 mL (¼ c)	28 g
Filbert hazelnut, dry	½ protein + 3½ fats	50 mL (¼ c)	30 g
Macadamia nuts, dried	½ protein + 4 fats	50 mL (¼ c)	28 g
Peanuts, raw	1 protein + 2 fats	50 mL (¼ c)	30 g
Pecans, dry roasted	½ fruits & vegetables + 3 fats	50 mL (¼ c)	22 g
Pine nuts, pignolia dried	1 protein + 3 fats	50 mL (¼ c)	34 g
Pistachio nuts, dried	½ fruits & vegetables + ½ protein + 2 ½ fats	50 mL (¼ c)	27 g
Pumpkin seeds, roasted	2 proteins + 2½ fats	50 mL (¼ c)	47 g
Sesame seeds, whole dried	½ fruits & vegetables + ½ protein + 2½ fats	50 mL (¼ c)	30 g
Sunflower kernel, dried	½ protein + 1½ fats	50 mL (¼ c)	17 g
Walnuts, dried chopped	½ protein + 3 fats	50 mL (¼ c)	26 g
Perogies	2 starches + 1 protein + 1 fat	3	
Pie, fruit	1 starch + 1 fruits & vegetables + 2 sugars + 3 fats	1 piece	120 g
Pizza, cheese	1 starch + 1 protein + 1 fat	1 slice (⅛ of a 12″)	50 g
Pork stir fry	½ to 1 fruits & vegetables + 3 proteins	200 mL (¾ c)	
Potato salad	1 starch + 1 fat	125 mL (½ c)	130 g
Potatoes, scalloped	2 starches + 1 milk + 1–2 fats	200 mL (¾ c)	210 g
Pudding, bread or rice	1 starch + 1 sugar +1 fat	125 mL (½ c)	
Pudding, vanilla	1 milk + 2 sugars	125 mL (½ c)	
Raisin bran cereal	1 starch + ½ fruits & vegetables + ½ sugar	175 mL (⅔ c)	40 g
Rice krispie squares	½ starch + 1½ sugars + ½ fat	1 square	30 g
Shepherd's pie	2 starches + 1 fruits & vegetables + 3 proteins	325 mL (1⅓ c)	
Sherbet, orange	3 sugars + ½ fat	125 mL (½ c)	
Spaghetti and meat sauce	2 starches + 1 fruits & vegetables + 2 proteins + 3 fats	250 mL (1 c)	
Stew	2 starches + 2 fruits & vegetables + 3 proteins + ½ fat	200 mL (¾ c)	
Sundae	4 sugars + 3 fats	125 mL (½ c)	
Tuna casserole	1 starch + 2 proteins + ½ fat	125 mL (½ c)	
Yogurt, fruit bottom	1 fruits & vegetables + 1 milk + 1 sugar	125 mL (½ c)	125 g
Yogurt, frozen	1 milk + 1 sugar	125 mL (½ c)	125 g

FOOD LABELS

◆

Consumers can gather a lot of information from a nutrition label. Figure I–1 demonstrates the reading of a food label and Table I–11 defines terms.

Figure I–1

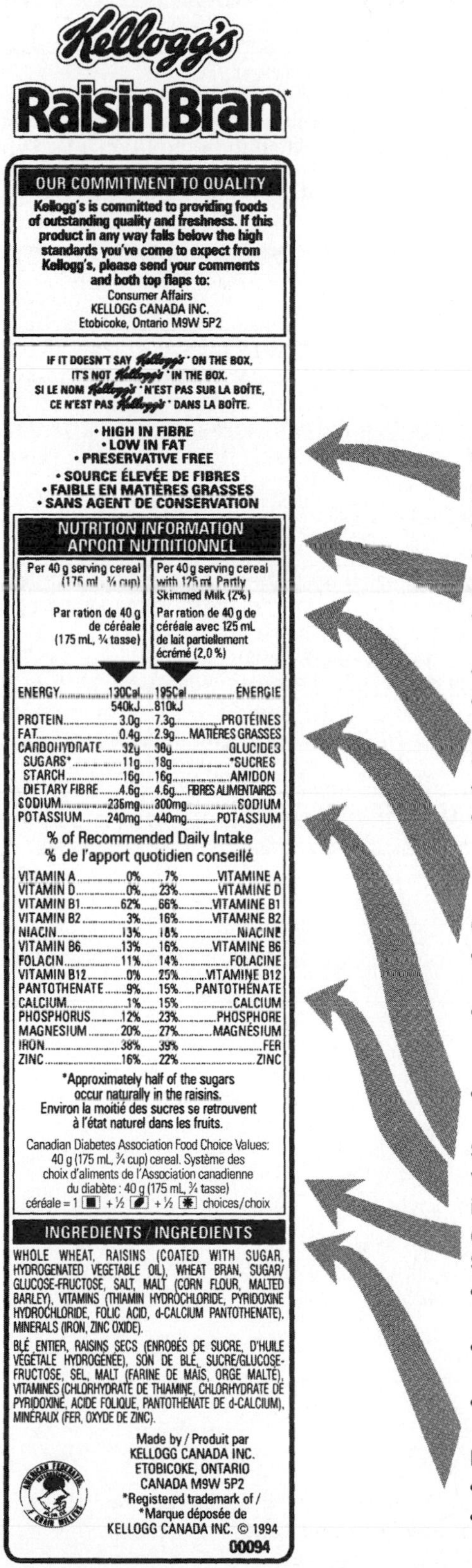
Kellogg's
RaisinBran*
OUR COMMITMENT TO QUALITY
Kellogg's is committed to providing foods of outstanding quality and freshness. If this product in any way falls below the high standards you've come to expect from Kellogg's, please send your comments and both top flaps to:
Consumer Affairs
KELLOGG CANADA INC.
Etobicoke, Ontario M9W 5P2
IF IT DOESN'T SAY Kellogg's ON THE BOX, IT'S NOT Kellogg's IN THE BOX.
SI LE NOM Kellogg's N'EST PAS SUR LA BOÎTE, CE N'EST PAS Kellogg's DANS LA BOÎTE.
• HIGH IN FIBRE
• LOW IN FAT
• PRESERVATIVE FREE
• SOURCE ÉLEVÉE DE FIBRES
• FAIBLE EN MATIÈRES GRASSES
• SANS AGENT DE CONSERVATION
NUTRITION INFORMATION
APPORT NUTRITIONNEL
Per 40 g serving cereal (175 mL, ¾ cup)
Par ration de 40 g de céréale (175 mL, ¾ tasse)
Per 40 g serving cereal with 125 mL Partly Skimmed Milk (2%)
Par ration de 40 g de céréale avec 125 mL de lait partiellement écrémé (2,0 %)
ENERGY 130Cal 195Cal ÉNERGIE
540kJ 810kJ
PROTEIN 3.0g 7.3g PROTÉINES
FAT 0.4g 2.9g MATIÈRES GRASSES
CARBOHYDRATE 32g 38g GLUCIDES
SUGARS* 11g 18g *SUCRES
STARCH 16g 16g AMIDON
DIETARY FIBRE 4.6g 4.6g FIBRES ALIMENTAIRES
SODIUM 235mg 300mg SODIUM
POTASSIUM 240mg 440mg POTASSIUM
% of Recommended Daily Intake
% de l'apport quotidien conseillé
VITAMIN A 0% 7% VITAMINE A
VITAMIN D 0% 23% VITAMINE D
VITAMIN B1 62% 66% VITAMINE B1
VITAMIN B2 3% 16% VITAMINE B2
NIACIN 13% 18% NIACINE
VITAMIN B6 13% 16% VITAMINE B6
FOLACIN 11% 14% FOLACINE
VITAMIN B12 0% 25% VITAMINE B12
PANTOTHENATE 9% 15% PANTOTHÉNATE
CALCIUM 1% 15% CALCIUM
PHOSPHORUS 12% 23% PHOSPHORE
MAGNESIUM 20% 27% MAGNÉSIUM
IRON 38% 39% FER
ZINC 16% 22% ZINC
*Approximately half of the sugars occur naturally in the raisins.
Environ la moitié des sucres se retrouvent à l'état naturel dans les fruits.
Canadian Diabetes Association Food Choice Values: 40 g (175 mL, ¾ cup) cereal. Système des choix d'aliments de l'Association canadienne du diabète : 40 g (175 mL, ¾ tasse) céréale = 1 + ½ + ½ choices/choix
INGREDIENTS / INGREDIENTS
WHOLE WHEAT, RAISINS (COATED WITH SUGAR, HYDROGENATED VEGETABLE OIL), WHEAT BRAN, SUGAR/GLUCOSE-FRUCTOSE, SALT, MALT (CORN FLOUR, MALTED BARLEY), VITAMINS (THIAMIN HYDROCHLORIDE, PYRIDOXINE HYDROCHLORIDE, FOLIC ACID, d-CALCIUM PANTOTHENATE), MINERALS (IRON, ZINC OXIDE).
BLÉ ENTIER, RAISINS SECS (ENROBÉS DE SUCRE, D'HUILE VÉGÉTALE HYDROGÉNÉE), SON DE BLÉ, SUCRE/GLUCOSE-FRUCTOSE, SEL, MALT (FARINE DE MAÏS, ORGE MALTÉ), VITAMINES (CHLORHYDRATE DE THIAMINE, CHLORHYDRATE DE PYRIDOXINE, ACIDE FOLIQUE, PANTOTHÉNATE DE d-CALCIUM), MINÉRAUX (FER, OXYDE DE ZINC).
Made by / Produit par
KELLOGG CANADA INC.
ETOBICOKE, ONTARIO
CANADA M9W 5P2
*Registered trademark of / *Marque déposée de
KELLOGG CANADA INC. © 1994
00094

WHAT YOU WILL FIND ON A LABEL:

Nutrition Claims

- in Canada, it is optional for a company to decide to use claims,
- when claims appear on a label, they must follow government laws

Nutrition Information

- gives detailed nutrition facts about the product, including serving size and core list
- does not have to appear by law on food products in Canada
- refers to the food as packaged, so if you add milk, eggs or other food, the nutritional content of the food you eat can be very different

Serving Size

- the amount of food for which the information is given
- check the serving size: the serving size on the label may not be the same as the serving size you would actually eat (for example, the serving size of cereal may be ¾ cup, much smaller than your regular serving

Core List

- the energy (in Calories and kilojoules), grams of protein, fat and carbohydrate for each serving
- some products break down fat into monounsaturates, polyunsaturates, saturates, and cholesterol (to find out what these mean, look at the Fats & Oils section)
- carbohydrates may include the amount of sugars, starch and fibre, or may list these items separately

Sodium and Potassium (in milligrams)

Vitamins and Minerals (as percent of your recommended daily intake)

Canadian Diabetes Association Food Choice Values and Symbols

- the Values and Symbols are tools to help you fit the food into your meal plan, they are not an endorsement by CDA
- it is up to the food company to decide if they want their foods analyzed and assigned symbols
- when they are on a label, they have been assigned by a dietitian working for CDA, so you can be sure the information is correct

Ingredients

- must be found on all food labels by law
- ingredients are listed in decreasing order by weight, so what you see first is what you get the most of

Table I–11
Terms on Food Labels

Energy
kcalorie reduced: 50% or fewer kcalories than the regular version. **light:** term may be used to describe anything (for example, light in colour, texture, flavour, taste, or kcalories); read the label to find out what is "light" about the product. **low kcalorie:** kcalorie-reduced and no more than 15 kcalories per serving.
Fat and Cholesterol
low cholesterol: no more than 3 mg of cholesterol per 100 g of the food and low in saturated fat; *does not* always mean low in total fat. **low fat:** no more than 3 g of fat per serving; *does not* always mean low in kcalories. **lower fat:** at least 25% less fat than the comparison food; be aware that 80% fat-free still means the food is 20% fat.
Carbohydrates: Fibre and Sugar
carbohydrate reduced: not more than 50% of the carbohydrate found in the regular version; *does not* always mean the product is lower in kcalories because other ingredients such as fat may have increased. **source of dietary fibre:** a product that provides 2–4 g of fibre. **high source of dietary fibre:** a product that provides 4–6 g of fibre. **very high source of fibre:** a product that provides 6 g (or more) of fibre. **sugar free:** low in carbohydrates and kcalories; can be used as an extra food in the exchange system. **unsweetened or no sugar added:** no sugar was added to the product; sugar may be found naturally in the food (for example, fruit canned in its own juice).

I

MEASURES OF PROTEIN QUALITY

Contents

In a world where food is scarce and many people's diets contain marginal or inadequate amounts of protein, it is important to know which foods contain the highest-quality protein. Chapter 6 describes protein quality and the different measures researchers use to assess the quality of a food protein. This appendix provides a few more details.

AMINO ACID SCORING

Amino acid, or chemical, scoring allows researchers to determine the amino acid composition of any protein relatively inexpensively, but unfortunately, it does not always accurately reflect the way the body will use a protein. The advantages of amino acid scoring are that it is simple and inexpensive, it identifies in one step the limiting amino acid, and it can be used to score mixtures of different proportions of two or more proteins mathematically without having to make up a mixture and test it. Its chief weaknesses are that it fails to predict the digestibility of a protein, which may strongly affect the protein's quality; it relies on a chemical procedure in which certain amino acids may be destroyed, making the pattern that is analyzed inaccurate; and it is blind to other features of the protein (such as the presence of substances that may inhibit the digestion or utilization of the protein) that would only be revealed by a test in living animals. Table J–1 shows how to use a reference pattern for the nine essential amino acids.

PDCAAS

PDCAAS (protein-digestibility-corrected amino acid score) takes the amino acid scoring method a step further by correcting for the digestibility of the protein. To calculate the PDCAAS, researchers first determine the amino acid profile of the test protein (in this example, pinto beans). The second column of Table J–2 presents the essential amino acid profile for pinto beans. The third column presents the amino acid requirements of preschool-aged children for comparison. To determine how well the food protein meets human needs, researchers calculate the ratio by dividing the second column by the third column (for example, $30 \div 19 = 1.578$ or 1.58).

The amino acid with the lowest ratio is the first limiting amino acid—in this case, tryptophan. Its ratio is the amino acid score for the protein—in this case, 80. Remember, though, the amino acid score does not account for digestibility. Protein digestibility, as determined by rat balance studies, yields a value of 79 percent for pinto beans. Together, the amino acid score and the digestibility value determine the PDCAAS:

$$\text{PDCAAS} = \text{protein digestibility} \times \text{lowest amino acid ratio.}$$

$$\text{PDCAAS for pinto beans} = .79 \times .80 = 63\%.$$

Thus the PDCAAS for pinto beans is 63 percent (or 0.63).

The PDCAAS is used to determine the % Daily Value on food labels. To calculate the % Daily Value for protein for canned pinto beans, multiply the number of grams of protein in a standard serving (in this case, 7 grams per ½ cup) by the PDCAAS:

$$7\text{ g} \times .63 = 4.41.$$

This value is then divided by the RDI for protein (for children over age four and adults, the RDI is 50 grams):

$$4.41 \div 50 = 0.088 \text{ (or 8.8\%).}$$

The food label for this can of pinto beans would declare that one serving provides 7 grams protein, and if the label included a % Daily Value for protein, the value would be 9 percent.

BIOLOGICAL VALUE

To determine the actual value of a protein as it is used by the body, it is necessary to measure both urinary and fecal losses of nitrogen

Table J-1
A Reference Pattern for Amino Acid Scoring of Proteins

Essential Amino Acids	Reference Protein (Whole Egg) Mg Amino Acid per G Nitrogen
Histidine	145
Isoleucine	340
Leucine	540
Lysine	440
Methionine + cystine[a]	355
Phenylalanine + tyrosine[b]	580
Threonine	294
Tryptophan	106
Valine	410
Total	3210

[a]Methionine is essential and is also used to make cystine. Thus the methionine requirement is lower if cystine is supplied.

[b]Phenylalanine is essential and is also used to make tyrosine if not enough of the latter is available. Thus the phenylalanine requirement is lower if tyrosine is also supplied.

Note: To interpret the table, read, "For every 3210 units of essential amino acids, 145 must be histidine, 340 must be isoleucine, 540 must be leucine," and so on. To compare a test protein with the reference protein, the experimenter first obtains a chemical analysis of the test protein's amino acids. Then, taking 3210 units of the amino acids, the experimenter compares the amount of each amino acid to the amount found in 3210 units of essential amino acids in egg protein. For example, suppose the test protein contained (per 3210 units) 360 units of isoleucine; 500 units of leucine; 350 of lysine; and for each of the other amino acids, more units than egg protein contains. The two amino acids that are low are leucine (500 as compared with 540 in egg) and lysine (350 versus 440 in egg). The ratio, amino acid in the test protein divided by amino acid in egg, is 500/540 (or about 0.93) for leucine and 350/440 (or about 0.80) for lysine. Lysine is the limiting amino acid (lowest ratio compared with egg), so the test protein receives a chemical score of 80.

J

when that protein is actually fed to human beings under test conditions. Even then, small additional losses from sweat, shed skin, hair, and fingernails will be missed. This kind of experiment determines the biological value (BV) of proteins, a measure used internationally.

In a test of biological value, two nitrogen balance studies are done. In the first, no protein is fed, and nitrogen (N) excretions in the urine and feces are measured. It is assumed that under these conditions, N lost in the urine is the amount the body always necessarily loses by filtration into the urine each day, regardless of what protein is fed (endogenous N). The N lost in the feces (called metabolic N in the equation) is the amount the body invariably loses into the intestine each day, whether or not food protein is fed. (To help you remember the terms: endogenous N is "urinary N on a zero-protein diet"; metabolic N is "fecal N on a zero-protein diet.")

In the second study, an amount of protein slightly below the requirement is fed. Intake and losses are measured; then the BV is derived using this formula:

Table J-2
An Example of PDCAAS

Essential Amino Acids	Amino Acid Profile of Pinto Beans (mg/g protein)	Amino Acid Requirements for 2–5 yr (mg/g protein)	Ratio
Histidine	30.0	19	1.58
Isoleucine	42.5	28	1.52
Leucine	80.4	66	1.22
Lysine	69.0	58	1.19
Methionine + cystine	21.1	25	0.84
Phenylalanine + tyrosine	90.5	63	1.44
Threonine	43.7	34	1.28
Tryptophan	8.8	11	0.80
Valine	50.1	35	1.43

$$\text{BV} = \frac{\text{food N} - (\text{fecal N} - \text{metabolic N}) - (\text{urinary N} - \text{endogenous N})}{\text{food N} - (\text{fecal N} - \text{metabolic N})} \times 100.$$

The denominator of this equation expresses the amount of nitrogen *absorbed:* food N minus fecal N (excluding the N the body would lose in the feces anyway, even without food). The numerator expresses the amount of N *retained* from the N absorbed: absorbed N (as in the denominator) minus the N excreted in the urine (excluding the N the body would lose in the urine anyway, even without food). Thus it can be more simply expressed:

$$\text{BV} = \frac{\text{N retained}}{\text{N absorbed}} \times 100.$$

This method has the advantages of being based on experiments with human beings (it can be done with animals, too, of course) and of measuring actual nitrogen retention. But it is also cumbersome, expensive, and often impractical, and it is based on several assumptions that may not be valid. For example, the physiology, normal environment, or typical food intake of the subjects used for testing may not be similar to those for whom the test protein may ultimately be used. For another example, the retention of protein in the body does not necessarily mean that it is being well utilized. Considerable exchange of protein among tissues (protein turnover) occurs, but is hidden from view when only N intake and output are measured. The test of biological value wouldn't detect if one tissue were shorted.

NET PROTEIN UTILIZATION

Like measurements of BV, determinations of net protein utilization (NPU) involve two balance studies: one on zero nitrogen intake, and the other on submaximal intake. The formula for NPU is:

$$\text{NPU} = \frac{\text{food N} - (\text{fecal N} - \text{metabolic N}) - (\text{urinary N} - \text{endogenous N})}{\text{food N}} \times 100.$$

The numerator is the same as it is for BV, but the denominator represents food N intake only—not absorbed N. More simply exprssed:

$$\text{NPU} = \frac{\text{N retained}}{\text{N intake}} \times 100.$$

This method offers advantages similar to those of BV determinations and is used more frequently, with animals as the test subjects. A drawback is that if a low NPU is obtained, the test results offer no help in distinguishing between two possible causes: a poor amino acid composition of the test protein or poor digestibility. There is also a limit to the extent to which animal test results can be assumed to be applicable to human beings.

PROTEIN EFFICIENCY RATIO

The protein efficiency ratio (PER) is a widely used procedure for evaluating protein quality. Young rats are fed a measured amount of protein and weighed periodically as they grow. The PER is expressed as:

$$\text{PER} = \frac{\text{weight gain (g)}}{\text{protein intake (g)}}.$$

This method has the virtues of economy and simplicity, but it also has many drawbacks. The experiments are time-consuming; the amino acid needs of rats are not the same as those of human beings; and the amino acid needs for growth are not the same as for the maintenance of adult animals (growing animals need more lysine, for example).

CHAPTER 1: PROBLEM SET ANSWERS

1.

Food	Item No.	Weight (g)	Water (%)	Protein (g)	Carbo-hydrate (g)	Fiber (g)	Fat (g)
Swiss cheese, 1 oz	64	28	37	8	1	0	8
Fried egg, 1	153	46	69	6	1	0	7
Cauliflower, cooked, ½ c	839	62	93	1	3	1	<1

a. 1 oz swiss cheese: **37% of 28 g = 10 g water.**
1 fried egg: **69% of 46 g = 32 g water.**
½ c cooked cauliflower: **93% of 62 g = 58 g water.**

b. 1 oz swiss cheese: **28 g − 10 g water = 18 g solids.**
1 fried egg: **46 g − 32 g water = 14 g solids.**
½ c cooked cauliflower: **62 g − 58 g water = 4 g solids.**

c. 1 oz swiss cheese: **8 g protein + 1 g carbohydrate + 0 g fiber + 8 g fat = 17 g energy nutrients and fiber.**
1 fried egg: **6 g protein +1 g carbohydrate + 0 g fiber + 7 g fat = 14 g energy nutrients and fiber.**
½ c cooked cauliflower: **1 g protein + 3 g carbohydrate + 1 g fiber + <1 g fat = 5 g energy nutrients and fiber.**

d. 1 oz swiss cheese: **18 g solids − 17 g energy nutrients and fiber leaves 1 g unaccounted for.**
1 fried egg: **14 g solids − 14 g energy nutrients and fiber leaves 0 g unaccounted for.**
½ c cooked cauliflower: **4 g solids − 5 g energy nutrients and fiber leaves 0 g unaccounted for.** (The apparent excess of energy nutrients and fiber indicates a rounding error, and the answer is that no grams remain unaccounted for.)

2. a. (5 ft × 12 in/ft) + 9 in = 69 in.
69 in × 2.54 cm/in = 175 cm.

b. 170 lb × 1 kg/2.2 lb = 77 kg.

c. ½ liter water: **2 c.**
100 g minced onion: **½ c.**
5 g garlic: **1 tsp.**

d. 1 kJ = **0.24 kcal.**
1 kcal = **4.2 kJ.**
400 kJ × 0.24 kcal/kJ = 96 kcal.
80 kcal × 4.2 kJ/kcal = 336 kJ.

3. a. 5 g protein × 4 kcal/g = 20 kcal protein.
30 g carbohydrate × 4 kcal/g = 120 kcal carbohydrate.
11 g fat × 9 kcal/g = 99 kcal fat.
Total = 239 kcal.

b. 20 kcal/239 kcal × 100 = 8.4% from protein.
120 kcal/239 kcal × 100 = 50.2% from carbohydrate.
99 kcal/239 kcal × 100 = 41.4% from fat.
Total = 100.0%.

c. No. 15 g protein × 4 kcal/g = 60 kcal.

CHAPTER 2: PROBLEM SET ANSWERS

1. a.

Item No./Food		Energy (kcal)	Calcium (mg)	Iron (mg)	Vitamin C (mg)
#93	Whole milk, 1 c	149	290	0.12	2
#98	Nonfat milk, 1 c	85	301	0.10	2
#41	Cottage cheese, 1 c	216	126	0.29	0
#598	Ground beef patty, 4 oz	318	14	2.78	0
#876	Navy beans, cooked, 1 c	258	127	4.51	2
#269	Fresh orange juice, 1 c	111	27	0.50	124

Item No./Food		b. Calcium Density (mg/100 kcal)	d. Iron Density (mg/100 kcal)	h. Vitamin C Density (mg/100 kcal)
#93	Whole milk	195	0.08	1.3
#98	Nonfat milk	354	0.12	2.4
#41	Cottage cheese	58	0.13	0
#598	Ground beef patty	4	0.87	0
#876	Navy beans	49	1.75	0.8
#269	Orange juice	24	0.45	111.7

c. The nonfat milk.
e. The navy beans.
f. The whole milk.
g. Milk is dense in calcium, but not in iron.
i. The orange juice.

2. a.

"A" Meal Item No./Food		Energy (kcal)	Iron (mg)	Vitamin A (μg RE)	Vitamin C (mg)
#637	Fried, batter-dipped chicken thigh, 1	238	1.25	25	0
#715	Potato salad with mayonnaise and eggs, ½ c	179	0.81	41	12
#800	Snap beans cooked from fresh, 1 c	44	1.6	84	12
#211	Unsweetened applesauce, ½ c	52	0.15	4	2
Totals:		513	3.81	154	26

b.

"B" Meal Item No./Food	Energy (kcal)	Iron (mg)	Vitamin A (μg RE)	Vitamin C (mg)
Previous totals from "A" meal	513	3.81	154	26
Minus chicken from "A" meal	−238	−1.25	−25	−0
Plus #652 Dark-meat turkey, 4 oz	212	2.64	0	0
New totals:	487	5.2	129	26

c. It reduced the kcalories and added more iron.
d. 5.2 mg − 3.81 mg = 1.39 mg.
e. 1.39 mg/15 mg × 100 = 9.3%.
f. Yes.
g. 154 μg RE − 129 μg RE = 25 μg RE.
h. 25 μg RE/800 μg RE × 100 = about 3%.
i. Yes.
j.

"C" Meal Item No./Food	Energy (kcal)	Iron (mg)	Vitamin A (μg RE)	Vitamin C (mg)
Previous totals from "B" meal	487	5.2	129	26
Minus potato salad from "A" meal	−179	−0.81	−41	−12
Plus #797 lima beans, ½ c	85	1.16	16	11
New totals:	393	5.55	104	25

k. It reduced the kcalories further and added more iron.
l. The meal lost 41 μg RE of vitamin A and gained 16 μg RE. Total loss was 25 μg RE, which is less than 5% of the vitamin A RDA, and so is not significant. Vitamin C loss was 1 mg, not significiant compared with an RDA of 60 mg.

m.

"D" Meal Item No./Food	Energy (kcal)	Iron (mg)	Vitamin A (μg RE)	Vitamin C (mg)
Previous totals from "C" meal	393	5.55	104	25
Minus snap beans from "A" meal	−44	−1.6	−84	−12
Plus #822 chopped broccoli, 1 c	51	1.12	348	74
New totals:	400	5.07	368	87

n. Vitamins A and C.

o.

	Energy (kcal)	Iron (mg)	Vitamin A (μg RE)	Vitamin C (mg)
Meal "A"	513	3.81	154	26
Meal "D"	400	5.07	368	87
Change	Significantly less	Significantly more	Significantly more	Significantly more

CHAPTER 4: PROBLEM SET ANSWERS

1. a. One package of M&Ms contains 228 kcal, so you could eat about two packages.
   b. One peach has 37 kcal: 450/37 = 12.16. You could eat a dozen peaches.
   c. One piece of melba toast has 19 kcal: 450/19 = 23.68. You could eat about two dozen pieces of melba toast.
   d. One frozen fruit juice bar has 63 kcal: 450/63 = 7.14. You could eat about 7 fruit juice bars.
   e. One cup of this ice cream has 357 kcal: 450/357 = 1.26. You could eat almost 1⅓ c of rich vanilla ice cream.
2. a. Yes, because 33 g of carbohydrate are equal to 132 kcal, which is more than half of 200 kcal.
   b. ½ c; 94 kcal; 2 g; 2 g × 4 kcal/g = 8 kcal; no; no.
   c. 1 c; 166 kcal; 35 g; 140 kcal; yes (84%); yes.
3.

	5 Servings of Vegetables and Fruits	Serving Size (from Figure 2-1)	Carbohydrate per Serving (g)
a.	Banana (item #223)	1 ea	27
b.	Fresh orange juice (item #269)	¾ c	19.5
c.	Black-eyed peas (item #816)	½ c	20
d.	Corn (item #847)	½ c	17
e.	Mashed potatoes (item #910)	½ c	18
	6 Servings of Grains		
f.	English muffin (item #433)	½	13
g.	Cooked oatmeal (item #491)	½ c	12.5
h.	Sliced wheat bread (item #357)	1 slice	12
i.	Bagel (item #326)	½	18
j.	Brown rice (item #542)	½ c	22.5
k.	Macaroni (item #532)	½ c	20
l.	Total		199.5 g

m. About half of the energy, or 750 kcal, should come from carbohydrate. At 4 kcal/g, 750 kcal are equal to about 188 g of carbohydrate. These foods deliver 199.5 g of carbohydrate, so yes, these foods do meet the recommended intake and also confirm that 5 servings of fruits and vegetables and 6 servings of grains help a person meet carbohydrate needs.

CHAPTER 5: PROBLEM SET ANSWERS

1. a.

Item No./Food	Energy (kcal)	Fat (g)	Calcium (mg)	Iron (mg)	Vitamin C (mg)
#1262 2-pc chicken dinner	829	49	161	2.51	36
#1265 Mashed potatoes, ⅓ c	60	1	21	0.28	4
#1268 Corn-on-the-cob, 1	176	3	7	0.8	2
Totals:	1065	53	189	3.59	42

b. 1065 kcal ÷ 2000 kcal × 100 = 53% of the day's energy.
c. This meal delivers 53 g fat and the Daily Value for fat is 65 g. 53 g ÷ 65 g = 0.815 or 81.5% of the day's fat allowance.
d. The person has almost half of the day's kcalories still to consume, but has eaten a much higher percentage of fat in the first half than recommended. The person should choose low-fat or nonfat foods for the rest of the day.
e. 1065 kcal ÷ 6000 kcal × 100 = 18% of the day's energy. 30% of 6000 kcal = 1800 kcal of fat allowed. 53 g × 9 kcal/g = 477 kcal fat, 477 ÷ 1800 = 26.5% of the day's fat allowance. This person has about 80% of his day's kcalories still to eat and almost 75% of the day's fat.
f.

Item No./Food	Energy (kcal)	Fat (g)	Calcium (mg)	Iron (mg)	Vitamin C (mg)
#1262 2-pc chicken dinner	829	49	161	2.51	36
#1269 Coleslaw, ⅓ c	103	6	28	0.17	19
#1268 Corn-on-the-cob, 1	176	3	7	0.8	2
Totals:	1108	58	196	3.48	57

g. Yes/no; because potatoes are almost all carbohydrate, and the coleslaw has a high-fat dressing on it.
h. Vitamin C, because cabbage contains more vitamin C than potatoes and neither vegetable contributes much calcium or iron.
i.

Item No./Food	Energy (kcal)	Fat (g)	Calcium (mg)	Iron (mg)	Vitamin C (mg)
#1401 Chunky chicken salad, 1	147	4	39	1.06	26
#1269 Coleslaw, ⅓ c	103	6	28	0.17	19
#1268 Corn-on-the-cob, 1	176	3	7	0.8	2
Totals:	426	13	74	2.03	47

2. a.

Item No./Food	Energy (kcal)	Fat (g)	Acceptable? Yes	No
#1724 Ice cream, ½ c	230	17		X
# 133 Sherbet, ½ c	133	2	X	
# 147 Vanilla yogurt, 1 c	193	3	X	
#1584 Yogurt, frozen, low-fat, ½ c	138	5	X	
# 318 Strawberries fresh, whole, 1 c	45	1	X	
# 372 Angel food cake, 1 piece	137	<1	X	
# 384 Carrot cake, 1 piece	488	30		X
# 404 Brownie, homemade, 1	93	6		X
# 407 Chocolate chip cookies, 4	213	10		X
# 464 Pecan pie, 1 piece	552	25		X
# 778 Popsicle, 1	68	0	X	
#1131 Snickers candy bar, 1	278	14		X

K

b. The person needed to have eaten 25 fewer g of fat at earlier meals and so should have planned better and selected more low-fat, nutrient-dense options early in the day. Alternatively, the recipe on the carrot cake could have been modified to lower the fat.

3.

	Milk A	Milk B	Milk C
a.	3%	2%	0%
b.	72 kcal	45 kcal	0 kcal
c.	152 kcal	125 kcal	80 kcal
d.	47%	36%	0%
e.	whole	2% low-fat	skim or nonfat

4.

Item No./Food	Energy (kcal)	Fat (g)	Energy from Fat (g × 9 kcal/g)	% of kcal from Fat
#1414 Granola bar (soft), 1 ea	188	7	63	34%
# 426 Croissant, 1 ea	231	12	108	47%
#1271 Plain tortilla chips, 1 oz	142	7	63	44%
# 482 Waffle (home recipe), 1 ea	218	11	99	45%
#1318 Oat bran cereal, 1 c	229	9	81	35%
# 537 Chow mein, dry, 1 c	237	14	126	53%
# 583 Salmon, broiled or baked, 4 oz	245	12	108	44%
# 661 Turkey patty, breaded, fried, 2 oz	160	10	90	56%
# 682 Chicken à la king, 1 c	468	34	306	65%
# 220 Avocado, 1 ea	306	30	270	88%
# 927 Tofu (regular), ½ c	94	6	54	57%

a. Students might note that there is some irony in the fact that the popular "diet" foods, tofu and granola, are so high in fat relative to the recommendations; some breads such as croissants and waffles may be surprisingly high in fat; similarly, plain white turkey meat is low in fat, but when ground up with the skin, or when fried, it is a high-fat food.

b. Yes. The 30% recommendation applies to the *day's* kcalories—not to particular *foods*. Of course, it would not be wise for all of your selections to contribute more than 30% kcalories from fat because then your day's total is certain to be greater than 30%. But some of your choices can provide more than 30% kcalories from fat. When you select these foods, you simply need to be aware of their fat contribution, and balance it with other foods that are lower in fat.

5. a. 6.5 g ÷ 65 g = 10%. It means that one serving of food contributes about ⅒ of the day's fat allotment.

b. 6.5 g × 9 kcal/g = 59 kcal from fat.

c. 59 kcal from fat/200 kcal × 100 = 30% of kcalories from fat.

6. 46%; that almost half of the day's fat allotment would be used in this one dessert.

CHAPTER 6: PROBLEM SET ANSWERS

1. a. and b.

Item No./Food	Energy (kcal)	Protein (g)	Protein per 100 kcal (g)
# 602 Roast, oven cooked, prime rib, lean only, 4 oz	272	31	11
# 611 Lamb chop, loin, broiled, lean and fat, 1	202	16	8
# 617 Bacon (pork), 3 medium slices	109	6	6
# 646 Roasted chicken breast, 1	141	27	19
# 647 Roasted chicken, drumstick, 1	76	12	16
# 653 Roasted turkey (white meat), 4 oz	177	34	19
#1297 Beef bologna, 1 pce	72	3	4
# 720 Almonds (whole), dry roasted, 1 oz	167	6	4
# 740 Peanuts, oil roasted, 1 oz	165	7	4
# 854 Chickpeas (garbanzo beans), cooked, 1 c	267	14	5
# 860 Kidney beans, canned, 1 c	217	13	6
#1288 Lentils (sprouted), stir-fried, 4 oz	115	10	9
# 94 2% Low-fat milk, 1 c	121	8	7
# 144 Soy milk, 1 c	79	7	9
# 146 Plain, low-fat yogurt, 1 c	143	12	8
# 156 Egg, poached, 1	74	6	8
#1681 Egg substitute, ½ c (equivalent to about 1½ regular, whole eggs)	106	15	14
# 925 Soybeans, ½ c	149	14	9

c. Best protein buys:
Roasted turkey with white meat
Roasted chicken breast
Roasted chicken, drumstick
Worst protein buys:
Whole, dry-roasted almonds
Beef bologna
Peanuts, oil roasted

d. Egg substitute, soybeans, soy milk, and lentils.

2. a. She is 61 in tall. The midpoint weight for a woman this height is 54 kg. 0.8 g/kg × 54 kg = 43 g protein per day.

b. He is 76 in tall. The midpoint weight for a man this height is 87 kg. He is 18 years old, so use 0.9 g/kg. 0.9 g/kg × 87 kg = 78 g protein per day.

3. a. 10% of 3500 kcal = 350 kcal. 350 kcal divided by 4 kcal/g protein = 87.5 g protein per day.

b. An appropriate weight for a man 5 ft 10 in tall is 74 kg. Using the RDA guidelines of 0.8 g/kg, an appropriate protein intake for this man would be 59 g protein/day. His intake of 87.5 g protein per day falls between the RDA and twice the RDA, and so meets diet and health recommendations.

4.

Item No./Food	Weight (g)	Energy (kcal)	Fat (g)	Fiber (g)
#598 Hamburger, 3 oz	85	238.5	15	0
#474 Hamburger bun, 1	45	129	2	1
#968 Catsup, 1 tbs	15	16	0	0
Totals:	145	383.5	17	1

b.

Item No./Food	Weight (g)	Energy (kcal)	Fat (g)	Fiber (g)
# 796 Black beans, ½ c	86	114	0	8
# 544 White rice, regular long grain, 1 c	205	267	1	1
#1347 Salsa, 1 tbs	14	2	0	0
Totals:	305	383	1	9

c. 16; 16 g fat × 9 kcal/g = 144 kcal from fat.

d. 8 g.

e. 145 g; 305 g.

CHAPTER 8: PROBLEM SET ANSWERS

1. a. (12.2 × 34) + 746 = 1161 kcal/day; or (22.5 × 34) + 499 = 1264 kcal/day.
   b. (17.5 × 68) + 651 = 1841 kcal/day; or (15.3 × 68) + 679 = 1719 kcal/day.
   c. (11.6 × 91) + 879 = 1935 kcal/day.
   d. (8.7 × 52) + 829 = 1281 kcal/day.
2. a. 0.045 kcal/lb/min × 142 lb = 6.39 kcal/min. 6.39 kcal/min × 120 min = 767 kcal.
   b. 0.103 kcal/lb/min × 142 lb = 14.6 kcal/min. 14.6 kcal/min × 20 min = 293 kcal.
   c. 0.032 kcal/lb/min × 142 lb = 4.54 kcal/min. 4.54 kcal/min × 45 min = 204 kcal.
   d. 0.035 kcal/lb/min × 142 lb = 4.97 kcal/min. 4.97 kcal/min × 60 min = 298 kcal.
3. The infant has the faster BMR (500 kcal ÷ 20 lb = 25 kcal/lb and 1500 kcal ÷ 170 lb = 8.8 kcal/lb). Because the infant has a BMR of 25 kcal/lb whereas the adult has a BMR of 8.8 kcal/lb, the infant's BMR is almost 3 times faster than the adult's based on body weight.
4. a. BMR = (14.7 × 59.1) + 496 = 1365 kcal/day.
   b. With an activity factor of 1.5, her daily energy need is 1.5 × 1365 kcal/day = 2048 kcal/day or, with a weight of 59.1 kg, her daily energy need is 35 kcal/kg/day × 59.1 kg = 2069 kcal/day.
5. 21 ÷ 0.172 = 122 lb.
6. a. 120 lb × .01 = 1.2 lb/week.
   b. 250 lb × .01 = 2.5 lb/week.
7. a. 1300 kcal.
   b. 2500 kcal.
8. a. 45 lb.
   b. 3500 kcal/lb × 45 lb = 157,500 kcal of body fat.
   c. 30 lb. 30 lb fat/135 lb total body weight = 22% fat.
   d. 15 lb × 3500 kcal/lb = 52,500 kcal.
   e. 52,500 kcal ÷ 500 kcal/day = 105 days (about 3½ months).

CHAPTER 9: PROBLEM SET ANSWERS

1. a. Three milk shakes provide: 3 × 190 kcal = 570 kcal; 3 × 32 g carbohydrate = 96 g carbohydrate; 3 × 13 g protein = 39 g protein; and 3 × 1 g fat = 3 g fat.
   b. To meet this criteria, the plan needs *at least* an additional 630 kcalories, an additional 4 grams of carbohydrate, an additional 7 to 24 grams of protein (depending on the person's RDA based on sex and age), and some additional fat.
   c. Of course, there are many possible dinners that you could plan. One might be:
      Salad made with 1 c lettuce, 1 c chopped tomatoes and onions, ¼ c garbanzo beans, and 2 tbs low-fat dressing
      4 oz grilled chicken
      1 medium baked potato
      1 c summer squash and zucchini
      1 c melon cubes
      This meal brings the day's totals to 1215 kcalories, 90 g of protein, 192 g of carbohydrate, and 13 g of fat, which meets the goals for kcalories, protein, and carbohydrate. Because the milk shake has been fortified, all vitamin and mineral needs are covered as well. The only possible dietary shortcoming is that the day's percent kcalories from fat is low (only 10%), but because energy and nutrient recommendations have been met and the goal is weight loss, this may be acceptable.
   d. This weight-loss plan uses a liquid formula rather than foods, making clients dependent on a special device (the formula) rather than teaching them how to make good choices from the conventional food supply. It provides no information about dropout rates, the long-term success of clients, or weight maintenance after the program ends.
2. a. More than a pound.
   b. 541 kcal: 551 g = 0.98 kcal/g.
   c. More than another whole pound.
   d.

Item No./Food	Weight (g)	Energy (kcal)
Original totals:	551	541
Minus:		
#867 Lettuce, 1 c	56	−7
Plus:		
#603 Roast beef, 1 oz	+28	+68
# 39 Cheddar cheese, 1 oz	+28	+114
Totals:	551 g	716 kcal

   e. 716 kcal − 541 kcal = 175 kcal added.
   f. 551 g − 551 g = 0 more grams added.

CHAPTER 10: PROBLEM SET ANSWERS

1. a. Thiamin: **mg.**
      Riboflavin: **mg.**
      Niacin: **mg NE.**
      Vitamin B_6: **mg.**
      Folate: **µg**
      Vitamin B_{12} : **µg**
      Vitamin C: **mg.**
   b. A thousand times higher.
   c. 1 million µg = 1 g; about 5 g; about 5 million µg = 1 tsp; 2 µg.
2. a.

Item No./Food	Ener (kcal)	Thia (mg)	Ribo (mg)	Niacin (mg NE)	Vit B_6 (mg)	Folate (µg)	Vit C (mg)
Grains (6):							
#357 Wheat bread, 6 slices	6(64)	6(.11)	6(.08)	6(1.13)	6(.03)	6(11)	6(0)
Total in grains:	384	.66	.48	6.78	.18	66	0
Vegetables (3)							
#929 Spinach, cooked from fresh, ½ c	21	.09	.21	.44	.22	131	9
#891 Green peas, cooked from frozen, ½ c	62	.23	.08	1.18	.09	47	8
#834 Carrots, cooked from fresh, ½ c	35	.03	.04	.39	.19	11	2
Total in vegetables:	118	.35	.33	2.01	.50	189	19
Fruits (2)							
#269 Orange juice, fresh, 1 c	111	.22	.07	.99	.1	75	124
#264 Cantaloupe melon, ½	93	.1	.06	1.53	.31	45	113
Total in fruits:	204	.32	.13	2.52	.41	120	237

K

Item No./Food	Ener (kcal)	Thia (mg)	Ribo (mg)	Niacin (mg NE)	Vit B_6 (mg)	Folate (µg)	Vit C (mg)
Meats (2 to 3)							
#1045 Bass fish, baked, 4 oz	166	.1	.1	1.72	.16	19	0
#598 Hamburger, lean, 4 oz	318	.07	.27	6.77	.34	12	0
Total in meats:	484	.17	.37	8.49	.5	31	0
Milks (2)							
#98 Milk, nonfat, 2 c	2(85)	2(.09)	2(.34)	2(.22)	2(.1)	2(13)	2(2)
Total in milks:	170	.18	.68	.44	.2	26	4

b. Grains; milk; meats; vegetables and meats; vegetables; fruits.

c. Vitamin C and folate; thiamin and riboflavin.

3. a. She eats 90 g protein. Assume she uses 46 g as protein. This leaves 90 g − 46 g = 44 g protein "leftover."

44 g protein ÷ 100 = 0.44 g tryptophan.
0.44 g × 1000 = 440 mg tryptophan.
440 mg tryptophan ÷ 60 = 7.3 mg NE.
7.3 mg NE + 9 mg niacin = 16.3 mg NE.

b. Yes.

4. a.

Item No./Food	Energy (kcal)	Thiamin (mg)	Servings/kCalories
# 98 Nonfat milk, 1 c 85			1.5 ÷ .09 = 16.7 c .0917 c = 1445 kcal
#206 Apple, fresh, 3¼″	125	.04	1.5 ÷ .04 = 37.5 apples 38 apples = 4750 kcal
# 37 Cheddar cheese, 1 oz	114	.01	1.5 ÷ .01 = 150 oz 150 oz = 17,100 kcal
#820 Broccoli, cooked from fresh, chopped, 1 c	44	.09	1.5 ÷ .09 = 16.7 c 17 c = 748 kcal
#357 Whole-wheat bread, 1 slice	64	.11	1.5 ÷ .11 = 13.6 slices 14 slices = 896 kcal
#606 Sirloin steak lean, 4 oz	228	.15	1.5 ÷ .15 = 10 (4 oz) steaks 10 (4 oz) steaks = 2280 kcal
#871 Mushrooms, raw, sliced, ½ c	9	.04	1.5 ÷ .04 = 37.5 (½ c) svgs 38 (½ c) svgs = 342 kcal
#623 Pork chop, lean broiled, 1 ea	166	.83	1.5 ÷ .83 = 1.8 chops 2 chops = 332 kcal
#750 Sunflower seeds, dry, ¼ c	205	.82	1.5 ÷ .82 = 1.8 (¼ c) svgs 2 (¼ c) svgs = 410 kcal
#891 Green peas, cooked from frozen, ½ c	62	.23	1.5 ÷ .23 = 6.5 (½ c) svgs 7 (½ c) svgs = 434 kcal

b. No. In most cases you'd either have to eat much too much of the food (19 c of mushrooms), or the kcalorie count would be way too high to accommodate (17,100 kcal from cheese), or both. The pork chops are a possible exception—you could afford to eat two chops (332 kcal) every day, but then you'd lose out on the variety of other meats you should have. Another possible exception is the sunflower seeds, but 400-some kcal is a lot of energy to consume trying to get one nutrient.

c.

From the grains:	.66 mg
From the vegetables:	.35 mg
From the fruits:	.32 mg
From the meats:	.17 mg
From the milks:	.18 mg
Total thiamin:	1.68 mg

d. Yes.

CHAPTER 11: PROBLEM SET ANSWERS

1. Vitamin A: µg RE. Vitamin D: µg.
   Vitamin E: µg α-TE. Vitamin K: µg.
2. a.

Item No./Food	Energy (kcal)	Vitamin A (RE)
Grains (6):		
# 357 Wheat bread, 6 slices	6(64)	0
Total in grains:	384	0
Vegetables (3):		
# 929 Spinach, cooked from fresh, ½ c	21	737
# 891 Green peas, cooked from frozen ½ c	62	54
# 834 Carrots, cooked from fresh, ½ c	35	1913
Total in vegetables:	118	2704
Fruits (2):		
# 269 Orange juice, fresh, 1 c	111	50
# 264 Cantaloupe melon, ½	93	860
Total in fruits:	204	910
Meats (2 to 3):		
#1045 Bass fish, 4 oz	166	40
# 598 Hamburger, lean, 4 oz	318	0
Total in meats:	484	40
Milks (2):		
# 98 Milk, nonfat, 2 c	2(85)	2(149)
Total in milks:	170	298

b. The vegetables (and fruits).

c. The grains and the meats.

d. The meats and the milk.

e. The plant foods—fruits and vegetables.

f. Fast-food meals often lack the types of foods rich in vitamin A such as leafy green vegetables, carrots, and fruits.

3. a.

Item No./Food	Energy (kcal)	Vitamin A (RE)	Servings/KCalories
#939 Sweet potato, baked in skin, 1 ea	117	2486	875 ÷ 2486 = .4 potato ½ potato = 58.5 kcal
#834 Carrots, from fresh, ½ c	35	1913	875 ÷ 1913 = 0.5 (½ c) ¼ c = 18 kcal
#264 Cantaloupe melon, ½	93	860	875 ÷ 860 = 1 (½ melon) svg ½ melon = 93 kcal
#820 Broccoli, cooked from fresh, 1 c	44	217	875 ÷ 217 = 4 c 4 c = 176 kcal
# 98 Milk, nonfat, 1 c	85	149	875 ÷ 149 = 5.9 c 6 c = 510 kcal
# 37 Cheddar cheese, 1 oz	114	86	875 ÷ 86 = 10 oz 10 oz = 1140 kcal
#891 Green peas, cooked from frozen, ½ c	62	54	875 ÷ 54 = 16.2 (½ c) svgs 16 (½ c) svgs = 992 kcal
#206 Apple, fresh, 3 ¼″	125	11	875 ÷11 = 79.5 apples 80 apples = 10,000 kcal
#623 Pork chop, lean broiled, 1 ea	166	1	875 ÷ 1 = 875 chops 875 chops = 145,250 kcal
#606 Sirloin steak, lean, 4 oz	228	0	875 : 0 = infinity No vitamin A in steak
#357 Whole-wheat bread, 1 slice	64	0	875 ÷ 0 = infinity No vitamin A in bread

b. The sweet potato, carrots, and the cantaloupe.

c. Four best sources per kcalorie: carrots, sweet potato, cantaloupe, broccoli. Yes, this rank order is slightly different, but the same foods appear.

CHAPTER 12: PROBLEM SET ANSWERS

1. Calcium: **mg.** Magnesium: **mg.** Phosphorus: **mg.**
   Potassium: **mg.** Sodium: **mg.**

2. a.

Item No./Food	Ener (kcal)	Calc (mg)	Magn (mg)	Phos (mg)	Potas (mg)	Sod (mg)
Grains (6):						
# 357 Wheat bread, 6 slices	6(64)	6(21)	6(11)	6(46)	6(34)	6(135)
Total in grains:	384	126	66	276	204	810
Vegetables (3):						
# 929 Spinach, cooked from fresh, ½ c	21	122	78	50	419	63
# 891 Green peas, cooked from frozen, ½ c	62	19	23	72	134	70
#834 Carrots, cooked from fresh, ½ c	35	24	10	23	177	51
Total in vegetables:	118	165	111	145	730	184
Fruits (2):						
# 269 Orange juice, fresh, 1 c	111	27	27	42	496	2
# 264 Cantaloupe melon, ½	93	29	29	45	825	24
Total in fruits:	204	56	56	87	1321	26
Meats (2 to 3):						
#1045 Bass fish, 4 oz	166	117	43	290	517	102
# 598 Hamburger, lean, 4 oz	318	14	27	206	396	101
Total in meats:	484	131	70	496	913	203
Milks (2):						
# 98 Milk, nonfat, 2 c	2(85)	2(301)	2(28)	2(247)	2(404)	2(126)
Total in milks:	170	602	56	494	808	252

b. Milks; fruits.
c. Vegetables; fruits and milks.
d. Meats; fruits.
e. Fruits; grains.
f. Grains; fruits.
g. Milks, vegetables, meats, fruits, and grains.

3. a.

Item No./Food	Energy (kcal)	Calcium (mg)	Servings/KCalories
# 98 Milk, nonfat, 1 c	85	301	1000 ÷ 301 = 3.3 c 3 c = 255 kcal
# 37 Cheddar cheese, 1 oz	114	204	1000 ÷ 204 = 4.9 oz 5 oz = 570 kcal
#820 Broccoli, cooked from fresh, chopped, 1 c	44	72	1000 ÷ 72 = 13.9 c 14 c = 616 kcal
#939 Sweet potato, baked in skin, 1 ea	117	31	1000 ÷ 32 = 31.3 potatoes 31 potatoes = 3627 kcal
#264 Cantaloupe melon, ½	93	29	1000 ÷ 29 = 34.5 (½ melon) svgs 35 (½ melon) svgs = 3255 kcal
#834 Carrots, from fresh, ½ c	35	24	1000 ÷ 24 = 41.7 (½ c) svgs 42 (½ c) svgs = 1470 kcal
#357 Whole-wheat bread, 1 slice	64	21	1000 ÷ 21 = 47.6 slices 48 slices = 3072 kcal
#891 Green peas, cooked from frozen, ½ c	62	19	1000 ÷ 19 = 52.6 (½ c) svgs 53 (½ c) svgs = 3286 kcal
#206 Apple, fresh 3¼"	125	15	1000 ÷ 15 = 66.7 apples 67 apples = 8375 kcal
#606 Sirloin steak, lean, 4 oz	228	12	1000 ÷ 12 = 83.3 (4 oz) steaks 83 (4 oz) steaks = 18,924 kcal
#623 Pork chop, lean broiled, 1 ea	166	4	1000 ÷ 4 = 250 chops 250 chops = 41,500 kcal

b. Milk > cheese > broccoli; yes.

CHAPTER 13: PROBLEM SET ANSWERS

1. Iron: **mg.** Zinc: **mg.**

2. a.

Item No./Food	Energy (kcal)	Iron (mg)	Zinc (mg)
Grains (6):			
# 357 Wheat bread, 6 slices	6(64)	6(.87)	6(.26)
Total in grains:	384	5.22	1.56
Vegetables (3):			
# 929 Spinach, cooked from fresh, ½ c	21	3.21	.68
# 891 Green peas, cooked from frozen, ½ c	62	1.26	.75
# 834 Carrots, cooked from fresh, ½ c	35	.48	.23
Total in vegetables:	118	4.95	1.66
Fruits (2):			
# 269 Orange juice, fresh, 1 c	111	.5	.12
# 264 Cantaloupe melon, ½	93	.56	.43
Total in fruits:	204	1.06	.55
Meats (2 to 3):			
# 1045 Bass fish, 4 oz	166	2.17	.94
# 598 Hamburger, lean, 4 oz	318	2.78	7.03
Total in meats:	484	4.95	7.97
Milks (2):			
# 98 Milk, nonfat, 2 c	2(85)	2(0.1)	2(.98)
Total in milks:	170	0.2	1.96

b. Grains, vegetables, and meats; milks and fruits.
c. Meats; fruits.

3.

Item No./Food	Iron Density (mg/kcal)
# 98 Milk, nonfat, 1 c	.0012
# 37 Cheddar cheese, 1 oz	.0017
#820 Broccoli, cooked from fresh, chopped, 1 c	.0298
#939 Sweet potato, baked in skin, 1 ea	.0044
#264 Cantaloupe melon, ½	.0060
#834 Carrots, from fresh, ½ c	.0137
#357 Whole-wheat bread, 1 slice	.0136
#891 Green peas, cooked from frozen, ½ c	.0203
#206 Apple fresh, 3¼"	.0030
#606 Sirloin steak, lean, 4 oz	.0167
#623 Pork chop, lean, broiled, 1 ea	.0040

a. Sirloin steak > broccoli > green peas > bread > pork chop > cantaloupe > sweet potato > carrots > apple > cheese > milk.
b. Broccoli > green peas > sirloin steak > carrots > bread > cantaloupe > sweet potato > pork chop > apple > cheese > milk.
c. Broccoli, green peas, and carrots are all higher on the per-kcalorie list.
d. They are all vegetables.

4. a.

Item No./Food	Iron (mg)	Vitamin C (mg)
#606 Sirloin steak, lean, 4 oz	3.81	0
#891 Green peas, cooked from frozen, ½ c	1.26	8
#542 Brown rice, cooked, 1 c	.82	0
# 32 Iced tea, instant, sweetened, 1c	.05	0
Totals	5.94	8

K

b. Step 1: 3.81 mg; step 2: 3.81 mg × 0.40 = 1.5 mg heme iron; step 3: 2.13 mg; step 4: 2.13 mg + (3.81 mg × 0.60) = 4.42 mg nonheme iron; step 5: low vitamin C; step 6: high MFP. For heme iron, 1.5 mg × 0.23 = 0.35 mg heme iron absorbed. For nonheme iron, availability of nonheme iron was high; 4.42 × 0.08 = 0.35 mg nonheme iron absorbed. Total: 0.7 mg iron absorbed.

c. 0.7 mg absorbed ÷ 5.94 mg eaten × 100 = 12% absorbed.

d. Yes—the tannic acid in tea may interfere with the absorption of iron.

e. 0.7 mg absorbed/meal × 3 meals = 2.1 mg absorbed. According to the RDA calculation, a woman needs to absorb 1.5 mg per day, so she will meet her iron RDA.

5. Tuesday's meals provided:

6 grains (English muffin, bread, cookies)	=	10 points
2 vegetables (lettuce, potato)	=	6.6 points
0 fruits	=	0 points
6 meats (bacon, egg, peanut butter, steak)	=	10 points
2 milks (cheese, milk)	=	10 points
>45% kcal fat	=	0 points
>15% kcal saturated fat	=	0 points
>450 mg cholesterol	=	0 points
<2400 mg sodium	=	10 points
>8 foods for variety	=	10 points
Total	=	56.6 points

This day's meals need improvement. To improve Tuesday's meals, select grains without added sugar and fat (cookies are a sweet treat but are not a good foundation of a healthy diet); select more vegetables and fruits; select low-fat milks and meats.

Many medical terms have their origins in Latin or Greek. By learning a few common derivations, you can glean the meaning of words you have never heard of before. For example, once you know that "hyper" means above normal, "glyc" means glucose, and "emia" means blood, you can easily determine that "hyperglycemia" means high blood glucose. The following derivations will help you to learn many terms presented in this glossary.

GENERAL

a or *an* = not or without
anti = against
di = two
dys or *mal* = bad
endo = inside or within
exo or *extra* = outside
genesis = gives rise to, making
homeo = the same
hyper = over, above normal, excessive
hypo = below normal, under, beneath
inter = between, in the midst
intra = within
itis = infection or inflammation
lysis = break
macro = large
micro = tiny
mono = one
neo = new
osis = condition
peri = around
poly = many
pre or *pro* = before
stasis = staying
tri = three

BODY

arterio = artery
cardiac or *cardio* = heart
cyte = cell
emia or *hemo* = blood
enteron = intestine
gastro = stomach
hepatic = liver
myo = muscle
osteo = bone
pulmo = lung
renal = kidney
ure or *uria* = urine
vaso = vessel
vena = vein

CHEMISTRY

-al = aldehyde
-ase = enzyme
-ate = salt
glyc or *gluc* = glucose
hydro or *hydrate* = water
lipo = lipid
-ol = alcohol
-ose = sugar
saccharide = sugar

-ase (ACE): a word ending denoting an enzyme. Enzymes are often identified by the place they come from and the compounds they work on; gastric lipase, for example is a stomach enzyme that acts on lipids, whereas pancreatic lipase come from the pancreas (and also works on lipids).

-ate: word ending that denotes a salt of the mineral.

absorption: the taking up of nutrients into the intestinal cells.

accredited: approved; in the case of medical centers or universities, certified by an agency recognized by the U.S. Department of Education.

acesulfame (AY-see-sul-fame) **potassium:** a low-kcalorie sweetener recently approved by the FDA; also known as acesulfame-K, because K is the chemical symbol for potassium; approved in Canada.

acetaldehyde (ass-et-AL-duh-hide): an intermediate in alcohol metabolism.

acetyl CoA (ASS-eh-teel, or ah-SEET-il, coh-AY): a 2-carbon compound (acetate, or acetic acid, shown in Figure 5–2 on p. 155) to which a molecule of CoA is attached.

acid-base balance: the equilibrium in the body between acid and base concentrations.

acidosis (assi-DOE-sis): above-normal acidity in the blood and body fluids.

acids: compounds that release hydrogen ions in a solution.

acne: a chronic inflammation of the skin's follicles and oil-producing glands, which leads to an accumulation of oils inside the ducts that surround hairs; usually associated with the maturation of young adults.

acquired immune deficiency syndrome (AIDS): the end stage of HIV infection, in which severe complications are manifested. In the early, symptomless stages, the person is said to have an HIV infection.

active solar: use of photovoltaic panels to generate electricity from sunlight. (A passive solar home is built to minimize heating and cooling costs by taking advantage of the available sun and shade.)

acute PEM: protein-energy malnutrition caused by recent severe food restriction; characterized in children by thinness for height (wasting).

adaptive thermogenesis: adjustments in energy expenditure related to changes in environment such as cold and to physiological events such as overfeeding, trauma, and changes in hormone status.

additives: substances not normally consumed as foods but added to food either intentionally or by accident.

adequacy (dietary): providing all the essential nutrients, fiber, and energy in amounts sufficient to maintain health.

ADH: see antidiuretic hormone.

ADI (Acceptable Daily Intake): the amount of a sweetener that individuals can safely consume each day over the course of a lifetime without adverse effect. It includes a 100-fold safety factor.

adipose (ADD-ih-poce) **tissue:** the body's fat tissue, which consists of masses of fat-storing cells.

adolescence: the period from the beginning of puberty until maturity.

adrenal glands: glands adjacent to, and just above, each kidney.

adverse reactions: unusual responses to food (including intolerances and allergies).

aerobic (air-ROE-bic): requiring oxygen.

aflatoxin: potent cancer-causing toxin produced by the mold *Aspergillus flavus* that infects grains and peanuts. The USDA tests grains and peanuts grown in this country for aflatoxin contamination.

agribusiness: agriculture practiced on a massive scale by large corporations owning vast acreages and employing intensive technological, fuel, and chemical inputs.

AIDS: see acquired immune deficiency syndrome.

AIDS-related complex (ARC): a condition of mild AIDS symptoms that sometimes occurs early in the course of the disease AIDS.

alcohol dehydrogenase: an enzyme that converts ethanol to acetaldehyde. The MEOS also oxidizes alcohol (see MEOS).

alcohol: a class of organic compounds containing hydroxyl (OH) groups.

aldosterone (al-DOS-ter-own): a hormone secreted by the adrenal glands that stimulates the reabsorption of sodium by the kidneys; aldosterone also regulates chloride and potassium concentrations.

alitame (AL-ih-tame): a compound of two amino acids (alanine and aspartic acid) that is 2000 times sweeter than sucrose; FDA approval pending.

alkalosis (alka-LOE-sis): above-normal alkalinity (base) in the blood and body fluids.

alpha-lactalbumin (lact-AL-byoo-min): the chief protein in human breast milk, as opposed to casein (CAY-seen), the chief protein in cow's milk.

alpha-tocopherol: the most biologically active vitamin E compound.

alternative agriculture: agriculture practiced on a small scale using individualized approaches that vary with local conditions so as to minimize technological, fuel, and chemical inputs.

amenorrhea: the absence of or cessation of menstruation. Primary amenorrhea is menarche delayed beyond 16 years of age. Secondary amenorrhea is the absence of three to six consecutive menstrual cycles.

American Dietetic Association (ADA): the professional organization of dietitians in the United States.

amino (a-MEEN-oh) **acids:** building blocks of proteins; each contains an amino group, an acid group, a hydrogen atom, and a distinctive side group attached to a central carbon atom.

amino acid scoring: a method of evaluating protein quality by comparing a test protein's amino acid pattern with that of a reference protein; sometimes called chemical scoring.

ammonia: a compound with the chemical formula NH3; produced during the deamination of amino acids.

amniotic (am-nee-OTT-ic) **sac:** the "bag of waters" in the uterus, in which the fetus floats.

amylase (AM-ih-lace): an enzyme that hydrolyzes amylose (a form of starch). Amylase is a carbohydrase, an enzyme that breaks down carbohydrates.

anabolism (an-ABB-o-lism): reactions in which small molecules are put together to build larger ones. Anabolic reactions require energy.

anaerobic (AN-air-ROE-bic): not requiring oxygen.

anemia: literally, "too little blood." Anemia is any condition in which too few red blood cells are present, or the red blood cells are immature (and therefore large) or too small or contain too little hemoglobin to carry the normal amount of oxygen to the tissues. It is not a disease itself but can be a symptom of many different disease conditions, including many nutrient deficiencies, bleeding, excessive red blood cell destruction, and defective red blood cell formation.

angiotensin: a blood protein that helps to raise blood pressure. Its precursor protein is called angiotensinogen.

anions (AN-eye-uns): negatively charged ions.

anorexia nervosa: an eating disorder characterized by a refusal to maintain a minimally normal body weight and a distortion in perception of body shape and weight, most commonly seen in teenage girls and young women.

antagonist: a competing factor that counteracts the action of another factor. When a drug displaces a vitamin from its site of action, the drug renders the vitamin ineffective and thus acts as a vitamin antagonist.

anthropometric (AN-throw-poe-MET-rick): relating to measurement of the physical characteristics of the body, such as height and weight.

antibodies: large proteins of the blood and body fluids, produced by the immune system in response to the invasion of the body by foreign molecules (usually proteins called antigens); antibodies combine with and inactivate the foreign invaders, thus protecting the body.

antidiuretic hormone (ADH): a hormone produced by the pituitary gland in response to dehydration (or a high sodium concentration in the blood); it stimulates the kidneys to reabsorb more water and therefore to excrete less. In addition to its anti-diuretic effect, ADH also elevates blood pressure and is called vasopressin.

antigen: a substance that elicits the formation of antibodies or an inflammation reaction from the immune system. A bacterium, a virus, a toxin, and a protein in food that causes allergy are all examples of foreign antigens.

antimicrobial agents: preservatives that prevent microorganisms from growing.

antioxidant: a compound that protects others from oxidation by being oxidized itself. An antioxidant donates electrons to another substance; that substance becomes reduced as the antioxidant simultaneously becomes oxidized.

antipromoters: with respect to cancer, factors that oppose its development.

antiscorbutic factor: the original name for vitamin C.

antisense gene: the chemical opposite of a native gene that adheres to the native working gene and blocks its production of proteins.

anus (AY-nus): the terminal sphincter of the GI tract.

appendix: a narrow blind sac extending from the beginning of the colon; a vestigial organ with no known function.

appetite: the psychological desire to eat or an interest in food; a positive sensation that accompanies the sight, smell, or thought of food.

arachidonic (a-RACK-ih-DON-ic) **acid:** an omega-6 polyunsaturated fatty acid with 20 carbons and four double bonds (20:4); synthesized from linoleic acid.

artery: a vessel that carries blood away from the heart.

artesian water: water that is drawn from a well that taps a confined aquifer in which the water level stands above the natural water table.

arthritis: a usually painful inflammation of a joint caused by many conditions, including infections, metabolic disturbances, or injury; joint structure is usually altered, with loss of function.

artificial colors: certified food colors added to enhance appearance. (Certified means approved by the FDA.)

artificial flavors, flavor enhancers: chemicals that mimic natural flavors and those that enhance flavor.

artificial sweeteners: sugar substitutes that provide no energy; sometimes called nonnutritive sweeteners.

ascorbic acid: one of the two active forms of vitamin C (see Figure 10–12). Many people refer to vitamin C by this name.

aspartame (ah-SPAR-tame or ASS-par-tame): a compound of two amino acids (phenylalanine and aspartic acid) that tastes like the sugar sucrose but is much sweeter. It provides 4 kcalories per gram, as does protein, but because so little is used, it is virtually kcalorie-free. In powdered form it is sometimes mixed with lactose, however, so a 1-gram packet may contain 4 kcalories. It is used in both the United States and Canada.

asymptomatic allergy: adverse reaction that produces antibodies without symptoms.

atherosclerosis (ath-er-oh-scler-OH-sis): a type of artery disease characterized by accumulations of lipid-containing material on the inner walls of the arteries.

atom: the smallest component of an element that has all of the properties of the element.

ATP (adenosine triphosphate): a common high-energy compound composed of a purine (adenine), a sugar (ribose), and three phosphate groups.

atrophic gastritis: chronic inflammation of the stomach accompanied by a diminished size and functioning of the mucosa and glands.

atrophy (AT-ro-fee): of muscles, a decrease in size because of disuse, undernutrition, or wasting diseases.

available carbohydrates: starch and sugar (because human digestive enzymes make them available to the body).

avidin: the protein in egg whites that binds biotin.

B-cells: lymphocytes that produce antibodies.

balance (dietary): providing foods of a number of types in proportion to each other, such that foods rich in some nutrients do not crowd out of the diet foods that are rich in other nutrients.

basal metabolic rate (BMR): the rate of energy use for metabolism under basal conditions, usually expressed as kcalories per kilogram body weight per hour. (Table 8–3 on p. 285 provides equations for estimating BMR.)

basal metabolism: the energy needed to maintain life when a body is at complete rest after a 12-hour fast (to exclude the thermic effect of the previous meal).

bases: compounds that accept hydrogen ions in a solution.

beer: an alcoholic beverage brewed by fermenting malt and hops.

behavior modification: the changing of behavior by the manipulation of antecedents (cues or environmental factors that trigger behavior), the behavior itself, and consequences (the penalties or rewards attached to behavior).

beikost (BYE-cost): supplemental, or weaning, foods.

belch: the expulsion of gas from the stomach through the mouth.

beriberi: the thiamin-deficiency disease; it pointed the way to discovery of the first vitamin, thiamin.

beta-carotene (BAY-tah KARE-oh-teen): an orange pigment and vitamin A precursor found in plants.

BHA and BHT: preservatives commonly used to slow the development of off-flavors, odors, and color changes caused by oxidation.

bicarbonate: an alkaline secretion of the pancreas, part of the pancreatic juice. (Bicarbonate also occurs widely in all cell fluids.)

bifidus (BIFF-id-us, by-FEED-us) **factors:** factors in colostrum and breast milk that favor the growth of the "friendly" bacteria *Lactobacillus* (lack-toh-ba-SILL-us) *bifidus* in the infant's intestinal tract, so that other, less desirable intestinal inhabitants will not flourish.

bile: an emulsifier that prepares fats and oils for digestion; an exocrine secretion made by the liver, stored in the gallbladder, and released into the small intestine when needed.

binders: chemical compounds occurring in foods that can combine with nutrients (especially minerals) to form complexes the body cannot absorb. Examples of such binders include phytic (FIGHT-ic) acid and oxalic (ox-AL-ic) acid.

bioaccumulation: the accumulation of contaminants in the flesh of animals high on the food chain.

bioavailability: the rate and extent to which a nutrient is absorbed.

bioelectrical impedance: a method for estimating body fat using low-intensity electrical current.

biological value (BV): the amount of protein nitrogen that is retained for growth and maintenance, expressed as a percentage of the protein nitrogen that has been digested and absorbed; a measure of protein quality.

biosensor: a genetically altered microbe that provides a rapid, low-cost, and accurate test for the products of spoilage in foods.

biotechnology: the use of biological systems or organisms to create or modify products; also called biogenetic engineering.

biotin (BY-oh-tin): a B vitamin that functions as a coenzyme in the metabolism of carbohydrates and fats.

blind experiment: an experiment in which the subjects do not know whether they are members of the experimental group or the control group.

blood doping: the process of injecting red blood cells to enhance the blood's oxygen-carrying ability. Risks include dangerous blood clotting, especially in athletes who become dehydrated, infections from nonsterile equipment, transfusion reactions, and dangers of improperly transferred blood. Blood doping is banned in Olympic competitions.

blood lipid profile: results of blood tests that reveal a person's total cholesterol, triglycerides, and various lipoproteins.

body composition: the proportions of muscle, bone, fat, and other tissue that makes up a person's total body weight.

body mass index (BMI): an index of a person's weight in relation to height, determined by dividing the weight (in kilograms) by the square of the height (in meters).

bolus (BOH-lus): a portion; with respect to food, the amount swallowed at one time.

bomb calorimeter (KAL-oh-RIM-eh-ter): an instrument that measures the heat energy released when foods are burned, thus providing an estimate of the potential energy of foods.

botulism (BOT-chew-lism): an often fatal food-borne illness caused by the ingestion of foods containing a toxin produced by bacteria that grow in improperly canned acidic foods.

bovine growth hormone (BGH): a hormone produced naturally in the pituitary gland of a cow that promotes growth and milk production.

bran: the protective coating around the grain kernel similar in function to the shell of a nut; rich in nutrients and fiber.

brown sugar: refined white sugar crystals to which manufacturers have added molasses syrup with natural flavor and color; 91 to 96 percent pure sucrose.

buffers: compounds that help keep a solution's acidity or alkalinity constant.

bulimia nervosa: an eating disorder characterized by repeated episodes of binge eating usually followed by self-induced vomiting, misuse of laxatives or diuretics, fasting, or excessive exercise.

caffeine: a natural stimulant found in many common foods and beverages, including coffee, tea, and chocolate, that in small amounts may produce alertness and reduced reaction time in some people, but also causes fluid losses. Overdoses cause headaches, trembling, rapid heart rate, and other undesirable side effects.

calcitonin (KAL-see-TOE-nin): a hormone from the thyroid glands that lowers blood calcium by inhibiting release of calcium from bone.

calcium: the most abundant mineral in the body, found primarily in the body's bones and teeth.

calcium rigor: hardness or stiffness of the muscles caused by high blood calcium concentrations.

calcium tetany (TET-ah-nee): intermittent spasm of the extremities due to nervous and muscular excitability caused by low blood calcium concentrations.

calcium-binding protein: a protein in the intestinal cells, made with the help of vitamin D, that facilitates calcium absorption.

calmodulin (cal-MOD-you-lin): an inactive protein that becomes active when bound to calcium; then it becomes a messenger that tells other proteins what to do. The system serves as interpreter for hormone- and nerve-mediated messages arriving at cells.

calorie: a unit by which energy is measured. Food energy is measured in kilocalories (1000 calories equal 1 kilocalorie), abbreviated kcalories or kcal. A capitalized version is also sometimes used: Calories. One kcalorie is the amount of heat necessary to raise the temperature of 1 kilogram (kg) of water 1°C.

Canadian Dietetic Association (CDA): the professional organization of dietitians in Canada.

cancer: a disease in which abnormal cells multiply out of control and disrupt the normal functioning of the body's cells or organs.

capillary (CAP-ill-ary): a small vessel that branches from an artery. Capillaries connect arteries to veins. Exchange of oxygen, nutrients, and waste materials takes place across capillary walls.

carbohydrase (KAR-boe-HIGH-drase): an enzyme that hydrolyzes carbohydrates.

carbohydrate loading: a regimen of moderate exercise followed by consuming a high-carbohydrate diet that enables muscles to store glycogen beyond their normal capacity; also called glycogen loading or glycogen supercompensation.

carbohydrates: compounds composed of carbon, oxygen, and hydrogen arranged as monosaccharides or multiples of monosaccharides.

carbonic acid: a compound with the formula H_2CO_3 that results from the combination of carbon dioxide (CO_2) and water (H_2O), of particular importance in the body's buffer system.

carcinogen (car-SIN-oh-jen): a cancer-initiating substance. A carcinogen is one kind of initiator; radiation is another.

carcinoma (KAR-see-NO-mah): a cancer that develops from epithelial tissue.

cardiac output: the volume of blood discharged by the heart each minute.

cardiac sphincter (CARD-ee-ack SFINK-ter): the sphincter muscle at the junction between the esophagus and the stomach; also called the lower esophageal sphincter or the gastroesophageal sphincter.

cardiorespiratory conditioning: improvements in the heart and lung function and increased blood volume, brought about by aerobic training.

cardiorespiratory endurance: the ability to perform large-muscle, dynamic exercise of moderate-to-high intensity for prolonged periods.

cardiovascular disease (CVD): a general term for all diseases of the heart and blood vessels. Atherosclerosis is the main cause of CVD. When the arteries that carry blood to the heart muscle become occluded, the heart suffers damage known as coronary heart disease (CHD).

carotene: a vitamin A precursor found in plants; an orange pigment.

carotenoids: pigments commonly found in plants and animals, some of which have provitamin A activity. Carotenoids are among the best-known phytochemicals—plant chemicals that are not nutrients but have biological activity in the body.

carpal tunnel syndrome: a pinched nerve at the wrist, causing pain or numbness in the hand.

cash crops: crops grown for cash, as opposed to crops grown for food; examples include cotton and tobacco.

catabolism (ca-TAB-o-lism): reactions in which large molecules are broken down to smaller ones. Catabolic reactions usually release energy.

catalyst (CAT-uh-list): a compound that facilitates chemical reactions without itself being changed in the process.

cataracts: thickenings of the eye lenses that impair vision and can lead to blindness.

cathartic: a strong laxative.

cations (CAT-eye-uns): positively charged ions.

CDC (Centers for Disease Control): a branch of the Department of Health and Human Services that is responsible for, among other things, monitoring food-borne diseases.

cell-mediated immunity: immunity conferred by the reaction of T-cells to an invading organism.

cellulite (SELL-you-light or SELL-you-leet): supposedly, a lumpy form of fat; actually, a fraud. The lumpy appearance in fatty areas of the body is caused by strands of connective tissue that attach the skin to underlying muscles. These points of attachment may pull tight where the fat is thick, making lumps appear between them. The fat itself is not different from fat anywhere else in the body. So, if the fat in these areas is lost, the lumpy appearance disappears.

central obesity: excess fat around the trunk of the body; also called abdominal fat or upper-body fat.

cerebral cortex: the outer surface of the brain's cerebrum.

certification: the process in which a private laboratory inspects shipments of a product for selected chemicals and then, if the product is free of violative levels of those chemicals, issues a guarantee to that effect.

cesarean section: a surgically assisted birth involving removal of the fetus by an incision into the uterus, usually by way of the abdominal wall.

chelate (KEY-late): a substance that can grasp the positive ions of a metal.

Chinese restaurant syndrome: an intolerance reaction that may occur in 1 to 2 percent of the population 20 minutes after the ingestion of the additive MSG (monosodium glutamate). Symptoms include burning sensations, chest and facial flushing and pain, and throbbing headaches.

chloride: the major anion in the extracellular fluids of the body. Chloride is the ionic form of chlorine, Cl^-; see Appendix B for a description of the chlorine-to-chloride conversion.

chlorophyll: the green pigment of plants, which absorbs photons and transfers their energy to other molecules, thereby initiating photosynthesis.

cholecalciferol (KO-lee-kal-SIF-er-ol): vitamin D.

cholecystokinin (coal-ee-sis-toe-KINE-in), or CCK: a hormone produced by cells of the intestinal wall. Target organ: the gallbladder. Response: release of bile and slowing of GI motility.

cholesterol: one of the sterols.

choline (KOH-leen): a nitrogen-containing compound found in plant and animal tissues as part of the phospholipid lecithin and the neurotransmitter acetylcholine; a nonessential nutrient that can be made in the body from a amino acid.

chronic diseases: degenerative diseases characterized by deterioration of the body organs; also called chronic, noncommunicable diseases (NCD). Examples include heart disease, cancer, and diabetes.

chronic PEM: protein-energy malnutrition caused by long-term food deprivation; characterized in children by short height for age (stunting).

chronological age: a person's age in years from his or her date of birth.

chylomicrons (kye-lo-MY-cronz): the class of lipoproteins that transport lipids from the intestinal cells into the body.

chyme (KIME): the semiliquid mass of partly digested food expelled by the stomach into the duodenum.

cirrhosis (seer-OH-sis): advanced liver disease in which liver cells turn orange, die, and harden, permanently losing their function; often associated with alcoholism.

clinically severe obesity: a BMI of 40 or greater or 100 pounds or more overweight for an average adult. A less preferred term used to describe the same condition is morbid obesity.

CoA (coh-AY): coenzyme A; the coenzyme derived from the B vitamin pantothenic acid and central to the energy metabolism of nutrients.

coenzymes: small organic molecules that work with enzymes to facilitate the enzymes' activity. Many coenzymes have B vitamins as part of their structures (Figure 10–1 in Chapter 10 illustrates coenzyme action).

cofactor: a mineral element that, like a coenzyme, works with an enzyme to facilitate a chemical reaction. The cofactor maintains the structural integrity of the enzyme and may also facilitate the enzyme's catalytic activity.

collagen: the protein material from which connective tissues such as scars, tendons, ligaments, and the foundations of bones and teeth are made.

colonic irrigation: the popular, but potentially harmful practice of "washing" the large intestine with a powerful enema machine.

colostrum (co-LAHS-trum): a milklike secretion from the breast, present during the first day or so after delivery before milk appears; rich in protective factors.

complementary proteins: two or more proteins whose amino acid assortments complement each other in such a way that the essential amino acids missing from one are supplied by the other.

complete protein: a dietary protein containing all the amino acids essential in human nutrition in amounts adequate for human use.

complex carbohydrates (starches and fibers): polysaccharides composed of straight or branched chains of monosaccharides.

compound: a substance composed of two or more different atoms—for example, water (H_2O).

condensation: a chemical reaction in which two reactants combine to yield a larger product.

conditionally essential amino acid: an amino acid that is normally nonessential, but must be supplied by the diet in special circumstances when the need for it exceeds the body's ability to produce it.

conditioning: the physical effect of training; improved flexibility, strength, and endurance.

cones: the cells of the retina that respond to bright light and are responsible for color vision.

confectioners' sugar: finely powdered sucrose; 99.9 percent pure.

constipation: the condition of having painful or difficult bowel movements (elapsed time between movements is not relevant).

contaminant: a substance that does not normally occur in a food.

contamination iron: iron found in foods as the result of contamination by inorganic iron salts from iron cookware, iron-containing soils, and the like.

control group: a group of individuals similar in all possible respects to the experimental group except for the treatment. Ideally, the control group receives a placebo while the experimental group receives a real treatment.

cool-down: five to ten minutes of light activity following a vigorous workout to gradually cool the body's core to near-normal temperature.

Cori cycle: the path from muscle glycogen to glucose to pyruvate to lactic acid (which travels to the liver) to glucose (which can travel back to the muscle) to glycogen; named after the scientist who elucidated this pathway.

corn sweeteners: corn syrup and sugars derived from corn.

corn syrup: a syrup produced by the action of enzymes on cornstarch; contains mostly glucose. See also high-fructose corn syrup (HFCS).

cornea (KOR-nee-uh): the transparent membrane covering the outside of the eye.

correlation (CORE-ee-LAY-shun): the simultaneous increase, decrease, or change of two variables. If A increases as B increases, or if A decreases as B decreases, the correlation is positive. (This does not mean that A causes B or vice versa.) If A increases as B decreases, or if A decreases as B increases, the correlation is negative. (This does not mean that A prevents B or vice versa.) Some third factor may account for both A and B.

correspondence school: a school that offers courses and degrees by mail. Some correspondence schools are accredited; others are diploma mills.

coupled reactions: pairs of chemical reactions in which energy released from the breakdown of one compound is used to create a bond in the formation of another compound.

covert (KOH-vert): hidden, as if under covers.

cretinism (CREE-tin-ism): an iodine-deficiency disease characterized by mental and physical retardation.

critical periods: finite periods during development in which certain events may occur that will have irreversible effects on later developmental stages. In a body organ, a critical period is usually a period of rapid cell division.

crypts: tubular glands that lie between the intestinal villi and secrete intestinal juices into the small intestine.

cuisine (kwi-ZEEN): style of cooking or preparing food.

cyclamate (SIGH-klo-mate): a 0-kcalorie sweetener; FDA approval pending in the United States; available in Canada on grocery-store shelves but only as a tabletop sweetener, not as an additive.

cytokines (SIGH-toe-kines): proteins secreted by phagocytes that activate metabolic and immune responses to infections.

D, L: D stands for dextro, or "right-handed," and L, for levo, or "left-handed," referring to the shapes of the molecules, which are mirror images of each other.

Daily Reference Values (DRV): a set of standards for nutrients and food components (such as fat and fiber) that have important relationships with health; used on food labels as part of the Daily Values.

Daily Values (DV): reference values developed by the FDA specifically for use on food labels. The Daily Values represent two sets of standards: Reference Daily Intakes (RDI) and Daily Reference Values (DRV).

deamination: removal of the amino (NH_2) group from a compound such as an amino acid.

defecate (DEF-uh-cate): to move the bowels and eliminate waste.

deficient: the amount of a nutrient below which almost all healthy people can be expected, over time, to experience deficiency symptoms.

dehydration: the condition in which body water output exceeds water input.

Delaney Clause: a clause in the Food Additive Amendment to the Food, Drug, and Cosmetic Act that states that no substance that is known to cause cancer in animals or human beings at any dose level shall be added to foods.

denaturation: the change in a protein's shape brought about by heat, acid, base, alcohol, heavy metals, or other agents.

dental caries: decay of teeth.

dextrins: the short chains of glucose units that result from the breakdown of starch. The word sometimes appears on food labels because dextrins can be used as thickening agents in foods.

dextrose: an older name for glucose.

diabetes (DYE-uh-BEET-eez) **mellitus** (MELL-ih-tus or mell-EYE-tus): a metabolic disorder characterized by altered glucose regulation and utilization, usually caused by insufficient or relatively ineffective insulin.

diarrhea: the frequent passage of watery bowel movements.

diet: the foods and beverages a person eats and drinks.

dietetic technician registered (DTR): a person with an associate's degree and training in nutrition, food science, and diet planning who works under the guidance of an RD (registered dietitian).

dietitian: a person trained in nutrition, food science, and diet planning. See also registered dietitian.

differentiation: development of specific functions different from those of the original.

digestion: the process by which food is broken down into absorbable units.

digestive enzymes: proteins found in digestive juices that act on food substances, causing them to break down into simpler compounds.

diglyceride: a molecule of glycerol with two fatty acids attached.

diketopiperazine (dye-KEY-toe-pie-PER-a-zeen), or **DKP:** a product to which aspartame breaks down during metabolism.

dioxins: any of 75 structurally related compounds that contain both nitrogen and chlorine.

dipeptide: two amino acids bonded together.

direct calorimetry (cal-o-RIM-uh-tree): the measurement of energy output as heat energy.

disaccharide: a pair of monosaccharides linked together.

dissociation: the physical separation of a compound into ions.

distilled liquor: an alcoholic beverage made by fermenting and distilling grains; sometimes called distilled spirits or hard liquor.

distilled water: water that has been vaporized and recondensed, leaving it free of dissolved minerals.

diuretic (dye-you-RET-ic): a drug that promotes water excretion; popularly, a "water pill."

diverticula (dye-ver-TIC-you-la): a sac or pouch that develops in the weakened areas of the intestinal wall (like bulges in an inner tube where the tire wall is weak).

diverticulitis (DYE-ver-tic-you-LYE-tis): infected or inflamed diverticula.

diverticulosis (DYE-ver-tic-you-LOH-sis): the condition of having diverticula.

docosahexaenoic (DOE-cossa-HEXA-ee-NO-ic) **acid (DHA):** an omega-3 polyunsaturated fatty acid with 22 carbons and six double bonds (22:6); synthesized from linolenic acid.

double-blind experiment: an experiment in which neither the subjects nor the researchers know which subjects are members of the experimental group and which are serving as control subjects, until after the experiment is over.

drink: a dose of any alcoholic beverage that delivers ½ oz of pure ethanol.

drug: a substance that can modify one or more of the body's functions.

DTR: see dietetic technician registered.

duodenum (doo-oh-DEEN-um, doo-ODD-num): the top portion of the small intestine (about "12 fingers' breadth" long in ancient terminology).

duration: length of time (for example, the time spent in each exercise session).

dysentery (DISS-en-terry): an infection of the digestive tract that causes diarrhea.

eating disorder: a disturbance in eating behavior that jeopardizes a person's physical or psychological health.

eclampsia: a condition characterized by convulsions and coma that develops in some women with untreated preeclampsia.

edema (eh-DEEM-uh): the swelling of body tissue caused by excessive amounts of fluid in the interstitial spaces; seen in protein deficiency (among other conditions).

eicosanoids (eye-COSS-uh-noyds): derivatives of fatty acids; hormonelike compounds that regulate blood pressure, clotting, and other body functions. They include prostaglandins, thromboxanes, and leukotrienes.

eicosapentaenoic (EYE-cossa-PENTA-ee-NO-ic) **acid (EPA):** an omega-3 polyunsaturated fatty acid with 20 carbons and five double bonds (20:5); synthesized from linolenic acid.

electrolyte solutions: solutions that can conduct electricity due to the presence of ions.

electrolytes: salts that dissolve in water and dissociate.

element: a substance composed of atoms that are alike—for example, iron (Fe).

embolism: the obstruction of a blood vessel by an embolus.

embolus (EM-boh-luss): a thrombus or other material that breaks loose from accumulated matter in the circulatory system and travels through the system.

embryo (EM-bree-oh): the developing infant from two to eight weeks after conception.

emetic (em-ETT-ic): an agent that causes vomiting.

empty-kcalorie food: a popular term used to denote foods that contribute energy but lack protein, vitamins, and minerals. Empty-kcalorie foods are low-nutrient density foods. The most notorious empty-kcalorie foods are sugar, fat, and alcohol.

emulsifier (ee-MUL-sih-fire): a substance with both water-soluble and fat-soluble portions that promotes the mixing of oils and fats in a watery solution.

endogenous protein: protein in the body.

endosperm (EN-doe-sperm): the bulk of the edible part of the grain kernel containing starch and proteins.

energy-yielding nutrients: the nutrients that break down to yield energy the body can use—carbohydrates, fats, and proteins.

energy: the capacity to do work. The energy in food is chemical energy. The body can convert this chemical energy to mechanical, electrical, or heat energy.

energy metabolism: all the reactions by which the body obtains and spends the energy from food.

enriched: the addition of nutrients to a food to meet a specified standard; often used interchangeably with fortified.

enterogastrone (EN-ter-oh-GAS-trone): a gastrointestinal hormone.

enteropancreatic (EN-ter-oh-PAN-kree-AT-ik) **circulation:** the circulatory route from the pancreas to the intestine and back to the pancreas.

enzymes: proteins that facilitate chemical reactions without being changed in the process; protein catalysts.

EPA (Environmental Protection Agency): a federal agency that is responsible for, among other things, regulating pesticides and establishing water quality standards.

epiglottis (epp-ee-GLOTT-iss): cartilage in the throat that guards the entrance to the trachea and prevents fluid or food from entering it when a person swallows.

epinephrine (EP-ih-NEFF-rin): a hormone of the adrenal gland that modulates the stress response; formerly called adrenaline.

epithelial (ep-i-THEE-lee-ul) **cells:** cells on the surface of the skin and mucous membranes.

epithelial tissues: the layers of the body that serve as selective barriers between the body's interior and the environment (examples are the cornea, the skin, the respiratory lining, and the lining of the digestive tract).

epoetin (eh-poy-EE-tin): a drug derived from human erythropoietin and marketed under the trade name Epogen; illegally used to increase oxygen capacity.

ergocalciferol (er-go-kal-SIF-er-ol): the plant version of vitamin D.

ergogenic aids: the term implies "energy giving," but in fact, no products impart such a quality.

erythrocyte (eh-REETH-ro-cite): red blood cell.

erythrocyte hemolysis: the breaking open of red blood cells; a symptom of vitamin E–deficiency disease in human beings.

erythrocyte protoporphyrin (PRO-toe-PORE-fe-rin): a precursor to hemoglobin.

esophagus (e-SOFF-uh-gus): the food pipe; the conduit from the mouth to the stomach.

essential amino acids: amino acids that the body cannot synthesize in amounts sufficient to meet physiological needs (see Table 6–1). Some researchers refer to essential amino acids as indispensable and to nonessential amino acids as dispensable.

essential fatty acids: fatty acids needed by the body, but not made by the body in amounts sufficient to meet physiological needs.

essential nutrients: nutrients a person must obtain from food because the body cannot make them for itself in sufficient quantity to meet physiological needs; also called indispensable nutrients. About 40 nutrients are known to be essential for human beings.

ethanol: a particular type of alcohol found in beer, wine, and distilled spirits; also called ethyl alcohol (see Figure H7–1). Ethanol is the most widely used—and abused—drug in our society. It is also the only legal, nonprescription drug that produces euphoria.

ethnic diets: foodways and cuisines typical of national origins, cultural heritages, or geographic locations.

euphoria (you-FORE-eh-uh): a feeling of great well-being, which people often seek through the use of drugs such as alcohol.

exchange lists: diet-planning tools that organize foods by their proportions of carbohydrate, fat, and protein. Foods on any single list can be used interchangeably.

exogenous protein: protein in foods.

experimental group: a group of individuals similar in all possible respects to the control group except for the treatment. The experimental group receives the real treatment.

external cue theory: the theory that some people eat in response to such external factors as the presence of food or the time of day rather than to such internal factors as hunger.

externalities: hidden costs that are not reflected in the prices of things, such as the costs of environmental deterioration or subsidies that permit agribusiness foods to be sold at artificially low prices.

false negative: a test result indicating that a condition is not present (negative) when in fact it is present (therefore false).

false positive: a test result indicating that a condition is present (positive) when in fact it is not (therefore false).

FAO (Food and Agriculture Organization): an international agency (part of the United Nations) that has adopted standards to regulate pesticide use among other responsibilities.

FAO: the Food and Agriculture Organization (of the United Nations).

fast-twitch muscle fibers: muscle fibers best suited to producing energy by anaerobic processes for high-intensity, short-duration activity.

fat: the lipids in foods or body fat, both of which are composed mostly of triglycerides.

fatfold measure: a clinical estimate of total body fatness in which the thickness of a fold of skin on the back of the arm (over the triceps muscle), below the shoulder blade (subscapular), or in other places is measured with a caliper. (The older, less preferred, term is skinfold test.)

fatty acid oxidation: the metabolic breakdown of fatty acids to acetyl CoA.

fatty acid: an organic compound composed of a carbon chain with hydrogens attached and an acid group (COOH) at one end.

fatty liver: an early stage of liver deterioration seen in several diseases, including kwashiorkor and alcoholic liver disease. Fatty liver is characterized by an accumulation of fat in the liver cells.

FDA (Food and Drug Administration): a part of the Department of Health and Human Services' Public Health Service that is responsible for ensuring the safety and wholesomeness of all foods sold in interstate commerce except meat, poultry, and eggs (which are under the jurisdiction of the USDA); inspecting food plants and imported foods; and setting standards for food composition.

fermentation: the oxidation of carbohydrate in the absence of atmospheric oxygen, a process that yields alcohol as an end product.

ferritin (FERR-ih-tin): an iron storage protein.

fertility: the capacity of a woman to produce a normal ovum periodically and of a man to produce normal sperm; the ability to reproduce.

fetal alcohol effects (FAE): a subclinical version of FAS, with hidden defects including learning disabilities, behavioral abnormalities, and motor impairments; also called alcohol-related birth defects (ARBD).

fetal alcohol syndrome (FAS): the cluster of symptoms seen in an infant or child whose mother consumed excess alcohol during pregnancy, including retarded growth, impaired development of the central nervous system, and facial malformations.

fetus (FEET-us): the developing infant from eight weeks after conception until term.

fiber: a general term denoting in plant foods the nonstarch polysaccharides that are not digested by human digestive enzymes, although some are digested by GI tract bacteria; fibers include cellulose, hemicelluloses, pectins, gums, and mucilages and the nonpolysaccharides lignins, cutins, and tannins.

fibrocystic breast disease: a harmless condition in which the breasts develop lumps, sometimes associated with caffeine consumption. In some, it responds to treatment by abstinence from caffeine; in others, it can be treated with vitamin E.

fibrosis (fye-BROH-sis): an intermediate stage of liver deterioration seen in several diseases, including viral hepatitis and alcoholic liver disease. In fibrosis, the liver cells lose their function and assume the characteristics of connective tissue cells (fibers).

fitness: the characteristics that enable the body to perform physical activity; more broadly, the ability to meet routine physical demands with enough reserve energy to rise to a sudden challenge; or the body's ability to withstand stress of all kinds.

flexibility: the capacity of the joints to move through a full range of motion; the ability to bend and recover without injury.

fluid and electrolyte balance: maintenance of the proper types and amounts of fluid and minerals in each compartment of the body fluids.

fluorapatite (floor-APP-uh-tite): the stabilized form of bone and tooth crystal, in which fluoride has replaced the hydroxyl groups of hydroxyapatite.

fluoridated water: water that has been treated so as to contain at least 0.8 mg fluoride per liter.

fluorosis: discoloration of tooth enamel caused by excess fluoride.

folate (FOLE-ate): a B vitamin; also known as folic acid, folacin, or pteroylglutamic (tare-o-EEL-glue-TAM-ick) acid (PGA). The coenzyme forms are DHF (dihydrofolate) and THF (tetrahydrofolate).

food allergies: adverse reactions to foods that involve an immune response; also called food-hypersensitivity reactions.

food aversion: a strong desire to avoid a particular food.

food chain: the sequence in which living things depend on other living things for food.

food consumption survey: a survey that measures the amounts and kinds of foods people consume (using diet histories), estimates the nutrient intakes, and compares them with a standard such as the RDA.

food craving: a deep longing for a particular food.

food group plans: diet-planning tools that sort foods of similar origin and nutrient content into groups and then specify that people should eat certain numbers of servings from each group.

food insecurity: intermittent hunger caused by lack of money or lack of control over other resources needed to assure a reliable food supply; the predominant form of hunger in the United States today.

food intolerances: adverse reactions to foods that do not involve the immune system.

Food Stamp Program: a federal food assistance program. The USDA issues food stamp coupons through state social services or welfare agencies to households—people who buy and prepare food together. The number of stamps a household receives depends on the household's size and income. Recipients may use the coupons like cash to purchase food and seeds, but not to buy tobacco, cleaning items, alcohol, or other nonfood items.

food-borne illnesses: illnesses transmitted to human beings through food, caused by either an infectious agent (food-borne infection) or a poisonous substance (food intoxication); commonly known as food poisoning.

foods: products derived from plants or animals that can be taken into the body to yield nutrients for the maintenance of life and the growth and repair of tissues.

foodways: the sum of the food habits, customs, beliefs, and preferences of a culture.

fortified: the addition of nutrients that were either not originally present or present in insignificant amounts to a food. Fortification can be used to correct or prevent a widespread nutrient deficiency, to balance the total nutrient profile of a food, or to restore nutrients lost in processing.

fossil fuel: coal, oil, and natural gas; these are nonrenewable fuels that pollute. (Renewable or alternative fuels, such as solar and wind energy, pollute less or not at all.)

frame size: the size of a person's bones and musculature.

fraud or quackery: the promotion, for financial gain, of devices, treatments, services, plans, or products (including diets and supplements) that alter or claim to alter a human condition without proof of safety or effectiveness. (The word quackery comes from the term quacksalver, meaning a person who quacks loudly about a miracle product—a lotion or a salve.)

free radical: an atom or molecule that has one or more unpaired electron(s) in the outer orbital (see Appendix B for a review of basic chemistry concepts). This electron imbalance makes free radicals unstable and highly reactive. Radicals typically arise during oxidation reactions and readily attack other molecules with which they come in contact.

frequency: the number of occurrences per unit of time (for example, the number of exercise sessions per week).

fructose: a monosaccharide; sometimes known as fruit sugar or levulose, fructose is found abundantly in fruits, honey, and saps.

galactose: a monosaccharide; part of the disaccharide lactose.

gallbladder: the organ that stores and concentrates bile. When it receives the signal that fat is present in the duodenum, the gallbladder contracts and squirts bile through the bile duct into the duodenum.

galvanized: a term referring to metals that have been treated with a zinc-containing coating to prevent rust.

gangrene (GANG-green): the death of tissue, usually due to deficient blood supply.

gastric glands: exocrine glands in the stomach wall that secrete gastric juice into the stomach.

gastric juice: the digestive secretion of the gastric glands of the stomach.

gastric partitioning: a surgical procedure used to treat clinically severe obesity. The operation limits food intake by reducing the size of the stomach and delays gastric emptying by restricting the outlet.

gastric-inhibitory peptide: a hormone produced by the intestine. Target organ: the stomach. Response: slowing of the secretion of gastric juices and of GI motility.

gastrin: a hormone secreted by cells in the stomach wall. Target organ: the stomach. Response: secretion of gastric juice.

gatekeepers: with respect to nutrition, key people who control other people's access to foods and thereby exert profound impacts on their nutrition. Examples are the spouse who buys and cooks the food, the parent who feeds the children, and the caretaker in a day-care center.

germ: the nutrient-rich inner part of a grain. The germ is the seed that grows into a wheat plant, so it is especially rich in vitamins and minerals to support new life.

gestation (jes-TAY-shun): the period from conception to birth; for human beings gestation lasts from 38 to 42 weeks. Pregnancy is often divided into thirds, called trimesters.

gestational diabetes: the appearance of abnormal glucose tolerance during pregnancy, with subsequent return to normal postpartum.

GI tract: the gastrointestinal tract or digestive tract; the principal organs are the stomach and intestines.

gland: a cell or group of cells that secretes materials for special uses in the body. Glands may be exocrine (EKS-oh-crin) glands, secreting their materials "out" (into the digestive tract or onto the surface of the skin), or endocrine (EN-doe-crin) glands, secreting their materials "in" (into the blood).

glucagon (GLOO-ka-gon): a hormone secreted by special cells in the pancreas in response to low blood glucose concentration that elicits release of glucose from storage.

gluconeogenesis (gloo-co-nee-oh-GEN-ih-sis): the making of glucose from a non-carbohydrate source.

glucose polymers: compounds that supply glucose, not as single molecules, but linked in chains somewhat like starch. The objective is to attract less water from the body into the digestive tract (osmotic attraction depends on the number, not the size of particles).

glucose tolerance factor (GTF): a small organic compound that enhances insulin's action.

glucose: a monosaccharide; sometimes known as blood sugar or dextrose.

gluten (GLOO-ten): an elastic protein found in wheat and other grains that gives dough its structure and cohesiveness.

glycemic (gligh-SEEM-ic) **effect:** a measure of the extent to which a food, as compared with pure glucose, raises the blood glucose concentration and elicits an insulin response.

glycerol (GLISS-er-ol): an alcohol composed of a three-carbon chain, which can serve as the backbone for a triglyceride.

glycogen (GLY-co-gen): an animal polysaccharide composed of glucose; it is manufactured and stored in the liver and muscles as a storage form of glucose. Glycogen is not a significant food source of carbohydrate and is not counted as one of the complex carbohydrates in foods.

glycolysis (gligh-COLL-ih-sis): the metabolic breakdown of glucose to pyruvate. Glycolysis does not require oxygen (anaerobic).

goblet cells: cells of the GI tract (and lungs) that secrete mucus.

goiter (GOY-ter): an enlargement of the thyroid gland due to an iodine deficiency, malfunction of the gland, or overconsumption of a goitrogen. Goiter caused by iodine deficiency is called simple goiter.

goitrogen (GOY-troh-jen): a thyroid antagonist found in food; causes toxic goiter. Goitrogens are found in such foods as cabbage, kale, brussels sprouts, cauliflower, broccoli, and kohlrabi.

gout (GOWT): a painful condition in which uric acid crystals form in the joints.

granulated sugar: crystalline sucrose; 99.9 percent pure.

GRAS (generally recognized as safe) list: a list, established by the FDA in 1958, of food additives that had long been in use and were believed safe. The list is subject to revision as new facts become known.

hair follicle (FOLL-i-cul): a group of cells in the skin from which a hair grows.

hard water: water with a high calcium and magnesium concentration.

hazard: source of danger; used to refer to circumstances in which toxicity is possible under normal conditions of use.

HDL (high-density lipoprotein): the type of lipoprotein that transports cholesterol back to the liver from peripheral cells; composed primarily of protein.

health claim: any statement that characterizes the relationship between any nutrient or other substance in a food and a disease or health-related condition.

Healthy Eating Index: a standard developed by USDA for assessing overall dietary quality; a single numerical summary of degree of adherence to the recommendations of the Food Guide Pyramid and the Dietary Guidelines for Americans.

heartburn: a burning sensation in the chest area caused by backflow of stomach acid into the esophagus.

heat stroke: the dangerous accumulation of body heat with accompanying loss of body fluid.

heavy metal: any of a number of mineral ions such as mercury and lead, so called because they are of relatively high atomic weight. Many heavy metals are poisonous.

Heimlich maneuver: a technique for removing an object from the trachea of a choking person (see Figure H3-2).

hematocrit: measurement of the volume of the red blood cells packed by centrifuge in a given volume of blood; the volume reflects red blood cell size.

hematopoietic (HEE-ma-toe-poy-ET-ik) **neoplasm:** a cancer of the blood and immune system.

heme (HEEM): the iron-holding part of the hemoglobin and myoglobin proteins. About 40% of the iron in meat, fish, and poultry is bound into heme; the other 60% is nonheme iron.

hemochromatosis (heem-oh-crome-a-TOCE-iss): a hereditary defect in iron metabolism characterized by deposits of iron-containing pigment in many tissues, with tissue damage.

hemoglobin: the globular protein of the red blood cells that carries oxygen from the lungs to the cells throughout the body.

hemolysis (he-MOLL-uh-sis): bursting of red blood cells.

hemophilia: a hereditary disease that has no relation to vitamin K, but is caused by a genetic defect; the blood is unable to clot because it lacks the ability to synthesize certain clotting factors.

hemorrhagic (hem-o-RAJ-ik) **disease:** a disease characterized by excessive bleeding.

hemorrhoids: painful swelling of the veins surrounding the rectum.

hemosiderin (HE-mow-SID-er-in): an iron-storage compound.

hemosiderosis (HE-mow-sid-er-OH-sis): a condition characterized by the deposition of hemosiderin in the liver and other tissues.

hepatic vein: the vein that collects blood from the liver capillaries and returns it to the heart.

herpes virus: a virus that can lead to mouth lesions and may also affect the lower GI tract, causing diarrhea.

hGH (human growth hormone): a hormone produced by the brain's pituitary gland that regulates normal growth and development; also called somatotropin. Some athletes misuse this hormone to increase their height and strength.

hiccups: repeated cough-like sounds and jerks that are produced when an involuntary spasm of the diaphragm muscle sucks air down the windpipe; also spelled hiccoughs.

high-fructose corn syrup (HFCS): a corn-syrup sweetener made especially for use in processed foods and beverages, where it is the predominant sweetener. HFCS is mostly fructose; glucose makes up the balance.

high-quality protein: an easily digestible, complete protein.

high-risk pregnancy: a pregnancy characterized by indicators that make it likely the birth will be surrounded by problems such as premature delivery, difficult birth, retarded growth, birth defects, and early infant death.

histamine (HISS-tah-mean, or HISS-tah-men): a substance produced by cells of the immune system as part of a local immune reaction to an antigen; participates in causing inflammation.

homeostasis (HOME-ee-oh-STAY-sis): the maintenance of constant internal conditions (such as blood chemistry, temperature, and blood pressure) by the body's control systems. A homeostatic system is constantly reacting to external forces so as to maintain limits set by the body's needs.

honey: sugar (mostly sucrose) formed from nectar gathered by bees. An enzyme splits the sucrose into glucose and fructose. Composition and flavor vary, but honey always contains a mixture of sucrose, fructose, and glucose.

hormones: chemical messengers that are secreted by a variety of glands in response to altered conditions in the body. Each hormone travels to one or more specific target tissues or organs, where it elicits a specific response to restore normal conditions.

hormone-sensitive lipase: an enzyme inside adipose cells that responds to the body's need for fuel by hydrolyzing triglycerides so that their parts (glycerol and fatty acids) escape into the general circulation and thus become available to other cells as fuel. The signals to which this enzyme responds include epinephrine and glucagon, which oppose insulin.

human immunodeficiency virus (HIV): the virus that causes AIDS. The infection progresses to become an immune system disorder that leaves its victims defenseless against numerous infections.

humoral immunity: immunity conferred by antibodies secreted by B-cells and carried to the invaded area by way of the body fluids.

hunger: the physiological need to eat, experienced as a drive to obtain food; an unpleasant sensation.

husk: the outer, inedible part of a grain; also called the chaff.

hydrochloric acid: an acid composed of hydrogen and chloride atoms (HCl). The gastric glands normally produce this acid.

hydrodensitometry (HI-dro-DEN-see-TOM-eh-tree): a method of measuring body density in which the person is first weighed and then submerged in water.

hydrogenation (high-dro-gen-AY-shun): a chemical process by which hydrogens are added to monounsaturated or polyunsaturated fats to reduce the number of double bonds, making the fats more saturated (solid) and more resistant to oxidation (protecting against rancidity). Hydrogenation produces trans-fatty acids.

hydrolysis (high-DROL-ih-sis): a chemical reaction in which a major reactant is split into two products, with the addition of a hydrogen atom (H) to one and a hydroxyl group (OH) to the other (from water, H_2O).

hydrophilic: a term referring to water-loving, or water-soluble, substances.

hydrophobic: a term referring to water-fearing, or non-water-soluble, substances; also known as lipophilic (fat loving).

hyperactivity: a disorder characterized by chronic behavior and learning problems. Behavior problems include impulsiveness and restlessness that are inappropriate for a child's age. Learning problems reflect a short attention span. Professionals call this syndrome attention deficit hyperactivity disorder (ADHD).

hypercalcemia: high blood calcium that may develop from a variety of disorders, including vitamin D toxicity. It does not develop from a high calcium intake.

hyperkalemia (HIGH-per-ka-LEE-me-ah): high levels of potassium in the blood.

hypertension: higher-than-normal blood pressure. Hypertension that develops without an identifiable cause is known as essential or primary hypertension; hypertension that is caused by a specific disorder such as kidney disease is known as secondary hypertension.

hyperthermia: an above-normal body temperature.

hypertrophy (high-PER-tro-fee): of muscles, growing larger; an increase in size in response to use.

hypoglycemia: an abnormally low blood glucose concentration.

hypokalemia (HIGH-po-ka-LEE-me-ah): low levels of potassium in the blood.

hypothalamus (high-po-THAL-ah-mus): a brain center that controls activities such as maintenance of water balance and regulation of body temperature.

hypothermia: a below-normal body temperature.

ileocecal (ill-ee-oh-SEEK-ul) **valve:** the sphincter separating the small and large intestines.

ileum (ILL-ee-um): the last segment of the small intestine.

imitation food: a food that substitutes for and resembles another food and is nutritionally inferior to it with respect to vitamin, mineral, or protein content. If the substitute is not inferior to the food it resembles and it provides an accurate name for itself, it need not be labeled "imitation."

immune system: the body's natural defense system against foreign materials that have penetrated the skin or mucous membranes.

immunity: the body's ability to recognize and eliminate foreign invaders.

immunoglobulin: a protein capable of acting as an antibody.

implantation: the stage of development in which the zygote embeds itself in the wall of the uterus and begins to develop; occurs during the first two weeks after conception.

indirect additives: substances that can get into food as a result of contact with foods during growing, processing, packaging, storing, cooking, or some other stage before the foods are consumed; also called incidental or accidental additives.

indirect calorimetry: the estimation of energy output from measures of the amount of oxygen used and carbon dioxide eliminated.

initiation: an event caused by radiation or chemical reaction that can give rise to cancer.

inorganic: not containing carbon or pertaining to living things.

inositol (in-OSS-ih-tall): a nonessential nutrient that can be made in the body from glucose. Inositol is used in cell membranes.

insulin (IN-suh-lin): a hormone secreted by special cells in the pancreas in response to (among other things) increased blood glucose concentration. The primary role of insulin is to control the transport of glucose from the bloodstream into the cells.

insulin resistance: the condition of having a normal amount of insulin producing a subnormal effect; a metabolic consequence of obesity.

insulin-dependent diabetes mellitus (IDDM): the less common type of diabetes in which the person produces no insulin at all; also known as type I diabetes or juvenile-onset diabetes (because it frequently develops in childhood), although some cases arise in adulthood.

integrated pest management (IPM): management of pests using a combination of natural and biological controls rather than indiscriminate application of pesticides.

intensity: the degree of exertion while exercising (for example, the amount of weight lifted or the speed of running).

intentional additives: additives intentionally added to foods, such as nutrients, colors, and preservatives.

intermittent claudication: severe calf pain caused by inadequate blood supply, it occurs when walking and subsides during rest.

international units (IU): a measure of vitamin activity, determined by such biological methods as feeding a compound to vitamin-deprived animals and measuring growth. This system was used to measure fat-soluble vitamins before direct chemical analysis was possible.

interstitial (IN-ter-STISH-al) **fluid:** fluid between the cells, usually high in sodium and chloride. Interstitial fluid is a large component of extracellular fluid (fluid outside the cells), which also includes plasma and the water of structures such as the skin and bones. Extracellular fluid accounts for approximately one-third of the body's water.

intestinal flora: the bacterial inhabitants of the GI tract.

intra-abdominal fat: fat stored within the abdominal cavity in association with the internal abdominal organs, as opposed to the fat stored directly under the skin (subcutaneous fat).

intracellular fluid: fluid within the cells, usually high in potassium and phosphate. Intracellular fluid accounts for approximately two-thirds of the body's water.

intrinsic: inside the system.

intrinsic factor: a glycoprotein (a protein with short polysaccharide chains attached) made in the stomach that aids in the absorption of vitamin B_{12}.

invert sugar: a mixture of glucose and fructose formed by the hydrolysis of sucrose in a chemical process; sold only in liquid form and sweeter than sucrose. Invert sugar is used as a food additive to help preserve freshness and prevent shrinkage.

iodopsin (eye-o-DOP-sin): the light-sensitive pigment of the cones of the retina.

ions (EYE-uns): atoms or molecules that have gained or lost electrons and therefore have electrical charges. Examples include the positively charged sodium ion ($Na+$) and the negatively charged chloride ion (Cl^-).

iron deficiency: the state of having depleted iron stores.

iron overload: toxicity from excess iron.

iron-deficiency anemia: a blood iron deficiency that results in small, pale, red blood cells. Iron-deficiency anemia is a microcytic (my-cro-SIT-ic) hypochromic (high-po-KROME-ic) anemia.

jaundice: yellowing of the skin, due to spillover of the bile pigments bilirubin (bill-ee-ROO-bin) from the liver into the general circulation; also known as hyperbilirubinemia (HIGH-per-BILL-eh-roo-bin-EE-me-ah). When these pigments invade the brain, the condition is kernicterus (ker-NICK-ter-us). Jaundice may be caused by obstruction of bile passageways, hemolysis, or dysfunctional liver cells.

jejunum (je-JOON-um): the first two-fifths of the small intestine beyond the duodenum.

Kaposi's (cap-OH-seez) **sarcoma:** a type of cancer rare in the general population but common in people with HIV infections.

kcalorie: see calorie.

kcalorie (energy) control: management of food energy intake.

keratin (KERR-uh-tin): a water-insoluble protein; the normal protein of hair and nails. Keratin-producing cells may replace mucus-producing cells in vitamin A deficiency.

keratinization: accumulation of keratin in a tissue; a sign of vitamin A deficiency.

keratomalacia (KARE-ah-toe-ma-LAY-shia): softening of the cornea seen in severe vitamin A deficiency that leads to irreversible blindness.

Keshan disease: the heart disease associated with selenium deficiency, named for one of the provinces of China where it was studied. Keshan disease is characterized by heart enlargement and insufficiency; the middle layer of the walls of the heart, which are normally composed of muscle tissue, are replaced with fibrous tissue.

keto acid: an organic acid that contains a carbonyl group (C=O).

ketone (KEE-tone) **bodies:** the product of the incomplete breakdown of fat when glucose is not available in the cells.

ketosis (kee-TOE-sis): an undesirably high concentration of ketone bodies in the blood and urine.

kosher (KOE-sure): foods prepared according to Jewish dietary laws.

kwashiorkor (kwash-ee-OR-core, kwash-ee-or-CORE): a form of PEM that results from either inadequate protein intake or, more commonly, from infections.

lactase deficiency: a lack of the enzyme required to digest the disaccharide lactose into its component monosaccharides (glucose and galactose).

lactase: an enzyme that hydrolyzes lactose.

lactation: production and secretion of breast milk for the purpose of nourishing an infant.

lactic acid: an acid produced from pyruvate during anaerobic metabolism.

lacto-ovo-vegetarians: people who include milk, milk products, and eggs, but exclude meat, poultry, fish, and seafood from their diets.

lactoferrin (lak-toh-FERR-in): a factor in breast milk that binds iron and keeps it from supporting the growth of the infant's intestinal bacteria.

lactose intolerance: a condition that results from inability to digest the milk sugar lactose; characterized by bloating, gas, abdominal discomfort, and diarrhea. Lactose intolerance differs from milk allergy, which is caused by an immune reaction to the protein in milk.

lactose: a disaccharide composed of glucose and galactose; commonly known as milk sugar.

lactovegetarians: people who include milk and milk products, but exclude meat, poultry, fish, seafood, and eggs from their diets.

large intestine or **colon** (COAL-un): the lower portion of intestine that completes the digestive process; its segments are the ascending colon, the transverse colon, the descending colon, and the sigmoid colon.

larynx: the voice box (see Figure H3–1).

LDL (low-density lipoprotein): the type of lipoprotein derived from very-low-density lipoproteins (VLDL) as cells remove triglycerides from them; composed primarily of cholesterol.

lecithin (LESS-uh-thin): one of the phospholipids; a compound of glycerol to which are attached two fatty acids, a phosphate group, and a choline molecule. Both nature and the food industry use lecithin as an emulsifier to combine two ingredients that do not ordinarily mix, such as water and oil.

legumes (lay-GYOOMS, LEG-yooms): plants of the bean and pea family. Bacteria in the root nodules of legumes "fix" nitrogen by trapping nitrogen from the air into the soil and then making it a part of the protein in the beans. Thus legumes are rich in high-quality protein compared with other plant-derived foods. Ultimately, the plant leaves more nitrogen in the soil than it takes out (sparing the land). Farmers sometimes plow under legume plants to fertilize the soil.

levulose: an older name for fructose.

license to practice: permission under state or federal law, granted on meeting specified criteria, to use a certain title (such as dietitian) and offer certain services. Licensed dietitians may use the initials LD after their names.

life expectancy: the average number of years lived by people in a given society.

life span: the maximum number of years of life attainable by a member of a species.

limiting amino acid: the essential amino acid found in the shortest supply relative to the amounts needed for protein synthesis in the body.

linoleic (lin-oh-LAY-ick) **acid:** an essential fatty acid with 18 carbons and two double bonds (18:2).

linolenic (lin-oh-LEN-ick) **acid:** an essential fatty acid with 18 carbons and three double bonds (18:3).

lipase (LYE-pase): an enzyme that hydrolyzes lipids (fats).

lipids: a family of compounds that includes triglycerides (fats and oils), phospholipids, and sterols.

lipoic (lip-OH-ick) **acid:** a nonessential nutrient.

lipoprotein lipase (LPL): an enzyme mounted on the surface of fat cells (and other cells) that hydrolyzes triglycerides passing by in the bloodstream and directs their parts into the cells, where they can be metabolized or reassembled for storage.

lipoproteins (LIP-oh-PRO-teenz): clusters of lipids associated with proteins that serve as transport vehicles for lipids in the lymph and blood.

liver: the organ that manufactures bile and is the first to receive nutrients from the intestines. The liver's many other functions are described in Chapter 7.

longevity: long duration of life.

low birthweight (LBW): a birthweight of 5½ lb (2500 g) or less; indicates probable poor health in the newborn and poor nutrition status in the mother during pregnancy, before pregnancy, or both. Normal birthweight for a full-term baby is 6½ to 8¾ lb (about 3000 to 4000 g).

low-risk pregnancy: a pregnancy characterized by indicators that make a normal outcome likely.

lymph (LIMF): a clear yellowish fluid that resembles blood without the red blood cells; lymph from the GI tract transports fat and fat-soluble vitamins to the bloodstream via lymphatic vessels.

lymphatic (lim-FAT-ic) **system:** a loosely organized system of vessels and ducts that convey fluids toward the heart; the GI part of the lymphatic system carries the products of digestion into the bloodstream.

lymphocytes: white blood cells that participate in acquired immunity; B-cells and T-cells.

lysosomes (LYE-so-zomes): the sacs of degradative enzymes.

macrobiotic diets: extremely restrictive diets limited to a few cereals and fluids; based on metaphysical beliefs and not on nutrition.

macrocytic or **megaloblastic anemia**: the large-cell anemia of a folate deficiency.

magnesium: a cation within the body's cells, active in many enzyme systems.

major minerals: essential mineral nutrients found in the human body in amounts larger than 5 grams.

malnutrition: any condition caused by excess or deficient food energy or nutrient intake or by an imbalance of nutrients.

maltase: an enzyme that hydrolyzes maltose.

maltose: a disaccharide composed of two glucose units; sometimes known as malt sugar.

maple sugar: a sugar (mostly sucrose) purified from the concentrated sap of the sugar maple tree.

marasmus (ma-RAZ-mus): a form of PEM that results from a severe deprivation, or impaired absorption, of energy, protein, vitamins, and minerals.

margin of safety: when speaking of food additives, a zone between the concentration normally used and that at which a hazard exists. For common table salt, for example, the margin of safety is ⅕ (five times the amount normally used would be hazardous).

matrix (MAY-tricks): the basic substance that gives form to a developing structure; in the body, the formative cells from which teeth and bones grow.

meat replacement: products formulated to look and taste like meat, fish, or poultry; usually made of textured vegetable protein.

menadione (men-uh-DYE-own): a synthetic form of vitamin K.

MEOS (microsomal ethanol-oxidizing system): a system of enzymes in the liver that oxidize not only alcohol, but also several classes of drugs. (The microsomes are tiny particles of membranes with associated enzymes that can be collected from broken-up cells.)

metabolism: the sum total of all the chemical reactions that go on in living cells.

metalloenzyme (meh-tal-oh-EN-zime): an enzyme that contains one or more minerals as part of its structure.

metallothionein (meh-TAL-oh-THIGH-oh-neen): a sulfur-rich protein that avidly binds with metals such as zinc.

metastasize (me-TAS-tah-size): the movement of cancer cells from one part of the body to another.

MFP factor: a factor associated with the digestion of meat, fish, and poultry that enhances iron absorption.

micelles (MY-cells): tiny spherical complexes that arise during fat digestion; each carries about 20 fatty acids and/or monoglycerides into intestinal cells.

microvilli (MY-cro-VILL-ee, MY-cro-VILL-eye): tiny, hairlike projections on each cell of every villus that can trap nutrient particles and transport them into the cells; singular microvillus.

milk anemia: iron-deficiency anemia that develops when an excessive milk intake displaces iron-rich foods from the diet.

milliequivalents (mEq): the concentration of electrolytes in a volume of solution. The number of milliequivalents is a useful measure when considering ions, because the number of charges reveals characteristics about the solution that are not evident when expressed in terms of weight.

mineral water: water from a spring or well that typically contains 250 to 500 ppm of minerals. Minerals give water a distinctive flavor. Many mineral waters are high in sodium.

mineralization: the process in which calcium, phosphorus, and other minerals crystallize on the collagen matrix of a growing bone, hardening the bone.

minerals: inorganic elements; some minerals are essential nutrients required in small amounts. The major minerals are calcium, phosphorus, potassium, sodium, chloride, magnesium, and sulfur. The trace minerals are iron, iodine, zinc, chromium, selenium, fluoride, molybdenum, copper, and manganese.

misinformation: false or misleading information.

moderate exercise: activity that can be sustained comfortably for 60 minutes or so.

moderation: in relation to dietary intake, providing enough but not too much of a substance; in relation to alcohol consumption, not more than two drinks a day for the average-sized man and not more than one drink a day for the average-sized woman.

molasses: the thick brown syrup produced during sugar refining. Molasses retains residual sugar and other by-products and a few minerals; blackstrap molasses contains significant amounts of calcium and iron—the iron comes from the machinery used to process the sugar.

molecule: two or more atoms of the same or different elements joined by chemical bonds. Examples are molecules of the element oxygen, composed of two oxygen atoms (O_2), and molecules of the compound water, composed of two hydrogen atoms and one oxygen atom (H_2O).

molybdenum (mo-LIB-duh-num): a trace element.

monoglyceride: a molecule of glycerol with one fatty acid attached.

monosaccharide (mon-oh-SACK-uh-ride): a carbohydrate of the general formula $C_nH_{2n}O_n$ that consists of a single ring.

monounsaturated fatty acid: a fatty acid that lacks two hydrogen atoms and has one double bond between carbons—for example, oleic acid.

motility: the ability of the GI tract muscles to move.

mucosal ferritin (FERR-ih-tin): protein that holds iron in the intestinal cell.

mucosal transferrin (trans-FERR-in): protein that passes iron from mucosal ferritin on to blood transferrin.

mucous membranes: the membranes, composed of mucus-secreting cells, that line the surfaces of body tissues.

mucus (MYOO-cuss): a slippery substance secreted by goblet cells of the GI lining (and other body linings) that protects the cells from exposure to digestive juices (and other destructive agents). The lining of the GI tract with its coat of mucus is a mucous membrane. (The noun is mucus; the adjective is mucous.)

muscle endurance: the ability of a muscle to contract repeatedly without becoming exhausted.

muscle fibers: muscle cells.

muscle strength: the ability of muscles to work against resistance.

muscular dystrophy (DIS-tro-fee): a hereditary disease in which the muscles gradually weaken; its most debilitating effects arise in the lungs.

mutual supplementation: the strategy of combining two protein foods in a meal so that each food provides the essential amino acid(s) lacking in the other. Mutual supplementation is the dietary strategy that brings complementary proteins together in a meal.

myoglobin: the oxygen-holding protein of the muscle cells.

NAD (nicotinamide adenine dinucleotide): the main coenzyme form of the vitamin niacin; its reduced form is NADH.

narcotic (nor-KOT-ic): any drug that dulls the senses, induces sleep, and becomes addictive with prolonged use.

natural water: water obtained from a spring or well that is certified to be safe and sanitary. The mineral content may not be changed, but the water may be treated in other ways such as by filtration or ozonization.

NE: see niacin equivalents.

net protein utilization (NPU): the amount of protein nitrogen that is retained from a given amount of protein nitrogen eaten; a measure of protein quality.

neuron: a nerve cell; the structural and functional unit of the nervous system. Neurons initiate and conduct nerve transmissions.

neurotransmitters: chemicals that are released at the end of a nerve cell when a nerve impulse arrives there; they diffuse across the gap to the next cell and alter the membrane of that second cell to either inhibit or excite it.

niacin (NIGH-a-sin): a B vitamin. Niacin can be eaten preformed or made in the body from its precursor, tryptophan, one of the amino acids. The active coenzyme forms are NAD (nicotinamide adenine dinucleotide) and NADP (the phosphate form of NAD).

niacin equivalents (NE): the amount of niacin present in food, including the niacin that can theoretically be made from its precursor, tryptophan, present in the food.

night blindness: slow recovery of vision after flashes of bright light at night or an inability to see in dim light; an early symptom of vitamin A deficiency.

nitrates: salts that are converted to nitrites by bacteria.

nitrites: salts added to food to prevent botulism; one example is sodium nitrite, which is used to preserve meats.

nitrogen balance: the amount of nitrogen consumed (N in) as compared with the amount of nitrogen excreted (N out) in a given period of time.

nitrosamines (nigh-TROHS-uh-meens): derivatives of nitrites that may be formed in the stomach when nitrites combine with amines; nitrosamines are carcinogenic in animals.

noninsulin-dependent diabetes mellitus (NIDDM): the more common type of diabetes in which the fat cells resist insulin; also called type II diabetes or adult-onset diabetes. NIDDM is usually milder than IDDM and progresses more slowly.

nonnutrients: compounds in foods with no known nutritional value.

nonpoint water pollution: water pollution caused by runoff from all over an area rather than from discrete "point" sources. An example is the pollution caused by runoff from agricultural fields.

nonspecific immunity: immunity directed at many kinds of organisms (also called general or innate immunity). Phagocytes, the skin, and mucous membranes confer this type of immunity.

nursing bottle tooth decay: extensive tooth decay due to prolonged tooth contact with formula, milk, fruit juice, or other carbohydrate-rich liquid offered to an infant in a bottle.

nutraceuticals: substances that supposedly provide medical and health benefits; a term not recognized by the FDA.

nutrient additives: vitamins and minerals added to improve nutritive value.

nutrient density: a measure of the nutrients a food provides relative to the energy it provides. The more nutrients and the fewer kcalories, the higher the nutrient density.

nutrients: substances obtained from food and used in the body to provide energy and structural materials and to regulate growth, maintenance, and repair of the body's tissues; nutrients may also reduce the risks of some chronic diseases.

nutrition assessment: a comprehensive approach, completed by a registered dietitian, to defining nutrition status that uses health, socioeconomic, drug, and diet histories; anthropometric measurements; physical examinations; and laboratory tests.

nutrition status survey: a survey that evaluates people's nutrition status using diet histories, anthropometric measures, physical examinations, and laboratory tests.

nutritional yeast: a preparation of yeast cells grown especially as a nutrient supplement, particularly for vegetarian diets. The type of yeast used is brewer's yeast, not baker's yeast. Different species of yeasts produce different compounds; yeast cells used in brewing produce alcohol, proteins, and B vitamins as they grow. The nutrients are removed from beer and wine in the filtering process. Yeast cells used in baking produce mostly carbon dioxide, which causes bread dough to rise.

nutritionist: a person who specializes in the study of nutrition. Some nutritionists are registered dietitians, whereas others are self-described experts whose training is questionable. In states with responsible legislation, the term applies only to people who have MS or PhD degrees from properly accredited institutions.

nutritive sweeteners: sweeteners that yield energy, including both sugars and sugar alcohols.

obligatory (ah-BLIG-ah-TORE-ee) **water excretion:** the amount of water the body has to excrete each day to dispose of its wastes—about 500 ml, or a pint.

oligopeptide: an intermediate string of four to nine amino acids bonded together.

omega-3 fatty acid: a polyunsaturated fatty acid in which the first double bond is three carbons away from the methyl (CH_3) end of the carbon chain.

omega-6 fatty acid: a polyunsaturated fatty acid in which the first double bond is six carbons from the methyl (CH_3) end of the carbon chain.

omega: the last letter of the Greek alphabet (ω), used by chemists to refer to the position of the endmost double bond in a fatty acid.

omnivores: people who have no formal restriction on the eating of any foods.

opportunistic infections: infections from microorganisms that normally do not cause disease in the general population but can infect people once their immune systems are compromised (as in HIV infection).

opsin (OP-sin): the protein portion of the visual pigment molecule.

oral rehydration therapy (ORT): the administration of a simple solution of sugar, salt, and water, taken by mouth, to treat dehydration caused by diarrhea.

organic halogen: an organic compound containing one or more atoms of a halogen—fluorine, chlorine, iodine, or bromine.

organic: a substance or molecule containing carbon-carbon bonds or carbon-hydrogen bonds. Some farmers call their produce "organic" if it was grown without manufactured fertilizers and pesticides, but by the definition given here, all foods are organic.

osmotic pressure: the pressure that develops when two solutions of different concentrations are separated by a membrane that permits water, but not the solutes, to cross. Water flows toward the side of the membrane on which the solutes are more concentrated.

osteoblasts: cells that build bone.

osteoclasts: cells that destroy bone.

osteomalacia (os-tee-o-mal-AY-shuh): a bone disease characterized by softening of the bones; symptoms include bending of the spine and bowing of the legs. The disease occurs most often in adult women.

osteopenia: a metabolic bone disease common in preterm infants; also called rickets of prematurity.

osteoporosis (OSS-tee-oh-pore-OH-sis): a condition of older persons in which the bones become porous and fragile due to a loss of minerals; also called adult bone loss.

overnutrition: excess energy or nutrients.

overt (oh-VERT): out in the open and easy to observe.

overweight: body weight above some standard of acceptable weight that is usually defined in relation to height (such as the weight-for-height tables).

ovum: the female reproductive cell, capable of developing into a new organism upon fertilization; commonly referred to as an egg.

oxidant: a compound (such as oxygen itself) that oxidizes other compounds. Compounds that prevent oxidation are called antioxidants, whereas those that encourage it are called prooxidants.

oxidation (OK-see-day-shun): the process of a substance combining with oxygen.

oxidative stress: damage to biological systems caused by free-radical formation.

palatability: pleasing taste. When tasting foods, the tongue presses them against the palate (PAL-ut), or roof of the mouth.

pancreas: a gland that secretes digestive enzymes and juices into the duodenum.

pancreatic (pank-ree-AT-ic) **juice:** the exocrine secretion of the pancreas, containing enzymes for the digestion of carbohydrate, fat, and protein as well as bicarbonate, a neutralizing agent. The juice flows from the pancreas into the small intestine through the pancreatic duct. (The pancreas also has an endocrine function, the secretion of insulin and other hormones.)

pantothenic (PAN-toe-THEN-ick) **acid:** a B vitamin; the principal active form is part of coenzyme A, called "CoA" throughout Chapter 7.

parathormone (PAIR-ah-THOR-moan): a hormone from the parathyroid that raises blood calcium.

pasteurization: a process of heating milk sufficiently to kill many disease-causing microbes commonly transmitted through milk; not a sterilization process. Pasteurized milk retains bacteria that cause milk spoilage. Unpasteurized ("certified" raw) milk transmits many food-borne diseases to people each year and should be avoided.

pathogens (PATH-oh-jens): microorganisms or substances capable of producing disease.

PC, phosphocreatine (also called **creatine phosphate**): a high-energy compound in muscle cells that acts as a reservoir of energy that can maintain a steady supply of ATP; PC provides the energy for short bursts of activity.

peak bone mass: the highest attainable bone density for an individual, developed during the first three decades of life.

peer review: a process in which a panel of scientists rigorously evaluates a research study to assure that the scientific method was followed.

pellagra (pell-AY-gra): the niacin-deficiency disease.

PEM: see protein-energy malnutrition.

pepsin: a gastric protease. Pepsin is secreted in an inactive form, pepsinogen, which is activated by stomach acid.

peptic ulcer: an erosion in the mucous membrane of either the stomach (a gastric ulcer) or duodenum (a duodenal ulcer).

peptidase: a digestive enzyme that hydrolyzes peptide bonds. Tripeptidases cleave tripeptides; dipeptidases cleave dipeptides. Endopeptidases cleave peptide bonds within the chain to create smaller fragments, whereas exopeptidases cleave bonds at the ends to release free amino acids.

peptide bond: a bond that connects the acid end of one amino acid with the amino end of another, forming a link in a protein chain.

peripheral resistance: resistance to the flow of blood caused by the reduced diameter of the vessels at the periphery of the body—the smallest arteries and capillaries.

peristalsis (peri-STALL-sis): wavelike muscular contractions of the GI tract that push its contents along.

pernicious (per-NISH-us) **anemia:** a blood disorder that reflects a vitamin B_{12} deficiency caused by lack of intrinsic factor and characterized by a deficit of red blood cells, muscle weakness, and neurological disturbances.

peroxidation: the production of unstable molecules containing more than the usual amount of oxygen. Hydrogen peroxide, H_2O_2, for example, may be produced from water, H_2O.

persistence: stubborn or enduring continuance; with respect to food contaminants, the quality of persisting, rather than breaking down, in the bodies of animals and human beings.

pesticides: chemicals used to control insects, diseases, weeds, fungi, and other pests on plants, vegetables, fruits, and animals. Used broadly, the term includes herbicides (to kill weeds), insecticides (to kill insects), and fungicides (to kill fungi).

pH: the unit of measure expressing a substance's acidity or alkalinity; a measure of the concentration of H^+ ions (see Appendix B). The lower the pH, the stronger the acid. Thus at pH 2, a solution is a strong acid, and at pH 6, a solution is a weak acid (pH 7 is neutral). A pH above 7 is alkaline, or base (a solution in which OH^- ions predominate).

phagocytes: white blood cells that have the ability to ingest and destroy foreign substances.

phagocytosis (FAG-oh-sigh-TOE-sis): the process by which phagocytes engulf and destroy foreign materials.

pharmacological effect: the effect a large dose of a nutrient (two to ten times greater than the RDA) has when it overwhelms some body system and acts like a drug.

phospholipid: a compound similar to a triglyceride but having choline (or another nitrogen-containing compound) and a phosphate group (a phosphorus-containing salt) in place of one of the fatty acids.

phosphorus: a major mineral found mostly in the body's bones and teeth.

photon (FOE-ton): a unit of light energy. Depending on its wavelength, a photon conveys different colors of light.

photosynthesis: the process by which green plants make carbohydrates from carbon dioxide and water using the green pigment chlorophyll to trap the sun's energy.

photovoltaic (PV) panels: panels that convert light (photons) into electricity (volts).

physiological age: a person's age as estimated from her or his body's health and probable life expectancy.

physiological effect: the effect a normal dose of a nutrient (levels commonly found in foods and not exceeding 150% of the RDA) has in providing for a normal blood concentration.

physiological fuel value: the number of kcalories that the human body derives from a food, as contrasted with the number of kcalories determined by calorimetry.

phytic acid: a nonnutrient component of plant seeds; also called phytate (FYE-tate). Phytic acid occurs in the husks of grains, legumes, and seeds and is capable of binding minerals such as zinc, iron, calcium, magnesium, and copper in insoluble complexes in the intestine, which the body excretes unused.

phytochemicals: nonnutrient compounds found in plant-derived foods that have biological activity in the body.

pica (PIE-ka): a craving for nonfood substances. Also known as geophagia (gee-oh-FAY-gee-uh) when referring to clay eating and pagophagia (pag-oh-FAY-gee-uh) when referring to ice craving.

pigment: a molecule capable of absorbing certain wavelengths of light, so that it reflects only those that we perceive as a certain color.

placebo (pla-SEE-bo): an inert, harmless medication given to provide comfort and hope; a sham treatment used in controlled research studies.

placebo effect: the healing effect that faith in medicine, even inert medicine, often has.

placenta (plah-SEN-tuh): the organ that develops inside the uterus early in pregnancy, in which maternal and fetal blood circulate in close proximity so that materials can be exchanged between them. The fetus receives nutrients and oxygen across the placenta; the mother's blood picks up carbon dioxide and other waste products to be excreted.

plaques, atheromatous: mounds of lipid material, mixed with smooth muscle cells and calcium, which develop in the artery walls in atherosclerosis.

plaque, dental: a gummy mass of bacteria that grows on teeth and can lead to dental caries and gum disease.

platelets: tiny, disc-shaped bodies in the blood, important in blood clot formation.

point of unsaturation: the double bond of a fatty acid, where hydrogen atoms can easily be added to the structure.

polar: describes a neutral molecule that has opposite charges spatially separated within the molecule; see Appendix B for more details.

polypeptide: many (ten or more) amino acids bonded together.

polysaccharide: many monosaccharides linked together.

polyunsaturated fatty acid (PUFA): a fatty acid that lacks four or more hydrogen atoms and has two or more double bonds between carbons—for example, linoleic acid (two double bonds) and linolenic acid (three double bonds). A polyunsaturated fat is composed of triglycerides containing a high percentage of PUFA.

portal vein: the vein that collects blood from the GI tract and conducts it to capillaries in the liver.

post term (infant): an infant born after the 42nd week of pregnancy.

postpartum amenorrhea: the normal temporary absence of menstrual periods immediately following childbirth.

potable (POTE-ah-bul): water that is suitable for drinking.

potassium: the principal cation within the body's cells, critical to the maintenance of fluid balance, nerve transmissions, and muscle contractions.

precursors: substances that precede others; with regard to vitamins, compounds that can be converted into active vitamins; also known as provitamins.

preeclampsia: a condition characterized by hypertension, fluid retention, and protein in the urine.

preformed vitamin A: dietary vitamin A in its active form.

pregnancy-induced hypertension (PIH): high blood pressure that develops in the second half of pregnancy.

preservatives: antimicrobial agents, antioxidants, and other additives that retard spoilage or maintain desired qualities, such as softness in baked goods.

preterm (infant): an infant born prior to the 38th week of pregnancy; also called a premature infant.

primary deficiency: a nutrient deficiency caused by inadequate dietary intake of a nutrient.

proenzyme: the inactive form of an enzyme.

progressive overload principle: the training principle that a body system, in order to improve, must be worked at frequencies, durations, or intensities that gradually increase physical demands.

promoters: with respect to cancer, factors that favor its development once the initiating event has taken place.

proof: a way of stating the percentage of alcohol in distilled liquor. Liquor that is 100 proof is 50% alcohol; 90 proof is 45%, and so forth.

prostaglandins (PROS-tah-GLAND-ins): eicosanoid compounds with a multitude of diverse effects on the body, including contraction of blood vessels, transmission of nerve impulses, immune assistance, and hormone responses.

protease (PRO-tee-ase): an enzyme that hydrolyzes proteins.

protein digestibility: a measure of the amount of amino acids absorbed from a given protein intake.

protein efficiency ratio (PER): a measure of protein quality assessed by determining how well a given protein supports weight gain in growing rats; used to establish the protein quality for infant formulas and baby foods.

protein turnover: the degradation and synthesis of endogenous protein.

protein-digestibility-corrected amino acid score (PDCAAS): a measure of protein quality assessed by comparing the amino acid balance of a food protein with the amino acid requirements of preschool-aged children and then correcting for the true digestibility of the protein; recommended by the FAO/WHO and used to establish protein quality of foods for Daily Value percentages on food labels.

protein-energy malnutrition (PEM), also called **protein-kcalorie malnutrition (PCM):** a deficiency of both protein and energy; the world's most widespread malnutrition problem, including kwashiorkor, marasmus, and instances in which they overlap.

protein-sparing action: the action of carbohydrate (and fat) in providing energy that allows protein to be used for other purposes.

proteins: compounds composed of carbon, hydrogen, oxygen, and nitrogen atoms, arranged into amino acids linked in a chain. Some amino acids also contain sulfur atoms.

puberty: the period in life in which a person becomes physically capable of reproduction.

public health nutritionist: a dietitian who specializes in public health nutrition.

public water: water from a municipal or county water system that has been treated and disinfected.

purgative: a strong laxative.

purified water: water that has been processed through distillation, deionization, or reverse osmosis and meets U.S. Pharmacopoeia standards for medical and research purposes.

pyloric (pie-LORE-ic) **sphincter:** the circular muscle that separates the stomach from the small intestine and regulates the flow of partially digested food into the small intestine (also called pylorus or pyloric valve).

pyruvate (PIE-roo-vate): pyruvic acid, a 3-carbon compound that, in metabolism, can be derived from glucose, certain amino acids, or glycerol. The term pyruvate means a salt of pyruvic acid.

radiation: ionizing rays used to sterilize and protect food.

radiolytic (RAY-dee-oh-LIT-ic) **products:** chemicals formed during the irradiation of food.

randomization (RAN-dom-ih-ZAY-shun): a process of choosing the members of the experimental and control groups without bias.

raw sugar: the first crop of crystals harvested during sugar processing. Raw sugar cannot be sold in the United States because it contains too much filth (dirt, insect fragments, and the like). Sugar sold as "raw sugar" domestically has actually gone through over half of the refining steps.

RD: see registered dietitian.

RDA: see Recommended Dietary Allowances.

RE (retinol equivalent): a measure of vitamin A activity; the amount of retinol that the body will derive from a food containing preformed retinol or its precursor beta-carotene.

recombinant DNA technology: methods of joining (recombining) pieces of the genetic material DNA in order to change the proteins produced by the altered DNA.

Recommended Dietary Allowances (RDA): the amounts of selected nutrients considered adequate to meet the known nutrient needs of practically all healthy people.

rectum: the muscular terminal part of the intestine, extending from the sigmoid colon to the anus.

Reference Daily Intakes (RDI): a set of standards for protein, vitamins, and minerals used on food labels as part of the Daily Values; previously known as the U.S. RDA.

reference protein: standard against which to measure the quality of other proteins.

refined: the process by which the coarse parts of a food are removed. With respect to refining wheat into flour, the bran, germ, and husk have been removed, leaving only the endosperm.

reflux: a backward flow.

registered dietitian (RD): a dietitian who has graduated from a university or college after completing a program of dietetics that has been accredited by the American Dietetic Association (or Canadian Dietetic Association), has served in an internship or coordinated program to practice the necessary skills, has passed the association's registration examination, and maintains competency through continuing education. Many states require licensing for practicing dietitians.

registration: listing; with respect to health professionals, listing with a professional organization that requires specific course work, experience, and passing of an examination.

remodeling: the dismantling and reformation of a structure, such as bone.

renin: an enzyme from the kidneys that works by activating angiotensin.

rennin: an enzyme that coagulates milk; found in the gastric juice of cows, but not human beings.

replication (REP-lee-KAY-shun): repeating an experiment and getting the same results. The skeptical scientist, on hearing of a new, exciting finding, will ask, "Has it been replicated yet?" If it hasn't, the scientist will withhold judgment regarding the finding's validity.

requirement: the amount of a nutrient that will maintain normal biochemical and physiological functions and prevent the development of specific deficiency signs; distinguished from the RDA, which is a recommended and generous allowance that provides for variability among individuals.

residues: whatever remains. In the case of pesticides, those amounts that remain on or in foods when people buy and use them.

resistant starch: starch that is not absorbed in the small intestine of healthy people.

resting energy expenditure (REE): a measure of energy output that is usually less precise than the BMR because the criteria for rest and fasting are less strict, but the difference is usually less than 10% and can be discounted for most purposes.

retina (RET-in-uh): the layer of light-sensitive nerve cells lining the back of the inside of the eye; consists of rods and cones.

retinal (RET-ih-nal): the aldehyde form of vitamin A, active in the eye.

retinoic (RET-ih-no-ick) **acid:** the acid form of vitamin A.

retinoids: chemically related compounds with biologic activity similar to retinol; metabolites of retinol.

retinol (RET-ih-nol): the alcohol form of vitamin A.

retinol equivalents: see RE.

retinol-binding protein (RBP): the specific protein responsible for transporting retinol.

rhodopsin (ro-DOP-sin): the light-sensitive pigment of the rods in the retina; it contains the retinal form of vitamin A.

riboflavin (RYE-boh-flay-vin): a B vitamin; the coenzyme forms are FMN (flavin mononucleotide) and FAD (flavin adenine dinucleotide).

rickets: the vitamin D–deficiency disease in children characterized by inadequate mineralization of bone (manifested in bowed legs or knock-knees, outward-bowed chest, and knobs on ribs). A rare type of rickets, not caused by vitamin D deficiency, is known as vitamin D–refractory rickets.

risk: a measure of the probability and severity of harm.

risk factors: factors associated with an elevated frequency of a disease but not proven to be causal.

rods: the cells of the retina that respond to dim light and convey black-and-white vision.

saccharin (SAK-ah-ren): a 0-kcalorie sweetener used in the United States but available in Canada only in pharmacies and only as a sweetener, not as an additive.

safety: a judgment that considers the risks acceptable.

saliva: the secretion of the salivary glands; its principal enzyme begins carbohydrate digestion.

salivary glands: exocrine glands that secrete saliva into the mouth.

salts: compounds composed of a positive ion other than H^+ and a negative ion other than OH^-. An example is sodium chloride (Na^+Cl^-).

sarcoma (sar-KO-mah): a cancer that arises from muscle, bone, or other connective tissue.

satiety (sah-TIE-eh-tee): the feeling of satisfaction and fullness that food brings.

saturated fatty acid: a fatty acid carrying the maximum possible number of hydrogen atoms—for example, stearic acid. A saturated fat is composed of triglycerides in which all or virtually all of the fatty acids are saturated.

science of nutrition: the study of the nutrients in foods and of the body's handling of them (including ingestion, digestion, absorption, transport, metabolism, interaction, storage, and excretion). A broader definition includes the study of the environment and of human behavior as it relates to food.

scurvy: the vitamin C–deficiency disease.

secondary deficiency: a nutrient deficiency caused by something other than diet, such as a disease condition that reduces absorption, accelerates use, hastens excretion, or destroys the nutrient.

secretin (see-CREET-in): a hormone produced by cells in the duodenum wall. Target organ: the pancreas. Response: secretion of bicarbonate-rich pancreatic juice.

sedentary: physically inactive (literally, "sitting down a lot").

segmentation (SEG-men-TAY-shun): a periodic squeezing or partitioning of the intestine at intervals along its length by its circular muscles.

selenium (se-LEEN-ee-um): a trace element.

semivegetarians: people who include some, but not all, groups of animal-derived foods in their diets; they usually exclude red meat, but may occasionally include poultry, fish, and seafood; sometimes called partial vegetarians.

senile dementia: the loss of brain function beyond the normal loss of physical adeptness and memory that occurs with aging.

senile dementia of the Alzheimer's type (SDAT): a degenerative disease of the brain involving memory loss and major structural changes in neuron networks; also known as primary degenerative dementia of senile onset or chronic brain syndrome, but often simply called Alzheimer's disease.

serotonin (SER-oh-tone-in): a neurotransmitter important in sleep and sensory perception; it is synthesized from the amino acid tryptophan with the help of vitamin B_6.

set point: the point at which controls are set (for example, on a thermostat). The set-point theory proposes that the body tends to maintain a certain weight by means of its own internal controls.

sickle-cell anemia: a hereditary form of anemia characterized by abnormal sickle- or crescent-shaped red blood cells. Sickled cells interfere with oxygen transport and blood flow. Symptoms include hemolytic anemia (red blood cells burst), fever, and severe pain in the joints and abdomen; they are precipitated by dehydration and insufficient oxygen (as may occur at high altitudes).

simple carbohydrates (sugars): monosaccharides and disaccharides.

slow-twitch muscle fibers: muscle fibers best suited to producing energy by aerobic processes for prolonged endurance activity.

small intestine: a 10-foot length of small-diameter intestine that is the major site of digestion of food and absorption of nutrients; its segments are the duodenum, jejunum, and ileum.

sodium bicarbonate: baking soda; an alkaline salt believed to neutralize blood lactic acid and thereby reduce pain and enhance possible workload. "Soda loading" may cause intestinal bloating and diarrhea.

sodium: the principal cation in the extracellular fluids of the body, critical to the maintenance of fluid balance, nerve transmissions, and muscle contractions.

sodium-potassium pump: the activity that exchanges sodium for potassium across the cell membrane, maintaining a strong concentration gradient of each.

soft water: water with a high sodium concentration.

solanine (SO-lah-neen): a poisonous narcotic-like substance present in potato peels and sprouts.

solutes (SOLL-yutes): the substances that are dissolved in a solution.

specific immunity: immunity directed at specific organisms (also called acquired immunity). The lymphocytes mediate this type of immunity, which depends on prior exposure, recognition, and reaction to invading organisms. Two types of specific immunity are cell-mediated immunity and humoral immunity.

sperm: the male reproductive cell, capable of fertilizing an ovum.

sphincter: a circular muscle surrounding, and able to close, a body opening.

sports anemia: a transient condition of low hemoglobin in the blood, associated with the early stages of sports training or other strenuous activity.

spring water: water originating from an underground spring or well. It may be carbonated or not ("flat" or "still"). Brand names such as "Spring Pure" do not necessarily mean that the water comes from a spring.

starch: a plant polysaccharide composed of glucose that is digestible by human beings. For the structures of starch's two forms, amylose (straight chain) and amylopectin (branched chain), see Appendix C.

sterile: free of microorganisms, such as bacteria.

sterol: a compound composed of C, H, and O atoms arranged in rings, like those of cholesterol, with any of a variety of side chains attached.

stomach: a muscular, elastic, saclike portion of the digestive tract that grinds and churns swallowed food, mixing it with acid and enzymes to form chyme.

stools: waste matter discharged from the colon; also called feces (FEE-seez).

stress: any threat to a person's well-being; a demand placed on the body to adapt.

stress eating: eating in response to arousal.

stress fractures: bone damage or breaks caused by stress on bone surfaces during exercise.

stress response: the body's response to stress, mediated by both nerves and hormones initially; begins with an alarm reaction, proceeds through a stage of resistance, and then leads to recovery or, if prolonged, to exhaustion. This three-stage response has also been termed the general adaptation syndrome.

stressor: an environmental element, physical or psychological, that causes stress.

stroke volume: the amount of oxygenated blood the heart ejects toward the tissues at each beat.

subclavian vein: the vessel that connects the thoracic duct with the right upper chamber of the heart, providing a passageway by which lymph can be returned to the vascular system.

subclinical deficiency: a nutrient deficiency in the early stages, before the outward signs have appeared.

subsidies: government money, derived from taxes, used to support (subsidize) practices that otherwise would force recipients to price their products too high to compete successfully.

substitute food: a food that is designed to replace another.

sucralose (SUK-kra-lose): a 0-kcalorie sweetener that is 600 times sweeter than sucrose; FDA approval pending in the United States; approved in Canada.

sucrase: an enzyme that hydrolyzes sucrose.

sucrose: a disaccharide composed of glucose and fructose; commonly known as table sugar, beet sugar, or cane sugar. Sucrose also occurs in many fruits and some vegetables and grains.

sudden infant death syndrome (SIDS): the unexpected and unexplained death of an apparently well infant; the most common cause of death of infants between the second week and the end of the first year of life; also called crib death.

sugar alcohols: sugarlike compounds that can be derived from fruits or commercially produced from dextrose; also called polyols. Like sugars, sugar alcohols are sweet to taste and yield 4 kcalories per gram, but they are absorbed more slowly and metabolized differently than other sugars in the human body, and are not readily utilized by ordinary mouth bacteria. Examples are maltitol, mannitol, sorbitol, and xylitol.

sulfites: salts containing sulfur that are added to foods to prevent spoilage.

sulfur: a mineral present in the body as part of some amino acids.

supplements: pills, liquids, or powders that contain purified nutrients, or foods with purified nutrients added in amounts per serving greater than 50% above a standard considered sufficient for all healthy people.

sushi: vinegar-flavored rice and seafood, typically wrapped in seaweed and stuffed with colorful vegetables. Some sushi is stuffed with raw fish; other varieties contain only cooked ingredients.

sustainable: able to continue indefinitely; the use of resources at such a rate that the earth can keep on replacing them—for example, cutting trees no faster than new ones grow and producing pollutants at a rate with which the environment and human cleanup efforts can keep pace, so that no net accumulation of pollution occurs.

symptomatic allergy: adverse reaction that produces antibodies and symptoms.

synergistic: multiple factors operating together in such a way that their combined effects are greater than the sum of their individual effects.

synthetase (SIN-the-tase): an enzyme that enables two or more substances to form a more complex structure.

T-cells: lymphocytes that attack antigens.

tempeh (TEM-pay): a fermented soybean food, rich in protein and fiber.

tension-fatigue syndrome: apparent hyperactivity produced in a child by the combination of lack of sleep, overstimulation, and anxiety.

teratogenic (ter-AT-oh-jen-ik): causing abnormal fetal development and birth defects.

term (infant): an infant born between the 38th and 42nd week of pregnancy.

textured vegetable protein: processed soybean protein used in vegetarian products such as soy burgers.

thermic effect of food (TEF): an estimation of the energy required to process food (digest, absorb, transport, metabolize, and store ingested nutrients); also called diet-induced thermogenesis (DIT), the specific dynamic effect (SDE) of food, or the specific dynamic activity (SDA) of food.

thermogenesis: the generation of heat; used in physiology and nutrition studies as an index of how much energy the body is spending.

thiamin (THIGH-ah-min): a B vitamin; the coenzyme form is TPP (thiamin pyrophosphate).

thirst: a conscious desire to drink.

thoracic (thor-ASS-ic) **duct:** the duct that conveys lymph toward the heart.

thrombosis: the formation or development of a thrombus.

thromboxanes: eicosanoid compounds with effects on the blood-clotting system.

thrombus: a blood clot that may obstruct a blood vessel or the heart cavity.

thrush: a fungal infection of the mouth caused by *Candida albicans;* the technical term for this infection is candidiasis.

tocopherol (tuh-KOFF-er-all): a general term for several chemically related compounds, most of which have vitamin E activity (see Appendix C for chemical structures).

tocopherol equivalents (TE): the units in which vitamin E activity is measured. One TE equals the amount of vitamin E activity in 1 milligram of D-alpha-tocopherol.

tofu (TOE-foo): a curd made from soybeans, rich in protein and often fortified with calcium; used in many Asian and vegetarian dishes in place of meat.

tolerance level: the maximum amount of a residue permitted in a food when a pesticide is used according to label directions.

toxicity: the ability of a substance to harm living organisms. All substances are toxic if high enough concentrations are used.

trace minerals: essential mineral nutrients found in the human body in amounts less than 5 grams.

trachea (TRAKE-ee-uh): the windpipe; the passageway from the mouth and nose to the lungs.

training: practicing an activity regularly, which leads to conditioning. (Training is what you do; conditioning is what you get.)

trans-fatty acids: fatty acids with an unusual configuration around the double bond.

transamination: the transfer of an amino group from one amino acid to a keto acid, producing a new nonessential amino acid and a new keto acid.

transferrin: the iron carrier protein.

transgenic organism: an organism that grows from an embryonic, stem, or germ cell into which a gene is inserted; the organism then carries the new gene in all of its cells.

triglycerides (try-GLISS-er-rides): the chief form of fat in the diet and the major storage form of fat in the body; composed of a molecule of glycerol with three fatty acids attached; also called triacylglycerols (try-ay-seel-GLISS-er-ols).

tripeptide: three amino acids bonded together.

tumor: an unchecked new growth of tissue forming an abnormal mass with no function; also called a neoplasm (NEE-oh-plazm). Tumors that pose no problem are called benign (bee-NINE); those that resist treatment and are harmful are malignant.

turbinado (ter-bih-NOD-oh) **sugar:** sugar produced using the same refining process as white sugar, but without the bleaching and anti-caking treatment; traces of molasses give turbinado its sandy color.

ulcer: an erosion in the topmost, and sometimes underlying, layers of cells in an area. See also peptic ulcer.

ultrahigh temperature (UHT): a process that exposes milk to temperatures above those of pasteurization just long enough to sterilize it.

umbilical (um-BILL-ih-cul) **cord:** the ropelike structure through which the fetus's veins and arteries reach the placenta; the route of nourishment and oxygen into the fetus and the route of waste disposal from the fetus. The scar in the middle of the abdomen that marks the former attachment of the umbilical cord is the umbilicus (um-BILL-ih-cus), commonly known as the "belly button."

unavailable carbohydrates: fibers (because human digestive enzymes cannot break their bonds).

unbleached flour: a tan-colored endosperm flour with texture and nutritive qualities that approximate those of regular white flour.

undernutrition: deficiency of energy or nutrients.

underweight: body weight below some standard of acceptable weight that is usually defined in relation to height (such as the weight-for-height tables).

unsaturated fatty acid: a fatty acid that lacks hydrogen atoms and has at least one double bond between carbons (includes monounsaturated and polyunsaturated fatty acids). An unsaturated fat is composed of triglycerides in which some of the fatty acids are unsaturated.

upper safe: the amount of a nutrient that appears safe for most healthy people and beyond which there is concern that some people will experience toxicity symptoms.

urea (you-REE-uh): the principal nitrogen-excretion product of metabolism. Two ammonia fragments are combined with carbon dioxide to form urea.

urethra (you-REE-thruh): the tube through which urine from the bladder passes out of the body.

USDA (U.S. Department of Agriculture): the federal agency responsible for enforcing standards for the wholesomeness and quality of meat, poultry, and eggs produced in the United States; conducting nutrition research; and educating the public about nutrition.

uterus (YOU-ter-us): the muscular organ within which the infant develops before birth; the womb.

validity (va-LID-ih-tee): having the quality of being founded on fact or evidence.

variable: a factor that changes. A variable may depend on another variable (for example, a child's height depends on his age), or it may be independent (for example, a child's height does not depend on the color of her eyes). Sometimes both variables correlate with a third variable (a child's height and eye color both depend on genetics).

variety (dietary): eating a wide selection of foods within and among the major food groups (the opposite of monotony).

vasoconstrictor: a substance that constricts or narrows the blood vessels.

vegans (VAY-guns or VEJ-ans): people who exclude all animal-derived foods (including meat, poultry, fish, eggs, and dairy products) from their diets; also called pure vegetarians, strict vegetarians, or total vegetarians.

vegetarians: a general term used to describe people who exclude meat, poultry, fish, or other animal-derived foods from their diets.

vein: a vessel that carries blood back to the heart.

villi (VILL-ee, VILL-eye): fingerlike projections from the folds of the small intestine; singular villus.

vitamin A activity: a term useful for referring to both the preformed vitamin A and carotene contents of foods without distinguishing between them.

vitamin B_{12}: a B vitamin characterized by the presence of cobalt (see Figure 13–7 in Chapter 13); the active forms of coenzyme B_{12} are methylcobalamin and deoxyadenosylcobalamin.

vitamin B_6: a family of compounds—pyridoxal, pyridoxine, and pyridoxamine; the primary active coenzyme form is PLP (pyridoxal phosphate).

vitamins: organic, essential nutrients required in small amounts by the body for health. The water-soluble vitamins are vitamin C and the eight B vitamins: thiamin, riboflavin, niacin, vitamins B_6 and B_{12}, folate, biotin, and pantothenic acid. The fat-soluble vitamins are vitamins A, D, E, and K.

VLDL (very-low-density lipoprotein): the type of lipoprotein made primarily by liver cells to transport lipids to various tissues in the body; composed primarily of triglycerides.

VO_2 max: the maximum rate of oxygen consumption by an individual at sea level.

voluntary activities: the component of a person's daily energy expenditure that involves conscious and deliberate muscular work—walking, lifting, climbing, or other physical activity. In contrast, involuntary activities occur independently, without conscious will or knowledge—heart beating, lungs breathing, glands secreting, GI tract muscles contracting, and other activities critical to maintaining life.

vomiting: expulsion of the contents of the stomach up through the esophagus to the mouth.

warm-up: five to ten minutes of light activity, such as easy jogging or cycling, to warm up the body in preparation for more vigorous activity.

water balance: the balance between water intake and output (losses).

water intoxication: the condition in which body water contents are too high.

wean: to gradually replace breast milk with infant formula or other foods appropriate to an infant's diet.

weight cycling: repeated cycles of weight loss and gain. The weight-cycling pattern is popularly called the ratchet effect or yo-yo effect of dieting.

well water: water drawn from groundwater by tapping into an aquifer.

Wernicke-Korsakoff (VER-nee-key KORE-sah-koff) **syndrome:** a cluster of symptoms commonly seen in malnourished alcohol abusers that are similar to those seen in thiamin deficiency and that can be treated with thiamin supplements.

wheat flour: any flour made from wheat, including white flour; wheat flour has been refined whereas whole-wheat flour has not.

white flour: an endosperm flour that has been refined and bleached for maximum softness and whiteness.

white sugar: pure sucrose or "table sugar," produced by dissolving, concentrating, and recrystallizing raw sugar.

WHO (World Health Organization): an international agency that has adopted standards to regulate pesticide use among other responsibilities.

whole grain: a grain milled in its entirety (all but the husk), not refined.

whole-wheat flour: flour made from whole-wheat kernels; a whole-grain flour.

wine: an alcoholic beverage made by fermenting grape juice.

withdrawal reaction: a reaction to removal of a substance (usually of a drug) that reveals that the user has become dependent.

xanthophylls (ZAN-tho-fills): pigments found in plants; responsible for the color changes seen in autumn leaves.

xerophthalmia (zer-off-THAL-mee-uh): progressive blindness caused by vitamin A deficiency.

xerosis (zee-ROW-sis): drying of the cornea; a sign of vitamin A deficiency.

zygote (ZY-goat): the product of the union of ovum and sperm; so-called for the first two weeks after fertilization.

Index

Note: Bold face numbers indicate pages on which definitions appear; italic numbers indicate figures; numbers followed by a *t* refer to tables, and numbers followed by a *n* refer to footnotes.

Photo credits continued from page iv

34 © Marilynne Herbert; **36** (Far right) Thomas Harm and Tom Peterson/Quest Photographic Inc.; **38** © Michael Davidson; **40** Thomas Harm and Tom Peterson/Quest Photographic Inc.; **41** © Rosemary Weller/Tony Stone Worldwide; **42** Thomas Harm and Tom Peterson/Quest Photographic Inc.; **43** © Michael Dwyer/Stock, Boston; **44** Thomas Harm and Tom Peterson/Quest Photographic Inc.; **45** Thomas Harm and Tom Peterson/Quest Photographic Inc.; **50** Thomas Harm and Tom Peterson/Quest Photographic Inc.; **51** © Felicia Martinez/PhotoEdit; **52** Thomas Harm and Tom Peterson/Quest Photographic Inc.; **53** Thomas Harm and Tom Peterson/Quest Photographic Inc.; **55** © Tony Freeman/PhotoEdit; **56** Thomas Harm and Tom Peterson/Quest Photographic Inc.; **58** (Far left) Ray Stanyard; **58** © Felicia Martinez/PhotoEdit; **58** (Far right) © Michael Newman/PhotoEdit; **59** © Tony Freeman/PhotoEdit; **60** Courtesy of the FDA; **73** © David Simson/Stock, Boston; **76** © Merritt Vincent/PhotoEdit; **77** © Felicia Martinez/PhotoEdit; **78** © Michael Newman/PhotoEdit; **79** © Bill Aron/PhotoEdit; **81** © Michael Davidson; **83** © Felicia Martinez/PhotoEdit; **94** From D. W. Fawcett, The Cell, 2nd ed. (Philadelphia: Saunders, 1981); color by Kidd Company. **102** © Michael Newman/PhotoEdit; **108** Thomas Harm and Tom Peterson/Quest Photographic Inc.; **109** © Jeff Dunn/The Picture Cube, Inc.; **111** © Michael Davidson; **113** © David Young-Wolff/PhotoEdit; **126** © David Young-Wolff/PhotoEdit; **127** © Tony Freeman/PhotoEdit; **133** Thomas Harm and Tom Peterson/Quest Photographic Inc.; **136** © Felicia Martinez/PhotoEdit; **140** Thomas Harm and Tom Peterson/Quest Photographic Inc.; **146** © Sunette Division, Hoechst Celanese Corp.; **153** © Michael Davidson; **158** © Felicia Martinez/PhotoEdit; **161** © Peter Correz/Tony Stone Worldwide; **176** © John Neubauer/PhotoEdit; **177** Ray Stanyard; **178** © Tony Freeman/PhotoEdit; **179** Thomas Harm and Tom Peterson/Quest Photographic Inc.; **182** Thomas Harm and Tom Peterson/Quest Photographic Inc.; **184** Thomas Harm and Tom Peterson/Quest Photographic Inc.; **185** Thomas Harm and Tom Peterson/Quest Photographic Inc.; **185** (Bottom) © Felicia Martinez/PhotoEdit; **193** © Mary Kate Denny/PhotoEdit; **196** © Michael Davidson; **205** © Robert Finken/The Picture Cube; **213** Thomas Harm and Tom Peterson/Quest Photographic Inc.; **214** © Michael Newman/PhotoEdit; **216** © Alan Oddie/PhotoEdit; **217** Courtesy of Robert S. Goodhard, M.D.; **218** Courtesy of Robert S. Goodhard, M.D.; **223** Thomas Harm and Tom Peterson/Quest Photographic Inc.; **229** Thomas Harm and Tom Peterson/Quest Photographic Inc.; **236** Thomas Harm and Tom Peterson/Quest Photographic Inc.; **238** © Michael Davidson; **239** © Paul Mozell/Stock, Boston; **258** Michael Newman/PhotoEdit; **265** © Southern Living/Photo Researchers, Inc.; **276** © Michael Davidson; **286** © David Young-Wolff/PhotoEdit; **288** © John Bahlik; **292** © Lori Adamski Peek/Tony Stone Worldwide; **293** © David

Young-Wolff/PhotoEdit; **294** © David Young-Wolff/PhotoEdit; **300** © Jose Carillo/PhotoEdit; **304** © David Young-Wolff/PhotoEdit; **306** ©Michael Davidson; **308** © Tony Freeman/PhotoEdit; **311** © Frank Whitney/The Image Bank; **312** © AP/Wide World Photos; **323** © Peter L. Chapman/Stock, Boston; **324** © David Young-Wolff/PhotoEdit; **335** © Tony Freeman/PhotoEdit; **336** © Michael Newman/PhotoEdit; **340** © Michael Newman/PhotoEdit; **344** © Michael Davidson; **348** © L. V. Bergman & Associates, Inc.; **349** Thomas Harm and Tom Peterson/Quest Photographic Inc.; **352** Thomas Harm and Tom Peterson/Quest Photographic Inc.; **356** (Top) © L. V. Bergman & Associates, Inc.; **356** (Bottom) Thomas Harm and Tom Peterson/Quest Photographic Inc.; **360** Thomas Harm and Tom Peterson/Quest Photographic Inc.; **366** Thomas Harm and Tom Peterson/Quest Photographic Inc.; **369** © Martin M. Rotker; **374** © Science Photo Library/Photo Researchers, Inc.; **380** (Top) © L. V. Bergman & Associates; **380** (Bottom) From C. Conn, The Specialties in General Practice, 2nd ed. (Philadelphia: Saunders, 1957); **381** Thomas Harm and Tom Peterson/Quest Photographic Inc.; **387** © Tony Freeman/PhotoEdit; **393** © Michael Davidson; **402** © David Farr; **403** © Ken Greer/Visuals Unlimited; **404** Thomas Harm and Tom Peterson/Quest Photographic Inc.; **407** Courtesy of Parke-Davis and Company; **409** © David Young-Wolff/PhotoEdit; **410** © Daniel Brody/Stock, Boston; **411** © Tom Prerryman/PhotoEdit; **416** Thomas Harm and Tom Peterson/Quest Photographic Inc.; **421** © Mary Kate Denny/PhotoEdit; **426** (Left) Thomas Harm and Tom Peterson/Quest Photographic Inc.; **426** (Right) © Tom McCarthy/The Picture Cube; **429** © Michael Davidson; **430** © Lawrence Migdale/Stock, Boston; **437** © Bob Daemmrich/Stock, Boston; **442** © David Young-Wolff/PhotoEdit; **445** Thomas Harm and Tom Peterson/Quest Photographic Inc.; **451** Thomas Harm and Tom Peterson/Quest Photographic Inc.; **462** Courtesy of Gjon Mill; **463** With permission from Dempster et al., J. bone Min. Res I, 15–21, 1986; **472** © Michael Davidson; **478** Thomas Harm and Tom Peterson/Quest Photographic Inc.; **481** © Martin M. Rotker; **484** Thomas Harm and Tom Peterson/Quest Photographic Inc.; **489** Reproduced with permission of Nutrition Today Magazine, P. O. Box 1829, Annapolis, MD 21404, March 1968; **491** Thomas Harm and Tom Peterson/Quest Photographic Inc.; **493** © L. V. Bergman and Associates Inc.; **498** Courtesy of H. Kaplan and V. P. Robbach; **506** Thomas Harm and Tom Peterson/Quest Photographic Inc.; **509** © Michael Davidson; **512** © Jurgen Reisch/Tony Stone Images; **514** © Ulli Seer/Tony Stone Images; **515** (Left) © David Madison/Tony Stone Images; **515** (Right) Dennis MacDonald/PhotoEdit; **525** © Amy C. Etra/PhotoEdit; **526** © Tony Freeman/PhotoEdit; **529** © Lori Adamski Peek/Tony Stone Images; **531** © David Young-Wolff/PhotoEdit; **534** © Jim Pickerell/Stock, Boston; **536** Thomas Harm and Tom Peterson/Quest Photographic Inc.; **540** © Michael Newman/PhotoEdit; **546** © M. Grecco/Stock, Boston; **547** © Michael Davidson; **550** (Top and bottom left) © Petit Format/Nestle/Photo Researchers, Inc.; **550** (Bottom right) © Anthony M. Vanelli; **552** © Michael Newman/PhotoEdit; **553** © Bill Bachmann/Stock, Boston; **554** David J. Sams/Stock, Boston; **561** © Nik Kleinberg/Stock, Boston; **564** © Leslie Sponseller/Tony Stone Images; **566** © Myrleen Ferguson Cate/PhotoEdit; **567** © Harry Wilks/Stock, Boston; **568** © Myrleen Ferguson Cate/PhotoEdit; **575** © Streissguth, A. P., Clarren, S. K., & Jones, K. L. (1985, July) Natural History of the Fetal Alcohol Syndrome: A ten-year follow-up of eleven patients, Lauret II, 89–92; **576** © 1995 George Steinmetz; **577** © Michael Davidson; **578** © C. J. Allen/Stock, Boston; **582** © Owen Franken/Sygma; **585** (Top) © Mary Kate Denny/PhotoEdit; **585** (Bottom) Courtesy of H. Kamplan and V. P. Rabbach; **588** Thomas Harm and Tom Peterson/Quest Photographic Inc.; **589** © Tony Freeman/PhotoEdit; **591** © Anthony M. Vanelli; **594** © David Young-Wolff/PhotoEdit; **596** © Michael Newman/PhotoEdit; **597** Thomas Harm and Tom Peterson/Quest Photographic Inc.; **600** © David Young-Wolff/PhotoEdit; **604** © Phyllis Picardi/Stock, Boston; **610** © David Young-Wolff/Tony Stone Images; **611** Reproduced by permission of ICI Pharmaceuticals Division, Cheshire, England; **615** © Penny Tweedie/Tony Stone Images; **617** © Michael Davidson; **621** © Tom McCarthy/The Picture Cube; **622** © David Young-Wolff/PhotoEdit; **624** © Christopher Brown/Stock, Boston; **625** © Michael Newman/PhotoEdit; **631** © Bill Bachmann/PhotoEdit; **633** © D & I MacDonald/PhotoEdit; **634** © Bill Aron/PhotoEdit; **636** (Top) © Myrleen Ferguson/PhotoEdit; **636** (Bottom) © L. Druskis/Stock, Boston; **640** © Bob Daemmrich/Stock, Boston; **645** © Michael Davidson; **655** © Bob Daemmrich/Stock, Boston; **658** © Dennis MacDonald/PhotoEdit; **661** © Amy C. Etra/PhotoEdit; **663** © David Young-Wolff/PhotoEdit; **667** © Frank Siteman/The Picture Cube; **671** © PhotoEdit; **675** © Michael Newman/PhotoEdit; **676** © Michael Newman/PhotoEdit; **676** © Mark Richards/PhotoEdit; **677** © Marlene Karas/Atlanta Constitution; **678** © Michael Davidson; **679** © Bob Daemmrich/Stock, Boston; **683** © Felicia Martinez/PhotoEdit; **686** © Lawrence Migdale/Photo Researchers, Inc.; **692** © Myrleen Ferguson Cate/PhotoEdit; **693** © George Loun/Visuals Unlimited; **694** © Felicia Martinez/PhotoEdit; **695** © Richard Brown/Tony Stone Worldwide; **696** © Felicia Martinez/PhotoEdit; **698** Thomas Harm and Tom Peterson/Quest Photographic Inc.; **699** © Diane Graham-Henry/Tony Stone Images; **700** © Felicia Martinez/PhotoEdit; **705** Smithsonian photo by Antonio Montaner; **707** © Jeff Greenberg/PhotoEdit; **712** © Tony Freeman/PhotoEdit; **717** © Michael Davidson; **719** © Bob Daemmrich/Tony Stone Worldwide; **724** © Bob Daemmrich/Stock, Boston; **726** © Bob Daemmrich/Stock, Boston; **728** © Jerry Irwin/Photo Researchers, Inc.; **729** © Diane M. Lowe/Stock, Boston; **730** © David Austen/Stock, Boston; **732** © David Austen/Stock, Boston; **734** © David Young-Wolff/PhotoEdit; **738** © David Young-Wolff/PhotoEdit; **740** Courtesy of Sun Frost; **743** © Elizabeth Zuckerman/PhotoEdit; **744** NASA; **748** © Stephen R. Swinburne/Stock, Boston; **750** © David Young-Wolff/PhotoEdit; **I–15** Reproduced with permission by Canadian Diabetes Association, from Good Health Eating Guide Resource, Copyright 1994.